Normal Vital Sign Values by Age

Age (years)	Heart Rate (beats per minute)	Respiratory Rate (breaths per minute)	Blood Pressure	
			Systolic	Diastolic
Newborn	95–160	30–60	72	55
Infant	110–180	24–38	90	54
1	90–150	22–30	85	53
			86	40
2			88	42
			88	45
3			91	46
			89	49
4	65–135	20–24	93	50
			91	52
5			95	55
			93	54
6	60–130		96	55
			94	56
7		18–24	97	57
			96	57
8			99	57
			96	57
9	60–110		100	60
			100	59
10		16–22	102	61
			102	60
11			104	61
			103	61
12			106	62
			105	62
13			108	62
			107	63
14			111	63
			109	64
15		14–20	113	63
			110	65
16			116	65
			111	66
17	60–100		118	67
			111	66
18		12–20	120	80

*Blood pressure values are for 50th percentile pressure at 50th percentile height for age. Males listed first, females listed second.

Normal Arterial Blood Gas Values When Breathing Room Air (at 37°C)

Age	pH	$PaCO_2$ (mm Hg)	PaO_2 (mm Hg)	HCO_3 (mEq/L)
Premature infant (<28 weeks' gestation)	≥ 7.25	45–55	45–65	20–24
Newborn (birth)	7.26–7.29	55	60	19
Newborn (>24 hours)	7.37	33	70	20
Infant (1–24 months)	7.40	34	90	20
Child (7–19 years)	7.39	37	96	22
Adult (>19 years)	7.35–7.45	35–45	90–110	22–26

Neonatal and Pediatric Respiratory Care

A Patient Case Method

Neonatal and Pediatric Respiratory Care

A Patient Case Method

Julianne S. Perretta, MSEd, RRT-NPS, CHSE

*Manager, Manikin and Procedural Skills
Programs and Lead Educator*
The Johns Hopkins Medicine Simulation Center
The Johns Hopkins University School of Medicine
Baltimore, MD

Adjunct Faculty
College of Health Professions
Towson University
Towson, MD

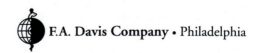

F.A. Davis Company • Philadelphia

F. A. Davis Company
1915 Arch Street
Philadelphia, PA 19103
www.fadavis.com

Copyright © 2014 by F. A. Davis Company

Printed in the United States of America

Last digit indicates print number: 10 9 8 7 6 5 4 3 2 1

Publisher: Quincy McDonald
Manager of Content Development: George W. Lang
Developmental Editor: Joanna Cain
Art and Design Manager: Carolyn O'Brien

As new scientific information becomes available through basic and clinical research, recommended treatments and drug therapies undergo changes. The author(s) and publisher have done everything possible to make this book accurate, up to date, and in accord with accepted standards at the time of publication. The author(s), editors, and publisher are not responsible for errors or omissions or for consequences from application of the book, and make no warranty, expressed or implied, in regard to the contents of the book. Any practice described in this book should be applied by the reader in accordance with professional standards of care used in regard to the unique circumstances that may apply in each situation. The reader is advised always to check product information (package inserts) for changes and new information regarding dose and contraindications before administering any drug. Caution is especially urged when using new or infrequently ordered drugs.

Library of Congress Cataloging-in-Publication Data

Neonatal and pediatric respiratory care (Perretta)
   Neonatal and pediatric respiratory care : a patient case method / [edited by] Julianne S. Perretta.
       p. ; cm.
   Includes bibliographical references and index.
   ISBN 978-0-8036-2831-1
   I. Perretta, Julianne S., editor of compilation. II. Title.
   [DNLM: 1. Respiratory Tract Diseases—therapy—Case Reports. 2. Child. 3. Infant. 4. Respiratory Therapy—methods—Case Reports. WS 280]
   RJ312
   618.92'2004636—dc23
                          2013022909

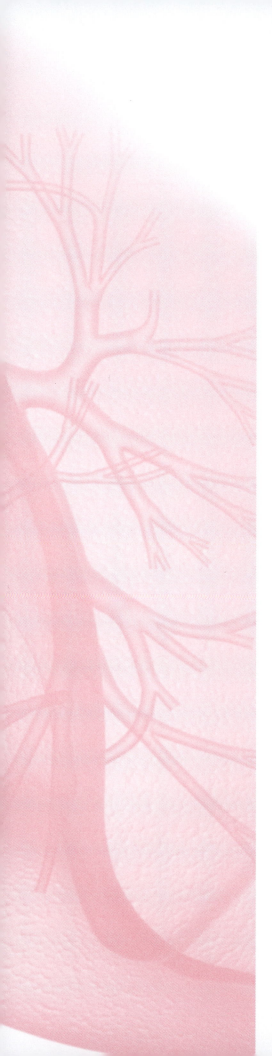

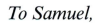

To Samuel,

The hardest working boy I've ever had the genuine pleasure to know. You have taught me that with hard work, anything is possible. I love you so much.

Preface

I knew from the moment I started my respiratory training at the Indiana University of Pennsylvania School of Respiratory Care that I wanted to focus on childhood cardiopulmonary management. I actively sought out extra clinical rotations in neonatal and pediatric units and spent all of my low-acuity clinical time interrogating neonatal and pediatric RTs about the clinical units, the equipment, and the role of the RT in interdisciplinary patient management. I was thrilled to secure a position upon graduation at the Johns Hopkins Neonatal Intensive Care Unit because it was one of the few places I knew that would hire a new RT into a pediatric specialty area.

My story is not a unique one. It is challenging for RT students who may want to specialize in caring for children, because neonatal and pediatric clinical rotations are inconsistent. Some students may not see a large portion of the patients, disease processes, or therapeutic modalities discussed in class, which means they graduate without first-hand experience. Nationally, the neonatal and pediatric exposure is different for graduates from different programs, and even classmates may have very different clinical experiences. In this text I hope to assist in giving students a cognitive understanding of pediatric and neonatal diseases, as well as a foundation of patient experiences that will help build a thorough understanding of how to translate that knowledge to the bedside. The clinical cases woven throughout this text provide readers with a context to understand the clinical information presented, as well as an opportunity to develop critical-thinking skills.

Running Case Studies

Each chapter begins with the introduction of a patient who is revisited at intervals throughout the chapter. This patient's story will reinforce key concepts such as laboratory values, clinical observations, and treatment modalities. At the end of the chapter, the patient is revisited to summarize his or her plan of care and outcomes, as well as to present some additional critical-thinking questions.

Consistent Format

Each disease chapter is presented in the same way and in the same order, including sections discussing background, pathophysiology, clinical manifestations, management and treatment, and course and prognosis.

Background information in each chapter seeks to answer questions such as: What is the frequency of the condition (how common is it)? What patient population does it most commonly affect (e.g., neonates, young children, males versus females)? Is it congenital? Is it an infectious disease? General causes and related descriptions are included.

Pathophysiology focuses on what happens physiologically in the body, how the disease progresses, and variants or different types of the disease. Clinical manifestations reveal clinical signs and symptoms such as vital signs, radiography, blood gas, and other physical findings, as well as other diagnostic tools. Management and treatment include surgical interventions, pharmacological therapies, respiratory and ventilatory interventions, and other multidisciplinary strategies. The course and prognosis section discusses morbidity and mortality rates, long-term complications, life span, projected course and hospital stay, as well as public burden and health-care costs.

At the end of each chapter, additional case studies for other diseases discussed within the chapter appear, incorporating critical-thinking questions. There are also multiple-choice questions that focus on the major learning objectives of the chapter.

Special Features

Throughout each chapter, special features introduce novel concepts in health-care teamwork, unique patient populations, and special care techniques.

- **Clinical Variations**: This feature presents a variation of the disease presentation, patient assessment, or diagnostic tool. It may be an atypical presentation or an uncommon manifestation or complication. It is something that does not seem to fit the normal assumptions of the disease and can be potentially misunderstood or even overlooked.
- **Evidence in Practice**: This feature introduces a new and/or upcoming way to manage a patient or disease. It may not yet be the current evidence-based standard of care, but research is currently under way, and it looks likely to become a common method of patient care in the near future.
- **Teamwork**: This feature introduces teamwork concepts and best practices throughout the text. The team approach is an important part of patient care. These features present the nomenclature and techniques of good teamwork.

- **Special Populations**: This feature identifies key patient demographics that may require you as the therapist to employ special care or considerations when caring for a patient with this disease.

Icons

Icons can be found throughout each chapter to help identify key information:

 Therapist Alert

Pharmacology

ABG

Mechanical Ventilation

Ancillaries

This textbook is supported by a rich collection of quality supplementary items available for both students and instructors on the Davis*Plus* website (http://davisplus.fadavis.com). Once students register on the Davis*Plus* site, using the Plus code included under a scratch off panel in the front of each new textbook, they will have access to study quizzes for each chapter, multi-stage interactive case studies, and a web-based e-version of their text (the Davis Digital Version), which they can use to search for important concepts, as well as to have access to reading assignments on their tablets or other computing devices.

Instructors also have ancillary support in the protected instructor's area of the Davis*Plus* site. Once registered, instructors have access to a full electronic test bank, PowerPoint presentations, an image resource, a dedicated instructor's manual (with sample simulations to run at the instructor's program), as well as the instructor's own Davis Digital Version of the textbook.

Contributors

JANE BENSON, MD
Assistant Professor
Pediatric Radiology
The Johns Hopkins School
 of Medicine
Baltimore, MD

RENEE BOSS, MD, MHS
*Assistant Professor, Division of
 Neonatology, Department
 of Pediatrics*
The Johns Hopkins School
 of Medicine
The Johns Hopkins Berman Institute
 of Bioethics
Baltimore, MD

MARISSA BRUNETTI, MD
Attending Intensivist
The Children's Hospital
 of Philadelphia
Philadelphia, PA

HEATHER CHANDLER, MD,
 MPH
*Assistant Professor, Pediatric
 Critical Care*
Emory University
Atlanta, GA

SHAWN COLBOURN, AS, RRT-NPS
Pediatric Respiratory Therapist
The Children's Hospital
 of Philadelphia
Philadelphia, PA

ELIZABETH CRISTOFALO, MD
Assistant Professor of Pediatrics
The Johns Hopkins School
 of Medicine
Baltimore, MD

ELLEN DEUTSCH, MD, FACS,
 FAAP
*Director, Simulation and Systems
 Integration*
Center for Simulation, Advanced
 Education, and Innovation
The Children's Hospital
 of Philadelphia
Philadelphia, PA

DHEERAJ GOSWAMI, MD
Pediatric Critical Care Fellow
The Johns Hopkins Hospital
Baltimore, MD

ROBERTA HALES, MHA,
 RRT-NPS, RN
Simulation Educator
Center for Simulation, Advanced
 Education and Innovation
The Children's Hospital
 of Philadelphia
Philadelphia, PA

ANDREA L. HONESTO,
 BS, RRT
Respiratory Care Practitioner II
Cystic Fibrosis Center
The Johns Hopkins Hospital
Baltimore, MD

ELIZABETH A. HUNT, MD,
 MPH, PHD
*Associate Professor of Anesthesiology
 and Critical Care Medicine*
Associate Professor of Pediatrics
The Johns Hopkins School
 of Medicine
Baltimore, MD

SAFEENA KHERANI, MD FRCSC
Assistant Professor
University of Ottawa
Ottawa, ON

HOLLY LOOSEN, PT
Physical Therapist II
Cystic Fibrosis Center
The Johns Hopkins Hospital
Baltimore, MD

STACEY MANN, BS, RRT
Manager, Pediatric Respiratory Care and ECMO Services
The Johns Hopkins Hospital
Baltimore, MD

MEGAN McCABE, MD, FAAP
Assistant Professor
Section of Pediatric Critical Care Medicine, Department of Pediatrics
Director, Pediatric Critical Care Fellowship Program
Yale University School of Medicine
New Haven, CT

SHARON McGRATH-MORROW, MD, MBA
Associate Professor of Pediatrics
Division of Pediatric Pulmonary
The Johns Hopkins School of Medicine
Baltimore, MD

PETER MOGAYZEL JR., MD, PhD
Associate Professor of Pediatrics
The Johns Hopkins School of Medicine
Director, Cystic Fibrosis Center
The Johns Hopkins Hospital
Baltimore, MD

SARAH JANN MOLA, MD
Assistant Professor of Pediatrics
Medical Director, Maryland Regional Neonatal Transport Program, University of Maryland School of Medicine
Baltimore, MD

WYNNE MORRISON, MD, MBE
Assistant Professor, Department of Anesthesiology and Critical Care, Perelman School of Medicine at the University of Pennsylvania
Children's Hospital of Philadelphia
Philadelphia, PA

VINAY NADKARNI, MD, MS
Endowed Chair, Pediatric Critical Care Medicine
Associate Professor, Anesthesia, Critical Care and Pediatrics, University of Pennsylvania School of Medicine
The Children's Hospital of Philadelphia
Philadelphia, PA

GARY OLDENBURG, RRT-NPS
ECMO and VAD Program Manager
Children's National Medical Center
Washington, DC

STACEY B. PEDDY, MD
Director of Simulation, Cardiac Intensive Care Unit
Assistant Professor, Anesthesiology and Critical Care Medicine
The Children's Hospital of Philadelphia
Philadelphia, PA

SHANNON POLING, BS, RRT
Simulation Educator
The Johns Hopkins Medicine Simulation Center
Baltimore, MD

SUZANNE PRESTWICH, MD
Medical Director, Inpatient Pediatric Rehabilitation Unit
Kennedy Krieger Institute
Baltimore, MD

WEBRA PRICE-DOUGLAS PhD, CRNP, IBCLC
Coordinator, Maryland Regional Neonatal Transport Program
Baltimore, MD

JENNIFER SCHUETTE, MD
Attending Physician, Cardiac ICU
Children's National Medical Center
Washington, DC

JAMIE McELRATH SCHWARTZ, MD
Medical Director, Cardiac Procedure Recovery Unit Anesthesiology and Pain Medicine
Children's National Medical Center
Washington, DC

THEODORA STAVROUDIS, MD
Assistant Professor of Pediatrics
University of Southern California
Los Angeles, CA

MATTHEW TROJANOWSKI, BA, RRT
Manager, Adult Respiratory Care Services
The Johns Hopkins Hospital
Baltimore, MD

KAREN VON BERG, PT
Physical Therapist II
Cystic Fibrosis Center
The Johns Hopkins Hospital
Baltimore, MD

Reviewers

TERI ALLEN, BSHA, RRT-NPS
*Neonatal/Pediatric Clinical Education
    Coordinator*
University of California–Irvine
Orange, CA

NICKI SUE BLY, BS, RRT-NPS
*Director of Clinical Education,
    Respiratory Care*
Highline Community College
Des Moines, WA

LISA CONRY, MA, RRT
Director of Clinical Education
Spartanburg Community College
Spartanburg, SC

HELEN S. CORNING, RRT
Registered Respiratory Therapist
Shands/UF Medical Center
Jacksonville, FL

JUANITA DAVIS, RRT
Faculty
Southern Alberta Institute of
    Technology
Alberta, Canada

MARTHA DeSILVA, MEd, RRT-
    AC-E
Program Director, Respiratory Care
Massasoit Community College
Brockton, MA

LEZLI HEYLAND, BS, RRT-NPS
*Program Director, Respiratory Care
    Program*
Oklahoma City Community College
Oklahoma City, OK

NANCY A. JOHNSON, RRT-NPS
*Pediatric Respiratory Education
    Coordinator*
University Hospitals of Cleveland
Rainbow Babies
Children's Hospital
Cleveland, OH

ROBERT L. JOYNER, JR., PhD,
    RRT, FAARC
*Associate Dean, Henson School of
    Science & Technology
Director, Respiratory Therapy
    Program*
Salisbury University
Salisbury, MD

CHRISTY J. KANE, PhD,
    RRT-NPS
*Department Chair, Respiratory
    Therapy Department*
Bellarmine University
Louisville, KY

ALETA KAY MARTIN, BSRC,
    RRT-NPS
Clinical Educator
Children's Medical Center
Dallas, TX

KERRY J. McNIVEN, MS, RRT
Professor, Director
Manchester Community College
Manchester, CT

LISA J. PIERCE, MSA, BS, RRT
Clinical Director, Respiratory Care
Augusta Technical College
Augusta, GA

GEORGETTE ROSENFELD, PhD,
    RRT, RN
Department Chair, Respiratory Care
Indian River State College
Fort Pierce, FL

MELISSA D. SMITH, BS, RRT
*Respiratory Care Education
    Coordinator
Chapter 8 President, Louisiana
    Society for Respiratory Care*
St. Tammany Parish Hospital
Covington, LA

Acknowledgments

I owe a great debt to many people who have made this book possible. First, I would like to thank all my contributing authors, whose expertise in neonatal and pediatric medicine was invaluable to the success of this text. Special thanks to Patricia Nolan for creating the test bank, Laura Shipp for creating the instructor presentations, and Dennise Stickley for compiling the glossary.

Thank you to Andy McPhee and Quincy McDonald from F. A. Davis for reaching out to me with the crazy idea to build a new and innovative pediatric respiratory care textbook. It was their leap of faith that started me on this path. A first-edition textbook takes a tremendous amount of editorial work and support. I'd like to thank Mackenzie Lawrence for her patience and guidance during the early stages of development and Joanna Cain and Pamela Speh of Auctorial Pursuits, Inc. for their direction during the completion of the manuscript.

I owe so much to my family for their patience, encouragement, and perseverance through this project. I give tremendous thanks to my parents and my mother-in-law, who helped provide a quiet home for research and development. When I started this project, I was a mother of one preschooler; now I have a second child. I am grateful for the special role that motherhood provides. Most importantly, I have tremendous gratitude for my husband, Jordan, who encouraged me to start this project and motivated me along the way until its completion. He also spent many single-dad weekends with the kids so Mommy could write her book.

Contents

Chapter 1

Making Sense of Caring for Kids: A Different Approach to Respiratory Care

Key Terms

Adverse drug event
Applicability
Capillary blood gas (CBG)
Cricoid pressure
Evidence-based medicine
Exclusivity
Expressive language
Functional residual capacity (FRC)
Medication error
Off-label use
Pharmacodynamic
Pharmacokinetic
Pores of Kohn
Proliferating
Receptive language
Sniffing position
Target effect
Transcutaneous monitoring
Validity

Chapter Objectives

After reading this chapter, you will be able to:

1. Discuss two reasons why all respiratory therapists should be able to care for pediatric patients.
2. Identify key differences in the anatomy of children compared to adults and the implications of those differences on the respiratory management of pediatric patients.
3. Describe how differences in neonatal and pediatric physiology affect work of breathing.
4. Identify three ways that pediatric patient assessment must be adjusted based on developmental milestones.
5. List normal and critical values for heart rate, respiratory rate, blood pressure, and arterial blood gas at different ages.
6. Discuss the ways to monitor oxygenation and ventilation in children.
7. List three ways to minimize the risk of medication errors in pediatric patients.
8. Describe how using target effect can drive the dosing of pediatric aerosol medications.
9. Choose a delivery method for a certain age when giving an aerosolized medication.
10. Select respiratory care equipment for a pediatric patient based on age or weight.
11. Differentiate among the three levels of neonatal intensive care units and between the two levels of pediatric intensive care units as proposed by the American Academy of Pediatrics.
12. Define *evidence-based medicine* and describe its implications on pediatric health care.

■■ Jamie Thibeaux

You are the respiratory therapist covering the emergency room in a rural hospital. It's 1330 and the triage nurse calls you to assess an 8-month-old girl, Jamie Thibeaux, who has been brought in. The nurse says the parents were driving her home from a cousin's birthday party when she started making high-pitched breathing noises from the backseat. The nurse thinks Jamie seems to be in respiratory distress, but because the hospital doesn't have a pediatric ward she's not exactly sure what to think. She has alerted the regional pediatric transport team, and the physician is on his way to see the baby. You hurry to the emergency room to assist with this new patient.

In its 2010 annual survey, the American Hospital Association listed the number of registered hospitals in the United States at 5,754 (1). Of this total, fewer than 5% were pediatric hospitals. For clinicians who work in the hospital setting, this means that the vast majority of jobs are caring for adult patients, not children. Why then is it important for respiratory therapists to know how to care for pediatric patients? First, most community hospitals have at least a pediatric in-patient unit. Second, pediatric long-term and respiratory care makes up a significant portion of home care services.

Many clinicians believe that the sickest patients are the most challenging to care for. However, it could be argued that stable patients who could deteriorate quickly and become critically ill are more challenging. Children fall into this category because they have less physiologic reserve and decompensate more rapidly than adults. Critical events in children are usually respiratory in origin, making the respiratory therapist an important member of any pediatric emergency team. A skilled respiratory therapist can save lives by identifying patients in a non-acute setting who need advanced levels of care. A valuable skill of experienced clinicians is how to recognize when a patient has outgrown the resources of his or her institution. Recognizing a child in distress early and requesting additional support takes confidence and dedication. It is a necessity when caring for children because they may need to be transported quickly to specialty pediatric hospitals that can offer advanced levels of care.

There are many things that make caring for children different from caring for adults, such as anatomical, physiological, and developmental differences. For example, children express themselves differently than adults, and communication evolves as children grow. Children come in different sizes, and equipment must be chosen accordingly. Expected normal vital signs are different based on age, and pediatric patient assessment, particularly the assessment of pain, may need to be modified based on age. Pharmacological dosing and responses are different for adults and children, and different delivery methods may need to be employed.

This chapter discusses these differences and how they affect how respiratory care is provided to children. The health-care services needed for children are extensive and are frequently available only in neonatal and pediatric inpatient settings and intensive care units. This chapter identifies current classification systems for neonatal and pediatric intensive care units recommended by the American Academy of Pediatrics (AAP). It also describes evidence-based medicine and its importance in current patient management. As research on children advances, it is the health-care community's responsibility to keep current on new recommendations and upcoming changes to practice.

Anatomical and Physiological Differences Between Children and Adults

Before identifying anatomical and physiological differences between different ages, it is important to first identify the age ranges used to describe pediatric patients. These terms are found in Box 1-1, and they will be used throughout the textbook to define time periods in childhood.

Many of the anatomical differences seen between children and adults are most pronounced in infancy. This is seen clearly when studying the nasopharynx, oropharynx, and pharynx, for example, because they continuously evolve throughout childhood. These changes have implications for airway management. See Table 1-1 for a summary of anatomical differences and their implications.

Beginning in the nasopharynx, differences include the following:

• Infants are considered obligate nose breathers. They are not totally dependent on nose breathing but breathe through their noses preferentially. Any obstruction, such as mucus or inflammation, can increase resistance to airflow and work of breathing (WOB).

Box 1-1 Childhood Age Ranges

Very/extremely preterm neonate	Less than 32 weeks gestational age
Moderate preterm neonate	32 to 36 weeks gestational age
Late preterm neonate	34 0/7 to 36 6/7 weeks gestational age
Full-term neonate	38 to 42 weeks gestational age, to first month of postnatal life
Infant	1 to 12 months
Toddler	12 to 36 months
Preschool-age child	4 to 5½ years
School-age child	5½ to 12 years
Adolescent	12 to 18 years
Adult	Greater than 18 years

• In children, the size of the tongue compared to the oral cavity is much larger, particularly in infancy. This makes the tongue a natural airway obstructer. An oral airway should be a first line of defense when beginning bag-mask ventilation on an unconscious child to avoid tissue airway obstruction.

• Children have large tonsils and adenoids and a large amount of lymphoid tissue in the pharynx. These are potential areas for swelling, which can cause upper airway obstruction. They may also bleed significantly during trauma or intubation, obstructing views and risking aspiration.

• An infant's epiglottis is larger, less flexible, and omega or U-shaped. It lies more horizontally than an adult's and is more susceptible to trauma.

• The angle between the epiglottis and laryngeal opening is more acute in an infant than in an adult, which makes blind nasal intubation difficult.

• In infancy, the glottis begins at the first cervical vertebrae (C1). As the thorax and trachea grow, the glottis moves to C3 to C4 by age 7 and is located at C5 to C6 in adulthood. This makes the glottis in children higher and more anterior than in adults.

• The cricoid ring is the smallest portion of a child's airway, whereas in adults the vocal cords are the smallest portion of the airway. An uncuffed endotracheal tube (ETT) provides an adequate seal in a small child because it fits snugly at the level of the cricoid ring. When using an uncuffed ETT, correct tube size is imperative because air can leak around an ETT that is too small, and tracheal damage can result from an ETT that is too large.

• Children have small cricothyroid membranes, and, in children younger than 3 years, it is virtually nonexistent. This means emergency surgical airway techniques such as needle cricothyrotomy and surgical cricothyrotomy are extremely difficult, if not impossible, in infants and small children.

• A child's trachea is smaller and more malleable than an adult's trachea, meaning it is more susceptible to changes in shape when under pressure. The newborn trachea is approximately 6 mm in diameter, and the cartilage is not fully developed, making it more compliant than the adult trachea. This means the trachea of a newborn collapses more easily, and in the presence of inflammation, airway resistance will increase exponentially. Increased inspiratory pressure during respiratory distress causes

Table 1-1	Anatomical Differences Between Adults and Children	
Anatomical Feature	**Presentation in Children (Compared with Adults)**	**Clinical Significance**
Tongue	Larger in relation to the oral cavity	Tongue is a natural airway obstructer
Tonsils, adenoids, and pharyngeal lymphoid tissue	Larger in size; large amount of lymphoid tissue in pharynx	These are potential areas for swelling, which can cause upper airway obstruction; they may also bleed significantly during trauma or intubation, obstructing views and risking aspiration
Epiglottis	Larger, less flexible, and omega shaped; lies more horizontally	Can make visualization difficult during intubation
Epiglottis and laryngeal opening	Angle between is more acute	Can make direct visualization difficult during intubation and blind nasal intubation
Glottis	Higher and more anterior	Can make direct visualization more difficult during intubation
Cricoid ring	Narrowest portion of the airway	Uncuffed tubes create seal at the cricoid ring
Cricothyroid membrane	Smaller; virtually nonexistent in children younger than 3 years	Needle cricothyrotomy and surgical cricothyrotomy are difficult in infants and small children
Extrathoracic trachea	More malleable	Increased risk of collapse during respiratory distress
Trachea	Shorter	Endotracheal tube misplacement and accidental extubation are more frequent
Airway	Smaller diameter	Airway obstruction is more common as a result of swelling
Thoracic cage	Ribs and sternum are mostly cartilage (infants); ribs lay more horizontal	The thoracic cage offers little stability; the chest wall will collapse with negative pressures; retractions are more pronounced in infants
Diaphragm	Main action for breathing in infants	Infants known as "belly breathers"; increases WOB when increasing tidal volume
Mainstem bronchus	Right mainstem angle lower	Right mainstem intubation and right foreign body obstruction are more frequent
Conducting airways	Smaller in diameter	More pronounced distress during reactive airways disease
Alveoli	Fewer at birth, increase in number during childhood	More respiratory distress during alveolar disease
	No pores of Kohn (infants)	Infants decompensate more rapidly during lower airway obstruction
Heart	Larger in relation to thoracic diameter	Less functional residual capacity
Lungs elastic recoil	Less than adult	
Abdominal contents	Proportionally larger and push up against the diaphragm	
Chest wall	Higher compliance	

increased negative intrathoracic pressure and can lead to collapse of the extrathoracic trachea. Caution should be taken when caring for pediatric patients with increased WOB because increased respiratory effort by patients to alleviate airway obstruction may instead exacerbate it.

• The diameter of children's airways is smaller than the airways of adults, making children more susceptible to airway obstruction caused by swelling.

• The shorter trachea of children makes tube misplacement and accidental extubation much more frequent than in adults. Small tube migrations due to head movement can cause ETT dislodgement (Fig. 1-1).

With both adults and children, an effective way of opening the airway is to place the patient in the **sniffing position**, in which the patient's head and chin are thrust slightly forward to keep the airway open.

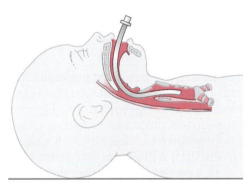
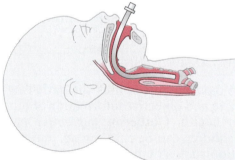
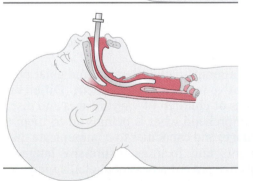

Figure 1-1 How Head Rotation Affects Endotracheal Tube Position Within the Trachea

However, the occiput (back part of the skull) is larger in children and may cause flexion of the neck and inadvertent obstruction of the airway. To align the airway in an adult, a roll can be placed under the head. In children this is not needed, and infants may need a shoulder roll to achieve sniffing position. See Figure 1-2 for an example of the proper sniffing position for an infant, child, and adult.

In summary, infants and toddlers (younger than 2 years) have higher anterior airways. Children older than 8 years have airways similar to adults. The age range of 2 to 8 years old marks a transition period, when the above-mentioned anatomical differences may have varying effects on airway management. On the positive side, the anatomical differences are consistent from one child to another, so they can be anticipated when managing a child's airway. This is not true in adults, however, in whom complex airway issues are related to body build, arthritis, and chronic disease.

Moving into the thoracic cavity, additional differences must be addressed.

• An infant's ribs and sternum are mostly cartilage, and the ribs lay more horizontally than do those of an adult. The thoracic cage thus offers little stability, and the chest wall will collapse with negative pressures. This makes retractions more pronounced in infants and most obvious in preterm infants. The cartilaginous ribs do, however, mean that closed-chest compressions from cardiopulmonary resuscitation do not usually cause rib fractures in children (2).

• Breathing for infants is mostly diaphragmatic, making them abdominal or "belly breathers." Instability of the thoracic cage makes it difficult to increase minute ventilation by increasing thoracic volume. Infants must drop the diaphragm more to increase tidal volume, which increases WOB. To avoid increased WOB, infants usually increase respiratory rate to increase minute ventilation.

• The angle of the right mainstem at the carina is lower in children than adults, making them more susceptible to right mainstem intubation and foreign body obstruction of the right lung.

• At birth, the number of conducting airways is completely developed. However, airway diameter increases with lung growth. This explains the phenomenon of children "outgrowing" reactive airways disease. It is less likely that the swelling and smooth muscles are no longer reactive; rather, the degree of airway obstruction is less pronounced as a result of the increased airway diameter.

• There is no effective way to measure number of alveoli in live humans. A recent electron microscopy study calculated that the adult

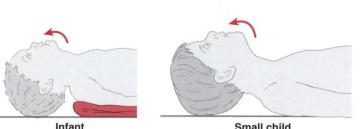
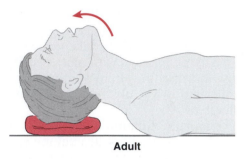

| Infant | Small child | Adult |

Figure 1-2 Sniffing Positions for an Infant, Child, and Adult

male lung has approximately 480 million to 500 million alveoli, with 1 cubic millimeter of lung parenchyma having approximately 170 alveoli (3). Between birth and adulthood, there is a 20-fold multiplication of alveolar surface area (4). There is no current consensus in the scientific community to say how or when the multiplication occurs. A 2006 article identifies different studies that list the age at which the alveoli stop **proliferating** (growing) as 2, 8, 11, and 20 years (4). To generalize on these studies, when body growth stops, so does lung growth, with a large portion of lung proliferation occurring in the first 3 years of life.

- The alveolar sacs in a newborn are structurally different from those of an adult. For the first several years of life, the lungs undergo a phase known as microvascular maturation, in which the septum between alveoli fuse and thin out, and after 2 to 3 years look like a smaller version of the adult lung. The alveoli in newborns also do not have **Pores of Kohn** (minute openings thought to exist between adjacent alveoli), which decreases a newborn's capacity for collateral circulation of air. The lack of collateral air circulation means that during lower airway obstruction, newborns and infants will be affected more significantly and decompensate more rapidly.

Compared to adults, infants and children have a lower pulmonary reserve, or **functional residual capacity (FRC),** which is the amount of air remaining in the lungs after a normal resting expiration. This is caused by several factors.

- Infants and children have larger hearts in proportion to the thoracic diameter, which imposes on the lungs and decreases lung capacity.
- An infant's chest wall is more compliant than an adult's chest.
- The elastic recoil of a child's lungs is less than that of an adult.
- Young children have proportionally large abdominal contents, which push up against the diaphragm. This can also make gastric insufflation during bag-mask ventilation more hazardous for children. Using **cricoid pressure**, also known as the Sellick maneuver (pushing the cricoid cartilage against the cervical spine, compressing the esophagus to prevent passive regurgitation), has been shown to decrease gastric insufflation in children, even when peak inspiratory pressures greater than 40 cm H_2O are used (5). It can also decrease the risk of aspiration. This is especially important for infants, in whom gastric distention can significantly compromise ventilation.

Furthermore, the basal oxygen consumption of children is twice that of adults: 6 mL O_2/kg for children versus 3 mL O_2/kg for adults. The clinical implication of lower pulmonary reserve and increased oxygen consumption is that children will desaturate more rapidly than will adults. Recommendations for airway management suggest that clinicians should be prepared to provide bag-mask ventilation with 1.0 F_IO_2 if a child's oxygen saturation falls below 90% (5).

Patient Assessment

Patient assessment requires the gathering of both subjective and objective information about past and current health. Gathering subjective information about children can be challenging, and objective information such as vital signs and blood gas values can differ based on age. Respiratory therapists need to be aware of these differences to accurately assess pediatric patients and make clinical decisions based on good evidence.

Obtaining a patient history and chief complaint is imperative in patient assessment. Differences in the abilities of children of varying ages and disease states to comprehend what is being said to them (**receptive language**) and capacities to communicate their current thoughts and feelings (**expressive language**) make subjective patient assessment challenging. Social and language developmental milestones are important to better communicate with and assess pediatric patients.

Developmental Milestones

The following list describes the typical progression of social and language developmental milestones from infancy up to 5 years. These are general guidelines, and typically developing children may reach these milestones before or after the stated time frames (2).

- At *3 months old,* an infant can begin to produce long, musical vowel sounds known as cooing. She will start to reach for familiar people or objects and will anticipate feeding.
- At *6 months old,* an infant will make more advanced noises (e.g., babbles, razz, and ah-goo noises) and can recognize when someone is a stranger. She has no expression of anticipatory fear, so the 6-month-old's level of anxiety will reflect that of the parent.
- At *9 months old,* an infant will start to say "mama" and "dada" indiscriminately, gesture, wave bye-bye, and understand the word "no." She will begin exploring the environment, frequently placing items in her mouth, so foreign body aspiration begins to be of concern.
- By *15 months old,* a toddler can use 4 to 6 words and follow one-step commands (e.g., "Go"). She can imitate actions, come when called, cooperate with dressing, and use a spoon and cup.
- At *18 months old,* a toddler says 7 to 10 words and knows five body parts. She can copy some daily tasks such as sweeping or dusting and play in the company of other children. Cooperating during assessments and asking questions may begin to occur during this age. A child at this age may be able to verbalize pain with words like "hurt" or "boo-boo."
- By *2 years old,* a toddler has a 50-word vocabulary, uses pronouns such as "I, you, me" (though not always appropriately), and begins using two-word sentences.
- Around *3 years old,* a toddler knows at least 250 words, knows all pronouns, and can repeat two digits. She knows her full name, age, and gender. She can assess how she feels physically but may still need visual cues to help localize sensory input such as pain (Special Populations 1-1).
- At *4 years old,* a child knows colors, can sing songs or a poem from memory, and asks questions. She can tell "tall tales" and play cooperatively with a group of children.
- At *5 years old,* a child can print her first name, abides by rules, and likes to help out in daily tasks such as household chores. Children around this age can begin to be physically involved in their own medical care, such as using their own metered dose inhaler. They also have an improved understanding of physical senses

● **Special Populations 1-1**

Autism Spectrum Disorders

Autism spectrum disorders (ASDs) are a group of neurodevelopmental disabilities that affect the way a child perceives the world and makes communication and social interaction difficult. These disorders affect 1 in 88 children in the United States (and 1 in 54 boys) and can have a serious impact on how children communicate with health-care providers (6). Signs of ASDs typically are apparent before age 3 and include delays in language and social development, as well as stereotypical and repetitive behaviors. No two children with ASD present with the same symptoms, so interacting with them can be challenging. Some children on the spectrum are nonverbal, whereas others have difficulty with the nuances of social language. Though a child with ASD may understand questions asked of him or her, the child may struggle to give you an appropriate answer, may not make eye contact, and may be sensitive to a stranger's touch. The child may also have hyper- or hyposensitivity to pain stimulus, which may make him or her more or less reactive to diagnostic procedures. Parents and other caregivers of a child with ASD should be able to offer insight for health-care providers on how to best interact with the child. Have parents and caregivers assist you in obtaining subjective information from the child and performing assessment and diagnostic procedures, and ask them for advice on how to interact effectively with the child.

such as pain and can cooperate during procedures and assessments.

Pain Assessment

Pain in particular is difficult to assess in young or noncommunicative children, and various tools have been designed to assist caregivers in evaluating and managing pain in children.

- **Infants:** The physiological response to acute pain includes increases in blood pressure, heart rate, and respiratory rate. Also seen are oxygen desaturations, crying, diaphoresis, flushing, and pallor. These are unreliable as indicators for chronic pain because the body no longer has a physiological response to pain. Behavioral responses can be observed by noting the characteristic and duration of the cry, facial expressions, visual tracking (following movement with the eyes), body movements, and response to stimuli. There is a behavioral assessment tool, known as the Neonatal Infant Pain Scale (NIPS) (7), which can be used to quantify pain in preterm neonates and full-term neonates up to 6 weeks old. Face, Legs, Activity, Cry,

Consolability (FLACC) is a pain scale for pre-verbal patients to evaluate the effectiveness of implemented pain interventions by quantifying pain behaviors such as facial expression, leg movement, activity, cry, and consolability by using a 0 to 10 scoring system (8).

- **Preschool-age children:** In addition to the same physiological and behavioral responses in infants, the Wong-Baker FACES pain rating scale is a self-assessment tool that children as young as 3 years old can use to express pain intensity (Fig. 1-3).
- **School-age children and adolescents:** In addition to noting physiological and behavioral responses, clinicians can also ask patients to describe, locate, and characterize pain. Starting at around age 7 to 8, children can use the standard pain rating scale, where 0 is no pain and 10 is the worst pain ever experienced.

Weight

Weight is one of the most important pieces of patient data for children, but it is not often available during emergencies. Medication dosages are based on weight, with length/height and age being secondary if weight is not known. The Centers for Disease Control and Prevention and the World Health Organization have created growth charts for infants, school-age children, and adolescents. These charts are used in preventive care to monitor growth and development and height versus weight discrepancies. In acute care settings, they can be used to help estimate weights or heights when age is known. See Figures 1-4 through 1-7 at the end of the chapter for male and female growth charts (9).

Studies have shown that visual estimations of patient weights are usually inaccurate and unreliable (10). Several methods have been developed to estimate a child's weight during emergencies. Three of these methods include the Leffler formula, Theron formula, and Broselow Tape. The Leffler and Theron formulas are used in children from 1 to 10 years of age. The UK-based Leffler formula is similar to the equations used in the American Heart Association (AHA) training program, Pediatric Advanced Life Support. The Theron formula was developed in the hopes of improving accuracy of weight estimations for overweight children (11) and works best in patients weighing greater than 40 kg. The formulas are

$$\text{Leffler: Weight (kg)} = (\text{age in months}/2) + 4$$

$$\text{Theron: Weight (kg)} = (\exp{[(0.175571 \times \text{age in years}) + 2.197099]}$$

The Broselow Tape is a long, durable tape measure used on a child during a medical emergency. It is designed for children 12 years or younger, with a maximum weight of roughly 80 pounds. Using a color-coded format, it provides specific medical instructions to health-care providers based on the height and then subsequent weight of the child. It has a tendency to underestimate weight in larger children but has been shown in younger children to be more accurate in determining equipment sizes.

Additional weight estimations are continuously being tested, particularly because height, age, and weight correlations in the United States are not transferrable to other countries. (See Evidence in Practice 1-1.)

Vital Signs

It is important to note that vital sign values are different for children than for adults, and they vary with age. Table 1-2 lists the normal values for heart rate (HR), respiratory rate (RR), and blood pressure (BP) based on age. Once blood pressure is obtained, the calculation to determine mean arterial blood pressure (MAP) is

$$\text{MAP} = 1/3 \text{ systolic pressure} + 2/3 \text{ diastolic pressure}$$

Wong-Baker FACES™ Pain Rating Scale

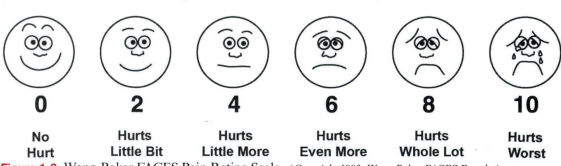

0	2	4	6	8	10
No Hurt	Hurts Little Bit	Hurts Little More	Hurts Even More	Hurts Whole Lot	Hurts Worst

Figure 1-3 Wong-Baker FACES Pain Rating Scale. *(Copyright 1983, Wong-Baker FACES Foundation, used with permission. www.WongBakerFACES.org. Originally published in* Whaley & Wong's Nursing Care of Infants and Children. *©Elsevier Inc.)*

Mid-Arm Circumference (12)

Mid-arm circumference has been used for many years in the assessment of malnutrition in the developing world. In primary schools and kindergartens in Hong Kong, the Healthy Children's Vital Signs and USCOM study recruited healthy Chinese children aged 1 to 11 years and took weight and mid-arm circumference measurements, along with other measurements. Mid-arm circumference was measured with the child's right arm relaxed in 90 degrees of flexion at the elbow. Landmarks were located to identify the midpoint of the arm, and the tape was wrapped around the arm there, taking care to ensure that the tape lay flat against the arm without pinching the underlying skin. Mid-arm circumference had a strong relationship with weight, and this relationship grew stronger with age. The formula, weight [kg] = (mid-arm circumference [cm] − 10) × 3, was at least as accurate and precise as the Broselow Tape method and outperformed the Leffler formula in school-age children, but was inadequate in preschool children. The conclusion of this study was that this weight-estimation formula based on mid-arm circumference is reliable for use in school-age children, and an arm tape could be considered as an alternative to the Broselow Tape in this population.

So, the normal male MAP at 12 years old would be 1/3 (106) + 2/3 (62) or 35.3 + 41.3, which is 76.6 mm Hg. MAP is often used in the pediatric setting to evaluate blood pressure stability and effectiveness of cardiac inotropic and sympathomimetic therapies.

The techniques for respiratory assessment are the same for children as for adults. Care must be taken, however, when assessing respiratory status and obtaining vital signs in children, because accurate measurement of HR, RR, pulse oximetry, and BP can all be affected by patient activity and irritability. In premature infants, it may be difficult to visualize respiratory rate, so a stethoscope is the best way to calculate spontaneous respiratory rate. However, as soon as an infant is touched, he or she will increase respirations, so it will take time and patience to obtain an accurate rate. Breath sounds may be more difficult to distinguish in very young children, and vocal noise transmissions are more common as a result of whining and crying during auscultation. Crying can also increase WOB in an infant up to 32-fold (5), so it is imperative to try to keep young children in respiratory distress as calm as possible. Keeping them in a quiet, comfortable environment with familiar people will help alleviate anxiety and minimize additional respiratory distress.

Table 1-2	Normal Vital Sign Values by Age (2, 13, 14)			
Age (years)	Heart Rate (beats per minute)	Respiratory Rate (breaths per minute)	Blood Pressure (mm Hg)* Systolic	Diastolic
Newborn	95–160	30–60	72	55
Infant	110–180	24–38	90	54
1			85	53
			86	40
2	90–150	22–30	88	42
			88	45
3			91	46
			89	49
4			93	50
	65–135	20–24	91	52
5			95	55
			93	54
6			96	55
			94	56
7	60–130		97	57
		18–24	96	57
8			99	57
			96	57

Continued

Table 1-2	Normal Vital Sign Values by Age (2, 13, 14)—cont'd			
Age (years)	Heart Rate (beats per minute)	Respiratory Rate (breaths per minute)	Blood Pressure (mm Hg)* Systolic	Diastolic
9			100	60
			100	59
10			102	61
			102	60
11			104	61
			103	61
12	60–110	16–22	106	62
			105	62
13			108	62
			107	63
14			111	63
			109	64
15			113	63
			110	65
16		14–20	116	65
			111	66
17			118	67
	60–100		111	66
18		12-20	120	80

● The 50th percentile pressure at 50th percentile height for age. Males listed first, females listed second.

Pulse Oximetry

Pulse oximetry has been advocated as an accurate, simple, and noninvasive method of measuring arterial oxygen saturation (SaO_2). Pulse oximetry (SpO_2) can accurately measure normal SaO_2 and reliably detect desaturation under a variety of conditions, and it may improve our ability to assess the cardiorespiratory status of infants and children. Similar to adults, healthy children breathing room air should have an SpO_2 reading greater than 97% (15).

Pulse oximetry offers more diagnostic information in pediatric patients than does observing respiratory rate alone. One study showed that despite having an SpO_2 reading of <90%, less than half the patients had a respiratory rate elevation above the 80th percentile for their age (16). This means that prior to pulse oximetry, hypoxemic patients without respiratory distress may have gone undiagnosed. Pulse oximetry, however, should not be the only method used to assess oxygenation in patients. Changes in cardiac output, cellular respiration or metabolism, and hemoglobin can all affect tissue hypoxia (Clinical Variations 1-1), and these are not assessed with pulse oximetry.

Blood Gas Monitoring

As with adults, arterial pH is the single best index of acid-base status in the body. Arterial blood gas (ABG) sampling is still the gold standard for assessment of pH, partial pressure of oxygen in the blood (PaO_2), partial pressure of carbon dioxide ($PaCO_2$), and bicarbonate (HCO_3). The indications for ABG sampling are the same in children as they are in adults: the need to evaluate the adequacy of the patient's ventilation, oxygenation, and acid-base status; the need to evaluate the patient's response to therapeutic intervention and/or diagnostic evaluation; and the need to monitor severity and progression of a documented disease process (18). Contraindications to ABG sampling normally apply to the location of the procedure, not to the entire procedure. These include a modified Allen's test result indicating lack of collateral circulation (another extremity should be chosen) or a lesion or surgical shunt proximal to the patient on the same limb. If there is evidence of infection or peripheral vascular disease involving the selected limb, an alternate site should be selected. A coagulopathy or high-dose anticoagulation therapy such as heparin or Coumadin may be a relative contraindication for

Clinical Variations 1-1

A Missing Link in Pulse Oximetry (17)

During the night, a 14-year-old girl hospitalized with leukemia required the attention of the on-call physician for dyspnea associated with tachycardia. General physical examination revealed pallor and tachycardia at 165 bpm. Her temperature was 98.6°F (37°C), respiratory rate was 50 breaths/min, blood pressure was 104/54 mm Hg, and oxygen saturation was 95%. A complete blood count performed in the afternoon revealed a hemoglobin (Hb) of 9 g/dL, but the patient reported that she had an episode of vomiting blood in the late evening. "Did you give oxygen?" the physician asked the nurse. ''No doctor, oxygen saturation is 95%. She called me for tachycardia; should I ask for the cardiologist?" Blood samples were drawn once more, showing a further decrease in the Hb level (6 g/dL). Blood was requested, and, in the meantime, colloid infusion was started. The nurse's reluctance was finally overcome, and oxygen was added at 10 L/min. Tachycardia and dyspnea gradually subsided.

Because this patient's hemoglobin was so low (normal values for adults are 12 to 16 g/dL), her body was attempting to compensate by increasing cardiac output and minute ventilation. She was moderately successful because the pulse oximeter reading was 95%. This is a prime example, however, of how one piece of patient data does not convey the whole patient picture. Increasing this patient's red blood cell count will improve her ability to transport oxygen to her tissues, allowing her ventilation and heart rate to return to normal.

arterial puncture. Slight variations in normal ABG values exist for children of different ages. Table 1-3 lists these variations, as well as the normal ABG range for adults.

ABG sample errors can be more pronounced in pediatric samples because they are usually smaller than adult samples owing to the smaller volume of blood available. Errors include the following:

- **Heparin dilution:** Because of the smaller sample size, neonatal and pediatric samples are more susceptible to liquid heparin dilution errors. Heparin has a lower pH than blood, so heparin will lower pH without affecting $PaCO_2$. This will make the ABG results trend toward a metabolic acidosis. This is most common in umbilical line sampling in neonates if all heparin is not removed from the line prior to collecting the ABG sample. Comparing the current values of pH and calculated bicarbonate with previous ABG results should help reveal this error should it occur.

- **Air in sample:** An air bubble consists of room air, which has a PO_2 of 158 mm Hg and a PCO_2 of approximately 0 mm Hg. $PaCO_2$ in the blood will decrease as CO_2 travels into the air bubble in an equilibrating manner because gases travel from areas of high pressure to areas of low pressure until they are equal. Room air will change the PaO_2 in the arterial sample in an attempt to equilibrate but will raise it or lower it based on the blood sample's starting PaO_2. If the sample PaO_2 is greater than 158 mm Hg, then oxygen will travel from the blood into the air sample and lower the PaO_2 of the blood sample. If the sample PaO_2 is less than 158 mm Hg, then additional oxygen molecules will travel into the blood sample and increase measured PaO_2. To avoid this, all air bubbles should be tapped to the end of the syringe and pushed out of the sample immediately after the sample is drawn.

- **Venous admixture:** This is an error that will occur with puncture sampling, not with arterial line sampling. Peripheral venous blood has different PvO_2, $PvCO_2$, and pH values based on local metabolism, perfusion, and tissue and organ function. So there is no direct correlation between any venous sample

Table 1-3	Normal Arterial Blood Gas Values When Breathing Room Air, at 37°C (14, 19–20)			
Age	**pH**	**PaCO₂ (mm Hg)**	**PaO₂ (mm Hg)**	**HCO₃⁻ (mEq/L)**
Premature infant (<28 weeks' gestation)	≥7.25	45–55	45–65	20–24
Newborn (birth)	7.26–7.29	55	60	19
Newborn (>24 hours)	7.37	33	70	20
Infant (1–24 months)	7.40	34	90	20
Child (7–19 years)	7.39	37	96	22
Adult (>19 years)	7.35–7.45	35–45	90–110	22–26

and an arterial one. In general, however, lower PO_2 and higher PCO_2 values should be expected. A mixed venous blood sample taken from the right atrium or ventricle of the heart can be correlated with an ABG and then subsequent samples used to trend changes in acid-base status. Normal mixed venous blood gas values are pH = 7.38, $PvCO_2$ = 48 mm Hg, and PvO_2 = 40 mm Hg.

- **Temperature:** Patient hypothermia or hyperthermia will cause the measured blood gas results to be less accurate. This is because the electrodes in a blood gas analyzer are heated to normal body temperature. In general, every 2°C decrease in body temperature will cause a drop in $PaCO_2$, causing a subsequent increase in pH of 0.03. Decrease in temperature will also cause a decrease in measured PaO_2. The reverse is true for increases in body temperature.
- **Metabolism:** Blood continues to metabolize when it is outside of the body. If a sample is left at room temperature, pH will decrease, CO_2 will increase, and PaO_2 will decrease. Icing samples have been used historically but are not effective when samples are stored in plastic syringes; therefore, the current recommendation is to run a sample immediately after it is obtained (19).

The complications from arterial puncture or catheterization force clinicians to look for suitable alternatives to multiple arterial samples. In neonatal and pediatric patients, there are several ways to monitor acid-base status. Table 1-4 lists the different techniques, along with their advantages and disadvantages. Two unique methods for measuring ventilation in infants and small children are transcutaneous monitoring and capillary blood gas sampling.

Transcutaneous Monitoring

Transcutaneous monitoring electrochemically measures skin-surface PO_2 and PCO_2 by heating localized areas of the skin to induce hyperperfusion. This provides a noninvasive estimate of arterial oxygen and carbon dioxide. Transcutaneous monitoring can decrease the number of invasive blood gas samples and can offer continuous monitoring of ventilation in infants and young children. Transcutaneous monitoring is considered a safe method of patient assessment, but validation of values is necessary to avoid false results and resulting inappropriate treatment of the patient. To validate transcutaneous measurements, an arterial blood sample should be drawn and compared with transcutaneous readings taken at the same time. Validation should occur at initiation of monitoring and at regular intervals. Though

transcutaneous monitoring is noninvasive, it is not without complications. In patients with poor skin integrity (e.g., extremely premature infants), tissue injury such as erythema, blisters, burns, and skin tears may occur at the measuring site (21). Patients with adhesive allergies can also be at risk for complications from the electrodes.

Capillary Blood Gas Sampling

Arterialized capillary blood can provide a rough estimate of arterial blood values. The physiological principle is that there is little time for oxygen and carbon dioxide exchange in blood flowing through a dilated capillary bed, so the sample drawn has approximately the same acid-base balance as that in the arteries. Oxygen values in capillary samples do not correlate with arterial samples, so the PO_2 values in capillary blood gases are of no clinical use (22). **Capillary blood gas (CBG)** samples can be drawn from a warmed heel or the sides of the tips of the fingers or toes. Sampling errors that can occur include the following:

- Inadequate warming of the site
- Clots within the sample tubing
- Excessive squeezing or "milking," which causes contamination with venous blood and interstitial fluid
- Exposure of blood to air during sampling

Complications from CBG sampling include calcified heel nodules, infection, hematoma, pain, and scarring and bruising at the sampling site. CBG samples are most helpful for neonatal patients, particularly those on mechanical ventilation, for whom serial blood draws are needed and no arterial access is available. They can be used for continuous monitoring and trending of pH and PCO_2.

■■ You arrive in the emergency room triage area and introduce yourself to Jamie's parents. You ask the parents for some history. She has no known allergies, has recently started eating finger foods, and uses the word "Dada" to describe any familiar adult. They were at a cousin's party and had just finished eating when Jamie started to get fussy. It was her naptime so they placed her in the car and left. On the drive she was cooing and babbling in the backseat for a while, then she started whining, then crying, then making a high-pitched squeaking noise. They saw the sign on the highway for the hospital and stopped in the emergency room. Mr. and Mrs. Thibeaux say Jamie has always been a healthy baby and deny any respiratory history.

You do a visual assessment of Jamie and notice that she is a chubby-looking infant, sitting

Table 1-4 Techniques for Monitoring Acid-Base Status and Oxygenation in Neonatal and Pediatric Patients

Modality	Description	Advantages	Disadvantages
Indwelling umbilical artery catheter	Catheter placed in one of two umbilical arteries	Can be easily placed and offers easy access once there Blood gases can be considered steady-state blood gases because patients are not manipulated during sampling Can continuously monitor blood pressure	Only for newborns There is a risk for major complications: • Embolism (air or clot) • Arterial occlusion • Bloodstream infection
Indwelling peripheral artery catheter	Catheter placed in one of several peripheral arteries (radial, femoral, brachial, posterior tibial arteries are all appropriate sites in small children)	Can continuously monitor blood pressure Offers easy access to steady-state samples once placed	Same major complications as with umbilical indwelling catheters when placed Complications also include • Anaphylaxis from local anesthetic • Arteriospasm • Vessel trauma • Pain • Vasovagal response When placed incorrectly or removed, a hematoma (a swelling composed of blood under the tissue that is caused by leaking from the artery at the puncture site) can form
Arterial puncture	One-time sampling of arterial blood from radial, brachial, posterior tibial, or femoral artery	Allows access when no catheter is in place	Technique of sampling may cause pain in patient, which can change minute ventilation and thus change blood gas values Complications may also include • Vessel trauma • Arteriospasm • Vasovagal response • Emboli (air or clot) • Arterial occlusion
Capillary sample	One-time sample from heel or finger Ideal technique for chronically ill patients	Low complication rate Easy to perform Fair estimates of pH and PCO_2	Values for PO_2 not reliable If peripheral perfusion is poor, then capillary samples are inaccurate
Transcutaneous monitor	Heated skin electrode used to measure PO_2 and PCO_2	Provides continuous monitoring Is noninvasive	Much more expensive than other sampling techniques Could be inaccurate with decreased patient perfusion

uncomfortably in her father's arms. She is kicking her legs and grimacing and doesn't seem to be able to settle. You can hear what sounds like a loud inspiratory "wheeze," similar to stridor. She is occasionally letting out a weak cry. Her cheeks are flushed pink and her skin is warm to touch. While you begin your assessment, the nurse places Jamie on the ECG monitor and pulse oximeter. HR is 180 bpm with a sinus rhythm, RR is 70 breaths/min, and SpO_2 is 90%. Blood pressure is 60/33 mm Hg. As you get your stethoscope to auscultate Jamie's lungs, you notice she begins to close her eyes, and her mouth relaxes from the grimace. She is no longer crying, but you still hear the wheezing noise during inspiration.

Pharmacology

Up until the 1990s, children were rarely included in studies of medical treatments. As a result, only 20% to 30% of drugs approved by, Food and Drug Administration (FDA) have been labeled for use in children. This means that the FDA did not have studies on how these products do or do not work in children; what different kinds of reactions children might have; or what the proper dose would be over the wide range of children's ages, weights, and developmental stages. In a 2011 study in a level II pediatric intensive care unit, researchers noted that 24% of medications dispensed by the pharmacy were not approved for use in any pediatric age group, 43% were approved for use in limited age groups, and 33% were approved for use in all pediatric age groups (23). Much is still unknown about how children respond to drugs, biologicals such as gene therapy, and medical devices. Strides have been taken, however, to remedy this situation. The FDA has the authority to require pediatric studies on a drug product for the product's approved indications "if there is substantial use in the pediatric population or the product would provide a meaningful therapeutic benefit—and the absence of adequate labeling could pose significant risk" (24).

Two initiatives have sought to encourage and support pharmaceutical companies in pediatric drug investigation: the Best Pharmaceuticals for Children Act (BPCA) and the Pediatric Research Equity Act (PREA). These acts offer incentives to corporations that include children in their testing, including **exclusivity** (patent protection that allows them to manufacture a drug without competition from other suppliers for a period of time). As of February 20, 2009, labeling changes had been made to more than 260 products that were studied in children under these acts. Of the more than 170 drugs studied under one incentive program within the BPCA, 159 have new pediatric labeling information, including 45 drugs with new or enhanced pediatric safety data that had not been known before, 27 drugs with new dosing or dosing changes, and 50 drugs with information stating that they were not found to be effective in children (25).

These initiatives, however, have not closed the gap for all medications that could potentially be beneficial in children, and there are still many drugs used frequently in pediatrics that are used "off-label." **Off-label use** (26) occurs when a medication is prescribed and delivered for an intended use, such as age group or condition, other than that indicated in the proposed labeling. Because the FDA cannot legally regulate how a drug is used, off-label use is allowable. When medication delivery is initiated for any indication, the following points should apply (27):

- The drug is prescribed in a manner that conforms to the community's standard of care.
- The therapy is considered reasonable; it is based on sound physiological principles and pathological need.
- The therapy is safe, meaning that the clinician is aware of known side effects, there are means for assessing toxicity, and generally any risk is acceptable and appropriate given the patient's situation.
- Before drug dosing begins, parameters to be used in monitoring for side effects and safety have been decided.

Medication Errors

The Institute of Medicine (IOM) defines an **adverse drug event** as an injury resulting from medical intervention related to a drug, which can be attributable to preventable and nonpreventable causes (28). Adverse reactions to medications include those that are usually unpredictable, such as unexpected allergic responses, and those that are predictable, such as adverse effects or toxic reactions related to the pharmacological properties of the drug. A **medication error** is any preventable event that occurs in the process of ordering or delivering a medication, regardless of whether an injury occurred or the potential for injury was present. Medication errors occur as a result of human mistakes or system flaws. For adults, the reported incidence of medication errors is about 5% of orders written, but in pediatrics this number has been reported to be three times as high (29). A 1995 to 1999 study by the U.S. Pharmacopeia (USP) Medication Errors Reporting Program demonstrated a significantly increased rate of medication error resulting in harm or death in pediatric patients (31%) compared with adults (13%) (30).

However, potential adverse drug events—those errors not causing harm—occurred in pediatric patients three times more often than in adults (29).

The lack of formal pediatric indications and dosing guidelines for many drugs increases the risk of medication errors and accounts for the significant difference in the frequency of errors in pediatric patients compared with adults (29). The 1999 IOM report implicates medication errors, at least in part, as a direct cause of up to 98,000 patient deaths annually (28) and an increase in inpatient health-care costs by an estimated $4,700 per hospital admission, or approximately $2.8 million annually for a 700-bed teaching hospital. Children vary in weight, body surface area, and organ system maturity, which affect their ability to metabolize and excrete medications. In addition, there are few standardized dosing regimens for children, with most medication dosing requiring body weight calculations.

The USP identified the following top 10 causes of pediatric medication errors for the 2-year period ending December 31, 2000:

1. Performance deficit
2. Procedure or protocol not followed
3. Miscommunication
4. Inaccurate or omitted transcription
5. Improper documentation
6. Drug distribution system error
7. Knowledge deficit
8. Calculation error
9. Computer entry error
10. Lack of system safeguards (30)

According to the same report, the top four causes of pediatric medication errors accounted for more than 50% of all errors. Distractions, workload increase, inexperienced staff, and insufficient staffing contributed to more than 70% of medication errors (30).

There are dozens of ways that health-care providers can attempt to decrease the number of adverse drug events in their institutions. Following are some actions and guidelines for decreasing pediatric medication errors suggested by the AAP (29):

- Provide a suitable work environment for safe, effective drug preparation.
- Standardize order sheets to include areas for patient weight, old and new allergies, prescriber name, signature, and contact number.
- Establish and maintain a functional pediatric formulary system with policies for drug evaluation, selection, and therapeutic use.
- Ensure that the weight-based dose does not exceed the recommended adult dose.
- Ensure that calculations are correct.
- Write weight on each order written.
- Include dose and volume when appropriate; specify exact dosage strength to be used.
- Spell out dosage units rather than using abbreviations (e.g., milligram or microgram rather than mg or µg; units rather than U).
- Stay current and knowledgeable concerning changes in medications and treatment of pediatric conditions.
- Consult with a pharmacist if available.
- Confirm patient identity before administration of each dose.

Aerosolized Medications

The dosing and delivery of aerosolized medication is particularly challenging in children when compared with adults. The differences in upper and lower airway anatomy affect drug deposition. There is therefore some variation in aerosolized drug dosing among institutions and potentially a lack of understanding among clinicians regarding how to dose aerosolized medications. This is further complicated by off-label use of many aerosolized medications. Few respiratory medications are FDA approved for use in neonates, though virtually all ß-agonists and corticosteroid formulations are approved by the FDA for use in patients older than 12 years of age (31). Aerosolization is a preferred delivery method and offers benefits over a systemic route. These include the following:

- Reduced systemic exposure and effects
- Potential for lower doses compared with intravenous or oral routes
- Painless and generally safe administration
- Ease of administration for very young children unable to use oral route with pills or tablets
- Avoidance of complicating **pharmacokinetic** (drug metabolism, particularly the duration of action, distribution in the body, and method of excretion) and **pharmacodynamic** (the action of drugs) factors in very young children
- Rapid onset of drug action

For most medications, pediatric dosage is calculated using body weight in kilograms. Aerosol dose, however, is not based on body size but rather on the amount of drug reaching the lungs. The strategy for determining dosage for inhaled medications should be based on finding **target effect**. Target effect is reached when a drug is dosed until the desired effect is achieved or until unacceptable side effects or toxicity occurs. Only a small portion of an aerosolized drug dose actually reaches the lower airways. The aerosol particle size range most likely to be deposited in an adult airway is 1 to 5, which is 10% to 15% of a delivered dose in a traditional jet nebulizer. For children, decreases in airway diameter coupled with smaller tidal volumes and lower inspiratory flows suggest that smaller size aerosol particles will reach the lower airways, and thus they receive a smaller percentage of the ordered dose. This is further reduced with the addition of inflammation and secretions common in respiratory diseases and infections present when children are prescribed aerosol therapy. Smaller tidal volumes mean that more drug is wasted during continuous jet nebulization. Young children are also frequently unable to follow commands and thus cannot perform a breath hold during aerosol delivery, shortening the amount of time an aerosol resides in the lower airway and decreasing absorption. Available data have suggested that the delivered dose could be as low as less than 1% (32) in neonates and infants, and around 2.7% in young children (33). Although the percentage is lower, it is possible that the amount of drug per kilogram of body weight delivered to the lungs is still higher than that found with adults. Using the target effect strategy, one study (34) compared a standard 2.5-mg dose of albuterol with a 0.1-mg/kg dose in children 4 to 12 years old in acute asthma and showed no difference in clinical improvement measured by flows, oxygen saturation, and clinical score. There was also no difference in cardiovascular and tremor side effects.

To maximize the effectiveness of aerosolized drug delivery, the device used to deliver medications to children should be chosen carefully. Delivery of one drug by an inhaler may differ from delivery of another drug by the same device. As with adult patients, proper education is also essential when prescribing an inhalation device to maximize therapy. For parents who are struggling to correctly deliver daily inhaled medications to young children, it is difficult to maintain compliance with ordered therapy. School-age children working with the complexities of medication delivery via dry powder inhalers and breath-actuated metered dose inhalers may not correctly manage their therapy. Pediatric compliance with correct pressurized metered dose inhaler (pMDI) inhalation technique ranges from 39% to 67% (35). A pMDI with a mask and spacer is the delivery method of choice for children younger than 5 years old (35). The spacer will eliminate loss of medication in the oropharynx and stomach, thus allowing for an effective dose delivered to the airways. Crying will break a facemask-face seal in both MDI and nebulizer delivery, eliminating almost all aerosol delivery (36). Infants seem to inhale through their nose regardless of whether their mouth is open, so care must be taken to aim aerosol delivery at the nose and not the mouth (33). By age 9, children should be able to manage using a mouthpiece with all devices and have a high enough inspiratory flow to activate any inspiratory demand delivery system.

External factors that can also affect the amount of MDI dose delivered to neonatal and pediatric patients include the following:

- Volume of spacer chamber
- Electrostatic charge on plastic spacers
- Presence and design of expiratory valves
- Presence of an inspiratory valve
- Amount of dead space in mask or mouthpiece

The choice of a delivery device should depend on the age of the patient, the drug to be administered, and the condition to be treated. It is also important for the respiratory therapist to remember that the optimal delivery device is one that a patient can and will use.

Equipment Selection

The selection of respiratory care equipment for pediatric patients should be based on age and/or weight. It is important to choose the right-sized equipment to best manage the airway, deliver appropriate oxygen and medications, and avoid unnecessary patient complications caused by ill-fitting or inappropriate supplies.

Because of the higher and more anterior glottic opening, floppy epiglottis, and large tongue in children younger than 3 years old, a straight (Miller) laryngoscope blade is recommended for these patients. It elevates the distensible airway and provides direct control of the epiglottis. Laryngoscope blade sizes and types are chosen based on patient weight.

- Size 0 Miller (straight): less than 3 kg
- Size 1 Miller: 6 to 11 kg
- Size 2 Miller: 12 to 31 kg
- Size 2 Macintosh (curved): 19 to 31 kg
- Size 3 Miller or Macintosh: greater than 31 kg

There are methods for selecting ETT sizes for pediatric patients of various ages. In neonates, ETTs are selected by either gestational age (when intubating at birth) or weight (once weight is known; see Table 1-5). Cuffless ETTs are preferred in infants. In children older than 1 year, selection of an ETT size should be based on the following calculation:

$$\text{ETT size (mm)} = (16 + \text{age in years})/4$$

Thus, a 6 year-old-child would require a tube size of (16 + 6)/4, or 22/4, which is a 5.5-cm ETT. The trachea becomes adult in size at approximately 12 to 14 years of age, at which time female ETT size is 7.0 to 8.5 mm and male ETT size is 8.0 to 10.0 mm. There is no evidence to support a specific age to use a cuffed versus an uncuffed ETT, so the AHA's Pediatric Advanced Life Support recommendations currently leave it up to the clinician whether to use a cuffed or uncuffed ETT (38).

Table 1-5	Endotracheal Tube Size Selection in Neonates (37)			
Gestational Age (weeks)	Weight	Tube Size (cm)	Location Marking at Lip (cm)	
<28	<1,000 g	2.5	7	
28–34	1,000–2,000 g	3.0	8	
34–38	2,000–3,000 g	3.5	9	
>38	>3,000 g	3.5–4.0	10	

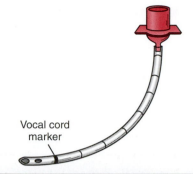

Vocal cord marker

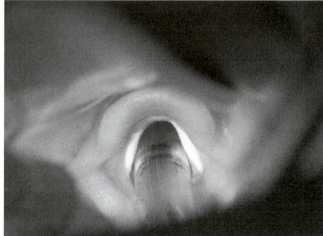

Figure 1-8 Vocal Cord Markers.

Because of the shorter length of the trachea, proper depth placement for a child's ETT is imperative. There are three main methods for determining depth placement of an ETT:

- For any age child, depth can be calculated by multiplying the internal diameter of the ETT by 3. This gives the provider the desired depth of the ETT, measured at the lip.
- For infants, depth can be calculated by adding 6 to the weight in kilograms. This gives the provider the desired depth of the ETT, measured at the lip.
- During intubation, the provider passes the ETT through the vocal cords until one of the vocal cord markers is visualized at the level of the cords (Fig. 1-8). The provider reads the number at the lip after intubation to document the correct depth.

The sizes for airway management and oxygen delivery devices can be found in Table 1-6 (39).

■■ The emergency room physician walks into the room and notices you and the nurse standing by the bedside. He introduces himself to Mr. and Mrs. Thibeaux and begins to ask them some questions about Jamie's medical history. You politely interrupt because you are concerned now that Jamie is no longer crying and seems to be less active than before. "Doctor, I'm concerned because Jamie just stopped crying," you say. "Her SpO$_2$ is only 90% and she has inspiratory wheezing. She seems less alert than she was just a few minutes ago. I'm not sure what's caused her distress, but I think we need to support her respirations right now." At that moment you notice that Jamie's respiratory rate is 25 breaths/min. The nurse carefully takes Jamie from Mr. Thibeaux's arms and lays her on the examination table. You take a portion of the bed sheet and roll it under Jamie's shoulders to keep her airway open, and while you are waiting for infant-sized equipment you place an adult non-rebreather mask over her mouth and nose. Her SpO$_2$ climbs to 93% but goes no higher. A Broselow Tape and color-coded pediatric equipment cart is pulled into the room. The triage nurse measures Jamie and estimates her weight to be 8 to 9 kg, which is the red section of the Broselow Tape. The charge nurse pulls the red equipment bin from the pediatric cart and hands you a newborn oxygen mask and infant resuscitation bag. Jamie's respiratory rate is now around 6 breaths/min. You connect the bag to 1.0 FIO$_2$ at 10 L and check to be sure the bag is working properly. You perform a head tilt–chin lift and begin manual ventilation at about 20 breaths/minute.

Intensive Care Unit Classifications

Hospitals differ in the type and quality of services they provide. The practice of pediatric and neonatal critical care is relatively young and has evolved over the past several decades. In order to understand the scope of practice available in intensive care units, AAP has developed guidelines for classifying neonatal intensive care units (NICUs) and pediatric intensive care units (PICUs). It is important to understand the services, monitoring, personnel, drugs, and equipment available based on the

Table 1-6	Respiratory Supplies by Patient Weight					
Equipment	**Patient Weight (kg)**					
	6–9	10–11	12–18	19–23	23–31	>31
Oral airway (mm)	50 mm	60 mm		70 mm	80 mm	
Nasal airway (French)	14	18	20–22	24	26	30
Oxygen mask	Infant	Child			Child/Adult	Adult
Laryngeal mask airway (LMA)	1.5	2	2–2.5	2.5	3	

ICU's designated level. These classifications will be used throughout the case studies in this text to qualify the services available to therapists and their patients. Table 1-7 lists the classification for NICUs, and Table 1-8 provides selected information for classification of PICUs.

Evidence-Based Medicine

Dr. David Sackett, a pioneer in evidence-based medicine, defines **evidence-based medicine** as the "conscientious, explicit and judicious use of current best evidence in making decisions about the care of the individual patient. It means integrating individual clinical expertise with the best available external clinical evidence from systematic research" (42). Evidence-based medicine is the integration of clinical expertise, patient values, and the best research evidence into patient care decision making. Clinical expertise refers to a clinician's experience, education, and skills. The best evidence is usually found in clinically relevant research that has been conducted using sound methodology (42). The steps for evidence-based practice are included in Box 1-2.

Table 1-7	Neonatal Intensive Care Unit Classifications (40)
Level I	Well-newborn nursery has the capabilities to do the following: • Provide neonatal resuscitation at every delivery • Evaluate and provide postnatal care to healthy newborn infants • Stabilize and provide care for infants born at 35 to 37 weeks' gestation who remain physiologically stable • Stabilize newborn infants who are ill and those born at ≤35 weeks' gestation until transfer to a facility that can provide the appropriate level of neonatal care
Level II	Level II NICUs are divided into two categories on the basis of the facility's ability to provide assisted ventilation, including continuous positive airway pressure
A	Has the capabilities to do the following: • Resuscitate and stabilize preterm and/or ill infants before transfer to a facility at which newborn intensive care is provided • Provide care for infants born at ≤32 weeks' gestation and weighing ≤1,500 g who (1) have physiological immaturity such as apnea of prematurity, inability to maintain body temperature, or inability to take oral feedings or (2) are moderately ill with problems that are anticipated to resolve rapidly and are not anticipated to need subspecialty services on an urgent basis • Provide care for infants who are convalescing after intensive care
B	Has the capabilities of a level IIA nursery and the additional capability to provide mechanical ventilation for brief durations (<24 hours) or continuous positive airway pressure
Level III	Level III NICUs are divided into three categories.
A	Has the capabilities to do the following: • Provide comprehensive care for infants born at >28 weeks' gestation and weighing 1,000 g

Table 1-7	Neonatal Intensive Care Unit Classifications (40)

	• Provide sustained life support limited to conventional mechanical ventilation • Perform minor surgical procedures such as placement of central venous catheter or inguinal hernia repair
B	Has the capabilities to provide the following: • Comprehensive care for extremely low birth weight infants (≤1,000 g and ≤28 weeks' gestation) • Advanced respiratory support such as high-frequency ventilation and inhaled nitric oxide for as long as required • Prompt and on-site access to a full range of pediatric medical subspecialists • Advanced imaging, with interpretation on an urgent basis, including computed tomography, magnetic resonance imaging, and echocardiography • Pediatric surgical specialists and pediatric anesthesiologists on site or at a closely related institution to perform major surgery such as ligation of patent ductus arteriosus and repair of abdominal wall defects, necrotizing enterocolitis with bowel perforation, tracheoesophageal fistula and/or esophageal atresia, and myelomeningocele
C	Has the capabilities of a level IIIB NICU and also is located within an institution that has the capability to provide extracorporeal membrane oxygenation and surgical repair of complex congenital cardiac malformations that require cardiopulmonary bypass

Table 1-8	Pediatric Intensive Care Unit Classifications (listing essential items only) (41)

Category	Level I	Level II
Physical Facility		
Two or more oxygen and air outlets each per bed	√	√
Easy, rapid access to head of bed	√	√
Television, radio, toys	√	√
Physician Staff		
Physician in house 24 hours a day	√	√
Pediatric physician or anesthesiologist (postgraduate year 3 or above) in house 24 hours per day	√	
Pediatric intensivist available in 30 minutes or less		
Available within 1 hour	√	
Anesthesiologist		
Pediatric anesthesiologist	√	√
General surgeon	√	
Pediatric surgeon	√	√
Neurosurgeon	√	
Pediatric neurosurgeon	√	√
Otolaryngologist	√	
Orthopedic surgeon	√	
Pediatric Subspecialists	√	
Pediatric intensivist		
Pediatric cardiologist	√	√
Pediatric nephrologist	√	
Neonatologist	√	
Neurologist	√	√
Radiologist	√	

Continued

Table 1-8	Pediatric Intensive Care Unit Classifications (listing essential items only) (41)—cont'd		
Category		**Level I**	**Level II**
Pediatric radiologist		√	√
Psychiatrist or psychologist		√	
		√	
Respiratory Therapy Staff			
Supervisor responsible for training registered respiratory therapist (RRT) staff		√	√
Maintenance of equipment and quality control and review		√	√
RT in house 24 hours per day assigned primarily to PICU		√	
RT in house 24 hours per day		√	√
RT familiar with management of pediatric patients with respiratory failure		√	√
RT competent with pediatric mechanical ventilators		√	√
Completion of pediatric advanced life support (PALS) training or an equivalent course (desirable but not essential)		√	√
Respiratory Support Equipment			
Bag-valve mask resuscitation devices		√	√
Oxygen cylinders		√	√
Respiratory gas humidifiers		√	√
Air compressor		√	√
Air-oxygen blenders		√	√
Ventilators of all sizes for pediatric patients		√	√
Inhalation therapy equipment		√	√
Chest physiotherapy and suctioning		√	√
Spirometers		√	√
Continuous oxygen analyzers with alarms		√	√

Box 1-2 Steps for Evidence-Based Practice

1. **Assess the patient:** Gather information from the patient about his or her primary problem, chief complaint, medical history, medications taken, vital signs, and other objective and subjective data.
2. **Ask a question:** Use the information you've gathered to build a clinical question for which the answer will improve the patient's care or help guide future treatment. A good clinical question should include four parts, known by the acronym PICO (40):
   • *Patient problem* or *Population:* Includes primary problem; main concern or chief complaint; disease or health status; and demographics such as age, race, gender, previous ailments, and current medications
   • *Intervention:* What you intend to do for the patient (e.g., diagnostic test, treatment, adjunctive therapy, medication)

   • *Comparison:* What other main alternative is being considered; this should include if no action is being taken
   • *Outcomes*: The result of what you plan to accomplish, improve, or affect
3. **Acquire the evidence:** Using appropriate resources, conduct a search of the current published data relating to the clinical question.
4. **Appraise the evidence:** Assess the research gathered for **validity** (closeness to the truth) and **applicability** (usefulness in clinical practice). Evidence with high validity that is not applicable is not useful, so be mindful of gathering data that may not help solve your particular patient's problem.
5. **Apply the evidence:** Integrate the new evidence with clinical expertise and patient preferences, and apply it to practice.
6. **Self-evaluate:** Assess your performance and results with the patient.

All published data are not equal. To help clinicians and scientists, different systems have been developed to classify the quality and validity of research evidence. The U.S. Preventive Services Task Force (USPSTF) is a panel of independent primary care providers who are experts in preventive and evidence-based medicine. The panel's purpose is to conduct scientific evidence reviews of a broad range of clinical preventive health-care services and develop recommendations for primary care clinicians and health systems. The USPSTF created a "hierarchy of research design" (44) (Box 1-3) because it recognizes that research design is an important component of the validity of the information in a study.

Box 1-3 USPSTF Hierarchy (44)

- I: Properly conducted randomized controlled trial; well-conducted systematic review or meta-analysis of homogeneous randomized control trials
- II-1: Well-designed controlled trial without randomization
- II-2: Well-designed cohort or case-control analytic study
- II-3: Multiple time series with or without the intervention; dramatic results from uncontrolled experiments
- III: Opinions of respected authorities based on clinical experience; descriptive studies or case reports; reports of expert committees

Once it has gathered data on a certain question and validated the research, the USPSTF assigns one of five letter grades (A, B, C, D, or I) to each of its recommendations and provides suggestions for practice and levels of certainty regarding net benefit (Table 1-9). This grading system is an example of how evidence-based practice has been implemented throughout the United States in a safe and effective manner. Well-known pediatric recommendations from the USPSTF currently include screening for newborn hearing loss, sickle cell disease, childhood obesity, speech and language delay, high blood pressure, and a variety of cancers (45). The task force has also made counseling recommendations for smoking and tobacco use in children and adolescents.

Prior to the initiation of a research study, investigators must meet rigorous international and federal guidelines, and their research must be approved through an internal review board. This is a particularly rigorous process if the study involves human subjects. Children are considered an especially vulnerable research subject population needing special protection against violation of individual rights and exposure to undue risk. Early research on children was done on those who were poor, mentally ill, institutionalized, or disabled (46). It was after discovering the work done by German physicians under the Nazi regime that an international set of standards was drafted. Established in 1947 at the end of World War II and known as the Nuremberg Code, they were the first regulations protecting human subjects. They are international standards that outline what are now considered to be the 10 basic principles governing the

Table 1-9 U.S. Preventive Services Task Force Grading Definitions (43)

Grade	Definition	Suggestions for Practice
A	The USPSTF recommends the service; there is high certainty that the net benefit is substantial	Offer or provide this service
B	The USPSTF recommends the service; there is high certainty that the net benefit is moderate or there is moderate certainty that the net benefit is moderate to substantial	Offer or provide this service
C	The USPSTF recommends against routinely providing the service; there may be considerations that support providing the service in an individual patient; there is at least moderate certainty that the net benefit is small	Offer or provide this service only if other considerations support the offering or providing of the service in an individual patient
D	The USPSTF recommends against the service; there is moderate or high certainty that the service has no net benefit or that the harms outweigh the benefits	Discourage the use of this service
I	The USPSTF concludes that the current evidence is insufficient to assess the balance of benefits and harms of the service; evidence is lacking, of poor quality, or conflicting, and the balance of benefits and harms cannot be determined	Read the clinical considerations section of USPSTF Recommendation Statement; if the service is offered, patients should understand the uncertainty of the balance between benefits and harms

ethical conduct of research on humans (47). Additional guidelines were initially created in 1983 by the National Commission for the Protection of Human Subjects of Biomedical and Behavioral Research, which further protect the interests, health, and safety of children involved in medical research (46). The current guidelines reside with the U.S. Department of Health and Human Services (48). These additional restrictions have resulted in significantly less published research in children compared to adults. For clinicians, this means a great deal more deliberation when evaluating smaller amounts of research available to guide health-care decisions. Often evidence-based practice in adults is transferred to children without assurance that results would be comparable in a different age population. Care must be taken to use the available evidence effectively and make informed decisions about patient care. Involving the child, parents, and other clinical team members in the decision-making process can assist in making the best decision for the patient.

■ ■ After about 1 minute of manual ventilation, you note that Jamie's SpO$_2$ is now 96%, but she is not making any spontaneous effort to breathe. Though you can see her chest rise with each breath, you're not confident that your efforts are as effective as they could be. You ask the physician his thoughts on intubation. He hesitates and asks the charge nurse to page the anesthesiologist on call and check the status of the pediatric transport team, who has been called and should be arriving to transport Jamie to the children's hospital approximately 30 miles away. The charge nurse notifies the team that the pediatric team from the children's hospital will arrive in about 10 minutes. The physician decides not to place an advanced airway before the team arrives because

you are able to move the chest, and oxygenation appears to have improved with your efforts. When the on-call anesthesiologist arrives in the room a few minutes later, the physician leaves Jamie's bedside to consult with the pediatric intensivist at the children's hospital. You and the anesthesiologist decide to place a nasogastric tube to eliminate gastric distention and use cricoid pressure to minimize any further gastric insufflation. The anesthesiologist determines that if at any point manual ventilation becomes difficult for you, the next step in the airway management plan will be to place an endotracheal tube.

You reassess Jamie and note that her HR is now 178 bpm, blood pressure is 55/30 mm Hg, and SpO$_2$ is 97%. Her skin is still flushed, and she seems to be developing a rash over her face and chest. You don't hear inspiratory wheezing when you squeeze the resuscitation bag, and she isn't taking any spontaneous breaths. The pediatric transport team has just arrived to take over Jamie's care.

■ ■ Critical Thinking Questions: Jamie Thibeaux

1. Based on her history, what could be the cause of Jamie's respiratory distress?
2. If your initial attempts at mask ventilation were unsuccessful and you were not able to see the chest rise, what would you do to improve your ventilations?
3. As a provider in a hospital that does not care for pediatric patients regularly, is there equipment that you would recommend having readily available in the emergency department as a result of your experience with Jamie?

Multiple-Choice Questions

1. Why should all respiratory therapists need to be able to care for pediatric patients?
   a. Every hospital has at least one pediatric unit, and therefore there will always be patients for whom to care.
   b. Children cannot communicate their symptoms to health-care providers.
   c. Pediatric critical events are frequently respiratory in origin and thus need the services of a skilled respiratory therapist.
   d. Inhaled medications have been approved for use in all age groups, so therapists must be competent in performing complex dose calculations for aerosolized medications.

2. Why are pediatric airways more difficult to intubate than adult airways?
   a. Pediatric patients have a large tongue in relation to the oropharynx.
   b. The cricoid ring is the smallest portion of the airway.
   c. Pediatric patients have large tonsils and adenoids.
   d. Pediatric patients have a higher and more anterior epiglottis.

Multiple-Choice Questions — cont'd

3. Which of the following anatomical features of children causes a decrease in functional residual capacity?
   I. Larger heart in proportion to the thoracic diameter, which imposes on the lungs
   II. Higher and more anterior glottis
   III. Decreased lung elastic recoil
   IV. Large abdominal contents pushing on the diaphragm
   a. I, II, III
   b. I, III, IV
   c. III, IV
   d. I, IV

4. Which would you use to assess pain in a 3-year-old?
   I. FACES pain scale
   II. FLACC
   III. NIPS
   IV. Physiological response
   a. III and IV
   b. II and IV
   c. I and IV
   d. IV

5. Which of the following is *not* a way to monitor oxygenation in an infant?
   a. Pulse oximetry
   b. Transcutaneous monitoring
   c. Umbilical artery catheter sample
   d. CBG sample

6. How is target effect used to determine the dosing of aerosol medications?
   a. Clinicians increase the dosage of a medication until the desired response is seen.
   b. Clinicians change the aerosol delivery device until the patient is comfortable and the correct response to the medication is seen.
   c. Clinicians begin with a high dose and decrease until a response is no longer seen.
   d. Clinicians calculate the dose of a medication by weight, then adjust up or down to achieve the desired results.

7. Which of the following are ways to minimize the risk of medication errors in pediatric patients?
   a. Be sure that a weight-based dose does not exceed the recommended adult dose.
   b. Write the patient's weight on each order.
   c. Stay current and knowledgeable concerning changes in medications and treatment of pediatric conditions.
   d. All of the above

8. Which of the following is *not* an appropriate method for delivering a bronchodilator to a 14-year-old?
   a. pMDI
   b. Jet nebulizer
   c. Oral syrup
   d. Dry powdered inhaler

9. Of the following resources, which would *not* be available to a therapist working in a level II PICU?
   a. Pediatric cardiologist
   b. Pediatric intensivist
   c. Two or more oxygen wall outlets
   d. Ventilators for pediatric patients

10. What does PICO stand for?
    a. Patient problem, Investigate, Conclude, Outcomes
    b. Population, Inspect, Complete, Originate
    c. Patient problem, Intervention, Comparison, Outcomes
    d. Plan, Interrogate, Conclude, Outcomes

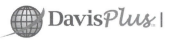

For additional resources login to Davis*Plus* (http://davisplus.fadavis.com/ keyword "Perretta") and click on the Premium tab. (Don't have a *Plus*Code to access Premium Resources? Just click the Purchase Access button on the book's Davis*Plus* page.)

REFERENCES

1. American Hospital Association. Fast facts on U.S. hospitals. http://www.aha.org/research/rc/stat-studies/101207 fastfacts.pdf. Accessed November 12, 2012.
2. Custer JW, Rau RE, eds. *The Harriet Lane Handbook*. Philadelphia, PA: Mosby Elsevier; 2009.
3. Hyde DM, Blozis SA, Avdalovic MV, et al. Alveoli increase in number but not size from birth to adulthood in rhesus monkeys. *Am J Physiol Lung Cell Mol Physiol*. 2007;293:L570-L579.
4. Burri PH. Structural aspects of postnatal lung development—alveolar formation and growth. *Biol Neonate*. 2006;89: 313-322.
5. Walls RM, Murphy MF. *Manual of Emergency Airway Management*. 3rd ed. Philadelphia, PA: Lippincot Williams & Wilkins; 2008.
6. Baio J. Centers for Disease Control. Prevalence of autism spectrum disorders—autism and developmental disabilities monitoring network, 14 sites, United States, 2008. http://www.cdc.gov/mmwr/preview/mmwrhtml/ss6103a1.htm?s_cid=ss6103a1_w, Accessed August 25, 2012.
7. Lawrence J, Alcock D, et al. The development of a tool to assess neonatal pain. *Neonatal Network*. 1993;12(6):59-66.
8. Merkel SI, Voepel-Lewis T, Shayevitz JR, et al. The FLACC: a behavioral scale for scoring postoperative pain in young children. *Paediatr Nurs*. 1997;23:293-297.
9. Centers for Disease Control, Department of Health and Human Services. *2000 growth charts for United States: methods and development*. May 2002;11(246).
10. Rosenberg M, Greenberger S, Rawal A, Latimer-Pierson J, Thundiyil J. Comparison of Broselow Tape measurements versus physician estimations of pediatric weights. *Am J Emerg Med*. 2011 Jun;29(5):482-488.
11. So TY, Farrington E, Absher RK. Evaluation of the accuracy of different methods used to estimate weights in the pediatric population. *Pediatrics*. 2009;123(6):1045-1051.
12. Cattermole GN, Leung PYM, Mak PSK, et al. Mid-arm circumference can be used to estimate children's weights. *Resuscitation*. 2010;81:1105-1110.
13. National Heart Lung and Blood Institute. National Institutes of Health. *Blood Pressure Tables for Children and Adolescents from the Fourth Report on the Diagnosis, Evaluation, and Treatment of High Blood Pressure in Children and Adolescents*. http://www.nhlbi.nih.gov/guidelines/hypertension/child_tbl.htm. Published May 2004. Accessed January 25, 2011.
14. Goldsmith JP, Karotkin EH. *Assisted Ventilation of the Neonate*. 5th ed. Philadelphia, PA: Saunders; 2011.
15. Malley WJ. *Clinical Blood Gases: Assessment and Intervention*. 2nd ed. St. Louis, MO: Elsevier Saunders; 2005.
16. Mower WR, Sachs C, Nicklin EL, Baraff LJ. Pulse oximetry as the fifth pediatric vital sign. *Pediatrics*. 1997;99(5):681-686.
17. Tozzetti C, Adembri C, Modesti PA. Pulse oximeter, the fifth vital sign: a safety belt or a prison of the mind? *Intern Emerg Med*. 2009;4:331-332.
18. AARC Clinical Practice Guideline. Blood gas analysis and hemoximetry. *Respir Care*. 2001;46(5):498-505.
19. Knowles TP, Mullin RA, Hunter JA, Douce FH. Effects of syringe material, sample storage time, and temperature on blood gases and oxygen saturation in arterialized human blood samples. *Respir Care*. 2006;51(7):732-736.
20. Rogers M. *Textbook of Pediatric Intensive Care*. 3rd ed. Baltimore, MD: Lippincott Williams and Wilkins, 1996.
21. AARC Clinical Practice Guideline. Transcutaneous blood gas monitoring for neonatal and pediatric patients—2004 revision and update. *Respir Care*. 2004; 49(9):1069-1072.
22. AARC Clinical Practice Guideline: Capillary blood gas sampling for neonatal & pediatric patients. *Respir Care*. 2001; 46(5):506–513.
23. Yang CP, Veltri MA, Anton B, Yaster M, Berkowitz ID. Food and Drug Administration approval for medications used in the pediatric intensive care unit: a continuing conundrum. *Pediatr Crit Care Med*. 2011 Sep;12(5):e195-9.
24. US Food and Drug Administration. Frequently asked questions on Pediatric Exclusivity (505A), the Pediatric "Rule," and their interaction. http://www.fda.gov/Drugs/DevelopmentApprovalProcess/DevelopmentResources/ucm077915.htm#the"Rule". Accessed February 1, 2011.
25. US Food and Drug Administration. Should your child be in a clinical trial? http://www.fda.gov/ForConsumers/ConsumerUpdates/ucm048699.htm. Accessed February 1, 2011.
26. US Department of Health and Human Services Food and Drug Administration Center for Devices and Radiological Health. *Determination of Intended Use for 510(k) Devices; Guidance for CDRH Staff (Update to K98-1)*. http://www.fda.gov/MedicalDevices/DeviceRegulationandGuidance/GuidanceDocuments/ucm082162.htm December 3, 2002.
27. Blumer JL. Off-label uses of drugs in children. *Pediatrics*. 1999;104(suppl 3):598.
28. Kohn LT, Corrigan JM, Donaldson MS, eds. *To Err Is Human: Building a Safer Health System*. Washington, DC: National Academy Press; 1999. http://books.nap.edu/openbook.php?record_id=9728. Accessed January 28, 2011.
29. American Academy of Pediatrics. Committee on Drugs and Committee on Hospital Care. Prevention of medical errors in the pediatric inpatient setting. *Pediatrics*. 2003; 112(2):431-436.
30. Cowley E, Williams R, Cousins D. Medication errors in children: a descriptive summary of medication error reports submitted to the United States Pharmacopeia. *Curr Ther Res*. 2001;62(9):627-640.
31. Gardenhire DS. *Rau's Respiratory Care Pharmacology*. 7th ed. St Louis, MO: Mosby Elsevier, 2008.
32. Rubin BK, Fink JB. The delivery of inhaled medication to the young child. *Pediatr Clin North Am*. 2003;50:717-731.
33. Chua HL, Collis GG, Newbury AM, et al. The influence of age on aerosol deposition in children with cystic fibrosis. *Eur Respir J*. 1994;7:2185-2191.
34. Oberklaid F, Mellis CM, Souef PN, et al. A comparison of bodyweight dose versus a fixed dose of nebulized salbutamol in acute asthma in children. *Med J Australia*. 1993;158:751.
35. Devadason SG. Recent advances in aerosol therapy for children with asthma. *J Aerosol Med*. 2006;19(1):61-66.
36. Nikander KN, Berg E, Smaldone GC. Jet nebulizers versus pressurized metered dose inhalers with valved holding chambers: effects of the facemask on aerosol delivery. *J Aerosol Med*. 2007;20(suppl 1):S46-S58.
37. American Heart Association/American Academy of Pediatrics. *Textbook of Neonatal Resuscitation*, 6th edition. Dallas, TX: American Heart Association; 2011.
38. Kleinman ME, Chameides L, Schexnayder SM, et al. Part 14: Pediatric advanced life support: 2010 American Heart Association guidelines for cardiopulmonary resuscitation and emergency cardiovascular care. *Circulation*. 2010; 122(suppl 3, pt.14):S876-S908.
39. Luten RC, Wears RL, Broselow J, et al. Length-based endotracheal tube and emergency equipment in pediatrics. *Ann Emerg Med*. 1992;21(8):900-904.
40. American Academy of Pediatrics. Committee on Fetus and Newborn. Policy statement. Levels of neonatal care. *Pediatrics*. 2004;114(5):1341-1347.
41. Rosenberg DI, Moss M. Section on critical care and committee on hospital care. Guidelines and levels of care for pediatric intensive care units. *Pediatrics*. 2004;114(4): 1114-1125.

42. Sackett D. Evidence-based medicine—what it is and what it isn't. *Clin Orthop Relat Res.* 2007;455:3-5. http://www.bmj.com/cgi/content/full/312/7023/71. Accessed January 26, 2011.

43. Balakas K, Sparks L. Teaching research and evidence-based practice using a service-learning approach. *J Nurs Educ.* 2010;49(12):691-695.

44. United States Public Health Service. United States Preventive Services Task Force. Procedure manual section 4: evidence report development. http://www.uspreventiveservicestaskforce.org/uspstf08/methods/procmanual4.htm Accessed January 28, 2011.

45. United States Public Health Service. United States Preventive Services Task Force. Child and adolescent recommendations. http://www.uspreventiveservicestaskforce.org/tfchildcat.htm. Accessed January 28, 2011.

46. Burns JP. Research in children. *Crit Care Med.* 2003;31(3)(suppl):S131-136.

47. National Institutes of Health, Office of Human Subjects Research. Directives for human experimentation. http://history.nih.gov/research/downloads/nuremberg.pdf. Accessed January 27, 2011.

48. National Institutes of Health, Office of Extramural Research. HHS regulatory requirements for research involving children. http://grants2.nih.gov/grants/policy/hs/children1.htm Accessed January 28, 2011.

Birth to 36 months: Boys
Length-for-age and Weight-for-age percentiles

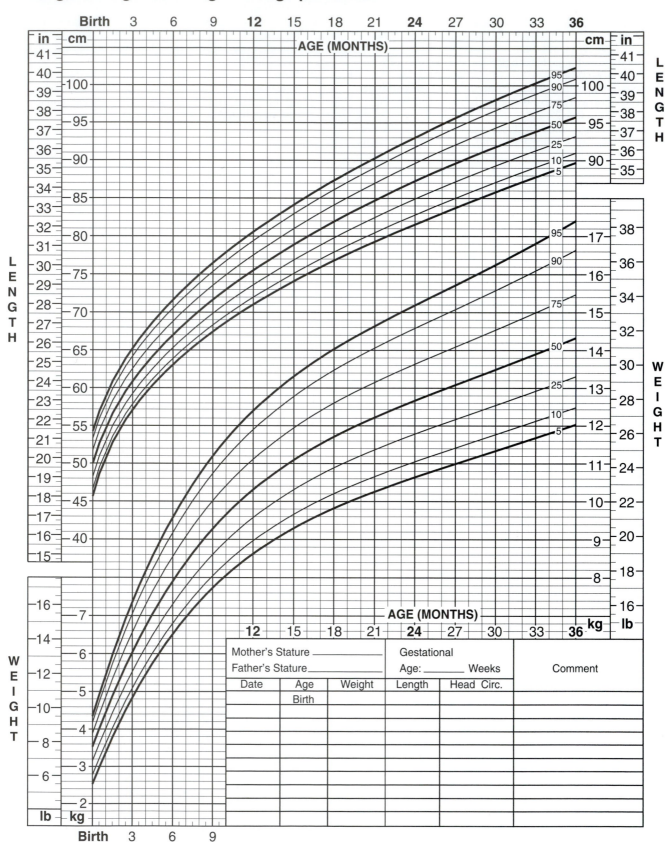

Figure 1-4 Boys Birth to 36 Months: Length-for-Age and Weight-for-Age Percentiles.
(*From: Kuczmarski RJ, Ogden CL, Guo SS, et al. 2000 CDC growth charts for the United States: methods and development. National Center for Health Statistics. Vital Health Stat 2002;11[246].*)

Birth to 36 months: Girls
Length-for-age and Weight-for-age percentiles

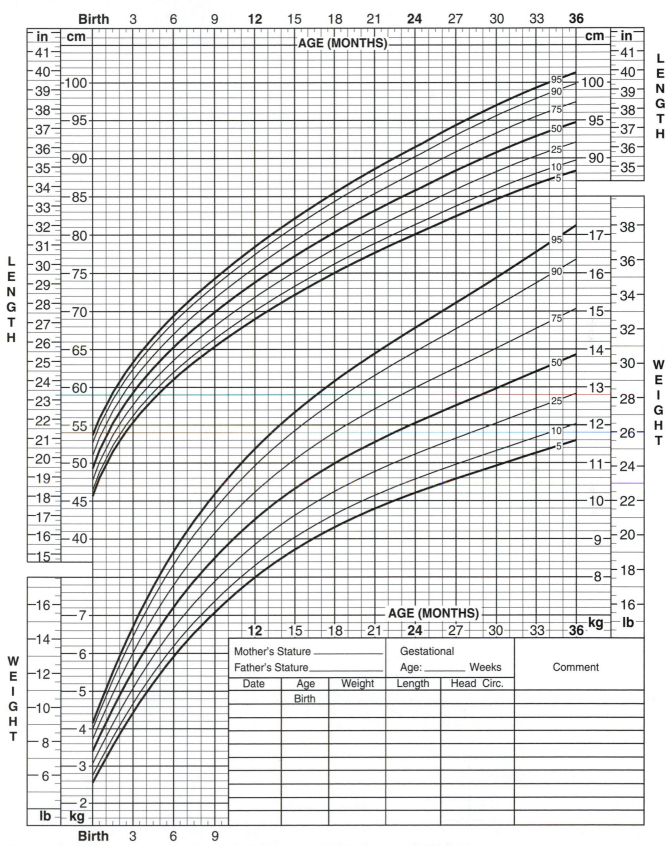

Figure 1-5 Girls Birth to 36 Months: Length-for-Age and Weight-for-Age Percentiles.
(From: Kuczmarski RJ, Ogden CL, Guo SS, et al. 2000 CDC growth charts for the United States: methods and development. National Center for Health Statistics. Vital Health Stat 2002;11[246].)

2 to 20 years: Boys
Stature-for-age and Weight-for-age percentiles

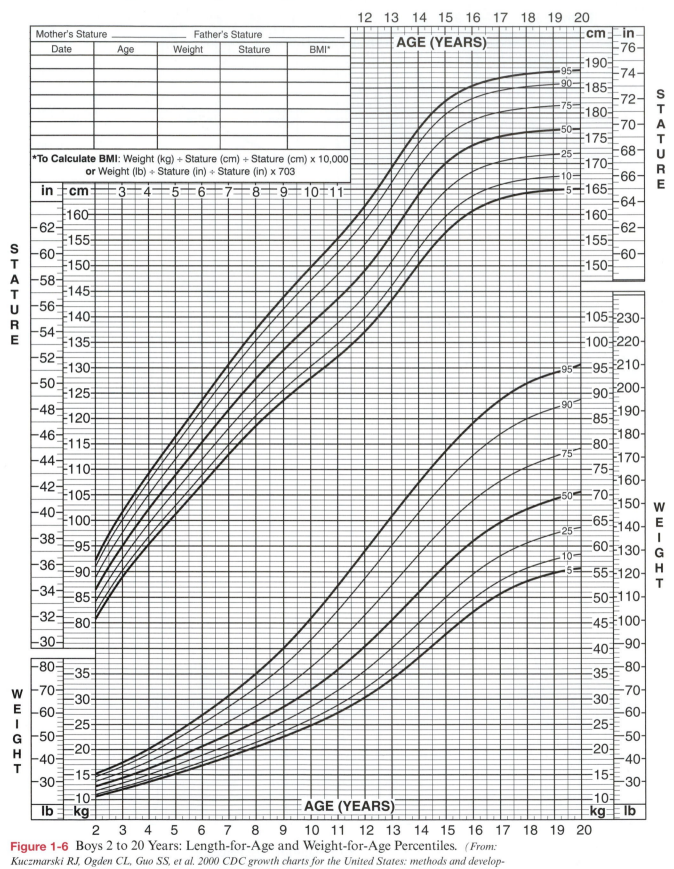

Figure 1-6 Boys 2 to 20 Years: Length-for-Age and Weight-for-Age Percentiles. *(From: Kuczmarski RJ, Ogden CL, Guo SS, et al. 2000 CDC growth charts for the United States: methods and development. National Center for Health Statistics. Vital Health Stat 2002;11[246].)*

2 to 20 years: Girls
Stature-for-age and Weight-for-age percentiles

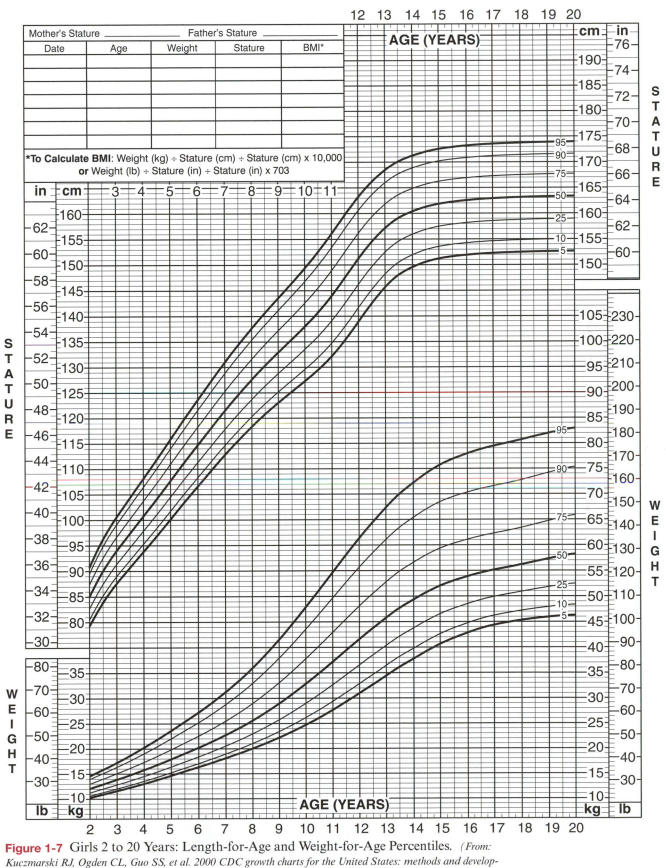

Figure 1-7 Girls 2 to 20 Years: Length-for-Age and Weight-for-Age Percentiles. *(From: Kuczmarski RJ, Ogden CL, Guo SS, et al. 2000 CDC growth charts for the United States: methods and development. National Center for Health Statistics. Vital Health Stat 2002;11[246].)*

Chapter 2

Fetal Cardiopulmonary Development

Key Terms

Acinar units
Alveolar phase
Canalicular phase
Cerebrum
Chorionic villi
Ductus arteriosus
Ductus venosus
Embryonic phase
Endoderm
Fetal circulation
Fetal lung fluid
Foramen ovale
Germinal matrix
Gestation
Gyri
Mesenchyme
Mesoderm
Morbidity
Myocardial cells
Phosphatidylcholine (PC)
Phosphatidylglycerol (PG)
Preterm
Pseudoglandular phase
Saccular phase
Saccules
Septa
Sulci
Surfactant
Tocolytic drugs
Type I cells
Type II cells
Viability

Chapter Objectives

After reading this chapter, you will be able to:

1. Identify two ways to calculate gestational age.
2. Compare the structure of the fetal lung at the embryonic, pseudoglandular, canalicular, saccular, and alveolar pulmonary development stages.
3. Describe the anatomical milestones for the embryonic, pseudoglandular, canalicular, saccular, and alveolar pulmonary development stages.
4. Explain the purpose of fetal lung fluid and its role in fetal development.
5. Describe the benefits of pulmonary surfactant, and note the gestational age of its initial appearance in the fetal lung.
6. Illustrate the timeline of fetal cardiac development.
7. Define the germinal matrix and describe its function in fetal neurological development.
8. Identify the structures and ducts that allow for fetal circulation.
9. Describe three changes to fetal circulation that occur during a normal delivery to assist the newborn in transition to extrauterine life.
10. Given a marginally premature fetus, select a method to assess fetal lung maturity.
11. Given a specific gestational age, describe the likelihood for survivability based on pulmonary, cardiac, and neurological development.

■■ Ann Wilson

You are a respiratory therapist working the day shift at a 200-bed community hospital with a level IIB neonatal intensive care unit (NICU). During your first patient rounds, you check in with the charge nurse and neonatologist in the NICU to assess potential deliveries and admissions for the day. The charge nurse informs you that labor and delivery called to give an update on a 41-year-old patient, Ann Wilson, who was admitted 3 hours ago for preterm contractions. She is pregnant with a single fetus. The fetus's estimated gestational age is 34 weeks, but the patient was unsure of the date of her last menstrual period, so the dates were confirmed using crown-to-rump measurements during fetal ultrasound at 9 weeks' gestation. An amniocentesis was done an hour ago to test for fetal lung maturity, but results are still pending. The neonatologist has already met with the mother to discuss the current diagnostic tests and possible risk to the fetus if it is born at this time. This is Ann's first pregnancy; she has no recent history of fever; and she denies smoking, alcohol consumption, or illicit drug use prior to or during pregnancy.

The human lungs serve the critical purpose of respiration, providing necessary oxygen to functioning tissues and preventing hypoxia and cell death. At no time is the importance of this function more evident than in the first few moments of life, when a newborn's first breath starts a cascade of physiological changes to transition the infant to life outside the uterus. For the newborn to take an effective first breath, the lungs must complete development during the period from conception to birth,

a time frame known as a **gestation**. Many infants, however, are born prior to a full term of 37 to 42 weeks' gestation. In the United States, about 12% of all live births occur before 37 week's gestation, placing them in the category of **preterm** (1). This is significantly higher than the less than 10% rate that occurs in most European countries (2).

Prematurity is the leading cause of neonatal death and is the leading contributing factor for other diseases and complications, such as respiratory distress syndrome, brain hemorrhage, developmental delays, neurological deficits, and chronic lung disease. In 2009, the number of preterm births was more than 528,000 (3), making this a significant population for U.S. health-care providers. Providers are focused on providing developmentally appropriate medical care for these small, premature neonates. To minimize infant death and **morbidity** (number of diseased infants), providers need to understand how gestational age and anatomical and physiological development are related and how this relationship affects the transition to normal extrauterine life. From there, providers can determine how fetal development affects an infant's survivability and his or her need for support after birth.

Pregnancy is broken into the following three stages of development:

1. **Conception:** First 2 weeks of pregnancy, when the female ovum and male sperm unite
2. **Embryonic stage**: Pregnancy weeks 3 to 12, encompassing 4 to 8 weeks of embryo development. This is when the major organs such as the central nervous system and heart begin development.
3. **Fetal development stage:** Encompasses the remaining weeks 13 to 40 for a full-term

delivery. Most lung development occurs during this phase.

For the respiratory therapist, assessment of fetal development is focused on pulmonary maturation, with additional attention to the cardiovascular and neurological systems. The level of development in these three systems at birth will determine the need for respiratory care and strategies for providing it.

Determining Gestational Age

Gestational time is a species-specific trait. In humans, the time from the start of the last menstrual period to birth typically is 280 days (40 weeks), with a normal range of 259 days (37 weeks) to 287 days (41 weeks). Accuracy of gestational age is important for estimating fetal maturity, particularly when lung development and immaturity are concerned. When the first day of the last menstrual period is not certain, other methods must be used to determine the start of gestation. Commonly used techniques are crown-to-rump measurement, biparietal diameter, and a combination of head circumference, abdominal circumference, and femur length. All measurements are taken using abdominal or intravaginal ultrasound.

Crown-to-rump measurement is used in the first trimester (up to week 12), and it is accurate starting at about 8 weeks. Measurement is taken from the top of the head, or crown, to the bottom of the buttocks, or rump. This tool is effective at young gestational ages because size variability is minimal. As gestational age advances, size variability increases, and this measurement is no longer an accurate estimate. Biparietal diameter, or the transverse diameter of the head, can be used as early at 13 weeks' gestation. At 20 weeks'

gestation, its accuracy is within about 1 week of gestational age. After 36 weeks' gestation, a combination of head circumference, abdominal circumference, and femur length will offer the best estimation of fetal age.

Once gestational age is determined, an accurate estimation of fetal maturity can be made, allowing neonatal risk to be determined. To calculate risk, clinicians need to be familiar with fetal development of the lungs as well as other organ systems, such as the heart and brain.

Fetal Lung Development

Lung development is divided into five phases: embryonic, pseudoglandular, canalicular, saccular, and alveolar. A list of these phases and their associated time frames and milestones is found in Table 2-1.

Embryonic Phase

The respiratory epithelium begins to grow during the **embryonic phase.** Growth begins around day 21 to 26, when the pharynx begins to form from the **endoderm**, or innermost germ layer of the embryo. During the next week, the lung bud appears as a small pouch on the pharynx, emerging at the laryngotracheal groove (Fig. 2-1). By the end of the week, the pouch has grown and branched into the right and left lung buds. The trachea has also formed, which is connected to the esophagus by means of the tracheoesophageal septum. Incomplete separation of the esophagus and trachea during this stage will result in esophageal atresia, which occurs in approximately 3,000 to 4,500 live births and is described in more detail in Chapter 10 (4). By about 31 days, the lobar bronchi form, two branching from the left bud

Table 2-1	Phases of Fetal Lung Development	
Phase	**Age Range**	**Key Development**
Embryonic	Conception to week 6	Right and left lung buds arise from esophagus Trachea forms Diaphragm completing development
Pseudoglandular	Weeks 7–16	Airways continue to branch Hard and soft palates grow Pulmonary vasculature develops Cilia and cartilage appear in large conducting airways
Canalicular	Weeks 17–26	Capillary network forms Airways complete branching Acinar units first seen Immature surfactant noted
Saccular	Weeks 27–35/36	Development of alveolar saccules End of structural lung formation
Alveolar	Week 36–term	Alveolar proliferation By birth ~50 million alveoli developed

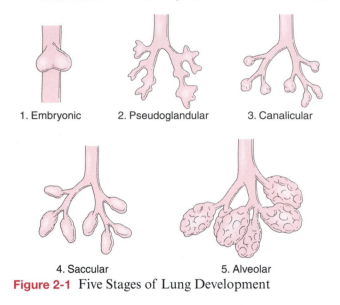

1. Embryonic   2. Pseudoglandular   3. Canalicular

4. Saccular   5. Alveolar

Figure 2-1 Five Stages of Lung Development

and three from the right. Embryonic connective tissue known as **mesenchyme**, which is part of the **mesoderm**, or middle germ layer of the embryo, will develop into the pulmonary interstitium, smooth muscle, blood vessels, and cartilage.

Starting at 31 days and ending at about 7 weeks, the diaphragm forms from five different elements within the mesoderm. Failure of the diaphragm to completely close during this phase results in a congenital diaphragmatic hernia, occurring in 2,000 to 4,000 live births (5).

Pseudoglandular Phase

The **pseudoglandular phase** is so named because of the gland-like appearance of the lung during this stage. This phase is notable for the large numbers of airway subdivisions. At week 7, the airway has branched to about four generations. By week 12, the major lobes of the lung (three on the right side and two on the left) are identifiable. Division of intrasegmental airways is fastest between weeks 10 and 24, by which time about 70% of the airway generation present at birth has formed (6).

During this phase, the epithelium of the airway will begin to develop cartilage, smooth muscle cells, and mucus glands. Smooth muscle around the airways begins developing around week 7, and in week 11 immature cartilage begins to form around the airways. Cilia appear on the surface of the lung epithelium starting at 10 weeks, beginning in the trachea and developing in the peripheral airways by 13 weeks. The presence of mucus can be found in the fetal lung starting at 13 weeks. Goblet cells begin proliferating mostly in the large airways and in small numbers in the lower airways. They are some of the cells responsible for creating mucus. Bronchial glands also begin to appear, which contain mucus-producing cells and serous cells. Pulmonary vasculature develops in

tandem with the airways. By week 12, the airways are similar in proportion to the adult lung, although not all the airways are developed and the alveoli they will supply are not yet present.

The larynx is also developing during this phase. The tissue that will form the epiglottis is present around week 7, and at the same time the arytenoid tissue begins to form. The vocal cords appear at about 8 weeks as small folds of connective tissue in the larynx.

The oropharynx and nasopharynx also undergo changes during the pseudoglandular phase. During week 7, the thin tissue membrane that separates the nasal cavity from the oropharynx disintegrates, creating a passage between the oral and nasal cavities. If this membrane remains at birth, it is known as choanal atresia. This defect causes early respiratory distress and is discussed in Chapter 10. The hard and soft palates, permanent structures that separate the oral and nasal cavities, develop during weeks 7 through 12.

Canalicular Phase

The **canalicular phase** of lung growth occurs during weeks 17 to 26. The end of the canalicular phase marks the beginning of survivability for infants born prematurely. During these weeks, the bronchioles continue to multiply, and the lung undergoes a vast amount of vascularization. This capillary network begins to grow around the airways, starting at about 20 weeks, in preparation for the arrival of alveoli. Gas exchange is not possible until the capillary network and alveoli have a sufficient surface area and until the two are close enough to each other to allow oxygen and carbon dioxide to cross the alveolar-capillary membrane. Both occur around 22 to 24 weeks' gestation. **Acinar units** are formed, consisting of a respiratory bronchiole, alveolar ducts, and alveolar sacs. Respiratory bronchioles contain no cartilage and are therefore sensitive to airway collapse in premature infants. **Fetal lung fluid** is secreted by epithelial cells of the lung to help maintain the patency of the airways and acinar units during their growth until delivery. Fetal lung fluid is different from amniotic fluid in composition, having very low pH, bicarbonate, and protein levels, but higher sodium and chloride concentrations. Fetal lungs secrete 250 to 300 mL of fluid per day. The volume of fetal lung fluid approximates the functional residual capacity of the lung.

In the primitive alveoli, epithelial tissue begins to differentiate into the two types of cells found in the adult lung. **Type I cells** form the structure of the alveolar capillary membrane. **Type II cells** make, store, and secrete matter such as type I cells, fetal lung fluid, and pulmonary surfactant. With the first appearance of type II cells comes the first appearance of pulmonary surfactant.

Surfactant is a surface-active agent that lowers surface tension at the air-liquid interface of the lungs. Lower alveolar surface tension improves lung compliance, thereby decreasing work of breathing. It eases the ability of the alveoli to stretch during inspiration and prevents alveolar collapse and eventual atelectasis during exhalation. Mature pulmonary surfactant is made up of lipids and glycoproteins. The main phospholipids that make up mature surfactant are **phosphatidylcholine (PC)** and **phosphatidylglycerol (PG)**. An immature form of surfactant that lacks PG is found in the alveoli beginning at approximately 24 weeks' gestation. It is less structurally stable and is inhibited by hypoxia, hyperthermia, and acidosis. Neonates born at this gestational age are very susceptible to surfactant deficiency, causing high surface tension and leading to increased work of breathing, respiratory distress, atelectasis, and pulmonary injury. PG appears at about 35 weeks' gestation (during the saccular phase, discussed next), and as a result, surfactant is much more stable. Chapter 4 discusses surface tension and its clinical significance in more depth, as well as strategies to improve outcomes for neonates with surfactant deficiencies.

Saccular Phase

The **saccular phase** of lung development is so named because true alveoli begin to appear at about 30 weeks in the airways distal to the terminal bronchioles, forming short, shallow sacs known as **saccules**. The alveoli of adults, by contrast, are deep and cup shaped (Fig. 2-2). It was thought that the saccular phase was the last stage of lung development before birth, but it is now known that true alveoli begin to develop prior to birth. The development of saccules at the end of the respiratory bronchioles marks the last generation of growth in the airway. Each saccule is made up of type I and type II cells and functions as an alveolar-capillary membrane; however, its structure is simple compared to an alveolar sac. Saccules are closely grouped, making the space between them, called the **septa**, twice as thick as an alveolar wall. The elastic fibers that constitute the walls are also small. These, in combination with immature surfactant, can increase work of breathing in neonates born prematurely.

Toward the end of this phase, at about week 35, mature surfactant begins to appear. A neonate born at this point is at minimal risk for pulmonary complications at birth caused by lung immaturity.

Alveolar Phase

The **alveolar phase** begins at about week 36, approximately 1 month before a full-term delivery. Alveoli are quickly proliferating during this phase, growing in number to the millions by the time of delivery. There is no clear distinction between the alveolar and

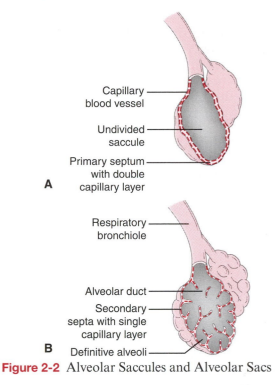

Figure 2-2 Alveolar Saccules and Alveolar Sacs

saccular phases, and the alveoli continue to proliferate in infancy and early childhood. The alveolar phase can be considered to end at about the first or second year of life, when the proliferation rate slows. There is published evidence to show that the number of alveoli present in the lungs at term range from zero to 50 million (7), with other data suggesting that this number may be too small and that individual numbers vary widely (8–10). Clinically, it is important to remember that neonates are born with only a small portion of the total number of alveoli that they will have in adulthood, and, during the first few years, alveoli grow and change shape rapidly; with each day, the numbers of gas exchange units will increase.

Fetal Cardiac Development

The heart is a complex organ, and it is the first major organ to develop. There are several phases of fetal heart development. Around gestational day 21, clumps of cells from the mesoderm begin to appear inside the forming pericardial cavity. By the end of the third week, they have formed two tubes surrounded by a sheath of **myocardial cells** (cardiac muscle cells). These two tubes fuse at the midline and form a single, continuous chamber. By the fourth week of development, this one-chambered heart is efficiently pumping blood to the embryo.

The top portion of the heart tube (the cranial portion) will dilate to form the aortic sac, which gives rise to the aortic arches. The middle portion (the caudal portion) dilates to form the early ventricle. The bottom portion of the tube develops in three distinct areas: One portion develops into the body of the right ventricle; another portion is called the *truncus arteriosus,* which develops into the aortic root and ascending aorta; and the midportion connects the first two portions. During this time, the ventricles are positioned above the atria, but the rapid growth of the heart tube forces it to bend upon itself. The ventricles will rotate into the correct anatomical position by bending into an S shape and moving down and to the right. The atria are then located behind and above the primitive ventricles and split into right and left at the center of the S shape around day 28. At about the same time, a single pulmonary artery grows from the outer wall of the left atrium. By early in week 8 of development, the truncus arteriosus has completely separated into the aorta and pulmonary trunk. During development, there are six pairs of aortic arches that supply blood to the developing brain. This creates a vascular ring that surrounds the developing esophagus and trachea. As the fetus develops, about half of the vascular system regresses, leaving the aortic arch, innominate artery, ductus arteriosus (which is described in the section on fetal circulation), pulmonary arteries, descending aorta, and subclavian arteries.

Between weeks 8 and 10, the valves begin to form between the atria and ventricles and at the root of the pulmonary artery and aorta. Around week 9 or 10, the heart begins biphasic pumping (11), similar to the function of an adult heart, and anatomical development of the heart is complete. See Figure 2-3 for a diagram of the embryological development of the heart. Deviations in cardiac development will lead to congenital cardiac defects, many of which are described in detail in Chapters 11 and 12.

Fetal Neurological Development

The neural system is the most complex structure within the embryo. Neural system development is one of the earliest to begin and is the last to be completed after birth. Its development begins at around

7 weeks' gestation, beginning with a neural plate that develops into a neural tube with an opening at each end. This new human brainstem continues to grow, forming the medulla, pons, and midbrain. The medulla mediates arousal, breathing, heart rate, and gross movement of the body and head, so that by week 9, the fetus will make spontaneous movements and 1 week later takes its first practice breath. By week 25, a fetus will display stimulus-induced heart rate accelerations. The pons mediates arousal, body movements, equilibrium, and perception of sound vibration; from around weeks 20 to 27, the fetus responds with arousal and body movements when sounds are delivered to the maternal abdomen. The midbrain auditory and visual system is the last to mature: In conjunction with the lower brainstem it makes fine auditory discriminations, and around week 36 it reacts to sound with fetal heart rate accelerations, head turning, and eye movements.

Within the developing brain, a **germinal matrix** is formed to assist in rapid cellular formation. It first appears around 9 weeks' gestation, and its volume increases exponentially until week 23 (12). This volume remains high until 28 weeks' gestation, when it begins to decrease sharply. It begins to disappear around 34 weeks and is no longer present in a full-term neonate. The germinal matrix is a weakly supported and highly vascularized area at the surface of the lateral ventricles and is prone to hypoxic-ischemic injury. The vessels of the germinal matrix are irregular and are prone to rupture. In addition to the structural instability of the germinal matrix, an increase in systemic blood pressure in a premature infant will increase cerebral blood flow, which can rupture the germinal matrix. This leads to a high incidence of intraventricular hemorrhage in premature neonates. Damage to the germinal matrix vessels may result in impairment of nerve and brain growth. High arterial carbon dioxide levels (hypercarbia) can also contribute to the risk of intraventricular hemorrhage. Intraventricular hemorrhage is described in more detail in Chapter 8.

Cerebral development also helps clinicians determine fetal **viability**, or capacity to live. The **cerebrum** is the largest portion of the brain, consisting of two

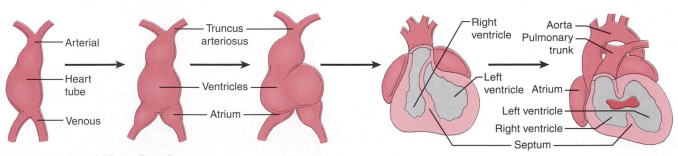

Figure 2-3 Fetal Heart Development

hemispheres separated by a deep fissure. It controls sensations, all voluntary muscular activities, consciousness, and higher mental functions such as memory, learning, reasoning, judgment, intelligence, and emotions. The surface of each hemisphere is covered by numerous folds called **gyri**, which are separated by furrows called **sulci**. The purpose of these gyri and sulci is to increase the surface area of the brain, which consists of gray matter (cell bodies) and white matter (nerve fibers). Until week 22 of fetal development, the brain appears smooth, with no gyri or sulci visible (13). The first major sulci begin to develop around 14 weeks' gestation, but the majority of their development is after 18 weeks. The presence of sulci and gyri is an indication of fetal viability. Sulci cannot be detected by ultrasound until around 18 to 26 weeks (13, 14), meaning that ultrasound identification of fetal brain development lags several weeks behind anatomical evidence. Identification using magnetic resonance imaging is more consistent, but there is still no feasible way to assess brain maturation before preterm delivery.

Fetal Circulation

The circulatory pathway for blood in a fetus is different from that of an adult. The addition of the placenta and lack of oxygen in the lungs make it necessary to divert blood flow through several alternate tracts. This system of shunts and differences in normal blood pressure is termed **fetal circulation**, and it is summarized in Box 2-1.

   To understand the differences between fetal circulation and normal circulation, it is important to understand how the vasculature of a developing fetus is different from that of an adult (Fig. 2-4). Moving toward the placenta, blood flows from the fetus through the two umbilical arteries. The blood then enters structures in the placenta that have tremendous surface areas, called **chorionic villi**. It is here that maternal and fetal blood passively exchange nutrients and waste through a thin epithelial layer within these branches. Blood returns to the fetus through one large umbilical vein. The vein connects to the body's circulation inside the liver, where it directs about half of the blood flow into the liver and the other half through the **ductus venosus**, the first shunt encountered from the placenta. This blood, because it has come directly from the placenta, is oxygenated, so it is reddish in appearance. The ductus venosus connects directly to the inferior vena cava, where it will travel to the right atrium. In an adult, the blood in the right atrium would be deoxygenated, so this is a major change in circulatory makeup for the fetus.

   Once blood enters the right atrium, it will encounter the second shunt. This is an opening between the right and left atria known as the **foramen**

Box 2-1 | Fetal Circulation

- The umbilical vein transports blood rich in O_2 and nutrients from the placenta to the fetal body via the liver and ductus venosus.
- Oxygenated blood from the placenta mixes with the deoxygenated blood from the body in the vena cava, continuing through the vena cava to the right atrium.
- A large proportion of this blood is shunted directly into the left atrium through an opening called the foramen ovale.
- The rest of the fetal blood entering the right atrium passes into the right ventricle and out through the pulmonary trunk.
- A minimal portion of the blood travels from the pulmonary trunk to the lungs.
- Most of the blood in the pulmonary trunk bypasses the lungs by entering a fetal vessel called the ductus arteriosus, which connects the pulmonary trunk to the descending portion of the aortic arch.
- The more highly oxygenated blood that enters the left atrium through the foramen ovale is mixed with a small amount of deoxygenated blood returning from the pulmonary veins.
- This mixture moves into the left ventricle and is pumped into the aorta. This feeds the upper regions of the body, and a portion reaches the myocardium through the coronary arteries and the brain through the carotid arteries.
- The blood is carried by the descending aorta to various parts of the lower regions of the body.
- A portion of the blood passes into the umbilical arteries to the placenta, where the blood is reoxygenated.

---

ovale. On the left atrial surface is a tissue flap that acts as a one-way valve that will close the foramen ovale after delivery. The right-side pressures within the fetus are higher than the left-side pressures, which keep the foramen ovale open. There are two reasons for the pressure difference. First, the placenta offers very little resistance to blood flow, which allows little back pressure on the left side of the heart and decreases expected systemic pressures. With 60% of blood flow circulating through the placenta, that leaves less than half of the circulating volume to perfuse the upper and lower portions of the body, feeding the growing tissue and returning to the heart via the superior and inferior vena cava. Second, the pulmonary vascular resistance is very high, which is a physiological response to the lack of oxygen in the lungs. Because of this high pressure, only about 10% of total blood flow circulates through the lung.

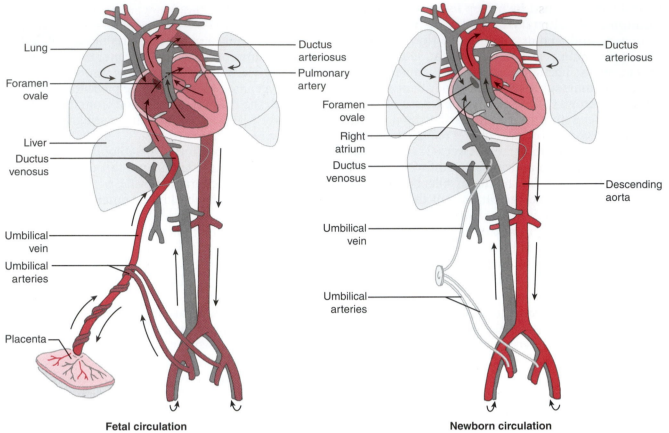

Fetal circulation

Newborn circulation

Figure 2-4 Fetal Circulation and Normal Circulation

This small volume of blood functions to feed the growing lung tissue. Without an escape, the remaining blood volume would back up dangerously into the right side of the heart, increasing its pressure. In addition to the foramen ovale, excess blood that enters the pulmonary system via the pulmonary artery is vented through the **ductus arteriosus** to the aorta, just after the right subclavian branch. Blood flowing through the ductus arteriosus will bypass the left side of the heart. Both the shunted blood and that from the left ventricle travel through the aorta, perfusing the upper and lower portions of the body. A portion passes through the umbilical arteries, which arise from the iliac arteries in the pelvis, and flows back to the placenta.

Changes to Fetal Circulation at Delivery

The change from intrauterine to extrauterine circulation occurs within minutes to hours after birth, and the first breaths a newborn takes help to make this transition possible. The first breath has to overcome the surface forces of the lung, and it helps create a gaseous functional residual capacity (FRC) to replace the fetal lung fluid initially held there.

There are several factors at play during delivery that stimulate a newborn to breathe. Chemoreceptors

in the aorta and carotid artery regulate ventilation in humans. As the fetus descends into the birth canal, he or she is cut off from the placenta. This causes a drop in the partial pressure of oxygen in the blood, or PaO_2 (commonly referred to as asphyxia), which is detected by the chemoreceptors and causes a chemical message to be sent to the brainstem to increase ventilation. The thorax is compressed through the birth canal during delivery, then expands to normal size at delivery, creating a negative intrathoracic pressure and causing air to enter the lungs. The environmental changes from a dark and warm uterus to a bright, cold, and noisy delivery room and the physical stimulation of the infant by handling will trigger his or her crying reflex.

Fetuses begin "practice breathing" during the second trimester (weeks 12 to 24) but refine the technique in the last 10 weeks of gestation. At delivery, the alveoli have no air in them. Fetal lung fluid is secreted by type II alveolar cells to stabilize the structure of the lung in utero. In late gestation and shortly before birth, fetal lungs convert from fluid secretion to fluid reabsorption. Epinephrine released during labor inhibits the chloride channel within type II cells, which causes the secretion of lung fluid. It simultaneously stimulates sodium channels, which absorb lung fluid. Through this mechanism, the lungs of a healthy term neonate after labor contain only a minimal amount of lung fluid. The majority of the fluid left is mechanically expelled during delivery, and any remaining fluid is reabsorbed by the lymphatic system during the first hours to days of extrauterine life. Once the fluid is reabsorbed or expelled, the newborn will have to overcome pressure in excess of -100 cm H_2O to inflate the alveoli. Surfactant will reduce this pressure and also prevent the alveoli from collapsing again during exhalation. Over the first few hours of life, FRC will gradually increase and stabilize the alveoli more permanently.

The first breath a newborn takes increases the amount of oxygen in the alveoli. When the oxygen crosses the alveolar-capillary membrane, it causes a decrease in pulmonary artery pressure and increases blood flow to the lungs. Around the same time, the umbilical cord is clamped, preventing blood from entering the placenta. This forces blood back into the lower extremities and increases pressure on the left side of the heart. This pressure forces the flap of tissue in the left atrium to close the foramen ovale. In the last few weeks of gestation, smooth muscle develops around the ductus arteriosus but remains relaxed as a result of hormones known as *prostaglandins* produced in utero. The increase in oxygen causes inhibition of ductal prostaglandins and constriction of the musculature in the ductus arteriosus, closing it off from blood flow. After the clamping of the umbilical cord, the ductus venosus vasoconstricts because of lack of blood flow. Over several months, the ductus venosus and umbilical arteries and vein become supporting ligaments in the body (Table 2-2).

Assessing Fetal Lung Maturity

A healthy neonatal period relies on proper fetal growth and a normal labor and delivery process. There is often no known cause for preterm labor, but there are many risk factors associated with premature labor and subsequent delivery (Box 2-2). Despite this knowledge and preventive care, 30% of all preterm births are unexplained and spontaneous (16). Recommendations have been set forth by the U.S. Department of Health and Human Services' Agency for Healthcare Research and Quality for the management of preterm labor (17), which include assessing for fetal lung maturity (FLM) prior to delivery if possible. The American College of Obstetricians and Gynecologists recommends testing for FLM between 34 and 39 weeks' gestation (18) when the safety of delivery and maturity of the lung are less certain. Prior to 32 weeks' gestation, most test results will indicate immaturity. At 39 weeks, the fetus is considered full term, and the risk of respiratory distress syndrome (RDS) is very low (Special Populations 2-1).

Box 2-2 Risk Factors for Preterm Labor (15)

- Previous preterm delivery
- Low socioeconomic status
- Non-white race
- Maternal age less than 18 years or more than 40 years
- Preterm premature rupture of the membranes
- Multiple gestations
- Maternal history of one or more spontaneous second-trimester abortions
- Maternal complications (medical or obstetric)
- Maternal behaviors
  - Smoking
  - Illicit drug use
  - Alcohol use
  - Lack of prenatal care
- Uterine causes
  - Myomata (muscle tissue tumor, particularly submucosal or subplacental)
  - Uterine septum
  - Bicornuate uterus
  - Cervical incompetence
  - Exposure to diethylstilbestrol (DES)
- Infectious causes
  - Chorioamnionitis
  - Bacterial vaginosis
  - Asymptomatic bacteriuria
  - Acute pyelonephritis
  - Cervical/vaginal colonization
- Fetal causes
  - Intrauterine fetal death
  - Intrauterine growth retardation
  - Congenital anomalies
- Abnormal placentation
- Presence of a retained intrauterine device

Table 2-2 Changes in Cardiovascular Structures After Birth

Fetal Structure	Adult Structure
Foramen ovale	Fossa ovalis
Umbilical vein (internal)	Ligamentum teres
Ductus venosus	Ligamentum venosum
Umbilical arteries and abdominal ligaments	Medial umbilical ligaments, superior vesicular artery (supplies bladder)
Ductus arteriosus	Ligamentum arteriosum

Gestational Diabetes

Gestational diabetes has many implications for the health of mother and fetus, but of particular importance is FLM. When glucose control is poor, the rate of surfactant delay is increased (19). At full term, the lung still seems to have matured, but prior to term, mothers with gestational diabetes are more likely to have FLM tests that show immature lungs when compared with expected results. This is complicated further by the fact that fetal size is usually larger than expected when mothers have gestational diabetes, giving false security to clinicians who think that a larger baby means more mature lungs.

Several tests for FLM are currently available, including the following:

- Lung profile test, consisting of
  - Lecithin-sphingomyelin (L/S) ratio
  - Presence of PG
- Shake test (also known as the foam test)
- Surfactant-albumin (S/A) ratio (also known as the TDx Fetal Lung Maturity test or FP test)
- Lamellar body concentration

These tests look at various characteristics of amniotic fluid and fetal lung fluid. Fetal lung fluid leaves the lung via the trachea and is excreted through the mouth, mixing with amniotic fluid. It is because of this mechanism that obtaining a sample of amniotic fluid can help assess lung maturity. No test has been conclusively found to be superior, so the type of test is usually chosen based on physician or institution preference.

Lung Profile Test

L/S Ratio

Developed in 1971, the L/S ratio is the most long-standing and well-known FLM test. It tests the ratio of lecithin, a principal active component of surfactant, also known as phosphatidylcholine (PC), to the level of sphingomyelin, a phospholipid found mostly in body tissues other than the lungs. Lecithin levels in the amniotic fluid increase in late gestation, whereas sphingomyelin remains constant throughout pregnancy. An L/S ratio at 31 to 32 weeks' gestation is usually around 1:1, and it increases to 2:1 by 35 weeks' gestation. An L/S ratio of 2:1 means that the lungs are mature, and there is only a 2% chance the fetus will develop RDS if delivered. An L/S ratio of 1.5:1 predicts a 50% chance of RDS if the fetus is delivered, whereas a less than 1.5:1 ratio predicts a 73% chance of RDS if delivered (20). When surveyed, 99% of obstetricians were familiar with the L/S ratio test, but only 42% list it as their test of choice for measuring FLM (21). The reasoning is that it is a costly test with a high turnaround time (5-6 hours) (22), and it requires highly trained laboratory personnel to perform.

PG Presence

PG appears first in amniotic fluid at around 35 weeks' gestation, when mature surfactant is produced, and levels increase at 37 to 40 weeks. The laboratory will report PG as either "present" or "absent," making it a useful marker late in pregnancy. This test is a good predictor of mature lungs, but it is a poorer predictor of occurrence of RDS when the result is "absent." A literature review found that in 25% to 63% of cases of an absent PG test, neonates developed RDS (21). However, this is the only currently available test that is not affected by sample contamination by blood or meconium, which are common contaminants in amniotic fluid sampling.

Shake Test

The shake test, also known as the foam test, is a simple test that can be used to indicate the need for further testing. A small sample of amniotic fluid is mixed with ethanol and shaken for 15 seconds. It is left to sit for 15 minutes, and then a reading is taken. The presence of a ring of bubbles in the ethanol shows that there is enough lecithin present to create stable foam. A negative result (no foam present) indicates that an L/S ratio should be performed.

SIA Ratio

The S/A ratio is more widely known by its brand name, TDx Fetal Lung Maturity test. It is FDA cleared and commercially available from Abbott Diagnostics (Abbott Park, Ill.). The test operates on the principle of fluorescence polarization (hence, it is also sometimes known as the FP test), and it is performed on the company's TDx instrument platforms. It measures the relative concentrations of surfactant and albumin (milligrams of surfactant per gram of albumin). This test provides a simple, automated, rapid test that is widely available; requires less technical expertise than the does the L/S ratio; varies minimally between laboratories; and requires only a small volume of amniotic fluid, typically 1 mL. A result showing more than 55 mg of surfactant per 1 g of albumin is considered mature; values of less than 40 mg surfactant per 1 g albumin are considered immature; and values of 40 mg to 54 mg surfactant per 1 g albumin are considered indeterminate. A 2010 survey showed that S/A ratio was the test of choice for 62% of physicians, and it was the test ordered clinically 72% of the time (21).

Lamellar Body Count

Surfactant is stored within type II cells in the form of lamellar bodies. These bodies are actively secreted into the alveolar space and end up in the amniotic fluid. Similar to tests for blood cell counts, a smear of amniotic fluid is used to count the number of lamellar bodies in a given specimen. There is no clear consensus on cutoff values that would predict absence of RDS, however. Some studies found success with lamellar body count (LBC) of greater than 50,000 (22). Testing must be conducted quickly to avoid negatively low results. The lack of consensus on maturity cutoffs and guidelines for test validation make this a less frequently ordered test (27% use in clinical practice) (21).

The use of FLM tests has diminished in recent years because of the close correlation between gestational age, rate of RDS, and accuracy of results at lower gestational ages. FLM tests are most useful when the decision to be made is for gestational ages less than 39 weeks but greater than 32 weeks. The decision regarding what test to use, however, is made by the ordering physician or is based on institutional availability.

■■ The initial results of the shake test on Ann Wilson's amniotic fluid samples showed no bubbles, so an S/A ratio and lung profile were obtained. The S/A ratio results were 52 mg surfactant per 1 g albumin, the L/S ratio was 1.9:1, and PG presence was positive. From these results, the obstetrician and neonatologist decide to allow Ann's labor to progress rather than try to pharmacologically stop the contractions. You now will wait until you are called to the delivery to assist with neonatal resuscitation if needed.

Tocolytics and Glucocorticoids During Preterm Labor

When gestational age or FLM tests suggest a high likelihood for lung immaturity, obstetricians have to make a choice regarding whether it is in the fetus's and/or the mother's best interest to proceed to delivery. If the decision is made to stop labor, this is attempted by use of **tocolytic drugs,** which are used to inhibit uterine contractions. These include betamimetics such as terbutaline and ritodrine, magnesium sulfate, calcium channel blockers, and nonsteroidal anti-inflammatory drugs (NSAIDs) such as indomethacin and sulindac (23). There is no recommendation for which tocolytic should be used first, so physician preference and the drug's availability will determine selection (24). These medications may prolong pregnancy for 2 to 7 days, which

is enough time to initiate treatment to accelerate FLM. These drugs are not indicated in all instances of preterm labor; contraindications to tocolytic therapy are listed in Box 2-3.

Glucocorticoids are a general class of adrenal cortical hormones that are primarily active in protecting against stress and metabolizing carbohydrates and proteins. They have also been shown to help speed up fetal lung growth and reduce the incidence of RDS, neonatal death, cerebroventricular hemorrhage, and neonatal morbidity when given to mothers prior to preterm delivery (24). They also do not seem to cause any short- or long-term side effects in the mothers. This therapy is most effective when administered to pregnant mothers between 26 and 35 weeks' gestation (25) and more than 24 hours but not more than 7 days before delivery (26). The positive effects of maternal glucocorticoid administration are discussed in more detail in Chapter 4.

Implications of Development on Neonatal Course

The gestational age at birth will directly influence the risk of lung disease, neurological injury, and other multisystem complications. It is thus important for neonatal clinicians to understand fetal development so that they will make safe clinical decisions. Once an infant is born, organ growth continues, but the baby is now subject to the hazards of extrauterine life. Hypoxia, hypercarbia, thermoregulation, and bradycardia can all contribute to complications for preterm infants during the neonatal period. Table 2-3 summarizes cardiopulmonary developmental milestones at various ages of fetal development. If clinicians consider a preterm neonate's neurological and lung development at delivery based on gestational age, clinicians can make changes to each individual patient's care plan based on his or her developmental needs. Clinicians must also know the normal process of the transition from fetal circulation to normal circulation. Difficulty in this process can lead to severe problems in oxygenation and critical illness in the first days or weeks after birth.

Box 2-3 Contraindications to Tocolytic Therapy (17)

Severe preeclampsia
Placental abruption
Intrauterine infection
Lethal congenital or chromosomal abnormalities
Advanced cervical dilation
Evidence of fetal compromise
Placental insufficiency

Table 2-3	Developmental Progress for Select Gestational Ages

Gestational Age (weeks)	Milestones
24	Structural airways developing, respiratory bronchioles still developing First appearance of immature surfactant (phosphatidylcholine); easily inactivated Capillaries close enough to begin gas exchange; beginning of acinar unit development Alveolar-capillary membrane thicker, may be several cell layers thick Cerebral sulci and gyri beginning to form Physiological response to physical stimulation Germinal matrix present; susceptible to injury from changes in cerebral blood flow
28	End of structural lung formation Alveolar saccules in development Immature surfactant present Physiological response to physical stimulation Volume of germinal matrix high
32	Increase in number of acinar units Immature surfactant present Volume of germinal matrix will begin to diminish over next few weeks
36	Mature pulmonary surfactant (with PG) should be present Auditory and visual systems in cerebrum developed Germinal matrix volume decreasing sharply
40	~50 million alveoli developed Mature surfactant present Fetal lung fluid volume decreasing Fetus practice breathing Germinal matrix disappeared

■■ Anne gives birth to a baby boy 14 hours after the lung profile results were shared with the neonatal team. Baby boy (BB) Wilson was born active and crying and only required supportive care in the delivery room. He was admitted to the NICU, and when you arrive to work you note that he is now 5 hours old and requires no respiratory support. His chest radiograph was clear, with no evidence of lung disease. He is sleeping comfortably, and Anne has been able to visit several times since he was born. He will spend the next several days attempting to feed, and if he is able to gain weight and shows no additional signs of respiratory immaturity, he will be discharged home.

■■ Critical Thinking Questions: Ann Wilson

1. What do you expect the implications would have been had Ann's estimated gestational age had been 28 weeks instead of 34?
2. How do you think the physician's decision would have changed if the results of the FLM tests had been as follows?
   a. S/A ratio 40 mg surfactant to 1 mg albumin
   b. L/S ratio 1.5:1
   c. PG presence negative
3. What may have caused this patient's preterm labor, based on your understanding of the risk factors and current patient history?
4. After delivery, what might you be able to assess regarding the infant to determine the accuracy of the FLM test results?

)● Case Studies and Critical Thinking Questions

■ Case 1: Jody Hayworth

You are working the night shift in a 20-bed level IIIC NICU and carrying the delivery room pager. You are occupied with discharge planning rounds for the following morning when labor and delivery pages you to attend a 26-week-gestation delivery. On the walk over to labor and delivery, you discuss the patient's history with the physician. Jody Hayworth is 16 years old, and this is her first pregnancy. She has been in the hospital on bed rest for 5 days for premature rupture of membranes. She denies drinking, smoking, or drug use. She has had no fever and no recent pain. When you arrive at labor and delivery, Jody is about to begin pushing. You review her current status with her nurse. She received a regimen of indomethacin and magnesium sulfate the previous morning, but it didn't stop labor. She received three doses of betamethasone (a glucocorticoid) beginning at admission to the hospital.

- *Should Jody have had FLM testing? Why or why not?*
- *How likely is it that Jody's newborn will have RDS?*
- *Currently, in what stage of pulmonary development is the fetus?*
- *What problems may arise from this fetus's current neurological development?*
- *Do you think Jody's newborn will have surfactant deficiency?*

■ Case 2: Maria Gonzalez

It is the end of the day shift at a rural community hospital. You are called to a 33-week-gestation delivery. Maria Gonzalez is 42 years old and is about to deliver her fourth child. She was just diagnosed last week with gestational diabetes. Maria was in a minor car accident today during the morning rush hour. She felt some abdominal cramping after the accident and was transported to the hospital via ambulance. She has had no bleeding, leaking of amniotic fluid, or obvious trauma, but her cramping was diagnosed as preterm contractions. Attempts were made to stop labor using indomethacin, but without success. A fetal ultrasound was done to assess any physical injury from the accident, but none

was evident. Fetal age was estimated at 35 weeks' gestation during prenatal visits and by ultrasound biparietal diameter. During the ultrasound, an amniocentesis was also obtained, and a lung profile was sent for analysis. L/S ratio is 1.5:1, and PG is absent.

- *What does the lung profile tell you about Maria's baby's lung maturity?*
- *Currently, in what stage of pulmonary development is the fetus?*
- *Are you concerned about the motor vehicle accident? If so, specifically what concerns you?*
- *Why do you think Maria's fetus is measuring larger than her predicted gestational age?*

Multiple-Choice Questions

1. What would be the best method to calculate gestational age for a woman who thinks it has been about 2 months since her last menstrual period, but she doesn't remember an exact date?
   a. Crown-to-rump measurement
   b. Biparietal diameter
   c. Abdominal circumference
   d. Femur length

2. During which fetal lung development stage does surfactant first appear?
   a. Pseudoglandular
   b. Canalicular
   c. Saccular
   d. Alveolar

3. Fetal lung fluid is designed to:
   a. Maintain patency of airways and alveoli during growth.
   b. Assist in newborns taking their first breath.
   c. Decrease surface tension.
   d. Provide nutrients for growing type I and type II cells.

4. The benefits of alveolar surfactant include:
   I. Lowering surface tension.
   II. Lowering airway resistance.
   III. Preventing alveolar collapse.
   IV. Higher lung compliance.
   a. I, II
   b. I, IV
   c. I, II, III
   d. I, III, IV

5. What is the function of the germinal matrix in cerebral development?
   a. Adds cellular stability to prevent intraventricular hemorrhage

   b. Develops gyri and sulci on the surface of the cerebellum
   c. Regulates the auditory and visual systems of the midbrain
   d. Assists in rapid cellular formation during fetal development

6. At what gestational age would a fetus display the following: immature surfactant, functional alveolar-capillary membranes, fully developed heart, and gyri and sulci in the cerebrum?
   a. 10 weeks
   b. 20 weeks
   c. 30 weeks
   d. 40 weeks

7. Returning from the placenta, which is the correct order of blood flow through fetal circulation?
   a. Umbilical artery, ductus arteriosus, ductus venosus, umbilical vein
   b. Umbilical vein, ductus venosus, foramen ovale, umbilical artery
   c. Umbilical vein, ductus venosus, ductus arteriosus, foramen ovale, umbilical artery
   d. Umbilical artery, ductus arteriosus, foramen ovale, ductus venosus, umbilical vein

8. Which of the following is *not* an event that occurs around the time of delivery that stimulates breathing in newborns?
   a. Aortic chemoreceptors responding to hypoxemia
   b. Reabsorption of fetal lung fluid in utero
   c. Negative intrathoracic pressure just after passing through the birth canal
   d. Environmental stimulation (e.g., delivery room noises, bright lights, cold room)

9. Which of the following patients has the lowest
   risk for RDS?
   a. 24 weeks' gestation
   b. 36 weeks' gestation with L/S ratio of 2:1
   c. 38 weeks' gestation with S/A ratio of 45 mg
      surfactant per 1 g albumin
   d. 31 weeks' gestation

10. Which of the following is the recommended
    treatment regimen for dosing with prenatal

glucocorticoids to accelerate fetal lung
development?
a. Within 24 hours of delivery
b. Not recommended before 35 weeks' gestation
c. More than 24 hours but not more than 7 days
   before delivery
d. Most effective at less than 26 weeks' gestation

DavisPlus | For additional resources login to Davis*Plus* (http://davisplus.fadavis.com/ keyword "Perretta") and click on the Premium tab. (Don't have a *Plus*Code to access Premium Resources? Just click the Purchase Access button on the book's Davis*Plus* page.)

REFERENCES

1. March of Dimes. March of Dimes 2011 premature birth report card. http://www.marchofdimes.com/peristats/pdflib/998/US.pdf. Accessed July 1, 2012.
2. MacDorman MF, Mathews TJ. Behind international rankings of infant mortality: how the United States compares with Europe. *NCHS Data Brief*. 2009;23(Nov):1-8. http://www.cdc.gov/nchs/data/databriefs/db23.pdf. Accessed February 10, 2011.
3. Hamilton BE, Martin JA, Ventura SJ. Births: preliminary data for 2009. *NVSR*. 2010;59(3):1-29.
4. Spitz L. Oesophageal atresia. *Orphanet J Rare Dis*. 2007; 2:24. http://www.ojrd.com/content/pdf/1750-1172-2-24.pdf. Accessed February 16, 2011.
5. Langham MR, Kays DW, Ledbetter DJ, Frentzen B, Sanford LL, Richards DS. Congenital diaphragmatic hernia: epidemiology and outcome. *Clin Perinat*. 1996; 23:671-688.
6. Jeffery PK. The development of large and small airways. *Am J Respir Crit Care Med*. 1998;157(suppl):S174-S180.
7. Burri PH. Structural aspects of postnatal lung development-alveolar formation and growth. *Biol Neonate*. 2006;89: 313-322.
8. Thurlbeck WM. Postnatal human lung growth. *Thorax*. 1982;37:564-571.
9. Hislop A, Wigglesworth JS, Desai R. Alveolar development in the human fetus and infant. *Early Hum Dev*. 1986;13:1-11.
10. Langston C, Kida K, Reed M, et al. Human lung growth in late gestation and in the neonate. *Am Rev Respir Dis*. 1984;97:237.
11. Makikillo K, Jouppila P, Räsänen J. Human fetal cardiac function in pregnancy. *Heart*. 2005;91:334-338.
12. Kinoshita Y, Okudera T, Tsuru E, Yokota A. Volumetric analysis of the germinal matrix and ventricles performed using MR images of postmortem fetuses. *Am J Neuroradiol*. 2001;22(Feb):382-388.
13. Cohen-Sacher B, Lerman-Sagie T, Lev D, Malinger G. Sonographic developmental milestones of the fetal cerebral cortex: a longitudinal study. *Ultrasound Obstet Gynecol*. 2006;27:494-502.
14. Menteagudo A, Timor-Tritsch IE. Development of fetal gyri, sulci and fissures: a transvaginal sonographic study. *Ultrasound Obstet Gynecol*. 1997;9:222-228.

15. Weismiller DG. Preterm labor. *Am Fam Physician*. 1999; 59(3):593-602.
16. Haas DM. Preterm birth. *Clin Evid (Online)*. 2011;Apr 4. doi: pii:1404.
17. Agency for Healthcare Research and Quality. Management of preterm labor. National Guidelines Clearinghouse. Guideline Summary NGC-3130. http://www.guideline.gov/content.aspx?id=3993. Accessed February 12, 2011.
18. American College of Obstetricians and Gynecologists. Fetal lung maturity. *Clinical Management Guidelines for Obstetrician-Gynecology*. 2008;112(3):717-726.
19. De Luca AKC, Nakazawa CY, Azevedo BC, et al. Influence of glycemic control on fetal lung maturity in gestations affected by diabetes or mild hyperglycemia. *Acta Obstet Gynecol Scand*. 2009;88(9):1036-1040.
20. Gomella TL. *Neonatology: Management, Procedures, On-call Problems, Diseases, and Drugs*. New York: McGraw-Hill; 2004.
21. Grenache DG, Wilson AR, Gross GA, Gronowski AM. Clinical and laboratory trends in fetal lung maturity testing. *Clinica Chimica Acta*. 2010;411:1746-1749.
22. Field NT, Gilbert WM. Current status of amniotic fluid tests of fetal maturity. *Clin Obstet Gynecol*. 1997;40(2): 366-386, http://ovidsp.tx.ovid.com.ezproxy.welch.jhmi.edu/sp-3.3.1a/ovidweb.cgi. Accessed February 15
23. American College of Obstetricians and Gynecologists. Management of preterm labor. *Clinical Management Guidelines for Obstetrician-Gynecology*. 2003;101(5): 1039-1047.
24. Agency for Healthcare Research and Quality. Preterm prelabour rupture of membranes. National Guideline Clearinghouse. Guideline Summary NGC-5920. http://www.guideline.gov/content.aspx?id=11383. Accessed February 11, 2011.
25. Roberts RD, Dalziel S. Antenatal corticosteroids for accelerating fetal lung maturation for women at risk of preterm birth. *Cochrane Database Syst Rev* 2006;Jul 19(3):CD004454.
26. Hallman M, Peltoneimi O, Kari MA. Enhancing functional maturity before preterm birth. *Neonatology*. 2010;97:373-378.

Chapter 3

Resuscitation of the Newborn During Transition to Extrauterine Life

Theodora A. Stavroudis, MD

Key Terms cont.

T-piece resuscitator

Variable decelerations

Withholding resuscitation efforts

Chapter Objectives

After reading this chapter, you will be able to:

1. Describe the three stages of labor.
2. Identify two methods used in assessing fetal well-being during labor and delivery.
3. Describe the normal transition to the extrauterine world.
4. Name antepartum and intrapartum risk factors associated with the need for neonatal resuscitation.
5. List the equipment needed for the resuscitation of the newborn.
6. List the three questions of rapid assessment at the time of birth.
7. Discuss measures that must be taken to ensure that adequate warmth is being provided to the newborn in the delivery room.
8. Determine when to provide oxygen and/or positive pressure ventilation during an infant's transition to extrauterine life.
9. Identify when to administer chest compressions and epinephrine to a newborn according to the Neonatal Resuscitation Program (NRP) guidelines.
10. Discuss special considerations during neonatal resuscitations, such as when not to initiate or stop resuscitation measures and how to take care of newborns with congenital anomalies.
11. Assign Apgar scores to an infant during neonatal resuscitation.

■■ BG Zacharian

You are working the night shift in the level IIIB neonatal intensive care unit (NICU) of a large teaching hospital when you are called to labor room 3 for a vaginal vacuum-assist delivery at 40 weeks' gestation. Estimated fetal weight is 4,200 grams. This is the first pregnancy and first live birth for a 33-year-old woman. She is 10 cm dilated and 100% effaced. She has been pushing for approximately 2 hours. Fetal heart tracings are significant for early decelerations, and a fetal scalp blood sample is being obtained.

In 2010, 3.99 million babies were born in the United States (1). About 90% of these babies made the transition to extrauterine life without difficulty, and fewer than 1% needed extensive resuscitative measures to survive (2). This translates to about 400,000 newborns who required some type of neonatal resuscitation and 40,000 who required extensive resuscitation. There are specific risk factors and signs present prior to delivery that can help obstetric teams identify which newborns will require resuscitation, including prenatal or perinatal risk factors or fetal heart rate (FHR) changes during labor. However, the obstetric team must always be prepared to resuscitate an infant because even newborns with no risk factors may require it. The outcomes of thousands of newborn lives can be improved by appropriate assessment during delivery and rapid neonatal resuscitation, which can prevent injury from birth asphyxia. In many hospitals, the respiratory therapist (RT) is an active member of the neonatal resuscitation team and assists team members in delivery room resuscitations. For newborns admitted to a neonatal special care or intensive care nursery, RTs will care for any respiratory difficulties encountered during the neonatal period; thus, it is imperative to understand how the problems babies have during labor and delivery translate into difficulties after delivery.

The Three Stages of Labor

Childbirth, also known as **labor**, is the passage of the fetus and the **placenta** from the uterus to the extrauterine world, and it is divided into three stages (3). The first stage of labor is the process by which the cervix reaches full dilatation to 10 cm. It is made up of three phases: the latent phase, the active phase, and the deceleration phase. In the **latent phase**, contractions become more coordinated, and the cervix reaches 4 cm dilatation. The latent phase can last as long as 12 hours for women who have given birth previously (multiparous) and as long as 20 hours for women who have never given birth (nulliparous). Membranes may spontaneously rupture during this phase of labor. In the **active phase**, the cervix dilates to approximately 8 to 9 cm, and it is the phase of the most rapid cervical dilatation. It lasts about 5 hours in nulliparous women and about 2 hours in multiparous women. Finally, in the **deceleration phase**, also known as transition, the cervix reaches complete dilatation, and the presenting part of the fetus (usually the head) descends into the midpelvis. The second stage of labor is the time between full cervical dilatation and the delivery of the fetus to the extrauterine world. It can last for approximately 2 hours in nulliparous women and about 1 hour for multiparous women. Finally, the third stage of labor is characterized by the delivery of the placenta, and this stage can take up to 30 minutes.

Fetal Monitoring During Labor and Delivery

Various methods can be used to assess fetal well-being during labor and delivery. Two such methods are FHR monitoring and fetal scalp blood sampling.

Intrapartum Fetal Heart Rate Monitoring

Continuous electronic **fetal heart rate (FHR) monitoring** has been used for intrapartum fetal surveillance since 1970 (4). Though never shown to improve neonatal outcomes when compared with intermittent auscultations of heart rate, FHR has become the standard of care in the United States. Trends in FHR are used to estimate a fetus's tolerance of the labor process and to assist the team in making decisions on the method and speed of delivery. Baseline heart rate, beat-to-beat variability, and chronic variability such as accelerations and decelerations are measured:

- Normal baseline FHR is 120 to 160 beats per minute (bpm). FHR less than 110 bpm is considered **bradycardia**. FHR greater than 160 bpm is considered **tachycardia**.
- Normal beat-to-beat variability is defined as deviation of FHR from a baseline of greater than 6 bpm. Moderate FHR variability (6 to 25 bpm) is associated with an umbilical cord pH of greater than 7.15.
- Absence of variability is defined as less than 2 bpm from baseline and is a sign of potential fetal distress.
- **Accelerations** in FHR are associated with fetal movement and are a sign of fetal well-being.
- **Early decelerations** (Fig. 3-1A) are benign and represent head compression or changes in vagal tone after brief hypoxic episodes. They begin with the onset of a contraction, reach a nadir (their lowest point) at the peak of the contraction, and return to baseline FHR as the contraction ends.
- **Variable decelerations** (Fig. 3-1B) are the most common form of decelerations and represent umbilical cord compression. They have no temporal relationship to the onset of the contraction. They are considered severe when the FHR is less than 60 bpm for 60 seconds or longer and are slow to recover.
- **Late decelerations** (Fig. 3-1C) are indicative of uteroplacental insufficiency and, if recurrent, are considered to demonstrate fetal compromise and need further evaluation for delivery. The temporal relationship is varies with the onset of the contraction, occurring after the peak of the contraction, persisting after the contraction stops, and gradually returning to baseline.
- **A sinusoidal FHR pattern** (Fig. 3-1D) is an ominous sign in that it is associated with severe fetal hypoxia, acidosis, or anemia. It consists of regular, smooth oscillations of the baseline variability and typically lasts for at least 10 minutes.

Fetal Scalp Blood Sampling

Fetal scalp blood sampling is used during labor when FHR is nonreassuring to determine the acid-base status of the fetus. The blood sample is obtained from the scalp after the membranes have been ruptured. A fetal scalp pH greater than 7.25 is considered reassuring (5). A low pH suggests that the baby may not be tolerating labor well. Fetal scalp blood sampling may need to be repeated during labor, and the context under which the sample is obtained should be taken into account during interpretation of the results. Contraindications to fetal scalp blood sampling include maternal herpes simplex virus and HIV infections, as well as fetal blood dyscrasias or scalp anomalies.

■■ You arrive at delivery room 3, and the obstetrics team informs you that the fetal scalp pH is 7.2 and that the variability is normal. They tell you that the pregnancy is significant for gestational diabetes. Serology test results are unremarkable, and the membranes were ruptured approximately 12 hours ago. The mother has not received any medications. The baby's head begins to crown, and you contact the NICU to call the doctor to delivery room 3.

Transition to the Extrauterine World

As described in Chapter 2, in utero the fetus depends on the placenta for gas exchange. As the fetus transitions to the extrauterine world, the lungs take over as the primary organ of gas exchange. Transition to the extrauterine world consists of a chain of rapid physiological events that ultimately result in the expansion of the lungs; the establishment of respirations; and the transition of fetal circulation, which functions parallel to that of the adult (which operates in series) (6). As described in Chapter 2, these

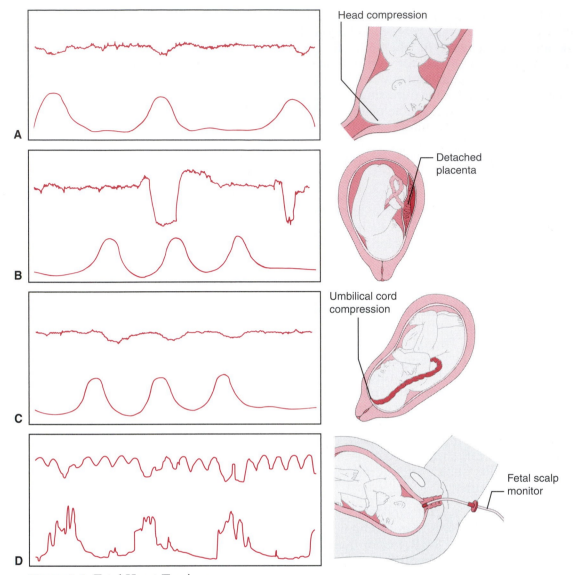

Figure 3-1 Fetal Heart Tracings

physiological events during the transitional period include the following:

- Clearance of fetal lung fluid
- Filling of the lungs with air
- Secretion of surfactant
- Establishment of functional residual capacity
- Vasodilatation of the pulmonary vasculature and decrease in pulmonary vascular resistance
- Removal of the placenta and increase in **systemic vascular resistance**
- Functional closure of two fetal channels (foramen ovale and ductus arteriosus)
- Increase in pulmonary blood flow

Anticipating Neonatal Resuscitation

A newborn may have difficulty transitioning to extrauterine life for a variety of reasons, including problems with fetal health, maternal health, or the placenta. It is extremely important that RTs recognize a newborn at risk for interruption of normal transitional physiology and in need of resuscitation. Box 3-1 presents a list of antepartum (prior to labor and delivery) and intrapartum (during labor and delivery) risk factors associated with neonatal depression and asphyxia. These factors may interfere with a newborn's ability to do the following:

- Fill the lungs with air
- Release surfactant
- Maintain cardiac output and systemic blood pressure
- Maintain sufficient oxygen-carrying capacity
- Vasodilate the pulmonary vascular bed

Problems with any or all of these functions prevent oxygen from reaching body tissues and may warrant the need for newborn resuscitation.

Box 3-1 Factors Associated With Neonatal Depression and Asphyxia

Antepartum Risk Factors
- Maternal diabetes
- Pregnancy-induced hypertension
- Chronic hypertension
- Anemia or isoimmunization
- Previous fetal or neonatal death
- Bleeding in second or third trimester
- Maternal infection
- Maternal disease
  - Cardiac
  - Renal
  - Pulmonary
  - Thyroid
  - Neurological
- Polyhydramnios
- Oligohydramnios
- Premature rupture of membranes
- Post-term gestation
- Multiple gestation
- Size-dates discrepancy
- Drug therapy
  - Lithium carbonate
  - Magnesium
  - Adrenergic-blocking drugs
- Maternal substance abuse
- Fetal malformation
- Diminished fetal activity

- No prenatal care
- Maternal age younger than 16 or older than 35

Intrapartum Risk Factors
- Emergency cesarean section
- Forceps or vacuum-assisted delivery
- Breech or other abnormal presentation
- Premature labor
- Precipitous labor
- Chorioamnionitis
- Prolonged rupture of membranes (more than 18 hours before delivery)
- Prolonged labor (more than 24 hours)
- Prolonged second stage of labor (more than 2 hours)
- Fetal bradycardia
- Nonreassuring FHR patterns
- Use of general anesthesia
- Uterine tetany
- Narcotics administered to mother within 4 hours of delivery
- Meconium-stained amniotic fluid
- Prolapsed cord
- Abruptio placentae
- Placenta previa

Anticipating the need for possible resuscitation and assembling the appropriate personnel in the delivery room are key elements in preparing for resuscitation. Communicating with the obstetrics team regarding the antepartum and intrapartum risk factors and the timing of birth is essential for the RT to ensure that the necessary neonatal team responds in a timely and effective manner. Birthing centers typically develop internal protocols indicating the graded response needed for neonatal resuscitation. However, there should be at least one person who is skilled in providing neonatal resuscitation at every delivery, with primary responsibility for the newborn. In addition, the personnel assembled in the delivery room should be capable of working together as a team (7).

■ ■ The pediatric delivery room team (pediatrician, RT, and neonatal nurse) has now assembled in labor room 3, and the doctor asks you to prepare and set up the equipment for neonatal resuscitation. As you gather your equipment, the baby is delivered. You hear a spontaneous cry as the obstetrician brings the newborn to the radiant heat warmer.

The Neonatal Resuscitation Program

Every year, an estimated 4 million infants around the world die during the neonatal period, and perinatal depression/birth asphyxia accounts for approximately 23% of neonatal mortality. It is postulated that effective resuscitation of the newborn baby could prevent and reduce approximately 42% of these deaths (8, 9). In 1987, the American Academy of Pediatrics and the American Heart Association developed the **Neonatal Resuscitation Program (NRP)**, an educational program designed to train clinicians in newborn resuscitation methods (1). More recently, behavioral skills such as teamwork and communication have been cited to be critically important to the effective resuscitation of the newborn (7, 10, 11).

Although the majority of newborns do not require assistance as they transition to extrauterine life, it is estimated that approximately 10% require some assistance to breathe, and fewer than 1% require extensive resuscitation measures (1). Thus, it is critical for the neonatal RT to be trained in NRP. An RT must be able to prepare for resuscitation of the newborn, perform rapid assessment of the newborn at the time of delivery, and provide the necessary interventions to assist the newborn in transitioning to extrauterine life.

Resuscitation begins with anticipating the management needs of the newborn during resuscitation. The two major components of preparation are assembling the equipment for resuscitation and providing an environment to prevent neonatal heat loss.

Preparation and Equipment

Having the proper equipment available and ready at the time of delivery is a critical step in the resuscitation of the newborn. Often, preparing the equipment is the RT's responsibility. An area of the delivery room should be designated for the resuscitation of the newborn and should be supplied with the necessary equipment for suctioning, bag-mask ventilating, intubating, administering medications, and providing warmth to the newborn. A checklist of neonatal resuscitation equipment and supplies is provided in Box 3-2.

Temperature Regulation

Preventing heat loss in the newborn is essential to providing effective resuscitation and decreasing morbidity. In addition to drying the newborn with a dry linen under a radiant heat warmer, other techniques used to prevent heat loss and achieve **normothermia** (12) include the following (10):

- Prewarming the delivery room to 26°C
- Prewarming the linens
- Drying and swaddling
- Offering skin-to-skin contact with the mother and covering both with a blanket
- Placing a hat on the newborn's head
- Placing the baby on a thermal warming mattress
- Covering the baby in plastic wrapping (food or medical grade, heat-resistant plastic) if he or she weighs less than 1,500 grams (Special Population 3-1)

Recent randomized, controlled, multicenter trials have shown that **induced hypothermia** of newborns 36 weeks' gestational age or older with moderate to severe hypoxic-ischemic encephalopathy may protect against brain injury (12–14). Strict criteria are used for eligibility, and induction of hypothermia must begin within 6 hours after birth. Infants with evidence of moderate to severe **hypoxic-ischemic encephalopathy** (acute or subacute brain injury as a result of hypoxia and acidosis) should be offered therapeutic hypothermia in a timely manner, and

---

Box 3-2 Standard Neonatal Resuscitation Equipment and Supplies Checklist*

Suction Equipment
- Bulb syringe
- Mechanical suction and tubing
- Suction catheters: 5F to 12F
- 8F feeding tube and 20-mL syringe
- Meconium aspirator

Bag-Mask Equipment
- Neonatal resuscitation bag with pressure-release valve or pressure manometer
- Face masks (term and preterm sizes)
- Oxygen source with flowmeter and oxygen blender

Intubation Equipment
- Laryngoscope with straight blades: No. 0 (preterm), No. 1 (term)
- Extra bulbs and batteries for laryngoscope
- ETTs (stylet optional): 2.5-, 3.0-, 3.5-, 4.0-mm internal diameter
- Tape
- Scissors
- Alcohol sponges

- CO_2 detector
- Laryngeal mask airway

Medications
- Epinephrine 1:10,000 (0.1 mg/mL) ampules
- Isotonic crystalloid (normal saline or lactated Ringer's solution)
- Normal saline for flushes
- Umbilical vessel catheter: 3.5F, 5F
- Sterile gloves
- Scalpel or scissors
- Povidone-iodine solution
- Umbilical tape
- Three-way stopcock

Miscellaneous
- Radiant heat warmer
- Plastic bag
- Hat
- Stethoscope
- Cardiac monitor or pulse oximeter
- Oropharyngeal airways (0, 00, and 000 sizes or 30-, 40-, and 50-mm lengths)

*Additional supplies may be needed for resuscitation of newborns with congenital anomalies.

Source: Modified from American Heart Association/American Academy of Pediatrics. *Textbook of Neonatal Resuscitation*. 6th ed. Dallas, TX: American Heart Association; 2011.

thus RTs must be aware of their institution's policies and nearest referral center with the capabilities and appropriate follow-up care for this therapy.

Initial Assessment and Interventions: The Golden Minute

Rapid assessment of the newborn at the time of birth involves asking the following four questions:

1. Is the newborn term or preterm?
2. Is the newborn crying or breathing?
3. Does the newborn have good muscle tone?
4. Is there meconium? (Special Population 3-2)

If a newborn is term, has an adequate cry, and has good muscle tone, then the baby should not be separated from the mother, and skin-to-skin contact with the mother should be encouraged as the newborn is dried, covered with dry linens, and observed for breathing, color, and activity.

If the infant is not term, not crying, or does not have good muscle tone, then initial resuscitation maneuvers may be needed and can include the following:

- Intubating the newborn and suctioning for meconium if meconium is present and the newborn is nonvigorous

- Suctioning the mouth
- Drying and stimulating the baby
- Providing positive pressure ventilation
- Calling for additional help from other members of the neonatal team
- Intubating the baby
- Administering chest compressions
- Placing an umbilical venous line to administer epinephrine and/or infuse volume expanders

NRP providers have approximately 60 seconds to complete the initial assessment and interventions of resuscitation (Fig. 3-2) (10). During this **golden minute**, the newborn should be placed on the back or side and then warmed, dried, and stimulated. The head should be placed in the sniffing position, a position that extends the neck to facilitate opening the airway. Care must be taken not to hyperextend or flex the newborn's neck, because these positions may restrict air entry. A shoulder roll, in which a rolled towel or blanket is placed under the shoulders, may be helpful in situations in which a newborn has a large occiput from molding or edema.

If necessary, suctioning of the mouth and nose may be done through a bulb syringe or suction

---

● **Special Populations 3-1**

Extreme Prematurity

Babies born prior to 32 weeks' gestation have many physiological differences that make them more susceptible to injury or complications in the period immediately following birth. These include the following:

- Immature tissue that is more susceptible to oxygen toxicity
- Weak thoracic musculature that may cause ineffective breaths
- Immature nervous system, which may not provide enough stimulation to breathe
- Surfactant-deficient lungs, making ventilation difficult and more likely to be injured by positive-pressure ventilation
- Thin skin, large skin surface area related to body mass, and decreased fat, which make babies more susceptible to rapidly losing body heat
- Immature immune system, which increases the risk of infection
- Fragile capillaries within the brain, which are at higher risk for rupture and bleeding
- Small blood volume, making them more susceptible to hypovolemic effects of blood loss

Delivery room intervention considerations to minimize these risks include the following:

- Additional trained personnel who are prepared to perform a complex resuscitation
- Increased temperature in the delivery room, 77° to 79°F
- Use of a chemically activated warming pad and prewarmed radiant warmer
- Immediate placement of newborn in a reclosable, food-grade polyethylene bag
- Use of a transport incubator when moving the newborn to a special care nursery
- Use of an air-oxygen blender to provide oxygen
- Use of pulse oximetry to adjust oxygen delivery and ventilation
- Use of noninvasive CPAP at 4 to 6 cm H_2O
- Initiation of ventilation at 20 to 25 cm H_2O, with cautious increases if no positive response is seen; avoid excessive positive pressures
- Once intubated, PEEP provided at 2 to 5 cm H_2O
- Early administration of surfactant
- Gentle handling of baby
- Avoiding Trendelenburg (head-down) placement
- Avoiding rapid infusion of fluid

catheter attached to mechanical suction (suction pressure should read −100 mm Hg when the suction catheter is blocked). The mouth is suctioned first to ensure that the newborn does not aspirate anything should he or she gasp when the nose is suctioned. Turning the head to the side facilitates suctioning, allowing secretions to collect in the cheek and to be easily removed. Suctioning immediately after birth should be done for those newborns who need positive-pressure ventilation or who have obstruction to breathing because suctioning of the nasopharynx can lead to bradycardia during resuscitation (15, 16).

Often, positioning, drying, and suctioning provide enough stimulation to initiate a newborn's breathing. Other techniques used to provide tactile stimulation include flicking the soles of the feet and gentle rubbing of the newborn's back or extremities. Care should be taken to not overstimulate the newborn because harmful sequelae may result.

Primary Versus Secondary Apnea

Although tactile stimulation is helpful in facilitating the first breaths a newborn takes, when a baby has persistent apnea continued tactile stimulation is not useful and only delays effective resuscitation. A skilled provider of newborn resuscitation must be able to determine the difference between **primary** and **secondary apnea** (Fig. 3-3). In primary apnea, stimulation results in resumption of breathing. In secondary apnea, no amount of stimulation will restart breathing. An NRP provider must initiate positive-pressure ventilation (PPV) to reverse the physiological characteristics of low heart rate and blood pressure when a newborn is in the state of secondary apnea.

At 30 seconds of life and continuing every 30 seconds, the NRP provider must reassess respirations and check the heart rate, because these two vital signs will guide every step of neonatal resuscitation. Heart rate detection can be accomplished by the following (Fig. 3-4):

- Auscultation of the precordial pulse using a stethoscope
- Palpation of the umbilical cord stump pulse
- Placement of a pulse oximeter if perfusion to the extremities is adequate

If the newborn is breathing well and the heart rate is greater than100 bpm by 30 seconds, then routine care is provided through suctioning, drying, and tactile stimulation. If the heart rate is greater than 100 bpm but respirations are labored, then ongoing pulmonary care is undertaken and may include continued suctioning, saturation of arterial blood with

---

● Special Populations 3-2

Meconium Aspiration

Direct suctioning of the trachea helps reduce the baby's risk of developing meconium aspiration syndrome. NRP recommends performing endotracheal suctioning of nonvigorous babies when meconium is present. When the baby is deemed nonvigorous (depressed respirations, depressed tone, and/or heart rate less than 100 bpm), an RT may be asked to assist the physician with endotracheal intubation and tracheal suctioning for meconium or, in some circumstances, perform the procedure alone. In this case, after an ETT has been inserted, the following steps should be taken:

- Connect the ETT to a meconium aspirator that has been connected to a suction source.
- Occlude the suction port on the aspirator and gradually pull out the ETT.
- If meconium is present, repeat intubation and meconium suctioning. If meconium is not present, proceed with resuscitation.

However, if intubation is prolonged or unsuccessful, or if there is persistent bradycardia, positive-pressure ventilation should be initiated.

---

oxygen (SpO_2) monitoring, and continuous positive airway pressure (CPAP). If the heart rate is less than 100 bpm and/or the newborn is gasping or apneic, then positive-pressure ventilation and SpO_2 monitoring must be provided.

When Meconium Is Present

Direct suctioning of the trachea may help reduce the risk of developing meconium aspiration syndrome (see Chapter 6 for more information on meconium aspiration syndrome). NRP recommends performing endotracheal suctioning of nonvigorous babies when meconium is present. When the baby is deemed nonvigorous (depressed respirations, depressed tone, and/or heart rate less than 100 bpm), an RT may be asked to assist the physician with endotracheal intubation immediately after birth so that tracheal suctioning for meconium can be provided. In some circumstances, the RT may be asked to perform this procedure. After an endotracheal tube has been inserted, the following steps should be taken:

- Connect the endotracheal tube to a meconium aspirator that has been connected to a suction source.
- Occlude the suction port on the aspirator and gradually pull out the endotracheal tube.

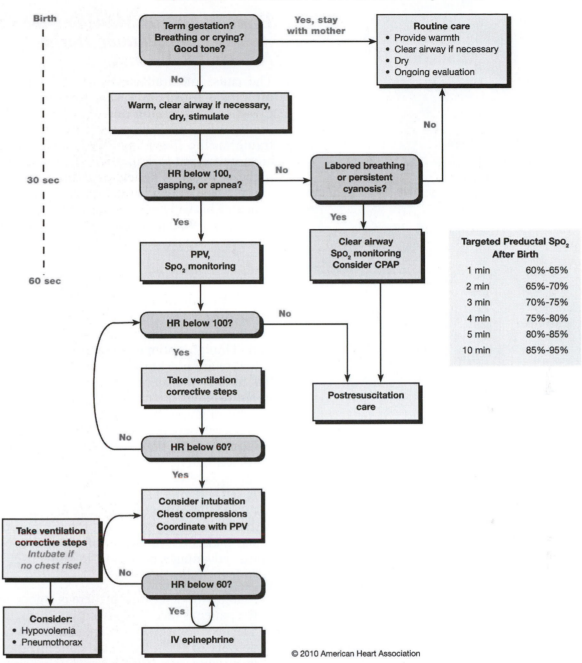

Figure 3-2 NRP Algorithm (*Used with permission of the American Academy of Pediatrics, Textbook of Neonatal Resuscitation, 6th ed, 2011.*)

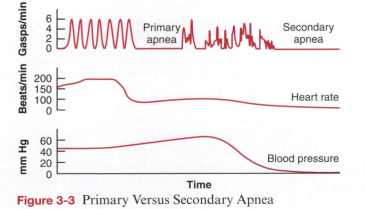

Figure 3-3 Primary Versus Secondary Apnea

• If meconium is present, repeat intubation and meconium suctioning. If meconium is not present, proceed with resuscitation.

However, if intubation is prolonged or unsuccessful, or if there is persistent bradycardia, positive-pressure ventilation should be initiated.

■■ Baby girl (BG) Zacharian is brought to the radiant warmer and is placed on her side by the obstetrician. The doctor begins to dry the baby as you bulb suction her mouth and then her nose. Meconium

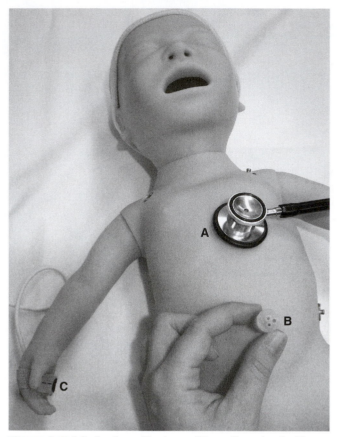

Figure 3-4 Methods to Evaluate Heart Rate in the Delivery Room

is not present. The first wet linen is removed, and the team continues to dry the baby with warm linens. You alert the team that 30 seconds have passed. The physician palpates the umbilical stump pulse and taps out the heart rate on the bed with his hand. The heart rate is 80 bpm. The team agrees with you that the newborn is gasping. The physician asks you to provide positive-pressure ventilation.

Establishing and Managing the Airway and Breathing During Neonatal Resuscitation

The cause of bradycardia in most newborns is prolonged apnea and/or asphyxia during delivery. Effective oxygenation and ventilation will reverse bradycardia and facilitate normal transition to extrauterine life. Providing PPV is therefore the single most important skill in NRP. It should be initiated if the newborn is apneic or if the baby is gasping and the heart rate is less than 100 bpm (secondary apnea). This will begin as noninvasive or mask ventilation and escalate to intubation if improvement is not seen or apnea continues.

Noninvasive Ventilation

Assisted ventilation should be given at a rate of 40 to 60 breaths per minute to achieve a heart rate greater than 100 bpm and movement of the chest wall. Though optimal pressure, inflating time, and flow rate are not known, some studies have shown that initial inflation pressures used to establish functional residual capacity may range between 20 cm and 40 cm H_2O (10, 17–19).

Devices used to provide PPV include the self-inflating bag, the flow-inflating bag, and the T-piece resuscitator. The key features, advantages, and disadvantages of each are included in Table 3-1.

A **self-inflating bag** does not need a compressed gas source in order to inflate. It fills spontaneously with air after being squeezed. It has a pop-off valve, which makes overinflation of the lungs less likely. The disadvantages of the self-inflating bag, however, include the following:

• Inability to determine if there is a good seal on the patient's face
• The need for a reservoir attachment to provide delivery of 100% fractional concentration of inspired oxygen (FIO_2)

Table 3-1	Devices for PPV		
Device	**Description**	**Advantages**	**Disadvantages**
Self-inflating bag	Mask-and-bag system designed to deliver tidal volumes during rescue breathing One-way valve at patient connection, to prevent exhaled gases from entering the bag Rapidly refills automatically after the bag is squeezed (during patient exhalation) • oxygen tubing and reservoir system to ensure reliable FIO_2 delivery when compressed gas is used • PIP controlled by how hard bag is squeezed	Can deliver PPV without a compressed gas source Pressure-release valve minimizes risk of lung overinflation and barotrauma	Hard to evaluate seal between face and mask Mask can't be used to deliver free-flow oxygen Requires a PEEP valve to deliver PEEP or CPAP

Table 3-1	Devices for PPV —cont'd		
Device	**Description**	**Advantages**	**Disadvantages**
Flow-inflating bag	Compliant bag that remains deflated until seal is made around mask Flow-control valve regulates how much gas enters bag, how much enters mask, and how much is vented from system. PIP controlled by flow rate, flow-control valve, and how hard the bag is squeezed Pressure manometer attached to monitor PIP	Reliable FIO_2 delivery Can deliver free-flow oxygen through mask Compliance of lungs can be "felt" when squeezing bag	Requires gas source to inflate bag Requires a tight seal between face and mask to inflate bag May not have pressure-relief valve
T-piece resuscitator	Compressed gas connected to resuscitation device PIP and PEEP preset using adjustable controls on resuscitator device Breath delivered by occluding expiratory opening on T-piece device at patient connection; released during exhalation Pressure manometer on device to monitor PIP and PEEP	Consistent PIP Reliable FIO_2 delivery	Requires gas source to inflate lungs Unable to "feel" compliance of lungs Pressures set before beginning PPV

- Inability to provide 100% FIO_2 free-flow oxygen dependably

The **flow-inflating bag** fills up with oxygen only when a compressed source of oxygen is attached, and it requires having a tight seal between the mask and the patient to remain inflated. The advantages of a flow-inflating bag (also known as the anesthesia bag) over a self-inflating bag include the following:

- Ease of determining if there is a seal on the patient's face
- Ability to feel the compliance of the lungs when squeezing the bag
- Ability to provide free-flow oxygen

A disadvantage of the flow-inflating bag, however, is that in addition to requiring the presence of a gas source, it usually does not have a pop-off valve. When preparing to use the flow-inflating bag, an RT must ensure that adequate flow (usually 5 to 10 L/min) is being provided to inflate the bag between manual breaths and that a 5 cm H_2O pressure is being delivered between bagged breaths.

The **T-piece resuscitator** is a mechanical device designed to deliver manual breaths at a set flow that provides consistent peak inspiratory pressure (PIP) and peak end expiratory pressure (PEEP). Similar to the flow-inflating bag, it requires a tight seal between the mask and the patient's face so that it will work well. Disadvantages of the T-piece resuscitator include the following:

- Having to preset PIP and PEEP prior to its use
- Inability to change PIP and PEEP easily during resuscitation
- Need for a gas source to operate the device

When providing PPV, an RT must ensure that the appropriate-sized mask is being used with a close seal around the newborn's mouth and nose (Fig. 3-5). In cases in which a tight seal is difficult to obtain, two NRP providers may need to deliver manual breaths; one provider holds the mask in place using a two-handed technique as the other squeezes the bag to

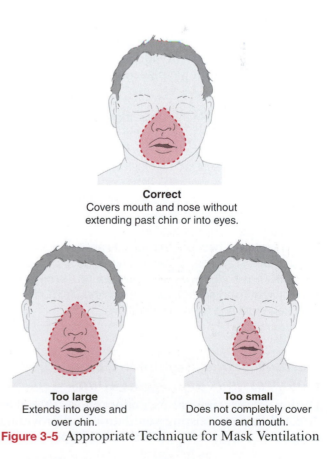

Correct
Covers mouth and nose without extending past chin or into eyes.

Too large
Extends into eyes and over chin.

Too small
Does not completely cover nose and mouth.

Figure 3-5 Appropriate Technique for Mask Ventilation

inflate the lungs. The newborn's stomach should be emptied during and after prolonged bag-mask ventilation through placement of an orogastric tube, because gastric distention can push on the diaphragm and make PPV less effective.

Endotracheal Intubation

Endotracheal intubation should be considered for cases in which there is prolonged bag-mask ventilation, meconium, or congenital defects such as congenital diaphragmatic hernia for which control of the airway is necessary. However, multiple unsuccessful attempts by inexperienced providers can be detrimental to the newborn. In these situations, it is best to continue bag-mask ventilation until experienced help arrives. In addition, use of a laryngeal mask airway (LMA) may be considered in situations in which intubation or bag-mask ventilation is unsuccessful and the newborn is 34 weeks or older or weighs more than 2,000 grams.

Often, RTs are asked to prepare the equipment for an anticipated endotracheal intubation. One way to quickly estimate endotracheal tube (ETT) size is to divide the gestational age by 10. For example, if the newborn is 35 weeks' gestation, a 3.5-mm ETT may be considered. When determining where to tape the ETT at the lip, adding 6 to the birth weight (in kilograms) provides a starting point for assessing the appropriate ETT placement. For instance, if the patient weighs 1.5 kg, taping the ETT at 7.5 cm at the upper lip is a reasonable starting point. When the tube is correctly placed, the tip of the ETT will be located in the mid-trachea, and breath sounds, when auscultated, should be equal bilaterally. Figure 3-6 provides an overview of landmarks for laryngoscopic placement of ETTs.

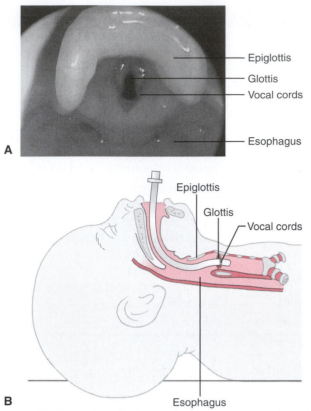

Figure 3-6 Landmarks for Endotracheal Intubation via Direct Laryngoscopy

You place BG Zacharian in the sniffing position and provide her with three breaths using a bag and mask. The resident physician squeezes the bag as you maintain a good seal on the mask with two hands. You see her chest rise with each bagged breath, and the nurse confirms that she can hear symmetric breath sounds with PPV. After 30 seconds, the nurse taps out the heart rate: 12 finger taps in 6 seconds. The team feels reassured, because this reflects an improved heart rate to 120 bpm. While you continue to provide PPV, the nurse places a pulse oximeter on the newborn's right hand so that you can continue to monitor her heart rate and oxygen saturations.

Cardiovascular Support: Chest Compressions and Medications

During delivery room resuscitation, efforts should be directed first to assisting ventilation and providing oxygen. If bradycardia of less than 60 bpm persists after 30 seconds of established effective ventilation, chest compressions should be initiated. Two techniques are described by NRP for cardiac massage:

1. The two-thumb encircling-hand technique (two thumbs with fingers encircling the chest and supporting the back)
2. The two-finger technique (compressing the chest with two fingers as the second hand supports the back)

The two-thumb encircling-hand technique is the method recommended by NRP because evidence suggests that it may generate higher peak systolic pressures (10). An RT may be asked to provide chest compressions or coordinate compressions and ventilations. Compressions should be delivered at the mid-sternum just below a line connecting the nipples to a depth of approximately one-third of the anterior-posterior diameter of the chest (Fig. 3-7). The provider's thumbs should not leave the chest between compressions, and frequent interruptions to chest compressions should be avoided. A ratio of three compressions to one breath should be delivered to achieve approximately 120 bpm (approximately one 4-event cycle every 2 seconds). The compressor should count the cadence out loud ("one-and-two-and-three-and-breathe") because this allows for a well-coordinated procedure. Compressions should

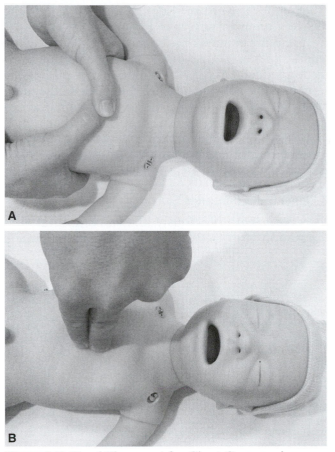

Figure 3-7 Hand Placement for Chest Compressions

continue until the heart rate recovers to greater than 60 bpm, reassessing the heart rate every 30 seconds for improvement. If a provider becomes fatigued when delivering compressions, he or she should alert the team so that resuscitation roles may be rotated.

Administration of medications in the delivery room for cardiovascular support is rarely needed because bradycardia typically can be reversed with adequate inflation and ventilation of the lungs. However, if bradycardia persists despite establishment of an airway, ventilation with 100% oxygen and chest compressions epinephrine and/or volume expanders should be administered. Epinephrine 1:10,000 (0.1 mg/mL) can be given via two routes: intravenously or endotracheally. Intravenous (IV) administration is the route preferred by NRP because it ensures entry into the bloodstream and use of the lower range of epinephrine dosing (0.01 to 0.03 mg/kg) (10). Because IV access must be established, the RT may be asked to give the first dose of epinephrine via ETT. In this case, higher doses of epinephrine may be considered (0.05 to 0.10 mg/kg). Epinephrine may be injected directly into the ETT and followed by a normal saline (0.5 to 1.0 mL) flush, or it may be diluted with normal saline to a 1-mL syringe volume before being injected into the ETT. If volume expansion is being considered

in the delivery room, the recommended dose is 10 mL/kg of an isotonic crystalloid solution or blood (O-negative, cytomegalovirus [CMV] irradiated).

Post-Resuscitation Care

■■ After she receives PPV for 60 seconds, BG Zacharian begins breathing spontaneously. You stop providing PPV, and at 2 minutes of postnatal life, you note that the oxygen saturation is 86% on room air (RA). You also notice that the newborn is jittery on physical examination. Given the mother's prenatal history of gestational diabetes, the physician decides to bring the newborn to the NICU for further management and care. You are asked to prepare the infant transport vehicle for the patient's transfer to a higher level of care.

Newborns who receive resuscitation maneuvers in the delivery room should be transferred to an environment where close monitoring and further evaluation and management can be provided. Although administration of glucose, sodium bicarbonate, calcium, atropine, sedation, and naloxone may be helpful during resuscitations, these interventions are not recommended for use in the delivery room; however, they may be considered during post-resuscitation care after the infant undergoes further evaluation. An RT may be asked to assist the transfer and to admit and manage the respiratory support of the newborn to the NICU as he or she continues to receive ongoing evaluation and medical interventions.

Special Considerations

There are some special considerations to be made during neonatal resuscitations. These include the use of supplemental oxygen, care of a newborn with a known congenital anomaly, discontinuing resuscitative measures, and calculating Apgar scores.

Use of Supplemental Oxygen

Optimal use of oxygen supplementation is an important aspect of neonatal resuscitation, because both excessive and insufficient oxygenation can be harmful to the newborn. Several studies have shown that it can take as long as 10 minutes following birth for an infant to reach 95% O_2 saturation (10). Resuscitation should be initiated with RA. However, when there is persistent cyanosis or bradycardia, or when positive-pressure ventilation is being administered during resuscitation, pulse oximetry should be used to facilitate the titration of blended oxygen (FIO_2). Goal oxygen saturations after birth are shown in Table 3-2. If blended oxygen is not available, 100% FIO_2 should be given after 90 seconds of bradycardia (heart rate less than 60 bpm) until the bradycardia has resolved.

Table 3-2	Goal Oxygen Saturation Values After Delivery (interquartile range of preductal saturations)
Time After Birth	**SpO$_2$**
1 minute	60%–65%
2 minutes	65%–70%
3 minutes	70%–75%
4 minutes	75%–80%
5 minutes	80%–85%
10 minutes	85%–95%

Source: Used with permission of the American Academy of Pediatrics for use from American Academy of Pediatrics/American Heart Association. *Textbook of Neonatal Resuscitation*. 6th ed. Dallas, TX: American Academy of Pediatrics; 2011. Copyright holder American Academy of Pediatrics, 2011.

Techniques used to provide free-flow oxygen in the delivery room are shown in Figure 3-8.

The pulse oximeter probe should be placed on the right upper extremity of the newborn so that it reflects preductal oxygen saturations. After placing the probe on the newborn, attach the probe to the pulse oximeter because this may hasten reception of a signal. It is important to note that the newborn must have normal cardiac anatomy as well as adequate cardiac output and perfusion for pulse oximetry to provide an accurate measurement.

Congenital Anomalies

Newborns with previously known congenital malformations are typically referred to birthing centers

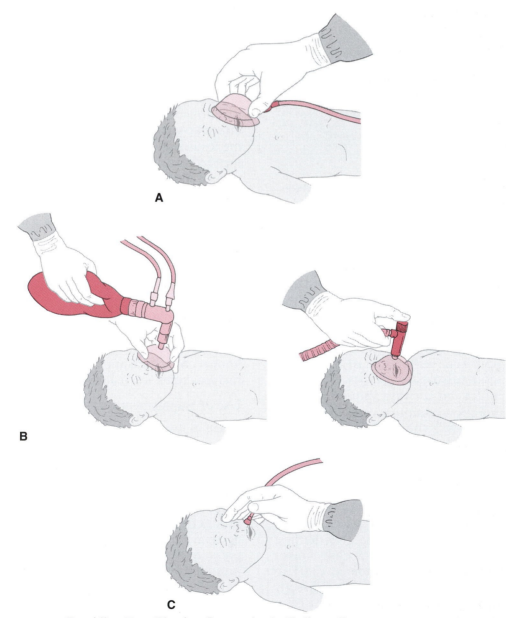

A

B

C

Figure 3-8 Providing Free-Flowing Oxygen in the Delivery Room

where multidisciplinary neonatal teams are available to assist these babies at birth. As an RT, you may work at one of these centers or come across a newborn in the delivery room with an undetected congenital anomaly during the prenatal period. Thus, recognizing how these conditions complicate transition to the extrauterine world is critical.

In cases in which establishing an airway has been unsuccessful and a congenital upper-airway obstruction is suspected (e.g., choanal atresia, Robin sequence, glottic web), use of oral airways, laryngeal mask airways, or emergency tracheostomy may be required. In cases in which establishment of ventilation has resulted in diminished or unequal breath sounds, shift of the precordial pulse, or no improvement in heart rate, conditions associated with impaired lung function should be considered (e.g., pneumothorax, congenital diaphragmatic hernia, pleural effusion, **pulmonary hypoplasia**, prematurity). Endotracheal intubation, transillumination of the chest, placement of a Replogle tube, and/or evacuation of the air leak by needle aspiration or chest tube placement may be necessary (see Chapter 7 for more information on treatment for pneumothorax). If premature delivery is suspected, these newborns may need higher inflation pressures and/or surfactant administration in the delivery room. Should an external anatomical defect be found (e.g., gastroschisis, omphalocele, **myelomeningocele**), the resuscitation team should handle the defect with care and place the baby in a sterile bag to protect and keep the defect moist until it can be further evaluated by pediatric subspecialists. Finally, **cyanotic congenital heart disease** should be suspected in cases in which oxygen saturations are low and the baby is cyanotic despite adequate ventilation and oxygenation. Confirmation by radiograph, electrocardiogram, and/or echocardiogram will be useful, and if a ductal-dependent heart lesion is found (e.g., hypoplastic left heart syndrome, pulmonic stenosis, tetralogy of Fallot), prostaglandin may be required, after which more definitive treatments can be initiated (see Chapter 12 for more information on management of cyanotic heart defects).

Many hospitals have protocols in place for organizing the delivery, medical care team, and anticipated resuscitation plan for newborns with congenital anomalies. Communication, teamwork, preparation, and delineation of the delivery room plan prior to delivery are necessary to ensure the safest and smoothest transition for these fragile babies (Teamwork 3-1).

Withholding and Discontinuing Resuscitation Efforts

Withholding resuscitation efforts may be appropriate in cases in which gestation, birth weight, and/or

---

Teamwork 3-1 Shared Cognition

Team performance is improved when team members continually assess their environment and update one another in a process called "shared cognition." Using shared cognition, team members make decisions based on current information and can have a shared mental model of the current state of affairs and an updated plan of action with contingencies. This includes the continuous sharing of information such as vital signs, current plan of care, the patient's diagnosis or working diagnosis, and requests by the team leader for information or suggestions from all members of the team.

---

congenital anomalies are associated with high mortality and poor outcomes (10). Some examples of these conditions include the following:

- Gestational age less than 23 weeks
- Birth weight less than 400 grams
- Anencephaly, a neural tube defect that results in the loss of a major portion of brain, skull, and scalp
- Trisomy 13, a chromosomal abnormality that manifests in problems of the nervous, musculoskeletal, cutaneous, and cardiovascular systems

In these cases, it is important to involve the parents in the discussion of resuscitation and outcomes prior to delivery and to attempt to obtain parental agreement regarding resuscitation as much as possible. In conditions in which prognosis and survival are uncertain, parental desires regarding resuscitation efforts should be supported. Discussions with parents and the medical team should highlight the benefits and disadvantages of aggressive resuscitation and comfort care measures. In addition, because prenatal data can be misleading regarding estimated fetal weight, gestational age, and congenital anomaly screening, it should be underscored that decisions to provide or withhold resuscitative efforts must be based on the examination of the baby by the health-care team after birth. In cases in which the heart rate remains undetectable for 10 minutes during a newborn resuscitation, it may be appropriate to discuss **discontinuing resuscitation efforts**. As an RT, discussing these decisions with the entire medical team is imperative as you anticipate and prepare for the delivery of these newborns.

Apgar Scores and Documentation

Devised by Dr. Virginia Apgar in 1952, the **Apgar score** is a tool used to describe the state of the newborn at various stages after birth (Table 3-3). It is a set of objective data used to help guide early post-resuscitative care and used by clinicians to assess the quality of their resuscitative efforts beyond heart rate and respiratory rate. It is based on five criteria, summarized by the acronym APGAR (appearance, pulse, grimace, activity, respirations). Each of the five criteria is awarded a value of 0, 1, or 2. They are then added together, and the sum becomes the Apgar score. Traditionally, Apgar scores are assigned at 1 and 5 minutes of age and repeated in 5-minute intervals until an Apgar score of at least 7 is reached. A neonatal resuscitation team should not wait to initiate resuscitation maneuvers while an Apgar score is assigned. Apgar scores should be documented in the medical record along with a narrative description of the resuscitation maneuvers performed and the initial newborn physical exam (21, 22).

■■ As you prepare for the transfer of BG Zacharian to the NICU, the physician has begun completing the resuscitation documentation for the newborn in the labor and delivery unit. He asks you if you agree with the Apgar scores, which he has assigned to be 4 and 8. You recall that, at 1 minute of postnatal life, the neonate was apneic without grimace, slightly limp, and peripherally cyanotic. Her heart rate was over 100 bpm. At 5 minutes of postnatal life, she had spontaneous respirations, vigorous cry, mild hypotonia, and heart rate greater than 100 bpm. She had peripheral cyanosis. You agree with the physician, and you cosign the paperwork.

Table 3-3	Apgar Scores (24)		
	Score		
Sign	**0**	**1**	**2**
Heart rate	Absent	<100 bpm	>100 bpm
Respiratory effort	Absent, irregular	Slow, crying	Good
Muscle tone	Limp	Some flexion of extremities	Active motion
Reflex irritability	No response	Grimace	Cough or sneeze
Color	Blue, pale trunk, lips, face	Acrocyanosis	Completely pink

■■ Critical Thinking Questions: BG Zacharian

1. What additional needs should be anticipated if BG Zacharian's mom received magnesium sulfate prior to delivery?
2. If BG Zacharian had a congenital heart defect, what would you do differently? What if you were told that she might have a congenital diaphragmatic hernia?
3. If BG Zacharian needed oxygen delivery for more than 5 minutes, do you think that would change your decision on where to send her after the delivery room? What if you only had to give oxygen, not PPV?

▶● Case Studies and Critical Thinking Questions

■ Case 1: BG Masiento

You are working in a level IIIC NICU when you are called by the obstetrics team; they inform you that they are anticipating the delivery of a 28-week-gestation infant within the next hour. Ms. Masiento is a 14-year-old female who is GBS positive. She was admitted in preterm labor and had premature rupture of membranes 1 week ago and received 2 doses of betamethasone. Fetal heart tracings have been reassuring. Despite administration of magnesium sulfate, she has progressed and is currently 10 cm dilated.

- *What information about this prenatal and perinatal history makes it a high-risk delivery?*
- *What equipment do you need to prepare in anticipation of this preterm delivery?*

The baby, a girl, is born limp, with poor respiratory effort, and is not responsive to stimulation from drying. The nurse applies the pulse oximeter to the right hand, and after 30 seconds you begin bag-mask ventilation with a T-piece resuscitator. You begin by using inflation pressure of 20 cm H_2O at a rate of about 40 breaths, FIO_2 0.70. At 1 minute of life, you are still ventilating using bag-mask ventilation, and you are achieving good chest rise and a heart rate of 100 bpm. BG Masiento is taking occasional gasping breaths, no more than five per minute, but is making no other spontaneous movements or responding to stimulation. Her lips and torso are pink, but hands and feet are blue. Mask ventilation is continued, and at about 2 minutes of life a 2.5 ETT is placed, with positive end-tidal CO_2 detector changes and bilateral breath sounds heard after placement. At 4 minutes of life, a dose of surfactant is given via ETT in four aliquots. At 5 minutes of life, BG Masiento's heart rate is 120 bpm, and she is breathing about 10 times per minute with substernal and intercostal retractions. Her skin is red all over, and she is making minor spontaneous movements. Her face scrunches into a grimace when her foot is flicked or her back is rubbed.

- *Using the Apgar scoring system, what are BG Masiento's 1-minute and 5-minute Apgar scores?*

■ Case 2: BB Diaz

A 38-year-old mother of three is admitted to the labor and delivery unit for induction of labor. She is 39 1/7 weeks' gestation and was diagnosed in her second trimester with preeclampsia. She had an artificial rupture of membranes 2 hours ago, which was meconium-stained. The fetal heart monitor shows early-onset early deceleration with each contraction.

- *What information about this prenatal and perinatal history makes it a high-risk delivery?*

You begin assembling your equipment as baby boy (BB) Diaz is delivered. The obstetrician says that there was a nuchal cord. The baby is apneic, limp, and covered in meconium.

- *What should you do?*

You assume the position at the head of the bed and intubate with a 3.5-cm ETT within 10 seconds of his placement on the warmer. You verbalize that you see meconium on the vocal cords. A meconium aspirator is used to suction moderate amounts of greenish-brown fluid from the lungs. You make a second attempt at intubation, while asking the RN to monitor the patient's heart rate at the umbilical stump. The ETT is placed a second time, and the meconium aspirator is used, but minimal amounts of fluid are returned during suctioning. The RN notes the heartbeat to be 60 bpm. The team begins drying, stimulating, and clearing the upper airway. At approximately 45 seconds of life, you begin bag-mask ventilation at a rate of 40 breaths per minute. Fifteen seconds later, the heartbeat is 110 bpm. BB Diaz's lips, trunk, hands, and feet are blue. He is limp and unresponsive to stimulation and is making no respiratory effort. An additional 30 seconds of positive-pressure ventilation is given, and after 30 seconds, he is breathing spontaneously at a rate of about 25 breaths per minute and has a weak cry. BB Diaz is moving

his extremities spontaneously and has an occasional grimace. You discontinue positive-pressure ventilation but start blow-by oxygen via small-bore oxygen tubing, which you maintain for about 2 minutes; then you remove the blow-by oxygen slowly, and BB Diaz maintains pink coloring of his lips and trunk, though his feet remain blue. At 5 minutes of life, an assessment is made. BB Diaz's respiratory rate is approximately 60 breaths per minute, and his heart rate is 140 bpm. He is moving actively, crying, and with every exhalation is making a grunting noise. He is pink through the torso and head, with a blue coloring of his hands and feet.

- *Using the Apgar scoring system, what are BB Diaz's 1- and 5-minute Apgar scores?*

■ Case 3: BB Dimitz

A 22-year-old, Jessica Dimitz, entered the emergency room fully dilated and in hard labor. She had no prenatal care and admits to frequent heroin use, the last time being 2 hours ago. The fetal heart monitor notes variable decelerations. A quick assessment by a physician notes that the baby is in frank breech position and appears to be "close to term." Dimitz is rushed for an emergency cesarean section, where the team from the level IIB nursery has assembled to care for the newborn.

- *What information about this prenatal and perinatal history makes it a high-risk delivery?*

A baby boy is born and given to the pediatrician. He is initially limp, with weak respiratory efforts. After about 30 seconds of drying and tactile stimulation, the baby begins screaming loudly. He appears long, but skinny, and is moving his extremities spontaneously. At 1 minute of life, his respiratory rate is 60 breaths per minute, and his heart rate is 160 bpm. BB Dimitz is kicking and screaming actively and pulls away from stimulation. His hands, feet, and lips are blue. You begin giving blow-by oxygen via small-bore oxygen tubing. His lips turn pink, but his hands and feet remain blue. At 3 minutes of life, you begin slowly removing the oxygen from his face and are able to turn it off at 4 minutes without his cyanosis returning. At 5 minutes of life, BB Dimitz is crying loudly, moving his extremities with and without stimulation, and his respiratory rate is 60 breaths per minute with a heart rate of 150 bpm.

- *Using the Apgar scoring system, what are BB Dimitz's 1- and 5-minute Apgar scores?*

Multiple-Choice Questions

1. During which stage of labor is the baby delivered into the extrauterine world?
   a. First stage
   b. Second stage
   c. Third stage
   d. Deceleration phase
   e. Active phase

2. Which of the following fetal heart tracings is a concern?
   a. Late heart rate deceleration
   b. Early heart rate deceleration
   c. Sinusoidal heart rate pattern
   d. B and C
   e. C and D

3. A 38-year-old mother of three is admitted to the labor and delivery unit for induction of labor. She is 39 1/7 weeks' gestation and was diagnosed in her second trimester with preeclampsia. She had an artificial rupture of membranes 2 hours ago, which was meconium-stained. The fetal heart monitor shows early onset early deceleration with each contraction. Which items are considered neonatal risk factors from the description above?
       I. Meconium-stained amniotic fluid
       II. Preeclampsia
       III. Maternal age
       IV. Early decelerations
       V. Prolonged rupture of membranes
       VI. Induction of labor
   a. I, II, III, IV, VI
   b. I, II, III
   c. I, II, IV, VI
   d. I, II, VI

4. Which of the following is *not* an assessment question that should be asked about a baby at the time of birth?
   a. Is the newborn term or preterm?
   b. Is the newborn crying or breathing?
   c. Does the newborn have good muscle tone?
   d. Is the baby cyanotic?

5. Which of the following should be done to ensure that adequate warmth is being provided to a newborn in the delivery room?
       I. Prewarming the delivery room to 37°C
       II. Prewarming the linens
       III. Drying and swaddling
       IV. Rubbing the newborn's back
       V. Placing a hat on the newborn's head
   a. I, II, III
   b. II, III, V
   c. I, II, III, V
   d. III, III, IV, V

6. You attend a cesarean section of a full-term baby in breech position. BB Byrd is born at 0823 and is handed to the neonatal resuscitation team by the surgeon. He is limp and blue and does not appear to be breathing. What is the initial step that should be completed by the team?
   a. Dry and stimulate
   b. Evaluate heart rate
   c. Provide PPV
   d. Provide blow-by oxygen

7. Thirty seconds later, BB Byrd is taking a few gasping breaths, has central cyanosis, and is still limp. The nurse palpates a heart rate of 80 bpm. What should be the team's next step?
   a. Blow-by oxygen
   b. Initiate PPV
   c. Continue to dry and stimulate
   d. Initiate chest compressions

8. You have been providing PPV to a 26 weeks gestation infant for 30 seconds. She is now 2 minutes old, and the heart rate via pulse oximeter is 55 bpm. She's limp and making no respiratory effort. What should be the next step in resuscitation?
   a. Reposition the airway
   b. Endotracheal intubation
   c. Continue PPV
   d. Begin chest compressions

9. Which of the following prenatal diagnoses would be a reason to withhold resuscitation measures?
       I. Trisomy 13
       II. Trisomy 21
       III. Anencephaly
       IV. 20 weeks' gestation
       V. 27 weeks' gestation
   a. II, III, IV
   b. I, III, IV
   c. I, II, III, IV
   d. I, II, IV

10. You are called to a full-term delivery and arrive after the baby is born. The delivery room nurse is providing stimulation and blow-by oxygen to the baby boy. At 1 minute, an alarm sounds to signify the need to evaluate the baby. The baby boy is moving actively, crying and grimacing, and has a bluish hue to his hands and feet, although his head and trunk are pink. You palpate the heart rate and count 12 beats in 6 seconds. Assign a 1-minute Apgar score to this infant.
   a. 10
   b. 9
   c. 8
   d. 7

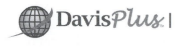 For additional resources login to Davis*Plus* (http://davisplus.fadavis.com/ keyword "Perretta") and click on the Premium tab. (Don't have a *Plus*Code to access Premium Resources? Just click the Purchase Access button on the book's Davis*Plus* page.)

REFERENCES

1. Martin JA, Hamilton BE, Ventura SJ, et al. Births: final data for 2010. *Natl Vital Stat Rep.* 2012;61(1). http://www.cdc.gov/nchs/data/nvsr/nvsr61/nvsr61_01.pdf - table01. Accessed November 20, 2012.
2. American Heart Association/American Academy of Pediatrics. *Textbook of Neonatal Resuscitation.* 6th ed. Dallas, TX: American Academy of Pediatrics; 2011.
3. Martin RJ, Fanaroff AA, Walsh MC. *Fanaroff and Martin's Neonatal-Perinatal Medicine: Diseases of the Fetus and Infant.* 9th ed. St. Louis, MO: Mosby; 2011.
4. McCrann JR, Schifrin BS. Fetal monitoring in high-risk pregnancy. *Clin Perinatol.* 1974;1(2):149, 229-252.
5. Boylan PC, Parisi VM, et al. Fetal acid base balance. In: Creasy RK, Reznik R, Iams J, eds. *Maternal-fetal Fetal Medicine.* Philadelphia, PA: Saunders; 1989.
6. Noori S, Stavroudis TA, Seri I. Systemic and cerebral hemodynamics during the transitional period after premature birth. *Clin Perinatol.* 2009;36(4):723-736.
7. Murphy AA, Halamek LP. Simulation-based training in neonatal resuscitation. *NeoReviews.* 2005;6(11):e489-e492.
8. Lawn JE, Cousens SN, Wilczynska K. *Estimating the Causes of Four Million Neonatal Deaths in the Year 2000: Statistical Annex—The World Health Report 2005.* Geneva, Switzerland: World Health Organization; 2005.
9. Darmstadt G, Zulfiqar AB, Cousens S, et al. Evidence-based, cost-effective interventions: how many newborn babies can we save? *Lancet* 2006;365(9463):977-988.
10. Kattwinkel J, Perlman JM, Aziz K, et al. 2010 American Heart Association guidelines for cardiopulmonary resuscitation and emergency cardiovascular care: neonatal resuscitation. *Circulation.* 2010;122(pt 15):S909-S919.
11. Thomas EJ, Sexton JB, Lasky RE, et al. Teamwork and quality during neonatal care in the delivery room. *J Perinatol.* 2006;26(3):163-169.
12. Gluckman PD, Wyatt JS, Azzopardi D, et al. Selective head cooling with mild systemic hypothermia after neonatal encephalopathy: multicentre randomised trial. *Lancet* 2005;365(9460):663-670.
13. Shankaran S, Laptook AR, Ehrekaraz RA, et al. Whole-body hypothermia for neonates with hypoxic-ischemic encephalopathy. *N Engl J Med.* 2005;353:1574-1584.
14. Azzopardi DV, Strohm B, Edwards AD, et al. Moderate hypothermia to treat perinatal asphyxia encephalopathy. *N Engl J Med.* 2009;361:1349-1358.
15. Gungor S, Kurt E, Teksoz E, et al. Oronasopharyngeal suction versus no suction in normal and term infants delivered by elective cesarean section: a prospective randomized controlled trial. *Gynecol Obstet Invest.* 2006;61(1):9-14.
16. Waltman PA, Brewer JM, Rogers BP, et al. Building evidence for practice: a pilot study of newborn bulb suctioning at birth. *J Midwifery Women's Health.* 2004;49(1):32-38.
17. Boon AW, Milner AD, Hopkin IE. Lung expansion, tidal exchange, and formation of the functional residual capacity during resuscitation of asphyxiated neonates. *J Pediatr.* 1979;95(6):1031-1036.
18. Vyas H, Milner AD, Hopkin IE, et al. Physiologic responses to prolonged and slow-rise inflation in the resuscitation of the asphyxiated newborn infant. *J Pediatr.* 1981;99(4):635-639.
19. Linder W, Vossbeck S, Hummler H, et al. Delivery room management of extremely low birth weight infants: spontaneous breathing or intubation? *Pediatrics.* 1999;103(5):961-967.
20. Wiswell TE, Gannon CM, Jacob J, et al. Delivery room management of the apparently vigorous meconium-stained neonate: results of the multicenter, international collaborative trial. *Pediatrics.* 2000;105(1 pt 1):1-7.
21. American Academy of Pediatrics, Committee on Fetus and Newborn, American College of Obstetricians and Gynecologists, Committee on Obstetric Practice. The Apgar score. *Pediatrics.* 2006;117(4):1444-1447.
22. Apgar V. A proposal for a new method of evaluation of the newborn infant. *Curr Res Anesth Analg.* 1953;32(4):260-267.

Chapter 4

Respiratory Distress Syndrome

Chapter Outline

Key Terms

Air-oxygen blender
Airway resistance
Analgesia
Assist-control (A/C) ventilation
Continuous positive airway
  pressure (CPAP)
Dead space ventilation
Gentle ventilation
Grunting
Heated, humidified, high-flow nasal
  cannula (HFNC)
High-frequency jet ventilation
  (HFJV)
High-frequency oscillatory
  ventilation (HFOV)
High-frequency ventilation
Hyaline membrane disease (HMD)
Hypoplasia
Intrapulmonary shunt
Incubator
Law of Laplace
Mean airway pressure (Paw)
Muscle relaxant
Noninvasive positive pressure
  ventilation (NIPPV)
Optimal peak end expiratory
  pressure (PEEP)
Oxygen hood
Patient-triggered ventilation
Poiseulle's law
Pressure control ventilation
Pressure support ventilation
Respiration
Respiratory distress syndrome (RDS)
Reticulogranular
See-saw breathing pattern

Key Terms cont.

Surfactant
Surfactant replacement therapy
Synchronized intermittent
  mandatory ventilation

Time-cycled, pressure-limited
  ventilation
Time-triggered breaths
Ventilation

Volume-control ventilation
Volume-targeted ventilation
Work of breathing (WOB)

Chapter Objectives

After reading this chapter, you will be able to:

1. Describe the pathological and clinical characteristics of neonatal respiratory distress syndrome (RDS).
2. Discuss how the chemical composition of surfactant improves lung compliance and its role in RDS.
3. List the changes to delivery room resuscitation that should be implemented for a very preterm infant.
4. Select initial respiratory support for a very preterm infant suspected of having RDS.
5. Assess the pulmonary status of a patient with worsening RDS and recommend changes in respiratory support.
6. Explain the role of surfactant replacement therapy in improving pulmonary function during RDS.
7. Determine when it is appropriate to initiate noninvasive versus invasive positive-pressure ventilation.
8. Describe the rationale for using synchronized and volume-targeted ventilation for patients with RDS.
9. Evaluate blood gas results for a neonate with RDS who is receiving mechanical ventilation (MV) and suggest changes to current ventilator settings.
10. Explain the benefits of high-frequency ventilation over conventional MV and recommend initial settings for high-frequency oscillatory or high-frequency jet ventilation (HFJV).

■■ Baby Girl (BG) Gibbs

You are working the evening shift in a 24-bed level IIIB neonatal intensive care unit (NICU). You are notified of a 25 2/7 weeks' gestation (wG) infant that is going to be delivered during your shift. Susan Gibbs, a 32-year-old woman, was admitted to the labor and delivery unit 4 days ago in premature labor. The neonatologist and NICU RN ask you to come with them to prepare the delivery room. You give a hand-off of your patients to your coworker and go to the delivery room to prepare for the baby's arrival.

In the United States in 2011, 1 in 8 babies (about 13%) were born prematurely. This rate has been on the rise, with a 6% increase from previous years (1). As many as 49% of NICU admissions are for prematurity and thus constitute a large portion of the intensive care population (1, 2). Care for premature infants first began in the 1880s in France, with the invention of an incubator to care for sick premature infants. It was designed by Alexandre Lion to keep the babies warm, similar to devices used to keep eggs warm until they hatched. In 1896, Martin Couney displayed actual premature babies at the Berlin World's Fair. It was a very popular attraction, but audiences didn't know what to make of it; at that time, society saw infant mortality as inevitable, and no resources were being put into pediatric medicine. The incubators became popular at

American fairs and carnivals, and a permanent exhibit was established at Coney Island in New York, which charged an entrance fee for vacationers to view the premature babies (3).

In 1898, Couney's incubator was used at the Chicago Lying-In Hospital, and in 1914 the first unit for premature babies was opened by Julius Hess at the Sarah Morris Hospital in Chicago. It incorporated incubators to regulate temperature, supplemental oxygen, and special feeding techniques to improve survival of newborns several weeks premature. Infant mortality dropped significantly, partly as a result of the improved medical care given to newborns. In the 1940s, doctors began to see a pattern of breathing difficulties in tinier, more premature babies, as they would struggle and gasp for breath, expending all their energy. They would eventually tire, stop breathing, and die. In the 1960s, the first trials of mechanical ventilation (MV) began to help these premature babies who had the characteristic "respiratory distress syndrome." In 1963, First Lady Jacqueline Kennedy gave birth to a premature baby boy. He was given high concentrations of oxygen that were not successful, and he died within hours of birth. This highly publicized premature death highlighted the need for more research for diseases of premature babies. Concurrently, in the mid-1960s, the March of Dimes changed its focus from polio to premature births, paving the way for rapid and significant advances in neonatal medicine and improved survivability of premature babies (3).

For nearly 40% of premature births, the cause is unknown; however, researchers have made some progress in learning the causes of prematurity. Reviews of the epidemiology of preterm birth have identified consistent associations with maternal and social adversity; multiple gestation; assisted conception; structural abnormalities of the uterus and cervix; serious medical, surgical, or gynecological conditions in the mother; stressful life events; "perceived" stress; poor psychological health; lack of family/social support; and tobacco and cocaine use (4, 5). Many of the known risk factors are rare, and others are difficult to modify. Studies suggest that there may be four main physiological causes that lead to spontaneous premature labor:

- **Infections/inflammation.** Studies suggest that premature labor is often triggered by the body's natural immune response to certain bacterial infections, such as those involving the genital and urinary tracts and fetal membranes. Even infections far away from the reproductive organs, such as periodontal disease, may contribute to premature delivery.
- **Maternal or fetal stress.** Chronic psychosocial stress in the mother or physical stress (such as insufficient blood flow from the placenta) in the fetus appears to result in production of a stress-related hormone called corticotropin-releasing hormone (CRH). CRH may stimulate production of a cascade of other hormones that trigger uterine contractions and premature delivery.
- **Bleeding.** The uterus may bleed because of problems such as placental abruption, in which the placenta peels away, partially or almost completely, from the uterine wall before delivery. Bleeding triggers the release of various proteins involved in blood clotting, which also appear to stimulate uterine contractions.
- **Stretching.** The uterus may become overstretched by the presence of two or more babies, excessive amounts of amniotic fluid, or uterine or placental abnormalities, leading to the release of chemicals that stimulate uterine contractions (6).

Delivery prior to 23 wG is considered too premature, and available data indicate that survival of appropriate-for-age infants less than 23 wG and less than 500 g birth weight is extremely unlikely, with virtually no chance for intact survival. This is mostly due to the extreme underdevelopment of the pulmonary and cerebral systems. In contrast, however, are preterm neonates born at 25 wG or more and 600 g or more, who have a survival rate of over 60% to 70%; as many as 50% or more of the survivors have no evidence of severe neurological disability (7). These statistics have allowed clinicians to provide better palliative care and delivery room decisions prior to presentation of a premature newborn and initiation of care (Teamwork 4-1).

Premature infants spend a significant amount of time in intensive care prior to their discharge home. The average length of stay for a newborn in the NICU is 13.2 days, with that number increasing to 46.2 days for infants less than 34 wG (9). The major complications of being born prematurely include brain injury, lung disease, and neurodevelopmental disorders caused by inadequate growth of the lungs and brain before delivery. One of the major roles that respiratory therapists (RTs) play in neonatal respiratory care is the management of premature infants. With the advent of advanced respiratory care techniques, survival has improved, particularly for very premature infants, who constitute 1.97% of live births (Box 4-1). The RT is responsible for managing acute severe illnesses such as respiratory distress syndrome (RDS), pneumonia, and air leaks (discussed in Chapter 7), as well as patients with acute complications that cause respiratory compromise, such as necrotizing enterocolitis (NEC) and intraventricular hemorrhage (IVH) (discussed in Chapter 8). RTs are also responsible for managing chronic respiratory illnesses, such as bronchopulmonary dysplasia (BPD) and apnea of prematurity (AOP).

Hyaline Membrane Disease/Respiratory Distress Syndrome

Respiratory distress syndrome (RDS) of the newborn is the leading cause of death in premature infants (11). It is characterized by severe impairment of respiratory function, which is caused by immaturity of the lungs, primarily due to lack of surfactant. The defining features of the pulmonary system during RDS include a decrease in surfactant production which causes low alveolar compliance; an overly compliant chest wall, which causes difficulty in improving ventilation; increased distance between alveolar spaces and capillaries, which worsens gas exchange; and lung tissue underdevelopment **(hypoplasia)** (Fig. 4-1). It was first characterized in the early 20th century as **hyaline membrane disease (HMD)** because of the unique cellular characteristics of the lung, but it was thought to be a rare form of pneumonia afflicting the premature infant and "causing a failure of the lungs to inflate normally" (12).

The incidence of RDS is as high as 60% for very preterm babies (9), but the likelihood of occurrence is inversely proportional to gestational age; that is, the closer to term a newborn is, the less likely the baby is to have RDS. Young gestational age and very low birth weight (VLBW) or extremely low birth weight (ELBW)—1,001 to 1,500 g and 500 to 1,000 g, respectively— are the biggest risk factors for RDS. Additional risk factors are listed in Box 4-2. Because of advancements in neonatal critical care medicine

Teamwork 4-1 Family-Centered Decision-Making in the Delivery Room (8)

When an infant is about to be born extremely prematurely, it can be difficult for physicians to predict for parents whether the infant will survive intact, with severe disability, or die soon after delivery. Because of this uncertainty, several management options are considered medically, ethically, and legally reasonable in the delivery room. These can range from aggressive resuscitation to compassionate care only. The American Academy of Pediatrics emphasizes the importance of including parents in decision-making. Time pressures, medical urgency, and lack of relationships between physicians and parents in these scenarios preclude comprehensive conversations, requiring physicians to prioritize what essential information to relay and to seek from parents.

Though there is a significant amount of objective data to help predict morbidity and death, parents have expressed that their decisions regarding delivery room resuscitation were not influenced by providers' grim predictions of death or disability. In contrast, parents' decisions were influenced by religion, spirituality, and hope. Regardless of the medical information, parents maintained hope that everything would be fine and were encouraged by friends and family members to pray for miracles or to trust that a miracle would happen despite the physicians' predictions.

Parents' own sense of the possibility of survival was nearly uniformly positive. Parents also described the reasons for not putting more stock in the physician's predictions as having difficulty understanding the information, feeling emotionally overwhelmed, and being preoccupied with enduring their own medical crises.

This emotional distress, cognitive difficulty with survivability predictions, and positive outlook from the parents are particularly important for RTs to acknowledge. Parents are active participants in the resuscitation process and the resultant ICU care, and it is easy to get frustrated with them for making the "wrong decision" regarding neonatal resuscitation. There is nothing inherently wrong with families having hope for a positive outcome or allowing their spirituality to help guide their decision-making, particularly when decisions need to be made quickly and there is a large degree of uncertainty regarding postnatal outcomes. Physicians often let family members know that having a plan is good, but revisiting a plan and changing it when new information presents itself is a valuable strategy. It may be useful to remember this prior to beginning resuscitation of a neonate at the threshold of viability and to acknowledge the emotional ties the family has to the work you are doing.

Box 4-1 Categories of Prematurity (1, 10)

- Late preterm: 34 0/7 to 36 6/7 wG
- Moderate preterm: 32 to 36 wG
- Very (extremely) preterm: less than 32 wG

in the 1980s and 1990s, the incidence of RDS and mortality has diminished significantly. Its incidence for infants less than 30 wG is 60%, but it decreases to 35% when corticosteroids are administered to the mother prior to delivery (13). Mortality dropped 14-fold between 1970 and 2007 (15), despite an

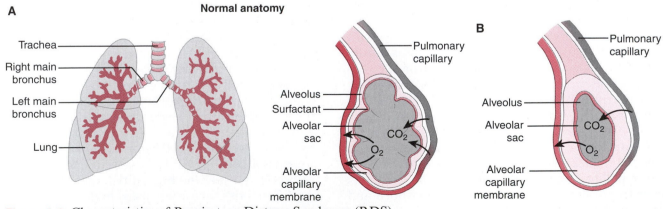

Figure 4-1 Characteristics of Respiratory Distress Syndrome (RDS)

<table>
<tr><td>

Box 4-2 Risk Factors for Developing RDS (13,14)

- Gestational age less than 37 weeks
- Maternal diabetes
- Multiple births
- Second twin
- Cesarean section with no prior labor
- Perinatal asphyxia
- Infants whose mothers have previously had RDS
- Male sex
- Chorioamnionitis
- Hydrops fetalis

</td></tr>
</table>

increase in preterm birth rates. The severity of the disease has also been restricted to the very preterm and ELBW babies, with an incidence as high as 74% for infants 501 g to 1,000 g (16, 17).

RDS does not, however, affect sex and races equally. It affects males more often than females, though the exact physiological cause is not yet understood. In one study, the incidence of RDS was more than three times higher in boys than in girls, and this is particularly noticeable at later gestational ages and at heavier weights (18). Black fetuses develop surfactant more rapidly than do white fetuses and thus historically have had a lower incidence of RDS (19).

Patients with RDS require extensive care from RTs, focusing on early establishment of functional residual capacity (FRC) using continuous positive airway pressure (CPAP), early surfactant delivery, appropriate ventilatory support with avoidance of volutrauma or atelectrauma, oxygen delivery to maintain adequate partial pressure of oxygen (PaO_2), and discontinuation of respiratory support as soon as possible to avoid long-term complications. Close monitoring and assessment, frequent changes in respiratory settings or modalities, and careful attention to changes in clinical presentation all contribute to improved outcomes for premature infants with RDS.

Pathophysiology

The primary cause of respiratory distress is underdevelopment of the lung. The biggest causative factor is surfactant deficiency, but it is compounded by other problems that result from lung hypoplasia, including decreased surface area for gas exchange, thick alveolar-capillary (A-C) membrane, and underdeveloped (and thus insufficient) vascularization. Neonates with RDS also have an increased likelihood for pulmonary edema. The mechanics of the thoracic cavity also cause problems, such as an overly compliant chest wall and decreased intrathoracic pressure. The end result is a very-low-compliance lung with normal airway resistance and poor maintenance of FRC.

When RDS was first being characterized in the early 20th century, it was known as HMD because of a unique lining, known as the hyaline membrane, found in the airway of these newborns upon postmortem examination. The hyaline membrane was characterized as an "eosinophilic layer of structureless, homogeneous material" in the bronchioles, alveolar ducts, and alveoli (20). The lungs were also abnormal, described in the 1950s as having the following characteristics:

- Dull red instead of pink
- Consistency of liver
- Congested and edematous
- Little evidence of aeration
- Engorged alveolar capillaries
- Most of the parenchyma collapsed
- Overdistended alveolar ducts and respiratory bronchioles

With the advent of advanced respiratory technologies such as CPAP, exogenous surfactant, and prenatal corticosteroid delivery, developed countries no longer see the pathological hyaline membranes. However, it is important to remember this resulting pathology because it reflects lung characteristics without necessary interventions.

Surfactant Deficiency

Surfactant is a chemically complex agent whose main function is to stabilize the air-liquid interface of the alveoli and bronchioles and to lower surface tension. Lower alveolar surface tension improves lung compliance, thereby decreasing work of breathing (WOB). Surfactant molecules are made and excreted by alveolar type II cells, which appear in fetal development during the canalicular phase (gestation weeks 17 to 26). Surfactant serves to ease the alveoli's ability to stretch during inspiration and prevents alveolar collapse and eventual atelectasis during exhalation or compression of the alveoli. Mature pulmonary surfactant is made of 90% lipids (mostly phospholipids) and 10% glycoproteins (Fig. 4-2).

There are many types of lipids, but surfactant is made mostly of phospholipids. They serve to interact with air in the alveolar space, helping to reduce the surface tension of the lungs upon compression or exhalation. The main phospholipids in the surfactant are phosphatidylcholine (PC), which makes up about 80% of lipids, and phosphatidylglycerol (PG), which makes up between 8% and 15% of the lipids (21, 22). Immature surfactant, found in the alveoli beginning at approximately 24 wG, lacks PG, and therefore is less structurally stable and is inhibited by hypoxia,

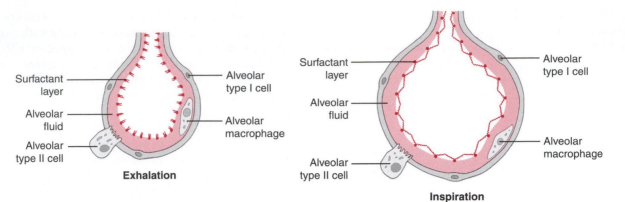

Figure 4-2 Chemical Composition of Surfactant

hyperthermia, and acidosis. Neonates born between 24 wG and 35 wG are very susceptible to surfactant deficiency, causing high surface tension and leading to increased WOB, respiratory distress, atelectasis, and pulmonary injury. PG appears at about 35 wG during the saccular phase of lung growth, and surfactant is then much more stable.

There are four surfactant proteins (SP)—A, B, C, and D—found in surfactant. They are mainly involved in promoting adsorption and the stabilization and respreading of surface film to decrease surface tension. Proteins make up about 6% to 8% of the total weight of surfactant (23).

- Surfactant proteins SP-A and SP-D are round, hydrophilic, and interface with the fluid portion of the alveolar membrane. Protein A is the major protein in surfactant, but both are associated with the body's host defense mechanisms; assist in clearing bronchioles and alveoli of inhaled pollution; and bind to pathogens such as bacteria, viruses, and fungi to assist with phagocytosis. These proteins also help prevent fluid from entering the alveolar space and help maintain the sterile conditions of the respiratory surface. Without these proteins, the lungs are highly susceptible to infection and pulmonary edema.
- Surfactant proteins SP-B and SP-C are very small hydrophobic proteins that are found in much smaller numbers in surfactant, but they play critical roles in the formation and stabilization of pulmonary surfactant films.

Surfactant is sensitive and is susceptible to inactivation by foreign bodies or changes in the content of the air-alveolar capillary interface. Box 4-3 lists the agents that can cause surfactant inactivation or dysfunction. Researchers have found that the most critical components for functional surfactant are the phospholipid DPPC (dipalmitoylphosphatidylcholine) and proteins SP-B and SP-C (23). DPPC

is the most commonly occurring type of PC phospholipid, comprising about 50% of the PC phospholipids. Both proteins enhance surface activity, in particular initial film formation and re-extension, which are important for proper dynamic behavior during the breathing cycle. Patients without these components are more susceptible to atelectasis, pneumonia, volutrauma from MV, and death.

Lung Hypoplasia

The gestational age of a newborn at birth significantly impacts how developed the lungs are and the potential for respiratory distress. Each stage of fetal pulmonary development is discussed in detail in Chapter 2. About 23 wG is the current agreed limit of viability (7), and a description of lung development after this stage is warranted to understand the potential for respiratory dysfunction:

- **24 to 28 wG:** Division of intrasegmental airways is fastest between weeks 10 and 24, by which time about 70% of the airway generations present at birth have formed (25). Gas exchange isn't possible until the capillary network and alveoli have a sufficient surface area and

---

Box 4-3 Agents Inhibiting Surfactant Function (24)

- Cholesterol
- Bilirubin
- Amniotic fluid
- Meconium
- Elastin
- Fibrin monomers
- Immunoglobulins
- Hemoglobin
- RBC membrane lipids
- Plasma/serum
- Albumin

until the two are close enough to each other to allow oxygen and carbon dioxide to cross the A-C membrane. Both occur around at 22 to 24 wG. Respiratory bronchioles contain no cartilage and therefore are sensitive to airway collapse in premature infants.

- **28 to 34 wG:** True alveoli begin to appear at about 30 weeks in the airways distal to the terminal bronchioles, forming short, shallow sacs known as saccules. Each saccule is made up of type I and type II cells and functions as an A-C membrane, but it is structurally simple compared with an alveolar sac. Saccules are close to one another, making the space between them, called the "septa," twice as thick as an alveolar wall. The elastic fibers that constitute the walls are also small. These, in combination with immature surfactant, can increase WOB in neonates born prematurely. The saccules themselves also have a much lower surface area for gas exchange when compared with alveolar sacs, which decreases the capacity for gas exchange.
- **34 to 40 wG:** At about week 35, mature surfactant begins to appear. A neonate born at this point is at minimal risk for pulmonary complications at birth caused by lung immaturity. Around week 36, alveoli begin quickly proliferating, growing in number daily to the millions by 40 wG.

Despite our ability to intubate and mechanically ventilate patients who may not be physiologically prepared to breathe independently, there is a critical difference between **ventilation** (the transport of gas in and out of the lungs) and **respiration** (the diffusion of oxygen [O_2] and elimination of carbon dioxide [CO_2] through the A-C membrane). The decreased surface area of the lungs and the increased distance between the alveoli and their associated capillaries during alveolar development (known as increased A-C membrane) make premature lungs much less efficient at respiration.

Local ventilation and capillary perfusion may not always be efficient, either. Known as ventilation/perfusion (V/Q) mismatch, it describes times when the distribution of ventilation throughout the lung and perfusion to the capillaries are not in synch. This is caused by either dead space ventilation or intrapulmonary shunt.

Dead Space Ventilation

Dead space ventilation occurs in an area of the lung that is being ventilated but not perfused. It can have many causes, but in infants with RDS it is frequently caused by insufficient vascularization, alveolar hyperinflation, or decreased cardiac output. Insufficient vascularization can occur when there is still an increased A-C membrane during extreme prematurity. This decreases available perfusion areas and, although ventilation can occur, O_2 and CO_2 are not exchanged. Alveoli that are over-inflated can directly compress their own capillary bed or those of neighboring alveolar units, decreasing local perfusion. Decreased cardiac output diminishes the amount of blood flow to the entire pulmonary system, causing relative dead space ventilation throughout. Pulmonary hypertension in infants with RDS is also a cause of V/Q mismatching in the first few days of life (26).

Intrapulmonary Shunt

An **intrapulmonary shunt** is perfusion without ventilation. Alveolar tissue underdevelopment, atelectasis, and pulmonary edema are common causes of shunt in patients with RDS and can occur regionally or globally in the lung, which significantly impact gas exchange.

Thoracic Mechanics and WOB

Each breath during RDS requires significant energy, and if this burden outstrips an infant's ability to overcome the mechanics of breathing, then progressive respiratory failure will be the result. **Work of breathing (WOB)** is the force generated by a patient to overcome the frictional resistance and static elastic forces that oppose lung expansion (27). Some characteristics of the chest wall in neonates also make them particularly susceptible to signs and symptoms of respiratory distress, as well as making them less able to overcome atelectasis and airway instability. These characteristics include a premature infant's overly compliant chest wall and lower than normal intrathoracic pressure. Surfactant deficiency was discussed above, and its effect of lowering lung compliance is an important component of distress.

Overly Compliant Chest Wall

When children and adults have areas of atelectasis, creating a large negative inspiration will assist them in opening poorly compliant alveoli. This mechanism is not effective for premature infants. Their overly compliant and unstable thoracic cavity will cause retraction and deformation of the chest wall, described clinically as retractions, instead of inflation of poorly compliant alveoli. Instability of the thoracic cage makes it difficult to increase minute ventilation (V_E) by increasing thoracic volume. Infants must drop the diaphragm more to increase tidal volume (V_T), which increases WOB. To avoid increased WOB, infants usually increase respiratory rate to increase V_E. This is not effective when the alveoli are collapsed because it may not improve alveolar gas exchange.

Decreased Intrathoracic Pressure

Infants with RDS must generate high negative intrapleural pressures to expand and stabilize their distal airways and alveoli. Neonates less than 30 wG are often unable to generate the high intrathoracic pressures necessary to inflate surfactant-deficient lungs (28). Any positive effect they may have in increasing lung volume with their high opening pressures is rapidly lost as the lung collapses to its original resting volume during expiration.

Oxygen Consumption

As described in Chapter 1, resting oxygen consumption for infants and children is twice that of adults. The average relative increase in energy expenditure, and thus oxygen consumption, with acute neonatal lung disease has been reported to be 36% (29). The diseased lung can be thought of as a metabolically hyperactive organ with increased oxygen consumption, which further increases WOB and worsens respiratory distress.

Clinical Manifestations

Clinical manifestations for RDS can be found prenatally as well as immediately after delivery. Prior to delivery, clinical manifestations of RDS are mainly found by assessing fetal lung maturity (FLM). Current recommendations from the American College of Obstetricians and Gynecologists recommend amniotic fluid testing for FLM between 34 and 39 wG (30), a time when the safety of delivery and maturity of the lung are less certain. Prior to 32 wG, most test results will indicate immaturity, but at 39 weeks the fetus is considered full term; thus, the risk of RDS is very low.

Descriptions of the tests for FLM can be found in Chapter 2. Results that support a diagnosis of RDS are as follows:

- Lung profile test, consisting of
  - Lecithin-sphingomyelin (L/S) ratio of 2:1
  - PG presence absent or negative
- Shake test negative
- Surfactant-albumin (S/A) ratio (TDx fetal lung maturity test or FP test) less than 40 mg surfactant per 1 g albumin

As the name describes, clinical features of RDS are related to severity of respiratory distress. Respiratory distress is nonspecific, meaning it includes many clinical symptoms that can be associated with many neonatal disorders. However, any preterm newborn displaying these symptoms should be considered highly suspect for having RDS:

- Abnormal breathing patterns, such as tachypnea or apnea
- Substernal and/or intercostal retractions

- Nasal flaring
- **Grunting** (the noise produced by breathing against a partially closed glottis, occurring during each exhalation)
- **See-saw breathing pattern**, in which the stomach and chest are moving out of synch with each other during breathing attempts
- Hypoxemia, usually monitored by pulse oximetry
- Cyanosis
- Hypercarbia
- Respiratory acidosis
- Atelectasis

Respiratory scoring systems are an objective way to assess respiratory distress. The Silverman-Andersen Scoring System was designed in 1956 as an objective means to quantify respiratory distress in premature infants (Fig. 4-3) (31). It allows clinicians to monitor distress over time and help guides decision-making.

Definitive diagnosis of RDS is made by chest radiograph, which will show a characteristic uniform **reticulogranular** pattern (network of rough, grainy-appearing lung tissue) and peripheral air bronchograms. Surfactant deficiency results in widespread alveolar collapse, which produces low lung volumes and generalized granular or reticular opacities, obscuring normal blood vessels (32). The abnormal lung opacity is also due to leaking of fluid from capillaries into the interstitium. The typical chest radiograph of a patient with RDS prior to MV is often described as a "ground glass appearance" because of the homogenous nature of the disease (Fig. 4-4). Once on MV, the central bronchi are usually distended by positive pressure because they are more compliant than surfactant-deficient alveoli. Clinicians will not see the classic pattern of radiographic evidence as frequently as in the past because treatment for patients at high risk for RDS begins in the delivery room before the first chest radiograph (CXR) is obtained.

The peak of symptoms for milder cases is normally seen in the first 12 to 72 hours of life, followed by gradual improvement of symptoms. Extremely premature infants may experience a "honeymoon" period within the first 72 hours, then progress to increased respiratory support.

Additional clinical symptoms of patients with RDS that can contribute to or compound respiratory distress may include low serum-glucose levels (hypoglycemia), low serum calcium levels (hypocalcemia), temperature instability, infection or sepsis, and temperature instability (see Table 4-1).

Management and Treatment

Without intervention, patients with RDS will lose lung volume, exhibit increased signs of respiratory distress, develop respiratory failure, and die. Since

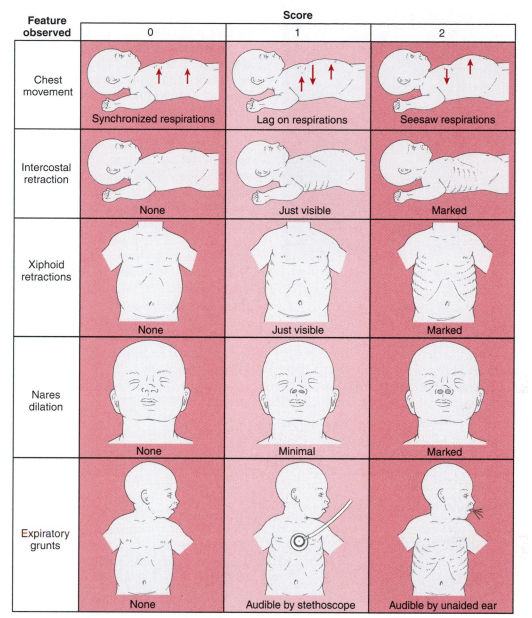

Feature observed	Score		
	0	1	2
Chest movement	Synchronized respirations	Lag on respirations	Seesaw respirations
Intercostal retraction	None	Just visible	Marked
Xiphoid retractions	None	Just visible	Marked
Nares dilation	None	Minimal	Marked
Expiratory grunts	None	Audible by stethoscope	Audible by unaided ear

Figure 4-3 Silverman-Andersen Scoring System

RDS was first studied and treated with oxygen in the 1950s, survival rates for the disease have improved, and its prevention has been particularly successful. Treatment begins from the moment labor starts until discharge from the NICU and focuses on surfactant replacement, establishing FRC, and supporting ventilation and oxygenation as necessary.

Prevention of RDS

The single best way to prevent RDS is to prevent preterm delivery. Preterm birth is a major public health problem worldwide, occurring in 6% to 10% of births in developed countries (33). The proportion of pregnancies that end prematurely, between 20 and 36 weeks, has not fallen in recent years. A successful plan to reduce the incidence of preterm birth would require first identifying which pregnant mothers are at high risk of delivering prematurely, then preventing preterm labor for these mothers, and if that fails, providing pharmacological therapies to increase lung maturation prior to delivery.

The ability to identify women whose pregnancies are at higher-than-average risk of preterm birth would allow clinicians to provide these women with a higher level of antenatal care, with the aim of preventing the preterm birth. Even though it is relatively easy to look retrospectively for common factors in women who delivered prematurely, there is not yet a useful and consistent scoring system to identify a woman at high risk for a preterm delivery. The risk

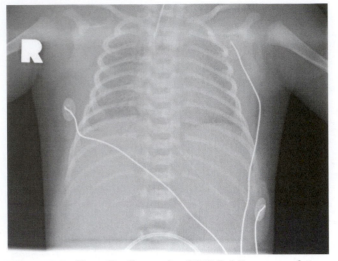

Figure 4-4 Chest Radiograph of RDS *(Courtesy of Jane Benson)*

factor found to be the most significant in predicting preterm birth is history of a previous preterm birth, which increases a woman's risk to 22.5% (34). Other prenatal considerations in the mother that have been consistently found to increase the risk for preterm delivery include the following:

- Consistent associations with material and social adversity
- Multiple gestation
- Assisted conception
- Structural abnormalities of the uterus and cervix
- Serious medical, surgical, or gynecological conditions
- Stressful life events
- Perceived stress
- Poor psychological health
- Lack of family or social support
- Tobacco and/or cocaine use (35)

Many of these risk factors are rare, and others are difficult to modify. It is also not certain that, just because a mother meets any of these criteria, she will deliver prematurely.

A number of strategies are used in an attempt to delay preterm birth. These include bedrest, drugs to dampen the contractions (tocolytics), insertion of a suture around the cervix to prevent it from opening (cervical suture), and antibiotics. The first two will be discussed below.

Bedrest, either at home or in the hospital, is considered a first line of defense to stop preterm contractions. This is based on the observation that hard work and hard physical activity during pregnancy could be associated with preterm birth and that bedrest could reduce uterine activity. Although bedrest in the hospital or at home is widely used as the first step of treatment, there is no evidence that this practice is beneficial. There are also potential adverse effects of bedrest on women and their families, such as an increased risk of venous thrombosis, muscle atrophy, maternal weight loss, stress for women and their families, and increasing costs to families and the health-care system. It has been suggested as recently as 2010 that clinicians should not routinely advise women to rest in bed to prevent preterm birth (36).

Drugs used to stop preterm labor are known as "tocolytics" (37). They include calcium channel blockers such as nifedipine (38), betamimetics such as terbutaline (39, 40), magnesium sulfate (41), and oxytocin receptor antagonists (37).

For those women with preterm labor who are treated with tocolytics and remain undelivered after 48 hours, maintenance treatment with a tocolytic is sometimes used to further delay delivery and to prolong pregnancy. Maintenance treatment regimens of differing duration and using a number of different tocolytics have been proposed; these include terbutaline, magnesium sulfate, calcium channel blockers, and progesterone. Studies to this point are not clear on the effectiveness of any of these interventions (38, 40–42), though progesterone seems to show promise at preventing delivery until close to 37 wG (43).

Table 4-1	Factors in Premature Infants That Can Increase Severity of Respiratory Distress (14)	
Clinical Symptom	**Cause in Premature Infants**	**How It Contributes to Worsened Respiratory Distress**
Hypoglycemia	Inability to manage own glucose levels; may be abnormal due to diabetic mother	Tachypnea and respiratory distress
Hypocalcemia	Common in sick, nonfed, preterm, or asphyxiated infants	Can contribute to tachypnea and other signs of respiratory distress
Infection/sepsis	Decreased effectiveness of immune system	Tachypnea or apnea; fever increases caloric needs
Hypothermia	Less brown fat to contain heat	Tachypnea or apnea

Corticosteroids

Antenatal corticosteroid therapy has become the mainstay of prophylactic RDS treatment and should be considered routine for preterm birth when it can be given at least 24 hours and no more than 7 days prior to delivery. In 1972, Liggins and Howie performed the first randomized controlled trial in humans of betamethasone for the prevention of RDS (44). Their hypothesis was that corticosteroids act to trigger the early synthesis of phospholipids, which will speed up surfactant development. This treatment has resulted in fewer neonatal deaths, as well as decreases in IVH (45) and NEC (46). There appear to be no negative effects of the corticosteroid on the mother. The evidence from a 2010 Cochrane review supports the continued use of a single course of antenatal corticosteroids to accelerate fetal lung maturation in women at risk of preterm birth. Reviews of the literature show that a repeat dose of prenatal corticosteroids given to women who remain at risk of an early birth helps the baby's lungs and reduces serious health problems in the first few weeks of life (47).

There are different types of corticosteroids, and they can be given in different ways and in different doses. There is currently no clear or agreed-upon best type or dose, and as a result, hospitals may vary in how they give them. The two most commonly used corticosteroids before early birth are dexamethasone and betamethasone, and in comparative trials they exhibit similar results (48).

Box 4-4 Factors That Put Preterm Babies at Risk After Delivery

- Immature tissue that is more susceptible to oxygen toxicity
- Weak thoracic musculature, which may cause ineffective breaths to be taken
- An immature nervous system, which may not provide enough stimulation to breathe
- Surfactant-deficient lungs, which make ventilation difficult and more likely to be injured by PPV
- More susceptibility to rapidly losing body heat owing to thin skin, a large surface area related to body mass, and decreased fat
- Immature immune systems, which increase the risk of infection
- Fragile capillaries within the brain, which are at higher risk for rupture and bleeding
- Small blood volume, which makes neonates more susceptible to hypovolemic effects of blood loss

---

Delivery Room Management

Care to preserve lung function and minimize pulmonary damage begins at the moment of birth. The delivery room team needs to be prepared to promptly resuscitate a preterm newborn, being mindful that all interventions involve risk. As discussed in Chapter 3, babies born preterm are at risk for a variety of complications following birth. Some are a direct result of anatomical and physiological immaturity, whereas others are a result of the cause of premature delivery. Specific issues of prematurity related to the pulmonary system are listed in Box 4-4.

The American Academy of Pediatrics recommends additional resources be present and interventions made during the resuscitation of a preterm newborn. These include the following (summarized in Box 4-5):

- Additional trained personnel should be available. There should be enough people present at the birth to perform a complex resuscitation, including someone skilled in endotracheal intubation and emergency umbilical venous catheterization (49).
- To minimize heat loss, the temperature in the delivery room should be increased to 25° to 26°C (77° to 79°F). The radiant warmer should be well preheated, and a chemically activated warming pad should also be made

---

Box 4-5 Delivery Room Intervention Considerations for Preterm Infants

- Adding trained personnel prepared to perform a complex resuscitation
- Increasing the temperature in the delivery room to 77° to 79°F
- Using a chemically activated warming pad and prewarmed radiant warmer
- Immediately placing the newborn in a reclosable, food-grade polyethylene bag
- Using a transport incubator when moving the newborn to the special care nursery
- Providing oxygen using an air-oxygen blender
- Using pulse oximetry to adjust oxygen delivery and ventilation
- Providing noninvasive CPAP at 4 to 6 cm H_2O
- Initiating PPV at 20 to 25 cm H_2O and increasing cautiously if no positive response is seen (avoiding excessive positive pressures)
- Once intubated, providing PEEP at 2 to 5 cm H_2O
- Giving surfactant early
- Handling the baby gently
- Avoiding Trendelenburg placement
- Avoiding rapid infusion of fluid

ready. Infants less than 29 wG should be immediately placed in a reclosable food-grade polyethylene bag rather than dried with towels because they are more susceptible to the effects of evaporative heat loss (50). A transport incubator should be used to maintain the newborn's temperature during the move to the nursery after resuscitation.

- An air-oxygen blender and pulse oximeter should be available for all preterm births. There is a large body of evidence showing that blood oxygen levels in uncompromised babies generally do not reach extrauterine values until approximately 10 minutes after birth. Oxyhemoglobin saturation may normally remain in the 70% to 80% range for several minutes following birth, thus resulting in the appearance of cyanosis during that time. Other studies have shown that clinical assessment of skin color is a very poor indicator of oxyhemoglobin saturation during the immediate neonatal period and that lack of cyanosis appears to be a very poor indicator of the state of oxygenation of uncompromised babies following birth (51). Until more information is available on appropriate saturation levels for preterm infants immediately after birth, clinicians should continue to follow the recommended SpO_2 levels for term babies, as described in Chapter 3 and listed in Table 4-2. Pulse oximetry and use of an air-oxygen blender to more accurately treat hypoxemia are particularly critical for infants born less than 32 wG.
- After birth, if a preterm baby is breathing spontaneously and has a heart rate (HR) greater than 100 bpm, allow the baby to progress through the first few minutes of life without additional assistance. Consider the following interventions:
  - Provide CPAP if respirations and HR are adequate, but the baby still has labored respirations, cyanosis, or a low SpO_2. CPAP will

provide alveolar stability and increase FRC for babies with a surfactant deficiency. In the delivery room, this is achieved by using a mask or nasal prongs connected to a flow-inflating resuscitation bag or a T-piece resuscitator held tightly to the baby's face or nose. A self-inflating bag cannot be used to deliver noninvasive CPAP. A CPAP setting of 4 to 6 cm H_2O is a safe and adequate amount of pressure in the delivery room until additional information about lung function is available. Several studies have shown that using CPAP in the delivery room for extremely premature infants, rather than prophylactic intubation and MV, can reduce the length of time on MV and decrease the incidence of lung injury.

- Positive-pressure ventilation (PPV) will be needed if spontaneous respiration and CPAP can't provide adequate oxygenation. Use the lowest inflation pressure necessary to achieve a positive response (HR greater than 100 bpm and improving SpO_2). Generally speaking, 20 to 25 cm H_2O is an adequate peak airway pressure for a premature infant, but clinicians may need to increase the pressure cautiously if improvement is not observed.
- If intubated, provide positive end expiratory pressure (PEEP) at 2 to 5 cm H_2O.
- Consider giving surfactant in the delivery room if the baby is significantly premature (less than 30 wG). Studies have shown that earlier delivery of surfactant is better, even if a baby is exhibiting no signs of respiratory distress (52, 53). However, indications for and timing of surfactant administration remain controversial (49).
- Prior to 32 wG, a portion of the brain called the germinal matrix has within it a fragile network of capillaries that are prone to rupture and bleeding (see Chapter 8 for more information). Physiological events that can cause rupture include rapid changes in $PaCO_2$, blood pressure, or blood volume. Inadequate blood flow to the brain can cause damage to its white matter, resulting in cerebral palsy. Measures that can be taken in the delivery room to minimize the risk of this type of brain injury include the following:
  - Handling the baby gently
  - Avoiding Trendelenburg (head down) placement
  - Avoiding delivering excessive positive pressure during manual ventilation or CPAP
  - Using pulse oximetry and blood gas values when available to adjust ventilation and oxygenation gradually and appropriately
  - Avoiding rapid infusions of fluid

Table 4-2	Pulse Oximetry Level Recommendations Based on Age in Minutes (49)
Time After Birth	**SpO_2**
1 minute	60% to 65%
2 minutes	65% to 70%
3 minutes	70% to 75%
4 minutes	75% to 80%
5 minutes	80% to 85%
10 minutes	85% to 95%

■ ■ On the way to the delivery room, the neonatologist briefs you on the information she has regarding Susan's pregnancy. She has no fever or signs of infection and no significant bleeding or placental abnormalities. Initial treatment with terbutaline was successful at stopping contractions, and she has received three doses of corticosteroids. The father of the baby was deployed for active military duty 2 weeks ago, and she has admitted to having a hard time coping since his departure. The neonatologist discussed the potential outcomes for delivery of Susan's daughter at this early stage in development. She acknowledges the potential poor outcomes and would like to have a full resuscitation provided at delivery. If new information arises in the delivery room, she would like the neonatologist to share that information with her so she can adjust the care plan if necessary. The neonatologist recommends that Susan bring in a family member or close friend as support for her, and she agrees to have her sister with her at the delivery. Contractions began again 12 hours ago, and Susan progressed to full cervical dilation. Her rupture of membranes was 5 hours ago, and there are no confounding factors to indicate it will be a stressful delivery course. You and the team prepare the room: You increase the temperature of the delivery room, preheat the radiant warmer, and place a polyethylene bag at the foot of the mattress. You set up the T-piece resuscitator and turn the fractional concentration of inspired oxygen (FIO_2) on the air-oxygen blender to 0.21. Your hospital's protocol is to administer surfactant in the delivery room for all infants born less than 26 wG, so you warm the surfactant to body temperature and place it in the warmer in preparation for delivery.

Surfactant Replacement Therapy

One of the biggest successes in the treatment of RDS was the U.S. Food and Drug Administration (FDA) approval of the first formulas for surfactant-replacement therapy in 1991 (54). **Surfactant replacement therapy** involves the instillation of artificially derived surfactant directly into the lungs. Surfactant administration early in the course of RDS can rapidly improve lung compliance, FRC, and V_T and prevent lung injury that is otherwise characteristic of surfactant-deficient lungs.

The timing of surfactant replacement therapy has been a topic of much debate and research. In general, there are two main strategies for initiation of surfactant replacement:

- **Prophylactic:** This form of therapy occurs as soon as possible in a newborn at high risk for developing RDS. Frequently, this involves instillation of surfactant in the delivery room, within minutes of birth. This early treatment should help prevent iatrogenic lung injury and improve oxygenation and ventilation. Prophylactic therapy has been shown to decrease the need for MV and lower the incidence of air leak syndromes, BPD, and death (52, 53, 55, 56). The definition of "high risk" is not standardized, but the American Association for Respiratory Care (AARC) clinical practice guidelines suggest using a gestational age of less than 32 weeks or a birth weight less than 1,300 g (57).

- **Rescue:** Also described as "selective" surfactant replacement therapy, rescue surfactant replacement involves waiting to deliver surfactant until evidence of RDS is seen. Evidence includes a chest radiograph with characteristic RDS features, increased WOB, or increased oxygen requirements. Though studies in the early 2000s showed an improvement in patient mortality and morbidity with prophylactic therapy, the use of early CPAP combined with rescue therapy results in equal improvement in outcomes, and its use may be increasing (Evidence in Practice 4-1). The benefit of rescue therapy includes less time on MV, the potential to avoid intubation for some patients, and a reduction in costs as a result of providing therapy only to those patients who require it.

● **Evidence in Practice 4-1**

Surfactant Versus CPAP in the Delivery Room (58)

Research in the 2000s clearly showed an improvement in neonatal outcomes when intubation and early use of surfactant occur in the delivery room. In the late 2000s, research on the use of nasal continuous positive airway pressure (NCPAP) in the delivery room (with or without surfactant therapy) has shown patient outcomes similar to those of prophylactic surfactant therapy. Results of the patient-management strategy of early NCPAP and rescue surfactant appears to be equal to prophylactic surfactant treatment. More research is ongoing to determine exactly which management strategy offers the best lung protection, lowest morbidity, and lowest incidence of BPD:

- Prophylactic surfactant therapy in the delivery room
- Prophylactic surfactant therapy, then extubation to NCPAP
- NCPAP and rescue surfactant therapy

There are two types of exogenous surfactant (surfactant that originates outside the lungs). One is natural surfactant, which is obtained from animal lungs, usually bovine or porcine. Natural surfactant can be obtained from pulverized lung or from a lung lavage. Pulverizing the lung has the potential for destroying some of the surfactant proteins A, B, C, and D, which makes it less capable of protecting the alveoli from infection or fluid entry when compared with native surfactant. Lung lavage is a more gentle extraction technique, leaving more of these proteins intact to perform effectively at the A-C membrane. Surfactant can also be made synthetically and will have the physiological properties of surfactant without the proteins. The dosage for exogenous surfactant is manufacturer dependent and is described in Table 4-3.

Equipment necessary for surfactant replacement therapy includes (57) the following:

- A 5- to 10-mL syringe containing the entire surfactant dose, warmed to room temperature
- A catheter for delivery of surfactant, which can be either a sterile 5 French (Fr) size feeding tube or a specially designed catheter for surfactant delivery
- A resuscitation bag
- Suctioning equipment
- Intubation supplies, if the patient does not already have an endotracheal tube

Additional supplies standard to neonatal respiratory care that should be available include a ventilator that can measure delivered or exhaled V_T and inspiratory pressure, a blended gas source, electrocardiogram (ECG) monitor, pulse oximeter, CO_2 monitor, radiant warmer or incubator, and resuscitation equipment.

The technique for surfactant delivery is designed to promote even distribution of surfactant within the lungs and is usually based on manufacturer recommendations. The dose is normally broken into two or four equal parts known as aliquots, and each is delivered to a lung region—left (left upper lobe, left lower lobe) and right (right upper and middle lobes, right lower lobe)—with a short break between aliquot delivery to ensure instillation into the alveoli. The patient is also positioned to promote equal distribution throughout the lungs:

- Head up, right side-lying
- Head up, left side-lying
- Head slightly down, left side-lying
- Head slightly down, right side-lying

The neonate should be suctioned prior to instillation of exogenous surfactant to clear the airway. The feeding tube or catheter is connected on one end to the full surfactant dose. The patient is positioned for the first dose, and the catheter is advanced into the endotracheal tube (ETT) using sterile technique until the tip is flush with the end of the ETT. The first aliquot is delivered, and the catheter is removed from the airway. PPV is initiated via resuscitation bag or mechanical ventilator to aid passage into the alveoli and prevent occlusion of the ETT or large airways with surfactant. PPV is continued for at least 1 minute or until the patient is stable and not experiencing bradycardia or hypoxemia, which would suggest airway occlusion. This procedure is repeated for the remaining aliquots. The RT must stay near the patient to ensure that excessive V_T delivery does not occur after surfactant replacement therapy and will need to wean the ventilator settings if it appears that lung overdistention is occurring. Suctioning of the

Table 4-3 Dosage for Surfactant Replacement Therapy (13)		
Surfactant	**Dosage**	**Repeat Dosage**
Beractant (Survanta)—minced bovine lung surfactant	4 mL/kg in four aliquots	Every 6 hours, up to a maximum of four doses during the first 24 hours of life
Calfactant (Infasurf)—lavaged bovine lung surfactant	3 mL/kg in two aliquots	Every 12 hours, up to a maximum of three doses
Poractant alfa (Curosurf)—porcine lung surfactant	First dose: 2.5 mL/kg in two aliquots Repeat dose: 1.25 mL/kg in two aliquots	Every 12 hours, up to a maximum of three doses
Colfosceril palmitate (Exosurf)	5 mL/kg in two aliquots	Every 12 hours, up to a maximum of three doses
Lucinactant (Surfaxin)*	5.8 mL/kg in four aliquots	Every 6 hours, up to a maximum of four doses

*Information from the Surfaxin package insert (59).

airway after surfactant delivery should be avoided unless necessary so that the surfactant isn't inadvertently removed from the lungs.

A positive response to surfactant replacement therapy includes the following:

- Improvement in saturation with oxygen (SpO_2) and/or reduction in FIO_2 requirement
- Decreased WOB
- Improvement in lung volumes, as seen by an increase in V_T during pressure ventilation or improved aeration on CXR (Fig. 4-5). This may occur very rapidly and requires close monitoring by the RT to avoid overventilation and lung injury in the period of time directly after surfactant replacement therapy.

Complications during surfactant administration include airway occlusion or endotracheal tube plugging, hypoxemia, or bradycardia. Late complications may include pulmonary hemorrhage and barotrauma caused by excessive MV after therapy.

Surfactant replacement therapy can be repeated, but the timing between doses and the number of repeat doses are based on manufacturer guidelines (see Table 4-3). Generally, they are at least 6 to 12 hours apart and should be given if the patient displays continuing signs of respiratory distress after the initial dose, requires an increase in ventilator support, or shows no improvement after the initial dose.

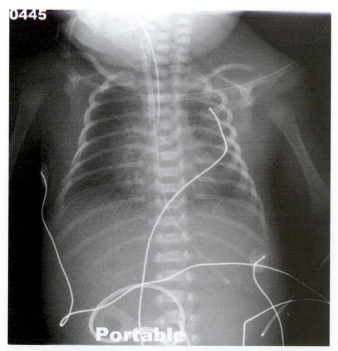

Figure 4-5 Chest Radiograph of Same Patient After Surfactant Replacement Therapy. Note the improved aeration. *(Courtesy of Jane Benson)*

■ ■ BG Gibbs is born 10 minutes later and is placed immediately in the polyethylene bag. She is initially breathing irregularly and has nasal flaring, substernal and intercostal retractions, and a weak cry. You note her respiratory rate (RR) to be about 20 breaths/min, and heart rate is about 120 bpm. At 1 minute, she has central cyanosis, and her SpO_2 reads 60% on her right hand. Initiation of blow-by O_2 at 0.40 FIO_2 does not improve her respirations or cyanosis. You provide mask CPAP, and the physician agrees to intubate so you can deliver the initial dose of surfactant. At 3 minutes, she is intubated with a 2.5-cm ETT, and by 6 minutes you have completed giving your fourth aliquot of surfactant. BG Gibbs is now breathing 60 times per minute, SpO_2 is 88% on FIO_2 0.30, and she is making spontaneous movements. The physician requests that she be extubated, and you initiate nasal CPAP (NCPAP) plus 5 cm H_2O prior to transport to the NICU. Susan is able to see her daughter and touches her before you place her in the transport incubator.

Oxygen Therapy

One of the first manifestations of respiratory distress is hypoxemia, as observed by low SpO_2 values on pulse oximetry or low PaO_2 on arterial blood gas. The administration of supplemental oxygen is a standard therapy that has been used in neonatal care since at least the 1940s, and it has improved survival in preterm and low-birth-weight infants (60).

Delivery devices are carefully selected for spontaneously breathing patients to maximize efficiency and comfort. Oxygen is delivered through noninvasive and invasive ventilation, and the strategies for managing FIO_2 are the same regardless of delivery modality. There are several reasons to avoid excessive oxygen delivery to premature infants. These include the increased risk of brain injury because of the instability of blood vessels in the germinal matrix, increased risk of retinal damage and retinopathy of prematurity due to excessive PaO_2 (see Chapter 8 for more details), and permanent structural damage to type I cells in the alveoli caused by toxic levels of oxygen in the lungs.

Titrating FIO_2 During Oxygen Delivery

Clinicians agree that the amount of oxygen delivered to premature infants should be closely monitored, excess oxygen delivery should be avoided, and weaning from supplemental oxygen therapy should be done as early as possible. However, institutions differ regarding how to define appropriate FIO_2 levels or SpO_2 ranges. Strategies that have been employed to minimize hyperoxemia in premature infants include the following (see Evidence in Practice 4-2):

- Minimizing abrupt changes in FIO_2. When SpO_2 is outside of normal range, make small changes in FIO_2 (0.01 to 0.05 at a time), and wait several minutes before making additional changes (61, 62).
- Ordering supplemental oxygen in an acceptable SpO_2 alarm limit range. The most commonly suggested ranges in studies have been 85% to 93% (62–66) and 89% to 94% (67).
- Assessing the patient for the cause of hypoxemia before increasing FIO_2 levels to avoid hyperoxemia. This will prevent cerebral blood pressure swings, rapid changes in retinal perfusion, and hemodynamic instability by opening and closing the ductus arteriosus (68) (see Chapter 8 for more information on patent ductus arteriosus). Assessment should include evaluating proper pulse oximetry function, degree of respiratory distress, presence of apnea, and duration of desaturation (62).
- Connecting both the oxygen-delivery device and resuscitation bag to an air-oxygen blender. An **air-oxygen blender** brings compressed air and oxygen from a high-pressure source into a chamber and then sends the gases to a metering device that controls the mixing of the two gases. An oxygen flow meter is usually connected to the gas outlet so that a patient device (such as a nasal cannula, oxygen hood, or resuscitation bag) can be connected. The use of a blender ensures that, when manual ventilation occurs, infants will receive the same FIO_2 they received via their oxygen-delivery device, avoiding abrupt changes in FIO_2 (62).
- Weaning oxygen as soon as SpO_2 rises above the preset value and then in small increments until SpO_2 is again in an acceptable range.

Oxygen-Delivery Devices for Spontaneously Breathing Neonates

Many different devices have been designed to treat hypoxemia in spontaneously breathing patients. They are classified as either low-flow devices or high-flow devices.

- Low-flow or variable-performance oxygen-delivery devices provide oxygen at flow rates that are lower than a patient's inspiratory demand. Patients are therefore required to inspire room air to achieve their desired V_T. Consequently, the FIO_2 delivered to the alveoli will vary based on inspiratory flow, V_T, and set FIO_2 and flow rate. The larger the V_T, the more room air has to be entrained and the lower the delivered FIO_2. Low-flow devices for neonates

---

● **Evidence in Practice 4-2**

Oxygen Administration Protocols for Preterm Infants (61, 62, 67)

Many neonatal units have developed protocols for more organized management of FIO_2 to minimize the harmful effects of hyperoxia in premature infants. Protocols and algorithms for managing oxygen delivery may include information about the following:

- Order requirements for oxygen delivery, which should include target SpO_2 or PaO_2 ranges. For premature infants (less than 36 wG), these ranges have been suggested as 85% to 93%, 89% to 94% (67), and 82% to 94% (61). The protocol may also include the high and low SpO_2 alarm limit ranges that should be set on the pulse oximeter.
- Assessment of a patient exhibiting desaturation to be completed *before* adjusting FIO_2:
  - Evidence of cyanosis
  - Validity of pulse oximeter value (correlation of HR on pulse oximeter to ECG, signal strength if available, or motion artifact)
  - Patient's respiratory status (apnea, retractions, tachypnea, WOB, nasal flaring, grunting)
  - Properly functioning oxygen-delivery equipment
  - Patency/adequacy of patient interface with oxygen-delivery equipment
- Strategies for changing FIO_2, including the allowable fraction of change, usually 0.01 to 0.05.
- Additional strategies to improve oxygenation *instead of* increasing F_IO_2, such as the following:
  - Manual breaths via mechanical ventilator or manual resuscitation bag
  - Tactile stimulation
  - Suctioning of the airway
- Description of an adequate observation period—3 minutes of observation during desaturation to allow the patient time to spontaneously recover from hypoxemia before making an F_IO_2 change
- Documentation of any desaturation event and the necessary intervention and guidelines for when to notify an authorized prescriber, such as whether the FIO_2 has been adjusted greater than 0.10 above baseline

---

include nasal cannulas (NCs), simple oxygen masks, and non-rebreather masks.
- High-flow or fixed-performance devices provide oxygen at flow rates that are higher than a patient's inspiratory demands. This means that they will deliver a fixed FIO_2 to the alveoli, regardless of changes in the patient's breathing patterns. High-flow devices for neonates include oxygen hoods, incubators, and high-flow NCs.

Delivery of supplemental oxygen in premature infants can be done via traditional NC, heated high-flow NC, mask, oxygen hood, or an environmental delivery system such as an incubator (Table 4-4). When selecting an oxygen-delivery device, clinicians should evaluate the size of the patient, goals of oxygen therapy, current FIO_2 requirements, patient comfort, and tolerance of the chosen device.

Like the adult version, a neonatal NC is a small-bore, soft plastic tube that contains two prongs that fit into the patient's external nares. The prongs, which are approximately a centimeter long, provide oxygen flow into the nasopharynx, which acts as an anatomical reservoir. It is the most commonly used device for oxygen delivery; is relatively comfortable; and allows the baby to be held, fed, or given bedside care without interrupting oxygen delivery. Oxygen delivered to the patient varies based on the set flow rate, FIO_2 set on the air-oxygen blender, variances in patient inspiratory flows, and nasal versus oral breathing (see Table 4-5). Long-term NC delivery can cause nasopharyngeal-mucosal irritation, skin irritation at pressure points where tubing touches the face and head, and inadvertent positive airway

Table 4-5 — FIO_2 Levels Delivered to the Neonatal Airway via Nasal Cannula (69)

FIO_2 (set on air-oxygen blender)	Delivered FIO_2 by Flow Rate (LPM)			
	0.25	0.50	0.75	1.0
0.40	0.22	0.23	0.25	0.26
0.60	0.26	0.31	0.35	0.37
0.80	0.31	0.36	0.41	0.49
1.0	0.35	0.45	0.61	0.66

pressure if the nares are completely occluded by the prongs. In neonates, the cannula should be placed in the nares, taking care that the prongs do not completely occlude them. Position the tubing past the ears and secure the plastic notch on the cannula behind the head to prevent airway obstruction. Secure the NC to the face using an adhesive device. Adhesive tape can cause skin irritation or epidermal stripping, so several manufacturers have designed cannula or tubing holders to minimize facial damage.

Table 4-4 — Oxygen-Delivery Devices for Premature Infants

Device	Benefits	Disadvantages	FIO_2 range
Nasal cannula	• Provides tactile stimulation while delivering oxygen • Can feed and care for patient without interrupting oxygen delivery • Allows patient greater mobility	• FIO_2 varies with changes in inspiratory flow and V_T • Cannula prongs can become occluded by secretions	0.21–0.70 at flows of 0.25–2 LPM
High-flow nasal cannula	• Delivers accurate FIO_2 at higher flows (>6.0 LPM) • Keeps patient comfortable • Delivers gas at body temperature, 100% relative humidity	• Incorrect cannula size can provide inadvertent positive distending pressure, similar to CPAP	0.21–1, at flows of 1–8 LPM
Face mask	• Can provide moderate concentrations of oxygen • Provides oxygen to nose and mouth	• FIO_2 can vary significantly • Must be removed for feeding • Can cause skin irritation	0.35–0.50 (FIO_2 data from studies in children and adults) at flows of 5–10 LPM
Oxygen hood	• Maintains a relatively constant FIO_2 • Does not need to be attached to patient's skin	• Higher FIO_2 may be found at bottom of hood • High noise levels inside • Must be set at 5–10 LPM to flush out exhaled CO_2 • Baby unable to be held or nursed when hood in place	0.21–1
Incubator (environmental delivery system)	• Requires no additional device to attach to patient • Displays set and measure FIO_2 continuously on new model incubators	• When care ports are open, FIO_2 may vary widely	0.21–0.65

These devices use microporous tape that adheres to the face and a clear tab with an adhesive backing that will secure the cannula to the tape.

• In 2000, the first **heated, humidified, high-flow nasal cannula (HFNC)** was approved for use in the United States by the FDA (70). HFNC produces a high flow of highly humidified air, virtually free of droplets, at body temperature or above. This high humidity allows for much higher flow rates (1 to 8 liters per minute [LPM]) to be tolerated by neonatal patients without the risk of nasal mucosal drying or bleeding. HFNC has been suggested as a high-flow (fixed-performance) oxygen-delivery device because, when set to higher flows, it can meet or exceed inspiratory demand. It can also flush carbon dioxide from the nasopharyngeal anatomical dead space, which creates a reservoir of fresh gas for early inspiration, improving the accuracy of delivered FIO_2. Several HFNC devices are now available for neonatal use and vary in their design and setup, but all have a traditional patient-cannula interface connected to a humidifier and air-oxygen delivery system, which will regulate gas flow, temperature, percent relative humidity, and set FIO_2. Data from NICUs suggest that patients are more comfortable using HFNC than any other high-flow oxygen-delivery device (71) (oxygen hood, mask, nasal CPAP, or MV). Several studies have suggested that the higher flows from NCs can increase esophageal and pharyngeal pressures in neonates, providing a distending pressure similar to CPAP (72–74). To avoid inadvertent positive airway pressure during HFNC delivery, nasal prongs should be selected that do not significantly occlude the nares (73, 75, 76).

Oxygen masks are cone-shaped devices that fit over the patient's nose and mouth and are held in place with an elastic band that fits around the patient's head. Oxygen is delivered through small-bore tubing connected to the base of the mask. During inspiration, the patient draws gas from the oxygen flowing into the mask and from room air through ports on the sides of the mask. Oxygen flow rates into the mask must be sufficient to wash out exhaled carbon dioxide that can accumulate in the mask. Delivered FIO_2 values by mask have not been studied in infants or neonates, but in children and adults they can range from 0.35 to 0.50. Delivered FIO_2 varies based on the flow of oxygen to the mask, the size of mask, and the patient's breathing pattern. The mask must be removed for feeding or nursing, may be restrictive, and can cause skin irritation where it touches the skin. In the NICU, masks are frequently used as an alternative to oxygen hoods when use of the latter is not possible, such as for transport or when the infant is being swaddled and held by a family member.

An **oxygen hood** or "oxyhood" is a clear plastic enclosure that is placed around a neonate's head and connected to a humidified gas source to provide a fixed oxygen concentration. An oxygen hood is an ideal method of oxygen delivery for neonates who require higher FIO_2 but do not have additional respiratory support requirements. At gas flows of greater than 7 LPM, FIO_2 delivered via an oxygen hood can be maintained at 0.21 to 1. Gas flow must be maintained above 5 LPM to ensure that exhaled CO_2 is flushed out of the hood. The gas in the hood should be measured intermittently to ensure accurate F_IO_2 delivery to the patient, and an air-oxygen blender or air-entrainment device should be used to select and adjust the desired FIO_2. The sound within an oxyhood can be loud, and neonates can't be fed or held during its use.

Incubators provide large volumes of oxygen-enriched gas to the atmosphere immediately surrounding the patient. **Incubators** are used in the neonatal population to provide variable control of environmental temperature and humidity. They minimize heat loss through conduction and can promote a quiet, dark environment, which minimizes external stimuli that can be distressing to premature infants. Supplemental oxygen can be provided by connecting an oxygen source and heated humidifier directly to the incubator and using the incubator's control panel to set an F_IO_2. Set oxygen values can range from 0.21 to 0.65 on most incubator models, but the actual oxygen concentration delivered to the patient can vary widely because of the frequent entry of room air when the hand ports are opened for patient assessment and nursing care. New incubators have an FIO_2 analyzer built in that will continuously display the set and delivered oxygen concentration within the incubator. If this is not available, the air inside the incubator should be measured intermittently to ensure accuracy of delivered FIO_2.

Noninvasive Respiratory Support

CPAP has been used noninvasively in the neonatal population for over 40 years as a less-invasive form of pulmonary support. CPAP is the application of positive pressure to the airways of the spontaneously breathing patient, via nasal prongs or a mask, throughout the respiratory cycle. It provides a positive pressure that increases FRC and offers the following benefits:

• Alveolar and airway stabilization
• Decreased airway resistance
• Improved ventilation-perfusion matching, clinically exhibited as improvements in oxygenation and ventilation

- Decreased WOB
- Increased lung expansion
- Preservation of the patient's natural surfactant
- Increased lung compliance
- Stabilization of the patient's respiratory pattern (77)

Newborns are preferential nose breathers, so the use of nasal continuous positive airway pressure (NCPAP) has been very successful in patients with RDS to prevent intubation and MV, to decrease WOB in spontaneously breathing patients, to provide respiratory support once patients are weaned from MV and extubated, and to improve atelectasis (see Chapter 7 for more information).

Indications for NCPAP include the following (78):

- Increased WOB, as seen by an increase in RR greater than 30% of normal, substernal and suprasternal retractions, grunting, and/or nasal flaring. Cyanosis and agitation are other non-specific symptoms that may be present in tandem with increased WOB.
- Inability to maintain a PaO_2 greater than 50 mm Hg with FIO_2 less than 0.60
- $PaCO_2$ greater than 50 mm Hg and pH greater than or equal to 7.25
- Infiltrated lung fields or atelectasis on chest radiograph
- Extubation from MV

NCPAP should not be considered in infants who have already met the criteria for ventilatory failure ($PaCO_2$ greater than 60 mm Hg and pH less than 7.25) or those who have an unstable respiratory drive with frequent episodes of apnea that cause desaturation and bradycardia.

Newer modalities of noninvasive support for neonates also include noninvasive positive-pressure ventilation (NIPPV), which adds a second level of pressure delivery at regular intervals to the patient in an effort to improve success of NCPAP. This creates a higher mean arterial pressure (MAP) than traditional NCPAP, which helps recruit collapsed alveoli, maintain FRC, improve airway stability, and improve oxygenation.

Nasal Continuous Positive Airway Pressure (NCPAP)

NCPAP can be used as a rescue therapy for patients with RDS who are exhibiting signs of worsening respiratory distress, either as an early intervention started in the delivery room or as a weaning modality after extubation. Initial settings for NCPAP have been recommended by the AARC as 4 to 5 cm H_2O and may be increased up to 10 cm H_2O (78). Once initiated, evidence of NCPAP success is defined as decrease in WOB; improved aeration by chest radiograph;

improved oxygenation; and reduction in episodes of apnea, bradycardia, and hypoxemia (Box 4-6).

Research supports the use of early NCPAP, showing that CPAP initiated in the delivery room decreases the need for intubation and lowers the risk of other comorbidities of prematurity such as IVH, NEC, or prolonged oxygen delivery. This applies to all but the smallest premature infants (less than 25 wG) and thus should be considered as respiratory support prior to intubation for all patients with suspected RDS (79–82). Other studies have supported extubation and NCPAP immediately after surfactant delivery, showing that it prevents later need for MV (83–85). RTs competent in the use of NCPAP can use it to help decrease the need for prolonged ventilatory support for patients with RDS and potentially decrease the incidence of chronic lung disease (CLD).

NCPAP is delivered by affixing nasal prongs or fitting a nasal mask to the patient's face. The device will deliver heated and humidified gas through a circuit that is connected to a gas source. The components of any type of NCPAP device include these features:

- Heated and humidified gas source that has an internal FIO_2 regulating system or is connected to an air-oxygen blender

---

Box 4-6   Guidelines for NCPAP for RDS (78)

Settings should be 4 to 5 cm H_2O initially, increasing 1 to 2 cm H_2O, as needed, to a maximum setting of 10 cm H_2O. FIO_2 should remain on the previous setting.

Evidence of success is as follows:

- Decreased WOB, shown by decrease in RR, retractions, nasal flaring, and grunting, as well as increased patient comfort
- F_IO_2 weaned to less than 0.60 with PaO_2 greater than 50 mm Hg or SpO_2 within acceptable limits per NICU protocol (usually greater than 85%)
- Improved aeration on chest radiograph
- Reduction in apnea, bradycardia, and cyanosis

Evidence of need for intubation:

- pH less than 7.25 and $PaCO_2$ greater than 50 mm Hg
- Significant apneic spells with associated hypoxemia and/or bradycardia
- Continued respiratory distress despite increase in CPAP setting
- Inability to wean FIO_2 less than 0.60 despite increase in CPAP setting

- Nasal interface, consisting of a set of bi-nasal prongs or a nasal mask, held in place using a bonnet with a securing device such as Velcro, safety pins, or ties (Fig. 4-6)
- Patient circuit
- Pressure-generation apparatus (86)

There are three major types of NCPAP delivery devices for the neonatal population: ventilator CPAP (also known as continuous-flow CPAP), variable-flow CPAP, and bubble CPAP. A description of each is found next (Table 4-6).

Ventilator CPAP

The most simple and efficient system, often referred to as "conventional CPAP," the ventilator CPAP has been used since the 1970s (87). It requires little additional setup because it uses a neonatal ventilator and patient circuit adapted for NCPAP. A set of nasal prongs are provided, replacing the patient Y connector. This setup uses the ventilator's PEEP valve (usually an expiratory resistor valve) to set and regulate CPAP levels and allows release of excess circuit pressure. Smaller patients may find it uncomfortable to exhale against the high continuous flow in this circuit and thus may not show as much alleviation in WOB or general comfort. In the most serious cases, patients may experience CO_2 retention as a by-product of this expiratory resistance.

Variable-Flow CPAP

The design of variable-flow CPAP systems functions to provide adequate inspiratory flow, maintain stable pressure at the nares and large airway, and thus maintain a more consistent FRC. Variable-flow CPAP systems are able to maintain a low level of imposed WOB by minimizing the need for patients to exhale against incoming gas flow. This improves patient comfort and stabilizes lung function in infants with weak respiratory efforts and leaky nasal interfaces. Gas is regulated with a flow driver, which regulates flow to the patient or out through an exhalation tube (Infant Flow) or into a low-pressure area (ARABELLA). When the machine senses the back pressure from the patient interface, it diverts gas away from the nares, making it easier for the patient to exhale. The net effect of these systems is the prevention of excess CPAP pressures by venting unnecessary gas away from the patient. These systems require their own pressure generator, equipment circuit, and patient interface. Variable-flow systems have been shown to provide adequate CPAPs and have lower oxygen requirements and respiratory rates (88–90) and shorter duration of CPAP support (91) than do other CPAP designs.

Bubble CPAP

Bubble CPAP is an inexpensive, simple, and effective way to provide CPAP to premature infants, and its design has been used since the 1970s. There is a lot of interest in this method of CPAP delivery, particularly in resource-limited environments (Special Populations 4-1). Bubble CPAP consists of the following:

- Neonatal dual-limb ventilator circuit
- Humidifier connected to an air-oxygen blender, gas set to 4 to 10 LPM
- NCPAP prongs
- Pressure manometer attached at the nasal prong interface
- Water column filled to 10 cm with sterile water or a 0.25% acetic acid mixture

See Figure 4-6 for a schematic setup of bubble CPAP. The inspiratory limb is connected to the humidifier and then to the bi-nasal prongs. The expiratory limb is submerged in the water column;

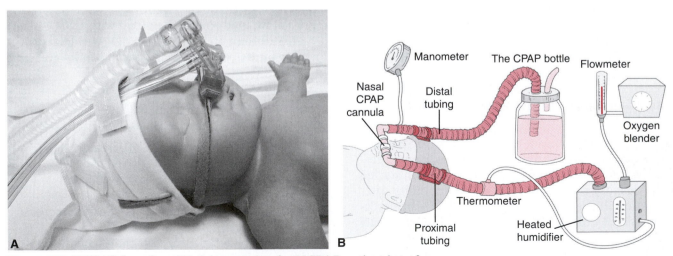

Figure 4-6 NCPAP Interface (A) An example of a NCPAP patient interface. (B) A schematic drawing of bubble CPAP.

Table 4-6	Methods for Delivering NCPAP and NIPPV			
Device	**Description**	**Benefits**	**Disadvantages or Limitations**	**Examples**
Ventilator CPAP	• Ventilator circuit with Y connector replaced with nasal prongs and adapter tubes, attached with a bonnet and connectors	• Simple and efficient after extubation • Requires little additional equipment to run • Has a built-in pop-off in case of excess pressure buildup	Pressure monitoring and pressure regulation less responsive to small patient efforts	• Hudson bi-nasal prongs • Argyle bi-nasal prongs
Variable-flow CPAP	• Gas flow determined by a flow driver, with excess gas diverted away from the patient when CPAP met and during exhalation	• Provides lower impedance to exhalation, decreasing WOB	Requires its own generator, circuit, and patient interface	• Cardinal Health Infant Flow CPAP • Hamilton ARABELLA
Bubble CPAP	• Neonatal dual-limb ventilator circuit • Humidifier and blender • NCPAP prongs • Pressure manometer • 10-cm water column	• Simple and inexpensive	Delivered CPAP may fluctuate based on water levels, gas flow, and resistance in circuit	• N/A
Noninvasive positive pressure	• Similar to variable flow CPAP, with a set rate and two levels of CPAP	• Improving alveolar recruitment and stimulation for apnea	Little guidance on how to select high CPAP settings, T_I, or rate	• SiPAP • NeoPAP

the depth of the circuit below surface of the water equals the delivered CPAP (e.g., –4 cm below the surface of the water equals 4 cm H_2O CPAP). The actual amount of CPAP delivered to the patient can vary based on resistance within the system; therefore, airway pressure should be monitored in the CPAP prongs to verify actual delivered pressure (93). Bubble CPAP has been shown to be as effective as ventilator CPAP (94, 95) and variable-flow CPAP (96) and may have the added benefit of shorter duration of CPAP and improved oxygenation.

Bubble CPAP in Resource-Limited Environments (92)

Use of a bubble CPAP system in a busy NICU in Fiji was associated with a 50% reduction in need for MV with no change in mortality, at a cost just 15% of that of the cheapest ventilator. Nurses were able to provide this care to neonates after 1 to 2 months of on-the-job training, improving the access to care for children in this region of Fiji. They found bubble CPAP to be a safe and affordable technique for respiratory support.

Complications

Most complications of NCPAP are due to overdistention of the lung caused by excessive CPAP settings. Overdistention can lead to the following problems:

- Poor ventilation/perfusion matching
- Increase in pulmonary vascular resistance
- Decrease in cardiac output
- Increase in $PaCO_2$
- Increased WOB
- Air leak syndrome
- Gastric insufflation, leading to aspiration if not corrected quickly

Patients on NCPAP may require increased levels of attention by bedside providers to assure proper fitting of NCPAP prongs or mask and headgear to confirm that the nasal prongs or mask remain in the nose and that minimal leakage occurs. Close monitoring will assure proper delivery of pressure to the alveoli and minimize nasal breakdown due to improper nasal prong or mask placement. Skin breakdown leading to nasal trauma is a serious complication of NCPAP delivery. When caring for patients with NCPAP prongs, providers should monitor for signs of nasal trauma, which include redness, bleeding, crusting, abrasion of the skin, or narrowing of the nasal passage (95).

Noninvasive Positive-Pressure Ventilation

NIPPV is used in an effort to improve the effectiveness of NCPAP as an initial form of therapy and as support to prevent extubation failure. The addition of positive-pressure breaths at a set rate creates a higher Paw than does traditional NCPAP, which helps recruit collapsed alveoli, maintain FRC, and improve oxygenation. NIPPV isn't a closed system, so not all breaths and full pressures are transmitted to the alveoli. As a result, it's not clear exactly why it is effective, but there are two potential physiological mechanisms. One is that NIPPV is providing some ventilation at the alveolar level. Another theory is that NIPPV works in a way that is similar to sigh breaths and recruits microatelectasis and improves airway stability. It has also been shown to be effective as a physical stimulus to breathing when treating AOP (see Chapter 5).

The delivery of NIPPV is similar to that of ventilator CPAP, with the addition of peak inspiratory pressure (PIP), inspiratory time (T_I), and inflation rate or RR. The management approach to NIPPV is not standardized, but the following settings have been suggested in different studies and are based on current practice:

- CPAP level similar to traditional NCPAP (4 to 6 cm H_2O)
- PIP 15 to 16 cm H_2O to start, with a maximum of 24 to 26 (98). In practice, the range of PIPs have been documented to be as wide as 7 to 20 cm H_2O (99).
- Inflation rate 50 to 60 (98), but practice ranges widely with rates from 10 to 60 (99)
- T_I set from 0.3 to 0.5 seconds (98, 100)

The wide variations in practice may be the result of the underlying physiological principle to which the provider prescribes. If the provider is attempting to deliver V_T-sized breaths to the lungs, using a traditional PIP and high RR would assist in ventilation of a neonate on NCPAP. The patient-CPAP interface at the nares is not a closed system, and the mouth can also work as a pop-off valve, preventing consistent delivery of breaths to the alveoli. It is also challenging to synchronize breaths with patient effort during NIPPV, and asynchronous breaths in particular are less effective (100).

An alternative principle is to use NIPPV to deliver alternating levels of CPAP (high and low) similar to adult BiPAP, thus providing bilevel nasal continuous positive airway pressure (bilevel NCPAP) or sigh NCPAP. There are now neonatal CPAP machines designed to deliver NIPPV in this way; they include the SiPAP and Infant Flow Advance. Recommended settings using the bilevel approach to NIPPV include a low-CPAP level of 4 to 6 cm H_2O and a high-CPAP level set 2 to 4 cm H_2O higher (101). One study using this method recommended a delta P (δP)—the change in pressure between low-CPAP and high-CPAP—of approximately 4 cm H_2O with a rate set at 30 per minute (102).

Despite the use of NCPAP and NIPPV in neonatal patients, there is still the risk of ventilatory failure and the need for intubation and MV. The rate of failure of initial NCPAP for patients with RDS is documented to be around 22% (103) to 36% (98), and NIPPV is slightly lower at 10% (101) to 13.5% (98). Failure in VLBW infants with RDS is much higher, and more than half will require intubation and MV (104–106).

■■ When BG Gibbs arrives in the NICU, she is placed on a variable-flow NCPAP machine at 6 cm H_2O and FIO_2 of 0.30, with a resultant SpO_2 of 88% and RR 48 breaths/min. A chest radiograph displays some reticulogranular patterns, but also shows moderate aeration that is suggestive of alveolar opening. Her admission weight is 700 g. At BG Gibb's sixth hour of life, you obtain an arterial blood gas (ABG) sample from the umbilical artery line, which reveals pH 7.25, $PaCO_2$ 52 mm Hg, PaO_2 60 mm Hg, and HCO_2 22.5 mEq/L on FIO_2 0.45. You take this information to the neonatologist and suggest intubation and another dose of surfactant. She agrees and orders you to leave the baby intubated after the surfactant to treat the respiratory acidosis.

Mechanical Ventilation

The use of maternal corticosteroids and surfactant replacement therapy, along with the improvement in noninvasive ventilatory support, has decreased the number of neonates with RDS requiring intubation and MV. However, 27% of all infants admitted to NICUs undergo MV, and most of those born at less than 28 wG need to be ventilated (107); in addition, it is still an independent risk factor for the development of lung injury and BPD (108, 109). The RT's goal in ventilator management is to closely monitor patients to assure appropriate ventilation, assess patient information to minimize overventilation, and wean patients as quickly as possible to extubation to avoid further lung injury.

Neonatal MV technology has been changing rapidly in the last several decades, and there are few randomized control trials to guide clinicians in the selection of the best ventilator modality, settings, or strategies to adjust ventilation. Historical data and expert opinions are driving factors in ventilator-management strategies, as is the use of data from adult and pediatric studies using similar ventilator strategies and technologies.

The goals of MV for neonates are the same as for any other patient: to facilitate alveolar ventilation and carbon dioxide removal, provide adequate tissue oxygenation, and reduce WOB (27). Additional goals for the RT should include the following:

- Support all spontaneous respiratory efforts
- Avoid pulmonary tissue injury
- Minimize interference of positive-pressure ventilation with cardiac circulation (Box 4-7)
- Liberate the patient from invasive ventilation

The optimal strategy for MV in RDS is not clear, based on research studies. Care should be taken to use minimal pressures and volumes to achieve adequate blood gases, CXR/lung inflation, oxygenation, and minimized WOB. **Mean airway pressure (Paw)** is a close reflection of mean alveolar pressure; it is calculated on all mechanical ventilators and can be used to evaluate the amount of support provided to mechanically ventilated patients. Higher Paw values indicate higher levels of support and a higher potential for lung injury. Likewise, lower Paw values are a reflection of lower levels of ventilatory support. Patients should be monitored closely and ventilator setting changes made frequently to minimize iatrogenic lung injury, and extubation should occur as soon as is reasonable.

MV management begins with intubation. Once an airway is established, selection of ventilator settings can occur. Clinicians should continually assess the adequacy of chosen settings, adjusting parameters whenever the patient is being inadequately or excessively ventilated. Over time, the patient will either meet criteria for weaning and extubation or fail conventional MV, at which time the RT will assist in transitioning the patient to a new respiratory support modality.

Intubation

Intubation is a skilled procedure that should be undertaken by a team of health-care professionals who are competent in the process. As few as 1 in 500 newborns may require intubation (111), and even fewer require emergent intubation. Intubation and airway stabilization in the delivery room are considered emergency procedures and were described in Chapter 3. Indications for emergency intubation for RDS patients include failure of airway control during mask ventilation, airway abnormalities, prolonged resuscitation, and instillation of surfactant. Indications for elective intubation include prolonged ventilation, airway instability, prematurity, and endotracheal tube change. All nonemergent or elective intubations should follow a similar algorithm that provides a controlled process for airway stabilization.

Equipment for an elective intubation should be collected and organized at the bedside prior to beginning the intubation attempt. Equipment should include the following:

Box 4-7 Side Effects of Mechanical Ventilation (110)

Air leak syndromes due to barotrauma and/
or volutrauma, including the following
(see Chapter 7):

- Pulmonary interstitial emphysema
- Pneumothorax
- Pneumomediastinum
- Pneumopericardium

  Bronchopulmonary dysplasia
  Nosocomial pneumonia
  Complications that occur when positive pressure applied to the lungs is transmitted to the cardiovascular system or the cerebral vasculature resulting in the following:

- Decreased venous return
- Decreased cardiac output
- Increased intracranial pressure leading to intraventricular hemorrhage (27, 33, 80)

  Excessive supplemental oxygen increasing risk of retinopathy of prematurity (see Chapter 8)
  Patient-ventilator asynchrony or inappropriate ventilator settings, both of which can lead to the following:

- Auto-PEEP
- Hypo- or hyperventilation
- Hypo- or hyperoxemia
- Increased WOB

  Rapid changes in lung compliance and airway resistance may result in alterations in V_T delivery that may significantly influence V_E.

- Infant resuscitation bag with premature or infant-size masks (correctly sized to patient)
- Gas source with air-oxygen blender
- Laryngoscope handle and a straight (Miller) blade: size 00 for extremely premature neonates, 0 for premature neonates. (Full-term-sized neonates may require a size 1 blade.)
- Appropriately sized oral or nasal airway to facilitate mask ventilation if necessary
- Correct size of ETT
  - Less than 1,000 g = 2.5 cm
  - 1,000 g to 2,000 g = 3.0 cm
  - 2,000 g to 3,000 g = 3.5 cm
- Stylet
- 5 and 6 French suction catheters
- Stethoscope

- Shoulder roll
- 1/2-inch cloth tape or Hy-Tape
- Scissors
- Carbon dioxide detector
- Pulse oximeter and ECG monitor
- Mechanical ventilator with neonatal dual-limb heated wire circuit

In 2010, the section on Anesthesiology and Pain Medicine, a part of the American Academy of Pediatrics' Committee on Fetus and Newborn, published recommendations for premedication of neonates prior to elective intubations. The goal was to provide analgesia to "eliminate the pain, discomfort, and physiological abnormalities of the procedure," as well as to help carry out a more expeditious intubation while minimizing the chance for traumatic injury to the newborn (112). A person skilled in noninvasive or bag-mask ventilation should be present to help maintain oxygenation and ventilation for the baby after the analgesic and/or muscle relaxant are given.

- **Analgesia** is the absence of a normal sense of pain. An analgesic medication will reduce the pain and discomfort of intubation. An ideal analgesic for intubation has a rapid onset with short duration and has no adverse effects on respiratory mechanics. Opioids are the most common analgesic used in the neonatal population, including morphine and fentanyl, and they should be given for any elective intubation. One of the side effects of fentanyl is acute chest wall rigidity, which can significantly impair ventilation. Slow infusion of the medication can prevent this effect, and it can be overcome by using a muscle relaxant.

- **Muscle relaxants** are used during intubation to eliminate a patient's spontaneous movement; in the neonatal population, muscle relaxants can minimize or eliminate the increase in intracranial pressure that occurs during awake intubation, which increases the risk of IVH. Muscle relaxants that have been studied and that are frequently used in the pediatric and neonatal population include succinylcholine, pancuronium, vecuronium, and rocuronium. Common side effects seen in young children include bradycardia, and therefore most institutions include a dose of a vagolytic agent such as atropine prior to the administration of a muscle relaxant to prevent it (112).

Begin the intubation procedure by preoxygenating the patient to maintain an adequate SpO_2. If the patient is spontaneously breathing, this can be accomplished initially by using blow-by oxygen or the patient's previous oxygen-delivery system. If the patient is apneic or breathing ineffectively, then bag-mask ventilation should be initiated at a rate of 30 to 40 breaths/minute. Placing the child in the sniffing position (see Chapter 1) and using a shoulder roll will facilitate opening of the airway and alignment of the oropharynx with the trachea. Once chest rise is seen during mask ventilation, a dose of analgesic should be given. Continue respiratory support via bag-mask ventilation for at least 1 to 2 minutes, until the medication takes effect. Several studies support beginning the first attempts at neonatal intubation without muscle relaxant (112, 113).

- Suction the mouth and pharynx and stabilize the head in the sniffing position.
- Hold the laryngoscope blade in the left hand. Open the mouth and gently insert the blade in the right side of the mouth, moving the blade midline to push the tongue to the left side of the mouth. Take care not to damage the gums.
- Lift the blade slightly, using a motion that raises the blade and jaw toward the ceiling, and look down the blade. Clear any secretions that may be obstructing the view. The tip of the Miller blade should be advanced until it is under the epiglottis, and then used to lift the epiglottis. If the blade is in correct position, the vocal cords should be in view, appearing as an inverted V. If the blade is too deep, only the soft tissue of the esophagus will be seen; if this is the case, then a slight withdrawal of the blade will cause the glottic structures to drop into view.
- Bring the tip of the ETT into view by sliding it along the right side of the mouth until it appears at the level of the vocal cords. Once the cords are open, slide the tube through the cords until the vocal cord guide marker is aligned with the cords.
- Hold the tube firmly against the hard palate while removing the laryngoscope blade and stylet.
- Begin bag tube ventilation. Look for signs of correct tube placement: Observe chest rise and misting of exhaled gas in the ETT, auscultate for equal bilateral breath sounds, verify end-tidal carbon dioxide using colorimetric or volumetric measures, and observe adequate HR and pulse oximetry after intubation. Once the tube is stabilized, a chest radiograph should be obtained to document exact tube placement, which should be 1 to 2 cm above the carina. When reviewing chest radiographs for tube placement, it is important to note that flexion (downward placement) of the neck causes a decrease in oral-carina distance, making the tube appear closer to the carina than it would be if the head were in neutral position. Likewise, extension of the neck causes an increase in

oral-carina distance, making the tube appear higher in the thorax than it would be if the head were in neutral position (114). Lateral rotation does not produce a significant change in tube placement (115).

- Verify centimeter marking at the lip and then secure the ETT to the neonate's upper lip using tape or a tube stabilization device.

Attempts at endotracheal intubation should be limited to 20 to 30 seconds (49, 111, 116), and the attempt should be terminated if the patient experiences bradycardia or significant hypoxemia prior to successful tube placement. Oxygenation and ventilation should precipitate all intubation attempts. One study recommends consideration of muscle relaxant with an accompanying vagolytic after two failed attempts at intubation, but only in the presence of a staff neonatologist or anesthesiologist (112, 113).

Side effects during endotracheal intubation include hypoxemia, bradycardia, intracranial hypertension, systemic hypertension, and pulmonary hypertension (112). Complications of long-term ETT placement can include the following (27, 110):

- Laryngotracheobronchomalacia
- Tracheal erosion
- Malpositioning of ETT, including unplanned extubation and main-stem intubation
- Obstruction of ETT by thickened secretions
- Air leak around uncuffed ETT
- Subglottic stenosis
- Pressure necrosis
- Pharyngeal, esophageal, or tracheal perforation
- Palatal grooving
- Interference with arrangement of primary teeth
- Increased WOB during spontaneous breaths caused by the high resistance of ETTs

The WOB for all intubated patients is higher during spontaneous breathing through an ETT because of a significant increase in airway resistance. **Airway resistance** is the friction that occurs between moving molecules in the gas stream and between these moving molecules and the wall of the respiratory system. In healthy, spontaneously breathing newborns, airway resistance is around 26 cm H_2O/L/sec (117)—in contrast, a normal healthy adult's airway resistance is around 1 cm H_2O/L/sec. The resistance produced by infant endotracheal tubes is equal to or higher than that in the upper airway of a normal newborn. ETT resistance can be calculated using **Poiseulle's law**, which states that resistance is a function of the tube length divided by the radius of the tube to the fourth power, or

$$R = L/r^4$$

Thus, a 2.5-cm ETT would generate a much higher resistance than a 3.0-cm ETT of the same length. This equation also illustrates that small obstructions within the ETT, such as mucus, will have a profound negative effect on airway resistance. The ventilator can generate the additional pressure needed to overcome the resistance due to the ETT, but when ventilator support is minimal (such as when weaning) or if the infant is disconnected from the ventilator with the ETT still in place, he or she may not be capable of generating sufficient effort to overcome the increase in upper-airway resistance. When reviewing patient comfort and airway resistance, it may be useful to consider prophylactically reintubating with a larger ETT if there is evidence that it will be well tolerated by the patient (Clinical Variations 4-1). Once placement of the ETT has been verified, conventional MV can be initiated.

Conventional Mechanical Ventilation

Successful use of MV for neonates was documented as early as the 1960s (118, 119) but was initially provided by using an adult ventilator adapted for neonatal use. The various causes of neonatal pulmonary disease were not well understood, and equipment was rudimentary, with monitoring limited to clinical assessment, intermittent radiography, and blood gas assessment (120). The options for ventilating neonates were limited, even with the introduction of neonatal targeted ventilators. Clinicians could control only FIO_2, PIP, PEEP, T_I, RR, and circuit flow rate. Patient-ventilator dyssynchrony was common, and iatrogenic lung injury was a major cause of morbidity. The introduction of the microprocessor into adult and then neonatal ventilators greatly improved the quality of neonatal ventilation. RTs are now also able to control mode of ventilation, select V_T, adjust the assist sensitivity, synchronize with spontaneous efforts, and accurately measure pulmonary mechanics.

Clinical Variations 4-1

Upsizing Endotracheal Tubes for Growing Babies

Regardless of RDS severity, premature infants are expected to gain weight while on MV. One milestone of prematurity is reaching the target weight of 1,000 g, or 1 kg. At this point, the RT should look for signs that an upgrade to a 3.0 ETT is needed, such as a greater than 40% leak as measured by the mechanical ventilator, an audible leak during mechanical ventilator breaths, or respiratory distress (i.e., retractions) during spontaneous breaths. Electively reintubating with a larger ETT should improve the comfort and effectiveness of spontaneous breaths, minimize airway resistance, and improve air leaks.

To understand how ventilators work, RTs and pulmonary clinicians must be familiar with a myriad of nomenclature for ventilator design and interaction. These terms will be defined as they are introduced, but it is important to review a few of them prior to discussing neonatal ventilation.

- Trigger: The ventilator parameter that begins inspiration
- Limit: The predetermined maximum that the ventilator will not exceed during inspiration
- Cycle: The ventilator parameter that terminates inspiration

The following sections include a description of the mechanics of neonatal ventilators; the available ventilator settings and features; and common strategies for initiation, management, and weaning for neonates with RDS.

Breath-Delivery Ventilator Types

The first neonatal ventilators could only provide **time-triggered breaths**, frequently described as mandatory ventilator breaths. These breaths occur at a regular frequency without regard to patient respiratory effort. For instance, if respiratory rate was set to 30 breaths/minute, the ventilator would give a breath every 2 seconds. Traditional neonatal mechanical ventilators were classified as continuous-flow, **time-cycled, pressure-limited (TCPL) ventilation**. Their simple design (Fig. 4-7) allowed clinicians to deliver a consistent pressure and a set number of breaths/minute to all ages of neonates. The ventilators consist of a flowmeter, an expiratory valve, and a ventilator circuit and have the following settings available:

- Respiratory rate
- Inspiratory time
- Pressure limit, or PIP
- PEEP

The flow rate allows continuous gas flow through the circuit and past the patient Y connector, making it readily available for the patient during spontaneous breathing. When a mechanical breath is delivered, the expiratory valve closes, allowing a buildup of pressure within the circuit and then into the patient. During inspiration, pressure within the circuit reaches the preset PIP, is maintained there during inspiration (causing a pressure plateau), and is not allowed to exceed the PIP setting. When the inspiratory time is reached, the expiratory valve reopens, and expiration occurs passively.

Patient-triggered ventilation is a generic term that refers to modes of ventilation in which a mechanical breath is provided in response to measured or presumed respiratory effort by the patient. Synchronized intermittent mandatory ventilation (SIMV), assist-control (A/C), and pressure support

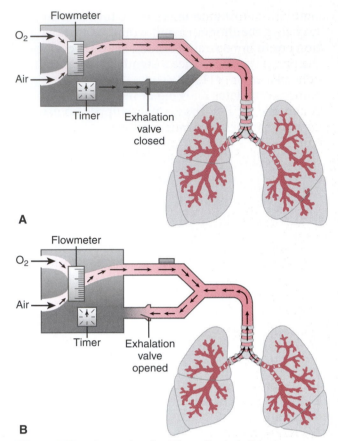

Figure 4-7 Schematic of a Time-Cycled, Pressure-Limited Ventilator

ventilation (PSV) are all forms of patient-triggered ventilation (120) and will be described later in the chapter.

Pressure Control Ventilation

Pressure control ventilation allows the pressure delivered to the lungs to remain constant, and volume delivery will change with lung characteristics. The underlying concept of pressure ventilation is that a volume of gas is delivered to the lungs over a specified time period until a clinician-chosen "safe" pressure is reached. Pressure ventilation can be used with either intermittent mandatory ventilation (IMV) or A/C modes of ventilation. Pressure support can also be incorporated. There are benefits of pressure ventilation:

- It minimizes barotrauma: By giving clinicians the ability to select a peak pressure, it will prevent excessive pressure changes in the lung in response to changes in airway resistance or lung compliance.
- It is not affected by the compressible volume of the circuit: During volume ventilation, a certain volume of gas is delivered to the ventilator circuit and does not make it to the patient. In adult ventilation, this amount may be a small percentage of the total V_T, but in neonatal

ventilation, this amount can be quite large and may significantly impact V_E. Pressure ventilation continues to deliver gas to the lungs until the preset pressure is reached, and thus V_T is delivered equally despite changes in circuit compressibility.

• It negates the challenge for ventilator technology to adequately deliver small V_T effectively: Initial ventilators did not have microprocessor technology or sophisticated flow sensors that could measure accurately the small tidal volumes required by extremely low-birth-weight infants. V_T delivered to the lungs for premature infants is frequently less than 10 mL, which adult ventilators were not capable of calculating. Thus, it was possible to inadvertently deliver two to three times the intended V_T to a neonate, which significantly increased the risk of overstretching the alveoli and causing lung injury.

• It has variable flow patterns: Newer ventilators have the ability to change the speed at which gas enters the lungs to improve volume delivery without excessive pressure spikes. In spontaneous breathing, gas flow begins slowly as the diaphragm drops, becoming greater as more gas moves into the lungs quickly. As the lungs begin to fill, flow slows down or decelerates, until it eventually terminates and exhalation begins. During pressure ventilation, gas flow is initially rapid as the ventilator fills the ETT and large airways with gas. Once gas reaches the alveoli, flows decelerate to prevent over-pressurizing the system, which allows a more even distribution of gas throughout the lungs. This flow pattern is known as a decelerating flow pattern, which can contribute to less

overdistention of the alveoli and prevent lung injury. Volume ventilation, by contrast, traditionally uses a constant flow pattern, delivering a set volume of gas to the lungs in an even pattern. This causes a continuous increase in inspiratory pressure until the volume is delivered.

During TCPL ventilation, the change in pressure (ΔP) during inspiration (PIP-PEEP) is the primary determinant of V_T. The larger the ΔP, the greater the potential V_T. However, there are many other factors that can affect the size of V_T during pressure ventilation. These factors are listed in Table 4-7 and include pulmonary characteristics as well as ventilator settings.

For more than 30 years, TCPL ventilation has been the technique most frequently applied to neonatal respiratory failure. It is easy to use and results in breaths that have a consistent PIP. However, the V_T delivered to the patient is dependent on pulmonary compliance (120).

Volume-Control Ventilation

Volume-control ventilation has been used traditionally in adult MV and is usually well understood by RTs. Volume-control ventilation delivers a consistent V_T with each breath, which allows better control of V_E. A downside of volume ventilation in RDS is illustrated by the **law of Laplace**, which states that volume will be preferentially delivered into segments of the lung that are partially open. In a surfactant-deficient lung, this means underventilating atelectatic alveoli and overventilating well-aerated ones, both of which contribute to iatrogenic lung injury. Other potential negative effects of volume ventilation in RDS include the following:

• A portion of the V_T delivered from the vent will be lost to compression of gas in the circuit

Table 4-7	Factors Affecting Tidal Volume During Pressure Ventilation		
	Factor		**Rationale**
Ventilator Settings	Inspiratory time (T_I)		Longer T_I allows more time for gas delivery, increasing V_T
	Inspiratory flow		Higher inspiratory flow delivers more volume without changing T_I
	ΔP	PIP	Higher PIP can increase the amount of gas delivered with each breath
		PEEP	Optimal PEEP will stabilize alveoli and improve gas delivery with each inspiration
Pulmonary Factors	TC	Lung compliance	Low compliance prevents adequate stretching of the alveoli during inspiration, decreasing V_T
		Airway resistance	High airway resistance restricts gas flow to the alveoli, decreasing delivered V_T

and humidifier and to stretching of elastic tubing. As discussed in the previous section, this may not have a significant impact in adult ventilation, but this volume loss is proportionally much larger for neonates and challenging to compensate for.

- A proportion of delivered V_T will be lost because of the leak around uncuffed ETTs. The amount lost is variable and therefore not easy to predict or treat. Ventilators are set to deliver a targeted V_T, but this V_T is measured within the machine prior to entering the circuit or the patient. A certain amount of this gas will be compressed within the ventilator, and this is referred to as "compressible volume loss." This is affected by the compliance of both the lungs and the ventilator circuit, in addition to other factors, such as humidification. Because of compressible volume loss, V_T measurement in neonates should occur as close to the airway as possible (120).
- Volume ventilation has usually used an accelerated or square waveform pattern, meaning that pressure will increase as volume is delivered to the lung, requiring higher PIPs to deliver a set V_T, which could increase the likelihood of pulmonary air leaks.

All of these features of volume-control ventilation make it challenging to use in neonates.

Volume-Targeted/Adaptive Ventilation

Volume-targeted ventilation allows clinicians to deliver a pressure-style breath while targeting a specific V_T. The ventilator adapts to changes in air leaks, patient effort, compliance, and resistance by adjusting inspiratory pressure or inspiratory time to stay within a target range. Randomized trials comparing pressure with volume-targeted ventilation suggest that the latter could reduce the duration of ventilation and reduce lung injury (121). The goal of volume-targeted ventilation is to avoid underventilation and overventilation, promote more uniform gas delivery, and respond to changing lung mechanics to wean pressures based on breath-by-breath characteristics, using the microprocessor to respond to wean ventilator settings faster than the clinician's capabilities. The following are examples of volume targeting designed by different manufacturers. This is not meant to be an exhaustive list but rather to illustrate the different ways that volume-targeted pressure ventilation can be achieved. Success for these modalities requires an accurate evaluation of V_T, measured as close to the patient as possible, preferably at the ETT and not at the expiratory limb (122).

Volume-Assured Pressure Support

Volume-assured pressure support (VAPS) is a mode on the Bird VIP Gold (Viasys Medical Systems, Conshohocken, PA) designed to volume target spontaneous breaths. The ventilator supports a spontaneous patient effort. When it senses the slowing of inspiratory flow, signaling the end of a breath, it compares the delivered volume with the set V_T. If it has exceeded the set V_T, the breath behaves like a pressure-supported breath and flow cycles off. If the measured V_T is less than the set V_T, the inspiratory time will be prolonged, and flow will continue until the desired volume is reached. If the breath is significantly below the set V_T, inspiratory pressure may be increased.

Pressure-Regulated Volume Control

Pressure-regulated volume control (PRVC) is a mode on the SERVO-i ventilator (Maquet Inc., Bridgewater, NJ). The clinician sets a target V_T and a maximum pressure (PIP). The ventilator delivers several test breaths to assess patient compliance and calculate how much pressure is needed to deliver the set V_T. The ventilator uses a decelerating flow pattern to minimize pressure and adjusts the delivered PIP based on the average volume of the previous four breaths. Pressures are adjusted in 3-cm H_2O increments to avoid large variations in V_T.

Volume Guarantee

Volume guarantee is a form of volume targeting available on the Dräger Babylog 8000 plus (Draeger Medical Inc., Telford, PA). It can be combined with A/C, SIMV, or PSV and allows the clinician to select a target V_T and maximum pressure limit, set by using the PIP knob. The ventilator will then increase or decrease the delivered PIP to achieve the target volume, using the previous exhaled V_T as a reference. It will adjust pressures over several consecutive breaths to avoid large swings in volume delivery. The ventilator will also cycle a breath if the inspiratory V_T exceeds 130% of the target.

Selecting Ventilator Settings

Once a patient is intubated, a selection of settings must be made: flow rate, mode of ventilation, PEEP and FIO_2, volume and/or pressure, and respiratory rate.

Flow Rate

The range of peak flow rates generated by spontaneously breathing newborns, including term and premature babies, is 0.6 to 9.9 LPM (27), but turbulent flow is generated in infant ETTs once ventilator flow rates exceed about 3 LPM through a 2.5-cm ETT or 7.5 LPM through a 3.0-cm ETT.

Flow conditions are likely to be at least partially turbulent when ventilator flow rates exceed 5 LPM in infants with a 2.5-cm ETT or 10 LPM with a 3.0-cm ETT. The bias flow needs to be sufficient to allow the ventilator to reach PIP in the allotted T_I but low enough to minimize turbulence (121). Rates of 5 to 8 LPM are commonly used for neonatal TCPL ventilation.

Mode

Initial time-cycled, pressure-limited ventilators were not able to "sense" neonatal respiratory effort, and thus the only mode available to this patient population was IMV. IMV allows the clinician to set an RR, PIP, and T_I that the ventilator will use to evenly space MV breaths. For instance, if the ventilator has a set rate of 20, PIP 15, and T_I 0.30 seconds, then every 3 seconds the ventilator will deliver a breath at a PIP of 15 cm H_2O for 0.30 seconds. This is done regardless of what the patient may have been doing at the time a breath is triggered, and irregular respiratory patterns of neonates can frequently lead to dyssynchrony between the ventilator and the patient. For instance, if the patient was in the middle of inspiration, the ventilator will give a breath into a lung already partially filled with gas. If the patient was exhaling, the ventilator will deliver a breath to a lung that was emptying. The former example will overdistend the lung, creating volutrauma and increasing the risk for iatrogenic lung injury. In the latter example, the ventilator will quickly reach the set PIP because it is attempting to deliver a breath when gas is being exhaled through the ETT, preventing the breath from being delivered to the lung. High airway pressure, poor oxygenation, and large fluctuations in intracranial pressures can result when a ventilator breath occurs as the infant exhales (123).

The lung injury that results from the inability to synchronize ventilator work and patient work prompted the design of sophisticated flow-sensing technology, which is used very successfully in neonatal ventilation. Flow sensors are placed between the ETT and the patient Y connector of the ventilator circuit, allowing the ventilator to monitor inspiratory and expiratory volumes and the smallest patient efforts. This technology allows the ventilator to calculate V_E and airway cuff leaks and can facilitate weaning of the ventilator by continuously assessing patient effort and spontaneous V_T. Patient-triggered ventilation was introduced to the neonatal population in the 1980s and promotes synchrony between the infant and ventilator inflations, which reduces air leaks and BPD (124). Current recommendations for neonatal ventilation include the use of patient-triggered modes to prevent patient-ventilator dyssynchrony (123, 125, 126). The introduction of patient-triggered, or synchronized, ventilation into neonatal care trailed behind its use in adults because of technological challenges imposed by the small size of preterm infants. The ideal synchronizing device must be sensitive enough to detect the effort of an extremely low-birth-weight infant, not auto-trigger (deliver a breath by reading erroneous data as patient effort), and have a quick response time to match the short T_I values and rapid RRs seen in small premature infants (123). The following section will describe the basic synchronized modes available in neonatal ventilators in the order of most support to least support. Studies show promise for both A/C and SIMV, with both pressure-controlled and volume-targeting systems. There is no clear evidence regarding which mode is superior, and it can be assumed that a single mode of ventilation would not be appropriate in every patient scenario. Selection of the mode should be based on patient characteristics and the current goals of ventilation.

Assist-control (A/C) ventilation is the least amount of work for the patient. It allows a ventilator breath to be either time triggered (initiated by the ventilator) or patient triggered, in which the ventilator senses a patient effort and initiates a ventilator breath at the T_I and PIP or V_T set by the respiratory therapist. RR set on the ventilator is a minimum or guaranteed rate that the ventilator will use in the event that no spontaneous effort is sensed. The ventilator will consider specified time periods in an attempt to evenly space ventilator breaths and prevent irregular breathing patterns. For instance, in Figure 4-8A, the ventilator is set to a rate of 30. The ventilator will look at 2-second windows of time. If the patient does not trigger the ventilator within the 2-second window, the ventilator will provide a mandatory breath at the beginning of the next 2-second window. This mode of ventilation assumes the majority of the WOB, requiring minimal effort from the patient. It is the mode that supplies the most ventilatory support, because the patient is only required to make an initial inspiratory effort and then will be provided with a full mechanical breath.

Synchronized intermittent mandatory ventilation (SIMV) will deliver the preset number of mechanical ventilator breaths. Any additional patient effort will be monitored by the ventilator but not supported in any way. The ventilator will attempt to synchronize ventilator breaths with patient efforts, but it will deliver a mandatory breath if none is sensed. To evenly space mandatory breaths and prevent irregular breathing patterns, the ventilator will observe the patient in predetermined time frames. For example, if the patient is set to an

RR of 30 breaths/minute, this would require the ventilator to deliver a breath every 2 seconds. In an attempt to synchronize these breaths, the ventilator will monitor the patient in 2-second "windows." The first respiratory effort the patient makes in that 2-second window will be a ventilator breath, while the remaining breaths will be unsupported by the ventilator. If no spontaneous effort is made within the 2-second window, then the ventilator will deliver a time-triggered (mandatory) breath at the very end of the window. See Figure 4-8B for a diagram of SIMV. This mode allows patient efforts between mechanical breaths and therefore requires the patient to assume some WOB.

Pressure support ventilation (PSV) is an assisted form of ventilation that provides a constant pressure during ventilation when it senses a patient's inspiratory effort. The patient controls T_I, RR, and inspiratory flow during PSV. V_T is determined by ΔP (PSV level – PEEP), time constant, and patient effort. The breath terminates when the ventilator senses a decrease in inspiratory flow, indicating that the patient is nearing completion of inspiration. The function of PSV is to overcome the resistance of the ventilator circuit and ETT during spontaneous ventilation, allowing lower WOB in a patient who is able to support some of his or her own ventilation. It can also be added to SIMV to support the spontaneous efforts between ventilator breaths. See Figure 4-8C for a schematic of PSV. This mode requires the patient to assume a significant portion of ventilation, and if set appropriately, will provide only enough support to overcome mechanical resistance to inspiration and to provide PEEP. One study that paired pressure support with SIMV revealed faster weaning and shorter duration of MV for preterm infants when compared with SIMV alone (127).

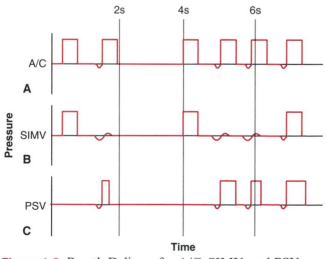

Figure 4-8 Breath Delivery for A/C, SIMV, and PSV

Oxygenation: PEEP and FIO₂

PEEP and FIO_2 are the two primary ventilator settings affecting oxygenation. PEEP should be set to help stabilize the alveoli and maintain FRC. The term "optimum" or **optimal PEEP**, is the pressure at which static lung compliance is maximized and oxygen transport is greatest. PEEP levels below optimal PEEP will cause atelectasis at end-exhalation. Levels above optimal PEEP cause some alveoli to become overexpanded, placing them on the flat upper part of the compliance curve and making them unable to accept additional volume during inspiration. Optimal PEEP will also evenly expand all alveoli at end-exhalation, allowing a more equal distribution of volumes during inspiration and maximizing the effectiveness of volume or volume-targeted ventilation.

Healthy newborns with normal lung compliance have a physiological PEEP around 3 cm H_2O, and matching that volume with the ventilator is an appropriate strategy. PEEP less than 2 cm H_2O is not recommended because the presence of an ETT bypasses the normal airway mechanics that typically provide a low-level end distending pressure during spontaneous breathing. However, a PEEP greater than 5 cm H_2O in a healthy neonate may overexpand the lungs, which could in turn impair venous return and decrease cardiac output. Patients with RDS will most often need medium levels of 4 to 7 cm H_2O, and those with severe disease may need PEEP levels of 8 to 10 cm H_2O or more to achieve adequate alveolar recruitment and improve ventilation/perfusion ratio (126). Care should be taken when selecting higher PEEP levels because greater than 8 cm H_2O can put patients with RDS at risk for pulmonary air leaks and reduction of cardiac output.

As previously discussed, FIO_2 should be adjusted to maintain an appropriate SpO_2, following a previously determined FIO_2 adjustment protocol. Oxygenation should be increased using FIO_2, and PEEP should be increased when there is evidence of derecruitment of alveoli during exhalation (see Table 4-8).

Ventilation: Pressure, Volume, and Respiratory Rate

Management of the relationship between RR and PIP in neonatal ventilation is ever evolving. These are the two parameters most commonly manipulated to maintain adequate ventilation. This is because the main determinant of gas exchange is V_E, which can be calculated by multiplying rate and volume. The equation is expressed as:

$$V_E = V_T \times RR$$

In neonatal pressure ventilation, V_T is most closely determined by PIP. In the past, several strategies of

Table 4-8 Preferred Ventilator Setting Changes to Adjust Blood Gas Values During Neonatal Mechanical Ventilation

Desired Change	FIO_2	Conventional Ventilation Volume (PIP/V_T)	Rate	PEEP	HFOV ΔP	Hz	Paw	HFJV PIP	Rate	PEEP	CMV Rate
↑ $PaCO_2$	—	↓	↓	—*	↓	↑	—	↓	—	—	—
↓ $PaCO_2$	—	↑	↑	—**	↑	↓	—	↑	↓	—**	—
↑ PaO_2	↑	—	—	↑	—	—	↑	—	—	↑	↑***
↓ PaO_2	↓	—	—	↓	—	—	↓	—	—	↓	—

*Increasing PEEP will decrease ΔP, so the RT can increase $PaCO_2$. It is not the preferred method to adjust $PaCO_2$ unless there is also radiographic evidence of atelectasis.

**Decreasing PEEP will decrease ΔP, so the RT can decrease $PaCO_2$. It is not the preferred method to adjust $PaCO_2$ unless there is also radiographic evidence of alveolar hyperinflation.

***Temporarily (15 to 30 minutes), in the presence of atelectasis, in tandem with increasing PEEP

ventilation have been described that manipulate rate and pressure relationally to maintain an appropriate acid-base balance, although no one strategy has been proven superior for patients with RDS. Normoventilation is a reasonable strategy (pH 7.35 to 7.45 and $PaCO_2$ 35 to 45 mm Hg), but the risks associated with hypocarbia in neonates is significant, causing an increase in the risk of IVH and BPD with recurrent $PaCO_2$ of less than 30 mm Hg (129, 130). There is also some evidence that hypercapnia may make VLBW infants more vulnerable to brain injury, particularly if it occurs within the first week of life (131).

Gentle ventilation was introduced in the mid-1980s as a lung-protective strategy in which a PIP is selected that provides adequate air entry and an IMV rate of 20 to 40 breaths/min is initiated and adjusted to maintain a $PaCO_2$ of 40 to 60 mm Hg (132). This type of ventilation, also described as "permissive hypercapnia," is a method in which slightly higher $PaCO_2$ or pCO_2s values are acceptable, in deference to avoiding or preventing lung injury. Initial publication of the gentle ventilation strategy occurred before synchronized ventilation or V_T monitoring capabilities, and therefore the published method of selecting ventilator settings is not consistent with current practice. It is, however, a frequently used method for patients with RDS.

Rate and Inspiration Time

Normal neonatal respiratory rate is 40 to 60 breaths/min, and normal I/E ratio (ratio of the duration of inspiration to the duration of expiration) in spontaneously breathing neonates is 1:3 to 1:4 (27). The characteristics of RDS indicate that most patients have a low lung compliance and normal airway resistance. This means that inspiratory times will be relatively short, around 0.25 to 0.40 seconds.

As with adult ventilation, ventilation for RDS can begin by supporting the majority of patient RR;

in the neonatal population, this equates to 30 to 60 breaths/min. RR should be adjusted in SIMV mode only after assessing whether alveolar recruitment is adequate and that delivered V_T is greater than 4 mL/kg (see Table 4-8). The rate should be increased in A/C if the patient is not making spontaneous respiratory effort above the minimum set ventilator rate. If a patient is consistently triggering additional ventilator breaths, increasing the rate will not result in changes to blood gas values.

Pressure

Selecting an adequate but not excessive PIP is one of the most important goals for RTs during MV for RDS. It can be challenging to find the perfect pressure, but by assessing the patient, it should be clear whether the chosen PIP is appropriate. Clinicians should continually evaluate exhaled V_T, cardiac output, pressure and volume measurements, and blood gas values to verify PIP selection. The lowest PIP that adequately ventilates the patient is the most appropriate and is seen by the following:

- Exhaled V_T greater than 3 mL/kg and less than 8 mL/kg
- pH 7.25 to 7.35 with $PaCO_2$ 45 to 55 mm Hg

Prior to having the ability to measure V_T delivered during TCPL ventilation, clinicians would select ventilator PIP based on visible chest rise and equal bilateral breath sounds. This practice is inexact and may lead to the selection of excessive pressures. It should be used only if other methods of patient assessment are not available.

Volume

Volumes for neonatal ventilation have been described differently in different studies and based on the specific modes used. The goals have ranged from 4 to 8 mL/kg, with most targeting around 4 to 6 mL/kg (102, 123, 133, 134). Lower V_T values (less than 4 mL/kg) may increase spontaneous ventilation but may also increase CO_2, lung inflammation, and WOB (128, 135).

Increases in ventilator settings may be necessary if oxygenation and ventilation fall outside the target range. When adjusting ventilator settings to decrease $PaCO_2$ and increase pH, PIP should be increased if the V_T is less than 4 mL/kg. Caution should be used if increasing PIP when V_T is between 4 and 7 mL/kg to avoid overstretching of the alveoli. If chest radiograph evidence shows atelectasis or pressure volume curves indicate that alveolar derecruitment occurs during exhalation, then PEEP and PIP should be increased incrementally (i.e., each should be increased by one unit at a time) to improve alveolar stability and maintain the previous ΔP (see Table 4-8).

Weaning

When weaning from MV, frequent small changes are preferable to occasional larger changes. To increase $PaCO_2$, decrease PIP by 1 to 2 cm H_2O (1 cm H_2O if P_aCO_2 is 35 to 40 mm Hg, 2 cm H_2O if less than 30 mm Hg) wean rate when PIP is at a minimal level of 12 to 15 cm H_2O or exhaled V_T is 4 mL/kg. Rate changes in SIMV can be made at 5- or 10-breaths/min increments, with special attention paid to how much respiratory support is being weaned. For instance, if the current RR is set at 40 breaths/min and the patient is breathing 20 additional times above the mandatory rate, decreasing the rate to 35 removes roughly 12% of the ventilator breaths supporting the patient and only 8% of the total RR for the patient. In contrast, decreasing the RR to 30 in the same patient removes 25% of ventilator-sized breaths and 17% of the total RR. Changing the RR in this patient by 5 breaths/min may not provide a significant change in CO_2 because it may not have a significant impact on V_E. However, the same patient may have ineffective spontaneous V_T, causing a small change in ventilator rate to have a larger effect on V_E.

Minimal ventilator settings in patients with RDS are not consistent from institution to institution. However, extubation should be considered when the multidisciplinary health-care team is confident that the patient can support his or her own V_E. Trials of ETT CPAP are not recommended in neonates because the high resistance to gas flow through the ETT causes very high WOB that may give the impression that the patient is "failing" a spontaneous breathing trial (136), when in fact the patient failed the ability to breathe through the ETT. Some publications have described using short trials of ETT CPAP lasting between 3 and 10 minutes. If the patient is able to support his or her own V_E without

bradycardia, hypoxemia (SpO_2 less than 85%), or an increase in FIO_2, then the patient is considered to be ready for extubation (137, 138). A patient can be considered to be on minimal ventilator settings when he or she is achieving normoventilation on the following:

- FIO_2 less than 0.40
- PIP 10 to 15 cm H_2O
- Rate 10 to 20 breaths/min

Extubation to NCPAP is a commonly used method of weaning in neonatal units (139), and a NCPAP level of 5 to 6 cm H_2O is usually appropriate.

Approximately 30% of intubated preterm infants fail an extubation attempt, requiring reintubation and MV. Extubation failure in ELBW infants is mainly caused by upper-airway instability, poor respiratory drive, and alveolar atelectasis or derecruitment (140). The rate of extubation failure using NCPAP is similar at 25% to 40% (139).

Failing Conventional Mechanical Ventilation

There are no standard guidelines for patients who have failed a course of conventional ventilation (CV), but failure can be considered if that patient's pH cannot be consistently maintained at more than 7.20 with $PaCO_2$ levels greater than 60 mm Hg. Ventilation that causes a significant impedance on cardiac output and any level of pulmonary air leaks during MV (see Chapter 7 for more information on pulmonary air leaks) should both be contributing factors in the decision to move to high-frequency ventilation.

■ ■ After delivery of an analgesic, you intubate BG Gibbs with a 2.5-cm ETT 7 cm at the lip, observing chest rise, misting in the tube, and colorimetric end-tidal CO_2, along with equal breath sounds. You deliver the surfactant dose and begin SIMV plus volume guarantee, PIP 20 cm H_2O, PEEP 5 cm H_2O, target V_T 3.5 mL, RR 40 breaths/min, T_I 0.30 sec, and FIO_2 0.40. A postintubation chest radiograph shows good ETT placement midway between the clavicles and carina, lung inflation to the eighth rib posteriorly, and minimal air bronchograms, although there are still some areas of atelectasis. A follow-up ABG 30 minutes after initiation of ventilation reveals a pH of 7.40, $PaCO_2$ of 38 mm Hg, P_aO_2 of 68 mm Hg, and HCO_3 of 23.2 mEq/L. Because of the recent surfactant delivery and a good spontaneous respiratory rate, you and the neonatologist agree to lower the rate to 35 breaths/min, and the follow-up gas is pH 7.37, $PaCO_2$ 41, PaO_2 64 mm Hg, and HCO_3 23.4 mEq/L.

High-Frequency Ventilation

High-frequency ventilation (HFV) uses rapid respiratory rates (greater than 150 breaths/min) and very small V_T (usually less than anatomical dead space) to provide ventilation and lung protection. HFV has been used both as an initial therapy for RDS and as a rescue modality for neonates who fail attempts at conventional methods of ventilation. When used appropriately, HFV improves oxygenation, CO_2 elimination, and circulation in infants with RDS (141). The theory of rapid shallow breathing was suggested in 1915 by a scientist named Yandell Henderson, who observed that dogs can pant indefinitely while still maintaining normocarbia. He did a series of experiments to illustrate the physiological mechanisms that make HFV an effective therapy (142). HFV sends a steady stream of very small volume into the airways at a high velocity, using relatively low pressures and using PEEP or Paw to maintain alveolar stability. Using higher Paw and small volumes allows minimizing of overdistention and underdistention of the lung and ventilating in the safe window (Fig. 4-9). The net effect of several breaths is that fresh gas will advance down the core of the airways to the alveoli, allowing diffusion of gas through the A-C membrane. Exhaled gas will move out along the airway walls, in a cyclic pattern around the incoming gas and out the large airways. This method of ventilation decouples oxygenation and ventilation, meaning that changes on the ventilator can be made that affect only oxygenation and that have little effect on CO_2, and vice versa. Changing the continuous distending pressure (CDP) will adjust oxygenation, and making changes in delivered volume will affect CO_2 clearance. In CV, $V_E = RR \times V_T$. In HFV, $V_E = RR \times V_T^2$. This means that small changes in volume will have a profound effect on CO_2 clearance. When adjusting HFV settings to improve CO_2 clearance, changes in volume will be more effective than changes in the rate. The leak around the ETT also helps to facilitate more effective CO_2 removal, with CO_2 escaping around the tube rather than having to move through it.

Higher ventilating pressures can be used during HFV because the pressure attenuates as it moves down the airway to the alveoli. At each point where the pressure waves hit an area of restriction or impedance, the pressure decreases, causing as much as a 90% drop in delivered pressure (143). HFV can overcome the complication of unequal gas distribution by using intra-alveolar communication to help more evenly distribute gas from well-inflated alveoli to adjacent atelectatic alveoli.

The complications of HFV are usually caused by the selection or continuance of inappropriate settings. They include the following:

- **Hypocarbia:** HFV, when used appropriately, is very effective at CO_2 clearance. This makes it easy to inadvertently cause hypocarbia, which can contribute to lung and brain injury. Blood gases should be followed closely, and HFV should be provided by clinicians familiar with its use to avoid this complication.
- **Air trapping:** With rapid rates, it is possible to allow inadequate time for exhalation, which will cause air trapping. This is most frequently manifested as auto-PEEP, which can be directly measured in high-frequency jet ventilation (HFJV) or can be presumed by observing chest radiographs and the presence of hypercarbia as seen in ABGs.
- **Excessive Paw:** This can occur when HFV is used in patients with very poor compliance. Once the alveoli are recruited, Paw needs to be reassessed and decreased if it is excessive. Paw that is left at a high setting will overstretch the alveoli and may interfere with gas exchange and cardiac output. Chest radiographs allow clinicians to visualize lung recruitment to determine when to decrease Paw.
- **Inadequate Paw:** Fear of barotrauma and lung injury makes it common for PEEP or Paw to be set too low during HFV, which will lead to alveolar derecruitment and poor oxygenation and ventilation.

There are two types of HFV: high-frequency oscillatory ventilation (HFOV) and HFJV (Fig. 4-10). The physiological mechanisms for the two forms of HFV are the same, but there are many differences between the two that make it challenging to understand and compare them.

HFOV allows the clinician to directly set Paw, which controls oxygenation along with FIO_2. During HFJV, PEEP and PIP are the primary factors that control Paw. Frequency, inspiratory time (T_I), and FIO_2 are set on both devices. During HFOV, amplitude ΔP) and Paw are set, whereas PIP and PEEP are set during HFJV. These differences limit the ability to extrapolate understanding of one device to the other or to compare management strategies during clinical research

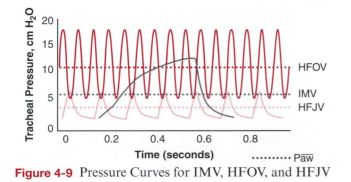

Figure 4-9 Pressure Curves for IMV, HFOV, and HFJV

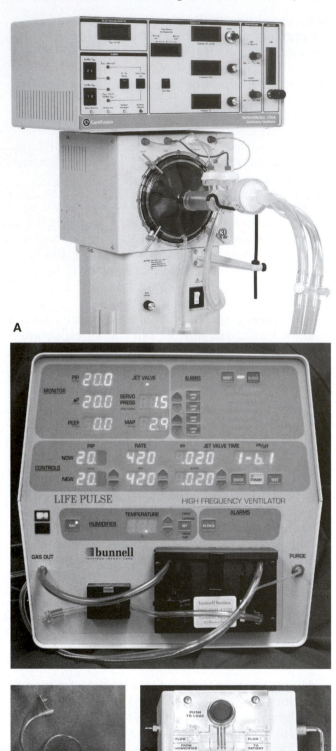

Figure 4-10 Sensormedics 3100A Oscillator (A) and Bunnell Jet Ventilator with Whisper Valve and Endotracheal Tube Adapter (B) *(Courtesy of CareFusion, Inc., and Bunnell, Inc.)*

(144). Large randomized studies of CV versus HFJV or HFOV have failed to show a difference in outcomes based on which initial ventilator modality is used in extremely premature infants (145, 146).

High-Frequency Oscillatory Ventilation

High-frequency oscillatory ventilation (HFOV) is a piston-diaphragm oscillator that uses rates of 180 to 900 coupled with a directly set Paw to manage oxygenation and ventilation. It has an active exhalation, meaning that it rapidly forces breaths into and pulls them out of the airway to facilitate CO_2 clearance. It was approved for use in 1991 in neonates with RDS who fail conventional MV (147). Patients provided with early HFOV may need fewer doses of surfactant than do those on CV (148), and at least one recent (2010) study is showing promise for HFOV to improve survival and lower incidence of lung injury over CV for VLBW infants (149).

The key difference between HFOV and other available modes of HFV is the active exhalation feature. The piston has an initial placement at the set Paw. During inhalation, the piston moves forward to displace gas into the ETT and down the airway to the alveoli. After reaching the peak of the inspiration, the piston reverses and actively pulls gas from the airway, providing an equal displacement below the Paw setting. The piston is continuously in motion, meaning that the oscillator is always in the act of either inspiration or exhalation; there is no time in the respiratory cycle without gas movement. The physiological result is that the volume of gas per breath, often called stroke volume, is increased when the HFOV rate is decreased, allowing a decrease in rate to significantly increase minute volume.

Initial settings for HFOV in patients with RDS who fail an initial trial of CV are (150) as follows:

- **Bias flow:** 10 to 15 LPM
- **Frequency (hertz):** 1 hertz (Hz) = 60 breaths. A range of 10 to 15 Hz has been found to be effective for both premature and near-term patients. In clinical practice, higher frequencies are associated with smaller patients, and as patient weight increases, the hertz value decreases.
- **Paw:** The initial setting should be slightly higher (1 to 2 cm H_2O) than the measured Paw on CV.
- **Percent of inspiratory time:** This should be set at 33%, which will provide an I/E ratio of 1:2.
- **Amplitude (ΔP):** Amplitude is adjusted using the "power" control knob. Higher power settings mean a larger displacement of the piston with each inhalation and exhalation. Start the power knob around 2 and increase the level until appropriate chest wiggle is seen. This continuous, visible vibration from the umbilicus to the nipple line is frequently referred to as "chest wiggle factor," and is used by clinicians to evaluate adequacy of amplitude during HFOV.

A blood gas should be obtained within 45 to 60 minutes and a chest radiograph obtained within 4 hours of initiating HFOV to assess acid-base status and lung inflation, respectively. Radiographic evidence should show observation of lung expansion to eight to nine posterior ribs or decreased opacification from previous radiographs.

Adjusting Settings

Ventilation should be primarily managed by adjusting the pressure amplitude. Increasing ΔP improves ventilation. At initiation of therapy, adjust ΔP just high enough to produce perceptible chest wiggle and adjust in 1- to 2-cm H_2O increments, increasing to improve CO_2 removal and decreasing if ventilation is excessive, similar to PIP on CV. If maximum ΔP is unable to sufficiently improve ventilation, reduce the frequency by 1 Hz to increase delivered V_T. A decrease in frequency equals increased V_T. An increase in frequency equals decreased V_T.

Oxygenation should be managed by maintaining Paw at the level necessary to obtain satisfactory pulmonary inflation. A chest radiograph that reveals lung inflation of nine posterior ribs above the level of the diaphragm has been used as an indication of satisfactory inflation.

If lung compliance improves, then Paw must be reduced to avoid lung overinflation. Place priority on weaning FIO_2 to less than 0.6 before weaning to lower Paws. Once FIO_2 is less than 0.6, shift the emphasis to weaning Paw, while still maintaining normal lung inflation and PaO_2 (143). If diaphragm expansion is nine rib levels or more, decrease the Paw 1 cm H_2O at a time. Serial chest radiographs should be obtained at least once a day within the first week of HFOV and more frequently in the first 24 hours. Any time that lung under- or overinflation is suspected or patient oxygenation has changed significantly, a chest radiograph is warranted.

Complications

HFOV has inherent risks in this patient population, which are similar to the risks of CV: under- or overventilation, under- or overhumidification, IVH, BPD, necrotizing tracheal bronchitis, atelectasis, hypotension, and air leak syndromes (143). The noncompliant nature of the circuit and the need for patients to be reasonably still to maintain airway patency also increase the risk of accidental extubation during HFOV.

Weaning

Patients with RDS who are on HFOV can be weaned to CV when all the following conditions have been satisfied:

- Paw has been weaned to the 6- to 12-cm H_2O range.
- Amplitude pressure has been weaned to less than 30 cm H_2O.

- Arterial blood gases have been stabilized in the following ranges:
pH = 7.25 to 7.45
$PaCO_2$ = 35 to 50 mm Hg
PaO_2 = 50 to 80 mm Hg

High-Frequency Jet Ventilation

High-frequency jet ventilation began to be studied in the 1970s as a method to safely ventilate premature lungs, and the strategy was refined over the next several decades. **High-frequency jet ventilation (HFJV)** uses a transitional flow pattern of gas delivery that allows fresh, oxygen-rich gas to travel down the center of the airways in small bursts at very high velocity, getting downstream from restricted portions of the airways reaching the alveoli and bypassing damaged portions of the lung without leaking. Exhalation is passive during HFJV, and CO_2 travels via the path of least resistance, which is against the airway walls in a counter-current helical flow pattern (151). Passive exhalation during HFJV allows effective ventilation and oxygenation at lower Paws than does HFOV. HFJV rates are about 10 times faster than CV, but V_T values are about five times smaller, making it less likely for volumes to be trapped during exhalation. Some small studies have supported its use to decrease the risk of BPD, but the long-term risks are unclear (152).

HFJV is used in tandem with a conventional ventilator. The purpose of the ventilator is threefold: (1) it provides fresh gas for a patient's spontaneous respiratory effort, (2) it maintains PEEP settings, and if necessary, (3) it provides "sigh breaths" to reexpand atelectatic lung units. The HFJV provides PIP, RR, and T_I.

Initiating and adjusting settings on the HFJV are straightforward. To begin, the patient's standard ETT adapter is replaced with the LifePort adapter, which is connected to the CV, traditionally, and to the HFJV through a side port on the LifePort adapter.

- **PIP:** Peak inspiratory pressure is approximately the same as that of the previous conventional ventilator.
- **Rate:** The RR is 420 breaths/min. Studies were done to show that rates of 320 to 520 produced approximately the same $PaCO_2$ in patients with RDS (153).
- **T_I:** Time is 0.02 seconds.
- **PEEP:** Start at 7 to 12 cm H_2O and increase until SpO_2 is stable in the prescribed range without an increase in FIO_2 (while the ventilator is in CPAP mode). This PEEP setting is known as the optimal PEEP in HFJV.
- **IMV settings:** The rate on the ventilator should only be used to reverse atelectasis. It is incorporated for short time frames, similar to sigh breaths, and is removed once alveolar recruitment is completed. The PIP should be adjusted to achieve visible chest rise, with a T_I of around

0.4 seconds and a rate of 5 to 10 breaths/min. Once O_2 saturation improves, lung recruitment using IMV breaths should be discontinued.

Adjusting Settings

To manage ventilation and oxygenation with HFJV, the following guidelines are helpful. The main determinant of CO_2 clearance is V_T, which is determined by ΔP. To increase CO_2 on blood gas, decreasing HFJV PIP is the best option. To lower CO_2, increase HFJV PIP. Changing HFJV rate will have a significant impact on CO_2 clearance only if the reason for hypercapnia is air trapping. In this case, decreasing rate will increase expiratory time, allowing time for more effective exhalation and thus decreasing CO_2.

Oxygenation is managed by adjusting PEEP and FIO_2. Initial PEEP should be set to maintain alveolar stability. With poor oxygenation and atelectasis, PEEP should be increased. Caution must be used when adjusting PEEP alone because it will also adjust ΔP, which will change CO_2. If CO_2 is adequate, incremental changes of PEEP and PIP will maintain ΔP while still giving the desired effect for PO_2. An example would be to change a patient with atelectasis from 18/5 to 19/6, maintaining a ΔP of 13 cm H_2O. In the absence of atelectasis, FIO_2 should be increased to improve PO_2.

An additional benefit when using HFJV is the ability to monitor servo pressure (154). Servo pressure is the driving pressure of the HFJV. It automatically regulates how much gas flow is needed to deliver a set PIP. Servo pressure changes can be an early warning of changes in the patient's condition. In general, increases in servo pressure mean an increase in lung compliance or improvement in lung function. A decrease in servo pressure indicates the following:

- Decrease in lung compliance (such as with a pneumothorax)
- Worsening lung resistance
- Obstructed ETT
- Mucus in the airway or that the patient needs suctioning

Weaning

Patients with RDS on HFJV can be weaned to CV when the following conditions have been satisfied:

- HFJV PIP has been weaned to a level comparable to an SIMV PIP
- Paw is less than 12 cm H_2O
- Servo pressure indicates an improvement in lung compliance

A short trial of CV can be achieved by placing the ventilator's neonatal flow sensor in line, increasing the RR on SIMV, and placing the HFJV in standby mode. If the patient tolerates SIMV for more than 1 hour and the result of a follow-up blood gas shows adequate ventilation, then the HFJV can be disconnected from the ETT and the patient can continue on SIMV.

Pain Management

Premature infants lack the autonomic and functional maturity to handle the noisy, chaotic, stressful, and painful extrauterine environment. Sick infants are also routinely exposed to a myriad of painful interventions, and the consequences include altered brain development and learning and behavioral difficulties in later childhood (155). Routine painful procedures that neonates experience include needle insertions, tape removal, diaper changes, physical examinations, nursing evaluations, and exposure to environmental stimuli (156). Procedures commonly provided by RTs are considered painful, including heel sticks for capillary blood gas (CBG) readings, arterial punctures, endotracheal suctioning, and prolonged MV.

Premature infants respond differently to pain, and their physiological response includes desaturation, bradycardia or tachycardia, apnea, or tachypnea. It has also been argued that acutely ill infants are less capable of manifesting behavioral responses to pain (155), meaning that it may not be clear to clinicians when neonates are feeling pain, although other physiological responses, such as alterations in cerebral blood flow and IVH (157), may still occur. There are several different tools designed to evaluate infant pain; an example is the premature infant pain profile (PIPP), which is a validated tool used in neonatal units internationally to assess behavioral and physiological indicators of pain in this population (158). It is important to treat a patient who is exhibiting signs of pain, but one of the most effective strategies is to prevent pain whenever possible (Clinical Variations 4-2). RTs should consider the following and discuss with the team how to best employ these strategies to minimize the number or effect of minor painful or stressful procedures:

1. Reduce the number of painful procedures performed by eliminating those that are unnecessary.
2. Bundle interventions together so that there are longer "hands-free" periods.
3. Use nonpharmacological pain prevention, such as oral sucrose or glucose (160), breastfeeding, nonnutritive sucking, skin-to-skin contact (known as "kangaroo care"), facilitated tuck (holding the arms and legs in a flexed position), and swaddling (161).
4. Apply topical anesthetics 30 minutes before procedures such as venipuncture, lumbar puncture, and intravenous catheter insertion.
5. Understand the perceived benefits of pain management for mechanically ventilated neonates, including improved patient-ventilator

Clinical Variations 4-2

The 10 Commandments of Pain Assessment and Management in Preterm Neonates (159)

Neonatal clinicians used to function under the myth that preterm infants couldn't feel pain because of the immaturity of their central nervous systems, even though observation of neonates during invasive procedures show a clear indication that they have both a physiological and behavioral response to pain. This, unfortunately, has historically caused clinicians to frequently undertreat pain in neonates, although the ethical principle of nonmaleficence obligates clinicians to care for patients in a way that causes no harm. Neonatal nurses have taken initiatives to improve the management of pain for premature infants and have created a set of 10 "commandments" for clinicians to follow, given from the perspective of the patient.

1. Take time to consider whether you can prevent me from experiencing pain as part of my medical care.
2. My signs of pain may be subtle or brief, but it does not mean that I don't have pain.
3. Take the time to manage my pain appropriately and put my needs ahead of your own.
4. Stay with me during painful procedures to help me cope with the pain and stress.
5. Use best pharmacological practices to manage my pain.
6. Make sure you know the side effects of pain medications and monitor me closely to keep me safe.
7. Be aware that, however you manage my pain, I will never forget it.
8. Please take care when you discontinue or wean my pain medications because I may have become dependent on these medications and need you to monitor my vital signs and behaviors for signs of opioid withdrawal.
9. Include my parents and other caregivers in decisions that affect my care.
10. If and when my death draws near, please stay with me and my parents.

synchrony, improved pulmonary function, and decreased catecholamine responses (162). Complications to treatment are associated with the selected analgesic and include hypotension from morphine and chest wall rigidity from fentanyl. Other complications include tolerance, dependence, and withdrawal. There is limited research in this area, but what is available shows that continuous opioid infusion for chronically ventilated preterm infants is associated with an

increase in ventilator settings (163) and prolonged duration of MV (164) without improving the long-term risk of brain injury (165, 166); therefore, their routine use is not recommended. Selective use of opioids has been recommended only after evaluation of pain, and morphine has been shown to be safer than midazolam in limited studies (167). Preliminary data also suggest that opioid infusion within the first 3 days of life may increase mortality and risk for long-term sequelae such as retinopathy of prematurity, BPD, and IVH (168).

Course and Prognosis

Survival of preterm neonates has steadily improved since the 1960s, with the gestational age at which at least half of the infants survive decreasing from 30 to 31 weeks in the 1960s to 23 to 24 weeks during the 2000s (169). Overall infant mortality in 2006 was 6.68 infants per 1,000 live births, with the second leading cause of death being disorders of preterm birth and low birth weight. Neonates born less than 32 wG comprised 2% of the infant population but constituted 54% of infant deaths (170). The mortality rate for infants with RDS has dropped significantly since the 1960s, from 236 per 100,000 live births in 1968 to 18.5 per 100,000 live births in 2007 (1). It is promising to note that, as of the 1990s, more than 50% of newborns 24 to 25 wG survive to hospital discharge (171). One study in Missouri, however, found a discrepancy between the diagnosis on medical records and those found on death certificates, suggesting that mortality of RDS may be underreported depending on where the data are derived (172).

The improvement in prenatal care has led to better neonatal survival, but has brought an increase in morbidity. For instance, a 2007 study showed a decrease in mortality from 52.1% to 31.8% in infants 25 to 27 wG, but an increase in incidence of BPD from 40.3% to 60% in the same age group (173). Short-term morbidities for premature infants include BPD (discussed in Chapter 5), persistent patent ductus arteriosus, IVH, periventricular leukomalacia, retinopathy of prematurity, and NEC (discussed in Chapter 8). Long-term morbidities consist of neurodevelopmental sequelae such as cerebral palsy, cognitive delay, blindness, and deafness; CLD; failure to thrive; feeding difficulties; and complications such as subglottic stenosis following prolonged endotracheal intubation (174).

Neurodevelopmental disability is a major cause of morbidity in extremely premature infants but is hard to quantify because many signs and symptoms do not manifest until school age or older. One longitudinal study assessed children who had been born at less than 25 wG at 6 years of age and found that 99% of those born at 23 wG had neurodevelopmental disability, and the incidence only decreased to 92% for children born at 25 wG (175). Cerebral palsy, a broad term for a group of motor-impairment syndromes, is not diagnosed until 3 to 5 years of age, so data currently available on its incidence in preterm infants may not accurately reflect recent changes in neonatal care. A 2005 study showed a decrease in mortality but an increase in cerebral palsy from 16% to 25%, with additional increases in the rate of deafness and general neurodevelopmental impairment (176). Infants surviving RDS will require more special education services and need to be followed closely through those services, particularly if they are living in poverty (177), because they may have less access to resources to improve cognitive and motor development.

The major long-term respiratory complication of a preterm birth is BPD, which occurs in about 20% of ventilated infants (178). Even in children who do not develop BPD, pulmonary function tests of those with RDS at school age show alterations in lung function (179, 180). Prematurity has been a risk factor for the development of reactive airway disease later in life, though studies are unclear on whether RDS alone will increase the risk for wheezing or if postneonatal health problems and environmental factors are more important determinants for its development (181). In a study of 126 preterm infants, cough occurred in 80%, wheeze in 44%, rehospitalization in 25%, and long-term inhalation therapy in those who wheeze occurred in 13%, even without being diagnosed with BPD (182).

One publication suggests five respiratory practices to improve neonatal outcomes and decrease costs for children born before 33 wG.

1. Exclusive use of bubble CPAP
2. Use of bubble CPAP in the delivery room
3. Strict intubation criteria for infants with recurrent apnea, hypoventilation, and $PaCO_2$ greater than 65 mm Hg for more than one ABG test
4. Strict extubation criteria within 1 hour of surfactant delivery or within 2 to 6 hours of reaching a predetermined extubation criteria
5. Prolonged CPAP without NC oxygen before 35 weeks postmenstrual age (183)

Early data from this initiative showed it has reduced the number of intubations, hypotension due to respiratory interventions, incidence of BPD, as well as earlier extubation, and has decreased equipment and surfactant costs.

Approximately 2% of the NICU population will develop sensorineural hearing loss (184). One 2011 study noted that hearing loss occurred in 5% of infants, and the largest noncongenital risk factor for hearing loss was being subjected to more than 5 days of MV (185).

Despite the improved survival, there are additional long-term factors for children and families

surviving RDS. For instance, health-care costs for infants less than 32 wG with morbidities are 4.4 times greater than for children without morbidities, which emphasizes the importance of preventing long-term sequelae for premature infants (186). Several therapies have been moderately successful in animal models when treating RDS or preventing CLD, but they are not currently recommended for routine use in preterm infants. These include the following:

- Antithrombin
- Thyroid hormone
- Inhaled nitric oxide (iNO)
- Digoxin
- Diuretics

■■ BG Gibbs remained on volume-guarantee SIMV for 9 days. She was extubated on day of life (DOL) 10 to NCPAP plus 5 cm H_2O until DOL 15, when she was placed on a HFNC for 1 week. She was then changed to an NC at 1 LPM for 9 days at an FIO_2 of 0.21 to 0.28. She is now 29 5/7 wG, and you have just discontinued her NC.

■■ Critical Thinking Questions: BG Gibbs

1. Do you think BG Gibbs should have been intubated so quickly after admission to the NICU? Were there other interventions you might have suggested to the physician?
2. How would you assess BG Gibbs for resolution of RDS? How would you know that she was no longer experiencing respiratory distress?
3. BG Gibbs seems to tolerate conventional ventilation well. What are some signs you should look for that would tell you she should be managed with HFV?

❯● Case Studies and Critical Thinking Questions

■ Case 1: Baby Boy (BB) Goldstein

You are the dayshift RT at a level IIIC NICU. Three days ago, you attended the delivery of BB Goldstein, a 550-g, 23 2/7 wG male born to a 22-year-old woman with chorioamnionitis. Apgar scores were 1 at 1 minute and 3 at 5 minutes. He showed no signs of respiratory effort in the delivery room, necessitating intubation and administration of exogenous surfactant by 5 minutes of age.

After transport to the NICU, he was placed on SIMV, PIP 22 cm H_2O, PEEP 4 cm H_2O, RR 30 breaths/min, T_I 0.35 sec, and FIO_2 0.60. Initial blood gas values were adequate. He has received three additional doses of surfactant in the last 48 hours and is now 72 hours old. You begin your shift and note in your report that BB Goldstein's RR has been increased to 60 breaths/min and PEEP to 6 cm H_2O to compensate for worsening respiratory acidosis. You are at the bedside 1 hour later and notice his retractions are more severe, and he is agitated and dusky.

- *What could be the cause for BB Goldstein's respiratory distress?*

You auscultate and hear equal breath sounds bilaterally with crackles at end-exhalation. Measured values on the ventilator include a spontaneous RR of 12 breaths/min, Paw of 11 cm H_2O, and exhaled V_T of 2 mL. Current SpO_2 is 87% on FIO_2 0.60, and BB Goldstein's mean arterial BP has

fallen from 42 to 35 mm Hg. You request a chest radiograph and obtain a blood sample for an ABG test from the umbilical artery catheter. The radiograph shows atelectasis and air bronchograms, as well as patchy infiltrates. ABG test results are pH 7.19, $PaCO_2$ 55 mm Hg, PaO_2 51 mm Hg, HCO_3 20.7 mEq/L.

- *Based on this information, what would you recommend?*

You discuss the options with the neonatologist, and you together agree to begin HFOV. While another RT pulls the ventilator to the bedside and does initial leak testing and pressure calibration, you discuss with the physician initial HFOV settings.

- *What are your recommended settings? How would you assess whether they are adequate?*

Multiple-Choice Questions

1. Which of the following are characteristics of RDS?
   I. Surfactant deficiency
   II. Lung hypoplasia
   III. Low-compliance chest wall
   IV. Reticulogranular pattern on chest radiograph
   V. Hypocarbia
   VI. See-saw breathing pattern
   a. I, II, III, IV, V, VI
   b. I, II, IV, VI
   c. I, II, IV, V, VI
   d. I, II, IV, V

2. You are in the delivery room preparing for the delivery of a 27 6/7 wG male. The team leader for the resuscitation requests that you provide respiratory support for the newborn upon delivery. Which of the following is your preferred plan?
   a. Begin immediate bag-mask ventilation after his arrival to the radiant warmer
   b. Provide NCPAP via T-piece resuscitator after verifying that he has spontaneous. respiratory effort
   c. Intubate and provide surfactant treatment within the first 3 minutes of life
   d. Observe the newborn and provide ventilatory or oxygen support as needed, based on his ability to support his own respiration

3. You are caring for a 28 wG boy, now 6 hours old. His HR is 140 bpm, RR 65 breaths/min, SpO_2 89% on 1 LPM NC, FIO_2 0.40. You are completing a respiratory assessment and note that he has see-saw respirations, mild intercostal retractions, visible xiphoid retractions, marked nasal flaring, and expiratory grunting when you listen with a stethoscope. What is his Silverman-Andersen score?
   a. 6
   b. 7
   c. 8
   d. 9

4. What change in respiratory support would you suggest for the above patient?
   a. Increase FIO_2 to 1
   b. Increase NC to 2 LPM
   c. Change to NCPAP plus 5 cm H_2O
   d. Intubate and place on A/C, V_T 6 mL/kg

5. Your NICU is rewriting its policy on surfactant-replacement therapy. You are asked to provide the description of expected positive response during this pharmacological therapy. Which of the following will you include in the policy?
   a. Improvement in SpO_2
   b. Reduction in FIO_2
   c. Decreased WOB
   d. Increased V_T during pressure ventilation
   e. All of the above

6. You are caring for a 4-day-old infant born at 24 5/7 wG. She was given a dose of surfactant in the delivery room and extubated to NCPAP of 5 cm H_2O, on which she has remained. She is now on a variable-flow NCPAP of 6 cm H_2O and FIO_2 0.70, and her CBG is pH 7.24, $PcCO_2$ 56 mm Hg, PcO_2 44 mm Hg, HCO_3 23.7 mEq/L. She has been having increased periods of apnea, with bradycardia and hypoxemia. What is your recommended course of action?
   a. Intubate and place on SIMV
   b. Intubate, give a second dose of surfactant, then resume NCPAP
   c. Continue on NCPAP of 6 cm H_2O and observe for 2 to 4 hours, assessing for signs of improvement in respiratory status
   d. Change to NIPPV at a rate of 5, with a PIP of 24 cm H_2O and a T_I of 0.6 seconds

7. Which of the following are benefits of using volume-targeted ventilation in neonates with RDS?
   VII. Avoiding overventilation
   VIII. Varying V_T based on lung compliance changes
   IX. Avoiding underventilation
   X. Promoting more uniform gas delivery
   XI. Providing a square waveform pattern
   a. I, IV
   b. I, II, III
   c. I, III, IV
   d. I, III, V

8. You are caring for BG Guthrie, a 25 6/7 wG girl who is now 4 days old. She is intubated with a 2.5-cm ETT taped 7.5 cm at the lip, on SIMV with volume guarantee: PEEP plus 5 cm H_2O, RR 35 breaths/min, PIP 18 cm H_2O, volume guarantee 3 mL, and FIO_2 0.40. You assess her at the beginning of your shift and note that her total HR is 142 bpm, RR is 50 breaths/min, and SpO_2 is 89%. Exhaled volumes are being met at 3 mL during SIMV breaths, with a PIP delivered at 17 to 19 cm H_2O; her exhaled V_T with spontaneous breaths is 3.7 mL. BG Guthrie's RN noted that today's weight is now 785 g, an increase from the last weight 2 days earlier. Her CXR shows lung inflation to seven ribs, and ABG values from umbilical artery catheter was pH 7.28, $PaCO_2$ 54 mm Hg, PaO_2 50 mm Hg, and HCO_3 25 mEq/L. Based on this information, what would you like to do?
   a. Nothing: Her vital signs, laboratory test data, and ventilator measurements are all within acceptable range
   b. Increase PEEP to plus 6 cm H_2O to improve lung inflation
   c. Increase PIP to 20 cm H_2O to increase V_T delivery
   d. Increase VG to 4.0 mL to improve exhaled V_T
   e. Increase rate to 40 breaths/min to better support her spontaneous respirations

9. How should Paw be chosen during initiation of HFOV?
   a. Set to the same value as the measured Paw on CV
   b. Use the optimal PEEP strategy to find what Paw is necessary to avoid hypoxemia
   c. Set 1 to 2 cm H_2O higher than the measured Paw on CV
   d. Set 2 to 3 cm H_2O below the PIP on CV

10. What is the correct initial rate for HFJV?
   a. Set to 420 breaths/min
   b. Select higher rates for smaller patients, up to a rate of 660 breaths/min
   c. Set the HFJV rate to 420 breaths/min and CMV to 5 or 10 breaths/min
   d. Multiply current rate on the ventilator by 10

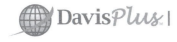

For additional resources login to Davis*Plus* (http://davisplus.fadavis.com/ keyword "Perretta") and click on the Premium tab. (Don't have a *Plus*Code to access Premium Resources? Just click the Purchase Access button on the book's Davis*Plus* page.)

REFERENCES

1. March of Dimes. *March of Dimes 2011 Premature Birth Report Card.* http://www.marchofdimes.com/peristats/pdflib/998/US.pdf. Accessed July 1, 2012.

2. March of Dimes. *National Perinatal Information System/Quality Analytic Services: Special Care Nursery Admissions.* http://www.marchofdimes.com/peristats/pdfdocs/nicu_summary_final.pdf. Accessed July 1, 2012.

3. Lantos JD. *The Lazarus Case: Life-and-Death Issues in Neonatal Intensive Care.* Baltimore, MD: The Johns Hopkins University Press; 2001.

4. Berkowitz GS, Papiernik E. Epidemiology of preterm birth. *Epidemiol Rev.* 1993;15(2):414-443.

5. Kramer MS, Goulet L, Lydon J, et al. Socio-economic disparities in preterm birth: causal pathways and mechanisms. *Paediatr Perinat Epidemiol.* 2001;15(suppl 2):104-123.

6. March of Dimes. *What we know about prematurity.* https://www.marchofdimes.com/mission/prematurity_indepth.html. Updated April 2012. Accessed July 4, 2012.

7. Seri I, Evans J. Limits of viability: definition of the gray zone. *J Perinatol.* 2008;28:S4-S8.

8. Boss RD, Hutton N, Sulpar LJ, et al. Values parents apply to decision-making regarding delivery room resuscitation of high-risk newborns. *Pediatrics.* 2008;122:583-589.

9. March of Dimes. *March of Dimes Perinatal Data Center: Special Care Nursery Admissions.* http://www.marchofdimes.com/peristats/pdfdocs/nicu_summary_final.pdf. 2011. Accessed September 28, 2012.

10. Raju TNK, Higgins RD, Stark AR, et al. Optimizing care and outcome for late preterm (near-term) infants: a summary of the workshop sponsored by the NICHD. *Pediatrics.* 2006;118:1207-1214.

11. Wilson-Costello D, Friedman H, Minich N, et al. Improved survival rates with increased neurodevelopmental disability for extremely low birth weight infants in the 1990s. *Pediatrics.* 2005;115:997-1003.

12. Claireaux AE. Hyaline membrane in the neonatal lung. *Lancet.* 1953;262(6789):749-753.

13. Custer JW, Rau RE, eds. *The Harriet Lane Handbook.* Philadelphia, PA: Mosby Elsevier; 2009:Box 4-3.

14. Gomella TL. *Neonatology: Management, Procedures, On-Call Problems, Diseases, Drugs.* New York: McGraw-Hill; 2004.

15. National Heart, Lung, and Blood Institute. *Morbidity and Mortality: 2012 Chart Book on Cardiovascular, Lung, and Blood Diseases.* Bethesda, MD: National Institutes of Health; 2012.

16. Horbar JD, Badger GJ, Carpenter JH, et al. Mortality and morbidity for very low birth weights infants, 1991-1999. *Pediatrics.* 2002;110:143-151.

17. Fehlman E, Tapia JL. Impact of respiratory distress syndrome in very low birth weight infants: a multicenter South-American study. *Arch Argent Pediatr.* 2010;108(5):393-400.

18. Miller HC, Futrakul P. Birth weight, gestational age, and sex as determining factors in the incidence of respiratory distress syndrome of prematurely born infants. *Pediatrics.* 1968;72(5):628-635.

19. Hamvas A, Wise PH, Yang RK, et al. The influence of the wider use of surfactant therapy on neonatal mortality among blacks and whites. *N Engl J Med.* 1996;334(25):1635-1640.

20. Hyaline membrane. *Lancet.* 1958;2(7053):945-946.

21. Serrano AC, Pérez-Gil J. Protein-lipid interactions and surface activity in the pulmonary surfactant system. *Chem Phys Lipids.* 2006;141(1-2):105-118.

22. Wüstneck R, Pérez-Gil J, Wüstneck N, et al. Interfacial properties of pulmonary surfactant layers. *Adv Colloid Interface Sci.* 2005;117(1-3):33-58.

23. Schürch D, Ospina OL, Cruz A, et al. Combined and independent action of proteins SP-B and SP-C in the surface behavior and mechanical stability of pulmonary surfactant films. *Biophys J.* 2010;99(10):3290-3299.

24. Petit K. *Surfactant Therapy for Conditions Other than Respiratory Distress Syndrome: An Analysis of the North American Pharmaceutical and Medical Sector with Perspectives on the Future.* London: Business Briefings Ltd.; 2004:1-4.

25. Jeffery PK. The development of large and small airways. *Am J Respir Crit Care Med.* 1998;157(5 pt 2):S174-S180.

26. Yeh TF. Persistent pulmonary hypertension in preterm infants with respiratory distress syndrome. *Pediatr Pulmonol.* 2001;(suppl 23):103-106.

27. Goldsmith JP, Karotkin EH. *Assisted Ventilation of the Neonate.* 5th ed. St. Louis: Elsevier Saunders; 2011.

28. Lyra PPR, Diniz EMA. The importance of surfactant on the development of neonatal pulmonary diseases. *Clinics.* 2007;62(2):181-190.

29. Schulze A, Abubakar K, Gill G, et al. Pulmonary oxygen consumption: a hypothesis to explain the increase in oxygen consumption of low birth weight infants with lung disease. *Intensive Care Med.* 2001;27(10):1636-1642.

30. American College of Obstetricians and Gynecologists (ACOG). *Clinical Management Guidelines for Obstetrician-Gynecology: Fetal Lung Maturity.* Washington, DC: ACOG; 2008.

31. Silverman WA, Andersen DH. A controlled clinical trial of effects of water mist on obstructive respiratory signs, death rate and necropsy findings among premature infants. *Pediatrics.* 1956;17(1):1-10.

32. Agrons GA, Courtney SE, Stocker JT, et al. From the archives of the AFIP: lung disease in premature neonates: radiologic-pathologic correlation. *Radiographics.* 2005;25(4):1047-1073.

33. Tracy SK, Tracy MB, Dean J, et al. Spontaneous preterm birth of liveborn infants in women at low risk in Australia over 10 years: a population-based study. *BJOG : An International Journal of Obstetrics and Gynaecology.* 2007;114(6):731-735.

34. Petrini J, Callaghan W, Klebanoff M. Estimated effect of 17 alpha-hydroxyprogesterone caproate on preterm birth in the United States. *Obstet Gynecol.* 2005;105(2):267-272.

35. Davey MA, Watson L, Rayner JA, et al. Risk scoring systems for predicting preterm birth with the aim of reducing associated adverse outcomes. *Cochrane Database System Rev.* 2011;11:CD004902.

36. Sosa C, Althabe F, Belizán JM, et al. Bed rest in singleton pregnancies for preventing preterm birth. *Cochrane Database System Rev.* 2004;1:CD003581.

37. Papatsonis D, Flenady V, Liley H. Maintenance therapy with oxytocin antagonists for inhibiting preterm birth after threatened preterm labour. *Cochrane Database System Rev.* 2009;1:CD005938.

38. Gaunekar N, Crowther CA. Maintenance therapy with calcium channel blockers for preventing preterm birth after threatened preterm labour. *Cochrane Database System Rev.* 2004;3:CD004071.

39. Dodd JM, Crowther CA, Dare MR, et al. Oral betamimetics for maintenance therapy after threatened preterm labour. *Cochrane Database System Rev.* 2006;1:CD003927.

40. Nanda K, Cook LA, Gallo MF, et al. Terbutaline pump maintenance therapy after threatened preterm labor for preventing preterm birth. *Cochrane Database System Rev.* 2002;4:CD003933.

41. Han S, Crowther CA, Moore V. Magnesium maintenance therapy for preventing preterm birth after threatened preterm labour. *Cochrane Database System Rev.* 2010;7:CD000940.

42. Gaunekar NN, Crowther CA. Maintenance therapy with calcium channel blockers for preventing preterm birth after threatened preterm labour. *Cochrane Database System Rev.* 2004;3:CD004071.

43. Van Os MA, van der Ven JA, Kleinrouweler CE, et al. Preventing preterm birth with progesterone: costs and effects of screening low risk women with a singleton pregnancy for short cervical length, the Triple P study. *BMC Pregnancy Childbirth.* 2011;11:77-81.

44. Liggins GC, Howie RN. A controlled trial of antepartum glucocorticoid treatment for prevention of the respiratory distress syndrome in premature infants. *Pediatrics.* 1972; 50(4):51-525.

45. Schwab M, Roedel M, Akhtar Anwar M, et al. Effects of betamethasone administration to the fetal sheep in late gestation on fetal cerebral blood flow. *J Physiol.* 2000;528(pt 3):619-632.

46. Crowley P, Chalmers I, Keirse MJNC. The effects of corticosteroid administration before preterm delivery: an overview of the evidence from controlled trials. *Br J Obstet Gynaecol.* 1990;97(1):11-25.

47. Crowther CA, McKinlay CJD, Middleton P, et al. Repeat doses of prenatal corticosteroids for women at risk of preterm birth for improving neonatal health outcomes. *Cochrane Database System Rev.* 2011;6:CD003935.

48. Brownfoot FC, Crowther CA, Middleton P. Different corticosteroids and regimens for accelerating fetal lung maturation for women at risk of preterm birth. *Cochrane Database System Rev.* 2008;4:CD006764.

49. American Heart Association/American Academy of Pediatrics. *Textbook of Neonatal Resuscitation.* 6th ed. Dallas, TX: American Heart Association; 2011.

50. Vohra S, Frent G, Campbell V, et al. Effect of polyethylene occlusive skin wrapping on heat loss in very low birth weight infants at delivery: a randomized trial. *J Pediatr.* 1999;134(5):547-551.

51. Kattwinkel J, Perlman JM, Aziz K, et al. 2010 American Heart Association Guidelines for Cardiopulmonary Resuscitation and Emergency Cardiovascular Care: neonatal resuscitation. *Circulation.* 2010;122(pt 15):S909-S919.

52. Rojas MA, Lozano JM, Rojas MX, et al. Very early surfactant without mandatory ventilation in premature infants treated with continuous positive airway pressure: a randomized control trial. *Pediatrics.* 2009;123(1):137-142.

53. Yost CC, Soll RF. Early versus delayed selective surfactant treatment for neonatal respiratory distress syndrome [review]. *The Cochrane Library.* 2009;1:1-30.

54. Engle WA. Surfactant-replacement therapy for respiratory distress in the preterm and term neonate. *Pediatrics.* 2008;121(2):419-432.

55. Stevens TP, Blennow M, Soll RF, et al. Early surfactant administration with brief ventilation vs. selective surfactant and continued mechanical ventilation for preterm infants with or at risk for respiratory distress syndrome [review]. *The Cochrane Library.* 2008;3:1-34.

56. Soll RF, Morley CJ. Prophylactic versus selective use of surfactant in preventing morbidity and mortality in preterm infants (review). *The Cochrane Library* 2009;1:1-33.

57. American Association for Respiratory Care. AARC clinical practice guideline: surfactant replacement therapy. *Respir Care.* 1994;39(8):824-829.

58. Rojas-Reyes MX, Morley CJ, Soll R. Prophylactic versus selective use of surfactant in preventing morbidity and mortality in preterm infants [review]. *The Cochrane Library.* 2012;3:1-73.

59. Surfaxin [package insert]. Warrington, PA: Discovery Laboratories, Inc.; 2012. http://www.surfaxin.com/prescribing-info.pdf. Accessed October 1, 2012.

60. Avery ME, Oppenheimer EH. Recent increase in mortality from hyaline membrane disease. *J Pediatr.* 1960;57(4):553-559.

61. The Johns Hopkins Hospital. NICU pulse oximetry protocol. http://www.hopkinschildrens.org/pulse-ox-screening-for-congenital-heart-disease.aspx. Accessed December 31, 2012.

62. Chow LC, Wright KW, Sola A. Can changes in clinical practice decrease the incidence of severe retinopathy of prematurity in very low birth weight infants? *Pediatrics.* 2003;111(2):339-345.

63. Finer N, Leone T. Oxygen saturation monitoring for the preterm infant: the evidence basis for current practice. *Pediatr Res.* 2009;65(4):375-380.

64. Wallace DK, Veness-Meehan KA, Miller WC. Incidence of severe retinopathy of prematurity before and after a modest reduction in target oxygen saturation levels. *J AAPOS.* 2007;11(2):170-174.

65. Vanderveen DK, Mansfield TA, Eichenwald EC. Lower oxygen saturation alarms limits decrease the severity of retinopathy of prematurity. *J AAPOS.* 2006;10(5):445-448.

66. Deulofeut R, Critz A, Adams-Chapman I, et al. Avoiding hyperoxia in infants < or = 1250 g is associated with improved short- and long-term outcomes. *J Perinatol.* 2006;26(11):700-705.

67. The STOP-ROP Multicenter Study Group. Supplemental therapeutic oxygen for prethreshold retinopathy of prematurity (STOP-ROP), a randomized, controlled trial. I: primary outcomes. *Pediatrics.* 2000;105(2):295-310.

68. Skinner JR, Hunter S, Poets CF, et al. Haemodynamic effects of altering arterial oxygen saturation in preterm infants with respiratory failure. *Arch Dis Child Fetal Neonatal Ed.* 1999;80(2):F81-F87.

69. Vain NE, Prudent LM, Stevens DP, et al. Regulation of oxygen concentrations delivered to infants by nasal cannulas. *Am J Dis Child.* 1989;143(12):1458-1460.

70. U.S. Food and Drug Administration. Medical devices: August 2000 510(k) clearances: Vapotherm. http://www.fda.gov/MedicalDevices/ProductsandMedicalProcedures/DeviceApprovalsandClearances/510kClearances/ucm093462.htm. Accessed October 1, 2012.

71. Holleman-Duray D, Kaupie D, Weiss MG. Heated humidified high-flow nasal cannula: use and a neonatal early extubation protocol. *J Perinatol.* 2007;27(12):776-781.

72. Wilkinson D, Andersen C, O'Donnell CP, et al. High flow nasal cannula for respiratory support in preterm infants. *Cochrane Database System Rev.* 2011;5:CD006405.

73. Locke RG, Wolfson MR, Shaffner TH, et al. Inadvertent administration of positive end-distending pressure during nasal cannula flow. *Pediatrics.* 1993;91(1):135-138.

74. Spence KL, Murphy D, Kilian C, et al. High-flow nasal cannula as a device to provide continuous positive airway pressure in infants. *J Perinatol.* 2007;27(12):772-775.

75. Kubicka ZJ, Limauro J, Darnall RA. Heated, humidified high-flow nasal cannula therapy: yet another way to deliver continuous positive airway pressure? *Pediatrics.* 2008;121(1):82-88.

76. Volsko T, Fedor K, Amadei J, et al. High flow through a nasal cannula and CPAP effect in a simulated infant model. *Respir Care.* 2011;56(12):1893-1900.

77. Morley CJ, Davis PG. Continuous positive airway pressure: scientific and clinical rationale. *Curr Opin Pediatr.* 2008;20(2):119-124.

78. American Association for Respiratory Care. AARC Clinical Practice Guideline: Application of Continuous Positive Airway Pressure to Neonates via Nasal Prongs, Nasopharyngeal Tube, or Nasal Mask—2004 Revision & Update. *Respir Care.* 2004;49(9):1100-1108.

79. Aly H, Massar AN, Patel K, et al. Is it safer to intubate premature infants in the delivery room? *Pediatrics.* 2005; 115(6):1660-1665.

80. Aly H, Massaro AN, Hammad TA, et al. Early continuous positive airway pressure and necrotizing enterocolitis. *Pediatrics.* 2009;124(1):205-210.

81. Ho JJ, Henderson-Smart DJ, Davis PG. Early versus delayed initiation of continuous distending pressure for respiratory distress syndrome in preterm infants [Review]. *The Cochrane Library.* 2010;3:1-29.

82. Finer, NN, Carlo WA, Walsh MC, et al.; SUPPORT Study Group of the Eunice Kennedy Shriver NICH Neonatal Research Network. Early CPAP versus surfactant in extremely preterm infants. *N Engl J Med.* 2010;362(21):1970-1979.

83. Reininger A, Khalak R, Kendig JW, et al. Surfactant administration by transient intubation in infants 29 to 35 weeks' gestation with respiratory distress syndrome decreases the likelihood of later mechanical ventilation: a randomized controlled trial. *J Perinatol.* 2005;25(11): 703-708.

84. Escobedo MB, Gunkel JH, Kennedy KA, et al. Early surfactant for neonates with mild to moderate respiratory distress syndrome: a multicenter, randomized trial. *J Pediatr.* 2004;144(6):804-808.

85. Thomson MA. Continuous positive airway pressure and surfactant; combined data from animal experiments and clinical trials. *Biol Neonate.* 2002;81(suppl 1):16-19.

86. Diblasi RM. Nasal continuous positive airway pressure for the respiratory care of the newborn. *Respir Care.* 2009;54(9):1209-1235.

87. Wung JT, Driscoll JM Jr, Epstein RA, et al. A new device for CPAP by nasal route. *Crit Care Med.* 1975;3(2):76-78.

88. Liptsen E, Aghai ZH, Pyon KH, et al. Work of breathing during nasal continuous positive airway pressure in preterm infants: a comparison of bubble vs variable-flow devices. *J Perinatol.* 2005;25(7):453-458.

89. Stefanescu BM, Murphy WP, Hansell BJ, et al. A randomized, controlled trial comparing two different continuous positive airway pressure systems for the successful extubation of extremely low birth weight infants. *Pediatrics.* 2003;112(5):1031-1038.

90. Mazzella M, Bellini C, Calevo MG, et al. A randomised control study comparing the Infant Flow Driver with nasal continuous positive airway pressure in preterm infants. *Arch Dis Child Fetal Neonatal Ed.* 2001;85(2):F86-F90.

91. Buettiker V, Hug MI, Baenziger O, et al. Advantages and disadvantages of different nasal CPAP systems in newborns. *Intensive Care Med.* 2004;30(5):926-930.

92. Koyamaibole L, Kado J, Qovu JD, et al. An evaluation of bubble-CPAP in a neonatal unit in a developing country: effective respiratory support that can be applied by nurses. *J Trop Pediatr.* 2005;52(4):249-253.

93. Kahn DJ, Courtney SE, Steele AM, et al. Unpredictability of delivered bubble nasal continuous positive airway pressure: role of bias flow magnitude and nares-prong air leaks. *Pediatr Res.* 2007;62(3):343-347.

94. Courtney SE, Kahn DJ, Sing R, et al. Bubble and ventilator-derived nasal continuous positive airway pressure in premature infants: work of breathing and gas exchange. *J Perinatol.* 2011;31(1):44-50.

95. Tagare A, Kadam S, Vaidya U, Pandit A, Patole S. A pilot study of comparison of BCPAP vs. VCPAP in preterm infants with early onset respiratory distress. *J Trop Pediatr.* 2010;56(3):191-194.

96. Gupta S, Sinha SK, Tin W, et al. A randomized controlled trial of post-extubation bubble continuous positive airway pressure versus Infant Flow driver continuous positive airway pressure in preterm infants with respiratory distress syndrome. *J Pediatr.* 2009;154(5):645-650.

97. Yong SC, Chen SJ, Boo NY. Incidence of nasal trauma associated with nasal prong versus nasal mask during continuous positive airway pressure treatment in very low birthweight infants: a randomised control study. *Arch Dis Child Fetal Neonatal Ed.* 2005;90(6): F480-F483.

98. Sai Sunil M, Kishore M, Dutta S, Kumar P. Early nasal intermittent positive pressure ventilation versus continuous positive airway pressure for respiratory distress syndrome. *Acta Paediatr.* 2009;98(9):1412-1415.

99. Owen LS, Morley CJ, Davis PG. Neonatal nasal intermittent positive pressure ventilation: a survey of practice in England. *Arch Dis Child Fetal Neonatal Ed.* 2008;93(2): F148-F150.

100. Davis PG, Morley CJ, Owen LS. Non-invasive respiratory support of preterm neonates with respiratory distress: continuous positive airway pressure and nasal intermittent positive pressure ventilation. *Semin Fetal Neonatal Med.* 2009;14(1):14-20.

101. DiBlasi RM. Neonatal noninvasive ventilation techniques: do we really need to intubate? *Respir Care.* 2011;56(9):1273-1294.

102. Lista G, Castoldi F, Fontana P, et al. Nasal continuous positive airway pressure (CPAP) versus bi-level nasal CPAP in preterm babies with respiratory distress syndrome: a randomised control trial. *Arch Dis Child Fetal Neonatal Ed.* 2010;95(2):F85-F89.

103. Meneses J, Bhandari V, Alves JG, et al. Noninvasive ventilation for respiratory distress syndrome: a randomized controlled trial. *Pediatrics.* 2011;127(2):300-307.

104. Morley CJ, Davis PG, Doyle LW, et al.; COIN Trial Investigators. Nasal CPAP or intubation at birth for very preterm infants. *N Engl J Med.* 2008;358(7):700-708.

105. Finer NN, Carlo WA, Duara S, et al. Delivery room continuous positive airway pressure/positive end-expiratory pressure in extremely low birth weight infants: a feasibility trial. *Pediatrics.* 2004;114(3):651-657.

106. Menon G, McIntosh N. How should we manage pain in ventilated neonates? *Neonatology.* 2008;93(4):316-323.

107. Avery ME, Tooley WH, Keller JB, et al. Is chronic lung disease in low birth weight infants preventable? A survey of eight centers. *Pediatrics.* 1987;79(1):26-30.

108. Ramanathan R, Sadesai S. Lung protective ventilatory strategies in very low birth weight infants. *J Perinatol.* 2008;28(suppl 1):S41-S46.

109. American Association for Respiratory Care. AARC Clinical Practice Guideline: Neonatal Time-Triggered, Pressure-Limited, Time-Cycled Mechanical Ventilation. *Respir Care.* 1994;39(8):808-816.

110. Wyllie JP. Neonatal endotracheal intubation. *Arch Dis Child Educ Pract Ed.* 2008;93:44-49.

111. Kumar P, Denson SE, Mancuso TJ.; Committee on Fetus and Newborn, Section on Anesthesiology and Pain Medicine. Premedication for nonemergency endotracheal intubation in the neonate. *Pediatrics.* 2010;125(3):608-615.

112. VanLooy JW, Schumacher RE, Bhatt-Mehta V. Efficacy of a premedication algorithm for nonemergent intubation in a neonatal intensive care unit. *Ann Pharmacother.* 2008;4(7):947-955.

113. Donn SM, Kuhns LR, Mechanism of endotracheal tube movement with change in head position in the neonate. *Pediatr Radiol.* 2008;9(1):37-40.

114. Rotschild A, Chitayat D, Puterman ML, et al. Optimal positioning for endotracheal tubes for ventilation of preterm infants. *Am J Dis Child.* 1991;145(9):doi 10071012.

115. O'Donnell CP, Kamlin CO, Davis PG, et al. Endotracheal intubation attempts during neonatal resuscitation: success rates, duration, and adverse effects. *Pediatrics.* 2006;117(1):e16-e21.

116. Swyer PR, Reiman RC, Wright JJ. Ventilation and ventilatory mechanics in the newborn: methods and results in 15 resting infants. *J Pediatrics.* 1960;56(5):612-622.

117. Delivoria-Papadopoulos M, Levison H, Swyer P. Intermittent positive pressure respiration as a treatment in severe respiratory distress syndrome. *Arch Dis Child.* 1965;40(213):474-478.

118. Glover WJ. Mechanical ventilation in respiratory insufficiency in infants. *Proc R Soc Med.* 1965;58(11 pt 1): 902-904.

119. Donn SM, Sinha SK. Invasive and noninvasive neonatal mechanical ventilation. *Respir Care.* 2003;48(4):426-439.

120. Wheeler K, Klingenberg C, McCallion N, et al. Volume-targeted versus pressure-limited ventilation in the neonate [review]. *The Cochrane Library.* 2011;6:1-86.

121. Cannon ML, Cornell J, Tripp-Hamel DS, et al. Tidal volumes for ventilated infants should be determined with a pneumotachometer placed at the endotracheal tube. *Am J Respir Care Crit Care Med.* 2000;162(6):2109-2112.

122. Keszler M. State of the art in conventional mechanical ventilation. *J Perinatol.* 2009;29(4):262-275.

123. Greenough A, Sharma A. What is new in ventilation strategies for the neonate? *Eur J Pediatr.* 2007;166(10): 991-996.

124 Brown MK, DiBlasi RM. Mechanical ventilation of the premature neonate. *Respir Care.* 2011;56(9):1298-1311.

125. Ramanathan R. Optimal ventilatory strategies and surfactant to protect the preterm lungs. *Neonatology.* 2008;93(4):302-308.

126. Reyes ZC, Claure N, Tauscher MK, et al. Randomized, controlled trial comparing synchronized intermittent mandatory ventilation and synchronized intermittent mandatory ventilation plus pressure support in preterm infants. *Pediatrics.* 2006;118(4):1409-1417.

127. Keszler M. Volume-targeted ventilation. *Early Human Dev.* 2006;82(12):811-818.

128. Erickson SJ, Grauaug A, Gurrin L, et al. Hypocarbia in the ventilated preterm infant and its effect on intraventricular haemorrhage and bronchopulmonary dysplasia. *J Paediatr Child Health.* 2002;38(6):560-562.

129. Okumura A, Hayakawa F, Kato T, et al. Hypocarbia in preterm infants with periventricular leukomalacia: the relation between hypocarbia and mechanical ventilation. *Pediatrics.* 2001;107(3):469-475.

130. Kaiser JR, Gauss CH, Williams DK. The effects of hypercapnia on cerebral autoregulation in ventilated very low birth weight infants. *Pediatr Res.* 2005;58(5):931-935.

131. Wung JT, James LS, Kilchevsky E, et al. Management of infants with severe respiratory failure and persistence of the fetal circulation, without hyperventilation. *Pediatrics.* 1985;76(4):488-494.

132. Sinha SK, Donn SM, Gavey J, et al. Randomised trial of volume controlled *versus* time cycled, pressure limited ventilation in preterm infants with respiratory distress. *Arch Dis Child Fetal Neonatal Ed.* 1997;77(3):F202-F205.

133. Singh J, Sinha S, Clarke P, et al. Mechanical ventilation of very low birth weight infants: is volume or pressure a better target variable? *J Pediatr.* 2006;149(3):308-313.

134. Herrera CM, Gerhardt T, Claure N, et al. Effects of volume-guaranteed synchronized intermittent mandatory ventilation in preterm infants recovering from respiratory failure. *Pediatrics.* 2002;110(3):529-533.

135. Davis PG, Henderson-Smart DJ. Extubation from low-rate intermittent positive airway pressure versus extubation after a trial of endotracheal continuous positive airway pressure in intubated preterm infants (Review). *The Cochrane Library.* 2009;2:1-16.

136. Kamlin COF, Davis PG, Morley CJ. Predicting successful extubation of very low birthweight infants. *Arch Dis Child Fetal Neonatal Ed.* 2006;91(3):F180-F183.

137. Gillespie LM, White SD, Sinha SK, et al. Usefulness of the minute ventilation test in predicting successful extubation in newborn infants: a randomized controlled trial. *J Perinatol.* 2003;23(3):205-207.

138. Davis PG, Henderson-Smart DJ. Nasal continuous positive airway pressure immediately after extubation for preventing morbidity in preterm infants [review]. *The Cochrane Library.* 2009;2:1-31.

139. Gizzi C, Moretti C, Agostino R. Weaning from mechanical ventilation. *J Matern Fetal Neonatal Med.* 2011; 24(suppl 1):61-63.

140. Nelle M, Zilow EP, Linderkamp O. Effects of high-frequency oscillatory ventilation on circulation in neonates with pulmonary interstitial emphysema or RDS. *Intensive Care Med.* 1997;23(6):671-676.

141. *High-Frequency Oscillatory Ventilation User's Manual.* www.fda.gov/ohrms/dockets/ac/01/briefing/3770b1_15 .doc. Accessed December 31, 2012.

142. Henderson Y, Chillingworth FP, Whitney JL. The respiratory dead space. *Am J Physiol.* 1915;38:1-19.

143. Bass AL, Gentile MA, Heinz JP, et al. Setting positive end-expiratory pressure during jet ventilation to replicate the mean airway pressure of oscillation. *Respir Care.* 2007;52(1):50-55.

144. Johnson AH, Peacock JL, Greenough A, et al.; the United Kingdom Oscillation Study Group. High-frequency oscillatory ventilation for the prevention of chronic lung disease of prematurity. *N Engl J Med.* 2002;347(9):633-642.

145. Marlow N, Greenough A, Peacock JL, et al. Randomised trial of high frequency oscillatory ventilation or conventional ventilation in babies of gestational age 28 weeks or less: respiratory and neurological outcomes at 2 years. *Arch Dis Child Fetal Neonatal Ed.* 2006;91(5):F320-F326.

146. Food and Drug Administration. *Summary of safety and effectiveness data: high-frequency ventilator.* http://www. accessdata.fda.gov/cdrh_docs/pdf/P890057S014b.pdf. Accessed July 21, 2012.

147. Tissières P, Myers P, Beghetti M, et al. Surfactant use based on the oxygenation response to lung recruitment during HFOV in VLBW infants. *Intensive Care Med.* 2010;36(7):1164-1170.

148. Kessel I, Waisman D, Barnet-Grinnes O, et al. Benefits of high frequency oscillatory ventilation for premature infants. *Isr Med Assoc J.* 2010;12(3):144-149.

149. VIASYS Healthcare-Critical Care Division. 3100A Quick Reference Card. http://www.carefusion.com/ pdf/Respiratory/HFOV/l23243100aquickrefcard775895_ 101.pdf. Accessed October 2, 2012.

150. Plavka R, Dokoupilova M, Pazderova L, et al. High-frequency jet ventilation improves gas exchange in extremely immature infants with evolving chronic lung disease. *Am J Perinatol.* 2006;23(8):467-472.

151. Bhuta T, Henderson-Smart DJ. Elective high frequency jet ventilation versus conventional ventilation for respiratory distress syndrome in preterm infants (Review). *The Cochrane Library.* 2009;1:1-34.

152. Keszler M, Modanlou HD, Brudno DS, et al. Multicenter controlled clinical trial of high frequency jet ventilation in preterm infants with uncomplicated respiratory distress syndrome. *Pediatrics* 1997;(4):593–599.

153. Chalak LF, Kaiser JR, Arrington RW. Resolution of pulmonary interstitial emphysema following selective left main stem intubation in a premature newborn: an old procedure revisited. *Pediatr Anesth.* 2007;17(2):183-186.

154. Badr LK, Abdallah B, Hawari M, et al. Determinants of premature infant pain responses to heel sticks. *Continuing Nurs Ed.* 2010;36(3):129-136.

155. American Academy of Pediatrics, Committee on Fetus and Newborn and Section on Surgery, Section on Anesthesiology and Pain Medicine, Canadian Paediatric Society and Fetus and Newborn Committee. Prevention and management of pain in the neonate: An update. *Pediatrics.* 2006;118(5);2231-2241.

156. Mainous RO, Looney SA. Pilot study of changes in cerebral blood flow velocity, resistance, and vital signs following a painful stimulus in the premature infant. *Adv Neonatal Care.* 2007;7(2):88-104.

157. Stevens B, Johnston C, Taddio A, et al. The premature infant pain profile: evaluation 13 years after development. *Clin J Pain.* 2010;26(9):813-830.

158. Walden M, Carrier C. The ten commandments of pain assessment and management in preterm neonates. *Crit Care Nurs Clin North Am.* 2009;21(2):235-252.

159. Okan F, Coban A, Ince Z, et al. Analgesia in preterm newborns: the comparative effects of sucrose and glucose. *Eur J Pediatr.* 2007;166(10):1017-1024.

160. Cignacco EL, Sellam G, Stoffel L, et al. Oral sucrose and "facilitated tucking" for repeated pain relief in preterms: a randomized control trial. *Pediatrics.* 2012;129(2):299-308.

161. Hall RW, Boyle E, Young T. Do ventilated neonates require pain management? *Semin Perinatol.* 2007;31(5):289-297.

162. Aranda JV, Carlo W, Hummel P, et al. Analgesia and sedation during mechanical ventilation in neonates. *Clin Ther.* 2005;27(6):877-899.

163. Bhandari V, Bergqvist L, Kronsberg S, et al.; NEOPAIN Trial Investigators Group. Morphine administration and short-term pulmonary outcomes among ventilated preterm infants. *Pediatrics.* 2005;116(2):352-359.

164. Simons SH, van Dijk M, van Lingen RA, et al. Routine morphine infusion in preterm newborns who received ventilatory support: a randomized controlled trial. *JAMA.* 2003;290(18):2419-2427.

165. Anand KJ, Hall RW, Desai N, et al. Effects of morphine analgesia in ventilated preterm neonates: primary outcomes from the NEOPAIN randomised trial. *Lancet.* 2004;363(9422):1673-1682.

166. Bellù R, de Waal KA, Zanini R. Opioids for neonates receiving mechanical ventilation [review]. *The Cochrane Library.* 2008;4:1-58.

167. Shah PS, Dunn M, Lee SK, et al.; Canadian Neonatal Network. Early opioid infusion and neonatal outcomes in preterm neonates < 27 weeks' gestation. *Am J Perinatol.* 2011;28(5):361-366.

168. Seri I, Evans J. Limits of viability: definition of the gray zone. *J Perinatol.* 2008;28(suppl 1):S4-S8.

169. Matthews TJ, MacDorman MF. Infant mortality statistics from the 2006 period linked birth/infant death data set. *National Vital Statistic Reports.* 2010;58(17):1-32.

170. Alexander G, Kogan M, Bader D, et al. US birth weight/gestational age-specific neonatal mortality: 1995-1997 rates for whites, Hispanics, and blacks. *Pediatrics.* 2003;111(1):e61-e66.

171. Hamvas A, Dwong P, DeBaun M, et al. Hyaline membrane disease is underreported in a linked birth-infant death certificate database. *Am J Public Health.* 1998;88(9):1387-1389.

172. de Kleine MJK, den Ouden AL, Kollée LAA, et al. Lower mortality but higher neonatal morbidity over a decade in very preterm infants. *Paediatr Perinat Epidemiol.* 2007;21(1):15-25.

173. Boat AC, Sadhasivam S, Loepke AW, et al. Outcome for the extremely premature neonate: how far do we push the edge? *Pediatr Anesth.* 2011;21:765-770.

174. Marlow N, Wolke D, Bracewell MA, et al. Neurologic and developmental disability at six years of age after extremely preterm birth. *N Engl J Med.* 2005;352:9-19.

175. Wilson-Costello D, Friedman H, Nimich N, et al. Improved survival rates with increased neurodevelopmental disability for extremely low birth weight infants in the 1990s. *Pediatrics.* 2005;115:997-1003.

176. Patrianakos-Hoobler AI, Msall ME, Huo D, et al. Predicting school readiness from neurodevelopmental assessments at age 2 years after respiratory distress syndrome in infants born preterm. *Dev Med Child Neurol.* 2010;52(4):379-385.

177. Kennedy JD. Lung function outcome in children of premature birth. *J Paediatr Child Health.* 1999;35(6):516-521.

178. Cano A, Payo F. Lung function and airway responsiveness in children and adolescents after hyaline membrane disease: a matched cohort study. *Eur Respir J.* 1997;10(4):880-885.

179. Fawke J, Lum S, Kirkby J, et al. Lung function and respiratory symptoms at 11 years in children born extremely preterm: the EPICure study. *Am J Respir Crit Care Med.* 2010;182(2):237-245.

180. Holditch-Davis D, Merrill P, Schwartz T, et al. Predictors of wheezing in prematurely born children. *J Obstet Gynecol Neonatal Nurs.* 2008;37(3):262-273.

181. Pramana IA, Latzin P, Schlapbach LJ, et al. Respiratory symptoms in preterm infants: burden of disease in the first year of life. *Eur J Med Res.* 2011;16(5):223-230.

182. Levesque BM, Kalish LA, LaPierre J, et al. Impact of implementing 5 potentially better respiratory practices on neonatal outcomes and costs. *Pediatrics.* 2011;128(1):e218-e226.

183. Coenraad S, Goedegebure A, van Goudoever JB, et al. Risk factors for sensorineural hearing loss in NICU infants compared to normal hearing NICU controls. *Int J Pediatr Otorhinolaryngol.* 2010;74(9):999-1002.

184. Bielecki I, Horbulewicz A, Wolan T. Risk factors associated with hearing loss in infants: an analysis of 5282 referred neonates. *Int J Pediatr Otorhinolaryngol.* 2011;75(7):925-930.

185. Korventranta E, Lehtonen L, Rautava L, et al.; PERFECT Preterm Infant Study Group. Impact of very preterm birth on health care costs at five years of age. *Pediatrics.* 2010;125950:e1109-e1114.

Chapter 5

Apnea of Prematurity and Bronchopulmonary Dysplasia

Key Terms

Apnea of prematurity (AOP)
Bronchopulmonary dysplasia (BPD)
Caffeine citrate
Central apnea
Central chemoreceptors
Chronic lung disease (CLD)
Corticosteroids
Methylxanthines
Mixed apnea
Obstructive apnea
Periodic breathing
Peripheral chemoreceptors
Vitamin A

Chapter Objectives

After reading this chapter, you will be able to:

1. Classify the clinical signs and symptoms of apnea of prematurity (AOP).
2. Differentiate between periodic breathing and AOP.
3. Recommend pharmacological and nonpharmacological treatment for AOP.
4. Assess discharge readiness for a patient diagnosed with AOP.
5. Describe the physiological mechanisms that contribute to the development of the "new bronchopulmonary dysplasia."
6. Classify the severity of bronchopulmonary dysplasia (BPD), given a set of patient criteria.
7. Suggest strategies to prevent severe BPD.
8. Describe how the currently recommended strategies for preventing BPD act to preserve pulmonary function.

■■■ Baby Girl (BG) Gibbs

You have been following BG Gibbs since her birth at your hospital 4 weeks ago. She is now 1,640 grams, on no respiratory support, and is feeding well via a nasogastric tube. Her respiratory support included two doses of surfactant, 9 days of invasive mechanical ventilation, 5 days of nasal continuous positive airway pressure, 7 days of a high-flow, heated nasal cannula, and 9 days on a traditional nasal cannula. You have just discontinued her nasal cannula, and she is now breathing room air.

Extremely premature infants are susceptible to more than just respiratory distress syndrome (RDS). After survival of the neonatal period, there are other significant respiratory disorders that can threaten survival without permanent sequelae. Apnea of prematurity can cause life-threatening bradycardia and hypoxemia and requires prompt intervention from health-care providers to prevent respiratory and cardiac arrest and neurological damage. Chronic lung disease has been described in the neonatal population for as long as mechanical ventilation has been used. Bronchopulmonary dysplasia is a form of chronic lung disease that was primarily caused by positive-pressure ventilation. Since the advent of surfactant replacement therapy and prenatal corticosteroids, this form of lung disease is rarely seen in infants other than extremely premature infants with severe RDS. As integral members of the neonatal clinical team, respiratory therapists (RTs) can positively affect the incidence and severity of these diseases early in a patient's clinical course by minimizing exposure to excessive oxygen and ventilation and making timely interventions when ventilation is insufficient.

Apnea of Prematurity

Apnea of prematurity (AOP) is defined as a sudden cessation of breathing that lasts for at least 20 seconds or is accompanied by bradycardia or oxygen desaturation (cyanosis) in an infant younger than 37 weeks' gestation (wG) (1). It usually ceases by 37 weeks postmenstrual age but may persist for several weeks beyond term, especially in infants born before 28 wG (2). Extreme episodes usually cease at approximately 43 weeks postconceptional age (3).

Apnea is common in preterm infants, particularly in those less than 30 wG. The incidence and severity increases with lower gestational age. The incidence of apnea is significantly greater in preterm infants, affecting 7% of infants born at 34 to 35 weeks, 14% born between 32 and 33 weeks, and increasing to 54% between 30 and 31 weeks and to 80% in neonates born at less than 30 wG (4).

There are many causes of apnea in premature infants. It typically results from a combination of incorrect neural signaling and airway obstruction, but it can also be a sign of underlying pathology (Box 5-1). AOP, specifically, is a developmental

Box 5-1 Causes of Neonatal Apnea (5, 8, 16)

- Sepsis
- Meningitis
- Necrotizing enterocolitis (NEC)
- Intracranial hemorrhage
- Seizures
- Asphyxia
- Congenital neurological malformations
- Hypoxemia
- RDS
- Pneumonia
- Aspiration
- Patent ductus arteriosus
- Hypovolemia
- Hypertension
- Heart failure
- Anemia
- Gastroesophageal reflux disease
- Abdominal distension
- Medications (opiate, magnesium, prostaglandin E_1)
- Pain
- Airway malformation
- Head and body position
- Hypoglycemia
- Hypocalcemia
- Hyponatremia

disorder. It is caused by the physiological immaturity of the neurological and chemical receptor systems of the body that regulate respiration and respond to hypoxemia and hypercapnia. Another common, but benign, form of abnormal breathing in neonates is called **periodic breathing**, which is characterized by cycles of hyperventilation followed by short apneic pauses of less than 3 seconds (6) (Clinical Variations 5-1).

AOP, like other forms of apnea, can be classified as central, obstructive, or mixed. **Central apnea** is caused by a dysfunction of the nerve centers in the brainstem to send signals to the muscles of respiration, and no attempt at inspiration can be observed. **Obstructive apnea** is characterized by some attempt to ventilate, resulting in chest wall movement but without gas entry, usually caused by an upper-airway obstruction. **Mixed apnea** consists of obstructed respiratory efforts, usually following central pauses, and is probably the most common type of apnea (6). Regardless of the type of apnea, neonates' low functional residual capacity (FRC) coupled with their relatively high metabolic rates will cause a rapid onset of hypoxemia following cessation of breathing (7).

It is imperative to treat AOP; otherwise, the associated bradycardia and hypoxemia may require aggressive resuscitation and may be associated with long-term adverse neurodevelopmental outcomes (8).

Pathophysiology

The primary role of the respiratory-control system is to regulate ventilation to supply the O_2 needs of the body and to remove CO_2. This control system is composed of neurons in the brainstem and higher brain centers, along with chemoreceptors in the brain and carotid body that provide feedback related to respiratory gas changes brought about by ventilation. Developmental dysfunction of the respiratory-control system appears to be the primary cause of the central apnea component of AOP (9). There are also anatomical and physiological characteristics of premature infants that put them at higher risk of obstructive apnea. These features include a large occiput and hypotonic neck muscles, along with smaller airways, which increase the risk of upper-airway obstruction. Premature infants also have reduced pulmonary reserves that make them more likely to tire and become hypoxemic more quickly than do other children and adults (8).

Control of ventilation occurs at the brainstem, which is developed early in fetal life and has completed construction around gestational week 9. Second-to-second changes in ventilation after birth are the result of the brainstem integrating and then responding to signals from the respiratory system. In addition to neural feedback from the upper airway and lung tissue, signals for respiratory control are also sent to the brainstem by the central and peripheral chemoreceptors to control the basic respiratory pattern.

Central chemoreceptors are found in the brainstem and increase ventilation in response to low cerebrospinal fluid (CSF) pH, which is affected by the amount of CO_2 crossing the blood-brain barrier. Carbon dioxide crosses the blood-brain barrier readily, so the pH of CSF is essentially the same as that of arterial blood. Therefore, high carbon dioxide partial pressures ($PaCO_2$) will also cause a high CSF CO_2, which in turn lowers CSF pH; this should stimulate the central chemoreceptors and increase ventilation.

Peripheral chemoreceptors are found in the carotid body between the internal and external carotid arteries and are sensitive to O_2, CO_2, pH, glucose, and temperature changes. They have cells within them that contain an oxygen sensor. In normal humans, if oxygen partial pressures (PaO_2) of the blood in the carotid body are less than 80 mm Hg or $PaCO_2$ greater than 40 mm Hg, the peripheral chemoreceptors send a signal to initiate an immediate and significant increase in breathing. Studies indicate that the peripheral arterial chemoreceptors contribute between 16% and 44% of premature infants' baseline ventilation (10–12); they are active from at least 28 wG; and their activity appears to be higher in neonates than in adults, indicating that they contribute more to breathing during the neonatal period (13, 14). The peripheral chemoreceptors' response to hypoxemia also includes bradycardia and peripheral vasoconstriction (15), which are compensatory mechanisms to ensure adequate cerebral blood flow during hypoxia and asphyxia. In term infants, children, and adults, the bradycardia is counterbalanced by tachycardia initiated by pulmonary

Clinical Variations 5-1

Periodic Breathing (6)

Fetal breathing is characterized by short bursts of breathing and apneic pauses, which are modulated by oxygen tension and glucose levels. Periodic breathing resembles fetal breathing, and cycles are characterized by hyperventilation followed by short apneic pauses. The hyperventilatory phase of periodic breathing reduces $PaCO_2$, which decreases the central drive to breathe, resulting in short apneic pauses which, in turn, allow $PaCO_2$ to rise and stimulate breathing again. Periodic breathing has been considered a benign breathing pattern in premature infants, which is not associated with significant desaturations or bradycardia. In children and adults, periodic breathing is classified as Cheyne-Stokes respiration and is often (but not always) caused by damage to the neurological centers of the brain.

stretch receptors that are activated when the lungs inflate (15), making the normal human response to hypoxia in the form of hyperventilation, tachycardia, and peripheral vasoconstriction. Premature infants, in contrast, respond to hypoxia with a brief increase in ventilation caused by stimulation of the peripheral chemoreceptors, followed by apnea and bradycardia, and they do not appear to increase respiratory rate in response to hypercapnia (16). This resultant apnea may be the result of hypersensitivity of the peripheral chemoreceptors to high PaO_2 or low $PaCO_2$, causing a significant decrease in respiratory rate (17). As bradycardia becomes more pronounced, both systolic and diastolic blood pressures may fall, which can be associated with a decrease in cerebral blood flow (6) and increase the infant's risk for hypoxic brain injury.

There is also speculation that certain neurotransmitters may be mediators for hypoxic depression, including adenosine, endorphins, gamma-aminobutyric acid (GABA), and serotonin. Cytokines involved in prostaglandin E_2 production have also been implicated. Knowledge of these chemicals may assist health-care teams in creating more specific pharmacological therapies for AOP, with fewer systemic side effects.

Regardless of the true cause of premature hypoxic respiratory depression, the clinical manifestations are essentially the same, and the care and course of AOP is similar for all infants.

Clinical Manifestations

The definition of AOP encompasses the clinical signs of the disease, including apneas of more than 20 seconds with bradycardia and hypoxemia for 4 seconds or more. Bradycardia is defined as a HR less than two-thirds of baseline, and hypoxemia is SpO_2 less than 80% (18). An easier method for rapidly evaluating apnea clinically was described by Finer et al. as cessation of breathing for greater than 20 seconds or cessation of breathing for greater than 10 seconds accompanied by either a heart rate (HR) of less than 100 beats per minute (bpm) or SpO_2 less than 80% (19) (Fig. 5-1). Either of these clinical signs needs immediate medical attention.

In an effort to better characterize the severity of apneic episodes and their effect on long-term outcomes, the CHIME study created advanced definitions of apneic episodes. They delineated between conventional apneic events and extreme apneic events: Conventional apneic events are those with a duration of 20 to 29 seconds or an HR of less than 50 to 80 bpm for 5 to15 seconds; extreme apneic events are those with a duration of 30 seconds or longer or an HR less than 50 to 60 bpm for 10 seconds or more (20).

Bradycardia does not always occur with apnea, although it is more likely with longer duration of

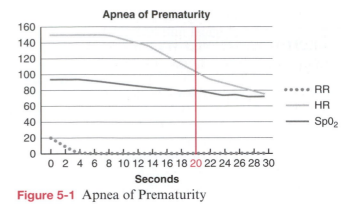

Figure 5-1 Apnea of Prematurity

apnea. Bradycardia occurs in 10% of apneic events lasting 10 to 14 seconds, in 34% of apnea lasting 15 to 20 seconds, and in 75% of apneas lasting greater than 20 seconds (21). Bradycardia usually occurs following apnea with associated desaturation, and once apnea ceases, recovery from bradycardia often precedes recovery of SpO_2.

Because the clinical picture of AOP relies heavily on bedside monitoring systems, it is essential to have sensitive systems that provide accurate information to the bedside clinicians, while also filtering out erroneous or incorrect data. There are many respiratory monitoring techniques available. The most simple is an abdominal pressure sensor: A diaphragm taped to the abdominal wall transmits a small pressure change to a sensor that sounds an alarm (or signals) if abdominal movement stops for a defined time period. Most neonatal unit cardiorespiratory monitors use transthoracic impedance pneumonography: Electrodes are placed on either side of the infant's chest above and below the diaphragm. As gas flows in and out of the lungs, the electrical impedance changes between the electrodes. The monitor can use that impedance data to display a live respiratory waveform and a calculated respiratory rate. Monitoring systems are continuously seeking to improve the technology for the smallest infants, and several quality-improvement plans have been published to minimize false alarms and improve accuracy in identifying central apnea (Evidence in Practice 5-1).

Every apneic episode should be monitored and documented in the patient's chart because respiratory or pharmacological treatment strategies and discharge decisions will be based on the frequency of apneic episodes and required interventions. Any care provider should intervene when clinically significant apneas are observed (i.e., provide tactile stimulation) and document any interventions necessary to reverse apnea. The patient's clinical picture surrounding an increase in apneic events will help clinicians determine the desired diagnostic testing and clinical intervention. Interventions may include a septic screen, full blood count,

Improving the Quality of Bedside Monitoring for AOP (22, 23)

A major problem with the current monitoring systems is that they are unable to identify obstructive apneas, which will exhibit chest and abdominal movement but an absence of upper-airway airflow. Another problem is that a strong blood pressure during bradycardia may cause the pulsatile activity of the heart to be read as a rapid, shallow respiratory rate, and the bedside monitor will therefore not identify the apnea. A third problem is the frequency of false alarms for apnea, causing staff to be desensitized to them and ignore the alarms when they occur, assuming them to be untrue.

One solution is the use of a nasal thermistor, which is a device that detects the temperature changes during inspiration and exhalation and quantifies the respiratory rate. It is attached above the upper lip and is surprisingly well tolerated (23). Another solution is to use an external device—in one study called a support vector machine (SVM)—to filter and evaluate the apnea alarm in combination with HR, RR, and SpO_2 from the monitor, as well as the quality of the monitored signals (22). The SVM will automate what all neonatal clinicians do as they are responding to an apnea alarm—survey all pertinent information to assist in determining which type of intervention is necessary.

chest radiograph, blood gas test, serum electrolytes and glucose tests, electroencephalogram (EEG), pH testing, and neurological imaging (8).

■■ You are by BG Gibbs's bedside several hours later and notice that she is having apneic spells with episodes of bradycardia and hypoxemia since you removed the nasal cannula (NC). When you ask BG Gibbs's bedside nurse about this, she tells you that BG Gibbs has been treated pharmacologically for AOP after her NCPAP was discontinued.

Management and Treatment

Apneas, by themselves, do not pose a threat to neonates. The associated bradycardia, hypoxemia, hypercarbia, and hypotension, however, can cause detrimental outcomes (23). Accurate diagnosis and management are important to ensure causes of apnea are appropriately treated and the consequences of severe apnea are minimized. The most immediate need for a patient experiencing a clinically significant apnea is to resume effective ventilation. This can be accomplished by providing some sort of stimulation

to breathe—usually tactile. Several other long-term treatment options, including pharmacological, respiratory, and environmental therapies, are available to treat or potentially prevent apnea. These include methylxanthines, blood transfusions, nasal cannula, noninvasive ventilation, invasive positive-pressure ventilation, and environmental interventions such as body positioning and kinesthetic stimulation.

Methylxanthines

Methylxanthines are stimulant medications, generally stimulating the central nervous system and cardiac muscles, and they have also been known to stimulate the respiratory drive, increase diaphragm activity, increase V_E, enhance chemoreceptor sensitivity to CO_2, reduce periodic breathing, reduce hypoxic respiratory depression, increase metabolic rate, increase oxygen consumption, and stimulate diuresis. Methylxanthines are nonspecific inhibitors of two of the four known adenosine receptors (24), and adenosine is recognized as being an important regulator of sleep and arousal states. Their exact mode of action is unclear. In older children and adults, methylxanthines such as theophylline have been proven to achieve bronchodilation for asthmatics. Theophylline, however, is well-known to have a narrow therapeutic range, with toxicity becoming evident when excessive serum levels were obtained greater than 20 mg/L (25). For neonates, there was concern that the therapeutic range for theophylline might be even narrower, observing control of apnea spells at plasma concentrations of theophylline of 6.6 mg/L but noting cardiovascular toxicity (HR greater than 180 bpm) with ranges between 13 and 32 mg/L (26). As a result, an alternative to methylxanthine, caffeine was considered to be safer than theophylline, demonstrating that blood levels of caffeine as low as 3 to 4 mg/L seemed to be effective in abolishing apnea (27).

Caffeine citrate has a very wide therapeutic index, is generally safe, and does not require routine serum therapeutic drug monitoring. Aranda et al. first showed the efficacy and safety of caffeine citrate in the management of neonatal apnea in 1977 (28), but randomized trials took nearly 20 more years to prove its safety and efficacy. In 1996, caffeine citrate was FDA approved for the short-term treatment of AOP in infants between 28 and 33 wG (29). In 1999, a multicenter, multinational, randomized controlled trial named Caffeine for Apnea of Prematurity (CAP trial) began to assess the performance of caffeine citrate. The study clearly showed substantial benefits from this drug in treating AOP, as well as a beneficial impact on neonatal short-term morbidities such as a decrease in incidence of bronchopulmonary dysplasia (BPD); the need for surgical ligation of patent ductus arteriosus (PDA); and long-term impairments such as cerebral palsy, severe retinopathy of prematurity, and neurocognitive defects (30). Caffeine also appears to be safer and more effective than other methods of treating apnea, such as kinesthetic stimulation (31) and pharmacological stimulants such as doxapram (32).

Caffeine citrate is a once-a-day therapy administered intravenously or orally, with a loading dose of 10 to 20 mg/kg and a daily maintenance dosage of 5 to 10 mg/kg (33). Caffeine citrate has a very long half-life, although it appears to vary with postmenstrual age and current weight. The half-life has ranged from 52 to 101 hours for patients between 30 and 33 wG (34–36), with a standard deviation of approximately 24 hours. This is important when weaning and discontinuing caffeine therapy, because it may take a week or more to return to subtherapeutic serum caffeine levels that will allow clinicians to observe true resolution of AOP without pharmacological therapy.

The side effects of methylxanthines include tachycardia, arrhythmias, irritability and crying, feeding intolerance, and seizures. These side effects, which are only evident when methylxanthine therapy reaches toxic levels, are rarely seen with caffeine because caffeine has a wide therapeutic margin. There were reports of an increased risk of necrotizing enterocolitis (NEC) with methylxanthine use in premature infants, which have not been substantiated for caffeine despite several large multicenter trials of caffeine citrate for treatment of AOP (37). The increased oxygen consumption has the potential to decrease weight gain in the short term (31), but it is not substantial in the long term.

Blood Transfusions

Anemia, another frequent problem in preterm infants, is a potential precipitating factor for AOP. Blood transfusions have been demonstrated to improve irregular breathing patterns in preterm infants, although the potential risk of blood transfusion has limited its use as treatment for apnea. The presumed physiological mechanism is that enhanced oxygen-carrying capacity, as with red cell transfusion, may decrease the likelihood of hypoxia-induced respiratory depression.

One study of 67 infants showed that transfusion was associated with fewer apneic events detected by the bedside monitor and that apneas were less frequent with higher hematocrit levels (38). Blood transfusions can be considered an appropriate therapy only in the presence of clinically significant apnea and with evidence of low hematocrit.

Nasal Cannula

The use of an NC to deliver pressure or gas flow to reduce the frequency of apnea and desaturation has not been tested adequately, although its use has become common for patients with AOP (39). The mechanism of action is thought to be twofold.

The first is delivery of mild positive pressure in the upper airway to prevent obstructive apnea; the second is tactile stimulation in the nares as a way to prevent central apnea. These can be prescribed without the addition of supplemental FIO_2. Additional oxygen delivery via NC can also serve to prolong the time period between apnea and desaturation. In a review of 52 infants prescribed an NC for oxygen delivery, 22 (11.8%) were prescribed room air through NC intentionally, presumably to treat AOP.

Noninvasive Ventilation

Nasal continuous positive airway pressure (NCPAP) is an established therapy for adult obstructive sleep apnea, and the mechanics and physiological mechanisms are the same in neonatal patients. During obstructive or mixed apnea, NCPAP provides a positive pressure throughout the respiratory cycle that increases pharyngeal pressure, which can splint the upper airway with positive pressure and reduce the likelihood of upper-airway collapse leading to obstruction and subsequent apnea (40, 41). Tactile stimulation in the nares from the device itself may also contribute to the effect as well as to the improvement of oxygenation by providing alveolar stabilization and improved FRC. Higher FRC will also prolong the time period from apnea to desaturation and bradycardia. An NCPAP setting of 4 to 6 cm H_2O is usually adequate.

The patient interface and delivery devices for NCPAP are the same as those discussed in Chapter 4. It is not clear which type of NCPAP device is more effective at minimizing apneic episodes, although one small study showed evidence that a variable-flow NCPAP device may be superior (42). CPAP is only effective at alleviating obstructive apneas and will have no effect on central apnea.

Noninvasive positive-pressure ventilation (NIPPV) may be a useful method of augmenting the beneficial effects of NCPAP in preterm infants with apnea that is frequent or severe. It is delivered in a manner similar to that of NCPAP, with the addition of a peak inspiratory pressure (PIP), inspiratory time (T_I), and inflation rate or respiratory rate (breaths/min). Its use appears to reduce the frequency of apneas more effectively than NCPAP and may be more effective at reducing work of breathing (43).

Invasive Positive-Pressure Ventilation

Intubation and invasive mechanical ventilation (MV) may be required for those infants who do not respond to noninvasive forms of ventilation or pharmacological therapies or who are experiencing severe refractory episodes. As with other preterm infants, a synchronized ventilator mode and minimal ventilator settings should be used to allow spontaneous ventilatory efforts and to minimize the risk of ventilator-induced lung injury (VILI).

Body Positioning

Prone positioning can improve thoracoabdominal synchrony and stabilize the chest wall without affecting the breathing pattern or SpO_2. It may have a role in improving the obstructive portion of apnea, although there is conflicting evidence regarding whether positioning has a definitive effect on apnea, bradycardia, oxygen desaturation, and oxygen saturation (44). Other methods of body positioning have been suggested to improve episodes of apnea, such as "head elevated tilt position" and "three-stair-position," but there is no evidence so far of a clinically significant difference in episodes of apnea (45–47). However, body positioning is an inexpensive and easily reversible form of intervention with few side effects, and it should be considered whenever possible for preterm infants with AOP. Clinicians should explain to parents the reasoning for prone positioning within the monitored units of the hospital and the necessity to change to the supine position when at home; the supine position reduces the risk of sudden infant death syndrome (SIDS) upon resolution of apnea and sleeping without continuous monitoring (8).

Stimulation

Two different methods are considered for tactile or kinesthetic stimulation. First, gentle skin stimulation by clinical staff is commonly used to arouse the apneic infant and stimulate breathing. This raises the question of whether frequent physical stimuli might reduce the number of apneic events. Second, some believe that the preterm infant is deprived of the frequent stimuli felt in utero and that substituting an oscillating mattress or inflatable bed to provide recurring kinesthetic stimulation might improve growth and development. The potential downside to the bed system is that the infant might attenuate to the stimulus, even when it is made to occur at variable times, so that the effect on apnea is gradually lost. Continuous stimulation has not been found to be as effective as other methods of treatment, such as methylxanthines (48).

It has also been suggested that the audible tones on the hospital and home cardiorespiratory monitors may incidentally be enough of a sensory stimulation to arouse the infant and terminate an apneic episode (49).

■ ■ The daily dose of caffeine citrate does not seem to be enough to prevent BG Gibbs's apneas. You suspect that she may have had some tactile stimulation from the NC, and request to the neonatologist that it be reinitiated. After return to 1 LPM NC at FIO_2 0.21, BG Gibbs spends the rest of your 8-hour shift without having any apneic spells requiring tactile stimulation.

Course and Prognosis

Resolution of apnea and establishment of a normal respiratory pattern is a major developmental milestone for premature infants. The age at resolution of apnea varies. By the time most infants reach 37 weeks postmenstrual age, apneas have resolved; however, one study showed that 80% of very low birth weight (VLBW) infants still had significant apneas at 37 weeks (50). It could take until 43 to 44 weeks postmenstrual age for preterm infants' incidence of apnea to match that of term babies (51). Most preterm infants no longer have significant episodes of apnea by the time they are ready for hospital discharge, which generally occurs around the same time as temperature control and feeding pattern maturation. Neonatal units require an observation period prior to discharge to document an apnea-free time period, ranging from 3 to 8 days, usually after discontinuation of caffeine citrate (49). If the child is otherwise stable and ready for hospital discharge, but caffeine has not yet been discontinued, the infant can be sent home while remaining on caffeine and be provided with a home cardiorespiratory monitor for at least the time it takes for the caffeine to reach a subtherapeutic level (Fig. 5-2). If, after 10 days to 2 weeks, the home cardiorespiratory study is normal, then monitoring can be safely discontinued (27). Alternatively, discharge

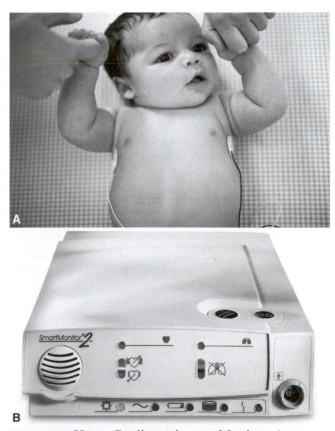

Figure 5-2 Home Cardiorespiratory Monitor *(Courtesy of Philips Healthcare, with permission)*

from the hospital can be delayed until caffeine is discontinued and serum tests verify it is at subtherapeutic levels, which will take at least 5 to 7 days. If apnea reappears after cessation of caffeine, caffeine should be reinstituted, and the process should be repeated in approximately 2 weeks' time. Discharge from the hospital should be delayed if there is persistence of apneic events with associated bradycardia and hypoxemia. An alternative to a prolonged hospital stay could include a discharge home with cardiorespiratory monitoring until 43 to 44 weeks postmenstrual age. The home monitor emits an alarm during a prolonged apneic episode, alerting a caregiver to a potentially dangerous condition so that the caregiver can intervene in a timely fashion.

Whatever the discharge care plan, family education and training is essential because apnea at home is a frightening event. Families may also be comforted by the cardiorespiratory monitors used in the hospital, which will be absent at home. Parents and caregivers should be instructed on the simple stimulatory techniques required to resolve apneic events and reassured that apneic events rarely result in death and do not put their child at an increased risk of SIDS (8, 23, 30). Their knowledge of access to emergency services should also be reviewed, and they should be provided with a basic life-support course before their infant is discharged.

Determining the long-term outcomes of AOP has been challenging because there are many other potential coexisting causes for neurological injury in premature infants (described in Chapter 8). Prolonged apnea and bradycardia are known to decrease systemic blood pressure and lead to cerebral hypoperfusion, which can contribute to hypoxic-ischemic injury of the immature brain (52). However, infants born prematurely have a higher rate of central nervous system injury such as periventricular leukomalacia and intraventricular hemorrhage (IVH), both of which cause apnea. It has been difficult for studies to establish whether apnea was a cause of a cerebral dysfunction or a result of it.

Premature infants have delayed mental and motor development regardless of the presence of AOP (53); some case comparisons reported no difference in outcome of infants with apnea, whereas others report evidence of a higher incidence of general neurodevelopmental delays, cerebral palsy, and blindness (32, 54, 55) in patients with frequent apnea. There was also concern that caffeine citrate may have a negative effect on neurodevelopmental outcome, but the CAP trial found no difference in outcomes at 18 months or 5 years in the rates of death, motor impairment, behavior problems, poor general health, deafness, or blindness (56). It also had the clear benefit of reducing the frequency of BPD, a chronic lung disease of prematurity discussed in the next section.

> ■ ■ At 35 3/7 wG, BG Gibbs is ready to be discharged to home. She has been on room air for 3 weeks and has been without caffeine therapy for 10 days without apneic incidence. Evaluation must now be made regarding her level of lung disease and need for support at home.

Bronchopulmonary Dysplasia

Any pulmonary disease that results from a neonatal respiratory disorder is called **chronic lung disease (CLD)** (57). **Bronchopulmonary dysplasia (BPD)** is a type of chronic lung disease, currently defined as the need for supplemental oxygen for at least 28 days after birth, assessed at discharge or when the baby is close to his or her estimated full-term age.

The first mention of lung disease caused by MV during hyaline membrane disease (HMD) was in 1967. The Stanford Premature Infant Research Center studied 30 patients with HMD with cyanosis and apnea who were not responsive to noninvasive oxygen therapy. The result of their findings, which they called *BPD*, was described as the "prolongation of the healing phase of RDS combined with a generalized pulmonary oxygen toxicity involving mucosal, alveolar, and vascular tissues" and was seen in infants receiving FIO_2 of 0.80– to 1.0 for more than 150 hours (58).

In 1985, it was described as occurring in 15% to 38% of infants weighing less than 1,500 g and requiring MV for RDS (59). The description of the cause of BPD in the 1980s included the iatrogenic injury from oxygen toxicity and barotrauma from MV, as well as compounding factors such as premature birth, fluid overload, PDA, damage from severe pulmonary disease, and familial asthma. The incidence of diagnosis of BPD decreased significantly between 1993 and 2006, but it appears that the care required for infants diagnosed with BPD increased (60). With the addition of surfactant replacement therapy and the use of antenatal glucocorticoids in the 1990s, the neonatal research community considered that the initial description and characteristics of BPD might no longer reflect what was seen in the patient population. The number of BPD diagnoses had decreased in older premature infants, but researchers noted an increase in the diagnoses of BPD in younger populations. Reports in the early 2000s indicated that almost two thirds of infants who acquire BPD weigh less than 1,000 g and are less than 28 wG at birth, and they frequently did not have a prior history of severe RDS. Clinical observation of extremely premature and extremely low birth weight (ELBW) infants who developed BPD showed they often required little supplemental oxygen during their initial postnatal course and rarely received MV with high inflation pressures or large V_T values (61). This new epidemiological data and clinical manifestation denoted a need to revisit the characteristics of BPD. A new term was suggested—chronic lung disease, or the "new BPD."

A National Institute of Child Health and Human Development/National Heart, Lung, and Blood Institute/Office of Rare Diseases Workshop, held in 2000, sought to better capture the nature of BPD after the advent of surfactant and steroid therapies. Gentler ventilation techniques, antenatal glucocorticoid therapy, and exogenous surfactant had minimized severe lung injury in larger and more mature infants (62), reserving it now for extremely premature ELBW infants nearing full-term age. The workshop team developed a working definition for new BPD, along with criteria for diagnosing it prior to an infant's discharge to home (see Table 5-1 for the diagnostic criteria), and this definition has since been validated using subsequent patient data (63).

The key physiological difference between "old BPD" and "new BPD" is that old BPD was considered a structural injury to lung tissue as a result of oxygen and MV. New BPD is considered a developmental delay or arrest of lung tissue. Premature infants born at a gestational age of 23 to 30 weeks—during the canalicular and saccular stages of lung development—are at the greatest risk for new BPD (64). Now, BPD rarely occurs in infants who are delivered at a gestational age greater than 30 weeks or who have a birth weight greater than 1,200 g (63, 65).

Table 5-1 Current Definition of Bronchopulmonary Dysplasia (62)

Severity of BPD	If Born <32 wG	If Born ≥32 wG
BPD is diagnosed by the need for oxygen >0.28 for at least 28 days, with respiratory support needed at a specified evaluation time, determined by degree of prematurity.		
When to evaluate	At 36 weeks postmenstrual age or discharge to home (whichever comes first)	At >28 days but <56 days postnatal age or discharge to home (whichever comes first)
Mild	No supplemental oxygen requirement at time of evaluation	
Moderate	Need for FIO_2 ≤ 0.30 and/or PPV or NCPAP at time of evaluation	
Severe	Need for ≥ 0.30 FIO_2 and/or PPV or NCPAP at time of evaluation	

The incidence of BPD is challenging to compare because different patient classifications, BPD criteria, and management strategies are used (Clinical Variations 5-2). Research data report the incidence for VLBW and extremely premature infants, using the new definition for BPD, as being between 52.8% and 77% (63, 67, 68), with 46% of those infants meeting the criteria for moderate or severe BPD (63). The incidence varies widely, with the Vermont Oxford Network data showing a variation of incidence between individual institutions from 5% to 65% (66).

There are multiple risk factors for the development of the new BPD. These are not, however, causative factors, and no one factor is considered a definitive link to BPD. The risk factors include the following:

- Gestational age 28 weeks or less
- Birth weight 1,000 g or less
- Hypothermia at admission to the neonatal intensive care unit (NICU)
- Hypotension at admission
- RDS
- The need for more than 2 hours of MV in preterm infants of greater than 26 wG. The need for prolonged MV could be an early marker for the development of BPD (69).
- Hypercarbia ($PaCO_2$ >50 mm Hg), particularly during the first 6 days of life in extremely premature, ELBW infants (70)
- The need for exogenous surfactant therapy
- Higher fluid therapy (71)
- Nosocomial infection (67)
- More than two packed red blood cell transfusions (72)
- Chorioamnionitis, which can increase the risk of BPD even in the absence of RDS (71, 73)
- Preeclampsia (74)

Clinical Variations 5-2

Variations in the Incidence of Bronchopulmonary Dysplasia (66)

The incidence of new BPD varies widely between countries, regions, and local health-care institutions. Many factors affect an institution's BPD rates: delivery room resuscitation practices for ELBW infants, invasive and noninvasive MV strategies, early versus rescue surfactant use, criteria for weaning and extubation, and acceptable pulse oximetry ranges. Geographical characteristics can also come into play because the incidence of new BPD is much greater at high altitudes than at sea level.

There are certain risk factors that increase the likelihood for more severe BPD, which include the following:

- Acidosis at admission
- Surfactant therapy
- Nosocomial infections
- PDA/BPD occurs more often in infants in whom symptomatic PDA develops, and the association is thought to be due to the excessive pulmonary blood flow caused by left-to-right shunting of blood through the PDA, leading to an increased need for supplemental oxygen and ventilatory support (67, 75).
- Oligohydramnios (76)
- An Apgar score less than 6 at 5 minutes (76)

Pathophysiology

Though the pathology of lung disease observed with old BPD is no longer seen in developed countries, it is imperative for RTs to understand the mechanics of lung injury that can occur in this patient population. The pathological features of old BPD have essentially been eliminated because of improvements in ventilator technology and patient management, but misuse of MV and improper patient assessment could still allow old BPD to occur.

The pathophysiology of old BPD was caused by volutrauma during positive-pressure ventilation, oxygen toxicity, and other compounding factors such as PDA, fluid overload, and prematurity. The pathophysiology of new BPD is thought to be caused by alveolar hypoplasia—abnormal pulmonary vascular and airway development after premature delivery. Table 5-2 summarizes the characteristics of both old and new BPD.

The Old BPD

The overriding pathological characteristics of old BPD included fibroproliferative airway damage, generalized inflammation, and parenchymal fibrosis. Old BPD was described as developing in four stages, which seemed to closely mimic the vascular phase of chronic bronchitis (58):

- **Stage 1,** occurring at 2 to 3 days of life (DOL), was described as a period of acute respiratory distress syndrome, the same as seen in RDS. Chest radiographs would show the generalized reticulogranular pattern, an increase in pulmonary density consistent with widespread atelectasis, and air bronchograms, similar to RDS. In 1980, this stage was termed "hyaline membrane disease."
- **Stage 2,** during DOL 4 to 10, would begin to show necrosis and repair of the alveolar epithelium, but there were also persisting hyaline membranes and merging of alveoli similar to

Table 5-2	Characteristics of Old and New BPD	
	Old BPD	**New BPD**
Airway	• Fibroproliferative airway injury • Smooth muscle hyperplasia	Varying amounts of smooth muscle Minimal damage present
Alveoli	• Fibrosis of alveolar tissue • Emphysematous changes • Heterogeneous pattern of atelectasis and overinflation	Alveolar hypoplasia Fewer and larger Less evidence of direct damage to alveolar tissue
Pulmonary Vasculature	• Thickening of the basement membrane, subsequently increasing A-C membrane distance	Decreased vasculature Lower A-C surface area
Inflammation	• Present	Less prominent

that which is seen in adult emphysema. There was a thickening of capillary basement membranes, as well as bronchiolar necrosis and exudate (fluid with high concentrations of cellular debris) in the airway. This stage was later termed "patent ductus arteriosus."

- **Stage 3,** at 10 to 20 DOL, presented with radiographic changes from nearly complete lung opacification with air bronchograms to small, rounded areas of radiolucency, resembling bullae, distributed throughout the lungs, alternating with areas of irregular density and resembling a sponge. Later, the air bronchograms disappeared, as did any apparent radiographic cardiomegaly. There were fewer hyaline membranes, but there was persisting injury to alveolar epithelia and focal thickening of the alveolar and airway basement membranes, as well as widespread bronchial and bronchiolar mucosal cellular changes. There were, at this stage, groups of emphysematous alveoli with surrounding atelectasis. This stage was termed "transition."
- **Stage 4** is seen beyond 1 month of life. Clinically, the surviving patients were still on supplemental oxygen, with CXR showing enlargement of the previously described rounded lucent areas, alternating with thinner strands of radiodensity. Cardiomegaly was seen in patients with right-sided congestive heart failure. Autopsy material showed groups of emphysematous alveoli

associated with hypertrophy of peribronchial smooth muscle and atelectatic areas associated with ordinary-looking bronchioles. Changes in alveolar epithelial cells included increased numbers of macrophages taking up residence in the airway, suggesting increased amounts of foreign material there. There was also a thick basement membrane, with an increase in alveolar-capillary (A-C) membrane distance. This stage was later classified as "chronic pulmonary disease."

The clinical cause of old BPD was thought to be multifaceted:

- The result of pulmonary healing in infants with severe RDS
- Toxic effects of oxygen on the lung superimposed upon pulmonary healing. In animal studies, oxygen free radicals caused damage to the endothelial cells of the pulmonary capillaries, followed by leakage of fluid into the interstitial spaces. With more exposure to oxygen, there is gross hemorrhage into the interstitial spaces and damage to the epithelial cells lining the airways. With continued exposure, interstitial edema is replaced by fibrosis, and permanent cellular changes to the bronchiolar and bronchial epithelium are found (77).
- Injury during MV, particularly seen with peak inspiratory pressure greater than 35 cm H_2O (77) or in patients who develop air leaks such as pneumothoraces (59, 78)
- Poor bronchial drainage secondary to intubation
- PDA because the increased FIO_2 and ventilator settings necessary to support the infant through the pulmonary complications of a PDA result in increased oxygen toxicity and barotrauma. Also, increased pulmonary blood flow during PDA may cause additional pulmonary damage (59, 79).
- Excessive fluid delivery. Brown et al. (80) found that infants who developed BPD had received significantly more fluid during the first 5 DOL than did infants who did not develop BPD. These investigators suggested that fluid overload might potentiate the other factors and increase the risk of BPD.

The New BPD

The new BPD seems to show a different pathological picture. There is less fibrosis and more uniform lung inflation. The large and small airways are remarkably free of epithelial cellular changes, smooth-muscle hypertrophy, and fibrosis, giving an appearance that they have been spared from injury (64). There are, however, fewer and larger alveoli, as well as decreased pulmonary-capillary vascularization (62). These features are thought to manifest because of subsequent changes in lung development upon birth at a young gestational age. At 24 weeks, the lung is in the canalicular stage of development, meaning that true alveoli have yet to develop, there is a low amount of alveolar surface area for gas exchange to occur, and there is no surfactant developed. The development of the lung from weeks 24 to 32 is significant, when alveoli and capillaries start developing along with remodeling of the bronchioles, smooth muscle, and alveolar sacs. Premature birth and the initiation of pulmonary gas exchange at this early stage appear to interrupt the normal alveolar and distal vascular growth, thereby triggering the development of the major features of new BPD (81). The normal structural complexity of the lung can be lost as a result: fewer, larger alveoli develop, and the overall surface available for gas exchange is reduced (82).

The key features of new BPD include the following:

- Alveolar hypoplasia (83)
- Arrest of terminal airway, alveolar, and associated vascular and capillary development (81). This includes a reduction in pulmonary arteries and an altered distribution of pulmonary arteries within the pulmonary interstitium, leading to a reduction of the A-C surface area for gas exchange (84, 85).
- Abundant smooth muscle in pulmonary vasculature and small airways (61, 62, 85, 86)
- Interstitial changes, such as differences in amount of elastin and collagen and interstitial fluid accumulation (61, 62, 82)

MV and oxygenation can still be mitigating factors in this type of BPD. Animal models have demonstrated that MV, with and without oxygen delivery, will severely reduce the numbers of alveoli and interfere with saccular lung development (87, 88). Oxygen alone can arrest lung development when it is given during the saccular stage (89). There is also research to suggest that vascular injury is the triggering mechanism in the development of new BPD (90), caused by vascular spasms that are the result of hypercarbia or hyperoxemia shortly after preterm delivery (70). Hypoxia may also delay alveolar development (71). In addition, there is a hypothesis that low baseline serum cortisol concentrations in VLBW infants may cause exaggerated inflammatory response to lung injury and may contribute to BPD (75).

Clinical Manifestations

The clinical course of old BPD typically manifested with air leak syndromes, pulmonary edema, respiratory failure, airway hyperreactivity, and often right heart failure. The clinical manifestations of new BPD are less severe and are common symptoms of patients in respiratory distress. The definition of BPD describes some of the clinical manifestations that are present, although there may be additional symptoms that are not encapsulated within the BPD definition. Patient history also plays a part in the diagnosis of BPD, but its role is not as clear as it was with old BPD, when oxygen and positive-pressure ventilation (PPV) were the direct cause of lung pathology. The major predictors of BPD are consistent: lower gestational age and MV on day 7. However, one study showed that 33% of infants receiving MV at 14 days did not develop BPD and 17% of the infants in room air at 14 days of age developed BPD (91). This is evidence that there are no clear factors determining which patients will develop BPD; therefore, continuous monitoring and evaluation should be employed to minimize risk and prevent clinical manifestations of BPD.

Clinical manifestations of developing or established BPD include the following (59):

- Prolonged oxygen use, measured at 36 weeks postmenstrual age
- Prolonged invasive or noninvasive MV
- Wheezing
- Compensated respiratory acidosis on capillary or arterial blood gas samples. A 2008 study of patients with BPD found higher $PaCO_2$ with increasing severity of BPD, with average values of 45 mm Hg in patients with no BPD, 47 mm Hg with mild BPD, 54 mm Hg with moderate BPD, and 62 mm Hg with severe BPD (92).
- Cyanosis and hypoxemia on room air. The degree of hypoxemia is related to the degree of BPD. The same 2008 study found room air SpO_2 of 97% in infants with no BPD, 95% with mild BPD, and less than 80% in moderate and severe BPD (92).
- Retractions
- Excessive sputum production
- Hyperinflation and atelectasis on chest radiograph (Fig. 5-3)
- Pulmonary artery hypertension in a subset of patients as a result of the increased pulmonary vascular tone (76)

Care must be taken when evaluating oxgyen requirements in this patient population. As described in Chapter 4, different institutions have different standards for pulse oximetry and oxygen delivery. One published study distinguished between "clinical BPD," which was an infant with oxygen use at 36 weeks, and "physiological BPD," which they described as SpO_2 less than 90% on room air. In their study of 1,598 patients, 35% had clinical BPD, whereas only 25% had physiological BPD (93). These results illustrate the importance of continued respiratory evaluation in this population of patients and removal of oxygen when it is no longer required to maintain adequate oxygenation.

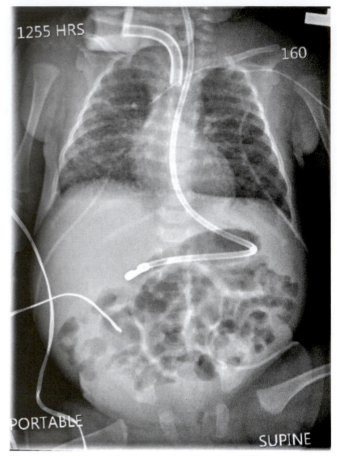

Figure 5-3 Chest Radiograph of Patient With Bronchopulmonary Dysplasia (Courtesy of Jane Benson, MD)

■ ■ Based on the current definition of BPD, BG Gibbs has mild BPD because she required oxygen for more than 28 days, but not at discharge. Because she has been free of supplemental oxygen for 3 weeks, she will not be sent home with any respiratory support. She will, however, be discharged with a home cardiorespiratory monitor, which will observe for apneas for 1 week, until she is 37 weeks postmenstrual age. At that time, if there are no documented apneas, the monitor will be discontinued.

Management and Treatment

The focus of therapy for BPD is on prevention of its development, and many of these strategies are considered routine treatment for RDS, such as minimal oxygen use, exogenous surfactant, open lung ventilation, and gentle ventilation strategies. Therapies that have been suggested to prevent BPD also include permissive hypercapnia, corticosteroids, mast cell stabilizers, vitamin A, inositol, antioxidants, inhaled nitric oxide (iNO), fluid intake restrictions, diuretics, and caffeine. The evidence of effectiveness of these therapies varies widely, and many are not recommended for routine use. A list of the currently recommended evidence-based strategies can be found in Box 5-2.

Treatment for the respiratory symptoms of ongoing BPD is mainly supportive, with the use of oxygen, ventilation, and bronchodilators used as needed to minimize symptoms.

Prevention Strategies

Currently, the only way to prevent BPD is to prevent premature birth. The strategies to prevent preterm delivery were discussed in the management and treatment section in Chapter 4.

Oxygen Therapy

Oxidative stress is a known cause of lung injury in preterm infants, and though supplemental oxygen is necessary to prevent tissue hypoxia, hyperoxemia should be avoided. Optimal strategies for supplemental oxygen use in infants at risk for BPD are still unclear and are the subject of ongoing clinical trials (71). As discussed in detail in Chapter 4, consensus has not been reached on the optimal oxygen saturation range; however, it is probably appropriate to maintain the oxygen saturation at less than 95% and the arterial oxygen tension at less than 90 mm Hg. If BPD is already established, higher targets may be prudent to avoid the development of cor pulmonale (66).

Surfactant Therapy

Early surfactant administration with less than an hour of MV, followed by extubation to NCPAP, has been associated with a lower incidence of BPD (94). Clinicians believe that the evidence showing that surfactant decreases BPD should be greater but that the

---

Box 5-2 Recommended Prevention Strategies for BPD

- Minimal oxygen use
- Exogenous surfactant
- Open-lung ventilation and gentle ventilation strategies
- Permissive hypercapnia
- Corticosteroids
- Mast cell stabilizers
- Vitamin A
- Inositol
- Antioxidants
- Inhaled nitric oxide
- Fluid intake restrictions
- Diuretics
- Caffeine citrate
- Stem cells
- H_2 blockers

---

lack of significant evidence may be due to the increased survival of very immature infants at high risk of BPD (74). This causes an increase in survival rates for extremely premature infants with RDS, but an unchanged incidence of BPD.

Later surfactant therapy has been proposed to treat surfactant inactivation that may occur in patients with RDS as a result of oxidative stress, pulmonary edema, inflammation, or other physiological mechanisms after the first week of life. An initial study showed transient improvement in oxygenation and ventilation, but there is currently no evidence that additional late surfactant therapy will decrease the incidence of BPD (95, 96).

Mechanical Ventilation Strategies

The need for even small amounts of MV can predict the development of BPD in preterm infants less than 26 wG (69), and prolonged MV has been suggested as a marker for the development of BPD. Extubation to NIPPV or NCPAP in the first week of life is associated with decreased probability of BPD (97), and preferential use of NIPPV over intubation and continuous mandatory ventilation (CMV) has been shown to decrease the incidence of BPD (60, 98). These outcomes, though promising, have not been consistently reproduced, suggesting that there may be more to consider than just avoidance of MV (74). In patients who require intubation, volume-targeted ventilation has been shown to reduce death and CLD over traditional pressure-limited ventilation (99) (Fig. 5-4). More generally, when ventilating premature infants, using adequate positive end expiratory pressure (PEEP) and avoiding overdistention of the lung will minimize VILI and decrease the risk for BPD. The goal is lung-protective ventilation aimed at reducing V_T values and stabilizing atelectatic lung units. Though HFV is an efficient open-lung and lung-protective strategy, evidence has not shown HFV to have a clear benefit over CMV in preventing BPD (100).

Permissive hypercapnia is a strategy for the management of patients receiving assisted ventilation in which relatively higher $PaCO_2$ levels (45 to 55 mm Hg) are accepted during MV to avoid VILI caused by excessive ventilation (101). There is not yet sufficient evidence to demonstrate that this ventilation strategy reduces the incidence of BPD (102). Retrospective reviews have shown that hypercapnia in the first 3 DOL is associated with IVH (103), suggesting that this strategy should be used cautiously, particularly early in the course of RDS.

It is probable that each of these interventions is not as effective alone as it is when bundled with other interventions to change management of patients with RDS. One institution was able to show an improvement in BPD rates for infants less than

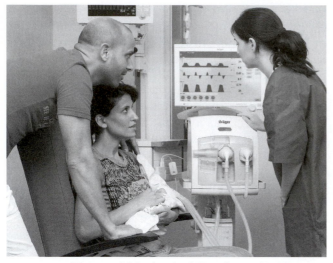

Figure 5-4 Neonatal Mechanical Ventilator (Dräger Babylog® VN500). *(© Drägerwerk AG & Co. KGaA, Lubeck. All rights reserved. No portion hereof may be reproduced, saved, or stored in a data processing system, electronically or mechanically copied or otherwise recorded by any other means without our express prior written permission.)*

1,500 g when initiating a quality-improvement process that included avoidance of intubation, pulse oximetry limits, and early NCPAP (104).

As with management of RDS, no clear pattern of MV was superior in preventing BPD, but minimizing oxygen and volume to the lungs will reduce the lung injury seen in old BPD.

Corticosteroids

Corticosteroids are a group of hormones secreted by the adrenal cortex in the brain, but they can also be manufactured synthetically. They acutely improve lung mechanics and gas exchange and reduce inflammatory cells and their products in tracheal samples of patients with BPD (105). Many questions exist regarding the risk-benefit relationship in the use of steroids because there are important concerns regarding increased mortality and adverse effects on head growth, neurodevelopmental outcomes, and lung structure (93,106). The first randomized controlled studies of the use of corticosteroids for BPD were published in 1983 (107) and 1985 (108). The most influential study appeared in 1989, which explored earlier administration and a prolonged weaning course (109). Corticosteroid use became more popular, until concerns about long-term sequelae were expressed, specifically, an increased risk for cerebral palsy with early, high doses of dexamethasone (110). Early corticosteroid treatment (within the first week of life) facilitates extubation and reduces the risk of CLD and PDA, but it causes short-term adverse effects including infection, gastrointestinal bleeding, intestinal perforation, hyperglycemia, hypertension, hypertrophic cardiomyopathy, and growth failure. Long-term follow-up studies report an increased risk of abnormal

neurological examination and cerebral palsy, and there is not yet significant data on neurological outcomes at school age or beyond. The benefits of early postnatal corticosteroid treatment, particularly dexamethasone, are not clear and may not outweigh the known or potential adverse effects of this treatment; therefore, early corticosteroid treatment is not recommended (111, 112). In 2010, the American Academy of Pediatrics restated its previous recommendations regarding corticosteroid use in premature infants (113) (Box 5-3). As a result, the use of steroids beyond the first week of life at lower doses and for shorter durations (5 to 7 days) is usually reserved for ventilator-dependent infants with severe, persistent lung disease who cannot be weaned from MV (114). Because of the observed side effects of dexamethasone, postnatal steroid administration using hydrocortisone has been adopted for the prevention of BPD. Whereas no study has shown clear benefit with hydrocortisone administration, results favor hydrocortisone in all studies (74). In one study of ventilator-dependent infants with established BPD, hydrocortisone administered at a dose of 5 mg/kg/day, tapered over 3 weeks, was as effective as dexamethasone for weaning infants from the ventilator and decreasing supplemental oxygen therapy, with fewer short-term and no long-term adverse effects (115).

Although early inhaled steroids have been studied, there is no evidence that they confer important advantages over systemic steroids in the management of ventilator-dependent preterm infants to

---

Box 5-3 American Academy of Pediatrics Recommendations for Corticosteroid Use for Premature Infants to Prevent or Treat BPD (113)

1. In the absence of randomized trial results showing improved short- and long-term outcomes, therapy with high-dose dexamethasone (0.5 mg/kg/day) cannot be recommended.
2. There is insufficient evidence to make a recommendation regarding treatment with low-dose dexamethasone (less than 0.2 mg/kg/day).
3. Early hydrocortisone treatment (1 mg/kg/day) may be beneficial in a specific population of patients; however, there is insufficient evidence to recommend its use for all infants at risk of BPD.
4. Existing data are insufficient to make a recommendation regarding treatment with high-dose hydrocortisone (3 to 6 mg/kg/day).

Evidence is insufficient to make a recommendation regarding other glucocorticoid doses and preparations.

either prevent (116) or treat (117) CLD. Because inhaled steroids might have fewer adverse effects than do systemic steroids, further research may offer additional insight into the benefits of the inhaled method of delivery.

Caffeine

Caffeine citrate is used as a stimulant to treat AOP and is discussed in the previous section. In a large multicenter trial, caffeine citrate was administered to infants with birth weight of 500 to 1,250 g beginning in the first 10 days after birth, and it decreased the rate of BPD when compared with placebo (36% vs. 47%). This reduction may be secondary to the shorter duration of exposure to MV observed in the caffeine-treated infants, or it may improve lung mechanics through its diuretic effects. Because many preterm infants have been exposed to caffeine and there has been no evidence of harm, routine use of this regimen appears warranted (2).

Mast Cell Stabilizers

Mast cells are concentrated beneath the mucous membranes of the respiratory tract, which release chemical mediators that trigger airway smooth muscle constriction, tissue swelling, mucus production, and vasodilation. Mast cell stabilizers such as cromolyn sodium prevent the release of chemical mediators, thus theoretically they should help prevent the inflammation in the lungs seen in the early stages of RDS. In studies of patients with established BPD, cromolyn sodium improved lung compliance and reduced MV requirements (118), but prophylactic treatment with it did not result in a statistically significant reduction in CLD and is therefore not recommended for the prevention of CLD in preterm infants (119).

Vitamin A

Vitamin A, or retinol, is essential for the optimal growth of cells and tissues. Evidence for low levels of vitamin A in BPD patients, along with its role in tissue differentiation and growth, support the hypothesis that vitamin A deficiency may contribute to the development of BPD. Some NICUs have adopted vitamin A supplementation prophylaxis because of the reduction of oxygen dependence at 36 weeks postmenstrual age and the incidence of BPD in VLBW infants, but supplementation does not change long-term respiratory outcomes (120). Despite the data on the potential benefits of vitamin A, its clinical use is inconsistent, and no general recommendations have been made. Although the response has been minimal despite a well-characterized mechanism of action and proven deficiency of vitamin A, optimal supplementation may potentially complement a host of other measures to reduce BPD (2).

Inositol

Inositol is a phospholipid that enhances the synthesis and secretion of surfactant phospholipids, thereby improving pulmonary function. Maintaining inositol concentrations similar to those occurring naturally in utero may reduce the rates of retinopathy of prematurity (ROP) and BPD in preterm infants. Studies of inositol early in the 1990s found a significant improvement in survival without BPD (121), but more current studies after the advent of surfactant are ongoing; thus, no recommendation is made at this time (122).

Antioxidants

Free radicals have been implicated in the pathogenesis of BPD. Premature infants are susceptible to oxidant injury because they are relatively deficient in antioxidant enzymes while being exposed to toxic oxygen levels (123). Pharmacological antioxidants have been suggested to decrease lung injury; these include superoxide dismutase (SOD), N acetylcysteine, vitamins E and C, and allopurinol (123). Studies so far have not shown antioxidant therapies to be effective in decreasing the incidence of BPD, but the current data on small numbers of infants suggest that it is well tolerated and has no serious adverse effects. As a result, further studies are warranted (124).

Inhaled Nitric Oxide

Elevated pulmonary vascular resistance and poor ventilation-perfusion matching are commonly found in preterm infants with severe RDS and respiratory failure, leading to high oxygen requirements and MV. This will contribute to oxidative injury and VILI. Inhaled NO is a selective pulmonary vasodilator that can improve gas exchange and decrease pulmonary vascular resistance. It is an inhaled gas with a half-life of less than 30 seconds, making it ideal for treatment of pulmonary-specific hypertension. Its use in full-term infants with persistent pulmonary hypertension of the newborn (PPHN) is well established, but data on the effectiveness and safety of iNO for preterm infants are less conclusive. Some premature newborns have critical hypoxemia associated with pulmonary hypertension, and iNO is the optimal treatment. Some research estimates that high doses of nitric oxide in preterm infants with birth weights less than 750 g in the first days of life may be associated with increased risk of IVH (125).

In addition, iNO has been shown to be effective in improving lung structure in experimental models of BPD (74), but studies in humans have shown conflicting results. One large study using low-dose iNO of 5 parts per million (ppm) showed a significant decrease in the incidence of BPD and brain injury in neonates with a birth weight greater than 1,000 g (126). A subsequent study found that the early initiation of low-dose nitric oxide does not prevent the subsequent development of BPD (127).

In an effort to better understand the risks and benefits of iNO, a recent multicenter randomized, double-blind, placebo-controlled trial of iNO for preterm infants weighing less than or equal to 1,250 g and who required ventilatory support between 7 and 21 days of age was conducted. Infants initially received 20 ppm of study gas for 48 to 96 hours, and the doses were subsequently decreased to 10, 5, and 2 ppm at weekly intervals, with minimum treatment duration of 24 days. The primary outcome was survival without BPD at 36 weeks postmenstrual age. The rate of survival without BPD was higher in the iNO-treated group, and there was a shorter duration of hospital stay and less need for supplemental oxygen therapy (128). There were no short-term safety concerns. Follow-up of these infants at 1 year showed that those treated with iNO received significantly fewer bronchodilators, inhaled steroids, systemic steroids, diuretics, and supplemental oxygen after discharge from the NICU (129). Follow-up at 2 years of age showed no significant increase in neurodevelopmental impairment when compared with placebo-treated infants (130). These recent findings may affect the use of iNO in premature infants at high risk for BPD.

Despite these studies, there is insufficient consistent evidence to support the routine use of iNO as a rescue therapy for the treatment of RDS, although it appears that there is no increased risk of IVH or neurodevelopmental impairment with its use. Its use to prevent BPD is promising, but further evidence is needed (131, 132).

Treatment of Pulmonary Edema

BPD is complicated by alveolar edema. Increase in fluid intake, capillary leak from inflammation caused by infection or from VILI, or volume overload caused by left-to-right shunting through a PDA can all contribute to pulmonary edema. Restriction of fluids and diuretics is a commonly used strategy to prevent and treat pulmonary edema.

Fluid Restriction

Standard management of infants with BPD usually includes moderate fluid restriction (120 to 130 mL/kg/day) to help prevent interstitial alveolar edema. Fluid management needs to be monitored closely to ensure adequate caloric intake for growth (75).

Diuretics

Diuretics potentially benefit pulmonary edema by increasing reabsorption of fluid from the lung. The two most common diuretics used in BPD, loop diuretics and thiazides, differ in their primary site of action on the nephron. Despite few randomized controlled trials, thiazides are the diuretics of choice in ventilator-dependent infants with evolving or established BPD (133). Loop diuretics, such as furosemide, carry additional risks when used sparingly to acutely treat pulmonary edema; these include hearing dysfunction, calcium deposition in the renal tubules, higher incidence of PDA, and low bone marrow density support (134). Furosemide can also be aerosolized, with a one-time dose of 1 mg/kg used to transiently improve pulmonary mechanics in preterm neonates with established CLD. However, there is not enough information available regarding oxygenation and pulmonary mechanics to support chronic administration of aerosolized furosemide (135). Regardless of the type or method of diuretics delivery, care should be taken to prevent electrolyte imbalance when using them.

Bronchodilators

Patients with BPD have increased airway resistance caused by smooth muscle hypertrophy and hyperreactivity. Adrenergic bronchodilators stimulate $ß_2$-adrenergic receptors on airway smooth muscles, thus relaxing the muscle and reversing the airflow obstruction. Albuterol and salbutamol are the most commonly used bronchodilators in the neonatal population. The side effects most seen with bronchodilators are tremors, tachycardia, and hypertension. The use of bronchodilators does not show a significant improvement in mortality or prevention of CLD (136). As with other patient populations, bronchodilator therapy should be limited to infants with evidence of bronchospasm and continued only if there is a clinical response to therapy (123).

Course and Prognosis

The prognosis for individual patients with BPD is relatively unpredictable, and the course can vary widely. Extremely premature infants treated with surfactant and corticosteroids are just beginning to reach adulthood, so there has not been time for an adequate evaluation of respiratory outcome. The benefits that should be evident as the result of better care may be obscured by the improvement in the survival of extremely premature and ELBW infants. Infants with BPD exhibit some degree of obstructive lung disease that can persist into adolescence and young adulthood. Evidence for this in early in childhood is repeat hospitalizations, abnormal pulmonary function results, and the need for home supplemental oxygen. For some, pulmonary dysfunction will continue to manifest into school age and adolescence as airway hypersensitivity; wheezing; and abnormalities in pulmonary function, radiographic evidence, and emphysematous symptoms comparable to chronic obstructive pulmonary disease (COPD).

Pulmonary Function

Initial pulmonary function results show that children with moderate and severe BPD have pulmonary function abnormalities that do not improve within the first 2 years of life (137). Spirometric values reflecting airflow (forced expiratory volume in 1 second [FEV_1], forced vital capacity [FVC], and forced expiratory flow at 25% to 75% of FVC [$FEF_{25-75\%}$]) are significantly and consistently lower in survivors of BPD at any age than in controls born at term or preterm, with substantial airway obstruction and alveolar hyperinflation (64, 138–141). Compared with earlier in childhood, the FEV_1/FVC ratio deteriorated more in BPD subjects between the ages of 8 and 18 years, suggesting that their lung function may also deteriorate more rapidly than that in other children (139).

Using pulmonary function tests to evaluate BPD lung dysfunction is challenging because they are designed to evaluate small airway abnormalities, whereas BPD causes changes in alveolar development not usually evident in flow measurements. Balinotti et al. designed techniques incorporating carbon monoxide diffusion to evaluate alveolar volume, and they found decreased gas diffusion capacities but normal alveolar gas volumes for infants with BPD. This suggests a persistence of impaired alveolar development at 1 year of age. Longitudinal studies show that survivors of BPD will have improved pulmonary compliance over time, although improvement may not be seen until after age 2 (82).

Computed tomography (CT) scans of the chests of patients with BPD have demonstrated that the majority have abnormalities that persist through childhood and young adulthood (142, 143). These include multifocal areas of hyperinflation, linear opacities, and subpleural opacities.

Home Oxygen

One study reported that 40% of preterm infants diagnosed with BPD required supplemental home oxygen (144). Although these infants may require oxygen at home for many months, few remain oxygen-dependent beyond 2 years of age (145, 144). Home supplemental oxygen allows infants to be discharged earlier from the neonatal unit (146). Early discharge is associated with reduced total health-related cost of care.

Respiratory Exacerbations

Infants with BPD after discharge have frequent "sick" office visits, emergency department visits, and rehospitalizations for respiratory symptoms and infections. They often require outpatient subspecialty care from pulmonologists and neonatologists as well as oxygen, diuretics, and/or respiratory medications (147).

Respiratory symptoms provoked by exercise, use of inhaled medications, regular follow-up visits and hospitalizations, need for physiotherapy, occupational therapy, technical aids, and financial support from society are more common for VLBW children compared with those born at term. Children with BPD suffered respiratory infections and needed antibiotic courses more frequently than did term controls (148).

Symptoms resembling those of asthma and spirometric evidence of airflow limitation in children surviving with BPD cause them to be often imprecisely labeled as asthmatic (141), although available evidence suggests that BPD and asthma do not have the same underlying pathology. Another functional abnormality clearly associated with preterm birth is airway hyperresponsiveness, which may occur in about half of adolescents with BPD (138, 149), though airflow limitation is only partially reversed by β_2-agonists in children with BPD, suggesting a stabilized remodeling process (149). Airway inflammation does not appear to be as prevalent in patients with BPD, and they are frequently treated with inhaled corticosteroids even though there is no evidence to support this practice. Using CT scanning, thickening of airway walls may be seen in both diseases; scattered parenchymal fibrosis and architectural distortion are common in BPD but are unusual in children with asthma (141). Additionally, school-age children with BPD are no more likely than their peers to have atopy (150), although this is frequently found in children with asthma.

Readmission to the hospital is common, particularly for those who had BPD, but only in the first 2 years after preterm birth (151). In one study, 73% of infants with BPD required at least one readmission, and 27% had three or more readmissions (144). The readmissions are usually for respiratory problems, particularly respiratory syncytial virus bronchiolitis, and infants with BPD who require home oxygen require twice the number of hospital readmissions during the first 2 years of life (145). Respiratory symptoms remain common in preschoolers who had BPD. In a cohort of 190 patients with BPD, 28% coughed more than once a week, and 7% wheezed more than once a week (144). Recurrent respiratory symptoms requiring treatment are common, even at school age and in adolescence.

Some imaging studies have shown emphysematous lung changes in young adults who have survived BPD, which could be a result of ventilator-associated parenchymal injury sustained early in life (152) or reflect the enlargement of distal airspaces caused by incomplete alveolar septation; this is a feature reported in the only pathological sample currently available from a patient with long-term BPD (153).

Neurocognitive Dysfunction

BPD is a major predictor of poor neurodevelopmental outcomes, including increased rates of cerebral palsy and other neurosensory and motor abnormalities, as well as poor cognitive outcomes during early childhood and school age (154). Higher severity of BPD is correlated with the presence of developmental delay (151). BPD constitutes a major cause of poor neuromotor outcomes at 6 months of age, but improvements in motor outcomes are seen over time (155).

Economic Impact

Chronic health problems associated with BPD have a major impact on families' daily lives after the neonatal period. Compared with families of full-term babies, more parents of children with BPD felt that the child's health affected the pastimes of other family members and created a significant burden for families far beyond the neonatal period (148). Home oxygen can also adversely impact the quality of life of families (146) and incur greater costs, mostly for prescriptions and respiratory-related care, despite not making a significant difference in clinical manifestations (144).

In contrast to other chronic respiratory diseases of childhood, there seem to be minimal health disparities related to socioeconomic status, sex, and race/ethnicity (147), meaning that care and resources appear to be evenly distributed for patients with BPD.

■■ One year later, Susan Gibbs returns for the NICU graduation party. She has brought BG Gibbs and her father, who recently returned from deployment. BG Gibbs is now 18 pounds and has been relatively healthy. She required one overnight hospitalization during the winter months for difficulty breathing, which they attributed to some mild airway hyperreactivity. She was not given any additional home medications to treat her BPD. BG Gibbs's neurological and motor development is delayed, but she is meeting the developmental milestones within the normal limits if her age is adjusted to compensate for her prematurity. She is just starting to crawl and attempts to place your hospital identification badge in her mouth when you pick her up to hold her. Susan expresses her gratitude to the NICU team for all the work they did for her and her baby during their 10-week stay in the hospital.

■■ Critical Thinking Questions: BG Gibbs

1. What strategies were used with BG Gibbs during the early course of BPD that may have helped minimize its severity? What additional strategies could have been used? What things were done that could have contributed to her developing BPD?
2. What discharge training should her parents be provided, and what additional home care support might be needed? How might the NICU team assess parental readiness for discharge to home?

3. How might her course have been different had you provided early CPAP without intubation and early surfactant in the delivery room? How might it differed if she had been given corticosteroids to help facilitate weaning and extubation from MV?

Case Studies and Critical Thinking Questions

■ Case 1: BG Stock

You are the floating RT in a rural hospital with a level II special care nursery. You are called by the charge registered nurse (RN) in the special care nursery to help assess a late-term infant born yesterday. BG Stock is 33 2/7 wG. The RN called you because the baby seems to have had a string of desaturation episodes in the last several hours. You agree to come and stay in the nursery to observe BG Stock's behavior. As you are standing across the room, with her in a radiant warmer, you watch the monitor appear to show rapid breathing at 70 breaths/min and then the respiratory tracing flat lines. You look at the infant's chest and cannot see any movement. The monitor begins to alarm at 15 seconds of apnea, and the alarms are joined by additional alarms for desaturation. After another 5 seconds, BG Stock's HR drops from her baseline 140 to 100 bpm.

- *What should you do?*
- *Do you think this is AOP? Why or why not?*
- *What would be the best next course of action?*

■ Case 2: Baby Boy (BB) Ranger

You are working in the pediatric intensive care unit (PICU) of a large regional pediatric hospital and receive notification of a transfer arriving from a level IIIB NICU that is closely affiliated with your hospital. BB Ranger is being transferred to be evaluated by the pediatric pulmonary team for failure to wean from MV and evaluation for a tracheostomy tube. He is an ex-25 wG African-American baby who is now 94 days old. He has a history of RDS and received three doses of Infasurf. He has been extubated three times: The first extubation was on DOL 9; he was reintubated on DOL 14 for severe AOP; he was weaned and extubated again on DOL 27. He was reintubated on DOL 46 for suspected sepsis and extubated on DOL 60. On DOL 75, he was intubated in the operating room for an inguinal hernia repair operation and has not been extubated since his surgery.

- *Based on the information provided to you by the transport team, what is BB Ranger's BPD status?*

After BB Ranger arrives, a set of lab test results and admission data are obtained. An arterial blood gas (ABG) results show the following: pH 7.39, $PaCO_2$ 58 mm Hg, PaO_2 88 mm Hg, and HCO_3 34.6 mEq/L. His ventilator settings when this information was obtained were Pressure Control with Pressure Support, PIP 24 cm H_2O, PEEP 6 cm H_2O, Rate 30 Pressure Support plus 15 cm H_2O, FIO_2 0.45, and T_I 0.50 sec. His spontaneous respiratory rate ranges from 12 to 25 breaths/min. His chest radiograph shows a very heterogeneous picture, with dense areas of atelectasis alternating with areas of radiopacity. He has bilateral equal breath sounds with scattered crackles throughout. BB Ranger was quite agitated on arrival, fidgeting and crying, and you were able to hear muffled-sounding cries when he appeared to be most upset.

- *How would you classify the blood gas?*
- *What is your impression of this patient's respiratory status? What would you recommend for him while waiting for a pulmonary consultation?*

MULTIPLE-CHOICE QUESTIONS

1. Which of the following is **not** a characteristic of AOP?
   a. A sudden cessation of breathing
   b. Lasts for greater than 20 seconds
   c. Accompanied by bradycardia
   d. Accompanied by hypoxemia
   e. Occurs only in infants younger than 30 wG

2. What is the difference between periodic breathing and AOP?
   a. Periodic breathing is a benign breathing pattern; AOP is a significant breathing disorder.
   b. Periodic breathing is associated with an increase in $PaCO_2$ and no change in PaO_2; AOP is associated with a decrease in PaO_2 and no change in $PaCO_2$.
   c. Periodic breathing only occurs in full-term infants; AOP occurs in premature infants up to 37 weeks postmenstrual age.
   d. Periodic breathing resembles fetal breathing; AOP resembles Cheyne-Stokes respiration.

3. You respond to an apnea alarm on a patient who is 33 weeks postmenstrual age and on no supplemental oxygen. When you arrive at the bedside, her HR is 90 bpm, and the SpO_2 is 79%. What should you do first?
   a. Observe until the HR is less than 60 bpm
   b. Call the nurse and physician to the bedside
   c. Provide tactile stimulation
   d. Begin PPV

4. Your patient begins breathing again. You document this in the patient's chart and note that in the last 4 hours there were five episodes of apnea with bradycardia and hypoxemia. You notify the nurse of your intervention, and the nurse tells you that the patient is scheduled to go home tomorrow. What are your concerns for this patient?
   I. She likely has AOP
   II. She should be discharged on a home cardiorespiratory monitor
   III. She may be septic
   IV. She should be prescribed caffeine citrate
   V. She should not be discharged tomorrow
   a. I, III, IV, V
   b. I, II, IV
   c. I, V
   d. III, V

5. What are characteristics of the "new BPD" that make it different from the traditional form of BPD, described in 1967?
   a. Overwhelming evidence of alveolar hypoplasia
   b. Dysfunction of the alveolar capillary membrane
   c. Emphysematous changes to the alveoli typical of lung injury
   d. Airway injury present

6. You are caring for a baby boy, born at 24 3/7 wG, who is now 36 weeks postmenstrual age. He was intubated and on supplemental oxygen for the first 35 days of life. He is now on NCPAP plus 7 cm H2O at 0.28 FIO_2. Classify the severity of his BPD.
   a. Mild
   b. Moderate
   c. Severe
   d. He doesn't have BPD

7. Which of the following patients should be considered to receive corticosteroid therapy?
   a. A 3-day-old neonate, born at 26 wG, currently on SIMV
   b. A 14-day-old neonate, born at 34 wG, on NC 0.40 FIO_2
   c. A 28-day-old neonate, born at 24 wG, currently on SIMV
   d. A 5-day-old neonate, born at 27 wG, currently on NCPAP

8. Which of the following respiratory care strategies should be avoided to minimize the risk of severe BPD when caring for extremely preterm infants?
    a. Use the lowest FIO_2 possible to achieve adequate oxygenation
    b. Provide low PEEP levels to prevent overdistention and damage to the alveoli
    c. Attempt to target V_T of 4 to 7 mL/kg to avoid excessive ventilation
    d. Use surfactant-replacement therapy
    e. Use NCPAP when possible to avoid invasive MV

9. Which of the following is an established pharmacological strategy that has been shown to reduce the risk of BPD:
    a. Corticosteroids
    b. Mast cell stabilizers
    c. Inositol
    d. Inhaled nitric oxide

DavisPlus | For additional resources login to DavisPlus (http://davisplus.fadavis.com/ keyword "Perretta") and click on the Premium tab. (Don't have a PlusCode to access Premium Resources? Just click the Purchase Access button on the book's DavisPlus page.)

REFERENCES

1. Daily WJ, Klaus M, Meyer HB. Apnea in premature infants: monitoring, incidence, heart rate changes, and an effect of environmental temperature. *Pediatrics*. 1969;43 (4):510-518.
2. Eichenwald EC, Aina A, Stark AR. Apnea frequently persists beyond term gestation in infants delivered at 24 to 28 weeks. *Pediatrics*. 1997;100(3, pt 1):354-359.
3. Hoffman HJ, Damus K, Hillman L, et al. Risk factors for SIDS: results of the National Institute of Child Health and Human Development SIDS Cooperative Epidemiological Study. *Ann N Y Acad Sci*. 1988;533:13-30.
4. Barrington K, Finer N. The natural history of the appearance of apnea of prematurity. *Pediatr Res*. 1991;29(4, pt 1): 372-375.
5. Martin RJ, Abu-Shaweesh JM, Baird TM. Apnoea of prematurity. *Paediatr Respir Rev*. 2004;5(5, suppl A):S377-S382.
6. Gauda EB, McLemore GL, Tolosa J, et al. Maturation of peripheral arterial chemoreceptors in relation to neonatal apnoea. *Semin Neonatol*. 2004;9(3):181-194.
7. Zhao J, Gonzalez F, Mu D. Apnea of prematurity: from cause to treatment. *Eur J Pediatr*. 2011;170(9):1097-1105.
8. Atkinson E, Fenton AC. Management of apnoea and bradycardia in neonates. *Paediatr Child Health*. 2009;19(12): 550-554.
9. Edwards BA, Sands SA, Berger PJ. Postnatal maturation of breathing stability and loop gain: the role of carotid chemoreceptor development [published online ahead of print June 13, 2012]. *Respir Physiol Neurobiol*. doi.org/ 10.1016/j.resp.2012.06.003.
10. Aizad T, Bodani J, Cates D, et al. Effect of a single breath of 100% oxygen on respiration in neonates during sleep. *J Appl Physiol*. 1984;57(5):1531-1535.
11. Cross KW, Oppe TE. The effect of inhalation of high and low concentrations of oxygen on the respiration of the premature infant. *J Physiol*. 1952;117(1):38-55.
12. Krauss AN, Tori CA, Brown J, et al. Oxygen chemoreceptors in low birth weight infants. *Pediatr Res*. 1973;7:569-574.
13. Rigatto H, Brady JP, de la Torre Verduzco R. Chemoreceptor reflexes in preterm infants, I: the effect of gestational and postnatal age on the ventilatory response to inhalation of 100% and 15% oxygen. *Pediatrics*. 1975;55(5):604-613.
14. Kutbi I, Al-Matary A, Kwiatkowski K, et al. Increased peripheral chemoreceptor contribution to respiration early in life: a major destabilizing factor in the control of breathing [abstract]. *Pediatr Res*. 2003;53:436A-437A.
15. Daly MD, Angell-James JE, Elsner R. Role of carotid-body chemoreceptors and their reflex interactions in bradycardia and cardiac arrest. *Lancet*. 1979;1:764-767.
16. Bayley G, Walker I. Special considerations in the premature and ex-premature infant. *Anaesth Intensive Care Med*. 2007;9(3):89-92.
17. Macfarlane PM, Ribeiro AP, Martin RJ. Carotid chemoreceptor development and neonatal apnea [published online ahead of print July 25, 2012]. *Respir Physiol Neurobiol*. doi.org/10.1016/j.resp.2012.07.017.
18. Moriette G, Lescure S, El Ayoubi M, et al. Apnea of prematurity: what's new? *Arch Pediatr*. 2010;17(2): 186-190.
19. Finer NN, Higgins R, Kattwinkel J, Martin RJ. Summary proceedings from the apnea-of-prematurity group. *Pediatr*. 2006;117:S47.
20. Ramanathan R, Corwin MJ, Hunt CE, et al. Cardiorespiratory events recorded on home monitors: comparison of healthy infants with those at increased risk for SIDS. *JAMA*. 2001;285(17):2199-2207.
21. Poets CF. Apnea of prematurity: what can observational studies tell us about pathophysiology? *Sleep Med*. 2010;11 (7):701-707.
22. Monasterio V, Burgess F, Clifford GD. Robust classification of neonatal apnoea-related desaturations. *Physiol Meas*. 2012;33(9):1503-1516.
23. Sale SM. Neonatal apnoea. *Best Pract Res Clin Anaesthesiol*. 2010;24(3):323-336.
24. Dunwiddie TV, Masino SA. The role and regulation of adenosine in the central nervous system. *Ann Rev Neurosci*. 2001;24:31-55.
25. Gardenhire DS. *Rau's Respiratory Care Pharmacology*. St. Louis: Mosby-Elsevier; 2008.
26. Shannon DC, Gotay F, Stein IM, et al. Prevention of apnea and bradycardia in low-birthweight infants. *Pediatrics*. 1975; 55(5):589-594.
27. Spitzer AR. Evidence-based methylxanthine use in the NICU. *Clin Perinatol*. 2012;39(1):137-148.
28. Aranda JV, Gorman W, Bergsteinsson H, et al. Efficacy of caffeine in treatment of apnea in the low-birth-weight infant. *J Pediatr*. 1977;90:467-472.
29. Center for Drug Evaluation and Research. Application Number 20-793. Caffeine citrate [approval letter]. Rockville, MD: Food and Drug Administration; September 21, 1999. http://www.accessdata.fda.gov/drugsatfda_docs/nda/99/ 020793_000_Cafcit_AP.pdf. Accessed October 2, 2012.

30. Schmidt B, Roberts RS, Davis P, et al. Caffeine therapy for apnea of prematurity. *N Engl J Med.* 2006;354(20): 2112-2121.

31. Osborn DA, Henderson-Smart DJ. Kinesthetic stimulation versus methylxanthine for apnea in preterm infants. *Cochrane Database System Rev.* 1998;2:CD000502.

32. Henderson-Smart DJ, Steer PA. Doxapram treatment for apnea in preterm infants. *Cochrane Database System Rev.* 2004;4:CD000074.

33. Custer JW, Rau RE, eds. *The Harriet Lane Handbook.* Philadelphia, PA: Mosby Elsevier; 2009:Box 4-3.

34. Pearlman SA, Duran C, Wood MA, et al. Caffeine pharmacokinetics in preterm infants older than 2 weeks. *Dev Pharmacol Ther.* 1989;12(2):65-69.

35. Ahn HW, Shin WG, Park KJ, et al. Pharmacokinetics of theophylline and caffeine after intravenous administration of aminophylline to premature infants in Korea. *Res Commun Mol Pathol Pharmacol.* 1999;105(1-2):105-113.

36. Charles BG, Townsend SR, Steer PA, et al. Caffeine citrate treatment for extremely premature infants with apnea: population pharmacokinetics, absolute bioavailability, and implications for therapeutic drug monitoring. *Ther Drug Monit.* 2008;30(6):709-716.

37. Davis JM, Stefano JL, Bhutani VK, et al. Changes in pulmonary mechanics following caffeine administration in infants with BPD. *Pediatr Pulmonol.* 1989;6(1):49-52.

38. Zagol K, Lake DE, Vergales B, et al. Anemia, apnea of prematurity, and blood transfusions. *J Pediatr.* 2012; 161(3):417-421.

39. Walsh M, Engle W, Laptook A, et al.; National Institute of Child Health and Human Development Neonatal Research Network. Oxygen delivery through nasal cannulae to preterm infants: can practice be improved? *Pediatrics.* 2005;116(4):857-861.

40. American Association for Respiratory Care. AARC Clinical Practice Guideline: Application of Continuous Positive Airway Pressure to Neonates via Nasal Prongs, Nasopharyngeal Tube, or Nasal Mask—2004 revision & update. *Respir Care.* 2004;49(9):1100-1108.

41. Diblasi RM. Nasal continuous positive airway pressure for the respiratory care of the newborn. *Respir Care.* 2009;54(9): 1209-1235.

42. Pantalitschka T, Sievers J, Urschitz MS, et al. Randomised crossover trial of four nasal respiratory support systems for apnoea of prematurity in very low birthweight infants. *Arch Dis Child Fetal Neonatal Ed.* 2009;94(4):F245-F248.

43. Lemyre B, Davis PG, De Paoli AG, et al. Nasal intermittent positive pressure ventilation (NIPPV) versus nasal continuous positive airway pressure (NCPAP) for apnea of prematurity. *Cochrane Database System Rev.* 2002;1: CD002272.

44. Bredemeyer SL, Foster JP. Body positioning for spontaneously breathing preterm infants with apnoea. *Cochrane Database System Rev.* 2012;6:CD004951.

45. Bauschatz AS, Kaufmann CM, Haensse D, et al. A preliminary report of nursing in the three-stair-position to prevent apnoea of prematurity. *Acta Paediatr.* 2008;97(12): 1743-1745.

46. Reher C, Kuny KD, Pantalitschka T, et al. Randomised crossover trial of different postural interventions on bradycardia and intermittent hypoxia in preterm infants. *Arch Dis Child Fetal Neonatal Ed.* 2008;93(4):289-291.

47. Sher TR. Effect of nursing in the head elevated tilt position (15 degrees) on the incidence of bradycardic and hypoxemic episodes in preterm infants. *Pediatr Phys Ther.* 2002;14(2): 112-113.

48. Osborn DA, Henderson-Smart DJ. Kinesthetic stimulation for treating apnea in preterm infants. *Cochrane Database System Rev.* 1999;1:CD000499.

49. Baird TM. Clinical correlates, natural history and outcome of neonatal apnoea. *Semin Neonatol.* 2004;9(3):205-211.

50. Cheung PY, Barrington KJ, Finer NN, et al. Early childhood neurodevelopment in very low birth weight infants with predischarge apnea. *Pediatr Pulmonol.* 1999;27(1): 14-20.

51. Ramanathan R, Corwin MJ, Hunt CE, et al.; Collaborative Home Infant Monitoring Evaluation [CHIME] Study Group. Cardiorespiratory events recorded on home monitors: comparison of healthy infants with those at increased risk for SIDS. *JAMA.* 2001;285(17):2199-2207.

52. Pilcher G, Urlesberger B, Muller W. Impact of bradycardia on cerebral oxygenation and cerebral blood volume during apnoea in preterm infants. *Physiol Meas.* 2003;24(3):671-680.

53. Koons AH, Mojica N, Jadeja N, et al. Neurodevelopmental outcome of infants with apnea of infancy. *Am J Perinatol.* 1993;10(3):208-211.

54. Janvier A, Khairy M, Kokkotis A, et al. Apnea is associated with neurodevelopmental impairment in very low birth weight infants. *J Perinatol.* 2004;24(12):763-768.

55. Sreenan C, Etches PC, Demianczuk N, et al. Isolated mental developmental delay in very low birth weight infants: association with prolonged doxapram therapy for apnea. *J Pediatr.* 2001;139(6):832-837.

56. Schmidt B, Anderson PJ, Doyle LW, et al. Survival without disability to age 5 after neonatal caffeine therapy for apnea of prematurity. *JAMA.* 2012;307(3):275-282.

57. Allen J, Zwerdling R, Ehrenkranz R, et al. Statement on the care of the child with chronic lung disease of infancy and childhood. *Am J Respir Crit Care Med.* 2003;168(3): 356-396.

58. Northway WH, Rosan RC, Porter DY. Pulmonary disease following respiratory therapy of hyaline-membrane disease: bronchopulmonary dysplasia. *N Engl J Med.* 1967;276(7): 357-368.

59. Nickerson BG. Bronchopulmonary dysplasia. Chronic pulmonary disease following neonatal respiratory failure. *Chest.* 1985;87(4);528-535.

60. Stroustrup A, Trasande L. Epidemiological characteristics and resource use in neonates with bronchopulmonary dysplasia. *Pediatrics.* 2010;126(2):e291-e297.

61. Bland RD. Neonatal chronic lung disease in the post-surfactant era. *Biol Neonate.* 2005;88(3):181-191.

62. Jobe AH, Bancalari E. Bronchopulmonary dysplasia. *Am J Respir Crit Care Med.* 2001;163(7):1723-1729.

63. Ehrenkranz RA, Walsh MC, Vohr BR, et al. Validation of the National Institutes of Health consensus definition of bronchopulmonary dysplasia. *Pediatrics.* 2005;116(6): 1353-1360.

64. Baraldi E, Filippone M. Chronic lung disease after premature birth. *N Engl J Med.* 2007;357:1946-1955.

65. Walsh MC, Szefler S, Davis J, et al. Summary proceedings from the Bronchopulmonary Dysplasia Group. *Pediatrics.* 2006;117(3, pt 2):S52-S56.

66. Pfister RH, Goldsmith JP. Quality improvement in respiratory care: decreasing bronchopulmonary dysplasia. *Clin Perinatol.* 2010;37(1):273-293.

67. Demirel N, Bas AY, Zenciroglu A. Bronchopulmonary dysplasia in very low birth weight infants. *Indian J Pediatr.* 2009;76(7):695-698.

68. Stoll BJ, Hansen NI, Bell EF, et al. Neonatal outcomes of extremely preterm infants from the NICHD Neonatal Research Network. *Pediatrics.* 2010;126(3):443-456.

69. Lopez ES, Rodriguez EM, Navarro CR, et al. Initial respiratory management in preterm infants and bronchopulmonary dysplasia. *Clinics (Sao Paulo).* 2011;66(5):823-827.

70. Subramanian S, El-Mohandes A, Dhanireddy R, et al. Association of bronchopulmonary dysplasia and hypercapnia

in ventilated infants with birth weights of 500-1,499 g. *Matern Child Health J.* 2011;15(suppl 1):S17-S26.

71. Chess PR, D'Angio CT, Pryhuber GS, et al. Pathogenesis of bronchopulmonary dysplasia. *Semin Perinatol.* 2006; 30(4):171-178.

72. Valieva OA, Strandjord TP, Mayock DE, et al. Effects of transfusions in extremely low birth weight infants: a retrospective study. *J Pediatr.* 2009;155(3):331-337.e1.

73. Lacaze-Masmonteil L, Hartling Y, Liang C, et al. A systematic review and meta-analysis of studies evaluating chorioamnionitis as a risk factor for bronchopulmonary dysplasia in preterm infants. *Paediatr Child Health.* 2007; 12(suppl A).

74. Gien J, Kinsella JP. Pathogenesis and treatment of bronchopulmonary dysplasia. *Curr Opin Pediatr.* 2011;23(3): 305-313.

75. Eichenwald EC, Stark AR. Management of bronchopulmonary dysplasia. *Paediatr Child Health.* 2009;19(12): 559-564.

76. Kim D, Kim H, Choi CW, et al. Risk factors for pulmonary artery hypertension in preterm infants with moderate or severe bronchopulmonary dysplasia. *Neonatology.* 2012; 101:40-46.

77. Taghizadeh A, Reynolds EO. Pathogenesis of bronchopulmonary dysplasia following hyaline membrane disease. *Am J Pathol.* 1976;82(2):241-264.

78. Moylan RMB, Walker A, Dramer SS, et al. Alveolar rupture as an independent predictor of bronchopulmonary dysplasia. *Crit Care Med.* 1978;6(1):10-13.

79. Gay JH, Daily WJR, Meyer BHP. Ligation of the patent ductus arteriosus in premature infants: report of 45 cases. *J Pediatr Surg.* 1973;8(5):677-683.

80. Brown ER, Stark A, Sosenko I, et al. Bronchopulmonary dysplasia: possible relationship to pulmonary edema. *J Pediatr.* 1978;92(6):982-984.

81. Coalson JJ. Pathology of new bronchopulmonary dysplasia. *Semin Neonatol.* 2003;8(1):73-81. 82. Balinotti JE, Chakr VC, Tiller C, et al. Growth of lung parenchyma in infants and toddlers with chronic lung disease of infancy. *Am J Respir Crit Care Med.* 2010;181(10):1093-1097.

83. Kramer BW, Kallapur S, Newnham J, et al. Prenatal inflammation and lung development. *Semin Fetal Neonatal Med.* 2009;14(1):2-7.

84. De Paepe ME, Mao Q, Powell J, et al. Growth of pulmonary microvasculature in ventilated preterm infants. *Am J Respir Crit Care Med.* 2006;173(2):204-211.

85. Hussain AN, Siddiqui NH, Stocker JT. Pathology of arrested acinar development in postsurfactant bronchopulmonary dysplasia. *Hum Pathol.* 1998;29(7):710-717.

86. Hislop AA, Wigglesworth JS, Desai R, et al. The effects of preterm delivery and mechanical ventilation on human lung growth. *Early Hum Dev.* 1987;15(3):147-164.

87. Coalson JJ, Winter VT, Siler-Khodr T, et al. Neonatal chronic lung disease in extremely immature baboons. *Am J Respir Crit Care Med.* 1999;160(4):1333-1346.

88. Mokres LM, Parai K, Hilgendorff A, et al. Prolonged mechanical ventilation with air induces apoptosis and causes failure of alveolar septation and angiogenesis in lungs of newborn mice. *Am J Physiol Lung Cell Mol Physiol.* 2010;298(1):L23-L35.

89. Warner BB, Stuart LA, Papes RA, et al. Functional and pathological effects of prolonged hyperoxia in neonatal mice. *Am J Physiol.* 1998;275(1, pt 1):L110-L117.

90. Thebaud B, Abman SH. Bronchopulmonary dysplasia: where have all the vessels gone? Roles of angiogenic growth factors in chronic lung disease. *Am J Respir Crit Care Med.* 2007;175(10):978-985.

91. Laughon M, Allred EN, Bose C, et al. Patterns of respiratory disease during the first 2 postnatal weeks in extremely premature infants. *Pediatrics.* 2009;123(4): 1124-1131.

92. Kaempf JW, Campbell B, Brown A, et al. PCO_2 and room air saturation values in premature infants at risk for bronchopulmonary dysplasia. *J Perinatol.* 2008; 28(1):48-54.

93. Philip AGS. Chronic lung disease of prematurity: A short history. *Semin Fetal Neonatal Med.* 2009;14(6):333-338.

94. Stevens TP, Blennow M, Soll RF, et al. Early surfactant administration with brief ventilation vs. selective surfactant and continued mechanical ventilation for preterm infants with or at risk for respiratory distress syndrome (review). *The Cochrane Library.* 2008;3:1-34.

95. Stevens TP, Harrington EW, Blennow M, et al. Early surfactant administration with brief ventilation vs. selective surfactant and continued mechanical ventilation for preterm infants with or at risk for respiratory distress syndrome. *Cochrane Database Syst Rev.* 2007;4:CD003063.

96. Donn SM, Dalton J. Surfactant replacement therapy in the neonate: beyond respiratory distress syndrome. *Respir Care.* 2009;54(9):1203-1208.

97. Dumpa V, Northrup V, Bhandari V. Type and timing of ventilation in the first postnatal week is associated with bronchopulmonary dysplasia/death. *Am J Perinatol.* 2011;28(4):321-330.

98. Kulkarni A, Ehrenkranz RA, Bhandari V. Effect of introduction of synchronized nasal intermittent positive-pressure ventilation in a neonatal intensive care unit on bronchopulmonary dysplasia and growth in preterm infants. *Am J Perinatol.* 2006;23(4):233-240.

99. Wheeler K, Klingenberg C, McCallion N, et al. Volume-targeted versus pressure-limited ventilation in the neonate (review). *The Cochrane Library.* 2011;6:1-86.

100. van Kaam A. Lung-protective ventilation in neonatology. *Neonatology.* 2011;99(4):338-341.

101. Thome UH, Carlo WA. Permissive hypercapnia. *Semin Neonatol.* 2002;7(5):409-419.

102. Kugelman A, Durand M. A comprehensive approach to the prevention of bronchopulmonary dysplasia. *Pediatr Pulmonol.* 2011;46(12):1153-1165.

103. Kaiser JR, Gauss CH, Pont MM, et al. Hypercapnia during the first 3 days of life is associated with severe intraventricular hemorrhage in very low birth weight infants. *J Perinatol.* 2006;26(5):279-285.

104. Birenbaum HF, Dentry A, Cirelli J, et al. Reduction in the incidence of chronic lung disease in very low birth weight infants: results of a quality improvement process in a tertiary neonatal intensive care unit. *Pediatrics.* 2009;123(1):44-50.

105. Yoder MC, Chua R, Tepper R. Effect of dexamethasone on pulmonary inflammation and pulmonary function of ventilator-dependent infants with bronchopulmonary dysplasia. *Am Rev Respir Dis.* 1991;143(5, pt 1): 1044-1048.

106. Garland JS, Alex CP, Pauly TH, et al. A three-day course of dexamethasone therapy to prevent chronic lung disease in ventilated neonates: a randomized trial. *Pediatrics.* 1999;104(1, pt 1):91-99.

107. Mammel MC, Green TP, Johnson DE, et al. Controlled trial of dexamethasone therapy in infants with bronchopulmonary dysplasia. *Lancet.* 1983;1(8338):1356-1358.

108. Avery GB, Fletcher AB, Kaplan M, et al. Controlled trial of dexamethasone in respirator-dependent infants with bronchopulmonary dysplasia. *Pediatrics.* 1985; 75(1):106-111.

109. Cummings JJ, D'Eugenio DB, Gross SJ. A controlled trial of dexamethasone in preterm infants at high risk for bronchopulmonary dysplasia. *N Engl J Med.* 1989; 320(23):1505-1510.

110. Stark AR. Risks and benefits of post-natal corticosteroids. *NeoReviews.* 2005;6(2):e99e103.

111. Shah VS, Ohlsson A, Halliday HL, et al. Early administration of inhaled corticosteroids for preventing chronic lung disease in ventilated very low birth weight preterm neonates. *Cochrane Database of System Rev.* 2007;4: CD001969.

112. Halliday HL, Ehrenkranz RA, Doyle LW. Early (< 8 days) postnatal corticosteroids for preventing chronic lung disease in preterm infants. *Cochrane Database System Rev.* 2009;1:CD001146.

113. Watterberg KL; Committee on Fetus and Newborn. Postnatal corticosteroids to prevent or treat bronchopulmonary dysplasia. *Pediatrics.* 2010;126(4):800-808.

114. Onland W, Offringa M, van Kaam A. Late (> 7 days) inhalation corticosteroids to reduce bronchopulmonary dysplasia in preterm infants. *Cochrane Database System Rev.* 2012;4:CD002311.

115. Rademaker KJ, Uiterwaal CS, Groenendaal F, et al. Neonatal hydrocortisone treatment: neurodevelopmental outcome and MRI at school age in preterm-born children. *J Pediatr.* 2007;150(4):351-357.

116. Shah SS, Ohlsson A, Halliday HL, et al. Inhaled versus systemic corticosteroids for preventing chronic lung disease in ventilated very low birth weight preterm neonates. *Cochrane Database System Rev.* 2003;1:CD002058.

117. Shah SS, Ohlsson A, Halliday HL, et al. Inhaled versus systemic corticosteroids for the treatment of chronic lung disease in ventilated very low birth weight preterm infants. *Cochrane Database System Rev.* 2007;4:CD002057.

118. Viscardi RM, Adeniyi-Jones SC. Retrospective study of the effectiveness of cromolyn sodium in bronchopulmonary dysplasia. *Neonatal Intensive Care.* 1994;7: 18-20.

119. Ng G, Ohlsson A. Cromolyn sodium for the prevention of chronic lung disease in preterm infants. *Cochrane Database System Rev.* 2001;1:CD003059.

120. Darlow BA, Graham PJ. Vitamin A supplementation to prevent mortality and short- and long-term morbidity in very low birthweight infants. *Cochrane Database Syst Rev.* 2007;4:CD000501.

121. Hallman M, Bry K, Hoppu K, et al. Inositol supplementation in premature infants with respiratory distress syndrome. *N Engl J Med.* 1992;326:1233-1239.

122. Howlett A, Ohlsson A, Plakkal N. Inositol for respiratory distress syndrome in preterm infants. *Cochrane Database System Rev.* 2012;3:CD000366.306.

123. Baveja R, Christou H. Pharmacological strategies in the prevention and management of bronchopulmonary dysplasia. *Semin Perinatol.* 2006;30(4):209-218.

124. Suresh G, Davis JM, Soll R. Superoxide dismutase for preventing chronic lung disease in mechanically ventilated preterm infants. *Cochrane Database System Rev.* 2001;1:CD001968.

125. Van Meurs KP, Wright LL, Ehrenkranz RA, et al. Inhaled nitric oxide for premature infants with severe respiratory failure. *N Engl J Med.* 2005;353(1):13-22.

126. Kinsella JP, Cutter GR, Walsh WF, et al. Early inhaled nitric oxide therapy in premature newborns with respiratory failure. *N Engl J Med.* 2006;355(4):354-364.

127. Su PH, Chen JY. Inhaled nitric oxide in the management of preterm infants with severe respiratory failure. *J Perinatol.* 2008;28(2):112-116.

128. Ballard RA, Truog WE, Cnaan A, et al. Inhaled nitric oxide in preterm infants undergoing mechanical ventilation. *N Engl J Med.* 2006;355(4):343-353.

129. Hibbs AM, Walsh MC, Martin RJ, et al. One-year respiratory outcomes of preterm infants enrolled in the Nitric Oxide (to prevent) Chronic Lung Disease trial. *J Pediatr.* 2008;153(4):525-529.

130. Walsh MC, Hibbs AM, Martin CR, et al. Two-year neurodevelopmental outcomes of ventilated premature infants treated with inhaled nitric oxide. *J Pediatr.* 2010; 156(4):556-561.

131. Barrington KJ, Finer N. Inhaled nitric oxide for respiratory failure in preterm infants. *Cochrane Database System Rev.* 2010;12:CD000509.

132. Donohue PK, Gilmore MM, Cristofalo E, et al. Inhaled nitric oxide in preterm infants: a systematic review. *Pediatrics.* 2011;127(2):e414-e422.

133. Stewart A, Brion LP, Ambrosio-Perez I. Diuretics acting on the distal renal tubule for preterm infants with (or developing) chronic lung disease. *Cochrane Database System Rev.* 2011;9:CD001817.

134. Stewart A, Brion LP. Intravenous or enteral loop diuretics for preterm infants with (or developing) chronic lung disease. *Cochrane Database System Rev.* 2011;9: CD001453.

135. Brion LP, Primhak RA, Yong W. Aerosolized diuretics for preterm infants with (or developing) chronic lung disease. *Cochrane Database System Rev.* 2006;3:CD001694.

136. Ng G, da Silva O, Ohlsson A. Bronchodilators for the prevention and treatment of chronic lung disease in preterm infants. *Cochrane Database System Rev.* 2001;2: CD003214.

137. Fakhoury KF, Sellers C, Smith EO, et al. Serial measurements of lung function in a cohort of young children with bronchopulmonary dysplasia. *Pediatrics.* 2010;125: e1441-e1447.

138. Northway WH Jr, Moss RB, Carlisle KB, et al. Late pulmonary sequelae of bronchopulmonary dysplasia. *N Engl J Med.* 1990;323:1793-1799.

139. Doyle LW, Faber B, Callanan C, et al. Bronchopulmonary dysplasia in very low birth weight subjects and lung function in late adolescence. *Pediatrics.* 2006;118; 108-113.

140. Filippone M, Bonetto G, Cherubin E, et al. Childhood course of lung function in survivors of bronchopulmonary dysplasia. *JAMA.* 2009;302(13):1418-1420.

141. Baraldi E, Filippone M, Trevisanuto D, et al. Pulmonary function until two years of life in infants with bronchopulmonary dysplasia. *Am J Respir Crit Care Med.* 1997;155(1):149-155.

142. Oppenheim C, Mamou-Mani T, Sayegh N, et al. Bronchopulmonary dysplasia: value of CT in identifying pulmonary sequelae. *AJR Am J Roentgenol.* 1994;163(1): 169-172.

143. Aukland SM, Rosedahl K, Owens CM, et al. Neonatal bronchopulmonary dysplasia predicts abnormal pulmonary HRCT scans in long-term survivors of extreme preterm birth. *Thorax.* 2009;64(5):405-410.

144. Greenough A, Alexander J, Boorman J, et al. Respiratory morbidity, healthcare utilisation and cost of care at school age related to home oxygen status. *Eur J Pediatr.* 2011;170(8):969-975.

145. Ali K, Greenough A. Long-term respiratory outcome of babies born prematurely. *Ther Adv Respir Dis.* 2012; 6(2):115-120.

146. Mclean A, Townsend A, Clark J, et al. Quality of life of mothers and families caring for preterm infants requiring

home oxygen therapy: a brief report. *J Paediatr Child Health*. 2000;36(5):440-444.

147. Collaco JM, Choi SJ, Riekert KA, et al. Socio-economic factors and outcomes in chronic lung disease of prematurity. *Pediatr Pulmonol*. 2011;46(7):709-716.

148. Korhonen P, Koivisto AM, Ikonen S, et al. Very low birthweight, bronchopulmonary dysplasia and health in early childhood. *Acta Pædiatr*. 1999;88(12):1385-1391.

149. Halvorsen T, Skadberg BT, Eide GE, et al. Pulmonary outcome in adolescents of extreme preterm birth: a regional cohort study. *Acta Paediatr*. 2004;93(10):1294-1300.

150. Guimaraes H, Rocha G, Pissarra S, et al. Respiratory outcomes and atopy in school-age children who were preterm at birth, with and without bronchopulmonary dysplasia. *Clinics (Sao Paulo)*. 2011;66(3):425-430.

151. Landry JS, Chan T, Lands L, et al. Long-term impact of bronchopulmonary dysplasia on pulmonary function. *Can Respir J*. 2011;18(5):265-270.

152. Wong PM, Lees AN, Louw J, et al. Emphysema in young adult survivors of moderate-to-severe bronchopulmonary dysplasia. *Eur Respir J*. 2008;32(2):321-328.

153. Cutz E, Chiasson D. Chronic lung disease after premature birth. *N Engl J Med*. 2008;358:743-745.

154. Kobaly K, Schluchter M, Minich N, et al. Outcomes of extremely low birth weight (<1 kg) and extremely low gestational age (<28 weeks) infants with bronchopulmonary dysplasia: effects of practice changes in 2000 to 2003. *Pediatrics*. 2008;121(1):73-81.

155. Karagianni P, Tsakalidis C, Kyriakidou M, et al. Neuromotor outcomes in infants with bronchopulmonary dysplasia. *Pediatr Neurol*. 2011;44(1):40-46.

Chapter 6

Disease of Full-Term Infants

Sarah Mola, MD
Gary Oldenburg, RRT-NPS
Shannon Polin, BS, RRT
Webra Price-Douglas, PhD, CRNP, IBLC

Key Terms

Activated clotting time (ACT)
Amnioinfusion
Ball-valve obstruction
Cardiomegaly
Chemical pneumonitis
Decannulation
Extracorporeal life support (ECLS)
Extracorporeal membrane
  oxygenation (ECMO)
Extracorporeal membrane
  oxygenation (ECMO) pump
Extracorporeal membrane
  oxygenation (ECMO) heater
Maladaptation
Maldevelopment
Meconium
Meconium aspiration syndrome
  (MAS)
Meconium aspirator
Methemoglobin (MetHb)
Nitric oxide
Nonvigorous
Oxygenation index (OI)
Oxygenators
Partial obstruction
Persistent pulmonary hypertension
  of the newborn (PPHN)
Postductal SpO_2
Preductal SpO_2
Pulmonary hypertensive crisis
Starling's forces
Total obstruction
Transient tachypnea of the
  newborn (TTN)
Underdevelopment
Venoarterial ECMO
Venovenous ECMO

Chapter Objectives

After reading this chapter, you will be able to:

1. Describe the physiological mechanism that causes failure of the transition from fetal circulation to adult circulation at delivery.
2. Evaluate oxygenation in a patient with persistent pulmonary hypertension in the newborn (PPHN) and recommend strategies to improve hypoxemia.
3. Recommend therapies to decrease pulmonary vascular resistance (PVR) in a newborn with severe PPHN.
4. Assess the effectiveness of inhaled nitric oxide (iNO) therapy and recommend necessary changes.
5. Determine whether a patient in hypoxic respiratory failure should be cannulated and placed on extracorporeal life support (ECLS).
6. Explain the ventilator support needed for a patient receiving ECLS.
7. List five risk factors associated with increased risk of meconium-stained amniotic fluid (MSAF) and subsequent development of meconium aspiration syndrome (MAS).
8. Describe the changes to delivery room management needed for an infant with MSAF.
9. Specify the most common signs and symptoms of compromise in an infant with MSAF.
10. Recommend respiratory interventions for an infant with MAS.
11. Identify the common causes of decreased fetal lung fluid absorption at delivery.

■■ Baby Boy (BB) Porter

You arrive for an evening shift and receive a report on a 3.5-kg full-term male, BB Porter. He was admitted to your level IIID neonatal intensive care unit (NICU) 12 hours ago from a rural hospital for cyanosis, tachycardia, hypoxia, grunting, and retractions. He was placed on nasal continuous positive airway pressure (NCPAP) device, 5 cm H_2O for transport, with an umbilical arterial blood gas (ABG) value of pH 7.35, partial pressure of carbon dioxide ($PaCO_2$) of 42 mm Hg, HCO_3 of 22.9 mEq/L, partial pressure of oxygen (PaO_2) of 50 mm Hg. His oxygen saturation (SpO_2) was 89% on a fractional concentration of inspired oxygen (FIO_2) of 0.90.

Most babies make the transition to extrauterine life independently and without complications. Some (10%) need some sort of assistance. Full-term newborns (those delivered between 38 and 42 weeks of gestation [wG]) rarely require resuscitative efforts in the delivery room because they have less risk of complications than do preterm newborns. Those who do, particularly those who are admitted to a special care nursery, are usually prenatally diagnosed with congenital abnormalities, many of which are discussed in Chapters 9 to 12. Full-term babies admitted to the hospital for reasons not associated with congenital abnormalities usually present with some varying levels of respiratory distress that require close monitoring or intervention. This respiratory distress is usually caused by a failure to complete the normal transition from fetal to extrauterine cardiac and pulmonary function. The most severe of these is persistent pulmonary hypertension (PPHN), and the most common known cause is meconium aspiration syndrome (MAS). A less severe form of respiratory distress is transient tachypnea of the newborn (TTN). These disorders are challenging to predict and prevent, and their severity can vary widely. The role of the respiratory therapist (RT) who cares for these patients is assisting in maintaining oxygenation and ventilation, minimizing noxious stimulation, and assessing and adjusting support frequently to prevent hypoxemic respiratory failure.

Persistent Pulmonary Hypertension of the Newborn

Persistent pulmonary hypertension of the newborn (PPHN) is a syndrome with severe hypoxemia and high pulmonary artery pressures that occurs when the pulmonary vascular resistance (PVR), normally high in utero, fails to decrease at birth. The term originally used to describe this syndrome was persistent fetal circulation, which accurately describes the cause of PPHN but does not as accurately describe the pathophysiology of the disease. The condition usually presents at birth or shortly after and is characterized by a failure to establish adequate pulmonary and systemic oxygenation. Without treatment, this can cause severe cardiac dysfunction, multiorgan dysfunction, and death.

PPHN primarily affects full-term and near-term neonates, although some premature neonates at less than 32 wG show echocardiographic evidence of PPHN (Special Population 6-1). The incidence of

PPHN in Preterm Infants

PPHN can occur as a complication of RDS in near-term premature neonates, often in those delivered by cesarean section at 34 to 37 wG (1). The increasing reactivity of pulmonary arteries at this gestation period predisposes these neonates to pulmonary hypertension when gas exchange is impaired, such as with surfactant deficiency.

PPHN in term and near-term newborns is estimated to be 1 to 2 per 1000 live births (2–4).

MAS is the most common underlying diagnosis of PPHN, followed by primary or idiopathic PPHN (5). Other diagnoses associated with pulmonary hypertension can be found in Box 6-1.

Many risk factors have been suggested to increase the likelihood of PPHN:

- NSAID drug use (7)
- Male gender (8)
- Cesarean delivery prior to the onset of labor (4, 8)
- Maternal factors such as high prepregnancy body mass index, diabetes, and asthma
- Birth weight greater than 90th percentile
- Gestational age greater than 41 weeks (8)

The exact cause of PPHN, particularly idiopathic PPHN, is not well-known. The hypothesis is that, prior to and just after delivery, there is an interruption in the normal, complex process of chemical and physical signaling that regulates pulmonary vascular tone and lung inflation.

Pathophysiology

PPHN occurs as a result of a failure to transition from fetal circulation to adult circulation. It is a complex process that involves clearance of fetal lung fluid, a decrease in PVR, and closure of several fetal

Box 6-1 Diagnoses Associated With Pulmonary Hypertension (6)

Asphyxia
Meconium aspiration syndrome
Neonatal respiratory distress syndrome
Sepsis
Pneumonia
Congenital diaphragmatic hernia
Pulmonary hypoplasia
Total anomalous pulmonary venous return
Hypoplastic left heart syndrome
Left ventricular outflow tract obstruction

anatomical structures in order for newborns to oxygenate and exhale CO_2 (gas exchange). There are also several chemical mediators that have been implicated in the successful transition from fetal circulation, and a failure of one or several of these may prevent effective pulmonary circulation. Fetal circulation was discussed in Chapter 2, but a review is warranted here.

Fetal Circulation

Blood flows from the fetus to the placenta via the two umbilical arteries, where nutrients and oxygen are transferred into fetal blood and oxygen and waste are secreted. Oxygen-rich blood returns to the fetus through one large umbilical vein, which passes through the ductus venosus in the liver, into the inferior vena cava and the right atrium. Once blood enters the right atrium, less than 10% will travel through the right ventricle and into the pulmonary arteries, with the rest passing through the foramen ovale into the left atrium. PVR is very high, as a physiological response to pulmonary hypoxia, helping to prevent blood flow through the fluid-filled lungs. Excess blood that enters the pulmonary system via the pulmonary artery is shunted through the ductus arteriosus to the aorta just after the right subclavian branch. Blood flowing through the ductus arteriosus will bypass the left side of the heart. Both the shunted blood and that from the left ventricle travel through the aorta, perfusing the upper and lower portions of the body. A portion passes through the umbilical arteries, which arise from the iliac arteries in the pelvis, and then back to the placenta.

Normal Changes to Fetal Circulation at Delivery

The change from fetal to adult circulation requires a drop in PVR and a significant increase in systemic vascular resistance (SVR). This is facilitated by a newborn's first breaths, clamping of the umbilical cord, and the physical stimulus of the new extrauterine environment. These changes normally occur within minutes to hours after birth.

There are several factors at play during delivery that stimulate a newborn to breathe. Chemoreceptors in the aorta and carotid artery regulate ventilation in humans. As the fetus descends into the birth canal, he or she is cut off from the placenta. This causes a drop in PaO_2, which is detected by the chemoreceptors and sends a chemical message to the brainstem to increase ventilation. The thorax is compressed through the birth canal during delivery and then expands to normal size at delivery, generating a negative intrathoracic pressure and causing air to enter the lungs. The environmental changes from a dark and warm uterus to a bright, cold, and noisy delivery room and the physical stimulation of the infant by handling will trigger the infant's crying reflex. The successful transition to active breathing and increased pulmonary oxygenation causes a 10-fold increase in pulmonary blood flow, resulting in dilation of the pulmonary vessels and a decrease in PVR (9). Ventilation also increases pH within the pulmonary vascular bed, further decreasing PVR.

When the umbilical cord is clamped at birth, it removes the low-resistance placental circuit and greatly increases SVR. Other factors at delivery that increase SVR are a catecholamine surge associated with birth and cutaneous vasoconstriction from the cold extrauterine environment. The increased SVR forces blood back into the lower extremities and increases pressure on the left side of the heart. This pressure forces the flap of tissue in the left atrium to close the foramen ovale. Within the first 24 hours after birth, pulmonary pressures decrease to half that of systemic levels.

Changes to Fetal Circulation During PPHN

When certain conditions develop before, during, or after birth, the normal postnatal adaptation of the pulmonary vasculature may be impeded and result in sustained high pulmonary arterial pressure. When pulmonary pressure is higher than systemic pressure, blood will shunt from the right side of the heart to the left, as in fetal life, through the foramen ovale or ductus arteriosus, and result in systemic hypoxemia and cyanosis. Hypoxemia, hypercarbia, and acidosis all act to increase PVR, so right-to-left shunting will create a cycle that continues to increase pulmonary artery pressure, which becomes challenging to halt and reverse.

There are chemical mediators deriving from the pulmonary vascular cells, known as endothelium-derived mediators, which play important roles in the regulation of PVR at birth (10, 11). These include nitric oxide (NO), prostacyclin, and endothelin. NO is thought to be the most important regulator of vascular tone during the transition to extrauterine life; in PPHN, there appears to be limited endogenous synthesis of NO. Prostacyclin is a vasodilator produced by the pulmonary vessels and stimulated by the onset of breathing at birth. Endothelin is a potent vasoconstrictor found in high levels in the fetus and in neonates with PPHN.

Classifications of PPHN

In 1984, Geggel classified PPHN in three groups, distinguished by the underlying cause of pulmonary hypertension: underdevelopment, maldevelopment, and maladaptation (12).

- **Underdevelopment** is characterized by hypoplastic pulmonary vasculature from pulmonary hypoplasia, which produces a relatively fixed level of pulmonary hypertension. Typical lesions include congenital diaphragmatic hernia (discussed in

Chapter 9), congenital cystic adenomatoid malformation of the lung (CCAM), renal agenesis (failure of one or both kidneys to develop), some instances of oligohydramnios (low levels of amniotic fluid), and intrauterine growth restriction.

- **Maldevelopment** refers to the situation in which the lungs develop normally, but the pulmonary arteriole muscle layer is abnormally thick and grows in smaller vessels that normally have no muscle cells. It appears that vascular mediators stimulate maldevelopment of the pulmonary vasculature. When compared with healthy control patients, infants with severe PPHN have higher plasma concentrations of vasoconstrictor chemical mediators and lower concentrations of vasodilator mediators (13). Conditions associated with PPHN caused by vascular maldevelopment include post-term delivery and MAS. In these disorders, the pulmonary vasculature responds poorly to oxygen and ventilation, which normally produce a decrease in PVR. Excessive perfusion of the lung during fetal development because of constriction of the ductus arteriosus or obstruction of the pulmonary veins may also predispose fetuses to maldevelopment PPHN.

- In **maladaptation**, the pulmonary vascular bed is normally developed. However, adverse perinatal conditions cause active vasoconstriction and interfere with the normal postnatal reduction in PVR. These conditions include perinatal depression, pulmonary parenchymal diseases, and bacterial infections, such as group B *Streptococcus* pneumonia (discussed in Chapter 7), and other less common malformations, such as vein of Galen arteriovenous malformations (14). It may also be caused by perinatal stressors including hypoxia, hypoglycemia, and cold stress (15).

Clinical Manifestations

PPHN should be suspected in any newborn infant who exhibits instability in oxygenation or progressive cyanosis shortly after delivery, usually within the first 12 to 24 hours of life. The diagnosis is confirmed with the history, physical examination, chest radiograph, preductal and postductal blood gases, hyperoxia test, and echocardiogram. Typically, PPHN should be suspected if there is no history or other pulmonary symptoms, making hypoxemia seem out of proportion to the degree of lung disease. Differentiation between lung disease, PPHN, and cyanotic congenital heart disease can be difficult, so a systematic approach to hypoxemic neonates is needed for a timely and accurate diagnosis of PPHN.

Patients are usually term or near term, with no previously diagnosed signs of congenital respiratory or cardiac disease. PPHN frequently occurs in conjunction with meconium aspiration and congenital diaphragmatic hernia, and if a newborn has any of the clinical diagnoses listed in Box 6-1, he or she should be considered highly suspect for PPHN.

A respiratory exam will show tachypnea, retractions, grunting, and cyanosis. Auscultation may be normal, or there may be abnormal cardiac sounds such as systolic murmur, loud P2, prominent or split S2, or diastolic murmur. The electrocardiogram (ECG) is usually normal but may have ST segment elevation. The systemic blood pressure (BP) may be normal, or there may be signs of congestive heart failure and low BP (16).

A chest radiograph result is nonspecific. It may be normal or there may be mild to moderate parenchymal disease. **Cardiomegaly** is possible, as defined by a heart silhouette occupying greater than 60% of the thoracic diameter. There may also be prominent vascular markings or pulmonary congestion. The radiograph is most useful to rule out or diagnose other causes of acute pulmonary decline, such as pneumothorax, MAS, pneumonia, or a congenital abnormality. Radiographic signs of PPHN include right ventricular enlargement and enlarged main and hilar pulmonary arterial shadows.

PPHN can be suspected when the preductal SpO_2 and postductal SpO_2 show a greater than 10% difference. A **preductal SpO_2** is an oxygen saturation taken from an area of the body for which the arterial blood supply comes prior to the ductus arteriosus, including the head and the right upper limb. A preductal SpO_2 sensor is commonly placed on the right hand. A **postductal SpO_2** is taken from an area of the body whose arterial blood supply is after the ductus arteriosus, which is typically taken from the lower limbs. Preductal and postductal S_pO_2 values will differ when right ventricular pressure exceeds left ventricular pressure, thus opening the ductus arteriosus and forcing deoxygenated blood to flow from the pulmonary artery into the aorta (Fig. 6-1). This occurs in approximately half of babies with PPHN (17).

A hyperoxia test should also be performed, in which arterial blood gases are obtained on room air (RA) and 1.0 FIO$_2$ and then compared to assess a newborn's ability to oxygenate. Chapter 12 describes how to perform a hyperoxia test. Analysis of arterial blood gases on RA typically reveals hypoxemia with relatively normal PaCO$_2$. Oxygen is a potent and selective pulmonary vasodilator. PPHN should be suspected when an arterial blood gas shows a PaO$_2$ increase greater than 20 mm Hg after 1.0 F$_I$O$_2$ is given. After diagnosis, PaO$_2$ is unstable and may show an intermittent and transient increase to greater than100 mm Hg with high FIO$_2$ and mechanical ventilation. If preductal and postductal arterial blood gases are obtained simultaneously, an arterial oxygen pressure gradient

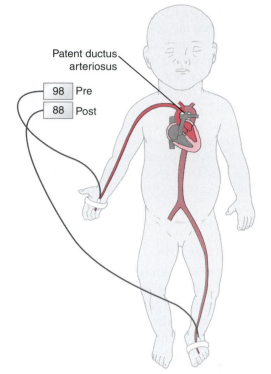

Figure 6-1 Placement of Pulse Oximeters to Measure Preductal and Postductal Saturations

of greater than 15 mm Hg suggests a right-to-left shunt at the level of the ductus arteriosus.

Once the clinical data are obtained and PPHN is suspected, a transthoracic echocardiogram is needed to make an accurate diagnosis and rule out congenital heart defects as the cause of hypoxia. Echocardiography can also document the presence and location of right-to-left shunts. It can also be used to accurately and noninvasively estimate pulmonary artery pressure. Diagnosis of PPHN will be based on the echocardiographic demonstration of normal cardiac anatomy, pulmonary artery pressures at or greater than systemic pressures, and right-to-left shunting of blood across the ductus arteriosus and/or foramen ovale.

The **oxygenation index (OI)** is an equation that assesses the severity of lung dysfunction and is used frequently to help determine the need for escalating care. It calculates how much pulmonary support is needed to maintain the patient's current PaO$_2$ using the following equation:

$$Paw \times FIO_2 \times 100/PaO_2$$

where Paw is mean airway pressures. A high numerator is indicative of a large amount of alveolar oxygen support, and a low denominator indicates poor tissue oxygenation. Taken together, the higher the OI, the worse a patient is able to oxygenate despite high levels of support. An OI at 20 is concerning, and an OI of greater than 40 is an indication of need for extracorporeal membrane oxygenation (ECMO).

■ ■ On admission, BB Porter was intubated and ventilated to maintain a $PaCO_2$ of 35 to 40 mm Hg and pH greater than 7.40 to reduce PVR. Settings are currently synchronized intermittent mandatory ventilation (SIMV), respiratory rate (RR) 40 breaths/min, inspiratory time (TI) 0.45 second, peak inspiratory pressure (PIP) 26 cm H_2O, peak end expiratory pressure (PEEP) 8 cm H_2O, and FIO_2 (Paw is 13.4 cm H_2O). Follow-up umbilical ABG results are as follows: pH 7.30, $PaCO_2$ of 55 mm Hg, HCO_3 of 26.7 mEq/L, and PaO_2 of 60 mm Hg. Pre- and post-SpO_2 are 96% and 85%, respectively. His OI is 22.

Management and Treatment

The objectives in managing PPHN are to correct the underlying disease, maintain adequate systemic blood pressure, decrease PVR, maintain optimal oxygen delivery to the tissues, normalize pH, and minimize ventilator-induced lung injury (VILI). Care should be tailored to the degree of hypoxemia and cardiopulmonary instability. Some patients with mild PPHN respond favorably to oxygen, whereas others require sedation and analgesia, mechanical ventilation, inotropes and pulmonary vasodilators, and complete cardiopulmonary support to prevent death. Because PPHN is often associated with parenchymal lung disease or systemic illness, respiratory therapy should target the underlying disease. Support should be provided as needed, as well as frequent assessment that focuses on restoring independent and normal cardiopulmonary function and avoiding lung injury or adverse effects on systemic perfusion. It is important to remember that the heart and lungs function as an integrated system, and changes to one will usually affect the other. The discussion that follows will focus on the management of patients with idiopathic PPHN who have no underlying disease or precipitating cause of PPHN. See Box 6-2 for a summary of treatment strategies for PPHN.

Box 6-2 Management Strategies for PPHN

- Oxygen to maintain preductal PaO_2 90 to 120 mm Hg
- CMV to produce normocapnia or mild hypocapnia
- HFOV when high pressures or rates are required with CMV
- Pulmonary vasodilators, such as iNO
- Maintain the hematocrit at 35% to 45%
- ECMO for patients who are unresponsive to above therapeutic measures with an OI greater than 40.

Oxygen Therapy

Oxygen is a first line of defense therapy for PPHN. It is a potent and selective pulmonary vasodilator (18), and neonates with mild respiratory distress may respond well to oxygen alone delivered via nasal cannula or face mask. Because of the risk of oxygen toxicity and absorption atelectasis, clinicians should strive for mild hyperoxemia, with PaO_2 kept between 90 and 120 mm Hg (5). Animal studies have shown evidence that prolonged use of high levels of oxygen can be counterproductive and may worsen PPHN, thus weaning FIO_2 should be encouraged whenever hyperoxemia is exhibited (19).

Respiratory Support

Neonates with moderate respiratory distress and hypoxemia may need ventilation support. Mechanical ventilation (MV) can support oxygen delivery, provide alveolar stability, and assist in ventilation during respiratory failure. The goal of MV should be normoxemia, normalization of pH, avoiding hypercapnia, and prevention of VILI. Recommendations for respiratory support can be found in Table 6-1.

Conventional Mechanical Ventilation

Typically, the strategy of mechanical ventilatory support depends on the degree of lung disease and the patient's response to treatment. In general, patients with less severe pulmonary impairment are treated with conventional mechanical ventilation (CMV) and ventilated to maintain $PaCO_2$ of 35 to 45 mm Hg. Studies of animal models and babies with PPHN demonstrated that low $PaCO_2$ and an increase in pH will cause pulmonary vasodilation (20, 21). These benefits are only temporary, however, and will increase the risk of VILI and other detrimental systemic effects (Box 6-3). The use of hyperventilation to treat PPHN is no longer recommended because of other methods of pulmonary vasodilation.

Synchronized ventilation should be used, and respiratory effort should be encouraged as long as it doesn't negatively impact oxygenation. PEEP is essential to stabilize alveoli and prevent atelectasis. Pressure ventilation is common in infants and should target a tidal volume (V_T) of at least 4 to 8 mL/kg body weight. PaO_2 should be used to adjust FIO_2 levels. Preductal and postductal SpO_2 should be used to monitor acute changes in oxygenation and to identify when right-to-left shunting of blood through the patent ductus arteriosus (PDA) occurs, as demonstrated by a difference of greater than 10% in preductal and postductal values.

Sedation may be necessary to provide comfort and decrease the oxygen consumption caused by agitation in hypoxemic neonates, though its use has not been tested in randomized trials (5). Opioid analgesics such

Table 6-1	Therapies for PPHN Based on Oxygenation Index	
Oxygenation Index	**Therapy**	**Recommended Settings**
<20	Supplemental oxygen	Adjust FIO_2 for PaO_2 90–120 mm Hg
	CMV	• SIMV • PEEP >4 cm H_2O • PIP for volume target 4–8 mL/kg • RR to maintain $PaCO_2$ 35–45 mm Hg (20–60 breaths/min)
	HFOV	• Bias flow 10–20 LPM • Hz 10–12 • T_I 33% • Paw 2–3 cm H_2O greater than CMV • P for visible chest wiggle
	HFJV	• Rate 420 (may need to lower; change in 60 breaths/min increments) • T_I 0.02 seconds • Optimal PEEP (see Chapter 4 for procedure); > 5 cm H_2O • PIP for normocapnia; begin with same as CMV
>20	iNO	Starting dose 20 ppm Wean FIO_2 when positive response seen Wean by cutting dose in half until 5 ppm, then discontinue
>40	ECMO	

as morphine or fentanyl may be administered if patient-ventilator asynchrony is a cause of hypoxemia. Prolonged use of opioids can cause hypotension, edema, and poor lung function. If asynchronous breathing continues without an identifiable cause, neuromuscular blockers can be used, but their use has been linked to an increased incidence of hearing impairment in survivors of PPHN (24). The use of sedation and paralytics should be reserved for patients who are unable to be effectively ventilated and oxygenated without them, and their use should be limited to less than 48 hours (5, 25). It is critical that infants with hypoxic respiratory failure for whom conventional ventilator therapy fails or is predicted to fail be

Although hyperventilation ($PaCO_2$ less than 35 mm Hg) has the potential to cause pulmonary vasodilation, this effect is due to the fact it increases pH. Unfortunately, hypocarbia and alkalosis also cause a decrease in cerebral perfusion, which has been associated with hearing loss and neurological injury in the follow-up studies of infants who survived PPHN (22, 23). Alkalosis also causes a left shift of the oxyhemoglobin dissociation curve, which means that oxygen molecules are more readily affixed to hemoglobin (Hb). This impedes the unloading of oxygen from Hb at the capillaries, which can potentially decrease oxygen delivery to the tissues and cause tissue hypoxia (44). The development of specific pulmonary vasodilators has made the practice of hyperventilation-induced alkalosis unnecessary, and it is no longer a supported practice.

cared for in institutions that have immediate availability of personnel, including physicians, nurses, and RTs, who are qualified to use multiple modes of ventilation and rescue therapies. The radiological and laboratory support required to manage the broad range of needs of these infants is also essential.

High-Frequency Ventilation

High peak pressures and FIO_2 on CMV increase the risk for volutrauma and are often not well tolerated by patients with PPHN. High-frequency ventilation (HFV) uses small V_T values at rapid rates, along with an "open lung" strategy to maximize lung inflation and oxygenation. Both high-frequency oscillatory ventilation (HFOV) and high-frequency jet ventilation (HFJV) can be used to improve oxygenation and ventilation of patients with PPHN who "fail" CMV. Significantly more published data are available on the use of HFOV specifically for this patient population, and thus the discussion here will focus on HFOV. Using the same mean airway pressures (Paw), HFOV has been shown to improve oxygenation faster than CMV without an increase in complications (26). This is most likely due to the early prioritization of lung recruitment during HFOV (27). Compared with CMV, HFV improves gas exchange, promotes more uniform lung inflation, decreases air leaks, and reduces inflammatory mediators in the lung (28). The effective use of inhaled pulmonary vasodilators, such as inhaled nitric oxide (iNO), requires adequate lung inflation to optimize alveolar drug delivery. HFOV causes safe and effective alveolar recruitment and has been shown to improve the response to iNO and decrease the risk of death or need for ECMO in infants with PPHN and parenchymal lung disease (29). Infants with more severe PPHN will more frequently require HFOV to improve ventilation; if this is used correctly, it is very effective. In fact, in one study, 23% of patients recovered from PPHN using HFOV, without requiring iNO (29). Some centers use HFV as an initial ventilation strategy for patients with PPHN, though there is no clear evidence that prophylactic HFV is better than other modes of ventilation.

The goals of therapy when using HFOV to treat PPHN are to rapidly recruit and stabilize alveoli using Paw, with amplitude (ΔP) providing visible chest wall movement (known as "chest wiggle factor") to clear $PaCO_2$, and adjusting FIO_2 to maintain normoxemia after alveolar recruitment. Recommended initial settings are as follows:

- Bias flow 10 to 20 LPM
- 10 to 12 Hz
- Inspiratory time 33%
- Paw 2 to 3 cm H_2O above that on CMV (29)
- ΔP for visible chest wiggle (30)

During HFV, minute ventilation is calculated using the formula: $f \times V_T^2$; small changes in delivered volume affect large changes in $PaCO_2$. Ventilation is therefore managed primarily by changing ΔP—increasing it to remove more $PaCO_2$ and decreasing it to increase $PaCO_2$. In HFOV, the ΔP setting is changed directly; during HFJV the PIP setting is adjusted. If maximum ΔP is unable to sufficiently improve ventilation, reducing the frequency by 1 Hz (60 breaths/min with HFJV) will improve alveolar gas exchange and increase delivered V_T. There are two reasons for this:

1. Lower rates allow for more relative time for exhalation, which will allow for better CO_2 clearance.
2. Pressure attenuation is less during lower HFV rates; this means that more of the set pressure will reach the alveoli, which creates a higher pressure gradient between inspiration and exhalation (ΔP) and more gas exchange per breath cycle.

Oxygenation is managed using Paw to recruit and stabilize alveoli, and the effectiveness of the current Paw should be assessed using both an ABG test and chest radiograph. If atelectasis is present on radiography, then Paw or PEEP should be increased by 1 cm H_2O until resolved, and FIO_2 may need to be increased transiently until PaO_2 is greater than 60 mm Hg.

Surfactant Therapy

Exogenous surfactant therapy can be used to facilitate alveolar expansion in parenchymal lung disease. It is most useful for patients who have surfactant deficiency or inactivation. It has not been shown to improve outcomes for patients with idiopathic PPHN, but it has been shown to improve oxygenation and decrease the need for ECMO when parenchymal lung disease was present, such as with sepsis or MAS (31–33). The use of surfactant in PPHN has increased over recent years, with nearly 80% of neonates with moderate-to-severe respiratory failure currently receiving this therapy (33, 34).

Cardiac Support

Reversal of right-to-left shunting through the PDA requires a reduction in pulmonary artery pressure and maintaining systemic blood pressure. Cardiac function can be supported in severely affected patients by using inotropes such as dopamine, dobutamine, and epinephrine, which will increase cardiac output by increasing heart rate and improving cardiac contractility (35). Norepinephrine has been shown to increase systemic pressure and oxygenation in neonates who have PPHN (5). Adequate vascular volume should be maintained with intravenous fluids (3), and transfusion of packed red blood cells is commonly required to keep hematocrit at 35% to 45%, to replace blood lost from sampling and to optimize tissue oxygen delivery.

Pulmonary Vasodilators

When supplemental oxygen and acid-base stabilization are not effective in reversing pulmonary hypertension, vasodilators that target the pulmonary circulation should be administered. The ideal pulmonary vasodilator would be delivered directly to the pulmonary vasculature, cause immediate vasodilation, and work selectively on the pulmonary system without systemic effect. The most frequently used pulmonary vasodilator for neonates is iNO, which has a short half-life and is administered by inhalation, making it very selective to the pulmonary system. Other vasodilators that have been used for PPHN include sildenafil, prostacyclin, milrinone, and magnesium sulfate. Improved methods of inhaled delivery to selectively target the pulmonary circulation are under development. Treatments for pulmonary hypertension under investigation include therapies based on combined mechanisms of action that can be administered by inhalation (36).

Inhaled Nitric Oxide

Nitric oxide is a substance produced by nearly every cell and organ in the human body. NO performs many functions, including vasodilation, platelet inhibition, immune regulation, enzyme regulation, and neurotransmission. Its main use in the medical environment focuses on the smooth muscle relaxation of the pulmonary vascular bed. Oxygenation (3) improves as pulmonary vessels are dilated in well-ventilated parts of the lung, thereby redistributing blood flow from regions with decreased ventilation and reducing intrapulmonary shunting. Inhaled NO selectively dilates the pulmonary vasculature adjacent to open lung units; alveoli that are atelectatic or fluid filled will not participate in iNO transfer. This makes it imperative for RTs to ensure alveolar stabilization and effective ventilation prior to initiating iNO, though it does not appear that mode of ventilation will significantly alter the effects of iNO (37). The half-life of iNO is less than 5 seconds because it combines with hemoglobin and is rapidly converted to methemoglobin (MetHb) and nitrate; therefore it has little effect on SVR and systemic blood pressure.

Inhaled NO should be used with U.S. Food and Drug Administration (FDA)–approved devices that are capable of administering it in constant concentration ranges in parts per million (ppm) throughout the respiratory cycle, such as that shown in Figure 6-2. Infants who receive iNO therapy should be monitored according to institutional protocols designed to avoid the potential toxic effects associated with iNO

administration (25). It has been FDA approved for use in conjunction with ventilatory support in the treatment of term and near-term neonates with hypoxic respiratory failure associated with clinical or echocardiographic evidence of pulmonary hypertension, where it improves oxygenation and reduces the need for ECMO (38).

The general indication for using iNO is a failure of ventilation to restore normal PVR. Many studies have used OI as an indication to begin iNO therapy. Many use an OI greater than 25 (17, 40, 41), but the numbers vary widely and can start as low as 10 or 15 (34, 41). The recommended starting dose for iNO is 20 ppm (42, 43), and treatment should be continued up to 14 days or until underlying hypoxemia is resolved and the infant is ready to be weaned. The Clinical Inhaled Nitric Oxide Research Group increased iNO dosage to 80 ppm for those who did not respond to 20 ppm, but no increase in effectiveness was seen (40). A positive response is evident by an increase in oxygenation (seen by SpO_2 and PaO_2), as well as a decrease in preductal and postductal SpO_2 gradient, indicating a reduction of right-to-left shunting of blood through the PDA, and is seen in approximately 50% of patients treated with iNO (43).

When PaO_2 is greater than 120 mm Hg and FIO_2 has been weaned, iNO dose should be halved until reaching 5 ppm. At this point, the dose can then either be weaned slowly until discontinued or turned to zero with tolerance assessed. Weaning is done slowly to prevent detrimental rebound hypoxemia and rapid increases in PVR with the removal of iNO.

The two most common side effects are rebound hypoxemia and methemoglobinemia. To prevent rebound hypoxemia, weaning is done incrementally, which avoids abrupt discontinuation of iNO. **Methemoglobin (MetHb)** is a red blood cell that loses an electron from the ferrous ion. It increases with the dose of iNO, and methemoglobinemia is defined as a MetHb concentration of greater than 2% (44), though treatment may not be initiated until the concentration is greater than 10% (45). MetHb is unable to participate in oxygen delivery and therefore is detrimental in PPHN. In clinical trials, maximum MetHb levels usually were reached approximately 8 hours after initiation of inhalation, although MetHb levels have peaked as late as 40 hours following initiation of iNO therapy (17, 40). Symptoms of methemoglobinemia include tachycardia, cyanosis, and increased respiratory distress, and leads to death if not treated (46). Following discontinuation or reduction of iNO, the MetHb levels returned to baseline over a period of hours. Once iNO is initiated, MetHb levels are monitored according to protocol, usually every 6 or 8 hours, and can be measured by blood gas spectrophotometry. Treatment for

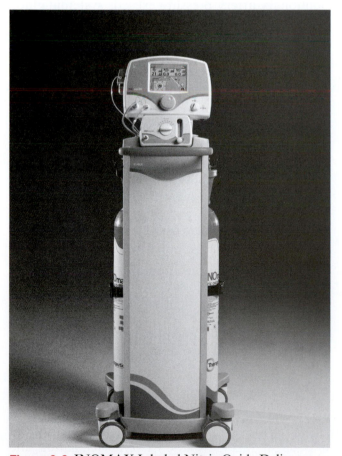

Figure 6-2 INOMAX Inhaled Nitric Oxide Delivery System *(Copyright Ikaria, Inc.)*

methemoglobinemia includes decreasing the dosage of iNO, IV methylene blue (44), ascorbic acid (47), hyperbaric oxygen (48), or exchange transfusion.

For infants who do not respond to iNO, other forms of pulmonary vasodilators can be attempted. If a decrease in PVR does not occur, ECMO must be readily available to prevent mortality. Centers that do not provide ECMO should establish treatment failure criteria for iNO in collaboration with the nearest ECMO center so that they can transfer a critically ill infant early, rather than wait for a response to iNO.

■■ The iNO is started at 20 ppm. A follow-up ABG test revealed a PaO_2 of 90 mm Hg and MetHb of 1.8%. HFOV is started to improve ventilation and oxygenation. MAP is 15 cm H_2O, T_I is 33%, 10 Hz, ΔP 35 mm Hg, and FIO_2 1.

Sildenafil

PPHN is associated with high mortality. Currently, the therapeutic mainstay for PPHN is assisted ventilation and administration of iNO. However, NO is costly and may not be appropriate in resource-poor settings. The evidence of high concentrations of phosphodiesterase (PDE) in the pulmonary vasculature during PPHN has led to the appeal of PDE inhibitors such as sildenafil (49). Sildenafil was introduced into clinical use for erectile dysfunction, but it was tested in adults with primary pulmonary hypertension and demonstrated efficacy and safety of oral dosing (5). Fetal lamb models showed a similar pathological mechanism of increased expression of PDE that contributes to impaired vasodilation (50). Sildenafil has been shown to decrease pulmonary artery pressure and prevent rebound pulmonary hypertension after iNO withdrawal in children with congenital heart defects (51).

A significant improvement in oxygenation occurred in the sildenafil-treated neonates with PPHN 6 to 12 hours after the first dose, without evidence of systemic hypotension (52). Oral sildenafil may be particularly useful for neonates with PPHN who are not responsive to iNO, who are experiencing rebound hypoxemia after withdrawal of iNO (54), or who are in low-resource or other environments where iNO is not available. The dosing for neonates and children is not yet clear, but oral dosage ranges from 0.3 to 1 mg/kg/dose every 6 to 8 hours (54), with a higher 3-mg/kg dose being used in another study to treat patients without access to iNO (55). Other pulmonary vasodilators have been suggested for use in PPHN, but their safety and efficacy have not yet been validated (Evidence in Practice 6-1).

● **Evidence in Practice 6-1**

Other Pulmonary Vasodilators— We Are Not There Yet...

Other pulmonary vasodilators that have been suggested for use in PPHN include other PDE inhibitors, such as milrinone, and prostaglandins, such as prostacyclin.

- No data from randomized control trials of milrinone have been able to establish its efficacy and safety for the neonatal population (56), though its benefits in terms of minimal effect on SVR and ability to deliver via inhalation make it a strong candidate for future research.
- Prostacyclin can be administered via inhalation and is a potent pulmonary vasodilator, increasing cAMP in vascular smooth muscle cells. Neonates may require higher doses than those conventionally used in older children, and systemic vasodilation may be a side effect that must be managed with inotropes (57).

Pulmonary Hypertensive Crisis

A **pulmonary hypertensive crisis** is characterized by a rapid increase in PVR, which results when the pulmonary artery pressure exceeds systemic blood pressure and right heart failure ensues. Several risk factors may contribute to a pulmonary hypertensive crisis:

- Hypoxemia
- Hypotension
- Hypoventilation
- Inadequate preload of the right ventricle
- Noxious stimulation

The management of a pulmonary hypertensive crisis consists of eliminating noxious stimuli that cause the increase of PVR, administering a pulmonary vasodilator, providing adequate preload, and supporting cardiac output. Treatment includes the following:

- Immediate administration of 1.0 FIO_2
- Correction of acidosis
- Increase in the depth of sedation or anesthesia using fentanyl
- Administration of pulmonary vasodilators
- Support of cardiac output with inotropes

■■ You arrive for a shift the following night. BB Porter is now on HFOV, with Paw of 18 cm H_2O, 9 Hz, ΔP of 40 mm Hg, and FIO_2 of 1.0; iNO is now at 40 ppm. Umbilical ABG values on these settings are pH 7.28, $PaCO_2$ 65 of mm Hg, HCO_2 of 30.1 mEq/L, PaO_2 of 35 mm Hg, and MetHb of 3%. OI is now 51.

He is on inotrope infusions of dopamine at 20 mcg/kg/hr, dobutamine at 20 mcg/kg/hr, and epinephrine at 0.3 mcg/kg/hr. He has also received two fluid boluses to improve systemic blood pressure and 10 mL/kg of packed red blood cells. The neonatologist has asked for activation of the ECMO team.

Extracorporeal Membrane Oxygenation

If all attempts at decreasing PVR using the methods described above are unsuccessful, this indicates an immediate need for ECMO therapy (39). Other indications may include persisting levels of OI greater than 20 or alveolar-arterial partial pressure oxygen (A-aO_2) gradients more than 600 after 4 hours of iNO therapy.

Extracorporeal life support (ECLS) is a technique used to support the heart and/or lungs externally when the native heart and/or lungs are no longer able to provide adequate support. This support was originally developed for use in the operating room (during open-heart surgery) and soon after was discovered to have use in the intensive care area for patients who developed respiratory and/or cardiac failure. ECLS, also known as **extracorporeal membrane oxygenation (ECMO)**, is the practice of placing an intensive care unit (ICU) patient on artificial support to give the native lungs and/or heart a period of rest (Fig. 6-3). For the lungs, the goal is to prevent iatrogenic damage caused by high Paw. For the heart, this period of rest prevents the use of high doses of toxic medications to keep the heart functioning. Once the disease process becomes more manageable for the native system to regain support, the ECLS system is weaned and removed.

John Gibbon invented the mechanical oxygenator, which allowed the first successful extracorporeal circulation in a human to be performed in 1953. Although more research developed over the years, it wasn't until 1975 that ECMO was successfully used at the University of California-Irvine in a neonate with MAS. The success of this first patient continued, and in 1982, Bartlett et al. reported 55% survival in a series of 45 neonates treated with ECMO (58). By the 1980s, two prospective randomized trials comparing ECMO with CMV were published. Bartlett's study reported 100% survival of 11 patients receiving ECMO and 0% survival in the control group (59). Although this study was met with scrutiny, the second trial performed by O'Rourke et al. confirmed similar data with 100% survival of nine ECMO patients compared with 33% survival for six patients treated with CMV (60).

Since the success of these trials, the number of ECMO centers has continued to grow, and now there are more than 160 active centers worldwide. The Extracorporeal Life Support Organization (ELSO) was formed in 1989 with the purpose of coordinating

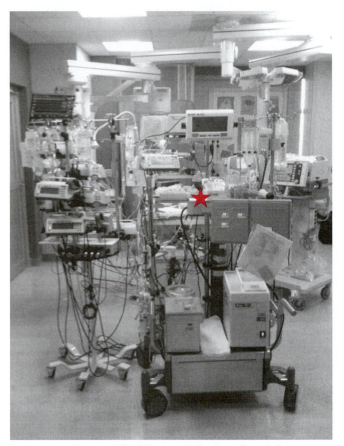

Figure 6-3 Image of a Neonatal Patient Receiving ECMO

clinical research, developing ECLS guidelines, and maintaining the ECMO National Registry Database, which include more than 40,000 patients.

Selection Criteria

The success of ECMO depends on proper patient selection criteria. Each institution governs its own criteria; however, the acceptable guidelines for patients with PPHN from the ELSO are listed in Box 6-4. Most patients with PPHN have a reversible process. However, the amount of lung damage incurred prior to ECMO may contribute to irreversible lung damage. Degree of lung damage becomes an important

---

Box 6-4 Neonatal ECMO Patient Selection Criteria

- OI greater than 40
- No major cardiac defect
- Reversible lung disease
- Gestation age greater than 33 weeks
- Mechanical ventilation less than 14 days
- No major intraventricular hemorrhage
- No significant coagulopathy or bleeding complications (relative contraindication)

indicator for escalating the process of moving a patient to ECMO prior to this irreversible point.

Types of Support

Delivery of ECMO can be accomplished with a variety of cannulation techniques to meet specific needs for ECMO support. The two cannulation approaches most commonly used are venoarterial and venovenous. The decision regarding which type of support to use should be based on the level of cardiac and pulmonary insufficiency and current patient status. A comparison of the advantages and disadvantages of each technique is found in Table 6-2.

During **venoarterial (VA) ECMO** support, two large cannulas are inserted by a surgeon, one into the right internal jugular vein and a second into the right common carotid artery. The cannulas are connected to the ECMO circuit, creating a cardiopulmonary bypass system that parallels the native cardiopulmonary system (Fig. 6-4). Blood is removed from the patient through the venous cannula, whose tip is placed in the right atrium. Blood is returned to the aorta via the right common carotid artery. This essentially bypasses the native heart and lungs and will support both the pulmonary and cardiac systems, allowing the heart and lung to rest. It is through this artificial system that the deoxygenated blood is cycled through the external ECLS artificial lung, which will provide oxygenation and ventilation. In addition, the ECMO pump will provide cardiac output suitable for the patient. VA ECMO offers the patient hemodynamic support, in addition to respiratory gas exchange.

In **venovenous (VV) ECMO** support, the surgeon places a double-lumen cannula in the right internal jugular vein. This will remove deoxygenated blood from the right atrium, cycle the blood though an artificial lung oxygenator, and then pump it back into the right atrium where the patient's native heart will be responsible for pumping the blood throughout the body. This type of ECMO provides respiratory gas exchange support (oxygen loading, CO_2 removal) in venous blood before it reaches the right ventricle. It is indicated in the management of severe respiratory failure when conventional means of support are unsuccessful. It does not, however, provide hemodynamic support, because blood is both drained and reinfused into the central venous system. Additionally, because both the drainage and reinfusion of the blood is in the right atrium, recirculation is common. Recirculation can occur when the blood is inadvertently siphoned back into the venous drainage cannulas after it has already gone through the ECMO circuit. The end result of the "arterial" blood mixing with venous blood from the body will invalidate the mixed venous oxygen saturation (SvO_2), which is a true marker of oxygenation support.

■ ■ The attending physician has determined that VA ECLS will be the mode of support. The physician discussed this option with the family, and they have decided they want "everything done." The family signed the informed consent. The ECLS, ICU, and surgical teams have been informed, and the patient is being prepped for cannulation.

Initiation

Once the decision is made to initiate ECMO, the team must move quickly because ECMO candidates are unstable and critically ill. The patient will need to be moved into a position in which the head is relocated to the foot of the bed, because the cannulas in the patient's neck need to be close to the ECMO equipment parked at the foot of the bed.

The head is rotated to the left, exposing the right side of the neck for cannulation. The chest and neck are prepared and draped using sterile technique. The RT secures the endotracheal tube (ETT) and

Table 6-2	Advantages and Disadvantages of VV- and VA-ECLS	
	Advantage	**Disadvantage**
Venovenous	• Sparing of the carotid artery • Preservation of pulsatile flow • Normal pulmonary flow • Perfusion of the native lungs • Perfusion of the coronary arteries • Potential emboli stays on venous side of patient	• No cardiac support • Lower systemic PaO_2 • Recirculation
Venoarterial	• Provides cardiac support • Excellent gas exchange • Rapid stabilization	• Carotid artery ligation • Nonpulsatile flow • Reduced pulmonary blood flow • Lower myocardial oxygen delivery • Potential emboli to atrial system

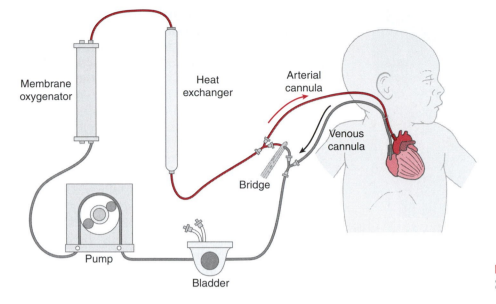

Figure 6-4 Diagram of VA-ECMO System

ventilator circuit to minimize the risk of extubation during the bedside surgery. Free-flowing oxygen, such as a resuscitation bag, should be removed from the bedside to prevent the risk of fire during the cautery process.

The intensivist and nursing team will monitor the patient's vital signs and continue to provide standard support therapy while the remaining ECMO team members prepare for cannulation and ECMO support.

While the surgeon and the surgical team are cannulating, the ECMO team will be preparing the ECMO circuit. The ECMO circuit has to be primed to connect to the cannulas that the surgeon will be placing. The first stage in preparing an ECMO circuit is to flush through the circuitry and replace air using carbon dioxide (CO_2). CO_2 is highly soluble in blood, decreasing the risk of microbubbles. Crystalloid solution is added and systematically expels CO_2 as each section of the circuit is primed with fluid. When the entire circuit is fluid primed, the debubbling process begins, during which any remaining air bubbles will be evacuated. When the circuit is air-free, the crystalloid may be replaced with packed red blood cells. The blood-primed circuit is then treated with bicarbonate to adjust for pH, heparin, and calcium chloride. Once the blood is circulating through the system, a blood sample is drawn from the circuit to evaluate the pump's blood gas, sodium, potassium, and ionized calcium levels, as well as the clotting time of blood in the circuit. These values need to be approximately equal to the patient's values. The blood is then heated to body temperature and is ready for connection to the cannulas.

Once the cannulas are placed, a chest radiograph is taken to visualize proper position. After the position is verified, the surgeon and a member of the ECMO team will make an air-free connection of the ECMO circuit to the patient cannulas. The patient is now considered "on-ECMO," and the native function of the patient's heart and lungs can begin to be reduced as the artificial system takes over pulmonary and cardiac functions.

- For VV-ECMO support, flow is increased slowly over 10 to 15 minutes to a level that is consistent with the needs of the patient, yet has low recirculation through the cannulas. Maximum flow for a VV-ECMO patient is generally 150 mL/kg/min.
- VA-ECMO support is initiated by slowly increasing pump flow and allowing the mixing of the oxygen-rich pump blood with that of the potentially anoxic, depressed patient. Flow is increased over the next 20 to 30 minutes to a support level consistent with the needs of the patient. Maximum flow for a VA-ECMO patient is generally 120 mL/kg/min.

ECMO Circuit and Equipment

Unlike ventilator circuits and other respiratory equipment, there is no standard ECMO setup or equipment. Each ECMO center may use many different setups, but all systems will incorporate some type of equipment described below:

- ECMO cannulas: Proper cannula size and location of the cannulas are crucial for successful ECMO support. VA-ECMO cannulas will have one venous cannula and one arterial cannula. As discussed earlier, the venous cannula is inserted through the right internal jugular vein downward into the right atrium. This cannula traditionally is wire reinforced to prevent kinking and to be visible on a chest radiograph (Fig. 6-5). In addition, multiple holes will be near the end of the cannula to allow for

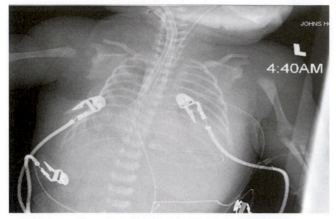

Figure 6-5 Chest Radiograph of Patient With VA-ECMO Cannulas Inserted *(Courtesy of Jane Benson, MD)*

maximum venous drainage. The tip of this cannula will have a radiopaque dot showing the exact end portion of the cannula. In addition, should venous drainage be a problem, a second venous cannula could be inserted to augment venous flow to the ECMO pump. This could be achieved through a femoral vein and would be wyed into the existing ECMO circuit. The arterial cannula is wire reinforced through to the lower portion of the cannula to prevent kinking, with one jet port at the tip directing flow to the descending aorta.

- **ECMO Pump:** The roller-head pump has traditionally been the pump of choice for smaller patients. It operates as a servo-controlled, positive-displacement pump and has two rollers that will optimally occlude or squeeze the tubing in the pump and direct blood through the tubing, creating pressure and flow through the system. Another type of pump that has been gaining popularity is the centrifugal pump. This type of kinetic pump uses the principle of a constrained vortex and spins inner cones, directing flow through the circuit. This energy is transferred to the blood by these rotating cones, and blood flows through the pump. Blood flow through this system is dependent on the preload and afterload conditions of the system. This means blood must be available from the patient to create forward flow. In addition, any increased pressure could reduce flow moving out of the pump.
- **Oxygenators:** Oxygenators play a critical role in any ECMO system by providing the artificial components that allow oxygenation and ventilation to take place. As blood passes through the polymethylpentene (PMP) hollow-fiber oxygenator, micropore hollow fibers allow gas exchange (sweep) to occur at the point at which these micropores are located. This design allows efficient and low-pressure gas exchange to take place. Oxygenation and

ventilation occur and can be adjusted to maintain appropriate blood gas values for the patient.

- **Heaters:** Because blood temporarily leaves the patient's body and moves through the ECMO circuit, it becomes necessary to heat the blood before reinfusing it into the patient to preserve thermal regulation. Artificial heat exchangers will be placed within the ECMO circuitry to allow for conduction of heat into the blood.
- **ECMO safety and monitoring devices:** Life-threatening mechanical and patient complications can occur while on ECMO. Preventing, managing, and minimizing these problems is important in any ECMO program. Types of safety monitoring include (1) venous and arterial line pressure monitoring, (2) bubble detection system, (3) blood and sweep gas flowmeters, (4) venous and arterial oxygenation saturation monitoring, (5) blood gas monitoring, (6) cerebral oximetry monitoring, and (7) bedside activated clotting time (ACT) monitoring.

Care of a Patient on ECMO

Once ECMO support has been initiated and the patient is stabilized, ventilator settings can be reduced. Because the ECMO system is now providing respiratory support, the potentially high barotraumatic ventilator settings will be adjusted to "lung rest" settings. These settings are typically a PIP of 20 cm H_2O, PEEP of 10 cm H_2O, RR 10 breaths/min, and FIO_2 of 0.30 to 0.40.

The patient will be continuously monitored throughout the ECMO course. Oxygenation, ventilation, and cardiac support are assessed, and the ECMO support will be adjusted to be adequate, with the goal of getting these settings to minimal support levels. Monitoring includes blood gases and coagulation and blood laboratory results assessed every 4 to 8 hours An ECMO specialist and a nurse will be at the bedside the entire time the patient is on ECMO. The ECMO specialist will ensure the ECMO machine operates safely and will be available should any problem occur that needs immediate attention.

Cardiovascular Support

The goal of ECMO is to provide adequate cardiorespiratory support for the infant. The ECMO pump will be adjusted based on many available values, including SvO_2 and pulse oximetry.

SvO_2 reflects the oxygen consumption of the tissues and should be 75%. Arterial oxygen saturation (SaO_2) and blood gas monitoring are also critical components to watch when caring for an ECMO patient. Pulse oximetry provides continuous assessment of SaO_2 and should be greater than 90%.

Once the patient is connected to the circuit by the cannulas the surgeon has placed, the ECMO pump flow is slowly increased while the arterial blood pressure is monitored. Flow is increased to a goal of 100 to 120 mL/kg/min or until the SvO_2 is greater than 75%, which correlates to approximately 70% to 80% of the patient's total cardiac output. In hypermetabolic states, the ECMO pump flow may exceed this to provide sufficient cardiac support. Once adequate support is achieved, the ventilator will be weaned to "rest settings." Typical rest settings are PIP 20 cm H_2O, PEEP 10 cm H_2O, RR 10 breaths/min, and F_IO_2 of 0.40. Rest settings are used to prevent atelectrauma, though some institutions may extubate their ECMO patients. Higher settings are not necessary, because the oxygenator in the ECMO system will provide efficient gas exchange for the patient.

If inotropic support was required during pre-ECMO management, this should no longer be needed because the ECMO pump is now providing cardiac support.

Anticoagulation System

Because the blood in the circuit will be exposed to this foreign surface, anticoagulation needs to occur. This is done by administering heparin to the blood, which prevents a thrombus from forming. To monitor the heparin effect, and therefore anticoagulation, a bedside laboratory test known as **activated clotting time (ACT)** will be performed. ACT detects how fast the blood will begin clotting once a sample of blood from the circuit is introduced into the device. The usual ACT is 180 to 220 seconds. Adjustments to the ACT range are made by increasing or decreasing the amount of heparin that is infusing into the circuit.

Fluid Balance

Due to the systemic inflammatory response after initiation of ECMO, and possible fluid resuscitation prior to ECMO, most patients become edematous. Restricting the daily intake to 60 to 80 mL/kg/day will assist in controlling this fluid overload. Diuretics will also facilitate the removal of excess fluid, which will improve cardiac output and lung consolidation.

Nutrition for ECMO patients occurs in the form of amino acids and total parenteral nutrition (TPN) for caloric intake. This will be monitored by the physician and adjusted per the patient's condition.

Often, oliguria or anuria (low urine output or no urine formation) can occur, necessitating the use of an ultrafiltration filter within the ECMO circuit. This system can enhance output and manage patients who may be fluid overloaded. In addition, dialysis can be added if the patient requires it.

Blood Products

ECMO circuits require many types of blood products to keep the patient hematologically stable. Packed red blood cells (PRBCs) are used to maintain the red blood cell count within normal range (hematocrit of 35% to 45% and hemoglobin of 12 to 16 g/dL).

Fresh frozen plasma (FFP) and cryoprecipitate are other important blood products that are administered to treat suboptimal values in a patient who has bleeding complications.

Platelets are continuously consumed by the circuit and need to be monitored and administered if the count drops below the normal range of greater than 100,000 μL (microliters).

■ ■ BB Porter has been placed on VA-ECMO support with the blender FIO_2 at 1 and pump flow at 120 mL/kg/min. The chest radiograph shows the venous cannula in good position in the right atrium, with the tip approximately 1 cm above the diaphragm. The arterial cannula is also in good position in the aortic arch, pointing toward the descending aorta at the level of the carina. Inotropic support has been weaned off. A heparin drip to maintain appropriate anticoagulation is running at 35 units/kg/hr with an ACT within range of 200 to 220 seconds. An umbilical ABG test shows pH 7.4 mm Hg, $PaCO_2$ 40 mm Hg, and PaO_2 200 mm Hg. The ventilator is changed from HFOV to a conventional ventilator with the following settings: PIP of 20 cm H_2O, PEEP of 10 mm Hg, RR of 10 breaths/min, and FIO_2 of 0.40.

BB Porter will have blood gases drawn every 4 to 8 hours; coagulation and blood laboratory test results will also be assessed every 4 to 8 hours during the entire ECMO procedure. An ECMO specialist and a nurse will be at the bedside the entire time he is on ECMO.

BB Porter's cardiovascular status has been assessed, and the inotropic support has been weaned off. The ECMO pump will provide any cardiac support necessary, and the patient will be continuously assessed, with the pump weaned as tolerated. He will be monitored for proper anticoagulation by the ACT each hour. The range will be 180 to 220 seconds, with adjustment to heparin as needed. BB Porter has neither bleeding complications from the cannula insertion site nor any other issues related to bleeding. Other laboratory test values for coagulation that will be monitored include activated partial thromboplastin time (aPTT), international normalized ratio (INR), fibrinogen, D-dimers, anti-factor Xa, and antithrombin III. He will be monitored for hemoglobin, hematocrit, and platelet count every 4 hours. Blood products have been given to maintain the range for each value.

Pulmonary Support

Once patients are placed on ECMO, it becomes important to wean the ventilator settings to "rest settings." These are typically a pressure control of 20 to 25 cm H_2O, RR of 5 to 10 breaths/min, PEEP of 4 to 10 cm H_2O, and FIO_2 of 0.21 to 0.30. These settings allow the lungs to heal and let the ECMO circuit provide the pulmonary support. Chest radiographs should be taken daily to observe opacification and the healing trend of the lungs, as well as to ensure that the ETT and ECMO cannulas remain in optimum position.

Lung recovery usually occurs over 3 to 5 days, which can be quantified by improvements in chest radiographs, lung compliance, and gas exchange.

Neurological Support

Sedation is usually required to help provide comfort to the patient and to keep the patient from moving too much, which could cause accidental decannulation. Paralysis is usually not a part of the maintenance of the ECMO patient except in cases of cannulation, decannulation, or other procedures requiring the patient to remain motionless.

Head ultrasounds will be performed routinely to rule out intraventricular hemorrhage (IVH). If IVH is identified, mean arterial blood pressure is reduced, and the ACT range should be lowered. Antifibrinolytic medication should be considered. As with any complication, the risk versus benefit of continuing ECLS should be carefully considered. Because ECLS systems are portable, a computed tomography (CT) scan should be considered to provide more detailed information regarding IVH.

Weaning ECMO Support and Decannulation

Weaning is a term used for slowly decreasing the ECMO support over time and assessing the patient's response to the wean. The amount of time a patient requires ECMO varies with the diagnosis. The average duration for a neonate with PPHN is 4 to 6 days. Patients are weaned from ECMO support as tolerated over several days. This includes lowering the FIO_2 of the ECLS blender and the ECMO pump flow to approximately 20 mL/kg/min. Once this level of support is reached, it is necessary to make moderate increases in ventilator support to compensate for the decrease in ECMO support. The patient circuit is then clamped off, which is known as a clamp trial. During a clamp trial, patients will be without ECMO support, and their native cardiorespiratory system can be assessed. While the circuit is clamped, blood gases and hemodynamics are monitored. If patients can successfully support themselves during this period, it is assumed they will do well when the cannulas are removed permanently. This is called "decannulating" the patient.

If patients are on VV-ECMO support, then the weaning trial is slightly different. In VV-ECMO support, weaning occurs by lowering the FIO_2 to the membrane to 0.21. The membrane gas ports are capped to eliminate the artificial lung as a source of oxygenation and ventilation. The ventilator settings are increased to a level that would be considered moderate and acceptable. Eventually, the blood entering and exiting the membrane achieves equilibrium and reflects typical venous values. Blood gases are monitored, and if they are acceptable, then the patient would be prepared for decannulation.

Decannulation is the process of removing the ECMO cannulas and ligating the vessels. This is a surgical procedure, so a sterile field will be created by the surgical team. Once the ECMO cannulas are removed, the vessels will be ligated and secured. Any bleeding will be assessed and controlled. A topical antibiotic will be applied along with a dressing to cover the area.

Complications

Many ECMO cases are without complications; however, this invasive procedure is not without problems. Complications of ECMO can be divided into patient issues and mechanical issues. All patient complications may be caused by two physiological alterations: changes in the blood-surface interaction and changes in the blood-flow pattern. Both of these variables can have adverse effects on all the organ systems. When blood comes into contact with any foreign surface, thrombus formation and platelet consumption will occur. This necessitates the use of heparin and consequently contributes to the bleeding complications of ECMO.

IVH is the primary concern for ECMO patients. These patients receive systemic heparin; IVH, as well as other physiological issues, could result if not monitored closely. In addition, blood-flow changes from the ligation of the right internal jugular vein and the right common carotid artery can create other concerns.

Mechanical complications of the ECMO system are listed in Box 6-5. It becomes imperative that an ECMO-trained provider is at the bedside of these patients at all times to provide emergent troubleshooting should the equipment have a mechanical problem.

■ ■ BB Porter remains intubated on "lung rest" settings. Suctioning is performed cautiously because he is being given anticoagulants. Radiographs are taken each day and reveal that the patient's lung fields are clear, with bilateral breath sounds. He is not medically paralyzed, but he does receive sedation medication as needed for comfort. BB Porter moves appropriately to stimulation and has reactive pupils. He is permitted to move slightly; however, he is monitored closely so the cannulas are not disturbed for fear of movement or dislodgement.

Complications of ECLS

Mechanical Complications of ECLS

- Clots in circuit
- Cannula problems
- Oxygenator failure
- Air in the circuit
- Pump malfunction
- Heat exchanger malfunction
- Tubing rupture

Patient Complications of ECLS

- Bleeding
- Cardiac dysrhythmias
- Dialysis/hemofiltration
- Hemolysis
- Hypertension
- Infection
- Intraventricular hemorrhage
- Myocardial stun
- Pneumothorax
- Seizures

Course and Prognosis

In the 1980s, one-third of full-term newborns diagnosed with PPHN were not expected to survive to hospital discharge (61, 62). The use of high-frequency ventilation, exogenous surfactant, ECMO, and iNO have reduced that number in developed countries to around 10% (34). Many of these interventions are expensive, however, and may not be readily available in developing countries.

Some causes of PPHN can increase mortality, such as alveolar-capillary dysplasia and mutations in the surfactant protein B gene (5), as well as congenital diaphragmatic hernias, discussed in Chapter 9.

Most recent studies reporting PPHN morbidities have identified a significant risk for hearing loss among survivors, which may not manifest for 18 to 24 months (63). Neurodevelopmental impairment is also seen in about 25% of survivors, which may include cerebral palsy, hearing or vision loss, and low scores on mental or psychomotor developmental indices (29). In a 2010 study evaluating survivors at school age, 24% had respiratory problems, 60% had abnormal chest radiographs, and 6.4% had some sensorineural hearing loss. Overall, survivors had average scores on cognitive and other neurological tests, but the cohort had a higher-than-expected percentage of IQ scores below 70 points (64). Hoskote et al. assessed pulmonary outcomes for infants with moderate-to-severe PPHN and found them to be similar to healthy peers at 1 year of age (65), though they did find some subclinical reductions in airway function in their study. This mild reduction supports the need for RTs to continue vigorous efforts to avoid VILI and encourage weaning and extubation when possible.

Meconium Aspiration Syndrome

Meconium is a baby's first bowel movement, and it usually occurs sometime shortly after delivery. In about 8% to 20% of deliveries, however, meconium is passed in utero and is identified by meconium-stained amniotic fluid (MSAF) (66–68). Of these fetuses who pass meconium in utero, about 3% to 5% will aspirate it into their airway before delivery (66–68), which can cause varying symptoms of respiratory distress and lung dysfunction. **Meconium aspiration syndrome (MAS)** is defined as respiratory distress occurring soon after delivery in a meconium-stained infant, which is not otherwise explicable and is associated with a typical radiographic appearance (69, 70). Wiswell reported 7% of infants born through amniotic-stained fluid developed respiratory distress and 3% developed MAS, with 4.2% having problems linked to other disorders (68). The reported incidence of infants with MAS requiring mechanical ventilation is 0.61 per 1,000 live births (71).

MAS is a disease process primarily affecting term and post-term infants. At 34 wG, the incidence of MSAF is 1.6%; it increases to 30% for infants 42 wG or more (67). Singh reports the rate of MAS increased from 1.1% of infants at 37 wG to 24% of infants 42 wG or more.

Factors associated with increased risk of meconium-stained fluid and subsequent development of MAS include the following:

- Post-term pregnancy (greater than 42 wG)
- Preeclampsia or eclampsia
- Maternal hypertension
- Maternal diabetes
- Intrauterine growth retardation
- Abnormal biophysical profile
- Oligohydramnios
- Maternal heavy smoking or chronic respiratory or cardiovascular disease
- Abnormal fetal heart rate and nonreassuring fetal heart rate tracing
- Presence of fetal distress
- Low 5-minute Apgar
- Ethnicity: Black Americans and Africans have increased risk when compared with other groups. Those of Pacific Islander and indigenous Australian ethnicity are also at increased risk.
- Home births

Pathophysiology

Meconium is the by-product or metabolic waste of gestation. It is the first intestinal discharge. Often, meconium-stained fluid is explained to parents as being the passage of stool prior to birth. Meconium is unlike the products of digestion; it consists of fetal hair, epithelial cells, bile salts, and mucus. Meconium is sticky, viscous, similar in consistency to tar, odorless, and almost sterile. Normally, over 90% of full-term infants pass meconium within the first 16 hours of life. Inability to pass meconium within the first day of life may be associated with other serious abnormalities (Special Populations 6-2). When the amniotic fluid is stained with meconium, estimates can be made on the timing of the exposure. Staining of the umbilical cord may begin within 15 minutes, the nails require 4 to 6 hours, and the vernix caseosa takes approximately 12 hours, depending on the amount/concentration of meconium released. The exact mechanism causing the release of meconium in utero is not well understood, but fetal hypoxia, fetal acidosis, and vagal stimulation by head or cord compression are suspected (67).

Once meconium is in the amniotic fluid, gasping or deep irregular respirations can result in aspiration. In utero, prior to labor, the thick fetal lung fluid prevents aspiration of MSAF. During labor and delivery and immediately after birth, as the fetal lung fluid is absorbed, there is an opportunity for meconium-stained fluid to be aspirated. Aspiration of meconium may result in airway obstruction, **chemical pneumonitis** (inflammation of the lungs caused by the inhalation of certain chemicals), atelectasis, and pulmonary hypertension. Meconium inhibits surfactant function (72) and is also directly toxic to the pulmonary epithelium (73).

The airway obstruction by meconium may vary in location and severity. **Partial obstruction** may allow some passage of air into and out of the alveolar space. A **ball-valve obstruction** will open during inspiration, allowing air to enter the alveoli, but close the airway during exhalation, causing localized air trapping (Fig. 6-6). **Total obstruction** will not

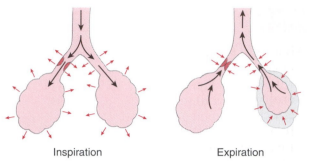

Inspiration   Expiration

Figure 6-6 Ball-Valve Effect Obstruction by Meconium in the Airway

allow for inhalation or exhalation and leads to atelectasis and hypoventilation. This may result in air trapping, alveolar hyperexpansion, air leaks, or atelectasis and ventilation-perfusion mismatch. Air leaks may occur during resuscitation.

Meconium is an irritant and results in an inflammatory response. Chemical pneumonitis may develop in infants with MAS. Within hours, the airways and lung parenchyma become infiltrated with large numbers of white blood cells such as polymorphonuclear leukocytes and macrophages. This intense inflammatory response produces direct local injury by release of inflammatory mediators-cytokines and oxygen-free radicals. Vascular leakage may result and cause toxic pneumonitis with hemorrhagic pulmonary edema. Meconium may also displace or inactivate surfactant, reducing surface tension and contributing to uneven ventilation, atelectasis, ventilation-perfusion mismatch, and poor oxygenation. Hypoxia, hyperinflation of the lungs, and acidosis cause increased PVR. Pulmonary hypertension, with or without atrial/ductal shunting, accelerates hypoxemia and respiratory acidosis and creates an unending cycle of deterioration, which may be referred to as "circling the drain."

Clinical Manifestations

Infants with MSAF may present with no symptoms or be in respiratory failure at birth. Most show some signs of respiratory distress (Box 6-6), including the following:

- Abnormal respiratory rate, which may initially manifest as tachypnea, but with fatigue may deteriorate to apnea
- Increased respiratory effort, seen as audible grunting, nasal flaring, and retractions
- Cyanosis

Auscultation may reveal diminished or unequal breath sounds, rales, rhonchi, or wheezing, depending on how meconium has affected the airway. Increased anterior-posterior diameter of the chest may be evident if the newborn has air trapping. Asymmetry of the chest is also common if air leaks develop.

● Special Populations 6-2

When Meconium Does Not Pass

A meconium plug is an intestinal obstruction in the lower colon and rectum, is associated with maternal diabetes, and may indicate Hirschsprung's disease. Hirschsprung's disease is a congenital defect of the colon causing bowel obstruction.

Meconium ileus, an intestinal obstruction in the terminal ileum, is the most common presentation for cystic fibrosis in the neonate. Ninety percent of infants with meconium ileus have cystic fibrosis (see Chapter 14 for more information on cystic fibrosis).

Meconium can also be used to detect tobacco, alcohol, and other drugs to which the infant has been exposed in utero.

Box 6-6 Clinical Symptoms of MAS

Abnormal breathing pattern (tachypnea or apnea)
Grunting
Nasal flaring
Retractions
Abnormal lung sounds (diminished, unequal, rales, rhonchi, wheezing)
Increased anterior–posterior chest diameter
Chest asymmetry
Cyanosis
Hypoxemia
Respiratory acidosis

Infants with MSAF and respiratory distress require monitoring of arterial blood gases, and an umbilical or peripheral arterial line may be essential. Blood gas results will typically reveal hypoxemia and hypercapnia.

An initial chest radiograph may show patchy infiltrates or irregular streaky, linear densities and consolidation throughout the lung fields. As the disease progresses (Fig. 6-7), hyperinflation, atelectasis, and pneumothorax may be present. The lungs typically appear hyperinflated, with flattening of the diaphragm, or diffuse patchy densities may alternate with areas of expansion. Low functional residual capacity and low lung compliance may be observed as a result of partial or complete atelectasis. In turn, increased functional residual capacity and low lung compliance may be due to hyperinflation (2).

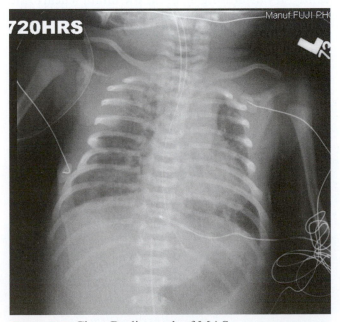

Figure 6-7 Chest Radiograph of MAS (*Courtesy of Jane Benson, MD*)

As with PPHN, preductal and postductal SpO_2 monitoring and echocardiogram will confirm, monitor, and evaluate the presence of pulmonary hypertension and shunting.

Initial laboratory evaluation must include the following:

• Complete blood count with differential
• Test for C-reactive protein, which assesses inflammation
• Blood cultures to evaluate for sepsis, particularly if sepsis was the cause of meconium release
• Coagulation studies and type and crossmatch

Any infant presenting with respiratory distress should be evaluated for sepsis and treated until sepsis is eliminated as a contributing factor to the respiratory distress. Bacterial sepsis should be suspected in infants with meconium-stained fluid. Ongoing evaluation will include electrolyte and metabolic evaluations. End-organ damage must be considered since these infants may have experienced perinatal asphyxia, hypoxemia, and hypoxia.

Management and Treatment

The focus of the management in MAS is respiratory support, and it may vary from supplemental oxygen via nasal cannula to HFOV, iNO, and ECMO, depending on the severity of disease. Singh reported the use of the following modalities in the first day after birth to treat more than 7,000 infants over a 10-year period: RA (11%); oxygen by hood (33%); nasal cannula (10%); continuous positive airway pressure (7%); CMV (28%); high-frequency ventilation (8%); surfactant (16%); iNO (6.1%), and extracorporeal oxygenation (1.4%). From 2000 to 2006, iNO and surfactant use increased. High-frequency ventilation use remained constant at 6% to 9%, and vasopressors and extracorporeal oxygenation use decreased. (66)

Care for newborns with MSAF begins in the delivery room and is adjusted based on the level of hypoxemia, physical respiratory distress, and respiratory acidosis. PPHN is treated as needed, using the strategies discussed in the previous section.

Delivery Room Interventions

Until 2005, all infants born through MSAF were routinely intubated and suctioned with a meconium aspirator repeatedly until no meconium was observed in the ETT (74). Several randomized studies, most recently published in 2004 by *Lancet*, concluded that, if meconium-stained fluid is observed during a delivery, the infant's oral and nasal pharynx may be suctioned by the obstetrician once the head is delivered to prevent the additional aspiration of meconium; however, intubation and tracheal suctioning should only be attempted if the infant is unresponsive immediately after birth (75, 76). Attempting an intubation on a vigorous newborn may cause vocal cord trauma or initiate a vagal response caused by the insertion of the laryngoscope. Care must always be taken when considering the condition of the newborn, and care should be adjusted to meet the patient's needs (70). Although the evidence is not strong regarding suctioning versus nonsuctioning, the American Academy of Pediatrics (AAP) still recommends endotracheal suctioning of nonvigorous babies with MSAF (Evidence in Practice 6-2). A **nonvigorous** baby is defined as having a depressed respiratory effort, poor muscle tone, and/or heart rate less than 100 bpm. In this instance, it is acceptable to perform an intubation to suction the trachea immediately after birth. Suction is limited to 5 seconds, and if no meconium is aspirated, no further intubations for suctioning are recommended. If meconium is aspirated and no bradycardia is present, a judgment is made whether to reintubate and suction a second time. If the heart rate is low, proceed to resuscitative efforts with drying, stimulating, repositioning, and administering oxygen or positive-pressure ventilation.

A vigorous baby is one with a normal respiratory effort, normal muscle tone, and heart rate greater than 100 bpm. Such a baby would not be intubated; instead, the mouth and nose may be suctioned with a bulb syringe or a large-bore suction catheter for remaining meconium before proceeding to neonatal resuscitative efforts with drying, stimulating, repositioning, and administering oxygen or positive-pressure ventilation.

To perform an intubation with intent to suction meconium from the trachea, an appropriate-sized ETT is used, with a **meconium aspirator** connected to it, which will allow attachment of wall suction and use of the ETT as a large-bore suction device within the trachea (Fig. 6-8). The infant should be placed in the sniffing position by the nurse, RT, or physician with a small neck roll under the infant's shoulders. This will create a straight view of the vocal cords. The laryngoscope is inserted with the left hand by gently opening the infant's mouth with thumb or finger and then gently sliding the blade into the mouth. The blade should be inserted only far enough to lift the epiglottis up out of the way to bring the chords into view. Care should be taken to not rock back onto the gums, which could cause damage and bleeding. Once the cords are visualized, the ETT is inserted down the right side of the mouth, being careful not to obstruct the view, only far enough to watch the glottis markings pass through the vocal cords. If a stylet was used to facilitate intubation, this is removed before the meconium aspirator is attached to the end of the ETT. The 15-mm adapter end of the meconium aspirator is attached to the ETT, and the nipple adapter is attached to suction tubing connected to a suction regulator. Occlude the thumb port on the meconium aspirator and withdraw the ETT. Assess the contents of the aspiration. If there was a large amount of meconium and the infant's heart rate has not dropped significantly, try aspirating again. If the infant's heart rate decreases or not much meconium was aspirated, proceed to resuscitative efforts with drying, stimulating, repositioning, and administering oxygen or positive-pressure ventilation.

There was also a time when performing an amnioinfusion to reduce the incidence of MAS was a common practice. **Amnioinfusion** is a procedure in which normal saline or lactated Ringer's solution is placed into the uterus after rupture of the amniotic sac. The thought is that a dilution of meconium with warm sterile saline will minimize the severity of

---

● **Evidence in Practice 6-2**

Suctioning at Delivery—What Is the Evidence?

The AAP Neonatal Resuscitation Program Steering Committee in 2010 recommended the following for newborns with MSAF (74):

- Obstetricians are not to routinely suction the oropharynx on delivery of the head but before the delivery of the shoulders because a randomized controlled trial demonstrated it to be of no value.
- There is no value to suctioning the trachea of vigorous babies.
- Tracheal suctioning of infants born to mothers with MSAF with poor tone and minimal respiratory effort is not associated with reductions in the incidence or mortality of these infants.
- There are no randomized, controlled trials comparing suctioning with nonsuctioning, and therefore the current practice of performing endotracheal suctioning of nonvigorous babies with MSAF will continue.
- If attempted intubation is prolonged and unsuccessful, bag-mask ventilation should be considered, particularly if there is persistent bradycardia.

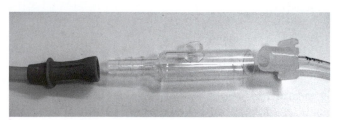

Figure 6-8 Meconium Aspirator

MAS. The evidence does not support amniofusion to prevent MAS, which may be because an infant may pass meconium in utero long before it is noted clinically, thus having no effect on the health outcomes for the baby (75).

Neonatal Management

There is currently no strategy to prevent MAS; therefore, treatment is mainly supportive. Therapy goals are to maintain normoxemia and ventilation, to assure adequate systemic blood pressure, and to correct acidosis and hypoglycemia when needed (77).

Oxygen Therapy

For mild cases of MAS, supplemental oxygen may be the only therapy required for stabilization. Oxygen should be titrated as needed to maintain higher SpO_2, preferably monitoring preductal SpO_2 for 94% to 98%. If a right arterial line is available (preductal), oxygen should be titrated to maintain a PaO_2 of 60 to 100 mm Hg (77). In mild cases, delivery devices may include a nasal cannula or oxygen hood. NCPAP can also be used to provide alveolar stabilization, airway stenting, and supplemental oxygen delivery. Approximately 10% to 20% of infants with MAS are able to be successfully treated with NCPAP alone (66, 78, 79). Pressures of 5 to 8 cm H_2O can be used, and patients should be monitored for agitation and discomfort while on NCPAP, which can exacerbate PPHN and necessitate intubation. If necessary, intubation and mechanical ventilation will be provided for hypoxemic and hypercarbic respiratory failure.

Mechanical Ventilation

Roughly 30% of newborns developing MAS will require some degree of ventilator support (78, 81). Indications for intubation and ventilation include the following:

- FIO_2 greater than 0.80
- Respiratory acidosis with pH less than 7.25 for several hours
- Pulmonary hypertension
- Poor systemic blood pressure and perfusion (77)

Initial management should focus on normalizing pH to 7.3 to 7.4 and maintaining $PaCO_2$ of 40 to 60 mm Hg (80, 81). There are few clinical trials regarding ventilator management for MAS, so few definitive recommendations are available. General guidelines for ventilator support are similar to those made for other neonates and include the following (see also Table 6-1):

- Use a synchronized mode of ventilation whenever possible.
- Monitor for ETT leak and avoid autotriggering.
- Use synchronized intermittent mandatory ventilation (SIMV) rather than assist/control (A/C)

to avoid air trapping and hyperinflation caused by inadvertent high respiratory rates.
- Use PEEP set at 4 to 7 cm H_2O (82), increasing it when atelectasis is present and decreasing it if significant overdistension is observed as flattened diaphragms on chest radiograph, or if the patient exhibits signs of hemodynamic instability indicative of decreased venous return.
- Set inspiratory time (T_I) around 0.5 seconds and use close monitoring to assure that T_I and expiratory time (T_E) settings are enough for full exhalation, as evidenced by expiratory flows returning to zero and end-expiratory pressures reaching set PEEP before the next breath begins. T_I may be increased to facilitate alveolar recruitment, but only if it does not cause air trapping. Normal RRs for a healthy neonate are 30 to 60 breaths/min, but patients with MAS should be maintained on a relatively low RR of less than 50 breaths/min.
- Target tidal volume at 4 to 6 mL/kg (77, 83). This may require high peak inspiratory pressures (PIP). If PIP must be maintained at greater than 30 cm H_2O, then high-frequency ventilation should be considered.

Correctly selected ventilator settings should allow the patient's work of breathing (WOB) to diminish, as evidenced by a resolution of hypoxemia and retractions and a decrease in spontaneous RR. As discussed previously, sedation may be needed to prevent agitation and hypoxemic crisis in patients with MAS and PPHN.

If the infant cannot be stabilized on a conventional ventilator as evidenced by blood gases that are not improving and/or hemodynamic instability, then HFOV is an alternative ventilation strategy to provide alveolar ventilation in patients with poor lung compliance. HFOV employs an open-lung strategy to minimize volutrauma and atelectrauma and may prevent air-leak syndrome in MAS patients (80). A combination of HFV and iNO administration has been linked to a greater improvement in oxygenation in severe MAS with PPHN (84).

Initiation of HFOV may require a high Paw to recruit atelectatic alveoli, and most infants with MAS should be able to be stabilized with a Paw of 16 to 20 cm H_2O (77). Paw should be weaned as tolerated to prevent interference with systemic blood pressure. Because of the risk of air trapping with MAS, hertz levels used are lower than those typical for other populations of neonates. An initial hertz of 10 is reasonable, and 8 or 6 may be necessary if $PaCO_2$ cannot be managed using ΔP. As previously recommended, T_I should be set to 33% and ΔP set to provide adequate chest wiggle factor (Table 6-3).

Hypoxia, acidosis, and hypoxia from increased pulmonary vascular resistance are common in this

Table 6-3	Recommended Settings for CMV and HFOV for MAS	
	CMV	HFOV
Mode	SIMV	—
Frequency	<50 breaths/min	10 Hz (can go to 6 Hz as needed)
Volume target	4–6 mL/kg (PIP < 30 cm H_2O)	—
Amplitude/ΔP	—	chest wiggle factor
T_I	0.50 seconds	33%
PEEP	4–7 cm H_2O	—
Paw	—	16–20 cm H_2O

patient population, and arterial blood gases are frequently monitored.

Surfactant-Replacement Therapy

Surfactant-replacement therapy is an appealing therapy for MAS because meconium can cause surfactant dysfunction and inactivation. Meconium may also outcompete for space in the alveoli, making it necessary to replace lost surfactant. The technique for instillation of exogenous surfactant for MAS is the same as that discussed in Chapter 4 for premature babies. Surfactant has not been shown to decrease the mortality rate in this population, but it has been demonstrated to reduce the severity of the disease and decrease hospital length of stay (84). It is presumed that surfactant administration may be more beneficial after the meconium is no longer in the airway. Disappointingly, one study found that as many as 40% of patients with MAS were "nonresponders" to bolus delivery of exogenous surfactant (85). In developed countries, this has become a relatively standard therapy for MAS, being used in 30% to 50% of ventilated patients with MAS (66, 79).

Pulmonary Vasodilators

Infants with MAS and PPHN can benefit from pulmonary vasodilators in the same way as newborns with idiopathic PPHN, and the most frequently used pulmonary vasodilator is iNO. Around one-quarter of all ventilated MAS newborns are treated with iNO (66, 79), with about half showing a positive response (29, 81). The focus of iNO therapy with MAS should be to optimize lung inflation prior to initiation to maximize the likelihood of a positive response. Gupta and colleagues used gentle CMV with permissive hypercapnia and iNO and reported an overall mortality rate of 9.8% in infants with MAS and PPHN (81).

Extracorporeal Membrane Oxygenation

MAS is one of the most common diagnoses among neonates treated with ECMO. MAS patients make up about 35% of patients requiring ECMO, and the initiation criteria are the same as for other causes of hypoxic respiratory failure (86). ECMO survival is high for MAS, nearing 95% (87), even with ECMO being used less frequently since the advent of iNO (80).

Cardiovascular Support

Cardiovascular support will include intravenous fluids and inotropic agents, such as dopamine, dobutamine, and epinephrine. This support should be provided when the patient exhibits a decreased cardiac output, as evidenced by hypotension, decreased pulses, and slow capillary refill. Fluid management will begin as clear fluids for initial resuscitation and stabilization. Total parenteral nutrition will begin after 12 to 24 hours, which will be based on electrolyte values.

In addition to respiratory and cardiovascular compromise (hypoxia and hypoxemia, hypotension), infants with MAS are also at risk for hypoglycemia, hypothermia, sepsis, and limited parental involvement (Teamwork 6-1).

Course and Prognosis

Mortality for ventilated infants with MAS varies widely and is found to be as low as zero and as high

---

Teamwork 6-1 Providing Parental Support

PARENTAL SUPPORT CANNOT BE OVEREMPHASIZED. Infants with MAS may require transport for additional care not provided in the birth hospital. The inability to function as a parent in the NICU can be devastating. Inability to hold or even touch their newborn is difficult for parents. Offer repeated explanations, encourage questions, recommend breast pumping, and acknowledge the stress of the NICU. Congratulate the parents on the birth of their child, referring to the infant by name, and use the words mother and father when speaking to the parents—a simple acknowledgment of the stress of the NICU and the separation from their baby. A willingness to listen and a familiar face can be comforting for parents. It is imperative to provide consistent information to parents. This can be accomplished with multidisciplinary rounds with the RT included. When parents ask questions, if you do not know an answer, offer to find out and return with the correct information.

as 37% (69). Mortality rates are influenced by the availability of alternative means of ventilation and adjunctive therapies such as iNO and ECMO. The two major causes of death in ventilated infants with MAS are pulmonary disease and hypoxic-ischemic encephalopathy. One-fourth to one-third of the deaths are caused by pulmonary disease (77).

Pneumothorax is a common side effect of MV, occurring in about 10% of all infants with MAS (79). Other short-term morbidities include other air-leak syndromes (pneumomediastinum, pulmonary interstitial edema) and pulmonary hemorrhage.

Up to half of infants discharged with MAS will have symptomatic wheezing and coughing in the first year of life, and evidence of airway hyperreactivity, airway obstruction, and hyperinflation may be seen in older children (77). As with idiopathic PPHN, there is an increase in the diagnosis of cerebral palsy and developmental delay in patients with MAS (88).

Transient Tachypnea of the Newborn

Transient tachypnea of the newborn (TTN) is a condition of term or near-term infants, characterized by mild respiratory distress during the first few hours of life. It is caused by failure to clear fetal lung fluid prior to delivery. It is a self-limiting disorder, typically resolving itself within 48 to 72 hours of life. At delivery, TTN maybe be difficult to differentiate from other causes of respiratory distress, such as sepsis, aspiration, and pneumonia. The exact incidence of TTN is not known, but a 2012 publication estimated that it occurs in 0.5% to 2.8% of live births and in as many as 30% of elective cesarean sections (89, 90).

The main risk factors associated with TTN include the following:

- Delivery by cesarean section
- Macrosomia (birth weight above the 90th percentile)
- Maternal asthma
- Maternal diabetes
- Male gender

Additional risk factors are listed in Box 6-7.

Pathophysiology

Fetal lung fluid is necessary for normal fetal lung development. It is secreted by type II alveolar cells to stabilize the structure of the lung in utero. In late gestation and shortly before birth, fetal lungs convert from fluid secretion to fluid reabsorption. Fetal adrenaline released during labor inhibits the chloride channel within type II cells, which causes the secretion of lung fluid. It simultaneously stimulates sodium channels, which absorb lung fluid. This signals the epithelial cells of the lung to stop secreting and start reabsorbing lung fluids. Through this

Box 6-7	Risk Factors for TTN

- Delivery via cesarean section
- Macrosomia (birth weight above the 90th percentile)
- Maternal asthma
- Maternal diabetes
- Male gender
- Negative PG presence test of amniotic fluid (see Chapter 2 for more information on this test)
- Maternal fluid overload
- Delayed clamping of umbilical cord
- Breech delivery
- Polycythemia
- Prematurity
- Very low birth weight (less than 1,500 g)
- Maternal drug dependence
- Exposure to B-mimetic agents
- Maternal sedation
- Perinatal depression
- Precipitous delivery
- Prolonged labor

mechanism, the lungs of a healthy term neonate at birth contain only a minimal amount of lung fluid. The majority of the fluid left is mechanically expelled during delivery, with additional clearance being facilitated by the ciliary escalator through the upper airway, mediastinum, and pleural space. Although **Starling's forces** or "vaginal squeeze" of the chest as it progresses through the birth canal was thought to account for the majority of fluid clearance, uterine contractions during labor create fetal postural changes that also compress the thorax; these two physical forces lead to the loss of about 25% to 35% of liquid from the lungs (89). Disruption of the physical or chemical components during this process can lead to retention of fluid in air spaces, setting the stage for alveolar hypoventilation. When infants are delivered near term, especially by cesarean section before the onset of spontaneous labor, the fetus is often deprived of these changes, making the neonatal transition more difficult. Failure of fluid clearance results in excess liquid filling the alveoli and moving into the interstitium, where it pools in perivascular tissues and interlobar fissures until it is cleared by the lymphatics or absorbed into small blood vessels over several days.

Pulmonary immaturity may play a role in the pathophysiology of TTN. A negative phosphatidylglycerol (PG) test (described in Chapter 2), even in the presence of a mature lecithin-sphingomyelin (L/S) ratio, is associated with an increased risk of TTN (91). Infants born closer to 36 wG than to 38 wG had an increased risk.

At least one study compared gastric secretions from healthy term newborns with secretions from newborns with TTN and found that those with TTN had low lamellar body counts associated with decreased surfactant function. This suggests that some cases of TTN are associated with surfactant abnormalities (92), but it is not clear whether this indicates surfactant deficiency, dysfunction, or both. Surfactant's effectiveness can be inhibited by pulmonary edema, and therefore fluid retention may decrease.

Clinical Manifestations

Obtaining a comprehensive history is essential to identify risk factors for TTN. Infants with TTN usually have respiratory distress within 6 hours of birth. Tachypnea (RR greater than 60 breaths/min), grunting, flaring, and retractions are most often noted.

A chest radiograph should be obtained (Fig. 6-9) and is characterized by the following:

- Diffuse parenchymal infiltrates
- A "wet silhouette" around the heart, or accumulation of fluid in the various intralobar spaces that indicate increased pulmonary interstitial, alveolar, or pleural water content
- The lungs normally displaying a homogenous pattern that may be difficult to distinguish from respiratory distress syndrome (RDS)
- A coarse interstitial pattern (exhibited in some cases of TTN), similar to pulmonary edema or an irregular opacification similar to MAS or neonatal pneumonia
- Possible transient slight cardiac enlargement

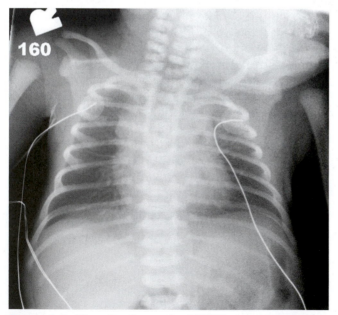

Figure 6-9 Chest Radiograph of TTN *(Courtesy of Jane Benson, MD)*

Most often, infants are hemodynamically stable, but they may have hypoproteinemia and/or elevated central venous pressure because of an overloaded thoracic lymphatic system. Mild asphyxia may occur, resulting in mild pulmonary capillary leak and myocardial dysfunction with elevated filling pressure.

Though not ideal, often the resolution of symptoms within the time frame is the definitive confirmation of a TTN diagnosis. If symptoms of TTN do not resolve within 72 hours or the FIO_2 requirement is greater than 0.40, then the working diagnosis of TTN has been proven to be incorrect, and additional patient evaluation must be done to determine the cause of respiratory distress.

Management and Treatment

Treatment of TTN is supportive, including supplemental oxygen, withholding of enteral feeds, and administration of intravenous fluids and antibiotics. Infants with TTN are also at risk for hypoglycemia, hypothermia, and sepsis, and support for these are given on an as-needed basis.

Oxygen therapy is a mainstay of care for newborns with TTN. Typical oxygen delivery includes an oxygen hood or nasal cannula connected to an air-oxygen blender, titrated to maintain SpO_2 90% to 96% (93). Moderate respiratory distress may require NCPAP of 4 to 6 cm H_2O to resolve grunting or retracting. Gradual improvement will be seen over 48 to 72 hours, and an FIO_2 of less than 0.40 is usually sufficient.

Armangil et al. attempted a trial of salbutamol, an inhaled beta-2 agonist, for the treatment of TTN and found that it improved blood gas values, decreased RR, and allowed for weaning of FIO_2 when compared with placebo (94).

Supportive care for thermoregulation, fluid, and nutrition is indicated. Nutritional status should be supported as needed because nursing or bottle feeding may initially be unsuccessful owing to tachypnea. Parental nutrition may be included, but continuous enteral feeds are often tolerated after initial stabilization. Hypothermia can be monitored and infants should be in a neutral thermal environment such as an incubator or radiant warmer. Evaluation is necessary to rule out sepsis as a cause of respiratory distress. Additional cardiovascular support is rarely indicated.

Maternal corticosteroids have been suggested to accelerate resorption of fetal lung fluid. A single, 2-day course of antenatal steroids 48 hours before elective cesarean at 37 to 38 weeks appears to improve respiratory morbidity from TTN (95). Its mechanism of action may be twofold: Antenatal steroids accelerate lung maturation and surfactant maturation, and they may also enhance sodium channel activity.

Course and Prognosis

TTN is a self-limiting disease and rarely causes mortality or long-term morbidity. One study showed that babies experiencing TTN have higher risk of physician-diagnosed preschool asthma, with this association being strongest for male infants (96). There is also some debate about whether TTN may cause pulmonary hypertension because of possible elevation in PVR associated with retained lung fluid (97). This would then follow the same clinical course as PPHN, discussed earlier in this chapter.

■ ■ After 5 days on VA-ECMO support, the radiograph is clear, and the patient has bilateral clear breath sounds. The ECMO pump flow is at 60 mL/kg/min, and the ECMO blender FIO_2 is at 0.30. The attending physician decides to wean BB Porter to 20 mL/kg/min and prepare for a clamp trial.

The clamp trial yields an ABG of pH 7.32, $PaCO_2$ of 46 mm Hg, PaO_2 of 150 mm Hg on ventilator settings of SIMV PIP of 24 cm H_2O, PEEP of 6 cm H_2O, RR of 25 breaths/min, and FIO_2 of 0.60 after being clamped for 1 hour. He has not required hemodynamic intervention and is stable. The surgeon is called, and BB Porter is decannulated.

■ ■ Critical Thinking Questions: BB Porter

1. Do you think that HFOV should have been started on BB Porter before starting iNO? On what do you base your decision?
2. Should preductal or postductal blood gases be used to monitor BB Porter's oxygenation status? What difference do you think it could make in his care?
3. Most research has shown little benefit to increasing iNO above 20 ppm. Why do you think the health-care team increased BB Porter's iNO setting to 40 ppm?

▶● Case Studies and Critical Thinking Questions

■ Case 1: BB Rogers

You are working in a level IIIC NICU and receiving shift reports. BB Rogers is a 41-wG newborn, now 2 days old. He was born via cesarean section, with Apgar scores of 3 and 6. An echocardiogram results in a diagnosis of idiopathic PPHN, and he is now being maintained on SIMV, respiratory rate 35 breaths/min, PIP of 25 cm H_2O, PEEP of 6 cm H_2O, T_I of 0.5 seconds, and FIO_2 of 0.90.

Paw is 11.5 cm H_2O. Most current ABG values are pH of 7.37, $PaCO_2$ of 44 mm Hg, HCO_3 of 25.1 mEq/L, and PaO_2 of 68 mm Hg. His HR is 125 bpm, BP is 50/30 mm Hg, spontaneous RR is 10 breaths/min, pre-SpO_2 is 98%, and post-S_pO_2 is 93%.

- *Do you think this patient is being well managed by his current therapy? Why or why not?*

The physician would like to change BB Rogers to HFOV. If that does not serve to improve ventilation and oxygenation, he would like to initiate iNO.

- *What would you suggest as initial settings for HFOV?*
- *Would you recommend iNO for this patient?*

■ Case 2: Baby Girl (BG) Fitzgerald

You and the delivery room team are called to a 41 6/7-wG delivery with MSAF. There is no other significant maternal history.

- *What additional equipment do you need to prepare for a delivery through MSAF?*

BG Fitzgerald is born and handed to the pediatrician. She is crying, actively moving her extremities, and has central cyanosis. You also observe meconium staining of her nail beds.

- *What is the appropriate delivery room intervention for BG Fitzgerald?*

You place the pulse oximeter on BG Fitzgerald's right hand, and it reads 55%. At 1 minute, she is still cyanotic, so you begin delivering 0.60 FIO_2 using blow-by oxygen. Her trunk and lips turn pink, and at 2 minutes her SpO_2 reads 70%. At 4 minutes, when you try to remove the blow-by oxygen, BG Fitzgerald's lips turn blue.

- *Where do you think BG Fitzgerald should be? Stay with her mother, go to the newborn nursery, or transfer to the NICU?*

After admission to the NICU, you place her on an oxygen hood at 1 and take pre- and post-ductal SpO_2 readings; they are 99% and 87%, respectively. Chest radiograph at admission is significant for hyperinflation and patchy infiltrates throughout the lungs. The physician places an arterial line and obtains an ABG test value from the umbilicus: pH of 7.29, $PaCO_2$ of 50 mm Hg, PaO_2 of 62 mm Hg.

- *Do you believe that BG Fitzgerald has PPHN? What information leads you to that conclusion?*
- *What respiratory measures would you suggest?*

■ Case 3: BB Kirkwood

You are called to the newborn nursery to help a baby in respiratory distress. BB Kirkwood is a 37 3/7-wG infant, born 3 hours ago via scheduled cesarean delivery for breech presentation. When you arrive, you note that BB Kirkwood is breathing 65 times a minute, with mild substernal retractions and nasal flaring. A pulse oximeter on his right foot reads 88%.

• *What would you like to do?*

You deliver blow-by oxygen and find BB Kirkwood's SpO_2 rapidly increases to 97%. You transfer him to the special care nursery and admit him for respiratory distress. Before the nurse begins the admission process, you quickly obtain an ABG reading on RA.

The results are pH 7.38, $PaCO_2$ of 34 mm Hg, HCO_3 of 19.8 mEq/L, and PaO_2 of 60 mm Hg. The physician agrees with your recommendation to begin oxygen therapy, so you start an oxygen hood at 0.40 FIO_2. You auscultate and hear end-expiratory crackles. A chest radiograph reveals diffuse parenchymal infiltrates with inflation to eight ribs posteriorly.

• *What do you believe is the cause of BB Kirkwood's respiratory distress? How can you definitively diagnose it?*

Multiple-Choice Questions

1. Which of the following is the best method to evaluate oxygenation in a patient with PPHN?
   a. Oxygenation index
   b. SpO_2
   c. PaO_2
   d. PcO_2

2. Which of the following are recommended therapies to decrease PVR in a newborn with severe PPHN?
      I. Oxygen
     II. Paralytic infusion
    III. Hyperventilation
    IV. HFOV
     V. iNO
   a. I, II, IV, V
   b. I, IV, V
   c. I, III, IV, V
   d. I, II, III, IV, V

3. What is the first clinical sign that iNO is effective in decreasing PVR?
   a. Increase in PaO_2
   b. Echocardiographic evidence of decreased pulmonary pressures
   c. Improved systemic blood pressure
   d. A narrowing gradient between preductal and postductal SpO_2

4. You are caring for a 3-day-old baby girl with idiopathic PPHN. She is intubated, on FIO_2 1, SIMV PIP of 30 cm H_2O, PEEP of 8 cm H_2O, RR of 45 breaths/ min (Paw = 16.25 cm H_2O). Her most recent blood gas is pH 7.39, $PaCO_2$ of 40 mm Hg, HCO_3 of 23.9 mEq/L, and PaO_2 40 mm Hg. Based on the patient's OI, what would you recommend as the next step in therapy for her?
   a. Increase PIP
   b. HFOV
   c. iNO
   d. ECMO

5. After initiation of ECMO, how should ventilator settings be managed?
   a. Patient should be left on the same ventilator settings.
   b. PIP and PEEP should be increased until patient is stabilized on ECMO.
   c. Patient should be placed on "lung rest" settings, to include a low RR, FIO_2, PIP of 20 cm H_2O, and PEEP of 10 cm H_2O
   d. Place on CPAP or extubate

6. Which of the following are risk factors associated with developing MSAF?
      VI. Polyhydramnios
     VII. Post-term pregnancy
    VIII. Preeclampsia
     IX. Congenital diaphragmatic hernia
      X. Low 5-minute Apgar
   a. I, II, III, V
   b. II, III, IV, V
   c. II, III, V
   d. I, II, V

7. You are called to the delivery of a 41 3/7-wG infant who was noted to have MSAF. The baby is delivered and handed to the neonatal nurse practitioner. The baby is not moving, is not crying, and has blue hands and trunk. Based on your assessment, what would be ideal treatment strategy?
   a. Quickly intubate and suction the airway using a meconium aspirator
   b. Dry, stimulate, and give oxygen
   c. Suction the mouth, then nose
   d. Begin positive-pressure ventilation

8. Specify the most common signs and symptoms of compromise in an infant with MSAF.

9. You are caring for a 4-hour-old infant MSAF on an oxygen hood at 1 FIO_2. You obtain a blood gas reading from the right wrist: pH 7.36, $PaCO_2$ of 41 mm Hg, and PaO_2 of 47 mm Hg. What respiratory therapy would you recommend?
   a. Stay on the current therapy
   b. Change to a 1 L nasal cannula
   c. Initiate NCPAP
   d. Intubate and initiate HFOV

10. A mother is scheduled for a repeat cesarean section today. She is 41 years old and has a history significant for asthma, gestational diabetes, and polyhydramnios. She gives birth to a baby boy who weighs 4,500 g. Which of these put this baby boy at an increased risk for TTN?
    I. Cesarean delivery
    II. Advanced maternal age
    III. Maternal asthma
    IV. Gestational diabetes
    V. Polyhydramnios
    VI. Male gender
    VII. Birth weight 4,500 g
    a. I, III, IV, V, VI
    b. II, III, V, VI
    c. I, III, IV, VI, VII
    d. I, II, III, VI, VII

DavisPlus | For additional resources login to Davis*Plus* (http://davisplus.fadavis.com/ keyword "Perretta") and click on the Premium tab. (Don't have a *Plus*Code to access Premium Resources? Just click the Purchase Access button on the book's Davis*Plus* page.)

REFERENCES

1. Heritage CK, Cunningham MD. Association of elective repeat cesarean delivery and persistent pulmonary hypertension of the newborn. *Am J Obstet Gynecol*. 1985;152 (6, pt 1):627-629.
2. Walsh-Sukys MC, Tyson JE, Wright LL, et al. Persistent pulmonary hypertension of the newborn in the era before nitric oxide: practice variation and outcomes. *Pediatrics*. 2000;105(1, pt 1):14-20.
3. Stayer SA, Liu Y. Pulmonary hypertension of the newborn. *Best Pract Res Clin Anaesthesiol*. 2010;24(3):375-386.
4. Wilson KL, Zelig CM, Harvey JP, et al. Persistent pulmonary hypertension of the newborn is associated with mode of delivery and not with maternal use of selective serotonin reuptake inhibitors. *Am J Perinatol*. 2011;28 (1):19-24.
5. Konduri G, Kim UO. Advances in the diagnosis and management of persistent pulmonary hypertension of the newborn. *Pediatr Clin North Am*. 2009;56(3):579-600.
6. Ostrea EM, Villanueva-Uy ET, Natarajan G, et al. Persistent pulmonary hypertension of the newborn: pathogenesis, etiology, and management. *Pediatr Drugs*. 2006;8(3):179-188.
7. Alano MA, Ngougmna E, Ostrea EM, et al. Analysis of nonsteroidal anti-inflammatory drugs in meconium and its relation to persistent pulmonary hypertension of the newborn. *Pediatrics*. 2001;107(3):519-523.
8. Hernandez-Diaz S, Van Marter LJ, Werler MM, et al. Risk factors for persistent pulmonary hypertension of the newborn. *Pediatrics*. 2007;120(2):e272-e282.
9. Rudolph A. Distribution and regulation of blood flow in the fetal and neonatal lamb. *Circ Res*. 1985;57:811-821.
10. Ziegler JW, Ivy DD, Kinsella JP, et al. The role of nitric oxide, endothelin, and prostaglandins in the transition of the pulmonary circulation. *Clin Perinatol*. 1995;22(2): 387-403.
11. Steinhorn RH, Millard SL, Morin FC III. Persistent pulmonary hypertension of the newborn: role of nitric oxide and endothelin in pathophysiology and treatment. *Clin Perinatol*. 1995;22(2):405-428.
12. Geggel RL, Reid LM. The structural basis of PPHN. *Clin Perinatol*. 1984;11(3):525-549.
13. Christou H, Adatia I, Van Marter LJ, et al. Effect of inhaled nitric oxide on endothelin-1 and cyclic guanosine 5'-monophosphate plasma concentrations in newborn infants with persistent pulmonary hypertension. *J Pediatr*. 1997;130(4):603-611.
14. Ashida Y, Miyahara H, Sawada H, et al. Anesthetic management of a neonate with vein of Galen aneurysmal malformations and severe pulmonary hypertension. *Paediatr Anaesthes*. 2005;15(6):525-528.
15. Dakshinamurti S. Pathophysiologic mechanisms of persistent pulmonary hypertension. *Pediatr Pulmonol*. 2005;39(6): 492-503.
16. Henry GW. Noninvasive assessment of cardiac function and pulmonary hypertension in persistent pulmonary hypertension of the newborn. *Clin Perinatol*. 1984;11(3):627-640.
17. The Neonatal Inhaled Nitric Oxide Study Group. Inhaled nitric oxide in full-term and nearly full-term infants with hypoxic respiratory failure. *N Engl J Med*. 1997;336:597-604.
18. Cornfield DN, Reeve HL, Tolarova S, et al. Oxygen causes fetal pulmonary vasodilation through activation of a calcium-dependent potassium channel. *Proc Natl Acad Sci USA*. 1996;93(15):8089-8094.
19. Lakshminrusimha S, Swartz DD, Gugino SF, et al. Oxygen concentration and pulmonary hemodynamics in newborn lambs with pulmonary hypertension. *Pediatr Res*. 2009;66 (5):539-544.
20. Drummond WH, Gregory GA, Heymann MA, et al. The independent effects of hyperventilation, tolazoline, and dopamine on infants with persistent pulmonary hypertension. *J Pediatr*. 1981;98(4):603-611.
21. Schreiber MD, Heymann MA, Soifer SJ. Increased arterial pH, not decreased $PaCO_2$, attenuates hypoxia-induced pulmonary vasoconstriction in newborn lambs. *Pediatr Res*. 1986;20(2):113-117.
22. Hendricks-Munoz KD, Walton JP. Hearing loss in infants with persistent fetal circulation. *Pediatrics*. 1988;81(5): 650-656.
23. Marron MJ, Crisafi MA, Driscoll JM Jr, et al. Hearing and neurodevelopmental outcome in survivors of persistent pulmonary hypertension of the newborn. *Pediatrics*. 1992;90(3):392-396.

24. Cheung PY, Tyebkhan JM, Peliowski A, et al. Prolonged use of pancuronium bromide and sensorineural hearing loss in childhood survivors of congenital diaphragmatic hernia. *J Pediatr*. 1999;135(2, pt 1):233-239.

25. Committee on Fetus and Newborn. Use of inhaled nitric oxide. *Pediatrics*. 2000;106(2):344-345.

26. Froese AB, Kinsella JP. High-frequency oscillatory ventilation: lessons from the neonatal/pediatric experience. *Crit Care Med*. 2005;33(suppl 3):S115-S121.

27. Kinsella JP, Abman SH. Inhaled nitric oxide and high frequency oscillatory ventilation in persistent pulmonary hypertension of the newborn. *Eur J Pediatr*. 1998;157 (suppl 1):S28-S30.

28. Yoder RA, Siler-Khodr T, Winter VT, et al. High-frequency oscillatory ventilation: effects on lung function, mechanics, and airway cytokines in the immature baboon model for neonatal chronic lung disease. *Am J Respir Crit Care Med*. 2000;162(5):1867-1876.

29. Kinsella JP, Truog WE, Walsh WF, et al. Randomized, multicenter trial of inhaled nitric oxide and high-frequency oscillatory ventilation in severe, persistent pulmonary hypertension of the newborn. *J Pediatr*. 1997;131(1, pt 1): 55-62.

30. SensorMedics Corporation. *High Frequency Oscillatory Ventilation User's Manual*. Homestead, FL: SensorMedics Corporation; 2001. Available at www.fda.gov/ohrms/dockets/ac/01/briefing/3770b1_15.doc. Accessed September 28, 2012.

31. Engle WA; Committee on Fetus and Newborn. Surfactant-replacement therapy for respiratory distress in the pre-term and term neonate. *Pediatrics*. 2008;121(2):419-432.

32. Finer NN. Surfactant use for neonatal lung injury: beyond respiratory distress syndrome. *Paediatr Respir Rev*. 2004; 5(suppl A):S289-S297.

33. Hintz SR, Suttner DM, Sheehan AM, et al. Decreased use of neonatal extracorporeal membrane oxygenation (ECMO): how new treatment modalities have affected ECMO utilization. *Pediatrics*. 2000;106(6):1339-1343.

34. Konduri GG, Solimano A, Sokol GM, et al. A randomized trial of early versus standard inhaled nitric oxide therapy in term and near-term newborn infants with hypoxic respiratory failure. *Pediatrics*. 2004;113(3, pt 1):559-564.

35. Seri I. Circulatory support of the sick preterm infant. *SeminNeonatol*. 2001;6(1):85-95.

36. Siobal MS. Pulmonary vasodilators. *Respir Care*. 2007; 52(7):885-899.

37. Coates EW, Klinepeter ME, O'Shea TM. Neonatal pulmonary hypertension treated with inhaled nitric oxide and high-frequency ventilation. *J Perinatol*. 2008;28(10):675-679.

38. Food and Drug Administration. *NDA 20-845 approval letter for INO Therapeutics, Inc*. Rockville, MD: Food and Drug Administration; 1999.

39. Fakioglu H, Totapally BR, Torbati D, et al. Hypoxic respiratory failure in term newborns: indications for inhaled nitric oxide and extracorporeal membrane oxygenation therapy. *J Crit Care*. 2005;20:288-295.

40. Clark RH, Kueser TJ, Walker MW, et al.; Clinical Inhaled Nitric Oxide Research Group. Low-dose nitric oxide therapy for persistent pulmonary hypertension of the newborn. *N Engl J Med*. 2000;342:469-474.

41. González A, Fabres J, D'Apremont I, et al. Randomized controlled trial of early compared with delayed use of inhaled nitric oxide in newborns with a moderate respiratory failure and pulmonary hypertension. *J Perinatol*. 2010;30 (6):420-424.

42. INOMax [label]. Clinton, NJ: INO Therapeutics, Inc.; 2012. Available at http://www.accessdata.fda.gov/drugsatfda_docs/label/1999/20845lbl.htm. Accessed October 18, 2012.

43. Finer N, Barrington KJ. Nitric oxide for respiratory failure in infants born at or near term. *Cochrane Database Syst Rev*. 2006;4:CD000399.

44. Malley WJ. *Clinical Blood Gases: Assessment and Intervention*. 2nd ed. St. Louis, MO: Elsevier Saunders; 2005.

45. Salguero KL, Cummings JJ. Inhaled nitric oxide and methemoglobin in full-term infants with persistent pulmonary hypertension of the newborn. *Pulm Pharmacol Ther*. 2002;15(1):1-5.

46. Verklan MT. Persistent pulmonary hypertension of the newborn: not a honeymoon anymore. *J Perinat Neonatal Nurs*. 2006;20(1):108-112.

47. Boran P, Tokuc G, Yegin Z. Methemoglobinemia due to application of prilocaine during circumcision and the effect of ascorbic acid. *J Pediatr Urol*. 2008;4(6):475-476.

48. Lindenmann J, Matzi V, Kaufmann P, et al. Hyperbaric oxygenation in the treatment of life-threatening isobutyl nitrite-induced methemoglobinemia—a case report. *Inhal Toxicol*. 2006;18(13):1047-1049.

49. Shah PS, Ohlsson A. Sildenafil for pulmonary hypertension in neonates. *Cochrane Database Syst Rev*. 2011;8: CD005494.

50. Hanson KA, Ziegler JW, Rybalkin SD, et al. Chronic pulmonary hypertension increases fetal lung cGMP phosphodiesterase activity. *Am J Physiol*. 1998;275 (5, pt 1):L931-L941.

51. Atz AM, Wessel DL. Sildenafil ameliorates effects of inhaled nitric oxide withdrawal. *Anesthesiology*. 1999;91 (1):307-310.

52. Baquero H, Soliz A, Neira F, et al. Oral sildenafil in infants with persistent pulmonary hypertension of the newborn: a pilot randomized blinded study. *Pediatrics*. 2006;117(4):1077-1083.

53. Huddleston AJ, Knoderer CA, Morris JL, et al. Sildenafil for the treatment of pulmonary hypertension in pediatric patients. *Pediatr Cardiol*. 2009;30(7):871-872.

54. Custer JW, Rau RE, eds. *The Harriet Lane Handbook*. Philadelphia, PA: Mosby Elsevier; 2009.

55. Vargas-Origel A, Gómez-Rodríguez G, Aldana-Valenzuela C, et al. The use of sildenafil in persistent pulmonary hypertension of the newborn. *Am J Perinatol*. 2010;27(3):225-230.

56. Bassler D, Kreutzer K, McNamara P, et al. Milrinone for persistent pulmonary hypertension of the newborn. *Cochrane Database Syst Rev*. 2010;11:CD007802.

57. Dhillon R. The management of neonatal pulmonary hypertension. *Arch Dis Child Fetal Neonatal Ed*. 2012;97 (3):F223-F228.

58. Bartlett RH, Andrews AF, Toomasian JM, et al. Extracorporeal membrane oxygenation for newborn respiratory failure: 45 cases. *Surgery*. 1982;92(2):425-433.

59. Bartlett RH, Roloff DW, Cornell RG, et al. Extracorporeal membrane oxygenation in neonates with respiratory failure: a prospective randomized study. *Pediatrics*. 1985;76(4): 479-487.

60. O'Rourke PP, Crone RK, Vacanti JP, et al. Extracorporeal membrane oxygenation and conventional medical therapy in neonates with persistent pulmonary hypertension of the newborn: a prospective randomized study. *Pediatrics*. 1989;84(6):957-963.

61. Hageman JR, Adams MA, Gardner TH. Persistent pulmonary hypertension of the newborn: trends in incidence, diagnosis, and management. *Am J Dis Child*. 1984;138(6):592-595.

62. Davis JM, Spitzer AR, Cox C, et al. Predicting survival in infants with persistent pulmonary hypertension of the newborn. *Pediatr Pulmonol*. 1988;5(1):6-9.

63. Robertson CM, Tyebkhan JM, Hagler ME, et al. Late-onset, progressive sensorineural hearing loss after severe neonatal respiratory failure. *Otol Neurotol*. 2002;23(3):353-356.

64. Rosenberg AA, Lee NR, Vaver KN, et al. School-age outcomes of newborns treated for persistent pulmonary hypertension. *J Perinatol.* 2010;30(2):127-134.

65. Hoskote AU, Castle RA, Hoo A, et al. Airway function in infants treated with inhaled nitric oxide for persistent pulmonary hypertension. *Pediatr Pulmonol.* 2008;43(3):224-235.

66. Singh BS, Clark RH, Powers RJ, et al. Meconium aspiration syndrome remains a significant problem in the NICU: outcomes and treatment patterns in term neonates admitted for intensive care during a ten-year period. *J Perinatol.* 2009;29(7):497-503.

67. Gomella TL, Cunningham MD, Eyal FG, et al, eds. *Neonatology: Management, Procedures, On-Call Problems, Diseases, and Drugs.* 6th ed. New York: McGraw Hill; 2009.

68. Wiswell TE, Knight GR, Finer NN, et al. A multi-center, randomized, controlled trial comparing Surfaxin (Lucinactant) lavage with standard care for treatment of meconium aspiration syndrome. *Pediatrics.* 2002;109(6):1081-1087.

69. Cleary GM, Wiswell TE. Meconium-stained amniotic fluid and the meconium aspiration syndrome: an update. *Pediatr Clin North Am.* 1998;45(3):511-529.

70. Fanaroff AA. Meconium aspiration syndrome: historical aspects. *J Perinatol.* 2008;28(suppl 3):s3-s7.

71. Gouyon JB, Ribakovsky C, Ferdynus C, et al. Severe respiratory disorders in term neonates. *Paediatr Perinat Epidemol.* 2008;22(1):22-30.

72. Herting E, Rauprich P, Stichtenoth G, et al. Resistance of different surfactant preparations to inactivation by meconium. *Pediatri Res.* 2001;50(1):44-49.

73. Oelberg DB, Downey SA, Flynn MM. Bile salt-induced intracellular Ca++ accumulation in type II pneumocytes. *Lung.* 1990;168(6):297-308.

74. Kattwinkel J, Perlman JM, Aziz K, et al. Neonatal resuscitation: 2010 American Heart Association Guidelines for Cardiopulmonary Resuscitation and Emergency Cardiovascular Care. *Circulation.* 2010;122:S909-S919.

75. The American Congress of Obstetricians and Gynecologists. ACOG Committee Opinion Number 379: Management of delivery of a newborn with meconium-stained amniotic fluid. *Obstet Gynecol.* 2007;110(3):739.

76. Vain NE, Szyld EG, Prudent LM, et al. Oropharyngeal and nasopharyngeal suctioning of meconium-stained neonates before delivery of their shoulders: multicentre, randomised controlled trial. *Lancet.* 2004;364(9434):597-602.

77. Dargaville PA. Respiratory support in meconium aspiration syndrome: a practical guide. *Int J Pediatr.* 2012;2012:965159.

78. Wiswell TE, Gannon CM, Jacob J, et al. Delivery room management of the apparently vigorous meconium-stained neonate: results of the multicenter, international collaborative trial. *Pediatrics.* 2000;105(1):1-7.

79. Dargaville, PA, Copnell B. The epidemiology of meconium aspiration syndrome: incidence, risk factors, therapies, and outcome. *Pediatrics.* 2006;117(5):1712-1721.

80. Yeh TF. Core concepts: meconium aspiration syndrome. *Neonatal Rev.* 2010;11(9):e503-e512.

81. Gupta A, Rastogi S, Sahni R, et al. Inhaled nitric oxide and gentle ventilation in the treatment of pulmonary hypertension of the newborn—a single-center, 5-year experience. *J Perinatol.* 2002;22(6):435-441.

82. Fox WW, Berman LS, Downes JJ Jr, et al. The therapeutic application of end expiratory pressure in the meconium aspiration syndrome. *Pediatrics.* 2004;56(2):198-204.

83. Dawson C, Davies MW. Volume-targeted ventilation and arterial carbon dioxide in neonates. *J PaediatrChild Health.* 2005;41(9-10):518-521.

84. Kinsella JP, Abman SH. Efficacy of inhalational nitric oxide therapy in the clinical management of persistent pulmonary hypertension of the newborn. *Chest.* 1994;105(suppl 3):92S-94S.

85. Halliday HL, Speer CP, Robertson B. Treatment of severe meconium aspiration syndrome with porcine surfactant Collaborative surfactant study group. *Eur J Pediatr.* 1996;155(12):1047-1051.

86. Swarnam K, Soraisham AS, Sivanandan S. Advances in the management of meconium aspiration syndrome. *Int J Pediatr.* 2012;2012:359571.

87. Short BL. Extracorporeal membrane oxygenation: use in meconium aspiration syndrome. *J Perinatol.* 2008;28(3):S79-S83.

88. Beligere N, Rao R. Neurodevelopmental outcome of infants with meconium aspiration syndrome: report of a study and literature review. *J Perinatol.* 2008;28(3):S93-S101.

89. Yurdakok M, Ozek E. Transient tachypnea of the newborn: the treatment strategies. *Curr Pharm Des.* 2012;18(21):3046-3049.

90. Yurdakok M. Transient tachypnea of the newborn: what is new? *J Matern Fetal Neonatal Med.* 2010;23(suppl 3):24-26.

91. Tennant C, Friedman AM, Pare E, et al. Performance of lecithin-sphingomyelin ratio as a reflex test for documenting fetal lung maturity in late preterm and term fetuses. *J Matern Fetal Neonatal Med.* 2012;25(8):1460-1462.

92. Machado LU, Fiori HH, Baldisserotto M, et al. Surfactant deficiency in transient tachypnea of the newborn. *J Pediatr.* 2011;159(5):750-754.

93. De La Roque ED, Bertrand C, Tandonnet O, et al. Nasal high frequency percussive ventilation versus nasal continuous positive airway pressure in transient tachypnea of the newborn: a pilot randomized controlled trial (NC T00556738). *Pediatr Pulmonol.* 2011;46(3):218-223.

94. Armangil D, Yurdakök M, Korkmaz A, et al. Inhaled beta-2 agonist salbutamol for the treatment of transient tachypnea of the newborn. *J Pediatr.* 2011;159(3):398-403.

95. Stutchfield P, Whitaker R, Russell I; Antenatal Steroids for Term Elective Caesarean Section (ASTECS) Research Team. Antenatal betamethasone and incidence of neonatal respiratory distress after elective caesarean section: pragmatic randomised trial. *BMJ.* 2005;331:662-667.

96. Birnkrant DJ, Picone C, Markowitz W, et al. Association of transient tachypnea of the newborn and childhood asthma. *Pediatr Pulmonol.* 2006;41(10):978-984.

97. Guglani L, Lakshminrusimha S, Ryan RM. Transient tachypnea of the newborn. *Pediatr Rev.* 2008;29(11):e59-e65.

Chapter 7

Pulmonary Complications

Chapter Outline cont.

Chapter Objectives

After reading this chapter, you will be able to:

1. List the four signs and symptoms a neonate will display when developing atelectasis.
2. Discuss the indications for nasal continuous positive airway pressure and its benefits to neonatal patients with atelectasis.
3. Identify two common causes of neonatal pulmonary air leak.
4. List three patient management techniques a respiratory therapist can employ to prevent pulmonary interstitial emphysema in preterm infants.
5. Differentiate between the radiographic findings of pulmonary interstitial emphysema, pneumothorax, pneumomediastinum, and pneumopericardium.
6. Choose initial ventilator settings for a patient with pulmonary interstitial emphysema being placed on high-frequency jet ventilation (HFJV).
7. Discuss the techniques for quick identification and emergency treatment of a tension pneumothorax.
8. List three common microorganisms that cause pneumonia in the neonatal population.
9. Identify one treatment and one preventive measure that neonatal intensive care units can initiate for the treatment of congenital pneumonia.

■■ Baby Girl (BG) Johnson

You begin working your night shift in the level IIIB neonatal intensive care unit (NICU) of a large teaching hospital. You are given a report on BG Johnson, a 25 wG premature infant, now 4 days old. She was the first pregnancy and first live birth for a 42-year-old woman. Delivery was significant for preeclampsia, preterm labor of unknown origin, and premature rupture of membranes (PROM). Apgar scores were 3, 5, and 6 at 1, 5, and 10 minutes, respectively. BG Johnson was intubated with a 2.5-cm endotracheal tube (ETT) taped 7.5 cm at the lip at 3 minutes of life, and she received a dose of surfactant in the delivery room before 10 minutes of life. She received two subsequent doses of surfactant 8 hours apart. Upon arrival in the NICU, she was placed on synchronized intermittent mandatory ventilation (SIMV), peak inspiratory pressure (PIP) was initiated at 19 cm H_2O and adjusted between 17 and 23 cm H_2O over 72 hours, using a tidal volume target of 4.0 mL. Peak end expiratory pressure (PEEP) was initiated and has remained at 4 cm H_2O. FIO_2 was initiated at 0.50, weaned to 0.35, and maintained in a range of 0.30 to 0.55 over the last 48 hours to maintain SpO_2 of 88% to 94%. Respiratory rate (RR) was initiated at 40 breaths/min, weaned to 30 breaths/min within 24 hours, and has been unchanged. Her current weight is 685 g.

Premature infants are predisposed to many different pulmonary complications. The underdeveloped lung tissue seen in respiratory distress syndrome (RDS) is easily damaged by under- and overdistension during positive-pressure ventilation, which can have serious and life-threatening effects. The immaturity of the immune system of preterm neonates increases the likelihood of infection, including pneumonias, during early infancy. For the non-preterm infant, there are other factors that can cause pulmonary complications. Neonatal health-care teams need to identify patients most at risk for atelectasis, air leaks (pulmonary interstitial emphysema, pneumothorax, pneumomediastinum, or pneumopericardium), or pneumonia, and monitor them closely for signs of respiratory distress. Recognition of the early warning signs and prompt initiation of treatment for these complications are fundamental skills for all respiratory therapists.

Atelectasis

■■ The shift report notes that BG Johnson has minimal spontaneous respiratory effort. Her last arterial blood gas (ABG) values as taken from the umbilical artery catheter (UAC) were 7.29/52/24.6/73, on the following vent settings: SIMV 20/4 with tidal volume (V_T) target of 4 mL, rate 30 breaths/min, FIO_2 of 0.55, inspiratory time (T_I) of 0.35 seconds, flow of 8 liters per minute

(LPM). Current vital signs are as follows: heart rate (HR), 150 to 165 bpm; blood pressure (BP) 57/32 (mean arterial blood pressure [MAP]), 40 mm Hg on 5 mcg of dopamine IV infusion; skin temperature 36°C managed in isolette, SpO_2 90% on FIO_2 0.55; RR 30 breaths/min from the mechanical ventilator. You are called to BG Johnson's bedside by the nurse because of an increase in the number of desaturations requiring increases in FIO_2.

Atelectasis is a collapsed or airless condition of the lung. It is caused by decreased lung compliance, inadequate tidal volume, or airway obstruction. Some common contributing factors for neonatal atelectasis include the following:

- Meconium obstruction in the terminal airways
- Lung compression from lung masses, tumors, or gastric contents (as in congenital diaphragmatic hernia)
- Respiratory failure and hypoventilation as a result of very low lung compliance and surfactant deficiency seen in RDS

Injury to the lung as a result of repeated collapse and re-expansion of alveoli, known as **atelectrauma**, is one of the major causes of lung injury in mechanically ventilated neonates.

Pathophysiology

There are several characteristics of premature infants' anatomy and physiology that predispose them to atelectasis. The chest wall of premature infants is more compliant than those of adults and offers little resistance to collapse during exhalation. This, compounded with surfactant deficiency that increases surface tension inside the alveoli and the preference of terminal air sacs to collapse on end exhalation as a result of structural instability, makes premature infants much more susceptible to atelectasis and atelectrauma (Fig. 7-1). Differences in neonatal chest shape also mean that intercostal muscles perform a less effective mechanical function during spontaneous breathing. See Box 7-1 for additional factors of neonatal anatomy that can contribute to atelectasis.

Another disadvantage for premature infants is that they must expend a tremendous amount of energy when effectively spontaneously breathing because of the high relative resistance in their smaller airways and low alveolar lung compliance. This puts them at high risk for respiratory failure. Progressive respiratory failure will manifest first in the lungs as atelectasis, because not enough energy is exerted with each breath to expand all alveoli. This results in ventilation/perfusion (V/Q) mismatching, in which blood is circulated to collapsed lung units and is unable to oxygenate. This shunting will not allow unloading of carbon dioxide

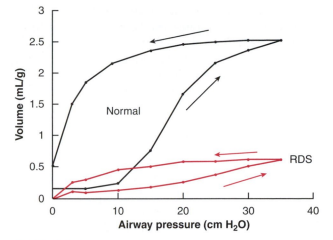

Figure 7-1 Pressure-Volume Curve

| Box 7-1 | Factors of Neonatal Anatomy That Contribute to the Development of Atelectasis |

- More compliant chest wall
- Surfactant deficiency
- Relatively low functional residual capacity
- Underdevelopment of structural support in conducting airways
- Diaphragm insertion causes ribs to move inward during inspiration, requiring more energy for effective ventilation

and loading of oxygen, which will manifest as respiratory failure and hypoxemia on blood gas.

Atelectrauma manifests from the repeated collapse and reopening of small airways and alveoli, which damages the cells of the airway and alveoli and causes inflammation. This begins a harmful cycle within the lungs, where inflammation increases the space between the oxygen within the alveoli and the capillaries (known as a diffusion barrier). This condition requires increased FIO_2 and mean airway pressure to overcome, causing more injury and further cellular dysfunction. Because the treatments for atelectasis, discussed later in this chapter, can cause further damage, prevention and quick and effective treatment are essential to avoid lung injury.

Clinical Manifestations

Neonates with RDS use two mechanisms to prevent atelectasis by counteracting their low lung compliance state. The first is **grunting**, a form of expiratory retard where neonates partially close their glottis at the end of expiration to create a back pressure in the lungs with the goal of stabilizing alveoli and terminal airways to prevent collapse. Grunting functions similarly to pursed-lip breathing taught to adult patients with chronic obstructive pulmonary disease. The second is tachypnea, in which neonates increase their respiratory rate until gas trapping results, bringing their functional residual capacity (FRC) to normal levels.

The condition of patients with atelectasis varies in severity, which will affect the extent of patients' clinical presentation. Clinical signs include the following:

- Cyanosis
- Tachypnea
- Nasal flaring
- Retractions
- Grunting
- Increasing FIO_2 requirements
- Decreasing trends in mechanical or spontaneous tidal volume despite unchanged peak inspiratory pressure (PIP) and peak end expiratory pressure (PEEP)
- Hypercapnia as evidenced by capillary blood gas (CBG) or arterial blood gas (ABG) values
- Hypoxemia on ABG
- Chest radiographs (CXR) will reveal areas of increased opacity where alveolar units have collapsed and are not air-filled (Fig. 7-2). If severe, the mediastinum may be shifted toward the side of collapse. If generalized, atelectasis is often described as "whiteout" on a radiograph, where little inflation is noted. In this case, elevation of the diaphragm may also be noted.

Management and Treatment

Prevention and early management of atelectasis is essential to prevent atelectrauma in neonates. It is important for respiratory therapists to identify patients at risk for atelectasis and to look for early

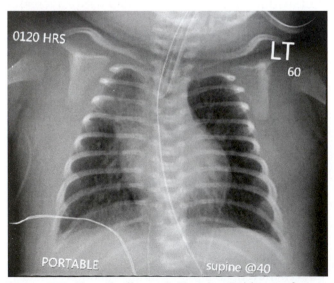

Figure 7-2 Chest Radiograph Showing Evidence of Right Upper Lobe Atelectasis *(Courtesy of Jane Benson, MD)*

■ ■ ■ You arrive at BG Johnson's bedside to note that her FIO_2 is now set at 0.80 and SpO_2 is reading 89%. You listen to breath sounds and find them to be diminished at bases and more diminished on the left side. You also notice that she is displaying substernal retractions with her spontaneous breaths. After monitoring the exhaled V_T read-out for over a minute, you observe an average of 2.2 mL V_T. When you check BG Johnson's chart, you see that the previous exhaled V_T, correlating with the time of the last ABG measurement, was documented as 4.1 mL. You call the physician to the bedside and request an ABG test and a CXR to assist in diagnosing the cause of BG Johnson's increase in respiratory distress. The physician agrees. ABG value is pH 7.27, $PaCO_2$ is 56 mm Hg, PaO_2 is 54 mm Hg, and HCO_3 is 25.3 mEq/L. CXR shows increased areas of opacity on the left side, consistent with atelectasis.

warning signs. Prevention of atelectasis includes the following:

- Early extubation and withdrawal of invasive mechanical ventilation (MV)
- Good airway clearance through adequate suctioning
- Frequent changes in patient positioning
- Prophylactic surfactant delivery for patients with RDS

When delivering surfactant, care must be taken to decrease inspiratory pressures during the rapid improvement of lung compliance, or lung overdistension can easily occur. This overdistension can cause lung tissue injury, known as **volutrauma**, and pulmonary air leaks (discussed later in this chapter). To prevent overdistension of the alveoli, respiratory therapists should stay at the patient's bedside during the 30 minutes following surfactant delivery and monitor the patient noninvasively. Changes in tidal volume, flow volume loops, and pressure volume loops will denote lung compliance changes and guide when to decrease inspiratory pressures. Improvement in SpO_2 is a characteristic sign of alveolar recruitment, so decrease FIO_2 with improvement in oxygenation. Do not wait for blood gas results to make ventilator setting changes because alveolar damage is possible before these results become available.

Respiratory therapists can minimize the risk of atelectrauma in intubated patients by using advanced patient monitoring tools available on modern neonatal ventilators. Using pressure-volume loops will help therapists recognize when excess pressure is being delivered to the lungs without the associated volume. Trends in exhaled volumes will help therapists assess ongoing changes in lung compliance and recognize the early formation of atelectasis.

Chest physiotherapy (CPT) has been suggested to prevent atelectasis, but there is no compelling data for neonates showing a benefit postextubation in preventing lobar collapse. However, a recent review of the literature showed no evidence of harm for babies who received active CPT (chest percussion and vibration) for a short time after extubation (1). Patient positioning is a frequently used mechanism to improve mucus clearance and prevention of atelectasis in all patient populations, and it is encouraged in the neonatal population both for its pulmonary and developmental benefits. Because of the high risk for intraventricular hemorrhage in premature infants, Trendelenburg positioning is to be avoided during postural drainage. Care must also be taken when repositioning intubated neonates to avoid accidental extubation.

Although mechanical ventilation is an invasive and potentially harmful respiratory care modality, proper ventilation management is a key component for treatment of atelectasis. In patients who are intubated, optimal PEEP is necessary to match the critical opening pressure of the lungs, which can be determined through pressure volume loops (see Fig. 7-1) or by clinical observation of FIO_2 requirements, alleviation of previously mentioned signs and symptoms, and radiographic evidence of alveolar recruitment.

In patients who are not currently intubated, nasal continuous positive airway pressure (NCPAP) is an effective method to recruiting collapsed alveoli and providing alveolar stability. NCPAP is the application of positive pressure to the airways of the spontaneously breathing patient, using nasal prongs or a mask, throughout the respiratory cycle (2). It provides a positive pressure that increases FRC and provides the following benefits (3):

- Splinting of airways
- Increasing lung expansion
- Preventing alveolar collapse
- Preserving patient's natural surfactant
- Improving V/Q matching
- Improving oxygenation
- Increasing lung compliance
- Decreasing airway resistance
- Decreasing work of breathing
- Stabilizing a patient's respiratory pattern

NCPAP's functions are similar to adult noninvasive ventilation and can be used with any lung disease that causes airway or alveolar instability that leads to atelectasis. The delivery device and settings vary widely throughout the world, but an initial NCPAP setting of 5 to 7 cm H_2O is generally thought to be reasonable. American Association for Respiratory Care Clinical Practice Guidelines recommend initial settings of 4 to 5 cm H_2O and gradual increases up to 10 cm H_2O as needed (2). Higher NCPAP levels may needed to recruit lungs with low compliance, but levels higher than 8 to 10 cm H_2O are more likely to result in pressure leakage through the mouth, and levels higher than 10 to 12 have been associated with increased risk of gastric insufflation (4). An orogastric tube should be placed to minimize gastric insufflation in patients receiving NCPAP.

Noninvasive positive-pressure ventilation (NIPPV), which delivers alternating levels of CPAP similar to adult bilevel positive airway pressure (BiPAP), may offer to neonates the additional benefit of recruiting unstable alveoli by switching between low CPAP and high CPAP levels. The results of a preliminary study showed that using NIPPV instead of traditional NCPAP may reduce the length of respiratory support and oxygen-dependent days without increasing the risk of lung damage, but there are currently no established standards on its use (5). The study recommended a delta P (δP, difference between low level and high level) of approximately 4 cm H_2O, with a rate set at 30 per minute. NIPPV is discussed in more detail in Chapter 4.

There are four basic categories of NCPAP delivery devices for neonates, which are listed in Table 7-1. NCPAP may require increased levels of attention by bedside providers to assure proper fitting of NCPAP prongs or mask and headgear and to confirm that the nasal prongs or mask remain in the nose and that minimal leakage occurs. This will assure proper delivery of pressure to the alveoli and the best patient outcome, as well as minimize nasal breakdown caused by improper nasal prong or mask placement. Skin breakdown leading to nasal trauma is a serious complication of NCPAP delivery. When caring for patients with

Table 7-1	Devices For Neonatal NCPAP Delivery
Device	**Description**
Bubble CPAP	Placing of the "expiratory limb" of the CPAP circuit under a known depth of water
Ventilator CPAP	Using a neonatal mechanical ventilator in CPAP mode, with adaptations to circuit to include nasal prongs or mask
Variable flow CPAP	Device in which pressure is generated by a high continuous gas flow through a tube with high resistance; often includes a bi-level support option
Nasal cannula	High gas flow delivered into the nares via a nasal cannula

NCPAP prongs, providers should monitor for the following five signs of nasal trauma (6):

1. Redness
2. Bleeding
3. Crusting
4. Excoriation (scaly abrasion of the skin)
5. Narrowing of the nasal passage

Prevention of nasal trauma should include vigilance of prong placement, avoiding excess pressure use, and continuous assessment by the health-care team, including pediatric otolaryngologists.

■■ Newly developing atelectasis seems to be the cause of BG Johnson's respiratory distress. You and the physician discuss and agree to do the following with BG Johnson's ventilator: increase PEEP to 5 cm H_2O and PIP to 21 cm H_2O. You will place BG Johnson with her left side up for the next 4 hours to encourage alveolar re-expansion in the most affected lung portions. After about 1 hour of new therapy, you and the nurse are able to wean the FIO_2 to 0.50, with a resulting SpO_2 of 91%.

Course and Prognosis

Because atelectasis is a common side effect or manifestation in many neonatal lung diseases, its recurrence is seen frequently and should always be monitored. Nontreatment of atelectasis will lead to respiratory failure and the need for intubation. However, inappropriate or overaggressive treatment can lead to an increased incidence of air leaks and increased risk for chronic lung disease (CLD). Using NCPAP to avoid intubation and mechanical ventilation can provide some lung protection and promote healthy lung development and should always be considered in the presence of atelectasis (4).

Reintubation and mechanical ventilation should be based on clinical deterioration, not on severity of radiographic evidence. Signs to look for include increases in the frequency of apnea, particularly those requiring bag mask ventilation; sustained increase in FIO_2; or respiratory failure by blood gas data (pH less than 7.20 or 7.25, based on institution standards) (7).

Pulmonary Interstitial Emphysema

■■ You return to the NICU 2 days later and are once again caring for BG Johnson. She seems to have tolerated the increase in ventilator settings well and has been unchanged in her respiratory settings since you left. Her atelectasis on CXR has resolved, and her FIO_2 has stayed in the 0.50 to 0.60 range.

She has been rotating between lying midline and left side up to encourage inflation of the left lung. Most recent ABG values are pH of 7.30, $PaCO_2$ of 52 mmHg, PaO_2 of 70 mmHg, HCO_3 of 25.2 mEq/L. BG Johnson's vital signs and medications are unchanged from 2 days previous.

Pulmonary interstitial emphysema (PIE) is dissection of air into the tissue of the lungs surrounding the pulmonary vasculature. It is an acute pulmonary complication seen most frequently in premature infants with RDS who require mechanical ventilation, for whom the rate of incidence has recently been noted to be as high as 3% (8). Most incidences occur within 96 hours of birth in babies receiving MV (9). A recent retrospective study suggests that extremely low birth weight (ELBW) infants who develop PIE suffer more severe respiratory distress than do infants who do not develop PIE, as indicated by increased doses of surfactant and more aggressive ventilator support during the first week of life (10).

Pathophysiology

PIE develops as a consequence of overdistension of the distal airways and alveoli. Distal airways have little structural support and a high compliance when compared with the low-compliance alveoli seen in RDS. When positive pressure is applied to the airway and lungs during MV, terminal bronchioles stretch and shear (Fig. 7-3). Tearing or rupture of the distal airways or air ducts provides the pathway for air leakage into the pulmonary vascular sheaths, which have the ability to stretch considerably. This can occur in a single lobe, unilaterally or bilaterally.

The advent of exogenous surfactant therapy and more sophisticated mechanical ventilators has decreased the incidence of PIE in NICUs, limiting it mostly to the smallest babies with the most immature lungs. PIE is normally slow to accumulate but may

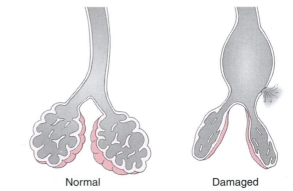

Normal   Damaged

Figure 7-3 Development of PIE in a Terminal Bronchiole

occasionally have acute onset, which will lead to more pronounced clinical manifestations.

Clinical Manifestations

The onset of abnormal clinical signs with PIE is usually gradual, worsening as the disease progresses. It normally manifests as:

- Hypoxemia and hypercapnia, which may or may not be responsive to an increase in ventilatory support
- Hypotension, which, if seen, is usually considered a late response
- Episodes of bradycardia that are usually responsive to traditional treatment

The CXR in the presence of PIE will reveal two radiolucent characteristics (Fig. 7-4):

1. Cyst-like formations 1 to 4 mm in diameter, which can appear oval or lobulated. If the cysts are numerous, they may appear spongy. If the cyst formations migrate into the pleura, they will present as blebs, which is characteristically seen prior to development of a pneumothorax.
2. Linear formations, irregular in form, are seen in the peripheral lung fields and the perihilar areas. They can be distinguished from air bronchograms, which are smooth and found branching from the hilum.

If PIE is unilateral and severe, CXR may also show mediastinal shift and atelectasis of the contralateral lung.

■ ■ Before your first ventilator check, you are called to BG Johnson's bedside by her nurse, Jane. Jane just began her shift and has noted three episodes of bradycardia, two of which required positive-pressure ventilation (PPV) with a manual resuscitator to alleviate them. She also notes that she was just about to call the pediatric resident to the bedside because BG Johnson's BPs have been drifting slowly over the last several hours, and she would like to increase the dopamine drip. The nurse on the previous shift also seems to have been increasing the FIO_2 to maintain adequate SpO_2, and the FIO_2 is now set at 0.70, increased from 0.40 three hours ago. You listen to breath sounds, which are diminished but seem equal bilaterally.

The resident arrives and asks for the patient's status, which you provide with the RN. You also recommend getting a CXR and ABG values from BG Johnson's UAC. The resident readily agrees. The ABG values are pH of 7.18, $PaCO_2$ of 65 mmHg, PaO_2 of 49 mmHg, and HCO_3 of 23.9 mEq/L. The CXR is shown in Figure 7-4.

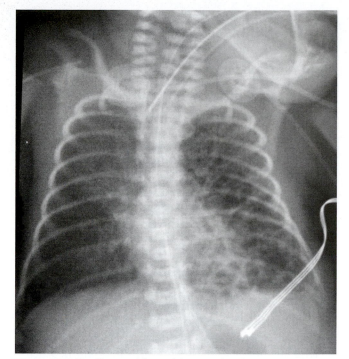

Figure 7-4 Radiographic Evidence of PIE *(Courtesy of Jane Benson, MD)*

Management and Treatment

Minimizing overdistension of the lungs in RDS patients is the best prevention for PIE. This includes using minimum pressure within the lungs and monitoring the effectiveness of chosen ventilator settings. An effective way of achieving this is to use volume-targeted ventilation, which can decrease the likelihood of air leaks in premature infants (11). Although high-frequency oscillatory ventilation (HFOV) is an effective mode to minimize positive-pressure delivery, a 2009 review of the literature suggests that it is no more effective at preventing PIE than is conventional mechanical ventilation (CMV) (12). Once PIE begins to form, treatment should focus on minimizing further damage to the lung and allowing time for the lung to heal.

Extubation is the ideal treatment, but often it is not feasible because of the patient's underlying disease process. If the patient cannot be extubated, minimize pressure delivered to the lungs. This can be achieved by doing the following:

- Lowering PIP, PEEP, and inspiratory T_I as tolerated by the patient. Monitor pressure-volume loops and decrease PIP and/or PEEP when there is evidence of pressure delivered by the ventilator without associated volume in the lungs.
- Using volume-targeted ventilation to minimize the risk of volutrauma (discussed in Chapter 4).
- Avoiding auto-PEEP, which causes overdistension during end exhalation. This is a risk for patients who have obstructive disease processes

or when high respiratory rates are used because there is not enough time for the patients to exhale fully. To avoid auto-PEEP, monitor flow loops for cessation of flow at end exhalation and monitor pressure and volume waveforms for values to return to baseline between breaths.

• Providing high-frequency ventilation (HFV), which is preferred to CMV.

• Evidence for high-frequency jet ventilation in this patient population makes it a particularly beneficial choice. High-frequency jet ventilation (HFJV) uses a transitional flow pattern of gas delivery, similar to the mechanism panting dogs use to effectively breathe with very small tidal volumes. It allows fresh, oxygen-rich gas to travel down the center of the airways at very high velocity in small bursts, getting downstream of restricted portions of the airways, reaching the alveoli, and bypassing damaged portions of the lung without leaking. Exhalation is passive during HFJV, and carbon dioxide (CO_2) travels by the path of least resistance, which is against the airway walls in a countercurrent helical flow pattern (13) (Fig. 7-5). Passive exhalation during HFJV also allows effective ventilation and oxygenation at lower mean airway pressures than does HFOV. HFJV rates are about 10 times faster than CMV, but tidal volumes are about 5 times smaller, making it less likely for volumes to be trapped during exhalation. Improved gas exchange has been shown using HFJV in patients with PIE and developing CLD (14).

HFJV is achieved in tandem with a conventional ventilator. The purpose of the conventional ventilator is threefold: (1) it provides fresh gas for patient's spontaneous respiratory effort, (2) it maintains PEEP settings, and if necessary, (3) it provides "sigh breaths" to re-expand atelectatic lung units. The HFJV provides PIP, RR, and T_I.

Initiating and adjusting settings on the HFJV are straightforward. To begin, the patient's standard ETT adapter is replaced with the LifePort adapter, which is connected to the CV traditionally and to the HFJV by a side port on the LifePort adapter. Guidelines for HFJV settings are in Table 7-2.

When managing blood gases in HFJV, the following guidelines are helpful (15):

• The main determinant of CO_2 clearance is tidal volume (V_T). As with HFOV, minute ventilation is determined by $f \times V_T^2$. Therefore, small changes in V_T will have exponentially larger changes in CO_2. Tidal volume is determined by δP, or PIP-PEEP. To increase CO_2 on blood gas, decreasing HFJV PIP is the best option. To lower CO_2, increase HFJV PIP. Changing HFJV rate will only have a significant impact on CO_2 clearance if the reason for hypercapnia is air trapping. In this case, decreasing rate will increase expiratory time, allowing time for more effective exhalation and thus decreasing CO_2.

• PEEP is the major determinate of oxygenation (PO_2). Initial setting of PEEP should be to maintain alveolar stability. Initial PEEP settings with HFJV can be 6 cm H_2O or higher, which is often more than CMV. This seems counterintuitive, given that one of the initial treatments for PIE is to lower PEEP. The short I-times of HFJV, however, mean long expiratory times, requiring higher PEEPs to maintain adequate mean airway pressure (Paw) and prevent atelectasis. If atelectasis develops, increasing PEEP and adding an intermittent mandatory ventilation (IMV) rate of 5 to 10 breaths/min temporarily will reverse atelectasis. Returning the IMV rate to 0 breaths/min once atelectasis has resolved will minimize the risk of volutrauma. In the absence of atelectasis, FIO_2 should be increased to improve PO_2. Caution must be used when adjusting PEEP alone, because it will

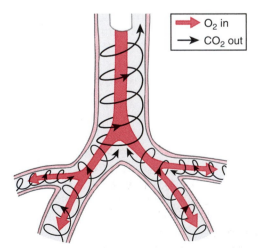

Figure 7-5 Inspiration and Exhalation With High-Frequency Jet Ventilation

Table 7-2	High-Frequency Jet Ventilator Settings For RDS, PIE (14)
Setting	**Recommendation**
HFJV PIP	Initiate approximately the same as previous conventional ventilation PIP; adjust for desired PaCO$_2$
HFJV rate	420 bpm (Hertz = 7)
HFJV I-time	0.02 seconds
IMV rate	0 bpm; only activate when recruiting atelectatic lung units
IMV PIP	Adjust to achieve visible chest rise
IMV I-time	Approximately 0.4 seconds
PEEP	Begin at 7–12 cm H$_2$O, adjust to optimal PEEP for alveolar stability. (Raise PEEP until SpO$_2$ stays constant in CV CPAP mode.)

also adjust δP, which will change CO_2. If CO_2 is adequate, incremental changes of PEEP and PIP will maintain at δP while still giving the desired effect for PO_2. An example would be to change a patient with atelectasis from 18/4 to 19/5, maintaining a δP of 14 cm H_2O and not affecting V_T.

- An additional benefit for patient monitoring on HFJV is servo pressure (16). Servo pressure is the driving pressure of the HFJV. It automatically regulates how much gas flow is needed to deliver a set PIP. Servo pressure changes can be an early warning of changes in patient condition. In general, increases in servo pressure mean an increase in lung compliance or improvement in lung function. A decrease in servo pressure indicates a change such as the following:
  - Decreased lung compliance (such as with a pneumothorax)
  - Worsened lung resistance
  - Obstructed ETT
  - Mucus in the airway, or a need for suctioning

Servo pressure can be useful in bedside assessment and management of a patient on HFJV.

For patients with unilateral PIE, two therapies have been suggested to promote lung tissue healing. The first therapy is to position the patient laterally, with the affected lung down, which will preferentially ventilate the superior, or uninjured, lung. The second and less frequently used therapy is to intubate the bronchus of the uninjured lung (known as the "contralateral bronchus") for a period of time, so only the uninjured lung participates in ventilation (Evidence in Practice 7-1).

● **Evidence in Practice 7-1**

An Old Procedure Revisited

A 2007 clinical case study (17) revisited a less-frequently used treatment for PIE: bronchial intubation. The clinicians selectively left mainstem intubated a 24 wG infant girl who developed right-sided PIE on day 4 of life that persisted through her second week of life despite right-side-down positioning and high-frequency ventilation with a low MAP strategy. To perform the procedure they turned her head to the right with the long bevel of the ETT along the left of the midtracheal wall (pointing to the normal lung). The ETT was advanced slowly until breath sounds were no longer heard over the right thorax, and confirmation was made using a CXR. Ventilation MAP and amplitude were adjusted for unilateral lung ventilation, and the right side was allowed to deflate completely for 24 hours. Before the ETT was returned to its previous position, a follow-up CXR was obtained that showed equal lung inflation with no evidence of PIE. The patient was extubated to nasal CPAP within 24 hours of PIE resolution.

The management chosen for PIE should be based on disease progression; thus, a combination of strategies specific to an individual patient will provide the best results.

■■ Based on BG Johnson's poor ABG results and cyst-like formation on the left side, you and the resident agree to initially change her ventilator settings: decrease PIP and PEEP to19/3, increase RR to 45 breaths/min, and decrease T_I to 0.30 seconds. You will follow up with an ABG test in 30 minutes. If you do not see significant improvement as shown by a pH greater than 7.25, then you agree that changing to HFJV is the best option. You have also placed the patient in the lateral position, left side down, to increase ventilation to the uninjured lung.

The follow-up ABG results are a pH of 7.22, $PaCO_2$ of 58 mm Hg, PaO_2 of 55 mm Hg, and HCO_3 of 23.4. The FIO_2 was weaned prior to the ABG test to 0.63, but BG Johnson won't tolerate an FIO_2 any lower. There was some improvement, so you and the resident agree to observe for 2 more hours to watch for clinical improvement. After 2 hours there is no significant change to exhaled V_T, SpO_2 or FIO_2, or blood pressure.

After discussion with the resident and the attending physician on call, you agree to start BG Johnson on HFJV: PIP of 19 cm H_2O, RR of 420 breaths/min, T_I of 0.02 seconds, FIO_2 of 0.65. You will start the PEEP at 4 cm H_2O and adjust as needed to find optimal PEEP. You have agreed to no rate from the CMV. You begin to gather the equipment for HFJV.

Course and Prognosis

One study focusing on ELBW infants showed that the mortality rate of patients with PIE was higher than for those without PIE (37% vs. 6%) (10). Death may be caused by circulatory embarrassment, as evidenced by hypotension and bradycardia, or by impaired gas exchange resulting from air between the alveoli and blood vessels. Another study demonstrated a strong association between patients diagnosed with PIE and subsequent development of type 2 chronic lung disease; however, the presence of PIE did not seem to alter outcome regarding mortality or duration of oxygen dependency (18). In those who are successfully treated, particularly those treated with HFV, PIE often resolves within 24 to 48 hours. If not treated, PIE can deteriorate into pneumothorax.

Pneumothorax

■ ■ As you get your HFJV and pull equipment from the supply closet, you and the resident are paged urgently to BG Johnson's bedside. When you arrive you note the nurse is providing PPV with the resuscitation bag at 1 FIO$_2$. The baby's heart rate is 80 bpm, SpO$_2$ is 60%, and BP is 37/15 mm Hg. BG Johnson's color is gray, and she is not moving. From your angle at the entrance of the room, you can't see chest rise with the PPV attempts, even though it appears that the nurse is squeezing the bag very hard. The resident runs in right behind you.

Pneumothorax is a collection of air in the pleural cavity. It is the most common of the air leaks, occurring in 2% of neonates (19) and 5% to 8% of infants with a birth weight less than 1,500 g (20). The incidence of pneumothorax in neonates has decreased dramatically as a result of surfactant therapy and lower ventilator pressures.

As with adults, a pneumothorax in neonates can occur spontaneously as a result of ventilator assistance or as a procedural complication. Spontaneous pneumothoraces affect 1% to 2% of all live births (21) and seem to affect full-term and post-term infants more than they do preterm infants (Clinical Variations 7-1). In neonatal patients, about 50% of pneumothoraces are preceded by radiographically apparent PIE (10).

Risk factors for pneumothorax include the following:

- RDS
- Mechanical ventilation
- Sepsis
- Pneumonia
- Aspiration of meconium, blood, or amniotic fluid
- Congenital malformations (20)

Pathophysiology

A pneumothorax occurs when extra-alveolar air ruptures into the pleural space. A **tension pneumothorax** occurs when each breath forces new air through the rupture, but air cannot escape through the route of entry. This causes increased pressure in the pleural space, resulting in lung collapse. An untreated tension pneumothorax will compress the heart, forcing the great vessels to shift toward the unaffected side and causing cardiac compromise. A tension pneumothorax is common during ventilatory assistance.

Clinical Manifestations

Respiratory distress is the initial response to a less severe pneumothorax and includes tachypnea and retractions. Definitive diagnosis of pneumothorax is

Clinical Variations 7-1

Spontaneous Pneumothorax

Even RTs who work in a hospital without a NICU may encounter an infant with spontaneous pneumothorax. Meconium aspiration and need for resuscitation at birth increase an otherwise healthy newborn's risk for a pneumothorax. It usually occurs within the first few breaths of life and is usually asymptomatic. If symptoms are present they may include the following:

- Tachypnea
- Grunting
- Retractions
- Cyanosis on RA
- Restlessness
- Irritability
- Chest bulge on the affected side

Many spontaneous pneumothoraces resolve without treatment, but they can also be treated with supplemental oxygen. Care must be taken, however, to avoid excess oxygen delivery if the baby is less than full term because of the risk of retinopathy of prematurity. Though some spontaneous pneumothoraces can be associated with more serious lung diseases such as meconium aspiration syndrome, RDS, TTN, pneumonia, pulmonary hypoplasia, and congenital diaphragmatic hernia, most occur in otherwise healthy lungs and resolve with no further complications or sequelae.

made with a CXR, which will be significant for a radiolucent band of air around the chest wall, with displacement of the lung on the affected side toward the hilar region.

A tension pneumothorax is an emergency that presents quickly, and patients decompensate rapidly. Patients will present with the following:

- Abrupt duskiness or cyanosis
- Hypotension
- Bradycardia
- Hypoventilation or apnea
- Decreased breath sounds on the affected side
- Decreased heart sounds
- Bulging of the affected hemithorax
- Mediastinal shift to the unaffected hemithorax
- Asymmetric chest wall movement

When a tension pneumothorax is suspected, there is not enough time to wait for a chest radiograph before immediate intervention is required. Diagnosis in neonates can be made quickly with transillumination. **Transillumination** of the chest is the placement of a high-intensity light source on the thorax. A healthy lung will create a small halo of light in the thoracic cavity, whereas a pneumothorax will cause the light to illuminate a large portion of the chest. A negative transillumination is not definitive evidence that no pneumothorax is present, and a CXR should be used to verify whether it is present if you are unsure. A positive transillumination with clinical signs of tension pneumothorax is a sign to begin immediate treatment to decompress the affected thoracic cavity.

■ ■ The resident runs to the bedside and uses a stethoscope to listen for breath sounds. She verbalizes that she hears breath sounds on the right but none on the left. Suspecting a tension pneumothorax, you suggest transillumination of the left chest wall, the location of the PIE. Transillumination "lights up" the entire left side of BG Johnson's chest. Bradycardia, hypotension, and SpO$_2$ have not improved.

Management and Treatment

A small, uncomplicated (or simple) pneumothorax will often resolve itself with observation alone. To speed the reabsorption of free air in the pleural cavity, high oxygen concentrations may be given using an oxyhood. Administering high oxygen concentrations is effective because room air is made up mostly of nitrogen, which is not metabolized by the body. Replacing the nitrogen with oxygen using a high FIO$_2$ delivery device (a procedure known as "nitrogen washout") will increase the pressure gradient between the air in the pleural space and the capillary blood. This encourages reabsorption of the gas in the pleural cavity during a pneumothorax. Care must be taken when delivering high oxygen to premature infants because of the increased risk of retinopathy of prematurity and lung tissue damage (discussed in Chapters 4 and 8).

A tension pneumothorax is an emergency situation that requires immediate intervention to prevent patient death. The immediate response to relieve air pressure is **needle decompression** of the thoracic space. Needle decompression is performed using a 19-, 21-, or 23-gauge IV or needle attached to a stopcock and 20-mL syringe. It is a two-person procedure, with one person inserting the needle over the top of the rib between the second and third intercostal space, midclavicular line. The second person pulls back on the syringe during the procedure. The needle is advanced just until air is withdrawn (21).

A more definitive treatment for a simple or tension pneumothorax is thoracostomy drainage. This drainage requires the insertion of a chest tube connected to continuous suction set at −10 to −25 cm H$_2$O. A more recent procedure involves the placement of a pigtail catheter in lieu of a chest tube. Pigtail catheters are made of a more compliant material, and insertion is less traumatic because it uses a guide

wire and dilator for placement rather than the blunt force required for chest tube placement (22).

Management of the drainage system after chest tube placement is often a respiratory therapist's responsibility. Most hospitals now use multifunction chest drainage systems, which contain three distinct chambers:

1. **Collection chamber:** Fluids drain directly from the thoracic cavity into this chamber and is measured in milliliters.
2. **Water seal chamber:** This chamber includes a one-way valve that monitors air leaks and changes in intrathoracic pressure.
3. **Suction control chamber:** This chamber serves as an atmospheric vent and fluid reservoir. A vacuum is connected by tubing to this chamber. The system is regulated to make controlling negative pressure easy. In some systems the level of water in the suction control chamber regulates the amount of negative pressure, whereas other systems include a suction regulation knob to set pressure. To supply gravity drainage without suction, suction is turned off to the control chamber or the suction tubing is disconnected. Follow the manufacturer's recommendations for setup and maintenance of multifunction chest drainage systems.

Analgesics should be administered to alleviate the pain and discomfort of the chest tube. CXR should be obtained regularly to verify tube placement and monitor lung expansion. The water seal chamber should be monitored for occasional bubbling, which is an indicator of air leaks. Absence of an air leak can indicate resolution of the pneumothorax or occlusion or misplacement of the chest tube. Clamping of chest tubes should be done when the chest drainage system is being changed, in the hours prior to tube removal, or when reconnecting an accidentally disconnected tube that resulted in loss of water seal.

■ ■ You, the resident, and the nurse all agree that BG Johnson's PIE has progressed to a tension pneumothorax. The nurse calls the neonatal rapid response team in anticipation of further decompensation. The resident also requests that the nurse call the radiology department for a CXR prior to any additional treatment (Fig. 7-6). You are worried because you know that if it is not treated within minutes, BG Johnson could die. You say to the resident: "I am concerned that if we wait for a radiograph, this patient could decompensate further and could die from lack of treatment. Needle decompression can be performed while we are waiting for radiology and can help stabilize the patient while we wait for the rapid response team to arrive. Have you ever done a needle decompression?" (Teamwork 7-1). She states that she has and that if you and the nurse will assist her, she will perform the needle decompression while another nurse contacts radiology. While you and the charge nurse gather the equipment for needle decompression, the resident reviews the procedure online and pages her attending physician to notify him directly of the emergency. After proper insertion of the needle and removal of 15 mL of air, BG Johnson's HR increases to 130 bpm, SpO_2 increases to 92%, and blood pressure returns to 50/30 mm Hg. The rapid response team arrives and assists in stabilization of the patient. After the attending physician arrives, a chest tube is placed and a multifunction chest drainage system is attached for continuous evacuation of air.

Course and Prognosis

Recurrence of tension pneumothoraces is frequent and requires either replacement of the chest tube if the current one is occluded or displaced or placement of a second tube if the first one is not blocked.

Pneumothorax has been associated with an increased risk of CLD in premature infants. One study showed that infants with a birth weight less than 1,500 g and diagnosed with pneumothorax during the first 24 hours of life were 13 times more likely to die or have CLD (23). Several initiatives in maternal and neonatal care have attempted to decrease the incidence of morbidity and mortality of ELBW infants, for which the rate of pneumothorax is an indicator of success. As an example, a clinical process improvement study showed that delivery of surfactant to all infants younger than 28 wG decreased the mortality of patients who suffered a pneumothorax from 62% to less than 17% (24).

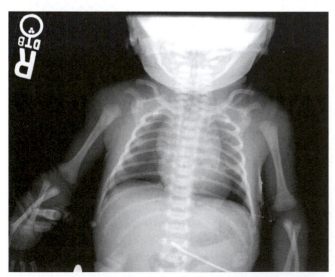

Figure 7-6 Chest Radiograph of Bilateral Pneumothorax *(Courtesy of Jane Benson, MD)*

Teamwork 7-1 Critical Language

When you are concerned about the care of a patient during a critical incident, it is important to have a communication strategy so that you are able to effectively share your concerns without being overlooked or offending other team members. One strategy of effective communication is *critical language,* in which where key words or phrases are used so the leader and other team members can focus on your communication as an important piece of information sharing. It includes strategies such as the following:

- Using the word "I" instead of "You"
- Stating objective data to support your view
- Focusing on the future
- Directly requesting or suggesting what you would like, rather than hinting and hoping someone will understand your meaning

For example, if you are worried that a delay in treatment could be detrimental to a patient, an appropriate way to express that would be to say, "Dr. Jones, I am concerned that if we wait for the test results before treatment, BB Johnson's bradycardia will become harder to treat and will require CPR. I believe we should intubate now and advance further treatment without waiting for test results."

Pneumomediastinum

A **pneumomediastinum** occurs when extra-alveolar air dissects through the lung interstitium and ruptures into the mediastinum. Spontaneous pneumomediastinum occurs in 25 out of 10,000 live births (12) and accounts for approximately 0.1% of NICU admissions (25). It is seen as a spontaneous occurrence in RDS, after resuscitation at birth, and with mechanical ventilation. It can also be a complication of traumatic deliveries or airway perforation during traumatic intubations. It often occurs in conjunction with other pulmonary air leaks such as pneumothorax or pneumopericardium.

Pathophysiology

Causes of pneumomediastinum include the following (25):

- Airway obstruction
- Mechanical ventilation
- Infections
- Obstructive lung disease
- Trauma
- Valsalva's maneuver, which increases intrathoracic pressure

Chapter Seven ■ Pulmonary Complications   177

Spontaneous occurrence of pneumomediastinum usually belies a healthy underlying lung. The air that leaks from alveoli into the interstitial tissue diffuses toward the tissue surrounding the lung vasculature and bronchioles, then toward the mediastinum and neck and into the subcutaneous tissue. The walls between the alveoli remain intact, and the lungs stay inflated.

Clinical Manifestations

Many patients with pneumomediastinum are asymptomatic. Clinical symptoms vary in frequency but can include the following:

- Tachypnea
- Bulging sternum
- Distant or crackly heart sounds
- Cyanosis
- Respiratory distress
- Subcutaneous (subQ) emphysema (if air moves into the cervical subcutaneous tissue)

Diagnosis is made using a CXR (Fig. 7-7), which will show free air in the mediastinal space that highlights the border of the heart but does not extend to the inferior border at the diaphragm. The mediastinal air in an infant can also elevate the thymus, which

produces what is known as the "spinnaker sail" sign. A lateral CXR will show air anterior to the heart.

Management and Treatment

Patients with pneumomediastinum without the presence of other pulmonary air leaks do not require aggressive therapy. Close observation and treatment of symptoms such as cyanosis are enough support. If the patient is intubated, lowering ventilator pressures will assist in resolution of the air leak.

Course and Prognosis

Pneumomediastinum usually resolves spontaneously within a few days with no long-term sequelae. If surgical intervention is required, then recovery is extended.

Pneumopericardium

Pneumopericardium is air within the pericardial sac. It is a rare and life-threatening event in the neonatal population, is almost always associated with mechanical ventilation, and is usually found in conjunction with another pulmonary air leak. Fewer than 2% of pulmonary air leaks in the neonatal population are found to be pneumopericardium (22).

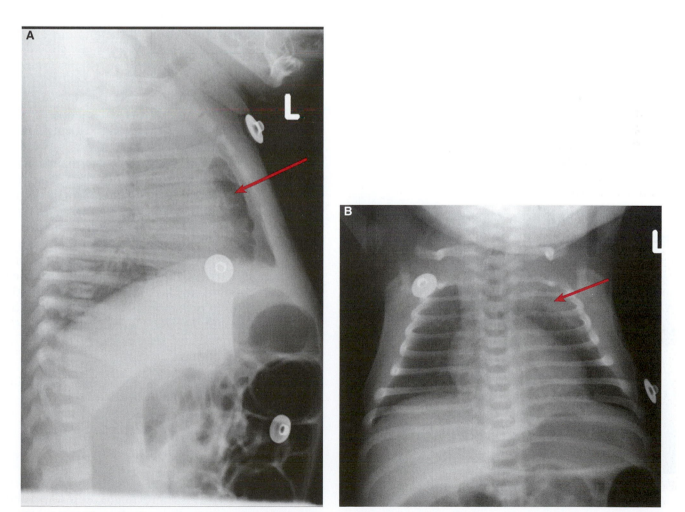

Figure 7-7 Chest Radiograph of Pneumomediastinum *(Courtesy of Jane Benson, MD)*

Pathophysiology

Pneumopericardium occurs during pulmonary air leaks when alveoli are ruptured and air passes down the perivascular sheaths and around the aorta or vena cava. The transmission of air can also pass from a pneumomediastinum near the pleural-pericardial connection. This injury frequently occurs in conjunction with very high ventilating pressures. If not resolved, air will continue to accumulate in the pericardial space and a life-threatening **tamponade** will develop, which impairs the filling of the heart during diastole and impedes cardiac output.

Clinical Manifestations

Sudden cyanosis and muffled or absent heart tones will be noted. As the pneumopericardium worsens, arterial blood pressure will fall, peripheral pulses will disappear, and bradycardia and hypoxia will worsen. When the situation worsens into tamponade, the patient will develop pulseless electrical activity (PEA). The patient will have abrupt cyanosis, hypotension, and inaudible heart sounds associated with decreased cardiac activity. Definitive diagnosis of pneumopericardium, like other forms of air leaks, is made by CXR (Fig. 7-8). There will be a broad radiolucent halo completely surrounding the heart. The thickness of the halo band depends on severity of the air leak.

Management and Treatment

The severity of pneumopericardium can vary widely. Occasionally, pericardial air can resolve spontaneously. Treatment should always include close observation, antibiotics to prevent infection, and support measures for hypotension and other clinical changes. A patient with tamponade requires CPR until a **pericardiocentesis**, a procedure in which a

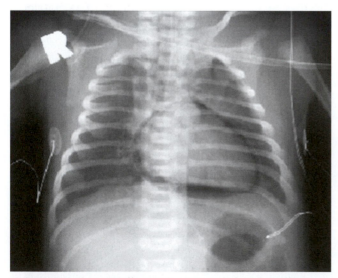

Figure 7-8 Chest Radiograph of Pneumopericardium
(Courtesy of Jane Benson, MD)

needle is inserted into the pericardial sac to evacuate air, can be performed. Multiple pericardial taps may be necessary to sustain life, or a pericardial tube may need to be placed for continuous drainage until the air leak can heal.

Course and Prognosis

Reaccumulation rates for pneumopericardium have been shown to be as high as 50% (9). The mortality rate for cardiac tamponade in neonates is high. In a review of 156 neonates, 73% survived the initial pneumopericardium, but only 32% ultimately survived to hospital discharge (26).

Pneumonia

Pneumonia is generally described as inflammation of the lung parenchyma, usually caused by infection with bacteria, viruses, or other pathogenic causes. In the most recent World Health Organization study, pneumonia was the single largest infectious disease killer of children worldwide, claiming 1.57 million children younger than 5 years old (27). The greatest risk of death from pneumonia in childhood is during the neonatal period. A study of late preterm infants (34 wG to 40 6/7 wG) determined a rate of pneumonia of 1.5% at 34 wG and 0.2% at 40 wG (28). There is some concern that neonatal pneumonias are underdiagnosed because their clinical signs and symptoms are nonspecific and mimic other common neonatal respiratory diseases, such as transient tachypnea of the newborn (TTN) and RDS.

Certain predisposing factors put neonates at a higher risk for pneumonia than other patient populations. Maternal factors include premature rupture of membranes, maternal fever, and **chorioamnionitis**, which is an infection of the amniotic fluid. The rates of pneumonia are higher for neonates born to women with chorioamnionitis, particularly for neonates older than 32 wG (29). Predisposing factors for preterm neonates include a decrease in effectiveness of the mucociliary escalator, immunocompromise, and compromised airway barriers such as the glottis and vocal cords. Birth weight and age strongly determine the mortality risk from pneumonia, with preterm and low birth weight neonates being at a much higher risk.

Common organisms that cause pneumonia in neonates are as follows:

- Group B streptococci (GBS)
- Gram-negative enteric bacteria
- *Cytomegalovirus*
- *Ureaplasma urealyticum*
- *Listeria monocytogenes*
- *Chlamydial trachomatis*

Less common organisms include *Staphylococcus pneumonia*, group D streptococcus, and anaerobes

(30). GBS is a significant cause of neonatal sepsis, pneumonia, and meningitis in the United States, and *C. trachomatis* has a very high risk of maternal-to-fetal infection, with a rate of pneumonia of about 30% (22).

Pathophysiology

Once the infectious microorganisms reach the lung tissue, they begin a reaction that causes an outpouring of fluid, inflammatory proteins, and white blood cells. The alveolar and interstitial spaces are filled with edema and exudative fluid (fluid with a high concentration of proteins, cells, or solid debris). This in turn makes distal lung spaces consolidated, creating localized areas of low lung compliance that prevent lung inflation and gas exchange. Surfactant inactivation and dysfunction also occurs, which causes pneumonia to mimic the clinical manifestations of RDS in preterm and term neonates. Pneumonias can affect localized areas or an entire lobe, a lung, or diffusely affect both lung regions.

Pneumonias are classified either as congenital or neonatal, differentiated when the infection or pathogen is acquired. Congenital pneumonias occur with maternal infection, such as with chorioamnionitis, GBS infection, or *C. trachomatis*. It usually occurs when infected amniotic fluid is aspirated in utero or during delivery. Neonatal pneumonia is categorized as early onset (within the first 48 hours of life up to 1 week of life) or late onset (1 to 3 weeks of life) (31). It can also be caused by nosocomial infection in the NICU.

Clinical Manifestations

Clinical manifestations of pneumonia are nonspecific, thus pneumonia should be suspected in any neonate with respiratory distress, as classified by rapid, noisy, or labored breathing; respiratory rate greater than 60 breaths/min; retractions; cough; and/or grunting (31). Other signs may include the following (32):

- Poor reflexes
- Lethargy
- Hyperthermia (more frequently seen with full-term neonates) or hypothermia (more common in preterm neonates)
- Abdominal distention

Both fever and feeding intolerance seem to occur in only about half of diagnosed cases of pneumonia (31). Pulmonary hemorrhage is commonly associated with gram-negative organism pneumonias. **Pleural effusion** (fluid between the pleura) or **empyema** (pus in the pleural cavity) may occur with any bacterial pneumonia.

CXR will assist in definitive diagnosis of pneumonia and may include nodular or coarse patchy infiltrates, diffuse haziness or granularity, air bronchograms, and

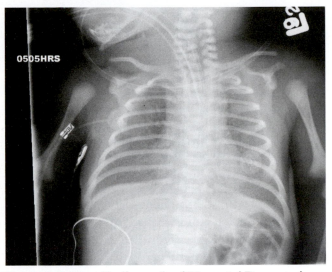

Figure 7-9 Chest Radiograph of Neonatal Pneumonia *(Courtesy of Jane Benson, MD)*

lobar or segmental consolidation (Fig. 7-9). GBS pneumonia has an appearance similar to that of RDS on chest radiographs.

Mucous culture and sensitivity screening is a useful diagnostic tool for pneumonia to facilitate identification of the infecting microorganism, though it is difficult to obtain an uncontaminated tracheal specimen.

Management and Treatment

Prevention of congenital pneumonia is a key initiative in the management of neonatal pneumonias. There have been some recent movements to decrease its incidence:

- Screening mothers for GBS and administering prophylactic antibiotics to mothers who are carriers. In 2002, the Centers for Disease Control and Prevention, the American College of Obstetricians, and the American Academy of Pediatrics revised the guidelines to prevent early-onset GBS disease. Recommendations include universal screening of all pregnant women in the United States for rectovaginal GBS colonization at 35 to 37 wG and administration of intrapartum antibiotic prophylaxis to carriers (33).
- Administering maternal and neonatal antibiotics as routine management for chorioamnionitis.
- Promoting hand hygiene. A 2009 study assessing a hand hygiene initiative in five NICUs showed a decrease in ventilator associated pneumonia of 38% after launch of the program (34).
- Promoting vigorous antibiotic treatment of mothers with rupture of membranes or premature labor between 22 and 26 wG, plus treatment of the infant immediately after delivery prophylactically because of frequent underdiagnosis of lung infection during the early neonatal period (35).

Most management of pneumonia is supportive: oxygen for hypoxemia, ventilation for apnea and hypercapnia, thermoregulation, and IV fluids and nutritional supplementations . Antimicrobial therapy should be based on the organism cultured and its sensitivity. Until sensitivity is determined, broad-spectrum antibiotics are often started, usually consisting of a penicillin (ampicillin) and an aminoglycoside (gentamicin). Exogenous surfactant delivery has been shown to increase gas exchange in GBS pneumonia, but clinically its response time was slower, and patients required more doses than did patients with RDS. There seems to be no harm, however, in implementing surfactant therapy for pneumonia, and it appears to improve respiratory symptoms about 70% of the time (36).

Course and Prognosis

The number of neonatal deaths worldwide in 2008 caused solely by pneumonia was 386,000 (36). Infection of amniotic fluid leading to pneumonia was a major cause of death in ELBW infants in one study; however, in 61% of the cases infection was not diagnosed until autopsy, and deaths were attributed clinically to RDS or immaturity (34). This suggests that clinicians may be missing infections in a significant number of premature infants with respiratory distress. Pneumonia has also been noted as a cause for the development of CLD in near-term infants (37). Prevention tactics have decreased the incidence of congenital and neonatal pneumonia, but it is still a significant cause of neonatal morbidity and mortality, even in developed countries.

■ ■ BG Johnson's chest tube remained in place for 3 days. After turning off suction and leaving the chest tube to water seal for 8 hours, the physician removed the tube, and her pneumothorax did not reaccumulate. BG Johnson continued on HFJV for 6 days, weaning PIP to 14 cm H_2O and FIO_2 as tolerated until you extubated her to NCPAP plus 5 cm H_2O and FIO_2 0.30 on day of life (DOL) 12. You and the other RTs continue to monitor her for apneas and desaturation, and assess for signs of nasal trauma from the NCPAP, but BG Johnson's respiratory status has stabilized and she has shown no signs of redeveloping atelectasis or air leaks.

■ ■ Critical Thinking Questions: BG Johnson

1. If the initial treatment for BG Johnson's atelectasis (increase in PIP and PEEP and repositioning) had been unsuccessful, what could you have recommended to the physician as a next step?

2. If you noticed a sharp drop in servo pressure while BG Johnson was on HFJV, what might be the cause?
3. If BG Johnson had not had a positive transillumination, what should have been the next step in her management?
4. How do you think BG Johnson may have presented differently if she had developed a simple pneumothorax instead of a tension pneumothorax?

▶● Case Studies and Critical Thinking Questions

■ Case 1: Baby Boy (BB) Adkinson

You are an RT in a 400-bed hospital working a shift in the level IIIA NICU. After completing your ventilator rounds, you stop by the bedside of BB Adkinson, a 28 wG infant now 1 week old, weighing 1,240 g. He was intubated in the delivery room and received two doses of exogenous surfactant. He was extubated on DOL 3 to nasal CPAP and weaned to a 1 LPM nasal cannula 2 days ago. BB Adkinson's nurse notes that he had had an increase in the frequency of apneas today that required stimulation. It does not seem to improve with changes in patient positioning. He is currently on caffeine citrate for apnea of prematurity, 5 mg/kg PO. His vital signs are as follows:

- *HR: 143 bpm*
- *BP: 51/33 mm Hg (MAP 39 mm Hg)*
- *RR: 76 breaths/min*
- *FIO_2 requirements noted in the shift report were 0.35 to 0.45 throughout the day.*

BB Adkinson is receiving full breast milk feedings via orogastric tube gavage with no gastric intolerance. The nurse is not sure if he is getting a little worse and asks for your opinion on his respiratory status.

You note bilaterally decreased breath sounds in BB Adkinson's bases, grunting, nasal flaring, and tachypnea (75 to 85 bpm) and note that his FIO_2 is increased on his nasal cannula. You suction the nares without obtaining any mucus. You decide to get a CBG and ask the physician t for a CXR, which shows radiolucent areas throughout both lung fields, with the diaphragm at the seventh ribs posteriorly. CBG results are 7.28/56/25.9, FIO_2 is set at 0.70, and SpO_2 is 90%. This morning's laboratory results showed a hemoglobin count of 14 g/dL and hematocrit of 55%.

- *What do you suspect is BB Adkinson's primary diagnosis?*
- *What would you do to reverse the process?*

Case 2: BB Martin

You are working the dayshift in a level IIIB NICU and are on patient rounds with the physicians. You are at the bedside of BB Martin, a 26 1/7 wG infant now 4 days old, weighing 780 g. In reviewing his daily laboratory and radiology results, it is noted that the CXR shows new cyst-like formations in his right middle lobe (RML). His vital signs are as follows:

- HR: 138 bpm
- BP: 51/25 (MAP 33.7)
- RR: 8 breaths/min (spontaneous rate)
- SpO_2 91% on FIO_2 0.47
- Morning CBG is pH 7.31, PCO_2 is 55 mm Hg, PO_2 is 47 mm Hg, HCO_3 is 27.3 mEq/L

Current ventilator settings are SIMV PIP at 20 cm H_2O, PEEP at 5 cm H_2O, rate at 25 breaths/min, T_I at 0.40 sec. The physicians ask you for recommendations to minimize further RML lung damage.

- How would you minimize further lung damage? How would you know if BB Martin tolerated it?

Case 3: BG Edwards

You are working as the floating RT in a small 200-bed community hospital. You and the pediatrician on call are called to newborn nursery to assess BG Edwards, a 39 3/7 wG newborn, now 3-hours-old, in respiratory distress. Delivery history is significant for clear amniotic fluid, second stage of labor (pushing phase) lasting 2.5 hours, Apgar scores of 9 and 10, and no distress noted immediately postdelivery. BG Edwards has been rooming with mom, but during a recent room check the nurse noted tachypnea, irritability, and trouble breastfeeding. The nurse took BG Edwards to the nursery to bottle feed, but she was too restless to latch and attempt feeding. The nurse placed a pulse oximeter on BG Edwards, and its reading was 91% on room air (RA).

- What do you suspect is BG Edward's primary diagnosis?
- What treatment would you recommend for this patient? How long do you anticipate she might need treatment?

Case 4: BB Thompson

You and the on-call pediatrician are called to the newborn nursery for an infant in respiratory distress. BB Thompson is a 41 3/7 wG infant weighing 4,057 g, now 20 minutes old. He was born by vaginal delivery with the complication of shoulder dystocia. Apgar scores were 7 and 8 at 1 and 5 minutes, respectively. The mother is 34 years old and had an uncomplicated pregnancy.

When you arrive, BB Thompson is audibly grunting, has intercostal and subcostal retractions, and has nasal flaring. You place a pulse oximeter on his foot and note a HR of 132 bpm and SpO_2 of 91%. Vital signs also include a RR of 75 breaths/min and BP 65/40 mm Hg (MAP 48.3). The physician would like to admit BB Thompson to the special care nursery for observation and more diagnostic testing.

BB Thompson is transferred to the special care nursery. Although there are no obvious signs of clavicular damage, the physician is concerned about structural damage during delivery. Upon palpation of the chest you feel crackling that you suspect may be subQ emphysema. Auscultation of the chest reveals equal bilateral breath sounds but muffled heart sounds. SpO_2 and BP are unchanged. BB Thompson appears irritable, and when crying and fussing, HR increases transiently from 135 to 155 bpm and RR from 65 to 90 breaths/min. CXR is obtained and shows free air in the mediastinal space and the "spinnaker sail" sign.

- What is causing BB Thompson's respiratory distress?
- What can you do to alleviate his symptoms?

Case 5: BB Cunningham

You are working in a 750-bed regional hospital's level IIIC NICU. About 3 hours into your night shift the charge nurse informs you of a critical transport from an outlying hospital that will be arriving within the next few minutes. The patient is a 28 wG, 1,150 g infant, BB Cunningham, now 3 days old. He was being cared for in a 14-bed level IIIA NICU and diagnosed with RDS. Maternal history was significant for premature rupture of membranes, oligohydramnios, and premature labor, which was unresponsive to terbutaline and magnesium sulfate. Mother was given two doses of antenatal corticosteroids prior to delivery. BB Cunningham was intubated for apnea with a 3.0 ETT, 8 cm at lip, at 5 minutes of life. Apgar scores were 5, 6, and 7 at 1, 5, and 10 minutes, respectively. He was given one dose of surfactant at 2 hours of life after radiological evidence of RDS and continued respiratory distress. Initial ventilator settings were IMV PIP at 22 cm H_2O, PEEP at 5 cm H_2O, RR at 50 breaths/min, FIO_2 at 0.80. Admission vital signs were HR of 173 bpm, BP of 48/24 (MAP of 32 mm Hg), SpO_2 of 90%, BrS decreased bilaterally, and moderate crackles documented. BB Cunningham has been maintained over the last 3 days on a dopamine drip, IV fluids, antibiotics, and mechanical ventilation. Last ABG values via UAC are 7.26/50/22.1/62 on IMV 27/5, rate 55, and FIO_2 0.75. Last vital signs include HR

145 bpm, BP 42/24 (MAP 30) with 20 mcg of dopamine, SpO_2 86%. The outlying hospital requested transport of the patient because they were unable to manage ventilation and perfusion despite maximum available therapy.

When BB Cunningham is wheeled through the doors of the NICU, the transport RN expresses his concern that the patient may have developed an air leak on transport. You quickly connect the patient to the ventilator waiting at the bedside and listen to breath sounds. You hear clear breath sounds bilaterally, but heart sounds seem very distant. The SpO_2 is 72% on FIO_2 1.0, BP is 30/15 mm Hg (MAP 20 mm Hg), and HR 90 bpm despite a 0.1 mL/kg dose of 1:10,000 solution of epinephrine upon arrival. A radiology technician is at the bedside and takes a chest radiograph as BB Cunningham is transferred from the transport isolette to the infant warmer. When the charge RN finishes connecting the bedside monitor, she notes that the arterial waveform does not appear to be working because it is now reading 10/10 mm Hg. You palpate for a brachial pulse but are unable to find one. You auscultate again for heart sounds but hear nothing.

- *What could be happening right now to BB Cunningham?*
- *What is the most important thing for the health-care team to do for him right now?*

Case 6: BG Davis

You are carrying the delivery room pager in an inner-city hospital and are called to respond to a precipitous delivery in the emergency room. You, the pediatrician, and a NICU nurse arrive and are given a 30-second report as the baby's head is being delivered. Mom, Ms. Davis, is a 22-year-old homeless woman with a history of cocaine use. She has had no obstetric care but thinks she is close to term. This is her first live birth, having had two previous spontaneous abortions. She has had increased vaginal discharge for the last 2 weeks and came to the emergency department when she felt she was in hard labor. Her last cocaine use was 2 hours ago, when labor started. You note a foul smell in the patient room that the emergency room nurse attributes to pus in the amniotic fluid. A baby girl is delivered and given to your team. She appears to be close to term, but you estimate her to be small for gestational age (SGA), probably weighing less than 2,000 g. She is covered in foul-smelling pus; is cyanotic, cool, and limp; and does not appear to be making any respiratory effort. You clear the airway while the team dries and

stimulates. Palpated HR is 80 bpm, and she has still not taken a spontaneous breath. You begin bag-mask ventilation (BMV), and after 30 seconds (approximately 1 minute of life), she still has central cyanosis, her HR is 120 bpm, but she still is not moving or breathing spontaneously.

Over the next minute her central cyanosis is gone and her lips and trunk are pink. The physician intubates with a 3.5 ETT, and after auscultating for equal breath sounds, you tape it 8.5 cm at the lip. At 5 minutes of life, BG Davis has still not made any spontaneous movement or respiratory effort, has made no reflexive movement or grimace with stimulation, and has acrocyanosis. HR is 130 bpm with bag-tube ventilation. You wrap her so mom can see her, then place her in an isolette and transport her upstairs to the NICU.

- *What do you suspect is causing her poor APGAR scores and respiratory distress?*

You arrive at the NICU and the team begins to admit BG Davis to the unit. Your coworker RT is having difficulty finding an available neonatal ventilator and was unable to set one up before you arrive. You continue manual ventilation with PIP at approximately 20 and the PEEP dial set at 5 while laboratory values are drawn and the radiographer shoots films. Results are below:

- *Skin temperature: 35°C*
- *Rectal temperature: 35.2°C*
- *HR: 180 bpm*
- *BP: 42/18 mm Hg (MAP 26)*
- *ABG values: pH 7.10, $PaCO_2$ 45 mm Hg, PaO_2 82 mm Hg, HCO_3 13.8 mEq/L*

CXR shows bilateral whiteout, there appears to be patchy infiltrates, and diaphragm level is obscured by infiltration but seems to be at the sixth ribs posterior

Your coworker arrives with the ventilator. The physician is preparing a sterile field to place umbilical lines in BG Davis and is unable to make recommendations for initial ventilator settings by observation, so he asks you to suggest settings and relay them to him.

- *What ventilator settings would you use for this patient?*
- *What do you suspect is BG Davis's primary problem? What additional underlying respiratory/pulmonary issues may also be contributing factors to her presentation? What additional suggestions can you make for patient management?*
- *Should you administer surfactant?*

Multiple-Choice Questions

1. Which of the following is not a contributing factor for neonatal atelectasis?
   a. Meconium obstruction in the terminal airways
   b. Lung compression caused by gastric contents
   c. Low lung compliance
   d. Repeated collapse and re-expansion of alveoli
   e. Surfactant deficiency

2. NCPAP provides which of the following patient benefits:
   I. Splinting of airways
   II. Preventing alveolar collapse
   III. Decreasing lung compliance
   IV. Decreasing airway resistance
   a. I, II
   b. III, IV
   c. I, II, III
   d. I, II, IV

3. Which of the following is the best choice to decrease CO_2 on a patient receiving HFJV?
   a. Decrease PIP
   b. Increase PIP
   c. Increase rate
   d. Decrease rate
   e. Increase PEEP

4. Which of the following are two causes of PIE in neonates?
   I. Traumatic delivery
   II. Excessive mechanical ventilation settings
   III. Surfactant deficiency
   IV. Meconium aspiration
   a. I, II
   b. II, III
   c. III, IV
   d. II, IV

5. What does a pneumothorax look like during transillumination?
   a. Small halo of light in the thoracic cavity
   b. Air bronchograms illuminated on affected side of chest
   c. Band of air around the chest wall
   d. Large portion of the chest is illuminated

6. Which of the following clinical signs and symptoms is specific only to tension pneumothorax?
   a. Cyanosis/hypoxemia
   b. Tachypnea
   c. Bradycardia
   d. Mediastinal shift to the unaffected hemithorax

7. What is the classic radiographic sign seen in neonates with pneumomediastinum?
   a. Halo sign
   b. Spinnaker sign
   c. Boot-shaped heart
   d. Ground-glass appearance

8. What is the treatment of cardiac tamponade?
   a. Needle decompression
   b. Transillumination
   c. Pericardiocentesis
   d. Pigtail catheter

9. Which of the following is not a microorganism that commonly causes neonatal pneumonia:
   a. Group B streptococcus
   b. *Chlamydial trachomatis*
   c. Cytomegalovirus
   d. *Pseudomonas aueroginosa*

10. What initiatives can be taken to minimize pneumonia in the neonatal population?
    a. GBS screening of mothers prior to delivery and prophylactic intrapartum delivery of antibiotics if she is a carrier
    b. Good hand hygiene
    c. Antibiotic treatment for mothers with premature prolonged rupture of membranes
    d. All of the above

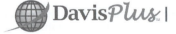 For additional resources login to Davis*Plus* (http://davisplus.fadavis.com/ keyword "Perretta") and click on the Premium tab. (Don't have a *Plus*Code to access Premium Resources? Just click the Purchase Access button on the book's Davis*Plus* page.)

REFERENCES

1. Flenady V, Gray PH. Chest physiotherapy for preventing morbidity in babies being extubated from mechanical ventilation. *Cochrane Database of Syst Rev.* 2002;2:CD000283.
2. AARC Clinical Practice Guideline. Application of continuous positive airway pressure to neonates via nasal prongs, nasopharyngeal tube, or nasal mask—2004 revision & update. *Respir Care.* 2004;49(9):1100-1108.
3. Morley CJ, Davis PG. Continuous positive airway pressure: scientific and clinical rationale. *Curr Opin Pediatr.* 2008;20:119-124.
4. DiBlasi R. Nasal continuous positive airway pressure (CPAP) for the respiratory care of the newborn infant. *Respir Care.* 2009;54(9):1209-1235.
5. Lista G, Castoldi F, Fontana P, et al. Nasal continuous positive airway pressure (CPAP) versus bi-level nasal CPAP in preterm babies with respiratory distress syndrome: a randomized control trial. *Arch Dis Child Fetal Neonatal Ed.* 2010;95(11):F85-F89.
6. Yang SC, Chen SJ, Boo NY. Incidence of nasal trauma associated with nasal prong versus nasal mask during continuous positive airway pressure treatment in very low birthweight infants: a randomized control study. *Arch Dis Child Fetal Neonatal Ed.* 2005;90(6):F480-F483.
7. Sandri F, Plavka R, Ancora G, et al. Prophylactic or early selective surfactant combined with NCPAP in very preterm infants. *Pediatrics.* 2010;125(5):e1402-e1409.
8. Muller W, Pichler G. Results of mechanical ventilation in premature infants with respiratory distress syndrome. Wien Med Wochenschr. 2002;152(1-2):5-8.
9. Goldsmith JP, Karotkin EH. *Assisted Ventilation of the Neonate.* 4th ed. Philadelphia, PA: Saunders; 2003:364.
10. Verma RP, Chandra S, Niwas R, Komaroff E. Risk factors and clinical outcomes of pulmonary interstitial emphysema in extremely low birth weight infants. *J Perinatol.* 2006;26(3):197-200.
11. Wheeler K, Klingenberg C, McCallion N, Morley CJ, Davis PG. Volume-targeted versus pressure-limited ventilation in the neonate. *Cochrane Database Syst Rev.* 2010;(11):CD003666.
12. Bhuta T, Henderson-Smart DJ. Elective high frequency jet ventilation versus conventional ventilation for respiratory distress syndrome in premature infants. *Cochrane Database Syst Rev.* 2000;(2):CD000328.
13. Bunnell Inspired Infant Care. The what, why, and how of high frequency jet ventilation. http://www.bunl.com/Support%20Materials/WhatWhyHow.pdf. Accessed August 22, 2010.
14. Plavka R, Dokoupilova M, Pazderova L, et al. High-frequency jet ventilation improves gas exchange in extremely immature infants with evolving chronic lung disease. *Am J Perinatol.* 2006;23(8):467-472.
15. Bunnell High Frequency Jet Ventilation. *General guidelines for Life Pulse HFV.* http://www.bunl.com/Patient%20Management/hfjvguidelines.pdf. Accessed August 22, 2010.
16. Bunnell High Frequency Jet Ventilation. *The importance of servo pressure.* http://www.bunl.com/Patient%20Management/ServoPressure.pdf. Accessed August 22, 2010.
17. Chalak LF, Kaiser JR, Arrington RW. Case report: resolution of pulmonary interstitial emphysema following selective left mainstem intubation in a premature newborn: an old procedure revisited. *Paediatr Anesth.* 2007;17(2):183-186.
18. Cochran DP, Pilling DW, Shaw NJ. The relationship of pulmonary interstitial emphysema to subsequent type of chronic lung disease. *Br J Radiol.* 1994;67(804):1155-1157.
19. Litmanovitz I, Waldemar AC. Expectant management of pneumothorax in ventilated neonates. *Pediatrics.* 2008;122(5):e975-e979.
20. Horbar JD, Badger GJ, Carpenter JH, et al. Trends in mortality and morbidity for very low birth weight infants, 1991-1999. *Pediatrics.* 2002;110(1):143-151.
21. Cates, LA. Pigtail catheters used in the treatment of pneumothoraces in the neonates. *Adv Neontal Care.* 2009;9(1):7-16.
22. Gomella TL. *Neonatology: Management, Procedures, On-Call Problems, Diseases, and Drugs.* 5th ed. New York: Lange Medical Books/McGraw-Hill; 2004.
23. Miller JD, Waldemar AC. Pulmonary complications of mechanical ventilation in neonates. *Clin Perinatol.* 2008;35(11):273-281.
24. Walker MW, Shoemaker MS, Riddle K, Crane MM, Clark R. Clinical process improvement: reduction of pneumothorax and mortality in high-risk preterm infants. *J Perinatol.* 2002;22(8):641-645.
25. Hauri-Hohl A, Baenziger O, Frey B. Pneumomediastinum in the neonatal and pediatric intensive care unit. *Eur J Pediatr.* 2008;167(4):415-418.
26. Mordue BC. A case report of the transport of an infant with a tension pnuemopericardium. *Adv Neonatal Care.* 2005;5(4):190-200.
27. Black RE, Cousens S, Johnson HL, et al. Global, regional, and national causes of child mortality in 2008: a systematic analysis. *Lancet.* 2010;375(9730):1969-1987.
28. The Consortium on Safe Labor. Respiratory morbidity in late preterm births. *JAMA.* 2010;304(4):419-425.
29. Aziz N, Cheng YW, Caughey AB. Neonatal outcomes in the setting of preterm premature rupture of membranes complicated by chorioanmionitis. *J Matern Fetal Neonatal Med.* 2009;22(9):780-784.
30. Ranganathan SC, Sonnappa SS. Pneumonia and other respiratory infections. *Pediatr Clin North Am.* 2009; 56(1):135-156.
31. Nissen MD. Congenital and neonatal pneumonia. *Paediatr Respir Rev.* 2007;8(3):195-203.
32. Mather NB, Garg K, Kumar S. Respiratory distress in neonates with special reference to pneumonia. *Indian Pediatr.* 2002;39(6):529-538.
33. Centers for Disease Control. Trends in perinatal group B streptococcal disease—United States, 2000-2006. *MMWR.* 2009;58(5):109-112.
34. Rogers E, Alderdice F, McCall E, Jenkins J, Craig S. *J Matern Fetal Neonatal Med.* 2010;23(9):1029-1046.
35. Barton L, Hodgman JE, Pavlova Z. Causes of death in the extremely low weight infant. *Pediatrics.* 1999; 103(2):446-451.
36. Wirbelauer J, Speer CP. The role of surfactant treatment in preterm infants and term newborns with acute respiratory distress syndrome. *J Perinatol.* 2009;29(6):s18-s22.
37. Baraldi E, Filippone M. Chronic lung disease after premature birth. *N Engl J Med* 2007;357(19):1946-1955.

Chapter 8

Multisystem Complications

Elizabeth Cristofalo, MD
Matthew Trojanowski, BA, RRT

Key Terms

Ascites
Asymptomatic
Catastrophic deterioration
Critical opening pressure
Disseminated intravascular
  coagulation (DIC)
Germinal matrix
High-frequency jet ventilation
High-frequency oscillatory
  ventilation
Intraventricular hemorrhage (IVH)
Ligation
Ostomies
Patent ductus arteriosis (PDA)
Pneumatosis
Pneumoperitoneum
Pulmonary edema
Pulse pressure
Retinopathy of prematurity (ROP)
Saltatory syndrome
Shock

Chapter Objectives

After reading this chapter, you will be able to:

1. Recognize some of the signs and symptoms characteristic of a patient developing necrotizing enterocolitis (NEC).
2. Adjust respiratory support for a patient with medical or surgical NEC to minimize complications.
3. Identify the preventable and unpreventable risk factors for intraventricular hemorrhage (IVH) in a neonate.
4. Provide ventilatory support to a very preterm infant to minimize the risk of IVH.
5. Describe how a patent ductus arteriosus (PDA) can complicate respiratory management of a premature infant.
6. Describe the factors that contribute to the development of retinopathy of prematurity (ROP).
7. Implement strategies to improve the quality of oxygen delivery to preterm infants to reduce the incidence of ROP.
8. Recognize the clinical signs and symptoms of a premature infant who is developing sepsis.

■ ■ Baby Girl (BG) Ray

You are a day shift respiratory therapist (RT) in a 45-bed level IIIC neonatal intensive care unit (NICU), and you assume care of BG Ray, a 2-day-old, 25 2/7 weeks' gestation (wG) neonate. She is currently on a conventional ventilator in synchronized intermittent mandatory ventilation (SIMV) mode, with the following settings: peak inspiratory pressure (PIP), 20 cm H_2O; positive end-expiratory pressure (PEEP), 6 cm H_2O; respiratory rate (RR), 35 breaths per minute; and fractional concentration of inspired oxygen (FIO_2) between 88% and 92%. She was diagnosed with respiratory distress syndrome (RDS) and received four doses of surfactant in the first 48 hours of life; her vent settings were weaned, with FIO_2 as low as 0.25. At 1000, the nurse calls you and the physician to the bedside because BG Ray had an acute drop in her blood pressure. You head to the bedside to assess her breath sounds and chest movement and to check the ventilator.

Because of improvements in perinatal and neonatal care, including important advances in respiratory management, the rate of survival of premature infants has increased over the last few decades, and the lower limit of gestational age that is considered viable has decreased. Extremely premature infants who survive resuscitation and proceed to the NICU require highly specialized and coordinated care for months. The risk of mortality during this period varies for each infant and depends on gestational age and birth weight, which is highly associated with their risk of developing complications of prematurity (1, 2). Prematurity is one of the most common causes of death during infancy and

for all children younger than 5 years of age. Only 12% of births in the United States are premature, but more than two-thirds of the infants who die within the first year of life were born prematurely (3, 4). Worldwide, it is the cause of approximately 12% of deaths before age 5, and this proportion is even greater in upper-middle and high-income countries, where prematurity is responsible for more than 30% the deaths in children younger than 5 years (5). Premature babies are susceptible to complications that can result from immaturity and inadequate function of any of their organ systems. Among those who survive, the risk of having complications increases as gestational age decreases.

All body systems are affected by prematurity, leaving them without appropriate protective and regulatory mechanisms that develop later in pregnancy. Because systems do not function independently, variations in ventilation and oxygenation can predispose premature infants to complications in other organ systems, and problems with other organ systems can adversely affect the respiratory system. Respiratory distress and premature lung development are only the beginning of potential system problems. The gastrointestinal system is not prepared to digest food until later in fetal development; the brain has not completely developed; fetal circulation may not make the transition smoothly; and the eyes are susceptible to injury. Premature infants are more likely to have injuries to the intestines, the brain, and retinas, as well as sepsis and a patent ductus arteriosus (PDA), which is necessary in utero, but results in complications if it persists after delivery. In some cases, these complications can impact the effectiveness of the pulmonary system; other times, respiratory management can generate or exacerbate complications with other body systems. Specifically, necrotizing enterocolitis (NEC) and PDA may make ventilation more challenging for the

RT, and intraventricular hemorrhage (IVH) and retinopathy of prematurity (ROP) can be caused by rapid changes in ventilation and excessive oxygenation, respectively. Neonatal RTs must understand how their interventions can help or hinder the progress of each of these conditions and recognize disease signs and symptoms to help provide timely and effective management of premature infants with multiple complex disease processes.

RDS and air leak syndromes are not the only complications that put premature infants at risk of injury. Very premature infants (<32 wG) are at high risk for neurological injury, particularly in the first few hours to days after delivery. Prematurity also puts infants at risk for cardiac complications, such as a failure to close the PDA, which can impair the function of both the pulmonary and cardiovascular systems. Within the neonatal period (the first 28 days of life), premature infants are also at risk of injury to intestinal tissue, known as necrotizing enterocolitis, which can be life threatening, especially if not promptly identified and treated. The oxygen given to treat hypoxemia has been known to cause injury to the developing retinas, known as ROP. This disease develops over time but often is not diagnosed until several weeks or even months after birth.

Each of these disorders can potentially complicate an already-complex patient care plan and may further complicate respiratory care. Inappropriate respiratory management can cause or exacerbate some of these disorders; good respiratory management, in contrast, can help minimize short-term symptoms and long-term sequelae. An RT should be closely involved in the interdisciplinary management of neonatal patients, which requires (1) an understanding of the roles that ventilation and oxygenation play in each of these disorders; (2) the ability to recognize the respiratory problems that accompany these disorders; and (3) familiarity with the most effective respiratory management when these complications occur to minimize the symptoms and provide a continuum of care despite other systemic complications. Just as children cannot be regarded as small adults, premature infants should not be managed as very small babies. Management of their respiratory issues can be very challenging, but vigilant attention to their complex and delicate nature can positively impact their outcome.

Intraventricular Hemorrhage

Germinal matrix-intraventricular hemorrhage (GM-IVH), commonly called **intraventricular hemorrhage** (IVH), is a neonatal complication that occurs most commonly in premature infants and is characterized by bleeding within the ventricles of the brain. The greatest risk factors for developing GM-IVH are gestational age and birth weight. The likelihood of developing GM-IVH decreases with more advanced gestational age at delivery and greater birth weight. Infants born at the lower limits of survival, considered to be 23 to 25 wG, have the highest risk of developing GM-IVH, especially the most severe hemorrhages that are associated with ongoing morbidity, higher mortality, and long-term neurodevelopmental problems.

The overall incidence of IVH in all neonates is 4.8%. Studies of very low birth weight (VLBW, birth weight <1,500 g) premature infants published over the past decade reveal that IVH complicates the early neonatal period of 15% to 20% of this group and is much more common in the smallest and most premature subset (1, 6–8). The Vermont Oxford Network's 2010 data reveal that 26% of VLBW premature infants develop IVH and 8.7% develop severe IVH (described below).

Pathophysiology

A grading system is commonly used to classify these hemorrhages by degree of severity. The two most widely used (9, 10), shown in Table 8-1, were developed in the late 1970s and 1980s. Given the advances made since then in the understanding of the pathophysiology of IVH and the improvements made in imaging techniques, these grading systems are simplistic. However, the majority of research about neurodevelopmental outcomes of premature infants refers to one or both of these grading systems.

Table 8-1	Grading Systems for IVH			
Papile, 1978 (9)			**Volpe, 1981 (10)**	
Grade I	Subependymal GM hemorrhage; not into the ventricles	Mild	GM hemorrhage with no or minimal IVH (<10% of ventricle)	
Grade II	Bleeding into the ventricles without dilatation	Moderate	IVH (10%–50% of ventricular area)	
Grade III	Bleeding into the ventricles, with dilatation of the ventricles	Severe	IVH (>50% of ventricular area)	
Grade IV	Hemorrhage into the brain parenchyma	Other	Blood in the periventricular area	

Premature infants are at risk for developing IVH because of the anatomical changes that occur in the brain prior to term. To support the rapid brain growth that occurs in utero (discussed in Chapter 2), a temporary blood supply called the **germinal matrix (GM)** emerges before 20 wG. This rich vascular bed provides support for developing neuroblasts (embryonic cells that will develop into neurons) through the second trimester. Involution of the GM begins at approximately 28 wG and is typically complete by 36 wG. This vascular structure is the primary source of bleeding in the brains of premature infants. In addition to being a very rich vascular bed with significant flow, the GM is a fragile structure. Unlike permanent vascular structures, there is no collagen support around the GM to prevent it from rupturing from physical injury or increased blood flow. It exists temporarily, during a period when, if a baby is not born prematurely, the impact of mechanical forces from outside the brain are absorbed by the amniotic fluid and blood flow to the brain is regulated by the placenta. Therefore, this support is not necessary when pregnancy continues to term. However, when a baby is born prematurely, this vascular bed is susceptible to damage by several mechanisms, most commonly by rapid changes in cerebral blood flow.

In premature infants, several factors can influence cerebral blood flow. The most premature infants have not yet developed cerebral autoregulation, which maintains a constant cerebral blood flow despite changes in systemic blood pressure. Without the ability to autoregulate, the vessels in the brain are even more susceptible to changes in physiological status that can alter the cerebral blood flow (Box 8-1). These

---

Box 8-1 Clinical Factors That Can Alter Cerebral Blood Flow

Sepsis
Patent ductus arteriosus with shunting
Adrenal insufficiency
Systemic blood pressure changes (such as
  hypovolemia and volume expansion)
Anemia and transfusion
Hypoglycemia
Hyperglycemia
Hypocarbia
Hypercarbia
Hypoxemia
Acidosis
Head positioning
High intrathoracic pressure
Coagulopathy

---

changes can include sepsis, PDA with shunting, adrenal insufficiency, hypovolemia, and volume expansion. Other factors that cause changes in cerebral blood flow, independent of systemic blood pressure, include anemia and transfusion, hypo- or hyperglycemia, hypo- or hypercarbia, hypoxemia, and acidosis. Positioning of the head can influence cerebral blood flow in small preterm infants, and neutral positioning has been associated with a lower risk of IVH (11). High intrathoracic pressure (caused by the high ventilator pressure needed for severe lung disease, or tension pneumothorax) can affect arterial blood flow to the brain by influencing cardiac output. Additionally, constant high intrathoracic pressure can interfere with venous return from the brain, resulting in elevated venous pressure and venous ischemia. Coagulopathy confers additional risk for developing IVH.

Clinical Manifestations

Premature infants are at highest risk of developing IVH within the first few days of delivery. It is very uncommon for a new bleed to appear beyond the first week of life. However, a bleed that occurs within the first few days can progress over subsequent days and become larger. This can sometimes result in a more severe intracranial lesion, such as hemorrhagic venous infarction or progressive posthemorrhagic hydrocephalus, which are beyond the scope of this text. There is a great deal of variability in the clinical presentation of IVH in premature infants, which can fall into one of three categories, as described by Volpe (12):

- **Catastrophic deterioration:** least frequent; sudden change in the status of the infant, which can include hypotension, shocky appearance, need for increased ventilatory support, seizures, acidosis, or anemia
- **Saltatory syndrome:** more gradual change in neurological status, tone, and spontaneous movements
- **Asymptomatic:** most frequent; 25% to 50% of IVH patients

Because there are often no symptoms associated with IVH, it is standard to perform routine cranial ultrasound studies in premature infants who are at the greatest risk, those born at up to 32 to 34 wG. Ultrasound can be performed at the bedside without moving or disrupting the care of vulnerable premature infants. Ultrasound is very sensitive for detecting IVH and monitoring evolution of the bleed. The IVH grading systems found in Table 8-1 also describe the clinical manifestations found on ultrasound. Figure 8-1 is illustrative of grades I, II, III, and IV IVH.

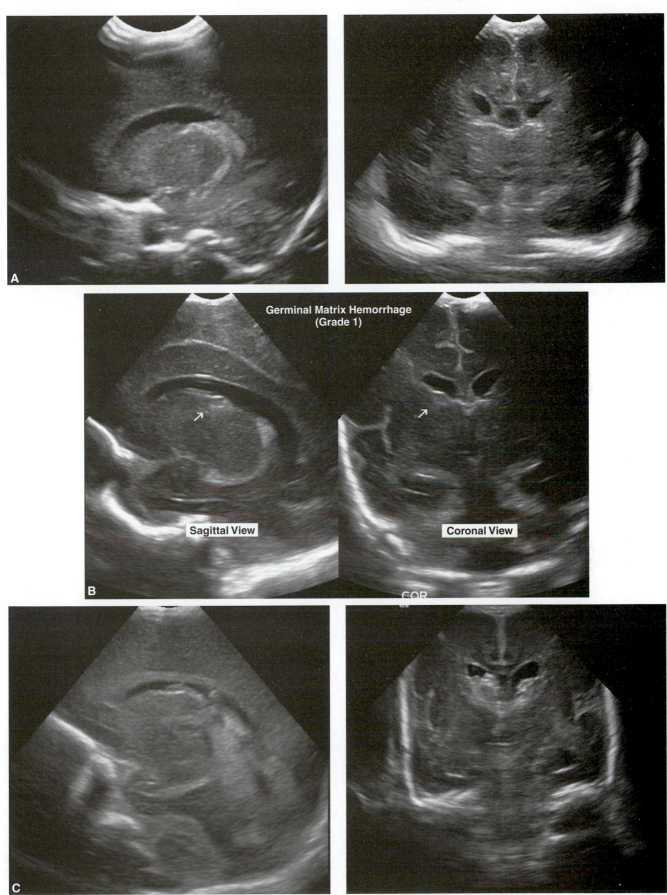

Germinal Matrix Hemorrhage
(Grade 1)

Sagittal View

Coronal View

Figure 8-1 Ultrasound Images of Intraventricular Hemorrhage

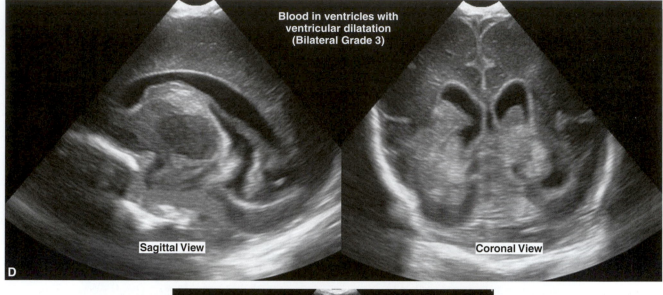

Blood in ventricles with
ventricular dilatation
(Bilateral Grade 3)

Sagittal View

Coronal View

D

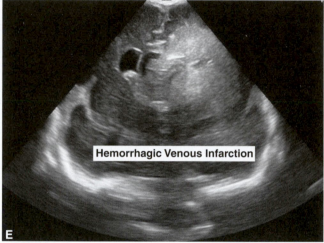

Hemorrhagic Venous Infarction

E

Figure 8-1—cont'd

■ ■ BG Ray's breath sounds are equal and clear bilaterally, her exhaled tidal volume (V_T) values are 5 cc/kg, and transillumination is negative for a pneumothorax. BG Ray's nurse is preparing to administer a normal saline bolus, while her doctor orders a dopamine drip. You notice that she looks quite pale, and she was not active during your assessment. You draw a sample for an arterial blood gas (ABG) test from her umbilical line and note that she has developed metabolic acidosis since her last lab check 3 hours ago, and her hemoglobin level has dropped significantly.

After BG Ray is transfused with packed red blood cells, her blood pressure becomes more stable, and the dopamine drip is weaned. Her next blood count shows improvement in her hemoglobin level, but it is still low. The team is concerned that BG Ray has ongoing blood loss. A STAT head ultrasound is ordered to evaluate for bleeding into the ventricles of the brain.

Management and Treatment

Prevention of IVH is the best management strategy. Preventive measures begin in the prenatal period; the most effective measure is prolonging pregnancy, and strategies to prevent preterm birth were described in Chapter 4. When this is not possible, obstetric interventions such as administration of antenatal steroids and antibiotics for chorioamnionitis have been associated with lower risk of IVH in the premature infant. In addition, there is a growing body of evidence showing that delaying cord clamping for 30 to 120 seconds after delivery improves the hemodynamics of premature infants and results in a lower incidence of IVH (13).

After delivery, close monitoring of the clinical systems that can alter cerebral blood flow has the potential to lower the risk of IVH. Maintaining a neutral head position and avoiding abrupt rotation of the head will decrease the likelihood of rupture to the GM from external stimuli. Prevention also includes monitoring and treatment when any of the following are out of the predetermined acceptable range:

- Glucose
- Blood pressure
- Hemoglobin and hematocrit
- Coagulation studies
- pH
- Partial pressure of carbon dioxide ($PaCO_2$)

From the moment of delivery, the RT can play a role in prevention of IVH. The selection and management of mechanical ventilation (MV) are key components. When considering respiratory management, it is essential to remember that there is interplay between all body systems and that the effects of interventions that support one system may have a significant and direct impact on another. The physiological changes that occur in response to changes in oxygenation and ventilation influence cerebral blood flow (14–16). Respiratory management can, therefore, impact the risk of developing GM-IVH (17).

Ventilatory Management

In the pulmonary vasculature, an increase in $PaCO_2$ causes vasoconstriction. In the brain, CO_2 has the opposite effect, causing vasodilatation. When hypoventilation occurs, the cerebral vasculature dilates, causing an increase in blood flow. Hyperventilation causes cerebral vasoconstriction and decreased cerebral blood flow, which are likely to be the first in a series of events that result in damage to the fragile GM vessels and subsequent bleeding. When cerebral blood flow decreases, in addition to hypoxic ischemic injury to the brain tissue, there can be hypoxic ischemic injury to the GM vessels. If this is followed by a rapid increase in cerebral blood flow, there is reperfusion injury to these vessels, which can result in rupture. When managing the ventilation of a premature infant, it is essential to consider the impact of wide *fluctuations* in $PaCO_2$, which lead to analogous fluctuations in cerebral blood flow (Table 8-2).

The relationship between CO_2 and cerebral blood flow has long been studied (14–16). Both extremes of ventilation, *hyper*ventilation and *hypo*ventilation, as well as wide fluctuations in CO_2, have been implicated as potential contributors to the development of IVH (17).

Pressure ventilation has been the standard in neonatal MV for decades, with its use emerging from the belief that barotrauma was the primary cause of lung injury and that it should be controlled by the clinician. This paradigm has persisted and has not changed despite a recent acceptance of volutrauma as an equal contributor to lung tissue damage. With recent advances in MV, neonatal ventilators are now capable of allowing clinician control over both volume and pressure and thus better management of $PaCO_2$.

Minute ventilation is the product of tidal volume (V_T) and respiratory rate ($f \times V_T$). During pressure ventilation, V_T is variable, which may increase the incidence of hyperventilation, hypoventilation, or both. Premature infants, particularly those with RDS, are susceptible to V_T variation because of changes that can occur in their lung compliance, as described in Chapter 4. When compliance changes occur during pressure ventilation, delivered V_T will change. An example is the increase in delivered V_T when exogenous surfactant treatment is given for RDS, which causes an abrupt improvement in lung compliance. If the ventilator peak inspiratory pressure (PIP) is not decreased, there is risk of hyperventilation. Conversely, unequal distribution of surfactant, atelectasis, air leak, and other pulmonary complications can cause heterogeneous lung characteristics and nonuniform ventilation, which can result in hypoventilation and hypercarbia.

Volume-targeted pressure ventilation may offer some benefits in very premature infants at risk of IVH. These modes were discussed in depth in Chapter 4; one such volume-targeted strategy that has been studied in this patient population is volume guarantee (VG) (Dräger Babylog, Dräger Medical Inc., Telford, PA) (18). It allows the clinician to set a PIP and target V_T, and the machine will adjust delivered PIP on a breath-by-breath basis, based on the previous three exhaled V_T values. This serves to avoid wide swings in delivered V_T values and subsequent $PaCO_2$ values. There is an emerging body of evidence that VG can reduce the incidence of hypo- or hypercapnia, reduce the incidence of wide fluctuations in CO_2, and reduce V_T variability (18–23). The evidence supporting the benefits of volume ventilation to decrease the risk of IVH and other complications of prematurity is growing (24, 25). Currently, pressure ventilation remains commonplace in NICUs, and there is a lack of consistency among practitioners who use volume ventilation with regard to their practice with this

Table 8-2	Effect of CO_2 on Perfusion	
	Hypercapnia	**Hypocapnia**
Pulmonary vasculature	Constricts (↓ blood flow to underventilated lung units)	Dilates (↑blood flow to well-ventilated lung units)
Cerebral vasculature	Dilates (↑ blood flow to brain)	Constricts (↓ blood flow to brain)
Implication on GM and hemorrhage	Reperfusion injury to vessels and rupture of GM	Can lead to hypoxic ischemic injury

mode (26). Research has revealed some unique pathophysiological features of premature infants, which provide an opportunity to decrease the risk of complications in the brain by optimizing ventilator management. It is important to continue to investigate modes of ventilation that might be particularly well suited to this population and develop guidelines for best practice. Data regarding selection of MV settings in premature infants with RDS also apply to infants at risk for IVH:

- Synchronized mode of ventilation
- PIP to allow for pH of 7.25 to 7.35 and $PaCO_2$ of 45 to 55 mm Hg and to keep V_T within prescribed limits
- V_T 4 to 7 mL/kg
- RR 30 to 60 breaths per minute
- Inspiratory time (T_I) 0.3 to 0.4 seconds
- Positive end-expiratory pressure (PEEP) 4 to 7 cm H_2O

Frequent assessment and early extubation can also play a part in improving the incidence of IVH, particularly the more severe bleeds. Some early evidence has also shown that using therapist-driven protocols in patients with RDS may significantly decrease the risk of IVH in extremely premature and extremely low birth weight (ELBW) neonates (Evidence in Practice 8-1) (27).

It is also important to discuss the role that high-frequency ventilation (HFV) may play in IVH. The use of HFV in premature neonates has been described in Chapter 4, and selecting settings should be based on the same criteria as for those with RDS:

High-Frequency Oscillatory Ventilation (HFOV) (28):

- Bias flow: Flow should be 10 to 15 LPM.
- Frequency (hertz): The frequency of 10 to 15 Hz is effective for both premature and near-term patients, with faster rates used more frequently in very premature infants.
- Mean airway pressure (Paw): The initial setting should be slightly higher (1 to 2 cm H_2O) than the last Paw settings on the conventional ventilator.
- Percentage of inspiratory time (T_I): The percentage should be 33%, which will provide an inspiration/expiration (I/E) ratio of 1:2.
- Amplitude (δP): Start the power knob around 2 and increase until chest wiggle is visible.

High-Frequency Jet Ventilation (HFJV) (29):

- PIP: The setting should be approximately the same as the previous conventional ventilator PIP.
- RR: The rate should be 420 breaths per minute.
- T_I: Inspiratory time should be 0.02 seconds.

● **Evidence in Practice 8-1**

Therapist-Driven Protocols: What Do They Help?

In 2004, McMaster University Hospital implemented an registered respiratory therapist–driven ventilation protocol in its neonatal unit, with the objective of providing greater consistency of care, optimal ventilatory support using evidence-based practice, maximal assistance to the health care team in ventilation management, minimal ventilation-related morbidity, and decreased time spent on the ventilator. The protocol was provided to premature infants with a birth weight of less than or equal to 1,250 g who were born within the center. In the first 4 days, the infants were maintained on SIMV with target pH of 7.22 to 7.35, PCO_2 of 45 to 55 mm Hg, and PaO_2 of 45 to 60 mm Hg. After 5 days of MV, the targets were changed to pH of 7.20 to 7.40 and PCO_2 of 50 to70 mm Hg. MV settings included V_T, 4 to 5 mL/kg; PIP, 12 to 25 cm H_2O; pressure support, 5 to 10 cm H_2O; PEEP, 4 to 8 cm H_2O; T_I, 0.25 to 0.45 seconds; and RR, 5 to 60 breaths per minute. Extubation occurred when FIO_2 was less than or equal to 0.30 and Paw was less than 7 cm H_2O or less than 8 cm H_2O for infants with birth weights less than 1,000 g or greater than 1,000 g, respectively.

During the study period, 301 patients were ventilated using this protocol. The incidence of IVH grades III and IV decreased from 31% to 18%, along with a significant decrease in amount of time on the ventilator before extubation.

- PEEP: Start at 7 to 12 cm H_2O and increase until SpO_2 is stable in the prescribed range without an increase in FIO_2 (while the ventilator is in continuous positive airway pressure, or CPAP, mode). This PEEP setting is known as the optimal PEEP in HFJV.
- Conventional ventilator: Set to CPAP unless atelectasis is present. See Chapters 4 and 7 for additional information on managing HFJV.

It has been speculated that the use of HFV may increase the risk of inadvertent hyperventilation (30). In addition, some studies suggest that the use of high frequency may actually increase the risk of developing IVH (31), although a few studies suggest that the cause of this increased risk may be a lack of familiarity with or improper use of HFV (32). Some studies also speculate that the relationship between HFV and hyperventilation is not as strong as once thought (33). The important distinction to make is whether it is the mode of ventilation itself that may contribute to IVH or whether hyperventilation, which may be more common when using HFV, is the actual culprit. This subject continues to be investigated. Clinicians should closely monitor pH and $PaCO_2$ and adjust respiratory support as often as necessary to maintain blood gases within desired parameters.

Regardless of the mode of ventilation chosen, the RT must be acutely aware of the critically ill neonate's ventilation and its potential impact on other body systems. Fluctuations in CO_2, and particularly hypocarbia, are known to affect cerebral blood flow and potentially contribute to the development of IVH in premature infants. It is imperative to closely monitor and regulate ventilation and explore alternative modes of ventilation and monitoring that might better facilitate such control.

■ ■ BG Ray's head ultrasound shows grade II IVH. The neonatologists have now requested daily serial ultrasounds to monitor changes and have asked you to change her mode of ventilation to a volume-targeted mode, with the goal of minimizing swings in $PaCO_2$ that may change cerebral blood flow. You adjust BG Ray to SIMV with VG at 4 cc/kg.

Course and Prognosis

Mortality for IVH is challenging to calculate because the cause of death for premature infants is normally reported as "prematurity" and not the complication that causes death. Mortality due to neurological devastation, however, is usually reserved for grade IV IVH. The overall incidence of grade III and IV IVH in survivors is 6% to 7% (34), with higher rates for grades I and II.

IVH is one of the main predictors of neurodevelopmental outcome (NDO) in preterm infants (35–37). Patients with grade III or IV are at a much higher risk for neurocognitive dysfunction and cerebral palsy (38) than are full-term infants or even other preterm infants without IVH. Cerebral palsy in children born at 23 to 27 weeks was reported in one 2012 study to be 60% and 100% for children with grade III and IV bleeds, respectively, and 100% of patients with grade IV IVH suffered from motor and cognitive delays when evaluated up to 3.5 years of age (39).

Even patients with low-grade (I and II) IVH show poorer NDOs than did infants with a normal cranial ultrasound, with rates of occurrence of around 8% (39, 40). The risk of cerebral palsy in patients with low-grade IVH is significantly higher for extremely premature infants (38, 40). Low scores in motor development evaluations were found in about one-third of patients with grades I and II IVH; this

finding decreased by age 2 (40). One study found an increased risk of severe (grades III and IV) IVH, hospital mortality, and moderate to severe functional disability for preterm males when compared with females (41).

Patent Ductus Arteriosus

■ ■ You are once again caring for BG Ray, who is now 11 days old. In his report, your night shift coworker, Dave, told you that the plan discussed during multidisciplinary rounds was to extubate her to NCPAP. Dave noted, however, that her status changed overnight. He increased her pressures (PIP/PEEP) from 16/4 cm H_2O to 20/4 cm H_2O because of respiratory acidosis and low delivered V_T with VG; he also had to increase her FIO_2 from 0.35 to 0.55. Dave also says the infant has frequent desaturation episodes, even with minor stimulation during assessment. You approach BG Ray's incubator and wonder what could have happened.

The **ductus arteriosus** is a blood vessel that connects the pulmonary artery and the aorta just past their origins on the right and left sides of the heart, respectively. This vessel is part of the normal structure of the fetal heart, and it is widely patent in utero to facilitate the appropriate flow of blood from the placenta to the organs to deliver oxygen and nutrients (described in detail in Chapter 2). A failure of this vessel causes a cardiac complication known as a **patent ductus arteriosus (PDA)**, which is one of the most common congenital heart defects found in preterm neonates. A PDA can spontaneously open and close, making it a transient problem that may be challenging to diagnose quickly. It changes the blood flow through the pulmonary system, which can cause ventilatory complications such as desaturations, hypercapnia, and pulmonary edema. Severe cases require surgical correction to improve cardiac output. The actual incidence of PDA is dependent upon infant maturity and birth weight. It is very uncommon in full-term infants, occurring in only 1 in 2,500 to 5,000 live births (0.04% to 0.02%) (42). In healthy term infants, functional closure of the ductus arteriosus occurs in almost 50% within 24 hours of life, in 90% by 48 hours of life, and in virtually all by 72 hours of life (43). As with many complications of prematurity, the likelihood of PDA closure correlates with gestational age at delivery; persistent patency is common in the smallest, most premature infants. PDA occurs in 30% of infants weighing less than 1,500 g at birth, possibly because of lower oxygen tension and immaturity of ductal closure mechanisms (44). This incidence increases dramatically in premature and low birth weight infants, with 79% of infants weighing less than 1,000 g having a PDA on the fourth day of life and 66% persisting past the first week of life (42). In a review of infants weighing less than 1,000 g, spontaneous closure of the ductus arteriosus occurred by 4 days of age in only about one-third of infants (43). Prematurity and RDS are both significant risk factors for PDA. Many congenital cardiac abnormalities also include a PDA or require one for survival; these are discussed in more detail in Chapters 11 and 12.

Pathophysiology

During fetal development, oxygenated blood travels from the placenta via the umbilical vein, through the inferior vena cava (IVC), and to the right side of the heart. A portion of this oxygenated blood is sent through the patent foramen ovale for delivery to the brain, and the remainder is pumped by the right ventricle through the main pulmonary artery. In adult circulation, this blood would continue to travel to the alveolar capillary membrane, where gas exchange would occur. Because the lungs are filled with fluid, gas exchange does not occur here; instead, the blood from the right ventricle needs to be diverted to provide oxygen to the rest of the organs. As a result, only a small fraction of the blood from the pulmonary artery (<10%) will travel through the lungs to provide oxygen and nutrients for lung tissue growth. The PDA provides a low-resistance pathway to the aorta, and the majority of the blood pumped from the right ventricle to the pulmonary artery will follow this route, delivering oxygen and nutrients from the placenta to the organs and tissues and then returning to the placenta through the umbilical arteries.

Normal Closure of the Ductus Arteriosus

At the time of delivery, fetal circulation must undergo a dramatic transition for babies to survive without the support of the placenta. With the initial expansion of the lungs, fluid clears to establish an area for gas exchange. Both the stretch of the lungs and the alveolar oxygen signal the pulmonary vessels to vasodilate, and pulmonary vascular resistance (PVR) decreases substantially, allowing blood from the right ventricle to travel preferentially to the pulmonary arteries and establish gas exchange. If this transition occurs properly, the blood flow through the pulmonary system increases by approximately 10-fold, and blood flow through the PDA will decrease significantly (Fig. 8-2). The PDA is still open, which may allow blood to flow from an area of high pressure to one of lower pressure. During this transition, in the first few hours of life, it is common for PVR to fluctuate, which can result in mild, temporary desaturations. If PVR increases transiently and becomes higher than systemic vascular resistance,

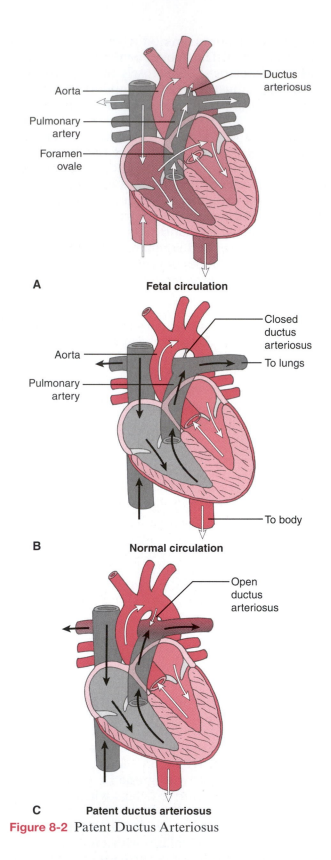

A　**Fetal circulation**

B　**Normal circulation**

C　**Patent ductus arteriosus**

Figure 8-2 Patent Ductus Arteriosus

deoxygenated blood from the right ventricle may be shunted across the PDA. When deoxygenated blood flows, or shunts from right to left (pulmonary artery to aorta), it mixes with oxygenated blood from the aorta, resulting in the delivery of partially oxygenated blood to the body.

In subsequent hours, as PVR continues to decrease, right-to-left shunting should stop, allowing the PDA to constrict and close. As flow through the PDA decreases, it begins to constrict and functionally close. Other signals that drive constriction of the ductus arteriosus include the increase in PaO_2 after delivery and the decrease in circulating prostaglandins. Complete and proper closure of the ductus arteriosus is caused by an increase in vasodilator substances such as bradykinin, an increase in PaO_2, a decrease in circulating prostaglandins, and an overall decrease in pulmonary pressure. Complete closure of the PDA and remodeling of this vascular structure occurs over subsequent days to weeks. Decreased flow across the ductus arteriosus results in hypoxia to the muscle, which is necessary to initiate the cascade of events leading to irreversible anatomical closure. During this process, the muscle of the vessel wall is replaced with a fibrous band of tissue. Definitive closure replaces the ductus arteriosus with the ligamentum arteriosum.

Failure of the Ductus Arteriosus to Close

Many factors may cause failure of PDA closure; these may include misinterpretation of chemical or environmental signals, failure to respond to oxygen, complications from disease processes, and underdeveloped smooth muscle.

- The signals that normally lead to constriction of the PDA and functional closure in the first days of life are not interpreted in the same way in premature infants. Throughout development, tissue responsiveness to different signals changes as the fetus matures. This process is programmed to help orchestrate the extremely complex series of events required for successful fetal development.
- When an infant is born prematurely, some tissues are not yet sensitive to the signals in the extrauterine environment that allow them to properly adapt.
- The tissue in the PDA has not yet developed optimal sensitivity to increased oxygen content in the blood, which is important for stimulating constriction.
- Instead, the PDA is still very sensitive to circulating prostaglandins that cause it to remain open. Circulating prostaglandins decrease significantly after delivery in both term and preterm infants. However, the premature ductal tissue may still respond, even to low concentrations of prostaglandins, causing a failure of constriction.
- Certain disease processes, such as sepsis and NEC, are accompanied by a surge of prostaglandins. This surge can cause a functionally closed, constricted PDA to reopen and further complicate the disease process.

- The musculature of the pulmonary vessels in premature infants has not yet fully developed, resulting in lower pulmonary vascular resistance, and left-to-right shunting is more likely to occur through the open ductus, which keeps it from constricting.

Exposure to antenatal glucocorticoids decreases the risk of persistent patency of the ductus arteriosus, which may be due to a maturation response to the steroids.

Some characteristics of the cardiopulmonary system of premature infants make them especially susceptible to problems from the PDA. As mentioned previously, the lower vascular tone of the pulmonary vessels at earlier gestational ages facilitates left-to-right shunting when the PDA is open, and this shunting perpetuates the failure of the ductus to constrict. Thus, when the PDA exists, premature infants are more likely than term infants to go into congestive heart failure. Additionally, the permeability of the capillaries in the pulmonary bed is greater in premature infants, leaving them more susceptible to developing pulmonary edema from the overcirculation that accompanies left-to-right shunting.

Complications of Pulmonary Overcirculation

When the PDA is open, regulation of blood flow from the great vessels relies largely on PVR and how that PVR compares with the vascular resistance in the rest of the body. PVR is very high in utero, causing blood to shunt through the PDA. PVR falls after delivery, minimizing blood flow across the PDA. Over the next few weeks of life, the PVR will continue to fall. In term infants, the PDA has constricted, so this is not a problem. However, if the ductus remains open, oxygenated blood from the aorta can shunt through the PDA into the pulmonary artery if the resistance of the systemic circulation exceeds that of the pulmonary circulation. This left-to-right shunting will not affect oxygenation and so does not cause abrupt desaturations as does right-to-left shunting. However, if allowed to continue, it will become problematic over time.

When oxygenated blood shunts from left to right, it travels through the pulmonary vascular system unnecessarily, instead of going directly to the organs to deliver oxygen. It will travel with deoxygenated blood through this system and return to the left heart to be pumped again. When this process is continuous, a fraction of the total blood volume will always be taking this route, and the heart performs extra work to deliver the same amount of oxygen to the organs. Congestive heart failure can develop when the heart cannot fully compensate and adequately keep up with the metabolic demands of the body.

Additionally, the pulmonary vascular bed has extra circulating blood volume, causing increased pressure within the pulmonary vessels. This increase in the hydrostatic forces within the pulmonary vessels can result in fluid leaking from the capillaries in the lungs into the interstitium, or **pulmonary edema**.

Fluid distribution within the body is frequently disrupted during illness, but it follows a consistent set of rules. Fluid moves either within the blood vessels (intravascular) or within the interstitial space (extravascular). Fluid has the potential to diffuse across the alveolar-capillary membrane. The direction in which fluid moves and is distributed depends upon four complementary forces: capillary pressure, interstitial fluid pressure, capillary osmotic (oncotic) pressure, and the interstitial fluid colloid osmotic (oncotic) pressure (Box 8-2).

- Capillary pressure tends to force fluid out through the capillary membrane into the interstitial space.
- Interstitial fluid pressure can be either positive or negative. When positive, it forces fluid into the capillaries. When negative, it draws fluid out into the interstitial space.
- Capillary osmotic pressure tends to draw fluid inward into the capillaries.
- Interstitial osmotic pressure tends to draw fluid outward into the interstitial space.

The overall movement of fluid is reflected by the net filtration pressure. Under normal conditions, net filtration pressure is slightly positive, so there is a normal tendency for fluid to diffuse across the capillary membrane into the interstitial space. In healthy conditions, the lymphatic system normally redistributes this interstitial fluid. When the net filtration exceeds the body's ability to eliminate the fluid, however, the result is edema. In the case of pulmonary edema caused by PDA, the increase in pulmonary blood flow due to left-to-right shunting causes an increase in capillary pressure, forcing blood into the alveolar air space.

Box 8-2 Movement of Fluid at the Alveolar-Capillary Membrane

Forces moving fluid from capillaries to the interstitial space:

Capillary pressure
Interstitial osmotic pressure

Forces moving fluid from the interstitial space into the capillaries:

Capillary osmotic pressure

Interstitial fluid pressure can cause fluid to move in either direction.

The lungs have unique properties that make them particularly susceptible to edema. First, the pulmonary capillaries tend to be more "leaky," meaning fluid is more easily absorbed into the interstitial space. Second, the alveolar epithelium is extremely thin, making it easily permeated. Pulmonary edema results from any factor that causes an increase in net filtration pressure subsequently filling the alveoli and interstitial space with fluid.

Clinical Manifestations

Premature infants with lung disease such as RDS have increased PVR because of hypoxemia and the immaturity of the pulmonary vascular bed. The PDA can become symptomatic after early pulmonary pathology improves and PVR decreases. Symptoms of a PDA usually present by the end of the first week of life.

The severity of symptoms depends on the degree of left-to-right shunting of blood. Vital sign symptoms may include the following:

- Tachypnea
- Tachycardia
- Persistently low SpO_2
- Hypotension
- Widened **pulse pressure** (difference between systemic and diastolic blood pressure)

Cardiovascular symptoms include a hyperactive precordium, increased left ventricular impulse, tachycardia from increased left ventricular load, and bounding pulses or palpable palmar pulses.

Infants with a PDA may have a systolic murmur that is best heard at the middle- to upper-left sternal border. It usually occurs on the third to fourth day of life. In 10% to 20% of infants with a PDA, there will be no murmur (42). The murmur occurs when the PDA is very wide and there is not much turbulent flow. The murmur may sound rough and irregular, or "rocky" in premature infants. As flow through the PDA increases, it continues through both systole and diastole, changing the murmur from systolic to a continuous murmur, described as a sound similar to machinery running; this "continuous machinery" murmur is more common in older infants.

Respiratory symptoms typically manifest as increased work of breathing (WOB), which can be challenging to distinguish as being cardiac versus pulmonary in origin. Respiratory distress is evidenced by the following:

- Tachypnea
- Nasal flaring
- Grunting
- Substernal or intercostal retractions
- Auscultation that reveals rales, crackles, or coarse breath sounds

Other symptoms may include feeding intolerance or hepatomegaly (enlarged liver), and oliguria (decreased urine output) may be present.

Laboratory test values include the following:

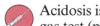

- Acidosis is seen in the results of a blood gas test (metabolic, respiratory, or mixed)
- Decreased CO_2 is seen in the results of a metabolic panel, with an elevated anion gap.
- Increased B-type natriuretic peptide (BNP), a value used to evaluate heart failure, is seen. Its increase is an indication of overworking of cardiac muscle (45, 46).

Chest radiograph may show cardiomegaly (heart silhouette is greater than 50% thoracic space), obscured angle of the carina, increased pulmonary vascular markings, and patchy infiltrates characteristic of pulmonary edema.

Echocardiogram will provide definitive diagnosis of a PDA. It allows clinicians to see the ductus and to measure the amount of blood flow across the PDA and when it occurs in the cardiac cycle. Echocardiogram will also provide an opportunity to measure changes in the heart volume; if the ratio of the left atrial diameter to aortic root diameter is increased (greater than 1.4:1), it indicates increase in left atrial volume secondary to the left-to-right shunt.

■■ As you prepare to assess BG Ray's breath sounds, her bedside nurse asks you to listen for a murmur because she is concerned that the infant has a PDA. You auscultate and note that breath sounds are significant for rales bilaterally, and you note a systolic murmur at the left sternal border. You report your findings to the physician and request a chest radiograph to evaluate the reason for the change in breath sounds. The radiograph shows increased pulmonary vascular markings and patchy infiltrates. The physician has further requested a cardiac ultrasound but agrees with the nurse that BG Ray's symptoms seem very characteristic of a PDA.

Management and Treatment

There is not currently a preferred, evidence-based method for management and treatment of PDA. Although there is evidence supporting several interventions, there is no consensus on whether to treat ELBW infants prophylactically or symptomatically based on the signs and symptoms of PDA. Neither technique has significantly affected outcomes or surgical rates for PDA ligation. The majority of symptomatic patients are candidates for intervention, which will involve a similar course of medications to support cardiac function and promote closure of the ductus arteriosus. The goals of nonsurgical management of a PDA include minimizing shunting across the ductus and promoting closure of the ductus arteriosus. If these are not successful, surgical ligation of the PDA may be necessary. Of primary importance to the RT is to treat the hypoxemia and pulmonary edema that manifest and complicate respiratory management and to understand how these edemas may affect current respiratory management.

Medical Management

Several techniques are used to decrease the amount of blood shunting across the PDA. Because they can be performed together, several methods are often used simultaneously to minimize the risk of pulmonary edema and heart failure. Techniques include restricting fluid and increasing hematocrit. Decreased fluid intake will decrease shunting as well as minimize pulmonary edema. Increasing the hematocrit above 40% to 45% may decrease the amount of blood able to pass through the PDA.

Pharmacological Management

Prostaglandins are known to play a critical role in PDA; thus, inhibiting the production of these vasoactive substances is the goal of pharmacological management (47).

Medical closure of the PDA is most frequently accomplished by using indomethacin, an NSAID that acts as prostaglandin inhibitor. Rates of initial ductus closure in infants born weighing less than 1,750 g range from 60% to 86% after a treatment course of indomethacin. An intravenous form of ibuprofen became available on the market in 2006 and has shown similar success in initial primary closure of a PDA (48). The dosing regimen, length of treatment, and timing of initial therapy has been challenging to determine and may depend on the size of the PDA and the degree of shunt. Both have been shown to decrease the need for surgical correction of a PDA, but a prolonged course of indomethacin has been associated with increased risk of NEC and therefore is not routinely recommended (49). Ibuprofen, by contrast, is as effective as indomethacin at closing a PDA and also reduces the risk of NEC; thus it currently appears to be the drug of choice for PDA closure. Long-term outcome studies have not been done, and these data are needed before a recommendation can be made (50).

Surgical Ligation

Surgical correction of a PDA includes severing the ductus arteriosus, known as **ligation.** Approximately 6% of patients with PDA require surgical ligation, after failing medical management and allowing time for spontaneous closure. It is performed by making a posteriolateral thoracic incision around the fourth intercostal space and placing a suture or band around the ductus arteriosus (Fig. 8-3). The lung, vagus nerve, and laryngeal nerve are all in close proximity to the surgical site and require careful protection to prevent injury. A chest tube is normally left in place to allow evacuation of any air, blood, or fluid postoperatively. Ligation provides definitive closure but has been associated with many risks, including the following:

- Pneumothorax
- Chylothorax
- Scoliosis
- Infection
- Unilateral vocal cord paralysis
- Diaphragm paralysis
- Profound postoperative hypotension
- Increased risk of bronchopulmonary dysplasia

Respiratory Management

In addition to medications, adjustment of mechanical ventilator settings can potentially alleviate respiratory compromise associated with pulmonary edema. Respiratory complications from PDA are most often associated with the pulmonary edema

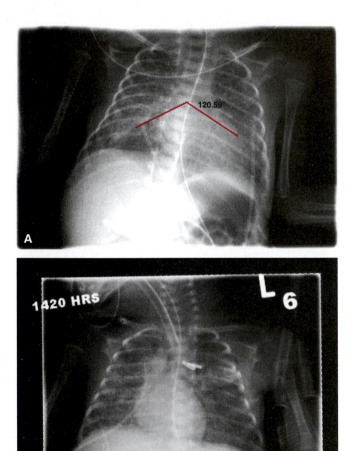

Figure 8-3 Chest Radiograph of a Patient Before and After Ligation of Patent Ductus Arteriosus

resulting from pulmonary overcirculation. Management of pulmonary edema can be challenging. A balance must be struck between reducing extravascular volume and maintaining adequate intravascular volume.

Continuous positive pressure can be used in the lung to alleviate capillary leakage, similar to the technique used to stop bleeding from a laceration. Applying pressure that opposes the movement of fluid into the interstitial space can help shift that fluid to the intravascular space. This is usually accomplished through the application of PEEP. PEEP provides a positive pressure that opposes the outward movement of fluid. Increasing end-expiratory lung volume has been a standard practice in managing pulmonary edema in neonates (51, 52). When pulmonary edema manifests, increasing PEEP in an intubated patient by 1 to 2 cm H_2O at a time and monitoring for positive response is a reasonable strategy. HFOV has also become a method for management of severe and/or hemorrhagic pulmonary edema because it is able to safely deliver higher Paws (53). Clinicians must be cautious because the application of *excessive* pressure to the lungs can cause additional complications such as air leaks, as discussed in the Chapter 7. The constant high intrathoracic pressure with HFOV, if delivered in excess, can compress the heart, which can impede venous return and decrease preload; this, in turn, will decrease cardiac output. The pressure from the HFOV can also cause external compression of the pulmonary vasculature, which can contribute to pulmonary arterial hypertension. When using these methods to manage pulmonary edema, it is important to monitor cardiorespiratory status closely and follow chest radiographs to evaluate for hyperexpansion or pneumothorax, especially if an increase in ventilator pressure results in decreased oxygen saturation or blood pressure.

Edema itself may induce an inflammatory response that can deactivate surfactant, which has led to some interest in the administration of exogenous surfactant to treat pulmonary edema (54, 55). Although this is not common practice, the practitioner must appreciate that, in addition to the pulmonary congestion caused by edema, gas exchange may also be inhibited by a secondary mechanism of surfactant deactivation.

Finally, the practitioner must be judicious in the administration of oxygen. Wide fluctuations in oxygen saturations are a hallmark of a PDA. These fluctuations come from a shift in the direction the blood is shunted through the PDA. Oxygen is a potent pulmonary vasodilator. As such, its administration in the presence of pulmonary edema can risk significant pulmonary circulation and subsequent worsening of pulmonary edema.

You suggest to the neonatologist that you increase PEEP to 6 cm H_2O in an effort to counteract the pulmonary edema shown on the radiograph. You decide not to change the PIP, but you are going to monitor whether the ventilator meets the target V_T. After 2 hours on the new PEEP, FIO_2 has decreased to 0.30, and breath sounds are equal bilaterally, with fine rales at bases.

Course and Prognosis

Spontaneous closure of the ductus arteriosus occurs without sequelae in at least 35% of ELBW infants and in up to 70% of infants greater than 28 wG (56). However, when patency of the ductus arteriosus complicates RDS in the preterm infant, mortality and serious morbidity rates are high (57). PDA that is not responsive to medical therapy is associated with a higher risk of death (58).

PDA has been related particularly to pulmonary problems. It is believed that a high blood shunt through the ductus is a risk factor for pulmonary hemorrhage (59), and surgical closing of a PDA may actually increase the expression of proinflammatory gene markers in the lungs (60). PDA in ventilated infants is also associated with increased risk of chronic lung disease (CLD) (61).

There are potential complications of medical PDA therapy, such as renal dysfunction and intestinal perforation, and PDA has also been considered a risk factor for the development of NEC (61).

Necrotizing Enterocolitis

BG Ray is now 3 weeks old. She is on a heated, humidified nasal cannula (HFNC), at 3 LPM and FIO_2 of 0.21 to 0.30. She has a capillary blood gas drawn with routine laboratory tests, and the results are as follows: pH, 7.31; $PcCO_2$, 54 mm Hg; PcO_2, 43 mm Hg; and HCO_3, 24 mEq/L. Halfway through your shift, while checking BG Ray's HFNC, you notice a small amount of formula around her mouth. You alert the nurse, who informs you that BG Ray has had some minor regurgitation with feeds, but the amount is small and not of concern. The nurse also informs you that BG Ray is receiving commercial formula because the mother is not interested in breastfeeding.

Necrotizing enterocolitis (NEC) is a very serious complication of prematurity that primarily affects the gastrointestinal (GI) tract. The process involves hypoxic-ischemic and inflammatory damage that can result in death of the tissues in almost any region of the GI tract. The severity of NEC is variable, and the progression of damage can be unpredictable, sometimes warranting surgical intervention. In addition to irreversible damage to the intestines, NEC can be complicated by acute cardiorespiratory collapse and death. In survivors of this condition, NEC and related sequelae can significantly impact long-term morbidity.

Among the general neonatal population in the United States, NEC affects fewer than 3 of 1,000 newborns (62–65). However, the incidence varies among medical centers and over time periods in unpredictable ways. Frequently, cases of NEC within centers occur in "waves," similar to epidemics of infections. However, no predisposing factors (such as season of the year or infectious agent) are consistently present when a series of episodes occurs. The infants most commonly affected by NEC are very premature with very low birth weight. Recently published data from the National Institute of Child Health and Development (NICHD) Neonatal Research Network reveal that in participating centers, 11% of infants born at 22 to 28 weeks' gestation with birth weights of 400 to 1,500 g developed NEC, and 52% with this complication were managed surgically (66). The reported mortality rates associated with NEC vary, depending on the characteristics of the infants affected, the stage of illness, and comorbidities. Generally, the smallest, most premature infants are least likely to survive NEC.

Pathophysiology

The etiology of NEC and specific pathophysiological mechanisms that result in NEC have not been well characterized. Risk factors that have been associated with NEC in premature and term infants have provided insight into the potential pathophysiological mechanisms. It has been proposed that a hypoxic ischemic insult to the GI tract and subsequent reperfusion injury can initiate an inflammatory cascade that further compromises gut integrity. The appearance of pathology specimens from intestines that have been damaged from NEC appear similar to those from adults with ischemic injury to the intestines. When NEC occurs in term infants, there is frequently a characteristic or circumstance that causes hypoperfusion to the intestinal tract in the prenatal or postnatal period. Some examples include maternal cocaine use and other maternal conditions that cause insufficient placental blood flow, which also results in intrauterine growth restriction of the fetus. Infants who are born small for gestational age at term are at higher risk of developing NEC than are infants who have not experienced growth restriction in utero, and both may be due to compromised placental blood flow affecting the GI tract. Perinatal and neonatal risk factors in term infants can be linked to compromised blood flow to the GI tract, as well. For example, perinatal asphyxia and low 5-minute Apgar scores are both consequences of poor systemic perfusion around the time of delivery, and both are associated with a higher risk of NEC. Congenital heart disease, umbilical catheters, exchange transfusions, and polycythemia with resultant intravascular sludging are all risk factors for inconsistent perfusion to the GI tract and associated with a greater risk of NEC in term infants.

In premature infants, NEC is not limited to those with distinct risk factors for hypoxic ischemic injury to the intestines. However, premature intestines are likely more susceptible to injury from subtle alterations in systemic perfusion. In addition, their immature host defenses and regulation of inflammatory responses can contribute significantly to the development of NEC. Some risk factors in premature infants that are associated with decreased intestinal perfusion include the presence of a PDA and treatment with indomethacin. There is evidence to suggest that perfusion to the intestines can be altered when a premature infant receives a transfusion for anemia. In addition, associations have been made between the timing of transfusions in premature infants and the onset of NEC (67–69). However, these studies are retrospective. The temporal association could represent several different factors and should not lead to the conclusion that transfusions increase the risk of NEC in premature infants.

Clinical Manifestations

There are numerous signs and symptoms of NEC, and the initial presentation can be subtle, with mild feeding intolerance, or be quite dramatic. Multiple body systems are affected by NEC, and symptoms can initially be broad and nonspecific, such as temperature instability. Respiratory symptoms can include tachypnea, increased WOB, hypopnea that can progress to apnea, hypoxia, and the need for increased respiratory support. Cardiovascular symptoms may include tachycardia and/or bradycardia and hypotension. Hypotension with decreased systemic perfusion, referred to as **shock**, can occur as part of the body's inflammatory response, which includes a decrease in vascular tone in addition to capillary leak; this can be generalized and lead to total body edema (anasarca), but it can be worst at the site of initial inflammation and cause bowel wall edema and **ascites** (fluid in the peritoneal cavity). Poor systemic perfusion can present as pale appearance of the skin with mottling and slow capillary refill. It can result in compromise to other organs as well and present with signs such as decreased urine output. Presenting signs and symptoms of NEC typically involve the GI system and can include feeding intolerance with increased volume of gastric aspirates that can be bilious, vomiting, or blood in stools. There are typically abnormalities seen in the abdominal examination in a baby with NEC, which can be subtle or profound. These babies can have abdominal distension, hypoactive or hyperactive bowel sounds, and a pain response with palpation, such as grimacing or flexing at the hips and bringing legs toward the abdomen. The skin of the abdomen can be reddened (erythema), discolored, or have a bruised appearance from venous stasis under the skin over the inflammatory site. NEC can also affect the neurological status of the baby and cause irritability or decreased tone and lethargy.

Because many of these signs and symptoms are nonspecific in premature infants, it is important to consider NEC in the differential diagnosis when checking laboratory test values to further investigate the source of illness. A complete blood count can reveal anemia and thrombocytopenia. In addition, the white blood cell count can be high, low, or within normal range. If there is a previous white blood cell count for comparison, it can be very helpful in determining whether the count has increased or decreased; either change can accompany NEC. The white blood cell differential can be valuable, as well. The C-reactive protein (CRP) can be elevated with NEC. However, this elevation can occur up to a day after the clinical onset, or it may not occur at all; a normal CRP does not rule out NEC. Metabolic acidosis can accompany NEC and is likely due to tissue damage to the intestines, but it can also occur in the setting of hypoperfusion of the body. When looking at an electrolyte panel, it is useful to check the anion gap $[Na^+ - (Cl^- + CO_2)]$. With an elevated anion gap (greater than 15) in the setting of acidosis (low pH or low serum CO_2), it is possible that tissue damage has occurred. Hyponatremia can also be seen with NEC. Laboratory analysis of the patient's stool frequently reveals the presence of heme (iron-containing portion of hemoglobin), although the blood can often be detected by the naked eye. With the development of sepsis and/or destruction of bowel, **disseminated intravascular coagulation (DIC)** can occur. This process consumes the factors that clot blood and can manifest as oozing or bleeding from any mucosal site or into the skin (petechiae). It can be confirmed with laboratory values that measure clotting function— prothrombin time (PT) and partial thromboplastin time (PTT)—and there is frequently a decrease in the number of platelets, which are consumed with the clotting factors.

An abdominal radiograph is indicated when there is suspicion of NEC, and it can help to confirm the diagnosis. NEC is characterized by the appearance of air within the intestinal wall, or **pneumatosis**. The appearance of pneumatosis on radiography varies depending on position of the bowel in relation to the direction of the radiograph. Air is lucent and appears darker than tissue on the radiograph. When air is confined within the layers of tissue of the bowel wall, it takes the appearance of small, narrow, linear lucencies, or a series of small, round lucencies. The radiograph in Figure 8-4A shows areas of pneumatosis in the right-lower and left-upper quadrants of the abdomen. When stool is mixed with air within the lumen of the bowel, it can have an appearance similar to pneumatosis. The area of small lucencies in the left-lower quadrant of Figure 8-5A could represent pneumatosis, stool, or both. Other characteristics that can indicate an unhealthy bowel can be seen in an abdominal radiograph and should be followed closely with a high index of suspicion for NEC. As in Figure 8-4A, the loops of intestine can appear featureless, distended, and stacked together in one area of the abdomen, whereas other areas do not have any bowel gas.

Even in the absence of pneumatosis, these findings should be followed with serial radiographs. Bowel gas patterns should change over time as the smooth muscle of the intestines moves; if the bowel gas pattern does not change, there is likely to be intestinal pathology. With more severe NEC, there may be lucent lines over the liver, indicating that air has tracked from the bowel wall into the portal venous system. In addition, it is possible to detect free air outside of the bowel wall, in the peritoneum, which is evidence of intestinal perforation. Because free air in the peritoneum typically rises to the most superior aspect of the abdominal cavity, it might not be evident on the standard anterior-posterior supine film, superimposed over the other bowel markings. It is necessary to take a lateral radiograph of the abdomen as a cross-table with the baby in the supine position or in the left-lateral decubitus position. Figure 8-4B shows free air that has risen above the liver when the baby is placed in the left decubitus position and a lateral film is taken. Throughout the course of NEC, it is important to obtain serial images of the abdomen to evaluate the degree of pneumatosis and detect portal or peritoneal free air (Fig. 8-4C), which is an indication for surgical intervention.

NEC can be characterized by stage, which indicates the severity of illness. The original staging criteria developed by Bell have been modified, as described in Table 8-3 (70).

■■ You return the next day, and the night shift RT informs you that there is some concern about BG Ray. The RT says that BG Ray has been vomiting after feeds. You mention that it was happening the previous day, and the team didn't seem too concerned about it. The RT then tells you that the patient is having discolored aspirate that almost

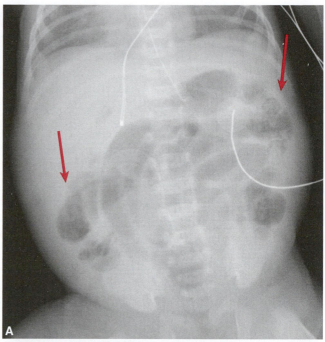
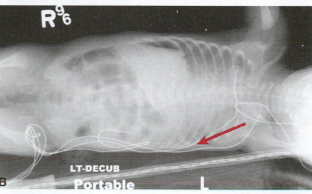
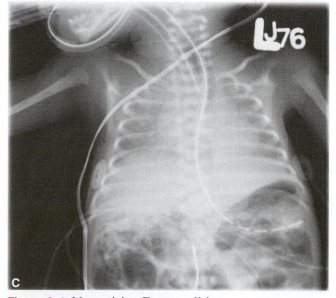

Figure 8-4 Necrotizing Enterocolitis

appears like coffee grounds. She informs you that BG Ray's feeds have been stopped, and the team planned to order an abdominal radiograph. You begin your rounds and notice that her abdomen is

Table 8-3			Modified Bell's Staging Criteria (72)			
Stage			Signs and Symptoms		Intestinal	Radiograph Findings
1	A	Suspected NEC	Temperature instability, apnea, bradycardia, lethargy		Prefeed residual, abdominal distension, emesis, heme plus stool	Normal or intestinal dilatation, mild ileus
	B	Suspected NEC	Same as above		Grossly bloody stool	Same as above
2	A	Definite NEC; mildly ill	Same as above		Absent bowel sounds with or without abdominal tenderness	Intestinal dilatation, ileus, pneumatosis intestinalis
	B	Definite NEC; moderately ill	Same as above plus mild metabolic acidosis, mild thrombocytopenia		Definite tenderness, peritonitis, possible abdominal celluliti	Same as above plus portal venous air plus or minus ascites
3	A	Advanced NEC; severely ill, bowel intact	Same as above plus hypotension, bradycardia, severe apnea, combined respiratory and metabolic acidosis, disseminated intravascular coagulation, neutropenia		Signs of peritonitis, marked tenderness and abdominal distension	Same as above plus definite ascites
	B	Advanced NEC; severely ill, bowel perforated	Same as above		Same as above	Pneumoperitoneum

distended and firm to the touch. You also notice that she is very tachypneic, and her color is seems gray. The nurse tells you that the doctors have ordered blood gas, CBC, and CRP tests. The results come back as follows: capillary gas: pH 7.11; $PcCO_2$, 61 mm Hg; PcO_2, 34 mm Hg; HCO_3, 13 mEq/L; CBC: white blood cell count, 50,800; hemoglobin; 10.1 g/dL; and the CRP, 9.1. The doctors inform you that BG Ray's abdominal radiograph shows dilated bowel loops and possible free air in the portal vein.

Management and Treatment

Little progress has been made in developing therapies that slow the progression of NEC. Management is generally supportive and varies widely depending on the degree of severity. It is important to have a high index of suspicion for NEC in premature infants who start to develop any of the symptoms because early while treating NEC, it is critical to very closely monitor the infant and watching for potential intestinal complications. The principles of management include bowel rest with decompression, parenteral nutrition, broad-spectrum antibiotics, correction of coagulopathy, replacement of blood products, and supportive cardiorespiratory therapy. The simplest cases can be managed with 7 to 10 days

of IV antibiotics and parenteral nutrition during bowel rest without enteral feeding.

Decompression of the bowel is also necessary because of poor peristalsis and can be achieved by placing a nasogastric (NG) or orogastric tube to suction. This keeps air and fluid from building up within the bowel lumen, which puts pressure on the bowel wall. Additionally, close monitoring for surgical complications is essential. Typically, this includes a physical exam and radiograph of the abdomen three to four times per day to detect increased abdominal girth or distension, worsening of pneumatosis, or the appearance of free air in the abdomen (**pneumoperitoneum**).

Surgical Management

Approximately 20% to 40% of infants who develop NEC require surgical intervention, mainly because of severe bowel necrosis with intestinal perforation. The degree of intestinal injury that occurs in relation to the perforation can vary. A small area of ischemic damage can result in a perforation, or a large portion of the bowel may be necrotic and require surgical excision. The extent of bowel removed during surgery has been shown to correlate with the likelihood of survival.

There are two surgical approaches for intestinal perforation from NEC: exploratory laparotomy and primary peritoneal drainage. Until recently, it was standard for surgeons to perform an exploratory laparotomy to identify the site of perforation and other compromised bowel and to remove it. With this approach, the ends from which the bowel was excised are externalized with the creation of **ostomies** (a surgically formed opening allowing a portion of the intestines to pass through a fistula to the skin surface). After NEC has been treated, intra-abdominal inflammation has subsided, and the infant has become more stable, another surgery (reanastomosis) can be performed to reconnect the ostomies and close the abdomen. The second approach, primary peritoneal drainage, was initially undertaken as a temporizing procedure for infants who were too hemodynamically unstable to undergo exploratory laparotomy. However, this procedure is now considered to be a reasonable alternative to laparotomy for infants with surgical NEC and has been the definitive surgical treatment for some infants who do not require additional procedures. Studies have compared some early outcomes of infants treated with primary peritoneal drainage with those who underwent primary laparotomy. Thus far, there is no substantial evidence to suggest that either procedure is more effective for preventing death or prolonged use of total parenteral nutrition. Ongoing studies will compare later outcomes, such as neurodevelopment of these infants, and may direct management in the future.

Respiratory Management

Babies who develop NEC may require increased respiratory support as a result of apnea and pulmonary edema. In addition, the gaseous distension in the abdominal cavity causes upward pressure on the diaphragm and results in decreased functional residual capacity. The goal of ventilatory support with NEC is to optimize oxygen delivery to the tissues.

NEC can impact respiratory status in two primary ways. First, it can create a systemic inflammatory cascade that has the potential to damage valuable lung tissue. Second, the increased abdominal pressure associated with NEC can create a physical opposition to the normal process of inspiration and subsequent lung inflation. Techniques for managing the physical impediment to lung inflation will be discussed here.

Increased abdominal pressure can affect both normal, spontaneous breathing and positive-pressure mechanical breaths. Spontaneous breathing requires the diaphragm to drop, allowing a negative pleural pressure and flow of gas into the lungs. Increased abdominal pressure may impede this physiological process. During MV, the ventilator uses positive pressure to inflate the lungs. It often requires a great amount of force to overcome the opposition of the intra-abdominal pressure that is impeding lung expansion, which may prevent the ventilator from adequately inflating the alveoli during inspiration without using excessive peak inspiratory pressures. Increased intra-abdominal pressure will also decrease the potential space for lung expansion, decrease compliance, and increase resistance by decreasing thoracic space and subsequent intrathoracic volume.

To overcome these challenges to ventilation, the RT must employ a ventilatory strategy that can recruit lung tissue and maintain an adequate level of inflation at exhalation, known as functional residual capacity (FRC). One way for RTs to assess the quality of lung inflation is to observe and evaluate pressure-volume loops as measured by the mechanical ventilator.

A flattened pressure-volume loop is a clear example of inadequate FRC, indicating that the pressure in the lungs at end exhalation falls below the critical opening pressure. **Critical opening pressure** is the pressure at which the lungs begin to expand or inflate. After exhalation, if the resting volume of the lungs falls below this critical opening pressure, the alveoli collapse, and the ventilator must deliver this pressure at the beginning of the next inspiration before any lung expansion occurs. In essence, the ventilator spends the first phase of inspiration trying to reach a resting level of inflation; this means that the beginning of inspiration involves delivering pressure with no gas exchange. For volume change to occur at the initiation of inhalation, the lungs must have an adequate FRC.

As the compliance of the lung improves, it is able to accept more volume with the same pressure from the ventilator. Volume delivery that occurs immediately at the start of inspiration is an indication that there is sufficient FRC at this point for a change in volume to occur. This is visualized by reviewing pressure-volume loops on the mechanical ventilator.

There are several possible options to improve lung compliance and gas delivery for a patient with NEC. If the baby is remaining on the conventional ventilator, it is reasonable to increase PEEP, which will act to stabilize alveoli at exhalation and promote adequate FRC. It will also serve to increase Paw, which is the average pressure in the lungs. Increasing Paw often serves to improve ventilation by increasing the delivered pressure to the lungs.

Patients with NEC often need an increase in Paw because of worsening compliance, loss of lung volume, increased oxygen requirement, and respiratory acidosis. Conventional mechanical ventilators do not allow RTs to directly set a Paw; rather, Paw is calculated based upon the set PIP, PEEP, T_I, and inspiratory flow rate and pattern. HFOV is an alternative to conventional ventilation that uses a set Paw along with smaller-than-dead-space delivered volumes to safely oxygenate and ventilate despite lower lung compliances. In this population, HFOV allows clinicians to safely apply an elevated Paw and provide little fluctuation in lung volume because of the very small V_T values. Fok and colleagues (71) published case reports of eight infants with a variety of pathologies that caused increased intra-abdominal pressure and sought to determine the short-term efficacy of HFOV in these patients. The general findings suggested that HFOV significantly improved oxygenation and ventilation in this group of patients. Although the study evaluated only a few patients, it did demonstrate an ability to manage the respiratory status of patients effectively with increased intra-abdominal pressure using HFOV.

■■ The attending physician is concerned that BG Ray is showing signs consistent with NEC and wishes to intubate her. You proceed with the intubation and place BG Ray on SIMV PIP at 18 cm H_2O; PEEP, 4 cm H_2O; T_I, 0.35 seconds; RR, 30 breaths per minute, and FIO_2, 0.45. Over the next few hours, BG Ray's oxygen requirement increases significantly. A blood gas value is obtained, and the results are pH 7.16; $PcCO_2$, 80 mm Hg; PcO_2, 55 mm Hg; and HCO_2, 22 mEq/L. A chest radiograph reveals overall hypoinflation of all lung fields.

You increase BG Ray's pressure settings to a PIP of 20 cm H_2O and PEEP of 6 cm H_2O. Over the next 20 minutes, you are able to wean FIO_2 from 0.80 to 0.55. After 3 hours, another chest and abdominal radiograph is taken. The abdomen is unchanged, but the lungs are showing equal aeration, with small patches of atelectasis and inflation to seven ribs posteriorly. BG Ray will be managed with parenteral nutrition, antibiotics, and decompression by NG tube.

Course and Prognosis

NEC is fatal in about 32% to 39% of diagnosed patients (72, 73); one study found that infants who die of NEC tend to die quickly, within 7 days of diagnosis (74). Factors that are associated with an increased risk of mortality include lower estimated gestational age, lower birth weight, lack of prenatal care, significant lung disease, and vasopressor use at the time of diagnosis.

For premature infants who survive, NEC can significantly increase the amount of time they are hospitalized. Patients who require surgical resection (called "surgical NEC"), have a significantly longer hospital stay, higher hospital charges, and greater mortality (75).

NEC may slightly increase the risk of neurodevelopmental delay for very preterm infants, but it does not seem to negatively impact growth by 2 years of age (76).

Retinopathy of Prematurity

■■ BG Ray is now 31 weeks' postmenstrual age. She completed her course of treatment for medical NEC and has been extubated for 2 weeks. She is now on a 1-liter nasal cannula (NC) at FIO_2 0.21. Today is BG Ray's ROP screening.

Retinopathy of prematurity (ROP) is a complication of prematurity and one of the major causes of blindness in children in the developed world. It is rapidly emerging in the developing world as neonatal intensive care advances and more premature infants are able to survive (77, 78). In simplest terms, ROP occurs when the normal development of retinal vessels is disrupted by premature delivery and the extrauterine environment. As with other disease processes discussed in this chapter, gestational age and birth weight are the strongest predictors of ROP. The incidence of ROP correlates inversely with gestational age and birth weight at delivery; the smallest, most premature infants are at highest risk for developing this complication, and with the greatest degree of severity. Additional factors that have been associated with ROP include duration of MV, requirement for supplemental oxygen, and several comorbidities of prematurity that could represent severity of illness and innate immaturity.

In developed countries, ROP occurs in 65% to 70% of premature infants with birth weights 1,250 g or less. This number has not changed despite the technological advances in neonatal care over the past 20 years (77–80).

Pathophysiology

Vascularization of the retina begins early in fetal development, around 14 to 18 wG. This process begins centrally, at the optic disc, and progresses outward as the retina differentiates; it is typically completed by 40 to 44 wG (81). Like many developmental processes, it is highly regulated and depends on a coordinated series of events that occur in response to complex signals. This process occurs optimally in the intrauterine environment. When an infant is born prematurely, the environment changes, and rapid adaptations are made to facilitate survival. The characteristics of the new environment and the survival responses of the neonate can interfere with retinal vascularization, which can result in ROP.

During the second trimester of gestation, the environment of the fetus in utero is hypoxic as compared with the extrauterine environment. As retinal differentiation progresses prior to approximately 30 wG, metabolic activity increases, which results in a greater degree of hypoxia relative to the metabolic demands. This prompts signals that promote an increase in local vasogenic growth factors (82), such as vascular endothelial growth factor (VEGF). The subsequent phase of retinal vascular development (32 to 34 wG) is characterized by reduced levels of VEGF and very specific and complex patterns of signals that result in apoptosis (programmed cell death) and cessation of development of some vessels but continued growth and differentiation of others (83). With premature delivery, the drastic environmental change disrupts these processes. Before 30 wG, there is a loss of the growth factors produced by the placenta that stimulate retinal vascularization, such as insulin-like growth factor-1 (82). In addition, the relative hyperoxia of the extrauterine environment reduces the levels of vasogenic factors, such as VEGF, resulting in stage 1 of ROP, characterized by incomplete blood vessel formation (vasculogenesis) and/or blood vessel destruction (vaso-obliteration) (84). During subsequent weeks, the relative hypoxia in the eye, resulting from poor vascularization, causes production of high levels of angiogenic factors, such as VEGF and erythropoietin (85), initiating stage 2 of ROP, which is characterized by uncontrolled vasoproliferation and pathological neovascularization of the retina (86). This new vascularization continues to proliferate in stage 3 ROP, and stages 4 and 5 begin partial and total retinal detachment, which can cause blindness.

Clinical Manifestation

Initially, the International Classification of Retinopathy of Prematurity was developed to provide consistent definitions among practitioners and researchers. At that time, it was published in two parts (in 1984 [87, 88] and 1987 [89, 90]), and then an updated version was published in 2005 (91). Box 8-3 lists the clinical manifestations used to diagnose ROP in infants. The diagnosis is usually made by an ophthalmologist during a dilated eye examination and documented on a retinal schematic such as the one shown in Figure 8-5. The American Academy of Pediatrics, in collaboration with the American Academy of Ophthalmology and the American Association for Pediatric Ophthalmology and Strabismus, created recommendations for ROP screening. They currently recommend screening examinations in infants with a birth weight of less than 1,500 g or a gestational age of 32 weeks or less. For infants less than 28 weeks, the first screening should be performed at 31 weeks postmenstrual age, with infants 28 to 32 wG at birth screened at 4 weeks of age. Examinations should be completed by an ophthalmologist who has sufficient knowledge and experience to enable accurate identification of the location and sequential retinal changes of ROP (92) (Special Populations 8-1).

Box 8-3 Stages of Retinopathy of Prematurity

Stage 1 Mildly abnormal growth with a sharp white line of demarcation; lies flat against the retina, marking the transitions between the vascular and avascular retina

Stage 2 Moderately abnormal blood vessel growth with a rolled ridge of scar tissue of variable length in the region of the white demarcation line. Small tufts of new blood vessels called ''popcorn'' may be found behind the ridge.

Stage 3 Severely abnormal blood vessel growth with neovascularization originating from the posterior aspect of the ridge and growing into the vitreous. Stage 3 can further be subdivided into mild, moderate, or severe, depending on the amount of new vessel growth projecting into the vitreous.

Stage 4 Subtotal retinal detachment caused by retraction or hardening of the scar tissue formed in earlier stages
 • Stage 4a is a partial detachment affecting the periphery of the retina.
 • Stage 4b is a subtotal or total detachment involving the macula and fovea, usually with a fold extending through zones I, II, and III.

Stage 5 Complete retinal detachment, with the retina assuming a closed or partially closed funnel from the optic nerve to the front of the eye.

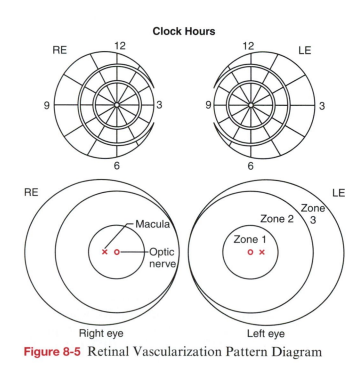

Figure 8-5 Retinal Vascularization Pattern Diagram

Retinal images of the stages of ROP can be seen in Figure 8-6. Care should be taken by the neonatal clinical team during screening examinations because they are uncomfortable and can cause immediate and prolonged physiological effects. Most commonly, apnea events and desaturations can increase significantly within 24 to 48 hours after eye examinations; this is more likely to manifest in patients who are not receiving ventilator support (94).

Management and Treatment

Treatment of all premature infants includes strategies to minimize the progression of ROP. This usually consists of judicious use of oxygen therapy and structured screening. Surgical intervention is provided prior to retinal detachment (stage 4), and the optimal treatment window is considered to be any point along the stage 2 ROP spectrum. Pharmacological therapy is also starting to show promising results to halt the course of ROP.

Oxygen Therapy

Supplemental oxygen therapy is one of the most documented risk factors for ROP and was first indicated as a cause of retrolental fibroplasia (a severe form of ROP) in the 1950s (95). Clinicians agree that the amount of oxygen delivered to premature infants should be closely monitored, excess oxygen delivery should be avoided, and weaning from supplemental oxygen therapy should be done as early as possible. However, there is no clear understanding of optimal blood oxygen ranges for safe retinal development. Thus, different strategies, FIO_2 levels, and SpO_2 ranges have been implemented and published, and practice can vary between institutions. However, a consensus of safe practices emerged in the 1990s and 2000s to minimize hyperoxemia in premature infants, and it includes the following:

- Minimizing abrupt changes in FIO_2. When SpO_2 is outside normal range, make small changes in FIO_2 (0.01 to 0.05 at a time) and wait several minutes before making additional changes (96).
- Making sure prescriber orders for supplemental oxygen include an acceptable SpO_2 alarm limit range. The most commonly suggested ranges in studies have been 85% to 93% (97–100) and 89% to 94% (101), though there is some concerning data published in 2010 stating that consistently lower SpO_2s may increase mortality (102).
- Assessing a neonate for the cause of hypoxemia before increasing FIO_2 levels to avoid hyperoxemia. This will prevent rapid changes in retinal perfusion (103).
- Using an air-oxygen blender. This ensures that infants will receive the same FIO_2 during manual ventilation that they received via their oxygen-delivery device, avoiding abrupt changes in FIO_2 (96).
- Weaning oxygen as soon as SpO_2 rises above the prescribed value, in small increments, until SpO_2 is again in an acceptable range.

Surgical Treatments

Surgical treatment for ROP is focused on halting further progression of the disease, not repairing current damage. Treatment is considered effective if it destroys the majority of the cells that produce VEGF in the retina, which is known to be the most important factor in the progression of ROP.

In 1988, cryotherapy was recommended for stage 3+ ROP that extends for a significant portion of retina as measured by clock face (104). Cryotherapy consists of freezing the sclera, the choroid, and the full thickness of the avascular retina from the external ocular surface. In the 1990s, transpupillary diode laser therapy was found to be a more elegant and accurate technique, causing fewer postoperative ocular and systemic complications. This therapy applies a laser through a dilated pupil to the internal retinal surface. The 810-nm diode laser therapy is now considered the technique of choice, but it causes permanent loss of the peripheral visual field (105).

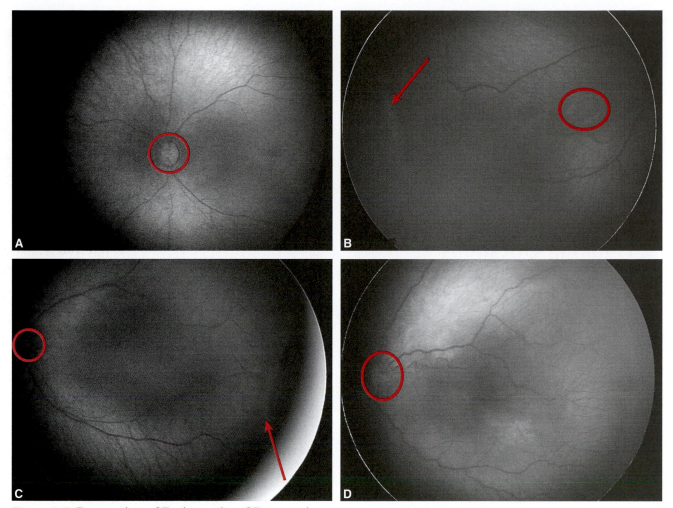

Figure 8-6 Progression of Retinopathy of Prematurity *(Courtesy of Michael Repka, MD.)*

VEGF Inhibitors

A VEGF inhibitor is an intravitreal (into the eye) medication that reduces the effect of VEGF on the developing retina, halting the development of ROP. It has been used in three different ways: (1) as a rescue therapy when surgery does not produce adequate regression; (2) as a combination therapy, used simultaneously with laser surgery; and (3) as an initial, solitary treatment. It shows promise for preserving peripheral vision but may not be as effective in all patient populations for all instances of ROP (106).

Course and Prognosis

ROP is one of the causes of severe morbidity in very preterm infants surviving to hospital discharge. Long-term follow-up by an ophthalmologist is required to monitor for continued visual complications. These can include the following:

- Myopia, or nearsightedness
- Strabismus, or an inability to align both eyes simultaneously (commonly thought of as being "cross-eyed")
- Amblyopia, the loss of one eye's ability to see details (commonly called "lazy eye")

- Glaucoma, a condition that leads to damage to the optic nerve, usually caused by increased intraocular pressure
- Late retinal detachment

If ROP progresses to retinal detachment, it usually results in poor visual prognosis. Even with timely and thorough treatments, some patients develop retinal detachment (107).

ROP frequently resolves itself, an event known as spontaneous regression. Up to 90% of cases of ROP stages 1 and 2 regress spontaneously, with no treatment or intervention (108). Even cases of stage 3+ ROP have the potential for spontaneous regression, although clinicians are currently unable to predict which patients will heal themselves and which will require surgical intervention to prevent retinal detachment and blindness.

■■ The ophthalmologist noted that BG Ray has stage 2 ROP. She will continue to be monitored until her discharge. Her PDA closed with indomethacin treatment, NEC resolved with bowel rest, and IVH did not progress beyond stage 2. She will continue to feed and grow until she is old enough to go home.

■■ Critical Thinking Questions: BG Ray

1. What would be a reasonable $PaCO_2$ range for BG Ray while you try to minimize the risk of worsening IVH?

2. If increasing BG Ray's PEEP after her NEC diagnosis hadn't improved FRC, what would your next recommendation have been?

3. Why do you think BG Ray was on a NC at 0.21 FIO_2?

▶● Case Studies and Critical Thinking Questions

■ Case 1: Baby Boy (BB) Miller

You are the day-shift RT in a level IIIC NICU. You are called to the bedside of BB Miller, a 27-wG boy, now 9 days old. He was intubated in the delivery room for presumed RDS/hyaline membrane disease (HMD). Extubated on day of life (DOL) 2 and weaned from nasal CPAP to NC 1 LPM on DOL 4, his feeding via NG tube has increased over the last 2 days. Over the last 3 hours, he had increasing episodes of apnea and bradycardia requiring alleviation with positive-pressure ventilation (PPV) using a resuscitation bag. You and the neonatologist intubate for apnea; postintubation chest and abdominal film is pending. Follow-up capillary blood gas after intubation is pH 7.20; PCO_2, 36 mm Hg; PO_2, 43 mm Hg; and HCO_3, 13 mEq/L.

You place BB Miller on SIMV; his RR is 35 breaths per minute, PIP is 18 cm H_2O, PEEP is 5 cm H_2O, and FIO_2 is 0.47.

- *The pediatric resident would like to improve the pH. What ventilator setting changes would you recommend to him?*

You notice that after intubation BB Miller is requiring a FIO_2 of 0.80 to 0.90. You request a chest radiograph, and the doctors at the bedside performing an arterial puncture to take blood for laboratory tests provide you with an ABG blood sample. The initial ABG result is pH 6.98; $PaCO_2$, 98 mm Hg; PaO_2, 51 mm Hg; and HCO_3, 12 mEq/L. You review the chest radiograph showing the endotracheal tube (ETT) is in good position, but BB Miller's lungs are only five ribs expanded and nearly completely whited out.

- *What would you like to do to improve ventilation?*

You place BB Miller on HFOV: Paw is 14 cm H_2O; P, 26 cm H_2O; and 15 Hz. The subsequent blood gas result is pH 7.21; $PaCO_2$, 55 mm Hg; PaO_2, 51 mm Hg; and HCO_3, 12 mEq/L. BB Miller is currently receiving packed red blood cells. A surgeon has been contacted to review BB Miller's status and decides BB Miller needs exploratory surgery to evaluate the condition of his intestines. The surgery is performed at bedside. Once BB Miller's abdominal contents are revealed, the surgeons note that much of his bowel is black. They estimate that BB Miller has lost 30% of his bowel. The surgeons remove the necrotic bowel and perform an ileostomy. As BB Miller recovers, you are subsequently able to wean the HFOV settings and transition back to conventional ventilation.

Multiple-Choice Questions

1. You are the only RT working in a 15-bed level IIIA NICU. Which of your patients, listed below, is at the highest risk for developing IVH?
   a. 23 4/7 wG infant, now 4 weeks old
   b. 25 3/7 wG, newly born, with no prenatal steroid treatment
   c. 27 1/7 wG infant, 2 days old, on NC
   d. 34 wG infant, now 2 days old, birth weight 1,750 g

2. Which of the following ventilatory strategies will minimize the risk of IVH in a very preterm infant?
   a. Minimize hyperoxemia
   b. Maintain mild hypercapnia
   c. Minimize swings in $PaCO_2$
   d. Provide mild hyperventilation

3. Which of the following symptoms in a patient being treated for RDS would make you suspect he had a PDA?
    I. Atelectasis
    II. Pulmonary edema
    III. Desaturation
    IV. Apnea
    V. Metabolic acidosis
a. I, II
b. I, III, IV
c. II, IV, V
d. II, III

4. A patient with metabolic acidosis, apnea, shock, and bilious aspirates should be evaluated for which of the following disorders?
a. IVH
b. NEC
c. RDS
d. PDA

5. One of your patients has just been diagnosed with medical NEC. The resident has been tasked with adjusting ventilator settings to minimize complications. Your patient is on SIMV with RR, 25 breaths per minute; PIP, 15 cm H_2O; PEEP, 4 cm H_2O; and FIO_2, 0.60. ABG from the radial line is pH 7.20; $PaCO_2$, 40 mm Hg; PaO_2, 56 mm Hg; and HCO_3, 15.4 mEq/L. What would you recommend?
a. Increase rate
b. Increase PIP
c. Increase PIP and PEEP
d. Do nothing

6. Which of the following factors can contribute to the development of ROP?
a. High SpO_2
b. Low SpO_2
c. Previous history of NEC
d. Grade IV IVH

7. Which of the following oxygen-delivery strategies for preterm infants can reduce the incidence of ROP?
    I. Use an air-oxygen blender during manual ventilation.
    II. Avoid large swings in PaO_2.
    III. Maintain SpO_2 greater than 94%.
    IV. Increase FIO_2 by 0.1 whenever the patient desaturates.
a. I, II
b. I, II, III
c. I, II, IV
d. I, II, III, IV

8. Which of the following SpO_2 values in a premature neonate requires the RT to adjust delivered FIO_2?
a. 89%
b. 91%
c. 93%
d. 95%

9. Pulmonary edema in premature infants is a symptom of which complication?
a. IVH
b. AOP
c. PDA
d. ROP

10. Which medication can be given to an infant to facilitate closure of a patent ductus arteriosus?
a. Prostaglandin
b. Indomethacin
c. Ibuprofen
d. a or b
e. b or c

Davis*Plus* | For additional resources login to Davis*Plus* (http://davisplus.fadavis.com/ keyword "Perretta") and click on the Premium tab. (Don't have a *Plus*Code to access Premium Resources? Just click the Purchase Access button on the book's Davis*Plus* page.)

REFERENCES

1. de Waal CG, Weisglas-Kuperus N, van Goudoever JB, Walther FJ. Mortality, neonatal morbidity and two-year follow-up of extremely preterm infants born in the Netherlands in 2007. *PLoS One.* 2012;7(7):e41302.
2. Fellman V, Hellstrom-Westas L, Norman M, et al. One-year survival of extremely preterm infants after active perinatal care in Sweden. *JAMA.* 2009;301(21):2225-2233.
3. Mathews TJ, MacDorman MF. Infant mortality statistics from the 2007 period linked birth/infant death data set. *Natl Vital Stat Rep.* 2011;59(6):1-30.
4. Mathews TJ, MacDorman MF; Division of Vital Statistics. Infant mortality statistics from the 2008 period linked birth/infant death data set. *Natl Vital Stat Rep.* 2012;60(5):1-28.
5. Boerma T, AbouZahr, C. *World Health Statistics 2010.* Geneva, Switzerland: World Health Organization; 2010.
6. Horbar JD, Badger GJ, Carpenter JH, et al. Trends in mortality and morbidity for very low birth weight infants, 1991-1999. *Pediatrics.* 2002;110(1, pt 1):143-151.
7. Larroque B, Marret S, Ancel PY, et al. White matter damage and intraventricular hemorrhage in very preterm infants: the EPIPAGE study. *J Pediatr.* 2003;143(4):477-483.

8. Cust AE, Darlow BA, Donoghue DA. Outcomes for high-risk New Zealand newborn infants in 1998-1999: a population-based, national study. *Arch Dis Child Fetal Neonatal Ed.* 2003;88(1):F15-F22.

9. Papile LA, Burstein J, Burstein R, Koffler H. Incidence and evolution of subependymal and intraventricular hemorrhage: a study of infants with birth weights less than 1,500 gm. *J Pediatr.* 1978;92(4):529-534.

10. Volpe JJ. Neonatal intraventricular hemorrhage. *N Engl J Med.* 1981;304(15):886-891.

11. Malusky S, Donze A. Neutral head positioning in premature infants for intraventricular hemorrhage prevention: an evidence-based review. *Neonatal Netw.* 2011;30(6):381-396.

12. Volpe JJ. *Neonatal Neurology.* 4th ed. Philadelphia, PA: WB Saunders; 2008.

13. Rabe H, Diaz-Rossello JL, Duley L, Dowswell T. Effect of timing of umbilical cord clamping and other strategies to influence placental transfusion at preterm birth on maternal and infant outcomes. *Cochrane Database Syst Rev.* 2012;8:CD003248.

14. Grubb RL Jr, Raichle ME, Eichling JO, Ter-Pogossian MM. The effects of changes in $PaCO_2$ on cerebral blood volume, blood flow, and vascular mean transit time. *Stroke.* 1974;5(5):630-639.

15. Leahy FA, Cates D, MacCallum M, Rigatto H. Effect of CO_2 and 100% O_2 on cerebral blood flow in preterm infants. *J Appl Physiol.* 1980;48(3):468-472.

16. Alberti E, Hoyer S, Hamer J, Stoeckel H, Packschiess P, Weinhardt F. The effect of carbon dioxide on cerebral blood flow and cerebral metabolism in dogs. *Br J Anaesth.* 1975;47(9):941-947.

17. Fabres J, Carlo WA, Phillips V, Howard G, Ambalavanan N. Both extremes of arterial carbon dioxide pressure and the magnitude of fluctuations in arterial carbon dioxide pressure are associated with severe intraventricular hemorrhage in preterm infants. *Pediatrics.* 2007;119(2):299-305.

18. Cheema IU, Sinha AK, Kempley ST, Ahluwalia JS. Impact of volume guarantee ventilation on arterial carbon dioxide tension in newborn infants: a randomised controlled trial. *Early Hum Dev.* 2007;83(3):183-189.

19. Abubakar KM, Keszler M. Patient-ventilator interactions in new modes of patient-triggered ventilation. *Pediatr Pulmonol.* 2001;32(1):71-75.

20. Cheema IU, Ahluwalia JS. Feasibility of tidal volume-guided ventilation in newborn infants: a randomized, crossover trial using the volume guarantee modality. *Pediatrics.* 2001;107(6):1323-1328.

21. Herrera CM, Gerhardt T, Claure N, et al. Effects of volume-guaranteed synchronized intermittent mandatory ventilation in preterm infants recovering from respiratory failure. *Pediatrics.* 2002;110(3):529-533.

22. Dawson C, Davies MW. Volume-targeted ventilation and arterial carbon dioxide in neonates. *J Paediatr Child Health.* 2005;41(9-10):518-521.

23. Keszler M, Abubakar K. Volume guarantee: stability of tidal volume and incidence of hypocarbia. *Pediatr Pulmonol.* 2004;38(3):240-245.

24. Wheeler KI, Klingenberg C, Morley CJ, Davis PG. Volume-targeted versus pressure-limited ventilation for preterm infants: a systematic review and meta-analysis. *Neonatology.* 2011;100(3):219-227.

25. Wheeler K, Klingenberg C, McCallion N, Morley CJ, Davis PG. Volume-targeted versus pressure-limited ventilation in the neonate. *Cochrane Database Syst Rev.* 2010(11):CD003666.

26. Klingenberg C, Wheeler KI, Owen LS, Kaaresen PI, Davis PG. An international survey of volume-targeted neonatal ventilation. *Arch Dis Child Fetal Neonatal Ed.* 2011;96(2): F146-F148.

27. Hermeto F, Bottino MN, Vaillancourt K, Sant'Anna GM. Implementation of a respiratory therapist-driven protocol for neonatal ventilation: impact on the premature population. *Pediatrics.* 2009;123(5):e907-e916.

28. IASYS Healthcare-Critical Care Division. 3100A Quick Reference Card. http://www.carefusion.com/pdf/Respiratory/ HFOV/l23243100aquickrefcard775895_101.pdf. Accessed October 2, 2012.

29. Bunnell International. General guidelines for LifePulse HFV: Bunnell High Frequency Jet Ventilation. http://www .bunl.com/Patient%20Management/hfjvguidelines.pdf. Accessed December 14, 2012.

30. Wiswell TE, Graziani LJ, Kornhauser MS, et al. Effects of hypocarbia on the development of cystic periventricular leukomalacia in premature infants treated with high-frequency jet ventilation. *Pediatrics.* 1996;98(5):918-924.

31. Cools F, Offringa M. Meta-analysis of elective high frequency ventilation in preterm infants with respiratory distress syndrome. *Arch Dis Child Fetal Neonatal Ed.* 1999;80(1):F15-F20.

32. Bollen CW, Uiterwaal CS, van Vught AJ. Cumulative meta-analysis of high-frequency versus conventional ventilation in premature neonates. *Am J Respir Crit Care Med.* 2003;168(10):1150-1155.

33. Clark RH, Dykes FD, Bachman TE, Ashurst JT. Intraventricular hemorrhage and high-frequency ventilation: a meta-analysis of prospective clinical trials. *Pediatrics.* 1996;98(6, pt 1):1058-1061.

34. Horbar JD, Carpenter JH, Badger GJ, et al. Mortality and neonatal morbidity among infants 501 to 1500 grams from 2000 to 2009. *Pediatrics.* 2012;129(6):1019-1026.

35. Linder N, Haskin O, Levit O, et al. Risk factors for intraventricular hemorrhage in very low birth weight premature infants: a retrospective case-control study. *J Pediatr.* 2003;111(5):e590-e595.

36. Mancini MC, Barbosa NE, Banwart D, Silveira S, Guerpelli JL, Leone CR. Intraventricular hemorrhage in very low birth weight infants: associated risk factors and outcome in the neonatal period. *Rev Hosp Clin Fac Med Sao Paulo.* 1999;54(5):151-154.

37. Stoinska B, Gadzinkowski J. Neurological and developmental disabilities in ELBW and VLBW: follow-up at 2 years of age. *J Perinatol.* 2011;31:137-142.

38. Klebermass-Schrehof K, Czaba C, Olischar M, et al. Impact of low-grade intraventricular hemorrhage on long-term neurodevelopmental outcome in preterm infants. *Childs Nerv Syst.* 2012;28(12):2085-2092.

39. Patra K, Wilson-Costello D, Taylor HG, Mercuri-Minich N, Hack M. Grades I–II intraventricular hemorrhage in extremely low birth weight infants: effects on neurodevelopment. *J Pediatr.* 2006;149(2):169-173.

40. Kent AL, Wright IM, Abdel-Latif ME. Mortality and adverse neurologic outcomes are greater in preterm male infants. *Pediatrics.* 2012;129(1):124-131.

41. Reller MD, Rice MJ, McDonald RW. Review of studies evaluating ductal patency in the premature infant. *J Pediatr.* 1993;122(6):S59-S62.

42. Hammerman C, Shchors I, Schimmel MS, Bromiker R, Kaplan M, Nir A. N-terminal-pro-B-type natriuretic peptide in premature patent ductus arteriosus: a physiologic biomarker, but is it a clinical tool? *Pediatr Cardiol.* 2010;31(1):62-65.

43. Clyman RI, Cuoto J, Murphy GM. Patent ductus arteriosus: are current neonatal treatment options better or worse than no treatment at all? *Semin Perinatol.* 2012;36(2):123-129.

44. Koch J, Hensley G, Roy L, Brown S, Ramaciotti C, Rosenfeld CR. Prevalence of spontaneous closure of the ductus arteriosus in neonates at a birth weight of 1000 grams or less. *Pediatrics.* 2006;117(4):1113-1121.

45. Hsu JH, Yang SN, Chen HL, Tseng HI, Dai ZK, Wu JR. B-type natriuretic peptide predicts responses to indomethacin in premature neonates with patent ductus arteriosus. *J Pediatr.* 2010;157(1):79-84.

46. Hammerman C. Patent ductus arteriosus. Clinical relevance of prostaglandins and prostaglandin inhibitors in PDA pathophysiology and treatment. *Clin Perinatol.* 1995;22(2):457-479.

47. Johnston PG, Gillam-Krakauer M, Fuller MP, Reese J. Evidence-based use of indomethacin and ibuprofen in the neonatal intensive care unit. *Clin Perinatol.* 2012;39(1):111-136.

48. Herrera C, Holberton J, Davis P. Prolonged versus short course of indomethacin for the treatment of patent ductus arteriosus in preterm infants. *Cochrane Database Syst Rev.* 2007;2:CD003480.

49. Ohlsson A, Walia R, Shah SS. Ibuprofen for the treatment of patent ductus arteriosus in preterm and/or low birth weight infants. *Cochrane Database Syst Rev.* 2010;4:CD003481

50. Tyler DC, Cheney FW. Comparison of positive end-expiratory pressure and inspiratory positive pressure plateau in ventilation of rabbits with experimental pulmonary edema. *Anesth Analg.* 1979;58(4):288-292.

51. Chakraborty M, McGreal EP, Kotecha S. Acute lung injury in preterm newborn infants: mechanisms and management. *Paediatr Respir Rev.* 2010;11(3):162-170.

52. Jackson JC, Truog WE, Standaert TA, et al. Effect of high-frequency ventilation on the development of alveolar edema in premature monkeys at risk for hyaline membrane disease. *Am Rev Respir Dis.* 1991;143(4, pt 1):865-871.

53. Kobayashi T, Nitta K, Ganzuka M, Inui S, Grossmann G, Robertson B. Inactivation of exogenous surfactant by pulmonary edema fluid. *Pediatr Res.* 1991;29(4, pt 1):353-356.

54. Willson DF, Thomas NJ, Markovitz BP, et al. Effect of exogenous surfactant (calfactant) in pediatric acute lung injury: a randomized controlled trial. *JAMA.* 2005;293(4):470-476.

55. Koch J, Hensley G, Roy L, Brown S, Ramaciotti C, Rosenfeld CR. Prevalence of spontaneous closure of the ductus arteriosus in neonates at a birth weight of 1000 grams or less. *Pediatrics.* 2006;117:1113-1121.

56. Nagle MG, Peyton MD, Harrison LH, Elkins RC. Ligation of patent ductus arteriosus in very low birth weight infants. *Am J Surg.* 1981;142(6):681-686.

57. Noori S, McCoy M, Friedlich P, et al. Failure of ductus arteriosus closure is associated with increased mortality in preterm infants. *Pediatrics.* 2009;123:e138-e144.

58. Kluckow M, Evans N. Ductal shunting, high pulmonary blood flow, and pulmonary hemorrhage. *J Pediatr.* 2000;137:68-72.

59. Waleh N, McCurnin DC, Yoder BA, Shaul PW, Clyman RI. Patent ductus arteriosus ligation alters pulmonary gene expression in preterm baboons. *Pediatr Res.* 2011;69(3):212-216.

60. Marshall DD, Kotelchuck M, Young TE, Bose CL, Kruyer L, O'Shea TM. Risk factors for chronic lung disease in the surfactant era: a North Carolina population-based study of very low birth weight infants. *Pediatrics.* 1999;104(6):1345-1350.

61. Dollberg S, Lusky A, Reichman B. Patent ductus arteriosus, indomethacin and necrotizing enterocolitis in very low birth weight infants: a population-based study. *J Pediatr Gastroenterol Nutr.* 2005;40:184-188.

62. Llanos AR, Moss ME, Pinzon MC, Dye T, Sinkin RA, Kendig JW. Epidemiology of neonatal necrotising enterocolitis: a population-based study. *Paediatr Perinat Epidemiol.* 2002;16(4):342-349.

63. Holman RC, Stoll BJ, Curns AT, Yorita KL, Steiner CA, Schonberger LB. Necrotising enterocolitis hospitalisations among neonates in the United States. *Paediatr Perinat Epidemiol.* 2006;20(6):498-506.

64. Lin PW, Stoll BJ. Necrotising enterocolitis. *Lancet.* 2006;368(9543):1271-1283.

65. Sankaran K, Puckett B, Lee DS, et al. Variations in incidence of necrotizing enterocolitis in Canadian neonatal intensive care units. *J Pediatr Gastroenterol Nutr.* 2004;39(4):366-372.

66. Stoll BJ, Hansen NI, Bell EF, et al. Neonatal outcomes of extremely preterm infants from the NICHD Neonatal Research Network. *Pediatrics.* 2010;126(3):443-456.

67. Gephart SM. Transfusion-associated necrotizing enterocolitis: evidence and uncertainty. *Adv Neonatal Care.* 2012;12(4):232-236.

68. Sellmer A, Tauris LH, Johansen A, Henriksen TB. Necrotizing enterocolitis after red blood cell transfusion in preterm infants with patent ductus arteriosus: a case series. *Acta Paediatr.* 2012;101(12):e570-572.

69. Amin SC, Remon JI, Subbarao GC, Maheshwari A. Association between red cell transfusions and necrotizing enterocolitis. *J Matern Fetal Neonatal Med.* 2012;25(suppl 5):85-89.

70. Neu J. Necrotizing enterocolitis: the search for a unifying pathogenic theory leading to prevention. *Pediatr Clin North Am.* 1996;43(2):409-432.

71. Fok TF, Ng PC, Wong W, Lee CH, So KW. High frequency oscillatory ventilation in infants with increased intra-abdominal pressure. *Arch Dis Child Fetal Neonatal Ed.* 1997;76(2):F123-F125.

72. Thyoka M, de Coppi P, Eaton S, et al. Advanced necrotizing enterocolitis part 1: mortality. *Eur J Pediatr Surg.* 2012;22(1):8-12.

73. Kelley-Quon LI, Tseng CH, Scott A, Jen HC, Calkins KL, Shew SB. Does hospital transfer predict mortality in very low birth weight infants requiring surgery for necrotizing enterocolitis? *Surgery.* 2012;152(3):337-343.

74. Clark RH, Gordon P, Walker WM, Laughon M, Smith PB, Spitzer AR. Characteristics of patients who die of necrotizing enterocolitis. *J Perinatol.* 2012;32(3):199-204.

75. Abdullah F, Zhang Y, Camp M, Mukherjee D, Gabre-Kidan A, Colombani PM, Chang DC. Necrotizing enterocolitis in 20,822 infants: analysis of medical and surgical treatments. *Clin Pediatr.* 2010;49(2):166-171.

76. Dilli D, Eras Z, Özkan Ulu H, Dilmen U, Durgut Sakrucu E. Does necrotizing enterocolitis affect growth and neurodevelopmental outcome in very low birth weight infants? *Pediatr Surg Int.* 2012;28(5):471-476.

77. Gilbert C. Retinopathy of prematurity: a global perspective of the epidemics, population of babies at risk and implications for control. *Early Hum Dev.* 2008;84(2):77-82.

78. Reynolds JD, Hardy RJ, Kennedy KA, et al; Light Reduction in Retinopathy of Prematurity (LIGHT-ROP) Cooperative Group. Lack of efficacy of light reduction in preventing retinopathy of prematurity. *N Engl J Med.* 1998;338:1572-1576.

79. Palmer EA, Flynn JT, Hardy RJ, et al; Cryotherapy for Retinopathy of Prematurity Cooperative Group. Incidence and early course of retinopathy of prematurity. *Ophthalmology.* 1991;98:1628-1640.

80. Early Treatment for Retinopathy of Prematurity Cooperative Group. Revised indications for the treatment of retinopathy of prematurity: results of the early treatment for retinopathy of prematurity randomized trial. *Arch Ophthalmol.* 2003;121:1684-1696.

81. Ashton N. Retinal angiogenesis in the human embryo. *Br Med Bull.* 1970;26(2):103-106.

82. Smith LE. Through the eyes of a child: understanding retinopathy through ROP. The Friedenwald lecture. *Invest Ophthalmol Vis Sci.* 2008;49(12):5177-5182.

83. Das A, McGuire PG. Retinal and choroidal angiogenesis: pathophysiology and strategies for inhibition. *Prog Retin Eye Res.* 2003;22(6):721-748.

84. McLeod DS, Brownstein R, Lutty GA. Vaso-obliteration in the canine model of oxygen-induced retinopathy. *Invest Ophthalmol Vis Sci.* 1996;37(2):300-311.

85. Kermorvant-Duchemin E, Sapieha P, Sirinyan M, et al. Understanding ischemic retinopathies: emerging concepts from oxygen-induced retinopathy. *Doc Ophthalmol.* 2010; 120(1):51-60.

86. Smith LE. Pathogenesis of retinopathy of prematurity. *Semin Neonatol.* 2003;8(6):469-473.

87. The Committee for the Classification of Retinopathy of Prematurity. An international classification of retinopathy of prematurity. *Arch Ophthalmol.* 1984;102(8): 1130-1134.

88. Patz A. The new international classification of retinopathy of prematurity. *Arch Ophthalmol.* 1984;102(8):1129.

89. An international classification of retinopathy of prematurity. II. The classification of retinal detachment. *Arch Ophthalmol.* 1987;105(7):906-912.

90. Patz A. An international classification of retinopathy of prematurity. II. The classification of retinal detachment. *Arch Ophthalmol.* 1987;105(7):905.

91. The International Committee for the Classification of the Late Stages of Retinopathy of Prematurity. The International Classification of Retinopathy of Prematurity revisited. *Arch Ophthalmol.* 2005;123(7):991-999.

92. American Academy of Pediatrics. Screening examination of premature infants for retinopathy of prematurity. *Pediatrics.* 2006;117:572-576.

93. Weaver DT, Murdock TJ. Telemedicine detection of type 1 ROP in a distant neonatal intensive care unit. *J AAPOS.* 2012;16:229-233.

94. Mitchell AJ, Green A, Jeffs DA, Roberson PK. Physiologic effects of retinopathy of prematurity screening examinations. *Adv Neonatal Care.* 2011;11(4):291-297.

95. Kinsey VE. Retrolental fibroplasia: cooperative study of retrolental fibroplasia and the use of oxygen. *Arch Ophthalmol.* 1956;56(4):481-543.

96. Chow LC, Wright KW, Sola A. Can changes in clinical practice decrease the incidence of severe retinopathy of prematurity in very low birth weight infants? *Pediatrics.* 2003;111(2):339-345.

97. Finer N, Leone T. Oxygen saturation monitoring for the preterm infant: the evidence basis for current practice. *Pediatr Res.* 2009;65(4):375-380.

98. Wallace DK, Veness-Meehan KA, Miller WC. Incidence of severe retinopathy of prematurity before and after a modest reduction in target oxygen saturation levels. *J AAPOS.* 2007;11(2):170-174.

99. Vanderveen DK, Mansfield TA, Eichenwald EC. Lower oxygen saturation alarm limits decrease the severity of retinopathy of prematurity. *J AAPOS.* 2006;10(5): 445-448.

100. Deulofeut R, Critz A, Adams-Chapman I, et al. Avoiding hyperoxia in infants < or = 1250 g is associated with improved short- and long-term outcomes. *J Perinatol.* 2006;26(11):700-705.

101. The STOP-ROP Multicenter Study Group. Supplemental Therapeutic Oxygen for Prethreshold Retinopathy Of Prematurity (STOP-ROP), a randomized, controlled trial. I: primary outcomes. *Pediatrics.* 2000;105(2): 295-310.

102. SUPPORT Study Group of the Eunice Kennedy Shriver NICHD Neonatal Research Network. Target ranges of oxygen saturation in extremely preterm infants. *N Engl J Med.* 2010;362:1959-1969.

103. Skinner JR, Hunter S, Poets CF, et al. Haemodynamic effects of altering arterial oxygen saturation in preterm infants with respiratory failure. *Arch Dis Child Fetal Neonatal Ed.* 1999;80(2):F81-F87.

104. Cryotherapy for Retinopathy of Prematurity Cooperative Group. Multicenter trial of cryotherapy for retinopathy of prematurity: preliminary results. *Arch Ophthalmol.* 1988;106:471-479.

105. Good WV; Early Treatment for Retinopathy of Prematurity Cooperative Group. Final results of the Early Treatment for Retinopathy of Prematurity (ETROP) randomized trial. *Trans Am Ophthalmol Soc.* 2004;102: 233-248.

106. Mintz-Hittner HA, Kennedy KA, Chuang AZ. Efficacy of intravitreal bevacizumab for Stage 3+ retinopathy of prematurity. *N Engl J Med.* 2011;364:603-615.

107. Clark D, Mandal K. Treatment of retinopathy of prematurity. *Early Hum Dev.* 2008;84(2):95-99.

108. Gomella TL. *Neonatology: Management, Procedures, On-Call Problems, Diseases, Drugs.* New York: McGraw-Hill; 2004.

Chapter 9

Abdominal Defects

Key Terms

Atresia
Congenital diaphragmatic hernia
  (CDH)
Disruption
Dysmotility
Echocardiogram
Epithelialization
Excision
Herniate
Hypoplasia
Iatrogenic
Inotropes
Malformation
Mesentery
Necrosis
Gastroschisis
Omphalocele
Perforation
Polyhydramnios
Resection
Scaphoid abdomen
Tracheal occlusion
Volvulus

Chapter Objectives
After reading this chapter, you will be able to:

1. Describe the fetal growth changes in a patient who develops a diaphragmatic hernia.
2. Describe the delivery room management of a patient with congenital diaphragmatic hernia.
3. Describe the preoperative respiratory management for a patient with a congenital diaphragmatic hernia, including ventilatory support, treatment for pulmonary hypertension, and extracorporeal membrane oxygenator (ECMO) therapies.
4. Identify key determinants for when to perform a surgical repair of a congenital diaphragmatic hernia.
5. Describe the most common surgical technique for a diaphragmatic hernia repair.
6. Identify the long-term outcomes for patients with a repaired congenital diaphragmatic hernia.
7. Describe the embryological time frame for when gastroschisis develops.
8. List two potential risk factors for gastroschisis.
9. Define the respiratory therapist's (RT's) role during surgical repair of a gastroschisis.
10. Describe the development of omphalocele in utero.
11. Identify three common abnormalities associated with omphalocele.
12. List three methods of repair used for patients with omphalocele.

■■ Baby Girl (BG) Hendricks

You arrive for a day shift at a level IIIC neonatal intensive care unit (NICU) and receive a report from the night-shift therapist, including the upcoming anticipated deliveries in obstetrics. She informs you of BG Hendricks, a 38 3/7 weeks' gestation (wG) neonate who was diagnosed by ultrasound with a left-sided diaphragmatic hernia at 20 wG. Prenatal counseling was offered to the family and a decision to monitor closely in utero was made, with no prenatal intervention. Labor was induced 16 hours ago, and delivery is anticipated within the next 2 hours. The respiratory therapist (RT) was not able to set up the room or meet with the delivery room team to anticipate and plan for this delivery, but the attending physician is expected to meet with the team in the next 15 minutes to delineate roles and prioritize management of the newborn.

Congenital abdominal defects occur when the abdominal contents are allowed to develop outside of the abdominal cavity. In a congenital diaphragmatic hernia, the abdominal contents grow and extend through a hole in the diaphragm and occupy space in the thoracic cavity. Ventral wall defects include several types of malformations, the most common of which include gastroschisis and omphalocele, whereby the intestines and other organs are outside of the abdominal wall at delivery. All of these defects require surgical interventions and often postoperative mechanical ventilation. The respiratory therapist's involvement relies heavily on the size and manifestation of the defect and its impediment on normal pulmonary development in utero or on natural inflation of the lung in the neonatal period.

Congenital Diaphragmatic Hernia

A **congenital diaphragmatic hernia (CDH)** occurs when the segments of the diaphragm fail to fuse by the eighth week of gestation, and the abdominal contents **herniate**, or protrude through the wall, into the thoracic cavity (Fig. 9-1). CDH is a serious congenital malformation that can cause severe problems beginning at delivery and has morbidities lasting through childhood. It is one of the more challenging neonatal problems for respiratory therapists to manage both before and after surgical correction.

CDH occurs in roughly 1 in 2,000 to 3,000 newborns (1). This is a wide range of incidence because the range includes both the prenatal diagnosis and the live birth rate. If the incidence of CDH was

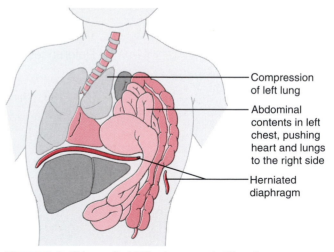

Figure 9-1 Congenital Diaphragmatic Hernia

Compression of left lung

Abdominal contents in left chest, pushing heart and lungs to the right side

Herniated diaphragm

calculated based only on live births, it would most likely underestimate the actual occurrence because some fetuses with hernias don't make it to delivery. One 20-year review study found that of the 130 patients who positively identified with CDH after death, 47% died before birth.

Seventy percent of diaphragmatic hernias occur on the posterolateral diaphragm, through what's known as the foramen of Bodchalek. Of these, about 85% are located on the left side, with 13% occurring on the right side and 2% occurring bilaterally (1). Approximately 27% occur anteriorly, known as Morgani type, and 2% to 3% are centrally located and are usually associated with early death. The size of the defect ranges from 2 mm to 3 mm to a complete absence of the diaphragm.

Pathophysiology

The pleural cavity of the chest and peritoneal cavity of the abdomen are normally separated by the diaphragm. During embryological development, the diaphragm is composed of five different elements that grow together between gestational weeks 4 and 7. The right side of the diaphragm closes before the left side. The left is the more common side to fail during closure. Although the gut is developing during the same time, at about week 6 it travels outside of the abdominal cavity and remains outside through week 10. If there is an opening in the diaphragm when the gut returns to the abdominal cavity, it will herniate through that opening and settle into thorax. The implications for this herniation are of concern because the gut's location in the thorax will begin to interfere with normal pulmonary development.

At 7 weeks, about the time the diaphragm should have closed completely, the airways have branched to about four generations. During the next 4 to 5 weeks, the five major lobes of the lung can be identified. During weeks 10 to 14, the proliferation of the intrasegmental airways is the fastest. Smooth muscle and cartilage also begin to form between weeks 7 and 11, respectively. The pulmonary tissue and capillary network don't begin developing until about week 20. By that time, the herniated intestines have settled into their place in the thorax and are competing with the developing lung for space.

The herniated contents will first cause compression of the lung bud on the same side as the defect. If the defect is big enough, it will shift the mediastinum and cause compression on the other side of the thorax as well. This will eventually manifest as airway compression as the lung continues to grow or cause reduced airway branching during development.

There is also lung **hypoplasia** (organ or tissue underdevelopment) on the affected side. Lung tissue and capillaries will fail to form based on the amount of space lost to the intestines. Decreased numbers of alveolar type II cells cause a decrease in the number of cells producing fetal lung fluid and surfactant, diminishing the amount of both in the developing lung (2). Studies also suggest that the lung begins abnormal development even before the development of the diaphragm defect, suggesting that a common genetic mechanism is causing not just one defect, but two—lung hypoplasia and diaphragmatic hernia (3, 4).

The pulmonary vasculature in patients with CDH has thicker arteriole musculature than that found in normal, healthy developing lungs. This makes the pulmonary vessels more sensitive to increases in arterial pressures and makes the patient more susceptible to persistent pulmonary hypertension after birth, sometimes known as persistent fetal circulation. The thicker musculature makes the vessels less responsive to traditional treatments for persistent pulmonary hypertension (discussed in Chapter 6), such as vasodilators or hyperventilation.

After birth, several clinical complications usually coexist with CDH and are collectively known as "CDH-syndrome." These include pulmonary hypoplasia, patent ductus arteriosus, patent foramen ovale, and malrotation. Pulmonary hypoplasia has already been discussed, but the remaining diagnoses warrant further description.

- **Patent ductus arteriosus:** In utero, the ductus arteriosus is a large vessel that connects the pulmonary trunk to the descending aorta. It serves to help divert blood flow away from the lungs in utero while they are fluid filled and are not participating in gas exchange. After delivery, the ductus arteriosus should close within hours of life because of an increase in partial pressure of oxygen in the blood (PaO_2). Because the ductus arteriosus is a vessel and not a valve, it can allow blood flow in both directions. Blood will flow from the area of higher pressure to one of lower pressure. In healthy infants, the aorta has a higher pressure than the pulmonary trunk, and thus oxygenated blood flows from the aorta and mixes with deoxygenated blood in the pulmonary arteries. In patients with pulmonary hypertension, the opposite is true, and blood flows from the high-pressure pulmonary arteries into the descending aorta and out to the body. This is a significant problem because it mixes deoxygenated blood with oxygenated blood and then lowers the PaO_2 traveling to the rest of the body, causing hypoxemia that can lead to tissue hypoxia.
- **Patent foramen ovale:** The foramen ovale is an opening between the two atria in the fetal heart. During normal transition after birth, the

increased blood pressure on the left side of the heart causes a tissue flap to close the foramen ovale. With CDH, the pulmonary vasculature may remain constricted, which keeps the pressure in the pulmonary arteries very high. This pressure backs into the right side of the heart, causing right heart pressures to equal or exceed left heart pressures. This prevents the foramen ovale from closing. This can cause deoxygenated blood from the right atrium to mix with oxygenated blood in the left atrium, potentially causing a lower PaO₂ to be ejected from the left ventricle to the aorta and out to the body, again causing hypoxemia and leading to tissue hypoxia.

• **Malrotation:** An incorrect rotation of the intestines during fetal development is called "malrotation." The intestines make a very distinct rotation pattern as they herniate into the umbilical cord and then return to the peritoneal cavity, beginning at week 5 and continuing until term. With an open channel into the thorax, the intestines will not move into their proper placement in the abdominal cavity. The intestines will also not be correctly affixed to the peritoneal cavity by the **mesentery** (peritoneal fold that encircles the small intestine and connects it to the posterior abdominal wall). With herniation into the thorax, the intestines have the ability to float freely, making them more susceptible to compression, twisting, or kinking of the small intestines. Kinking of the intestines can cause tissue death known as necrotizing enterocolitis (see Chapter 8 for more information), and without surgical correction, it can cause severe illness and even death.

Clinical Manifestations

The first clinical signs of a diaphragmatic hernia are usually seen in utero during a prenatal ultrasound. After delivery, patients will exhibit very significant signs of respiratory compromise, which will assist in dictating their care.

Prenatal Findings

Ultrasound diagnosis of CDH can be made as early as 15 weeks' gestation. A diagnosis earlier in gestation is associated with worse outcomes (5), because an earlier herniation often means a more severe defect and more pulmonary dysfunction and hypoplasia. The diagnosis is suspected when the stomach is not seen where it is supposed to be on ultrasound, and intestines are seen next to the heart. A right-sided CDH is harder to diagnose in utero because the liver is the organ that would herniate into the chest, and liver tissue appears very similar to lung tissue on ultrasound. The presence of the liver in the thorax (often called "liver up"), regardless of the location of the diaphragm opening, is associated with worse outcomes because it denotes a larger defect and more pulmonary dysfunction (6). Measurements of the lungs and head will be taken to calculate a lung/head ratio, or LHR. The lower the LHR, the more severe the defect. An LHR of less than 1 is associated with close to a 100% mortality rate, and an LHR greater than 1.4 is associated with an almost 0% mortality rate (6). **Polyhydramnios** (abnormally high volume of amniotic fluid) in a patient with CDH is a predictor of poor clinical outcomes (5). This is thought to be because of kinking of the esophagus where the stomach has relocated to the thorax, which obstructs fetal swallowing (7). This can also cause a small fetal stomach that's difficult to see on ultrasound, either in the chest or abdomen.

If a CDH is suspected, a fetal MRI may be recommended because it can better visualize all the developing organs and more accurately predict the severity of the defect. A fetal **echocardiogram** (ultrasound of the heart) may also be recommended to assess whether the herniation has affected the development of the heart.

Clinical Findings at Delivery

Most newborns have large, protruding bellies, so one of the most obvious physical findings for a newborn with CDH is a **scaphoid abdomen** (a hollowed out or convex belly; see Fig. 9-2) because the abdominal contents are in the thorax. CDH should be suspected in a tachypneic newborn with a scaphoid abdomen, but the diagnosis needs to be confirmed by chest and abdominal radiograph (Fig. 9-3).

At delivery, newborns with CDH may initially present with apnea or respiratory insufficiency. They are not as responsive to traditional interventions in the delivery room, such as supplemental oxygen or positive-pressure ventilation. Many patients with CDH will not transition well to extrauterine life, and fetal circulation will persist after birth.

Continuing with newborn assessment, the clinician will not hear lung sounds over both sides of the chest. Lung sounds will be heard on one side and bowel sounds on the affected side. Auscultation of

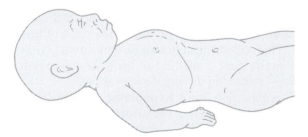

Figure 9-2 Scaphoid Abdomen

the heart may not be in the anatomically correct location because of a mediastinal shift. If mediastinal compression is severe, it could compromise venous return, which will manifest as poor perfusion and hypotension (7).

Clinical manifestations upon admission to the NICU will follow a fairly consistent pattern. Most clinical signs manifest from the respiratory failure caused by lung hypoplasia and pulmonary hypertension that are the defining characteristics of CDH.

Hypoxemia

One of the most commonly seen characteristics of lung disease in CDH is hypoxemia. This is caused by multiple factors. Neonates with CDH have pulmonary vascular abnormalities, which may prevent the normal decrease in pulmonary vascular resistance seen at birth in healthy, typically developing newborns (8). Their pulmonary vascular beds do not respond to increases in oxygen within the alveoli or to the change in systemic vascular resistance that is seen as the umbilical cord is clamped. This will cause a form of persistent pulmonary hypertension that directly causes hypoxemia. The amount of lung hypoplasia present at birth also contributes to hypoxemia. Compression of lung units by abdominal contents within the thoracic cavity will also cause atelectasis, further worsening hypoxemia.

One postmortem study also showed that 91% of infants showed hyaline membrane formation more prominently in the severely affected lung (9). This suggests that, despite being fully developed (greater than 37 wG), patients with CDH share characteristics of those with respiratory distress syndrome (RDS) (see Chapter 4).

Hypoxia

With continuing, untreatable hypoxemia, tissues throughout the body will not receive enough oxygen for metabolism and must revert to anaerobic metabolism to function. This will cause increases in blood lactate levels and metabolic acidosis (10).

Oxygenation Index

The **oxygenation index (OI)** is an equation used to assess the severity of lung dysfunction and is used frequently to help determine the need for extracorporeal membrane oxygenation (ECMO). The calculation assesses how much pulmonary support is needed to maintain the patient's current PaO_2. It is calculated using the following equation:

Mean airway pressure (Paw) $\times FIO_2 \times 100/PaO_2$

A high numerator is indicative of a large amount of alveolar oxygen support, and a low denominator indicates poor tissue oxygenation. Taken together, the higher the OI, the worse is a patient's ability to oxygenate despite high levels of support. An OI at 20 is a concern (11–13) and warrants transfer of a patient with CDH to a center capable of offering ECMO or inhaled nitric oxide (iNO). An OI of greater than 40 is an indication to initiate ECMO (12, 14–18).

Pulmonary Hypertension

Increased pulmonary vascular resistance is an almost universal finding in patients with CDH (8). Pulmonary hypertension (PHTN) can be suspected when the preductal oxygen saturation of arterial blood (SpO_2) and postductal SpO_2 show a greater than 10% difference. A preductal SpO_2 is an oxygen saturation taken from an area of the body whose arterial blood supply comes before the ductus arteriosus. The ductus arteriosus connects the aorta and pulmonary artery in fetal life and anatomically sits just after the right subclavian artery branches off of the aortic arch. Preductal areas of the body include the head and the right upper limb; thus, a preductal sample to determine SpO_2 is commonly taken from the right hand. A sample to determine postductal SpO_2 is typically taken from the lower limbs (right or left foot). Of note, an arterial blood gas blood sample taken from any area other than the right hand (including the umbilical artery) is considered to measure postductal blood gas. Pre- and postductal SpO_2 values will differ when right ventricular pressure exceeds left ventricular pressure, thus opening the ductus arteriosus and forcing deoxygenated blood to flow from the pulmonary artery into the aorta. Definitive diagnosis of PHTN should be calculated using echocardiography. A measurement of pulmonary artery pressure is taken and compared to systemic arterial blood pressure. A pulmonary artery pressure that is less than two-thirds of arterial blood pressure is clinically significant for PHTN (19).

Cardiac Insufficiency

Anatomical abnormalities in the thorax and PHTN are both contributing factors to cardiac insufficiency for patients with CDH. Echocardiography can be used to differentiate the causes of decreased cardiac output and heart failure, which can be a common preoperative issue. (20). Low systemic vascular resistance can aggravate PHTN and worsen hypoxemia and further tissue hypoxia as a result of ineffective blood delivery to vital organs.

Management and Treatment

Treatment options are offered to families from the moment that an in utero diagnosis is made. There are prenatal surgical options that may be implemented prior to delivery. If a child with a CDH makes it to delivery, then tailored treatment begins from the moment of birth to minimize lung damage and maximize ventilation and oxygenation. Quick initiation of therapy offers the best chance of survival with minimal long-term sequelae, and it is imperative for health-care teams to have a clear management plan so that they may maximize outcomes.

Prenatal Treatment Options

There are some general guidelines to assist clinicians in prenatal management of CDH, but there is no set standard of care. The first step once definitive diagnosis has been made is to begin counseling with a multidisciplinary team consisting of obstetricians, pediatric surgeons, and neonatologists. All team members should have experience in the management of CDH. Parents should be clearly informed of the potential for a poor outcome for their infant. These outcomes include the following:

• Death
• Neurological defect
• Pulmonary complications
• Gastrointestinal morbidities
• Low quality of life

Optimal prenatal counseling allows parents to anticipate and understand the events that are likely to occur after delivery. It also allows parents the opportunity for informed decision-making regarding termination of pregnancy or prenatal therapy. Care of the mother and fetus should be transferred to a tertiary medical center, and the baby should be delivered at a facility where ECMO is readily available after delivery.

It is difficult to know when prenatal treatment options should be offered. Prenatal options are most frequently aimed at those infants least likely to survive without treatment. Some factors used to make the determination of likelihood for survival are detection of CDH prior to 25 wG, polyhydramnios, presence of the stomach in the thorax, small lung-to-thorax ratio, and heart hypoplasia (14). Another sign that can be associated with outcomes is "liver-down" versus "liver-up" status in CDH. Liver-down denotes a liver that is still contained within the abdomen, whereas liver up denotes a liver that has migrated into the thorax, which is associated with worse outcomes. These have all been reported as potential determining factors for fetal surgery.

The initial prenatal intervention was in utero repair, first attempted in 1984 (21). This was an open fetal operation requiring surgical incisions in the mother's abdomen and uterus, and then in the abdomen and thorax of the fetus. The first successful case using this procedure was reported in 1990 (21), and a prospective randomized study in fetuses with liver-down CDH was started (22). Results showed, however, there was no difference in mortality and morbidity with this procedure when compared to postnatal conventional management, and thus it was not considered favorable as a definitive treatment for CDH.

The next attempted prenatal surgical procedure was the **tracheal occlusion**, where a fetus with CDH has his or her trachea plugged for a period of time to promote lung growth. Through clinical and research observations on animals it was noted that patients with tracheal **atresia** (closure or absence) had lung hyperplasia (23). If occluding the trachea can cause excessive lung tissue growth, perhaps a technique similar to tracheal atresia could be used to promote lung growth. The theory was that during normal fetal development, the lungs produce a continuous flow of fluid that exits the trachea into the amniotic space. In the presence of tracheal obstruction, the lungs grow, and for a fetus with CDH there is gradual return of the herniated intestines back into the abdomen. With tracheal occlusion, fetuses are given a period of intrauterine tracheal occlusion, with the use of vascular clips or a balloon, sufficient to reverse pulmonary hypoplasia, then the occlusion is reversed when lung growth is adequate (20). Although several surgical procedures have been used since the technique was first suggested in 1994, a single surgical technique for tracheal occlusion has not yet been established and randomized clinical trials

---

● **Evidence in Practice 9-1**

Fetoscope Endoluminal Tracheal Occlusion (FETO) (24)

Tracheal occlusion has yet to be proven as an effective treatment for CDH, although it is still offered in a number of hospitals throughout the world. It currently consists of placing and inflating a balloon in utero, which can then be popped when no longer needed. The detachable balloons were originally designed to treat aneurysms, but were found to be useful for treating CDH. Rather than a major surgical procedure, placement of the balloon in the trachea requires a single 10-Fr cannula and a 1.2-mm fetal endoscope under regional anesthesia, and it takes about 20 minutes. LHR was seen to improve when the procedure was complete, and studies show promising results, with some survival rates at 77%. Care is being taken with the use of this method, however, because clinical trials have not been done to prove the efficacy of this surgical procedure, although the surgical technique has been improved over the last decade or so and risk during the procedure has now been minimized. Two randomized control trials that have compared tracheal occlusion to conventional therapy have shown no benefit of surgery over traditional care. It is interesting, however, that the conventional therapy outcomes in these studies have been significantly better than the published retrospective data, and therefore both the surgery and control group have better survival rates than that which was predicted.

have yet to show its benefit over conventional postnatal care (Evidence in Practice 9-1) (25).

Delivery Room Management

In addition to standard neonatal resuscitation, some additional steps need to be taken when a CDH is suspected. Respiratory distress should always be anticipated. The pulmonary involvement of this disease gives newborns very small pulmonary reserve, so respiratory distress will occur early and patients will deteriorate rapidly. The delivery room team should prepare for immediate intubation prior to signs of hypoxia and hypercarbia (Teamwork 9-1). Bag-mask ventilation should be avoided to prevent air inadvertently being forced into the stomach and intestines, which would further compress the lung tissue and exacerbate respiratory distress. Intubation should be performed by someone proficient in the procedure to avoid an inadvertent esophageal intubation. In addition to early intubation, a nasogastric tube should be placed in the patient in the delivery room to remove any gastric air that may impede lung inflation. Because there is a high likelihood for patients with CDH to develop PHTN, an FIO_2 of 1 should be used during ventilation (Box 9-1).

Teamwork 9-1 Ten Seconds for 10 Minutes (26)

After 10 years of observation at the Tuebingen Center for Patient Safety and Simulation (TuPASS), instructors found that good healthcare teams made errors when they felt themselves to be under considerable pressure. The team felt if they did not do something quickly, the patient would die. Unfortunately, it often meant the team worked too quickly, making errors in decisions or execution and compromising patient safety. This is known as a speed/accuracy trade off, or "hurry up syndrome." If just a bit more time was taken by the team, patients would be safer because fewer errors would be made. Successful patient management relies not only on identification of the problem, but also on accurate assessment of the level of risk and time available. For patients whom you suspect you may need to resuscitate, taking a few seconds as a team to quickly agree on a plan of action for the next 10 minutes of emergency will allow everyone on the team to understand the primary problem, clarify facts, focus efforts, determine roles, and accept specific responsibilities during emergency management. It also gives each team member a chance to ask for clarification regarding diagnosis, time line for action, responsibilities, and resource needs.

Box 9-1 Delivery Room Management of Patients with CDH

Anticipate respiratory distress
Early intubation by a skilled clinician
No mask ventilation
Place nasogastric tube
Use 1 FIO_2

■ ■ The delivery room team meets for 10 minutes after you finish receiving the report. The attending physician assigns roles for the team: She will intubate immediately after delivery. You will be responsible for placing a pulse oximeter and managing ventilation and oxygenation after intubation. The nurse in attendance will monitor heart rate and activity, and a neonatal nurse practitioner will be an extra set of hands to place an umbilical line and deliver medications if needed.

You are called to Mrs. Hendrick's delivery room, and BG Hendricks is born 3 minutes after the team's arrival. The attending physician takes about 15 seconds to intubate, announcing "the tube passed through the vocal cords." You begin manual ventilation at 1 FIO_2 with a T-piece resuscitator at a PIP of 20 cm H_2O and observe chest rise over the left side, with minimal chest rise on the right. The nurse taps out a heart rate (HR) of 120 beats per minute (bpm). You see BG Hendricks take a few gasping breaths, but otherwise she is making little spontaneous movement. At 1 minute of the baby's life, you assess her to have acrocyanosis; she is limp and making a respiratory effort of less than 10 breaths/min; HR is 140 bpm; and she does not respond to stimulation. You continue ventilation, and the nurse practitioner prepares the transport isolette for the trip to the NICU. After placing BG Hendricks in the isolette, you push it over so her mother can see her, then you continue ventilation during the transport to the NICU.

Definitive diagnosis of CDH is made with a chest and abdominal radiograph (Fig. 9-3) showing bowel loops in the stomach and mediastinal shift.

Preoperative Management

The initial strategy for CDH management was immediate surgical intervention after birth, but the 1990s saw a shift to delayed operative management, with a focus on stabilization of cardiopulmonary systems preoperatively to improve mortality (27). One of the primary reasons for the shift in management from early to late surgical intervention is the understanding that "pulmonary hypoplasia and pulmonary hypertension caused by CDH represent a physiological emergency, not a surgical one" (7). Neither of these physiological findings is resolved by repairing the hernia, and thus the timing of repair is inconsequential to resolution of lung dysfunction.

The focus of preoperative management now is on hemodynamic stabilization and respiratory support, with avoidance of hypoxemia and acidemia and minimization of **iatrogenic** lung injury (lung injury caused by medical interventions, such as mechanical ventilation). This shift in the focus of care management to preoperative stabilization and delayed surgical repair is one of the biggest causes of the improved CDH survival rate for patients who did not undergo fetal intervention (28).

Previous Ventilation Strategies

Prior to the 1990s, the accepted method to treat PHTN and hypoxemia in CDH was chemical- and ventilator-induced alkalosis (17), with the goal of decreasing right-to-left shunting across the ductus arteriosus by decreasing pulmonary vascular resistance and pulmonary artery pressures. This usually meant hyperventilation and hyperoxygenation, with goal $PaCO_2$ values at less than 40 mm Hg and PaO_2 greater than 100 mm Hg. Postmortem data showed that 91% of patients with CDH who died had ventilator-induced lung injury (VILI) (9), which helped the neonatal community recognize the damage the then-current model of ventilation caused. VILI can also start a systemic inflammatory response similar to acute respiratory distress syndrome (ARDS), which can lead to multisystem organ failure (28). VILI can be caused by several mechanisms, including barotrauma, volutrauma, and atelectrauma. These are facilitated by the selection of excessive pressures, which overdistend the functional alveoli and cause parenchymal damage.

Conventional Ventilation

The method of mechanical ventilation that has been accepted as standard for CDH patients was termed "gentle ventilation" in 1985 (29). Many studies that were conducted and published in the 1990s and early 2000s to assess the effectiveness of gentle ventilation techniques were summarized in a 2007 publication (30). There are no national or international standards for what "gentle ventilation" entails, but several, more recent studies have suggested conventional ventilator settings and clinical targets (2, 11, 13, 15, 17, 19, 20, 31–35). Therapists should familiarize themselves with institutional preferences or standards for gentle ventilation.

- Peak inspiratory pressure (PIP) limitations seem to be one of the most accepted parameters to monitor and adjust to minimize VILI, although the maximum PIP may vary from institution to institution. Several studies have published promising results with a recommended pressure limit of less than 25 cm H_2O (13, 12, 36) or less than 26 mm Hg (35). One CDH treatment protocol recommends adjusting PIP to maintain $PaCO_2$ at 45 to 60 mm Hg (13) and another suggests $PaCO_2$ at less than 65 mm Hg (35).

  Of importance, most studies suggest a postductal pH greater than 7.2 (12) or 7.25 (11, 16, 35). One study in particular noted that the creation of target blood gases was associated with improved survival of CDH, though the blood gas targets were not consistent between study subjects. This suggests that it is the act of selecting and targeting the blood gas values that may improve outcomes and not necessarily the specific numerical values chosen (31).
- Peak end expiratory pressure (PEEP) has been suggested to stay in normal physiological range (4 to 6 cm H_2O) (16), or more specifically at 5 cm H_2O (11).
- **Normoxemia** has been suggested despite the presence of PHTN, which often responds favorably to hyperoxemia. Published data on oxygen targets suggest the following:
  - Preductal PaO_2 at greater than 90 mm Hg (when available) (15)
  - Postductal PaO_2 at 40 to 80 mm Hg (11)
  - Preductal SpO_2 at 85% to 95% (13), 90% to 98% (11)
  - Postductal SpO_2 at greater than 70% (13)
  - PEEP at 2 to 5 or less than 5 cm H_2O
- Frequency has been less specifically suggested in protocols because it has less of an effect on

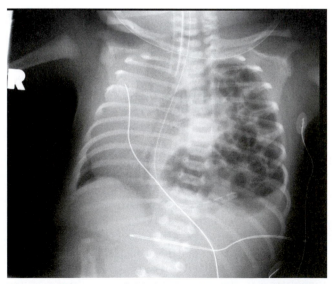

Figure 9-3 Chest and Abdominal Radiograph Showing a CDH

VILI if pressure and volume are maintained at appropriate levels. One protocol study used a range of 40 to 60 breaths/min. (13)

- Inspiratory time has also been suggested to stay at a 0.30 to 0.40 second range in at least one study (16).

Failure of conventional mechanical ventilation (CMV) is a clear indication for either high-frequency ventilation or ECMO. Failure of CMV has been suggested as:

- Requiring a PIP greater than 26 cm H_2O or Paw greater than 12 cm H_2O to achieve a $PaCO_2$ less than 65 mm Hg (16)
- Postductal PaO_2 less than 30 mm Hg (35)
- Inability to maintain pH greater than 7.25 despite reaching all maximal limits of therapy (11, 16, 35)

High-Frequency Ventilation

There is no consensus on whether high-frequency ventilation (HFV) should be used proactively as the primary and initial mode of ventilation or as a rescue therapy when traditional pressure-limited ventilation fails (15). Because HFV allows for less than dead-space tidal volumes at rates of 180 to 900 per minute, it avoids both over- and underventilation and should decrease the risk of VILI. One study showed data that suggest that in facilities without the availability of ECMO, high-frequency oscillatory ventilation (HFOV) with iNO increases survival over conventional ventilation and systemic vasodilation (33).

Several studies suggest the following approximate starting settings for HFOV:

- Mean airway pressure (Paw) should be 13 to 16 cm H_2O (18, 21, 37).
- Amplitude (ΔP) should be 30 to 45 cm H_2O (18, 37). Amplitude should be adjusted to maintain CO_2 values within the desired range.
- Hertz has been recommended to be between 10 and 15 (18, 20).

One prospective study used high-frequency jet ventilation (HFJV) as the rescue mode of ventilation for patients with CDH who failed conventional ventilation. HFJV was chosen because it has been shown in other patient populations to improve cardiovascular parameters, specifically pulmonary vascular resistance, more effectively than conventional ventilation or HFOV (16). Several studies have also shown that HFJV requires lower mean airway pressures than conventional ventilation and HFOV to achieve the same arterial blood gas values (38).

Surfactant

When compared with healthy neonates, the chemical composition of surfactant for infants with CDH who

---

■ ■ BG Hendricks is admitted to the NICU, and a weight of 3.1 kg is obtained. You begin ventilation at SIMV PIP of 20 cm H_2O, PEEP of 5 cm H_2O, respiratory rate of 30 breaths/min, inspiratory time (T_I) of 0.35 seconds, and an FIO_2 of 1. Preductal and postductal SpO_2 are 99% and 96%, respectively. Exhaled tidal volumes range from 11 to 14 mL. Noninvasive blood pressure is 55/32 mm Hg. You obtain a preductal blood gas sample from the right radial artery (7.30/42/90/20.4) while the physician places an umbilical artery catheter and obtains a postductal blood gas sample (7.29/44/60/20.9).

You maintain your current ventilator settings while awaiting a chest radiograph (CXR) and echocardiogram results for evidence of PHTN.

---

are on mechanical ventilation has been found to be "grossly abnormal" (39). The composition of alveolar type II cells may also be abnormal, which can affect the production of surfactant (40). There are several potential factors that may contribute to surfactant dysfunction in patients with CDH:

- Lung hypoplasia
- Primary surfactant deficiency—the lung produces less surfactant than does a healthy neonate
- Changes in surfactant composition as a direct result of VILI
- Decreased surfactant production in alveoli as a result of HFOV because the alveoli do not actively stretch during oscillation, which is a normal mechanism to stimulate surfactant production (39)

Despite the theoretical foundations for surfactant therapy for neonates with a CDH, no studies have been able to show its effectiveness in improving survival rates (41, 42). However, one 15-year retrospective study from 2006 found surfactant therapy used for 768 patients with CDH prior to cannulation for ECMO (42). This is evidence that surfactant is still a considered therapy, although it does not appear to be a primary choice for improving lung function. It is generally agreed that there is no benefit to exogenous surfactant therapy for full-term CDH (41). However, surfactant replacement therapy should be considered for preterm neonates (less than 34 wG at birth) with evidence of hyaline membrane disease, either manifesting as atelectasis or a ground-glass RDS appearance on chest radiograph (11, 14), and who those require high FIO_2 to maintain PaO_2 greater than 60 mm Hg (18).

Pulmonary Vasodilators

According to Logan and colleagues, "The most significant clinical dilemma continues to be the appropriate approach to pulmonary hypertension (PHTN) in CDH infants" (17). Lung hypoplasia and hypoxemia found in patients with CDH make them highly susceptible to PHTN. Neonates with CDH may also have functional pulmonary vascular abnormalities that prevent the natural decrease in pulmonary vascular resistance after birth (8). Their pulmonary vascular beds also do not seem to respond to vasodilators as do typically developed lungs (8).

The most commonly used vasodilator in use is iNO. It is a selective pulmonary vasodilator, meaning that it will dilate only the pulmonary vascular bed adjacent to the functioning alveoli. The half-life of iNO is less than 5 seconds, which makes it very unlikely to have an effect on the systemic vasculature. This makes it particularly useful for the treatment of PHTN in patients who have poor systemic vascular resistance because it will not cause a systemic vasodilation and a consequential drop in systemic blood pressure. Studies of iNO use in CDH patients, however, have failed to show consistent improvement in PHTN (17, 19). In the largest iNO randomized control trial to date, there was no difference in mortality rate or ECMO use over the control group for infants with CDH treated with iNO (43). Some studies have shown an early acute improvement in PHTN and oxygenation after initiation of iNO, but that is often transient (17). With PHTN being such a significant contributor to morbidity and mortality, iNO is still frequently ordered and used in CDH, without the evidence of consistent effectiveness. Treatment with iNO should be considered for persisting signs of PHTN, as seen by an oxygen index of equal to or greater than 20 or a difference in pre- and postductal SpO_2 of equal to or greater than 10% (13). Inhaled nitric oxide should be started at 20 parts per million (ppm) for all patients with echocardiographic evidence of PHTN (18), and responsiveness should be assessed in the same manner (8). The expected response would be some reduction in right ventricular pressure, not a complete resolution of PHTN (17, 37), and treatment can be suspected with an increase in postductal SpO_2 of greater than 10% (8). If responsiveness is seen, then therapy should continue. Right ventricular pressures should be assessed serially using echocardiography.

For patients who do not respond to iNO, other pulmonary vasodilators have been used empirically, and their use has not been validated in clinical trials of patients with CDH. They are mentioned here as possible treatments when attempting to wean patients from iNO, with recurrence of PHTN, or when reaching a chronic phase of PHTN.

It is possible that combinations of these drugs may be more effective than one particular agent. The following drugs are not as selective to pulmonary vasculature and thus could cause systemic vasodilation, which will further complicate cardiovascular management.

- *Sildenafil* is a type 5 phosphodiesterase (PDE) inhibitor, which has been used to treat PHTN in adults and children with congenital heart disease (Box 9-2). It has been used orally for CDH patients who do not respond to iNO or who have reached a chronic phase of PHTN (8, 13). It has a half-life of 4 hours, making it a more long-lasting medication and increasing the risk for systemic vasodilation.
- *Prostacyclin* is a potent vasodilator that can be given intravenously, orally, subcutaneously, or through a nebulizer. Nebulized prostacyclin delivers the medication directly to the lungs and is more likely to affect the pulmonary vasculature than the systemic vasculature. It has a half-life of 42 seconds, which may allow for less systemic response.
- Other recommended vasodilators if iNO is unsuccessful include bosentan and dipyridamole (8).

Inotropes

Placement of an umbilical artery catheter allows continuous blood pressure management and facilitates frequent arterial blood gas sampling. Systemic blood pressure should be maintained above 50 mm Hg. This will prevent tissue hypoxia caused by decreased perfusion and also minimize right-to-left shunting of blood seen with PHTN by not allowing left heart pressures to become lower than right heart pressures. If systemic pressure falls consistently below 50 mm Hg, treatment should include the following:

- Isotonic fluids such as normal saline or lactated Ringer's solution
- **Inotropes** (agents that improve cardiac contractility), such as dopamine and dobutamine, up to a maximum of 10 mcg/kg/min (18, 20, 36)
- Minimizing diuretic use, which decreases blood volume and consequentially blood pressure
- Daily echocardiography to monitor PHTN and direct right and left heart pressures

Analgesia and Paralysis

Because pain can cause hypoxemia and hypotension in patients who are critically ill and have little pulmonary reserve, analgesia is a common regimen for CDH patients in hypoxemic respiratory failure. Pain management varies among institutions, and the standard treatment protocol should be used in CDH patients. Several studies have recommended fentanyl at 2 to 5 mcg/kg or midazolam drips at 60 mcg/kg/hour (18, 20).

Treatment for patients on HFV can also include paralysis, although there is no consensus for recommending this therapy. For those who have published studies of this type of treatment, it is recommended as a bolus therapy as needed when respiratory resistance or "fighting" the ventilator is assumed to be causing episodes of hypoxemia. The recommended therapies have been pancuronium or vecuronium at 0.1 mg/kg (18, 20).

■ ■ BG Hendricks' postductal SpO$_2$ decreases to 82% (preductal was 96%), so fentanyl is started at 2 mcg/kg. An echocardiogram shows an arterial systolic pressure of 55 mm Hg, and the pulmonary systolic pressure is 40 mm Hg, which the cardiologist agrees are sufficient for a diagnosis of PHTN. Inhaled nitric oxide is ordered, and after setting it up and calibrating, you initiate therapy at 20 ppm. Pre- and postductal SpO$_2$ increase to 100%, so FIO$_2$ is weaned over the next 6 hours to maintain the postductal PaO$_2$ at 60 to 80 mm Hg.

ECMO

The first CDH survivor treated with ECMO was reported in 1977 (44). In a retrospective study from the Extracorporeal Life Support Organization database, from 1991 to 2006, a total of 4,115 neonates required ECMO for CDH (45), and ECMO was used as a rescue therapy when other interventions failed in up to 20% to 40% of cases. As pre-ECMO treatments such as HFOV and iNO have advanced, the incidence of ECMO use has decreased. One study found that the incidence of ECMO for CDH patients in 1998 was 18.2%, and by 2006 it had dropped to 11.4% (42).

ECMO is used to support oxygenation and allow for cardiovascular rest until surgery is possible, but is not a definitive treatment for CDH. Several criteria for ECMO initiation have been suggested and are summarized below (11, 13, 18):

- OI greater than 40 for greater than or equal to 4 hours
- PaO$_2$ less than 50 mm Hg on FIO$_2$ 1.0
- Preductal SpO$_2$ less than 85% or postductal SpO$_2$ less than 70%
- pH less than 7.15 and increase in CO$_2$ despite PIP greater than 28 cm H$_2$O (conventional ventilation) or Paw greater than 17 cm H$_2$O

1. Preservation of the ligation of the carotid artery
2. Selective perfusion of the pulmonary vasculature with enriched oxygenated blood
3. Delivery of oxygenated blood to the coronary arteries
4. Preservation of pulsatile blood flow
5. Decreased incidence of cardiac stun
6. Minimization of embolic risks to the brain

- Increase in blood lactate levels with pH less than 7.15 as evidence of cellular anaerobic metabolism because of tissue hypoxia
- Decrease in urine output

When initiated on ECMO, the majority of CDH patients (82%) are cannulated with venous-arterial (VA) cannulas (42). This allows full cardiopulmonary support; however, there is no compelling evidence that this method improves outcomes. Venovenous (VV) ECMO has advantages over VA ECMO (Box 9-3), but the use of one method has not been proven to improve mortality or risk of chronic lung disease.

Some institutions will allow surgical repair while the patient remains on ECMO support. However, many hospitals and surgical teams will delay repair until ECMO has been discontinued so the patient has better cardiac function and is no longer on large doses of heparin therapy. Heparin, which is required with ECMO, increases the risk for bleeding during and after surgery.

Surgical Management

Historically, it was believed that rushing to reduce the hernia and relieve lung compression would offer the best chance for patient survival. Evidence showed that this strategy worked for a brief period, and then high pulmonary vascular resistance would cause progressively worse hypoxemia and respiratory deterioration. The current patient management strategy is to allow a period of preoperative stabilization and delay surgical repair, waiting days or even weeks. Specific patient presurgical goals include the following (11, 18, 20):

- Radiographic clearing of lung fields
- Resolution of right-to-left shunting across PDA as a sign of improved PHTN
- Right ventricular pressures less than 2/3 of systemic pressures, with good right ventricular function on echocardiography

- Systemic blood pressure greater than 60 mm Hg consistently over previous 12 hours
- Stable urination of greater than 1 mL/kg/hr over previous 12 hours
- Tidal volume (V_T) greater than 4 mL/kg with PIP less than or equal to 25 cmH$_2$O and PEEP less than 5 cmH$_2$O
- Optimal ABG values were reached with FIO$_2$ less than 0.40 for at least the previous 24 hours.

Primary Repair Versus Reconstruction

The most commonly used surgical technique is an open laparotomy, involving a subcostal (below the rib cage) incision (27), although up to 21% of neonatal centers performing CDH repair have begun to use a minimally invasive surgery laparoscopic repair (27). In either technique, the abdominal contents are excised (removed) from the thoracic cavity, and the hernia is closed. If there is enough diaphragm muscle tissue, the defect can be closed primarily with a nonabsorbable suture. If there is not enough diaphragm to accomplish a primary repair, reconstruction with nearby musculature can be accomplished. If there is likelihood for postoperative ECMO, then nearby

musculature is contraindicated because of the risk of postoperative bleeding. A prosthetic material, such as Gortex, can be used for reconstruction and is preferred by most surgeons (Fig. 9-4) (7).

Closure of the abdominal wall after repair can result in very high intra-abdominal pressures, and surgeons may close the skin after surgery without closing the abdominal wall musculature; or, a silo (described in the following section on gastroschisis) can be used, and the contents of the abdominal cavity can be reduced into the abdomen over several days. Air may be seen in the pleural cavity on chest radiographs because of lung hypoplasia, but it does not need to be evacuated. Chest tubes are not routinely used, except for active thoracic bleeding or uncontrolled air leak from barotrauma.

Postoperative Management

Postoperative management of patients with CDH includes stabilization of the pulmonary and cardiovascular system, pain management, prevention of infection, and assessment of gastrointestinal function. Despite reduction of the abdominal contents, the pathophysiology of the lungs (lung hypoplasia and PHTN) remains, and cardiopulmonary management will continue with the same goals as presurgical management.

Weaning of mechanical ventilation is gradual, and the course will be determined based on clinical data such as exhaled tidal volumes, blood gas measurements, and spontaneous ventilatory effort. The removal of the abdominal contents will eradicate the mechanical compression of the lungs, and some improvement in ventilation should be seen. Serial chest radiographs will be useful in monitoring the growth of the lungs within the thoracic cavity and the return of the mediastinum to midline.

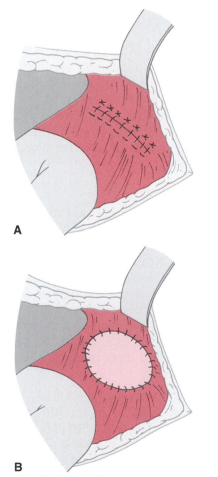

A

B

Figure 9-4 Surgical Repair of Diaphragmatic Hernia

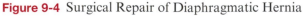

■ ■ BG Hendricks is maintained on dopamine, iNO, and conventional ventilation until day 9, when she is successfully weaned from inotropic therapy. On day 11, her iNO therapy is weaned and discontinued. Surgical repair is completed on day 16, and a primary closure with her own diaphragm muscle and sutures is performed. BG Hendricks returns to the NICU and begins postoperative ventilation at assist control (A/C) PIP, 22 cm H$_2$O; PEEP, 5 cm H$_2$O; respiratory rate, 30 breaths/min; and FIO$_2$, 1.0, to be weaned to maintain PaO$_2$ greater than 60 to 80 mm Hg.

Management of analgesia and the cardiovascular system should continue based on presurgical goals, with special attention paid to postoperative fluid management and the additional risk of bleeding.

Course and Prognosis

Survival rates for CDH vary widely, depending on the patient populations studied. If stillbirths are included in incidence and mortality rates, they are considered to be much higher than the current survival rate averages. Overall survival rates for live-born infants seem to range from 60% to 68% (46, 47), with some high-volume centers reaching survival rates as high as 90% (35). About 95% of those intrauterine deaths with CDH have major associated anomalies, most commonly cardiac, neural tube, and gastrointestinal (48). Infants with liver in the thoracic cavity have shown a survival rate of about 50% (21). Patients treated with ECMO survive at lower rates, which range from 46% to 67% (7, 47, 49, 50) (Special Populations 9-1).

Most patient deaths are associated with a combination of chronic parenchymal lung disease and PHTN (11). Even in survivors there seems to be a long-term risk of pulmonary disease, manifesting as wheezing episodes and pulmonary function results that are lower than predicted values (51). There is no consistency in study results to predict whether survivors will have restrictive, obstructive, or mixed lung disease.

The incidence of recurrence of the hernia is rare, with a range of 1.7% to 8.8% based on the type of surgical approach (27), but carries a potential risk that can occur months to years after the initial repair. The most important predictive factor is whether the defect was large and needed a patch to repair it. (51)

More than half of CDH survivors have gastrointestinal dysfunction, including gastroesophageal reflux disease (GERD) and foregut **dysmotility** (abnormality of smooth muscle function in gastrointestinal tract) (52). GERD has been seen in 22% to 81% of CDH survivors (53), and infants with patch repair are at higher risk than those with primary closures. GERD can cause aspiration and worsen pulmonary morbidity, and medical management mainly consists of antireflux medications. Esophageal motor function is usually preserved in CDH survivors despite the wide range of esophageal acid exposure in early infancy. Those with symptomatic GERD have been shown to outgrow it, unless it has been associated with advanced respiratory distress or neurological impairment (54).

Close nutritional monitoring is also needed to maximize growth for CDH survivors. Many infants with CDH fail to grow as well as healthy infants; one study showed that more than 40% have weights below the fifth percentile at 2 years of age (41). Factors for this include the following:

- Oral aversion
- Gastroesophageal reflux
- Poor oral feeding skills

Neurologically, CDH survivors are at a significantly high risk for delays and disorders. These include neurocognitive delay, delays in reaching developmental milestones, behavioral disorders, and hearing loss. The exact cause for the increased incidence is unclear, and it appears that the use of ECMO may contribute to an increased incidence (55). A literature review has suggested several possible causes for neurological delays (54):

- An intrinsic neurological abnormality
- Greater number and severity of morbidities that impair development in infants who require ECMO
- Greater number of ECMO-associated complications

● Special Populations 9-1

CDH in Prematurity (25)

Prematurity is the strongest influence on poor outcomes for all neonatal diseases. A database review found 30% of patients with CDH were premature, and they had a nearly 50% decrease in survival compared with term infants with CDH. Certain therapies such as ECMO and iNO are not established therapies in premature infants, although they are a mainstay of therapy for CDH. Premature infants may be more likely to require patch repair to close their defect, which puts them at additional risk for complications such as reherniation. However, even though survival of preterm infants born with CDH is lower compared with their term counterparts, overall survival is still greater than 50%, with approximately 31% survival of the infants less than or equal to 28 weeks estimated gestational age. Their high rate of associated anomalies may be responsible for this increased mortality, as well as their being ineligible for ECMO based on size limitations. Survival for premature infants depends on disease severity, comorbidities such as hyaline membrane disease, and efficacy of other therapeutic interventions. After adjusting for these factors, preterm infants still have increased odds of death.

■■ BG Hendricks continues on mechanical ventilation until day 38, when she is weaned and extubated to a high-flow nasal cannula at 6 LPM at FIO$_2$ 0.40. Three days after extubation she is weaned to a nasal cannula (NC) at 1 LPM and started on albuterol every 6 hours as needed for wheezing. She is being evaluated now for GERD. She is scheduled for hearing and vision assessments prior to discharge, and she will require an apnea monitor and gavage feeding at home.

Sensorineural hearing loss has been reported in 26% to 49% of CDH survivors (55). Hearing assessments are recommended, but the cause of hearing dysfunction is unclear. Contributing factors have included the duration of mechanical and HFOV, use of pancuronium for paralysis, and loop diuretic use.

Gastroschisis

Gastroschisis is an abdominal wall defect characterized by protrusion of the intestines through the abdominal wall not covered by amnion (Fig. 9-5). It is most commonly found on the right side of the umbilicus, occurring there 95% of the time. Occasionally, abdominal contents other than intestines, such as the liver or gall bladder, can be seen. It is likely that the cause of this defect is from a combination of genetic and environmental factors. The induction of the defect probably occurs between the end of the third week of gestation and end of the fourth week of gestation (56), with the defect developing between weeks 3 and 8 of gestation. There is a low risk of associated defects, and only 1.2% of infants with gastroschisis have chromosomal abnormalities (56), making this defect one that normally occurs in isolation.

The most current incidence rate of gastroschisis is 3.3 per 10,000 births (56). Unlike most congenital defects, the incidence of gastroschisis has increased 10-fold to 20-fold in the United States in recent years (57). Chabra and colleagues in Washington State showed an average increase of 10% annually between 1987 and 2006 (58). It has also been shown to have higher prevalence in regional areas and potentially a higher likelihood of recurrence in families (59). It is unclear exactly why this is, but several risk factors (listed below) have been suggested based on preliminary and early studies. Survival to reproductive age is more common, allowing for future assessment of familial links to this disease.

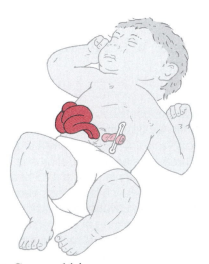

Figure 9-5 Gastroschisis

There is an established risk factor for maternal age younger than 20 years (56). This is the only well-established risk factor. Many of the studies assessing additional risk factors focus on subsets of the young maternal age groups, such as the following:

- Cigarette smoking, which increases carbon monoxide exposure and is associated with increased risk of gastroschisis, particularly in young mothers
- Malnourishment in young mothers, which has been associated with increased risk of gastroschisis, whereas high body mass index (BMI) has been associated with a lower risk (60)
- Recreational drug use in general, and methamphetamines specifically, which have both been associated as increasing the risk of gastroschisis (61, 62)
- White or Hispanic mothers, who are at higher risk than African American mothers (58, 63)

One study showed that infants of young mothers who complained of chest colds and sore throats in the first few weeks of pregnancy were at an increased risk of having gastroschisis (61). This suggests that early maternal infection may play a part in development.

Pathophysiology

Gastroschisis occurs when the umbilical cavity within the abdomen fails to form. The expanding gut is not contained in the peritoneal cavity and herniates, usually to the right of the umbilicus. It is unclear why the abdominal wall weakness is usually found on the right side, but in only 5% of cases is the herniation found on the left.

There is uncertainty about the cause of gastroschisis and its development in utero. There are several theories circulating about the embryological cause of this defect, without sufficient evidence to support any one theory. Traditionally, gastroschisis was thought of as a **disruption** in fetal development, meaning it was abnormally produced after normal development of the abdominal structures and wall. Now the assumption is that it is a **malformation**, meaning it abnormally occurs during early embryologic development (64). It is frequently thought to be vascular in origin and to be the malfunction or reabsorption of one of the fetal or embryonic vessels that causes a weakness in the right side of the abdominal wall, allowing for herniation. The two vessels considered are the umbilical vein and the yolk sac artery. Not enough evidence exists, however, to make a definitive determination of either of these as the cause. Another hypothesis is that during early embryologic development the lateral body-wall folds fail to close at the midline of the abdomen, leaving a hole where herniation can occur. The size of the hole determines the extent of the defect.

Clinical Manifestations

Diagnosis of gastroschisis is normally made during fetal ultrasound around week 20, depending on the size of the defect. At delivery the defect is obvious, as seen in Figure 9-5. It can be distinguished easily from omphalocele (discussed in the next section) because a gastroschisis is not covered by any membrane or fluid, whereas the omphalocele is located within the umbilicus, and is encapsulated in the umbilical sheath.

Intestines located outside of the abdominal wall are sensitive to various insults. Bowel damage occurs in utero because of exposure to amniotic fluid and constriction at the abdominal wall. Delivery can cause further complications by causing the following:

- **Volvulus**: twisting of the bowel on itself, causing obstruction
- Intestinal atresia: closure of part of the intestine
- Bowel **perforation**: formation of a hole in the large intestine; this portion of bowel will need **resection** (cut off or cut out a portion of organ)
- Bowel **necrosis**: death of bowel tissue; this portion of bowel will also need to be resected (65)

Affected infants frequently lose water through the exposed bowel, causing electrolyte imbalances and metabolic acidosis. Intestinal atresia, which is also a common occurrence, can cause bowel obstruction.

Management and Treatment

At delivery, the resuscitation team should immediately place the newborn in a sterile drawstring bag, known as a bowel bag, up to the axillae. This will protect the bowel from contamination or infection and prevent evaporative fluid loss. The GI tract should also be decompressed in the delivery room using a nasogastric tube to minimize distention and potential injury. Other resuscitative efforts should be focused on normal transition to extrauterine life. Temperature regulation is important because the increased intestinal surface area exposed to the environment makes these patients susceptible to hypothermia. To keep the intestines from drying out, a dry or moist protective dressing should be applied and then wrapped in cellophane. This will also prevent evaporative heat loss. Broad-spectrum antibiotics are necessary because contamination of the intestines must be assumed. Intravenous nutritional support must be given until the intestines begin normal function, as evidenced by peristalsis and appropriate absorption. This will not occur until after complete surgical repair. At this point enteral feeding can begin.

Once the infant is settled in the NICU, operative repair must begin. There is not yet an optimal surgical management protocol designated for patients with need of gastroschisis reduction. Treatment options are aimed at reducing the viscera back to the abdominal cavity and closing the abdominal wall defect. This can be accomplished with either a primary closure or staged closure, meaning it will take one or several surgical procedures to complete.

A primary closure is associated with the best outcomes, but is not always possible. An uncomplicated gastroschisis (one without volvulus, atresia, perforation, or necrosis) may qualify for a primary closure. It often is performed at the bedside in a NICU under sedation and paralysis. At this point, patients will be intubated and placed on mechanical ventilation. The mechanical ventilation course will be based on the presence of any pulmonary disease and severity of thoracic impairment. The aim of mechanical ventilation is to provide support during the surgical resection and to overcome newly decreased thoracic compliance. Atelectasis should be prevented when the abdomen pushes the diaphragm up and decreases functional residual capacity. Primary closure during a bowel resection will cause the intestines and other abdominal contents to elevate the diaphragm, anatomically decreasing thoracic cavity space. This can cause increased work of breathing, elevate PIPs on the mechanical ventilator, and decrease delivered tidal volume in pressure ventilation. Failure of traditional volume-targeted ventilation may require HFV or nontraditional methods to maintain oxygenation and ventilation in a low compliance state. The respiratory therapist will be responsible for monitoring pressures and delivered volumes. The team must ensure that primary repair does not significantly interfere with ventilation. If it does, then that is an indication for a staged approach.

Staged closure involves the use of a spring-loaded silo (SLS). The silo contains the affected bowel contents and allows for the gradual reduction of visceral contents over the course of several days or weeks. Potential benefits for gradual reduction over primary reduction include the following:

- Fewer days of ventilatory support because the thorax is not impeded by a large, rapid reduction
- Decreased incidence of pulmonary barotrauma
- Shorter time to begin enteral feeding. Patients often initially present with intestinal edema, which prevents enteral feedings. Delayed closure allows earlier resolution of edema and earlier enteral feeding. (66)
- Improved tissue perfusion and improved cosmetic outcome
- Decreased incidence of infectious complications
- Avoidance of emergency surgical intervention (66)

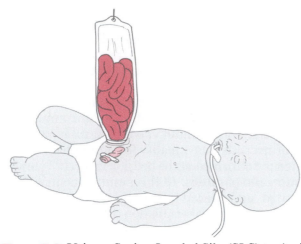

Figure 9-6 Using a Spring-Loaded Silo (SLS) to Assist in Staged Reduction of a Gastroschisis

The silo is sutured to the skin and sits upright from the abdomen (Fig. 9-6). The silo is then tightened sequentially to reduce the viscera until they are contained in the abdominal cavity. A respiratory therapist should be at the bedside during reductions in anticipation of respiratory complications because of pressure on the diaphragm. Once all reductions are complete, closure of the abdominal wall is necessary. If the wall is not large enough to be sutured closed, then a Tegaderm or mesh patch can be used. A sutureless closure is also possible, where the defect is covered with sterile dressings and allowed to heal, and this method has shown similar outcomes when compared to traditional closure techniques (67).

Course and Prognosis

The survival of infants with gastroschisis to discharge and adulthood is increasingly more common. Mortality rates in the United States from 2003 to 2008 were 3.6% (68). Several factors were associated with higher mortality, including large bowel resection, congenital circulatory or pulmonary disease, and bacterial sepsis (68). The most common complication was sepsis, which was diagnosed in 31% of patients. The median length of hospital stay is 35 days, the majority of which will be spent in intensive care. A key identifier of morbidity is the number of days the patient is using mechanical ventilation. This data can be misleading, however, because time between reductions, amount of sedative and paralytic, and ventilator management is not standard between institutions, or even surgeons, within one institution. For instance, one surgeon may require heavy sedation of the patient during the entire course of reduction, which necessitates intubation and ventilation throughout the several-week course. Another surgeon may encourage extubation between reductions or noninvasive management during reductions. Additionally, the rate of premature births with gastroschisis was 57% (69), increasing the likelihood for pulmonary disease and complications as well as other comorbidities associated with prematurity.

Omphalocele

An **omphalocele** is a midline defect with the umbilical cord rising from the middle (Fig. 9-7). The small intestines, liver, and stomach are frequently the herniated organs. An omphalocele is encapsulated by the peritoneal sac, although it is possible for the sac to rupture and thus expose the viscera. Discussions of omphalocele and gastroschisis are often paired together because their clinical course neonatally can be similar. However, their prevalence, causes, pathophysiology, and outcomes are very different. Omphalocele has a known cause, can be a much more significant defect, and has an increased risk for mortality.

Defining the rate of omphalocele is complex because many neonates with this defect do not make it to live delivery. The incidence of omphalocele as diagnosed by second trimester ultrasound is 1 per 1,100 fetuses (70), which drops to approximately 2.5 out of 10,000 births (56). It occurs within the first trimester of fetal development and in 76% of cases had associated abnormalities (71), with cardiac, cranial, and urogenital defects being most common (69). About one-third of fetuses also have trisomy 13 (2%), 18 (20%), or 21 (12%) (69). Premature births occur about 42% of the time, according to one study (70). The incidence of newborns presenting with omphalocele has decreased in recent years. This is most likely due to more prenatal diagnoses and genetic counseling for chromosomal abnormalities that are incompatible with life (71).

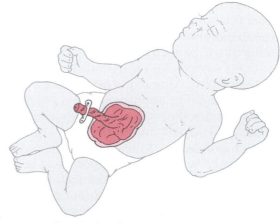

Figure 9-7 Omphalocele

Pathophysiology

There is a period of rapid intestinal growth from weeks 6 to 10 of gestation, and the intestines temporarily herniate into the umbilical cord during this period before migrating back into the peritoneal cavity. Failure of the intestines to make this migration results in an omphalocele (Fig. 9-7). This allows for a large variation in the size of the defect, based on the amount of intestines that fail to migrate. A "giant" omphalocele is loosely defined as being greater than 5 cm in size (70) and contains the liver or a large portion of intestines. The peritoneal cavity of infants with giant omphaloceles is very small because growth has proceeded without the solid organs in the correct position.

Clinical Manifestations

Diagnosis of omphalocele is most often made in utero by about gestational week 18 using fetal ultrasound. The size of the defect is not directly related to the likelihood of associated physical or chromosomal abnormalities. To determine size of the defect, the circumference of the omphalocele and the abdomen are determined and compared. Called the omphalocele circumference/abdominal circumference or OC/AC ratio, a higher ratio is associated with herniation of the liver and an increased risk of respiratory insufficiency at birth. If an amniocentesis is collected, increased levels of alpha fetoprotein are often present.

Management and Treatment

Initial management of a patient with omphalocele at delivery is similar to gastroschisis. Decompression of the GI tract with nasogastric suction should be done, and care must be taken to protect the defect from contamination should the sac rupture. If it is a large defect, it could contain the liver, and care must be taken to avoid hepatic vein injury or liver laceration.

The intact sac of an omphalocele makes it a less urgent surgical problem. The membrane of the sac conserves heat and in many cases allows effective peristalsis, allowing bowel function prior to surgical repair.

The choice of surgical closure is based on the size of the defect. In patients with small defects, a primary closure is feasible. Primary closures are normally associated with lower mortality, less mechanical ventilator time, and earlier return to full feeding with a shorter length of hospital stay (70). If the size of the defect is not amenable to primary closure, then a staged or delayed repair may be necessary. Patients with lower birth weights or who were born prematurely are more likely to have a staged repair.

Staged repairs may include one of several techniques to successfully reduce the omphalocele. An SLS can be used as it is with gastroschisis. Alternatively, the peritoneal sac can be used like a silo to gently reduce the herniated contents over time. Tissue expanders have been used with success (72). Tissue expanders are silicon balloons that are placed under the skin and gradually filled with saline to stretch the abdominal skin and increase space in the abdominal cavity for successful reduction, and they encourage the use of native tissue over synthetic patches.

Repair may be delayed for months or even years, depending on the size of the defect. Delayed closure allows for **epithelialization** (growth of skin) over the sac or cutting away (**excision**) of the sac and closing the defect after infancy. Patients will then be discharged and topical medications will be applied to encourage epithelialization. These may include mercurochrome, povidone-iodine, silver sulfadiazine, and neomycin-bacitracin ointments (70). There is, however, poor definition of when patients should be provided with a staged or delayed repair option, and the number of large or giant omphaloceles is low, making it difficult to create standards for care.

After repair, intragastric and airway pressures should be monitored to minimize damage to either the gastrointestinal or pulmonary systems. Once repair is complete, fluid and electrolyte management can progress to enteral feeds. The role of the respiratory therapist in management of omphalocele is the same as for gastroschisis. Ventilator management will be based on any primary pulmonary deficiency in conjunction with decreases in thoracic compliance. Monitoring of peak pressures and associated tidal volumes are essential to understanding respiratory insufficiency related to omphalocele repair.

Course and Prognosis

Outcomes for omphalocele are poor. In one study, 29% of patients died during the neonatal period, with an additional 14% dying after the neonatal period (71). All deaths in this study were patients with chromosomal or syndromic anomalies. In the same study, only 14% of patients were alive by publication time (71). In another study, the rate of survival to delivery was low. Spontaneous termination rate in this study was 13.5%, with an addition 16% electively terminated because of the unlikelihood of survival (69). In another study, the elective termination rate was 60%, with an additional 15% suffering intrauterine fetal death (71). It is reasonable to assume that the incidence of additional anomalies in this disease increases the mortality rate.

■■■ BG Hendricks was discharged home on day 67 (9 1/2 weeks old). She was feeding via a gastric tube and receiving anti-reflux medications. Her family brings her into the NICU for a social visit after an appointment with the gastrointestinal specialist, when she is about 4 months old. She is still on an NC 1/2 LPM, and her pulmonologist is concerned that she is aspirating gastric secretions in very small quantities when she sleeps; for this reason she will have a sleep study performed in the next month. Despite these struggles, she is gaining weight and is now 5.4 kg, has begun to smile spontaneously, and has begun to sleep in 6-hour stretches at night. Her parents are thrilled with her progress.

■■ Critical Thinking Questions: BB Hendricks

1. Although BG Hendricks was never placed on HFOV, what clinical signs and key interventions would make you consider recommending a switch from conventional to high-frequency ventilation?
2. What clinical signs would you look for when weaning iNO from BG Hendricks that tell you she is having rebound PHTN?
3. How would you expect her pulmonary status to change after her hernia repair?

▶● Case Studies and Critical Thinking Questions

■ Case 1: Baby Boy (BB) Garcia

You are working the night shift in the level IIIB NICU. You are called to the emergency room where a male infant was just born to a 32-year-old female at 39 weeks' gestation. Pregnancy, maternal history, and maternal serologies are unavailable. Mom does not speak English. The baby was delivered by the emergency room physician by precipitous vaginal delivery. Amniotic fluid was clear. The baby is apneic, pale, and limp, and appears to have a scaphoid abdomen. The physician asks you to begin positive-pressure ventilation. Despite appropriate head positioning, placement of a shoulder roll, adequate size and seal of the mask, and good inflation pressures, the physician auscultates diminished breath sounds on the left. Heart sounds are shifted to the right. Heart rate is 80 bpm.

- *What do you suspect is BB Garcia's primary diagnosis?*

- *How would you manage this condition?*
- *What would be reasonable HFOV settings?*

HFOV is started with a Paw of 15 and a CXR is obtained that confirms lung inflation to the eighth rib. Umbilical venous and arterial lines are placed. A fentanyl drip is started, and paralytics are administered. A CXR confirms the team's suspicion of a left CDH. An echocardiogram is ordered and shows elevated right-sided heart pressures. The first arterial blood gas is 7.36/43/32/20/–0.3 on 100% FIO_2. The physician asks you to initiate inhaled nitric oxide as he contacts the nearest ECMO referral center for further management.

- *What is an appropriate starting dose for iNO? What are the team's options if iNO does not work?*
- *What is BB Garcia's oxygen index? Would he be considered a candidate for ECMO?*

Case 2: BB Hathaway

You are preparing for a planned C-section delivery at a level IIIB NICU. Jennifer Hathaway is 16 years old, and this is her first pregnancy. Her pregnancy history is significant for smoking during the first trimester, but she quit around week 11 when she realized she was pregnant. Her parents, with whom she lives, continue to smoke in the house. A 21-week ultrasound showed a ventral wall defect consistent with gastroschisis. Jennifer has met with the neonatologist and a pediatric gastric surgeon and they discussed the care plan once the baby is born.

The decision was made at 38 4/7 weeks gestation to deliver via C-section. A lecithin/sphingomyelin (L/S) ratio was determined to be 2:1.

- *What does an L/S ratio of 2:1 indicate?*

The delivery room team is called to the operating room before the first incision is made. The neonatology fellow is the leader of the team and has decided to accept the baby from the obstetrician upon delivery. She will then step back to manage the baby. The resident is the second physician in attendance and will maintain the sterility of the intestines to minimize contamination. The NICU nurse will place BB Hathaway in the bowel bag after the resident and fellow have a quick initial assessment of the defect. She will then monitor vital signs. Your job will be the initial steps in resuscitation, to include drying, clearing the airway, and stimulation.

The resuscitation goes very smoothly. BB Hathaway makes initial attempts to breathe within the first few seconds of life, and by 1 minute is crying actively. His Apgar score at 1 minute was 7, with

2 points off for color and 1 point off for tone, and the score was 9 at 5 minutes, with one point off for color. In the first minute of life, he was placed in a bowel bag up to his nipples, and his heart rate remained above 130 bpm throughout the resuscitation. He is shown to mom quickly and then transported to the NICU.

The pediatric anesthesiologist and two surgeons are called to the bedside. The surgeons see a large defect with no obvious volvulus, perforations, necrosis, or atresia. The defect is, however, too large for a primary closure, so the anesthesiologist sedates and paralyzes the patient and intubates with a 3.5-cm ETT to prepare for initial reduction and silo placement. He asks you to place the baby on volume-targeted SIMV, with a PIP of 20 cm H_2O, PEEP of 6 cm H_2O, respiratory rate of 20, FIO_2 of 1 during the procedure, and target V_T of 10 mL. The neonatologist and anesthesiologist stay by the bedside while the patient is paralyzed and the SLS is placed. An initial reduction is completed. As the surgeons are reducing the bowel into the abdomen you notice that the ventilator is sounding an alarm for "tube occlusion" and "low volume" with each inspiration.

• *What do you think is happening?*

You relay this information to the anesthesiologist, who verifies that the patient is still paralyzed and notifies the surgeons. They stop the procedure and secure the silo. Concurrently the anesthesiologist gives you an order to increase the PIP to 23 cm H_2O for the duration of the procedure to maintain V_T. Approximately 2 hours after this first reduction you note that the V_T values are now consistently greater than 10 mL, and you request to titrate the PIP back down to 20 cm H_2O.

BB Hathaway requires two more silo reductions over the next 10 days before closure. He remained intubated, sedated, and paralyzed between the first two, but was allowed to wake up and was extubated for 3 days prior to the final reduction and closure. He had to be reintubated, however, for the closure. With each reduction, BB Hathaway required increased ventilator settings, specifically an increase in PIP by 3 to 4 cm H_2O to maintain VT.

• *Should you be concerned with the rapid increase in airway pressures that BB Hathaway must undergo during his silo reductions?*

Serial CXRs did not show any atelectasis after reductions. In each case, you or your coworkers were able to return PIP to baseline within 8 hours. BB Hathaway was in the NICU for an additional 3 weeks while waiting for bowel function to resume, and he was discharged at postnatal week 5

Case 3: BG McShea

You are covering for a coworker while he attends a delivery when you are called to BG McShea's bedside by a nurse for a "ventilator that won't stop alarming." You arrive at BG McShea's bedside and note that she appears to be less than 2 kg and has an SLS attached to the warmer. The ventilator is reading "low tidal volume," and BG McShea does not appear to be moving. You look at the monitor and note that she is saturating 86%. You disconnect the ventilator, begin bag ventilation, and ask the nurse to listen to breath sounds. You obtain minimal chest rise when squeezing the bag at the patient's set PIP (21 cm H_2O), and so increase the pressure until you see visible chest rise. The nurse notes that the breath sounds are diminished in the bases, but clear at the apices. SpO_2 has increased to 98%, so you return BG McShea to the ventilator. The father asks you, "Why is the ventilator alarming?"

• *What additional information do you want to know before answering Dad's question?*

The nurse informs you that a small reduction (BG McShea's third since birth 5 days ago) was performed about an hour ago. The surgeons did it quickly without calling the entire team to the bedside and left immediately after the procedure, signing out to the nurse the amount of bowel reduced and requesting a fentanyl bolus be given, which the nurse gave. A chest and abdominal film was taken about 5 minutes ago. The film shows bilateral basal atelectasis, lung inflation at six ribs' expansion, with the ETT 0.5 cm above the carina.

• *What do you think is the problem, and what plan would you suggest to the neonatologist?*

Multiple-Choice Questions

1. Which of the following ultrasound findings in a fetus with CDH is *not* associated with a poor clinical outcome?
   a. Liver in thorax
   b. Bowel next to heart
   c. LHR of 1
   d. Polyhydramnios

2. Determine which of the following should be part of the delivery room management for a newborn who has been diagnosed with a CDH as a fetus?
   - I. No mask ventilation
   - II. Use 1 FIO_2
   - III. Create a delivery room plan with team
   - IV. Paralytics in the delivery room
   - V. Early intubation
   a. I, II, III
   b. I, II, IV
   c. I, II, III, V
   d. I, II, III, IV, V

3. You have a patient who has been diagnosed with PHTN. Ventilator settings are:
   Mode: SIMV
   PIP: 20 cm H_2O
   PEEP: 5 cm H_2O
   Respiratory rate: 35 breaths/min
   FIO_2: 0.80

   The physician would like to increase ventilator settings to counteract the effect of PHTN on oxygenation and prevent hypoxia. Which of the following ventilator changes would you suggest to achieve his goal?
   a. Increase PIP to 23
   b. Increase rate to 40
   c. Decrease PEEP to 4
   d. Increase FIO_2 to 1

4. Which is not a possible presurgical treatment option for newborns with CDH?
   a. Inhaled nitric oxide
   b. Tracheal occlusion
   c. High-frequency ventilation
   d. Surfactant replacement therapy

5. Calculate the oxygen index (OI) for a patient with the following settings and ABG values:
   HFOV: Paw 25 cm H_2O, amplitude 30 cm H_2O, Hertz 12, I_T 33%
   ABG: 7.20/68/44/26.2. On FIO_2 0.95
   a. 54
   b. 167
   c. 83
   d. 45

6. Which of the following can RTs do to minimize morbidity for CDH patients?
   a. Gentle ventilation
   b. Avoid hypoxemia

   c. Minimize noise at the bedside to prevent hearing dysfunction
   d. Monitor PHTN via pre- and postductal SpO_2
   e. All of the above

7. At what point in embryologic development does gastroschisis form?
   a. 3 to 5 weeks' gestation
   b. 3 to 8 weeks' gestation
   c. 6 to 11 weeks' gestation
   d. By the seventh week of gestation

8. Which of the following are potential risk factors for gastroschisis?
   - I. Maternal age less than 20 years
   - II. High body mass index
   - III. Malnutrition
   - IV. Smoking
   a. I, IV
   b. I, II, IV
   c. I, III
   d. I, III, IV

9. During a primary closure, the RT should monitor the intubated patient for:
   a. Signs of wakefulness or pain.
   b. Tachypnea.
   c. High peak pressures or low tidal volumes.
   d. Low PEEP.

10. Omphalocele develops when portions of the bowel herniate:
    a. To the right of the umbilicus.
    b. Through the diaphragm.
    c. Into the umbilical cord.
    d. To the left of the umbilicus.

11. Which of the following is *not* an anomaly associated with omphalocele?
    a. Trisomy 21
    b. Trisomy 13
    c. Trisomy 18
    d. Trisomy 23

12. Which one of these is *not* a method used to assist in closure of an omphalocele defect?
    a. Tissue expanders
    b. Topical treatment for epithelialization
    c. Primary closure
    d. Genetic counseling

13. The benefits of alveolar surfactant include:
    - I. Lowering surface tension
    - II. Lowering airway resistance
    - III. Preventing alveolar collapse
    - IV. Higher lung compliance
    a. I, II
    b. I, III, IV
    c. I, II, III
    d. II, III, IV

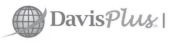 | For additional resources login to Davis*Plus* (http://davisplus.fadavis.com/ keyword "Perretta") and click on the Premium tab. (Don't have a *Plus*Code to access Premium Resources? Just click the Purchase Access button on the book's Davis*Plus* page.)

REFERENCES

1. Keijzer R, Puri P. Congenital diaphragmatic hernia. *Semin Pediatr Surg.* 2010;19:180-185.
2. Vitali SH, Arnold JH. Bench-to-bedside review: ventilator strategies to reduce lung injury—lessons from pediatric and neonatal intensive care. *Crit Care.* 2005;9:177-183.
3. Jesudason EC, Connell MG, Fernig DG, et al. Early lung malformations in congenital diaphragmatic hernia. *J Pediatr Surg.* 2000;35:124-127; discussion, 128.
4. Keijzer R, Liu J, Deimling J, et al. Dual-hit hypothesis explains pulmonary hypoplasia in the nitrogen model of congenital diaphragmatic hernia. *Am J Pathol.* 2000;156: 1299-1306.
5. Adzick NS, Vacanti JP, Lillehei CW, O'Rourke PP, Crone RK, Wilson JM. Fetal diaphragmatic hernia: ultrasound diagnosis and clinical outcome in 38 cases. *J Pediatr Surg.* 1989;124(7):654-658.
6. Hedrick HL, Danzer E, Merchant A, et al. Liver position and lung-to-head ratio for prediction of extracorporeal membrane oxygenation and survival in isolated left congenital diaphragmatic hernia. *Am J Obstet Gynecol.* 2007;197:422.e1-422.e4.
7. Skarsgard ED, Harrison MR. Congenital diaphragmatic hernia: the surgeon's perspective. *Pediatric Rev.* 1999;20: e71-e78.
8. Mohseni-Bod H, Bohn D. Pulmonary hypertension in congenital diaphragmatic hernia. *Semin Pediatr Surg.* 2007;16: 126-133.
9. Sakurai Y, Azarow K, Cutz E, Messineo A, Pearl R, Bohn D. Pulmonary barotrauma in congenital diaphragmatic hernia: a clinicopathological correlation. *J Pediatr Surg.* 1999;34(12):1813-1817.
10. van den Hout L, Reiss I, Felix JF, et al. Risk factors for chronic lung disease and mortality in newborns with congenital diaphragmatic hernia. *Neonatology* 2010;98: 370-380.
11. Antonoff MB, Hustead VA, Groth SS, Schmeling D. Protocolized management of infants with congenital diaphragmatic hernia: effect on survival. *J Pediatr Surg.* 2011;46:39-46.
12. Reiss J, Schaible T, van den Hout L, et al. Standardized postnatal management of infants with congenital diaphragmatic hernia in Europe: the CDH EURO consortium consensus. *Neonatology.* 2010;98:354-364.
13. Van den Hout L, Schaible T, Cohen-Overbeek TEC, et al. Actual outcomes in infants with congenital diaphragmatic hernia: the role of a standardized postnatal treatment protocol. *Fetal Diagn Ther.* 2011;29:55-63.
14. Hedrick HL. Management of prenatally diagnosed congenital diaphragmatic hernia. *Semin Fetal Neonatal Med.* 2010;15:21-27.
15. Jain V, Agarwala S, Bhatnagar S. Recent advances in the management of congenital diaphragmatic hernia. *Indian J Pediatr.* 2010;77:673-679.
16. Kuluz MA, Smith PB, Mears SP, et al. Preliminary observations of the use of high frequency jet ventilation as a rescue therapy in infants with congenital diaphragmatic hernia. *J Pediatr Surg.* 2010;45:698-702.
17. Logan JW, Cotton CM, Goldberg RN, Clark RH. Mechanical ventilation strategies in the management of congenital diaphragmatic hernia. *Semin Pediatr Surg.* 2007;16:115-125.
18. Migliazza L, Bellan C, Alberti D, Auriemma A, Burio G, Locatelli G. Retrospective study of 111 cases of congenital diaphragmatic hernia treated with early high-frequency oscillatory ventilation and presurgical stabilization. *J Pediatr Surg.* 2007;42:1526-1532.
19. Masumoto K, Teshiba R, Esumi G, et al. Improvement in the outcome of patients with antenatally diagnosed congenital diaphragmatic hernia using gentle ventilation and circulatory stabilization. *Pediatric Surg Int.* 2009;25: 487-492.
20. Kitano Y. Prenatal intervention for congenital diaphragmatic hernia. *Semin Pediatr Surg.* 2007;16:101-108.
21. Harrison MR, Adzick NS, Longaker MT, et al. Successful repair in utero of a fetal diaphragmatic hernia after removal of herniated viscera from the left thorax. *N Engl J Med.* 1990;322(22):1582-1584.
22. Harrison MR, Adzick NS, Bullard KM, et al. Correction of congenital diaphragmatic hernia in utero VII: a prospective trial. *J Pediatr Surg.* 1997;32:1637-1642.
23. Wigglesworth JS, Desai R, Hislop AA. Fetal lung growth in congenital laryngeal atresia. *Pediatr Pathol.* 1987;7: 515-525.
24. Depreste JA, Nicolaides K, Gratacos F. Fetal surgery for congenital diaphragmatic hernia is back from never gone. *Fetal Diagn Ther.* 2011;29:6-17.
25. Tsao K, Lally KP. Surgical management of the newborn with congenital diaphragmatic hernia. *Fetal Diagn Ther.* 2011;29:46-54.
26. Rall M, Glavin RJ, Flin R. The '10-seconds-for-10-minutes principle': why things go wrong and stopping them from getting worse. *Bull Roy Coll Anaesthetists.* 2008;51: 2613-2616.
27. De buys Roessingh AS, Dinh-Xuan AT. Congenital diaphragmatic hernia: current status and review. *Eur J Pediatr.* 2009;168:393-406.
28. Ranieri VM, Suter PM, Tortorella C, et al. Effect of mechanical ventilation on inflammatory mediators in patients with acute respiratory distress syndrome: a randomized controlled trial. *JAMA.* 1999:281(1):54-61.
29. Wung JT, James LS, Kilchevsky E, et al. Management of infants with severe respiratory failure and persistence of the fetal circulation, without hyperventilation. *Pediatrics.* 1985;76:488-494.
30. Logan JW, Rice HE, Goldberg RN, Cotton CM. Congenital diaphragmatic hernia: a systematic review and summary of best-evidence practice strategies. *J Perinatol.* 2007;27:535-549.
31. Brindle ME, Ma IWY, Skarsgard ED. Impact of target blood gases on outcome in congenital diaphragmatic hernia (CDH). *Eur J Pediatr Surg.* 2010;20:290-293.
32. Ng GYT, Derry C, Marston L, Choudhury M, Holmes K, Calvert SA. Reduction in ventilator-induced lung injury improves outcome in congenital diaphragmatic hernia. *Pediatric Surg Int.* 2008;24:145-150.

33. Sluiter I, van den Ven CP, Wijnen RMH, Tibboel D. Congenital diaphragmatic hernia: still a moving target. *Semin Fetal Neonatal Med.* 2011;16:139-144.

34. Tracy E, Mears SE, Smith PB, et al. Protocolized approach to management of congenital diaphragmatic hernia: benefits of reducing variability in care. *J Pediatr Surg.* 2010;45:1343-1348.

35. Hedrick HL, Chiu P. Postnatal management and long-term outcome for survivors with congenital diaphragmatic hernia. *Prenat Diagn.* 2008;28:592-603.

36. Bohn D. Congenital diaphragmatic hernia. *Am J Respir Crit Care Med.* 2002;166:911-915.

37. Bunnell High Frequency Jet Ventilation. Advantages of Life Pulse HFJV compared to other HFV. http://www.bunl.com/Support%20Materials/LifePulse Advantages.pdf. Accessed August 22, 2011.

38. Cogo PE, Zimmerman LJI, Meneghini L, et al. Pulmonary surfactant desaturate-phosphatidylcholine turnover and pool size in newborn infants with congenital diaphragmatic hernia (CDH). *Pediatr Res.* 2003;54(5):653-658.

39. Dargaville PA, South M, McDougall PN. Pulmonary surfactant concentration during transition from high frequency oscillator to conventional mechanical ventilation. *J Paediatr Child Health.* 1997;33:517-521.

40. Van Meurs KP, Robbins ST, Reed VL, et al. Congenital diaphragmatic hernia: long-term outcome in neonates treated with extracorporeal membrane oxygenation. *J Pediatr.* 1993;122(6):893-899.

41. The Congenital Diaphragmatic Hernia Study Group. Surfactant does not improve survival rate in preterm infants with congenital diaphragmatic hernia. *J Pediatr Surg.* 2004;39(6):829-833.

42. Guner Y, Robinder GK, Faisal GQ, et al. Outcome analysis of neonates with congenital diaphragmatic hernia treated with venovenous vs venoarterial extracorporeal membrane oxygenation. *J Pediatr Surg.* 2009:44:1691-1701.

43. Neonatal Inhaled Nitric Oxide Study Group. Inhaled nitric oxide and hypoxic respiratory failure in infants with congenital diaphragmatic respiratory failure. *Pediatrics.* 1997;99:838-845.

44. German JC, Gazzaniga AB, Amlie R, Huxtable RF, Bartlett RH. Management of pulmonary insufficiency in diaphragmatic hernia using extracorporeal circulation with a membrane oxygenator. *J Pediatric Surg.* 1977;12(6):905-912.

45. Raval MV, Wang X, Reynolds M, Fischer AC. Costs of congenital diaphragmatic hernia repair in the United States—extracorporeal membrane oxygenation foots the bill. *J Pediatr Surg.* 2011;46:617-624.

46. Sola JE, Bronson SN, Cheung MC, Ordonez B, Neville HL, Koniaris LG. Survival disparities in newborns with congenital diaphragmatic hernia: a national perspective. *J Pediatr Surg.* 2010;45:1336-1342.

47. Brownlee EM, Howatson AG, Davis CF, Sabharwal AJ. The hidden mortality of congenital diaphragmatic hernia: a 20-year review. *J Pediatr Surg.* 2009;44:317-320.

48. Seetharam R, Younger JG, Bartlett RH, Hirschl RB. Factors associated with survival in infants with congenital diaphragmatic hernia requiring extracorporeal membrane oxygenation: a report from the Congenital Diaphragmatic Hernia Study Group. *J Pediatr Surg.* 2009:44:1315-1321.

49. Stevens TP, Chess PR, McConnochie KM, et al. Survival in early- and late-term infants with congenital diaphragmatic hernia treated with extracorporeal membrane oxygenation. *Pediatrics.* 2002;110:590-596.

50. Basek P, Bajrami S, Straub D, et al. The pulmonary outcome of long-term survivors after congenital diaphragmatic hernia repair. *Swiss Med Wkly.* 2008;138(11-12):173-179.

51. Committee on Fetus and Newborn. Postdischarge follow-up of infants with congenital diaphragmatic hernia. *Pediatrics.* 2008;121:627-632.

52. Su W, Berry M, Puligandla PS, Asirot A, Flageole H, Laberge JM. Predictors of gastroesophageal reflux in neonates with congenital diaphragmatic hernia. *J Pediatr Surg.* 2007;42:1639-1643.

53. Kawahara H, Okuyama H, Nose K, et al. Physiological and clinical characteristics of gastroesophageal reflux after congenital diaphragmatic hernia repair. *J Pediatr Surg.* 2010;45:2346-2350.

54. McGahren ED, Mallik K, Rodgers BM. Neurological outcome is diminished in survivors of congenital diaphragmatic hernia requiring extracorporeal membrane oxygenation. *J Pediatr Surg.* 1997;32(8):1216-1220.

55. Morando C, Midrio P, Gamba P, Filippone M, Sgro A, Orzan E. Hearing assessment in high-risk congenital diaphragmatic hernia survivors. *Int J Pediatr Otorhinolaryngol.* 2010;74:1176-1179.

56. Sadler TW. The embryologic origin of ventral body wall defects. *Semin Pediatr Surg.* 2010;19(3):209-214.

57. Sadler TW, Rasmussen SA. 2010. Examining the evidence for vascular pathogenesis of selected birth defects. *Am J Med Genet.* Part A;152A:2426-2436.

58. Chabra S, Gleason CA, Seidel K, Williams MA. Rising prevalence of gastroschisis in Washington State. *J Toxicol Environ Health A.* 2011;74(5):336-345.

59. Kohl M, Wiesel A, Schier F. Familial recurrence of gastroschisis: literature review and data from the population-based birth registry "Mainz Model." *J Pediatr Surg.* 2010;45:1907-1912.

60. Lam PK, Torfs CP. Interaction between maternal smoking and malnutrition in infant risk of gastroschisis. *Birth Defects Res A Clin Mol Teratol.* 2006;76:182-186.

61. Elliott L, Loomis D, Lottritz L, Slotnick RN, Oki E, Todd R. Case-control study of a gastroschisis cluster in Nevada. *Arch Pediatr Adolesc Med.* 2009;163(11):1000-1006.

62. Draper ES, Rankin J, Tonks AM, et al. Recreational drug use: a major risk factor for gastroschisis? *Am J Epidemiol.* 2008;167:485-491.

63. Benjamin BG, Ethen MK, Van Hook CL, Myers CA, Canfield MA. Gastroschisis prevalence in Texas 1999-2003. *Birth Defects Res A Clin Mol Teratol.* 2010;88(3):178-185.

64. Feldkamp ML, Carey JC, Sadler TW. Development of gastroschisis: review of hypotheses, a novel hypothesis, and implications for research. *Am J of Med Genet.* 2007;143(A):639-652.

65. Lobo JD, Kim AC, Davis RP, et al. No free ride? The hidden costs of delayed operative management using a spring-loaded silo for gastroschisis. *J Pediatr Surg.* 2010;45:1426-1432.

66. Jensen AR, Waldhausen JHT, Kim SS. The use of a spring-loaded silo for gastroschisis: impact on practice patterns and outcomes. *Arch Surg.* 2009;144(6):516-519.

67. Riboh J, Abrajano CT, Garber K, et al. Outcomes of sutureless gastroschisis closure. *J Pediatr Surg.* 2009;44(10):1947-1951.

68. Lao OB, Larison C, Garrison MM, Waldhausen JHT, Goldin AB. Outcomes in neonates with gastroschisis in US children's hospitals. *Am J Perinatol.* 2010;27(1):97-101.

69. Hwang PJ, Kousseff BG. Omphalocele and gastroschisis: an 18-year review study. *Genet Med.* 2004;6(4):232-236.

70. Mortellaro VE, St. Peter SD, Fike FB, Islam S. Review of the evidence on the closure of abdominal wall defects. [published online ahead of print Dec. 15, 2010]. *Pediatr Surg Int.* http://www.springerlink.com/content/750nlhp 22gr15334/.

71. Kleinrouweler CE, Kuijper CF, van Zalen-Sprock MM, Mathijssen IB, Bilardo CM, Pajkrt E. Characteristics and outcome and the omphalocele circumference/abdominal circumference ratio in prenatally diagnosed fetal omphalocele. [published online ahead of print, Feb. 16, 2011]. *Fetal Diagn Ther.* http://content.karger.com.ezproxy.welch.jhmi. edu/produktedb/produkte.asp?DOI=000323326&typ=pdf.

72. Clifton MS, Heiss KF, Keating JJ, Macay G, Ricketts RR. Use of tissue expanders in the repair of complex abdominal wall defects. *J Pediatr Surg.* 2011;46:372-377.

Chapter 10

Airway Abnormalities

Ellen Deutch MD FACS, FAAP
Safeena Kherani MD, FRCSC

Chapter Outline cont.

Key Terms cont.

Tracheoesophageal fistula (TEF)
Tracheostomy
Tracheotomy
Valleculae
Vallecular cysts
Vestibular stenosis
Vocal fold paralysis
Vocal fold nodules
Vomer

Chapter Objectives

After reading this chapter, you will be able to:

1. List several pediatric airway abnormalities that may necessitate a tracheostomy.
2. Manage tracheostomy tube emergencies.
3. Provide airway stabilization for a patient recently diagnosed with choanal atresia.
4. Identify therapies given a newborn with Robin sequence to relieve airway obstruction before surgical reconstruction.
5. Recommend airway management techniques to minimize the risk of subglottic stenosis for premature infants requiring intubation and long-term mechanical ventilation.
6. Describe the different forms of tracheoesophageal fistulas.
7. Describe the respiratory management of laryngomalacia.

■■ Baby Girl (BG) Walters

You are the dayshift respiratory therapist (RT) working in a level 4 neonatal intensive care unit (NICU), and you are caring for BG Walters, a former 27-wG infant, now 5 months old. She has been diagnosed with respiratory distress syndrome (RDS) and bronchopulmonary dysplasia (BPD), is on minimal ventilator settings, and is spontaneously breathing 35 times a minute with tidal volumes ranging from 5 to 7 mL/kg. She has failed extubation three times in the last 2 weeks, each time being reintubated for increased work of breathing, stridor, and impending respiratory failure.

During multidisciplinary rounds this morning, the team discusses another extubation attempt for her. They ask for your recommendation to improve the chance of success during today's attempt.

The airway is a complex network of structures, and in children in particular there are many different causes for airway obstruction. Stridor is the most common clinical manifestation of airway abnormality, and it can be a challenge to determine the exact cause in children. The respiratory therapist's role for the majority of these abnormalities will be to maintain airway stabilization and oxygenation preoperatively, and ventilatory management postoperatively as needed.

When addressing airway abnormalities in the pediatric setting, it is helpful to consider signs and symptoms in an anatomical framework. The airway is an elegant system, composed of a number of specialized structures with varied but integrated functions. Understanding the anatomical location and the effects of compromising lesions helps shape an insightful differential diagnosis and an effective management strategy. With this in mind, the following sequential anatomical levels set the framework for this chapter's discussion of airway abnormalities:

- Nasal passages and nasopharynx
- Oral cavity and oropharynx
- Supraglottis
- Glottis (vocal folds)
- Subglottis
- Trachea and bronchi

A complete discussion of all abnormalities of the airway is beyond the scope of this chapter. Instead, a single disorder will be discussed for each level of the airway, with a discussion of other disorders that may require RT support briefly described at the end of each section. Most of these malformations are either self-limiting or completely correctable with surgical interventions, allowing a normal progression into adulthood without recurring airway distress. See Table 10-1 for a list of all disorders described in this chapter. After discussion of the disorders is a section regarding pediatric tracheotomy and subsequent tracheostomy management.

Airway Abnormalities of the Nasal Passages and Nasopharynx

An infant or child presenting with obstructed nares requires rapid assessment to facilitate effective ventilation. The causes for an obstructed nasopharynx in newborns are usually congenital, whereas abnormal tissue growth and foreign bodies are the more likely causes in toddlers and school-aged children. The most common pathology causing nasal obstruction is choanal atresia, which will be discussed in detail in this section. Other conditions that can affect the nasal passages and nasopharynx will be discussed at the end of the section.

Choanal Atresia

Choanal atresia is a congenital condition in which the posterior portion of the nasal passage ends in a blind pouch, with complete obstruction of the passageway between the nose and the nasopharynx. Choanal atresia can be unilateral or bilateral. Choanal atresia is the most common congenital nasal abnormality, with bilateral choanal atresia occurring in 1 out of every 5,000 to 8,000 births, and unilateral choanal atresia is twice as common (1).

Congenital choanal atresia can present as a single defect or a component of a larger complex of findings, such as **CHARGE syndrome**, in which coloboma, heart abnormalities, atresia choanae, retarded mental development, genital hypoplasia, and ear deformities may be present (2).

Table 10-1	Airway Abnormalities by Anatomical Level
Anatomical Level	**Abnormality**
Nasal Passages and Nasopharynx	Choanal atresia Choanal stenosis Cleft lip Intranasal mass Hamartomas Adenoid hypertrophy Vestibular stenosis
Oral Cavity and Oropharynx	Robin sequence Tonsillar hypertrophy Macroglossia Peritonsillar abscess Retropharyngeal abscess Congenital vascular malformations
Supraglottis	Laryngomalacia Epiglottitis Vallecular cysts Ectopic thyroid tissue Saccular cysts Laryngoceles
Glottis	Recurrent respiratory papillomatosis Vocal fold paralysis Glottic web Vocal fold nodules Laryngopharyngeal reflux
Subglottis	Subglottic stenosis Subglottic cysts Subglottic hemangiomas Laryngotracheobronchitis (croup)
Trachea and Bronchi	Tracheoesophageal fistula Exudative tracheitis Tracheal masses Tracheal compression

Pathophysiology

In choanal atresia, the normal opening at the back of the nares, called the choanae, is not patent; the obstructing "wall" is composed of a combination of bony and membranous tissue, making it difficult or impossible to breathe through the nose. This is important because up to 50% of newborns are obligate nose breathers, meaning that they cannot compensate by oral breathing if their nose is obstructed; they may not gain this ability until 6 weeks to 6 months of age (3).

The physiological or embryological mechanism that causes choanal atresia is not yet understood.

Several theories have been suggested related to failures early in embryological development, many within the foregut or mesoderm. It appears likely to occur between the fourth and 11th weeks of gestation (4). There is also a potential link between choanal atresia and maternal hypothyroidism (5).

Clinical Manifestations

Bilateral choanal atresia normally presents at birth, as the airway obstruction could constitute a medical emergency. The usual presentation includes obvious airway obstruction, stridor, and paradoxical cyanosis, in which infants turn pink when crying as they begin to breathe through an open mouth and relieve their own airway obstruction. Unilateral choanal atresia typically presents later, usually by 5 to 24 months of age, and will have unilateral nasal obstruction and persistent nasal discharge (5).

A variety of inexpensive and painless evaluation methods can be used for preliminary identification of choanal atresia. For instance, in a **tissue test**, the practitioner holds a piece of tissue or wisp of cotton (easily obtained from a cotton applicator) in front of each nare: If choanal atresia is present, the tissue (or cotton wisp) will not move with respiration. Similarly, a mirror held under the nares will not fog up with respiration, and auscultation with a stethoscope will not detect the sound of airflow from either nare during respiration. A more traditional technique is to attempt to pass a lubricated, narrow-gauge suction catheter through each nare; this technique is less comfortable for the child and can be misleading if the catheter is thought to have advanced through the choanae but is actually curled up in the nasopharynx. **Nasal endoscopy** at the bedside, using a narrow fiber optic or rigid telescope or even an otoscope, also may be helpful in evaluating choanal atresia.

Definitive assessment of choanal atresia is by computed tomography (CT) scan, which will show bony as well as soft tissue anatomy (Fig. 10-1). Obtaining the scan with a protocol that could be used for intraoperative image guidance equipment should be considered; this allows for minimally invasive endoscopic surgical techniques to be used, which can improve surgical management of choanal atresia (6). It is helpful to suction the nares before scanning so that retained secretions do not obscure the anatomical findings.

Management and Treatment

Short-term management of bilateral choanal atresia can be accomplished by propping the infant's mouth open with a device such as an oral airway or a feeding nipple with a large opening, which is secured in place. It may be more practical, however, to intubate the infant until surgery can be performed.

Definitive management is accomplished by creating choanal openings surgically. If the choanal

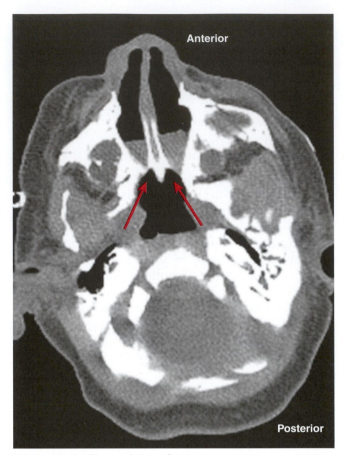

Figure 10-1 Choanal Atresia *(Courtesy of Ellen Deutch MD, FACS, FAAP)*

openings are able to be created in one surgery, it is known as a primary repair. Some patients may require several procedures, including dilation (stretching to increase the diameter of the openings). The risks of surgical repair include central nervous system (CNS) damage (7) and restenosis or subsequent closure of the choana, causing recurrence of airway obstruction.

Depending on the surgeon's preference, nasal stents may be placed to maintain patency of the nares. A variety of methods and materials are available to construct nasal stents (8, 9). Some may be entirely intranasal, and some project anterior to the nares. Some are secured with sutures; others are constructed to completely encircle the **vomer** (posterior aspect of the nasal septum) and the **collumella** (anterior, external aspect of the septum) and therefore cannot be dislodged with suctioning or other manipulation. All stents require meticulous suctioning to maintain patency; these narrow channels may be the child's only functional airway (Fig. 10-2). The nares and collumella should be monitored for injury and necrosis.

Although unilateral choanal atresia is twice as common as bilateral choanal atresia, it is generally minimally symptomatic and well tolerated by infants

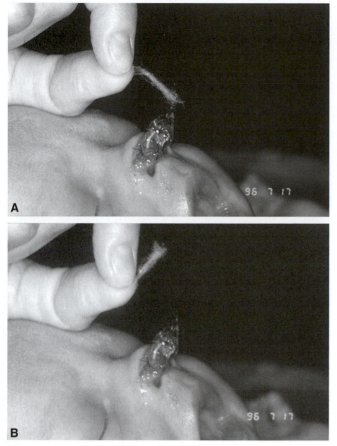

Figure 10-2 Choanal Atresia Repair *(Courtesy of Ellen Deutch MD FACS, FAAP)*

and children (10). Because of the milder manifestations, surgical repair of unilateral choanal atresia is often deferred until at least 1 year of age; there is not a consensus about exact timing, however (2).

Course and Prognosis

The most challenging complication of choanal atresia is restenosis, also known as refractory choanal atresia. One hospital found that 9.8% of their patients had restenosis that required as many as six surgeries to complete the repair (11). Neonates who undergo primary repair are intubated for the procedure, and most are extubated within 24 to 48 hours postoperatively with no lung complications (12). Once surgical repair is completed and there is no evidence of restenosis, there are no continued sequelae and children develop normally.

Other Conditions Affecting the Nasal Passages and Nasopharynx

Choanal stenosis occurs when the choanae are narrowed but not completely obstructed; management is usually surgical and will depend on the severity of the condition. An unrelated condition, anterior nasal stenosis, may occur at the most anterior bony opening

into the nare, known as the "pyriform aperture." Congenital pyriform aperture stenosis, if symptomatic, may be managed by surgically enlarging the pyriform aperture. Soft tissue stenosis, known as **vestibular stenosis**, can develop as an uncommon consequence of using nasal prongs. It can be difficult to identify on physical examination, and is difficult to repair. It is important that respiratory therapists monitor for damage resulting from a variety of nasal devices, including nasal stents, nasal prongs, noninvasive nasal masks, or other devices used in or on the nose.

A complete **cleft lip** (failure of parts of the lip to completely fuse together during the first 12 weeks' gestation) also involves the nose (Fig. 10-3) and can have an effect on the patency of a child's nasal passages and nasopharynx. Some congenital or syndromic conditions affecting the nose may also cause chronic nasal obstruction, particularly those that affect facial growth, and include midface hypoplasia, such as trisomy 21 (Down syndrome); Crouzon's disease; and craniosynostosis. There are also a variety of uncommon conditions that can cause diverse midface dysplasias, including a single nare and profound developmental delays (13).

Intranasal foreign bodies are not uncommon among young children; they are usually unilateral so that they typically present with unilateral rhinorrhea (mucous discharge from one nare) and excoriation

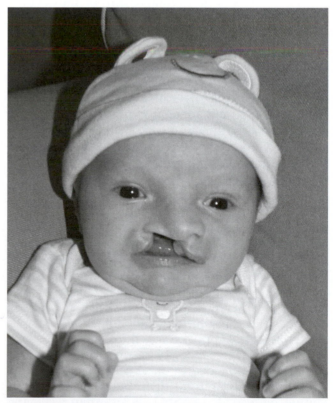

Figure 10-3 Photograph of a Child with Cleft Lip and Palate *(Courtesy of Kimberly A. Kimble BS, RRT-NPS, and Danny R. Kimble Jr, RRT-NPS)*

(breakdown of tissue caused by scratching or abrasion) of one nasal sill. They also are often accompanied by a foul odor. Button batteries, such as those found in toys and singing greeting cards, comprise a special case of foreign bodies that require emergent removal. Children may present with unilateral dark "chocolate" rhinorrhea; foreign bodies can erode into the nasal septum, causing permanent perforation.

Intranasal masses can cause nasal obstruction and should be considered in a thorough differential diagnosis. Nasal polyps are uncommon in children but do occur—and may be massive—in children with cystic fibrosis, for example. Occasionally antrochoanal polyps may occur; they generally arise from the maxillary sinus and enlarge posteriorly until they fill the choanae—they may even continue to expand so that they can be seen bulging below the free margin of the soft palate in the oropharynx. Dermoids, gliomas, encephaloceles, and teratomas are congenital abnormalities that tend to occur in the midline and can present as intra- or extranasal masses. Intracranial connections and content of the herniation vary depending on the type of lesion; it is important to consider that the lesion may include brain tissue.

Hamartomas, or "hairy polyps," are pedunculated congenital masses that may occur in the posterior of the nose, near the internal opening of the eustachian tube orifice (the eustachian tube connects the middle ear with the nasopharynx).

Adenoid hypertrophy (enlargement of the adenoid tissue) is probably the most common anatomical cause of nasal obstruction in children. Adenoids are lymphatic tissue located in the nasopharynx (Fig. 10-4), posterior to the choanae, which function as part of the immune system (14). They tend to enlarge until approximately 4 to 8 years of age and then begin to regress (15). Severe adenoid hypertrophy can cause obstructive sleep apnea.

Nonanatomical conditions, such as infectious and inflammatory conditions, should be considered when investigating causes of nasal obstruction. Viral infections of the nose and/or the paranasal sinuses are particularly common causes for temporary airway obstruction in children. Because of the smaller size of the nasopharynx, children (particularly during infancy) have significant increases in audible airway obstruction or "noisy breathing" during viral infections. This can cause distress in observers, but is usually benign and will disappear after resolution of the infection.

Respiratory support for each of these abnormal findings in the nasal cavity is supportive in nature, depending on the degree of airway obstruction and subsequent respiratory distress. Oxygen therapy should be provided if SpO$_2$ is less than 92%, and repositioning the airway to improve air entry are common nonsurgical interventions.

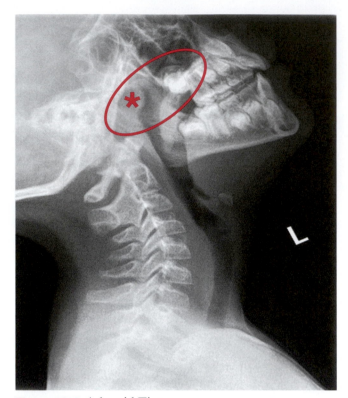

Figure 10-4 Adenoid Tissue *(Courtesy of Ellen Deutch MD FACS, FAAP)*

Airway Abnormalities of the Oral Cavity and Oropharynx

The oral cavity extends from the mouth to the soft palate. The oropharynx continues from the soft palate to the epiglottis. The oral cavity and oropharynx are shared by the respiratory and digestive tracts, and abnormalities in this region can negatively affect both systems. These include Robin sequence, tonsillar hypertrophy, macroglossia, and abscesses on various structures. Robin sequence requires the most RT intervention or support than other disorders of the oropharynx, and thus it will be discussed in more detail.

Robin Sequence

Robin sequence, previously known as Pierre-Robin syndrome, classically consists of a triad of a small mandible (**micrognathia** or retrognathia), **glossoptosis** (obstruction of the airway by the bulk of the tongue), and **cleft palate** (failure of parts of the hard palate to completely fuse together during the first 12 weeks' gestation, leaving a connection between the oral and nasal cavities). Robin sequence is normally diagnosed in utero and treated early in life, but it often causes airway obstruction that requires temporizing interventions from the health-care team prior to surgical interventions. Very few studies have examined the incidence of Robin sequence, but it was estimated in one Denmark study to occur in 1 in 14,000 live births (16). Common syndromes associated with Robin sequence include Stickler syndrome, velocardiofacial syndrome (also known as 22q11), and Treacher Collins syndrome, as well as facial and hemifacial microsomia (17). Children with a syndromic diagnosis are more likely to have developmental delays (17).

Pathophysiology

Embryologically, the small mandible causes relative glossoptosis. This prevents closure of palatal shelves, resulting in midline cleft palate (17) (Fig. 10-5). This occurs between weeks 4 and 8 of gestation (18). The cleft palate is not required for diagnosis of Robin sequence. The mandible abnormality can be caused by an inherent growth problem that may be genetic or syndromic.

Robin sequence can also be observed secondary to maldevelopment in utero that restricts mandible growth (16). Studies suggest that Robin sequence secondary to maldevelopment is more likely to resolve with conservative treatment from "catch-up" growth (Clinical Variations 10-1).

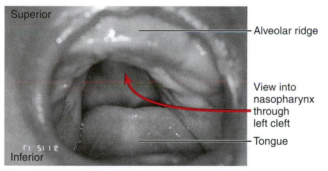

Figure 10-5 Cleft Palate *(Courtesy of Ellen Deutch MD FACS, FAAP)*

Clinical Variations 10-1

"Catch Up" Growth for Robin Sequence (16)

One of the potential causes of the small mandible found in Robin sequence may be a physical restriction on the mandible's ability to grow in utero. This may occur because of fetal head positioning in utero and may be restricted by oligohydramnios, multiple births, or cervical spine deformities. Most of these infants will have no other problems, and once the restriction is removed (e.g., by birth), the mandible is likely to grow quickly and alleviate the oropharyngeal obstruction. This group of infants usually requires minimal clinical interventions.

Clinical Manifestations

The main respiratory clinical symptom is airway obstruction from the glossoptosis and requires assessment to determine the degree of ventilatory impairment. Severe airway obstruction manifests as retractions and stridor. Assessment of the airway obstruction may include continuous vital sign monitoring because children with this condition may be symptomatic while awake as well as during sleep. Definitive diagnosis of obstructive sleep apnea is completed with a formal **polysomnogram** (sleep study), which can also be repeated posttreatment to assess for improvement in the obstructive sleep apnea (19).

Feeding may also be difficult for neonates with Robin sequence, mostly relating to a deficient mandible and difficulty swallowing effectively. This manifests as impaired feeding and failure to thrive.

Management and Treatment

Neonates with Robin sequence have varying degrees of respiratory and feeding difficulties, and the severity of mandibular deficiency will help determine the severity of symptoms. Glossoptosis requires some method to minimize obstruction of the oropharynx by the tongue. A simple jaw thrust is a physical intervention that respiratory therapists can perform that can immediately relieve airway obstruction, but it is not a long-term solution. Prone positioning is the initial intervention; in fact 70% of children suffering from Robin sequence may require only prone positioning to relieve airway obstruction (16). Additional options include using a nasopharyngeal airway, such as a nasal trumpet, modified nasal-tracheal tube, or even a nasogastric tube, to stent the tongue anteriorly, which will minimize the effect of glossoptosis and ultimately the airway obstruction.

The more challenging cases require a multidisciplinary approach, consisting of medical and surgical intervention (16, 17). Surgical management is necessary for severe cases and may include tongue-lip adhesion, mandibular advancement, or tracheostomy. Tongue-lip adhesion consists of tethering the anterior tongue to the inferior alveolar ridge in an attempt to pull the tongue forward. Mandibular advancement involves incising the mandible and attaching a fixation device, which is incrementally expanded to increase the size of the mandible and decompress the bulk of tissue in the posterior pharynx. Tracheostomy may be required in up to 10% of children suffering from Robin sequence, particularly if they have additional airway abnormalities (16).

Course and Prognosis

After surgical reconstruction of the mandible, airway obstruction is relieved, and in most patients accelerated growth and improved feeding success is noted. In a subset of patients, however, there may be impaired weight and length growth despite an increased calorie diet and additional feeding interventions. The mortality rate ranges from 0% to 13.6%, and the small number of children with this disorder relative to the general population and differences in long-term patient management are probably responsible for the wide mortality rate range (18).

Other Conditions Affecting the Oral Cavity and Oropharynx

In **tonsillar hypertrophy**, the palatine tonsils, commonly referred to as tonsils, which are situated between the anterior and posterior tonsillar pillars (palatoglossus and palatopharyngeus muscles, respectively), become enlarged, causing airway obstruction (Fig. 10-6). They can be enlarged secondary to acute infection by various pathogens including bacteria such as streptococcus pneumonia or viruses such as Epstein-Barr virus (EBV) and infectious mononucleosis. Chronic tonsillar hypertrophy can also occur without an inciting etiology and can be associated with adenoid hypertrophy (the adenoids are located in the nasopharynx). Symptoms of tonsil enlargement can include snoring with apnea, stertor (noisy snoring), and dysphagia. Management includes antimicrobials and/or surgical intervention such as

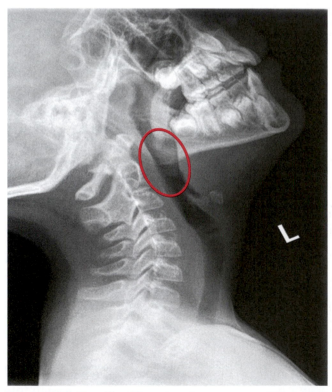

Figure 10-6 Tonsillar Hypertrophy *(Courtesy of Ellen Deutch MD FACS, FAAP)*

tonsillotomy (partial removal of the tonsils) or tonsillectomy (complete removal of the tonsils) as appropriate. Placement of a nasopharyngeal airway can be very effective acute management.

Macroglossia (enlarged tongue) is common in individuals with Down syndrome as well as other conditions such as mucopolysaccharidosis (an inherited disease that causes defects in bone, cartilage, and connective tissue). Macroglossia can contribute to airway obstruction, particularly during sleep when there is decreased muscle tone (20). The treatment for macroglossia is tongue reduction surgery.

A **peritonsillar abscess**, also referred to as quinsy, can develop in the potential space superolateral to the tonsil and is thought to be secondary to obstruction of the minor salivary glands in this region, known as "Weber's glands." Typical symptoms include unilateral soft palate swelling, deviation of the uvula away from the infected side caused by mass effect, hot potato voice (muffled speech), dysphagia (difficulty with swallowing), odynophagia (painful swallowing), trismus (decreased mouth opening from masticator muscle spasm), and in severe cases airway obstruction. Management options include antibiotics, incision and drainage, and possibly tonsillectomy (21).

A **retropharyngeal abscess** occurs when a pocket of purulence develops behind the posterior pharyngeal wall, causing symptoms of neck stiffness, neck pain, fever, and cervical adenopathy. Although intravenous antibiotic therapy can be sufficient to manage early forms of this condition, definitive treatment is surgical, often through an intraoral approach (22).

Congenital vascular malformations can be arterial, venous, lymphatic, or a combination of the three and can cause airway obstruction. Within the tongue, the most common vascular malformation is the microcystic lymphangioma (traditionally called a cystic hygroma); because of its location, presenting symptoms are often similar to those seen with macroglossia. Surgical removal may be necessary.

Airway Abnormalities of the Supraglottis

The **supraglottis** is the portion of the larynx just above the **glottis** (vocal folds); it includes the epiglottis, bilateral false vocal folds, bilateral arytenoids (containing the cuneiform and corniculate cartilages), and the bilateral aryepiglottic folds, which connect the epiglottis and the arytenoids (Figs. 10-7 and 10-8). The supraglottis is very dynamic and serves to protect the airway from drowning and from aspiration of ingested food. Abnormalities of the supraglottis include laryngomalacia, epiglottitis, vallecular cysts, ectopic thyroid tissue, saccular cysts, and laryngoceles.

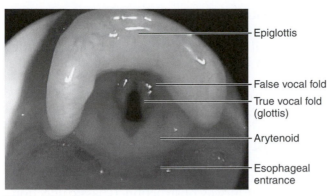

Figure 10-7 Larynx *(Courtesy of Ellen Deutch MD FACS, FAAP)*

Laryngomalacia

Laryngomalacia is the most common laryngeal anomaly and the most common congenital cause of stridor (23, 24). Although it is considered congenital if there has not been any airway manipulation or trauma, symptoms typically are not present until about 2 weeks of age (23).

Pathophysiology

The stridor is caused by supraglottic structures, such as the epiglottis and the arytenoids prolapsing or caving in toward the central airway during inspiration; this obstruction creates increased airway turbulence. Various combinations of a tubular or omega-shaped epiglottis, short aryepiglottic folds, and redundant mucosal tissue covering the arytenoids may contribute to the obstruction in particular patients. There is not yet consensus on whether the etiology is neurological or structural (e.g., immature cartilage) (23).

Clinical Manifestations

Laryngomalacia has a characteristic stridor, which is inspiratory, high-pitched, and has a vibratory quality. The stridor is best heard when the child is quietly awake, and it may not be present during exertion or crying. The pitch becomes lower over time, and in many cases, the stridor resolves completely by 12 to 24 months of age (24). The stridor typically worsens with feeding, excitement, agitation, crying, and supine positioning. Severe laryngomalacia may present with failure to thrive, feeding problems, aspiration, apnea, hypoxia, recurrent cyanosis, cor pulmonale, and other end-organ damage (25).

Diagnosis is confirmed by endoscopy. As this is a dynamic lesion, fiber-optic laryngoscopy while the child is calmly awake is the optimal way to observe prolapse of supraglottic structures occurring synchronously with stridor. If the child is agitated, the stridor may transiently resolve. Typically the stridor is more evident when the child is awake than asleep, unless it is severe.

The majority of infants with laryngomalacia have gastroesophageal reflux disease (GERD) and/or **laryngopharyngeal reflux (LPR)** (reflux of gastric acid into the pharynx and larynx) (24), and it is likely that laryngomalacia and reflux exacerbate each other.

Other variants of laryngomalacia affecting sleep, feeding, and exercise have also been described (26, 27) (Clinical Variations 10-2). The relationship between laryngomalacia and other airway lesions, such as subglottic stenosis or vocal fold paralysis, is controversial (29) and may be related to increased negative intrathoracic pressure.

Mild laryngomalacia has been described as inspiratory stridor with occasional feeding-related

Clinical Variations 10-2

Acquired Laryngomalacia (28)

Secondary or acquired laryngomalacia also involves supraglottic structures collapsing and obstructing the airway, but this condition typically occurs in school-aged and older children with significant neurological problems. In contrast to congenital laryngomalacia, these children and adolescents may have severely hypertrophied arytenoid mucosa, and the condition is expected to worsen over time.

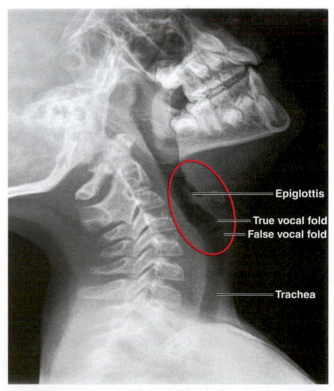

Figure 10-8 Supraglottic and Glottic Areas *(Courtesy of Ellen Deutch MD FACS, FAAP)*

symptoms of cough and choking or regurgitation. Moderate laryngomalacia is differentiated from mild symptoms by an increased frequency of feeding-related symptoms (29). Assessing the severity of laryngomalacia can be challenging. Patients with severe symptoms can have obstructive episodes with cyanosis, feeding difficulties, failure to thrive, and cor pulmonale (30). Continuous monitoring, similar to that used in a sleep study, may reveal episodes of obstructive apnea and oxygen desaturation.

Management and Treatment

Most children with congenital laryngomalacia can be managed expectantly. Respiratory management for mild and moderate laryngomalacia is usually minimal and will spontaneously resolve in the first year of life. Body positioning can often alleviate much of the airway obstruction. Upright positioning, such as in an infant seat during the daytime and a side-lying position at night in a crib is often helpful. If the obstruction is primarily from the epiglottis, prone positioning may provide airway relief. Intubation could be considered, but is not generally necessary. Many children with laryngomalacia also are treated for GERD or the feeding difficulties that arise from airway obstruction.

Surgical management should be considered for children with severe obstruction. Surgical procedures are designed to release or trim the affected structures using microlaryngoscopy and sharp dissection, microdebriders, or CO_2 laser. The procedures may be called "supraglottoplasty," "epiglottoplasty," or "aryepiglottoplasty" (26, 31). Tracheotomy is not commonly performed, but it may be necessary in a small subset of patients who have additional neurological problems that decrease airway tone, and may not be reversible.

Postoperatively, patients are generally managed in an intensive care setting and monitored for oxygen desaturation and symptoms of airway edema, such as increased work of breathing and inspiratory stridor. If intubated during surgery, they may be extubated immediately postoperatively, or they may remain intubated overnight. Steroids and racemic epinephrine may be prescribed after extubation. Initial postoperative feeding is begun cautiously because there is some risk of aspiration (32).

Course and Prognosis

The vast majority of infants will outgrow this disorder uneventfully (29) with no long-term sequelae. Associated comorbidities include GERD or LPR, neurological disease, congenital heart disease, congenital anomalies or a syndrome, or the presence of a secondary airway lesion. They are found more commonly in children with moderate and severe disease. Excluding GERD or LPR, 25% to 50% of

children with laryngomalacia will present with an additional comorbidity (25). To improve long-term outcomes, it is important to manage comorbidities as the team is able.

Other Conditions Affecting the Supraglottis

Epiglottitis, which anatomically is actually "supraglottitis," is an uncommon but very serious condition of swelling of the epiglottis that can cause sudden and complete airway obstruction. (Classic infectious epiglottitis is discussed in Chapter 16.) Epiglottitis may also be caused by thermal, chemical, allergic, caustic (33), or mechanical injury.

Both **vallecular cysts** and ectopic (abnormally located) thyroid tissue may present as masses at the base of tongue or in the **valleculae** (space between the base of tongue and the epiglottis) (Fig. 10-9). Both have the potential to cause feeding difficulties and airway obstruction. Two hypotheses about the etiology of vallecular cysts include obstruction of mucous gland ducts or embryological malformation (34). Most are successfully treated with marsupialization (unroofing the lesion) (34). Ectopic thyroid tissue can be confirmed by a thyroid scan (35, 36), which will also provide information about the presence or absence of functional thyroid tissue in

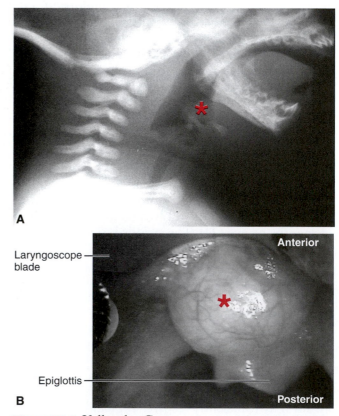

Figure 10-9 Vallecular Cysts *(Courtesy of Ellen Deutch MD FACS, FAAP)*

normal anatomical locations. Surgery for ectopic thyroid tissue is reserved for lingual thyroid tissue that fails medical management (37).

Saccular cysts and **laryngoceles** are abnormal outpouchings of the laryngeal mucosa in the laryngeal ventricle, originating between the true and false vocal folds. Both can cause significant airway obstruction, and management for either is surgical excision (38).

Airway Abnormalities of the Glottis

The glottis (vocal folds) is an elegant structure that opens to allow inspiration and closes to facilitate various functions, including speech, airway protection, and increasing intrathoracic pressure. The vocal folds are shaped in a V with the anterior commissure (apex) located anteriorly: They have a glistening white appearance. Any condition that impairs complete approximation of the vocal folds and prevents complete glottic closure will also interfere with the ability to seal the airway. This seal is necessary for increasing subglottic pressure in preparation for activities that require significant intrathoracic pressure changes, such as coughing and completing Valsalva's maneuver used to facilitate defecation. Conversely, conditions that interfere with the glottis opening, limiting airway patency, can contribute to stridor or respiratory distress. Some abnormalities associated with the glottis include recurrent respiratory papillomatosis, vocal fold paralysis, glottic web, vocal fold nodules, and laryngopharyngeal reflux.

Recurrent Respiratory Papillomatosis

Recurrent respiratory papillomatosis (RRP) is the most common benign neoplasm of the larynx. RRP is a viral disease caused by the human papillomavirus (HPV) and is generally transmitted from the child's mother, who may be asymptomatic (39). It causes tumor-like legions to grow on the larynx, and although RRP is histologically benign, it can obstruct the airway because of its mass effect, and can be fatal if adequate airway control is not accomplished (Fig. 10-10). Malignant degeneration is rare (40, 41).

Pathophysiology

The most common HPV subtypes manifesting in RRP are types 11 and 6; type 11 tends to be more virulent, with greater tendency for pulmonary involvement, obstructive symptoms, and need for a tracheostomy (39). Although RRP has a predilection for the glottis at the junction of the ciliated and squamous epithelium, these wart-like exophytic (outward growing) lesions can also occur at other sites within the larynx in addition to any site in the airway from the oral cavity and nasal vestibule to the trachea and distal bronchi (39, 41).

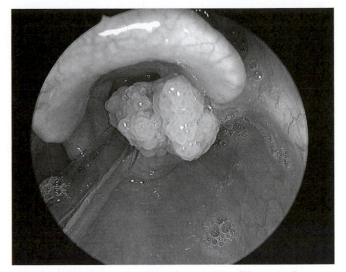

Figure 10-10 Recurrent Respiratory Papillomatosis (*Courtesy of Ellen Deutch MD FACS, FAAP*)

Clinical Manifestations

The presentation of RRP is variable, but often the initial sign is hoarseness. Hoarseness can be a nonspecific component of other infectious and noninfectious conditions affecting the larynx, but any child who has persistent hoarseness, especially when it is severe or progressive, requires a thorough investigation. RRP can also present with stridor, respiratory distress, chronic cough, dysphagia, choking episodes, recurrent pneumonia, and shortness of breath; all of these symptoms can easily be attributed to other conditions such as asthma, croup, allergy, bronchitis, and vocal cord nodules (42), but RRP should be considered in the differential diagnosis and verified with endoscopy.

Management and Treatment

The mainstay of treatment is repeated removal of new growth. Typically, RRP of the larynx is removed under general anesthesia, with the larynx stabilized using a rigid laryngoscope, and the papilloma are removed with microlaryngeal instruments, lasers, and/or microdebriders. Special care is taken to preserve the underlying structures. Ventilation intraoperatively can be accomplished through a variety of means, including a traditional or laser-safe endotracheal tube passed between the cords throughout the procedure, alternating extubation and reintubation, or even intermittent jet ventilation, although this modality entails a theoretic risk of HPV dissemination to the distal airway. Postoperatively there is a risk of edema, but generally the child's airway is significantly improved following surgical removal of the growth. RRP frequently recurs but the rate is variable even for the same child. Children who develop RRP before the age of 3 tend to have more frequent recurrences requiring more surgeries for removal (39). In more severe cases, a tracheotomy may be required. This step can be controversial because there is concern about potentiating disease.

A number of adjuvant medical therapies have been administered, often with initial promising results and variable long-term results (Evidence in Practice 10-1).

Course and Prognosis

Although there is no cure for RRP, it is a generally benign disease when treated in a timely manner. The major burden on patients is through voice dysfunction, although there is a significant social and economic burden on the patient and family. Children are frequently hospitalized for surgeries, and there is a negative social stigma regarding HPV that causes stress for families affected by RRP. It can recur throughout a patient's life span, sometimes after as much as a 20-year remission (45).

Other Conditions Affecting the Glottis

Vocal fold paralysis (also known as vocal cord paralysis) is the interruption of laryngeal nerve impulse, which controls vocal cord movement. It is the second most common laryngeal anomaly after laryngomalacia. It can be bilateral or unilateral and is often the result of a neurological abnormality. Bilateral vocal fold paralysis must always be investigated for a central source such as intracerebral hemorrhage, hydrocephalus, or even Arnold-Chiari malformation, which can result in herniation of the brainstem (30).

Bilateral vocal fold paralysis can result in cords that are in an abducted (spread apart or open) resting position or alternatively are in an adducted (apposed or closed) position. If the cords are abducted, then the child might present with a breathy voice or even aspiration from inability to close the glottis during swallowing. Children with adducted cords present with stridor and airway obstruction but may have a normal voice. This condition often requires a tracheostomy (46). Other surgical management of the adducted larynx is less common because some conditions will resolve after treatment or over time and procedures to improve airway patency can compromise voice quality.

Unilateral vocal fold paralysis requires investigation of the entire course of the recurrent laryngeal nerve that supplies most of the motor function and sensation to the larynx. This nerve is a branch of the vagus nerve, and extends from the neck into the chest, with portions circling around the aorta and right subclavian artery before rising back into the neck and innervating the larynx. A common cause of unilateral vocal fold paralysis is iatrogenic injury during cardiac or thyroid surgery. Like bilateral paralysis, the presentation can vary between stridor from airway obstruction when the cord is paralyzed in an adducted position and aspiration when the paralyzed cord has an overall abducted position. The paralyzed cord can recover spontaneously or, over time, the normal vocal cord may compensate for the weaker paralyzed one (47). In some cases, surgical interventions may be considered, such as injection of the vocal fold with a filler material if the cord is abducted or recurrent laryngeal nerve reinnervation (47).

Another condition that can affect the glottis is known a **glottic web**, which is a membrane spread between the vocal folds near the anterior commissure. This results from incomplete development of the laryngeal opening in utero and appears as a web just posterior to the anterior commissure, which is the anterior junction of the two vocal cords. This condition can occur as an isolated condition or can be associated with syndromes such as 22q11, formerly known as velocardiofacial syndrome (48). Webs can also develop iatrogenically after intubation trauma, aggressive removal of papillomatosis at the anterior commissure, or other interventions. Management may consist of endoscopic lysing of the web or surgical excision and/or laryngotracheal reconstruction, with the extent of surgery dependent on the thickness of the web.

Vocal fold nodules can also result in hoarseness and are thought to be caused by vocal abuse. Typically, these callus-like lesions develop at the junction between the anterior and middle third of the vocal folds. The nodules can be acute and soft, or chronic and more mature. Management typically targets the primary cause using speech language therapy. Surgical intervention is uncommon, but it may be warranted in selected cases.

The reflux of gastric contents superiorly through the esophagus to the pharynx (LPR) can cause inflammation of the posterior region of the larynx. The reflux can also cause laryngeal changes including swelling of the supraglottic and glottic structures and

---

● **Evidence in Practice 10-1**

Treatments for RRP

Recent examples of adjuvant medical therapies for RRP include interferon alpha, mumps vaccine, indole-3-carbinol, and intralesional cidofovir (41). Systemic propanolol is also under investigation (43). Gardasil prophylactic vaccinations are now recommended by the American Academy of Pediatrics for both boys and girls (44); the effect on airway lesions is not yet known.

result in voice hoarseness and dysphagia. Initial management is conservative, with positional and feeding changes and consideration of antireflux medications. In some severe cases, surgical intervention such as a fundoplication of the gastroesophageal junction may be necessary (49).

■■ After discussing BG Walters' previous extubations with some of your coworkers and reviewing RT notes in the chart, your biggest concern is her inspiratory stridor, which does not seem to respond to racemic epinephrine. You voice your concerns, and with the physician and bedside nurse, prepare to create an action plan for the baby postextubation.

Airway Abnormalities of the Subglottis

In infants and children, the subglottis is the narrowest portion of the airway, and it is therefore the area within the airway most susceptible to edema from trauma. The subglottis in a neonate should be at least 4 mm in diameter (50), and even small decreases in the radius of the airway will cause very large increases in work of breathing and air turbulence. The subglottis is also nondistensible because it corresponds externally to the cricoid cartilage. Although the tracheal "rings" are truly arches, the cricoid cartilage is a complete ring and therefore cannot distend to accommodate an endotracheal tube (51). This combination of a narrow diameter and nondistensible quality makes this area vulnerable to any inflammation, scar, or mass, which can cause significant respiratory compromise. The most common subglottic airway abnormality seen by RTs is subglottic stenosis; others include subglottic cysts, subglottic hemangiomas, and laryngotracheobronchitis (croup).

Subglottic Stenosis

Stridor caused by subglottic narrowing, known as **subglottic stenosis**, is predominantly inspiratory, but it can be biphasic if severe. Intubation is the most common cause of acquired subglottic stenosis (50), and premature infants are at particular risk for this because they may require prolonged intubation to manage BPD. Subglottic stenosis can also be congenital.

Pathophysiology

In patients who have congenital subglottic stenosis, the airway lumen is elliptical rather than round, and vocal fold function is normal (42, 50). In subglottic stenosis caused by endotracheal intubation, the endotracheal tube can damage the mucosa and underlying

cartilage, resulting in scarring that further narrows the lumen. The subglottic narrowing can progress from an acute, edematous, soft inflammatory phase to a chronic, firm, mature scar causing stenosis.

Clinical Manifestations

The clinical finding for subglottic stenosis is inspiratory stridor. When caused by intubation, it will be heard as inspiratory stridor occurring soon after extubation. It normally is not alleviated by typical treatments for upper airway edema, such as inhaled racemic epinephrine or intravenous corticosteroids.

The acuity and severity of narrowing is assessed endoscopically and can be classified based on the Cotton-Myer grading system: From least to most severe, grade I is 0% to 50% obstruction of the lumen, grade II is 51% to 70% obstruction, grade III is 71% to 99% obstruction, and grade IV indicates that there is no detectable lumen (52).

■■ The medical team collectively decides to continue with BG Walters' extubation, and the nurse delivers a dose of dexamethasone about 6 hours prior to extubation to help compensate for any airway edema caused during extubation. You prepare equipment for reintubation at the bedside and agree to provide the physician with updates on BG Walters' status every 30 minutes. You will extubate her to nasal continuous positive airway pressure to provide additional airway stabilization. The physician verbalizes his concern for subglottic stenosis and suggests that if BG Walters fails this attempt, then a pediatric otorhinolaryngology consult should be requested. You and the nurse agree.

Management and Treatment

A team approach is required after subglottis stenosis is suspected. In some cases, subglottic stenosis can be managed conservatively, by watchful waiting. In mild cases, the subglottic region may be managed endoscopically. Gentle balloon dilation and topical application of local agents may minimize subsequent narrowing. In other cases, the airway may still be quite compromised, and surgical intervention may be indicated. Surgical options include dilation, cricoid split, laryngotracheal reconstruction, cricotracheal resection, and tracheotomy.

■■ BG Walters initially tolerated extubation well, requiring CPAP at 7 cm H_2O and FIO_2 at 0.30. About 20 minutes postextubation, you begin to hear inspiratory stridor that does not improve by moving her to an upright position or administering a one-time inhaled racemic epinephrine treatment. You also note that she has moderate substernal retractions and nasal flaring. After another 20 minutes, BG Walters' FIO_2 has been increased to 0.60 to maintain her SpO_2 at greater than 90%. You call the physician back to the baby's bed to reevaluate her. You, the nurse, and the physician all agree that BG Walters' respiratory distress is unlikely to improve and decide to reintubate. The physician will attempt once and agrees to contact pediatric anesthesia if he has any difficulty during the procedure.

Several of the surgical procedures used to manage subglottic narrowing involve mechanically enlarging the cartilaginous framework of the airway. A cricoid split is based on the principle that the cricoid cartilage forms a complete ring, and incising the ring allows it open slightly more, thereby expanding the airway lumen. This procedure is completed in neonates who are medically stable and require only minimal ventilatory support (53). The procedure entails exposure and vertical incision of the most anterior midline portion of the cricoids, which allows the ring to spring open a small amount. Typically, the infant is extubated 7 to 10 days postoperatively.

Laryngotracheal reconstruction is generally an open procedure that involves expanding the laryngeal airway caliber with an anterior and possibly posterior cartilage graft, often taken from the thyroid cartilage or even more commonly the cartilaginous portion of a rib. It can be completed in one or two stages, plus follow-up endoscopic management. A single-stage procedure includes inserting the graft(s), removing the existing tracheostomy tube, and closing the tracheostomy defect. These children leave the operating room with an oral or nasal endotracheal tube in place and are extubated days later. In a two- or double-stage procedure, the airway is reconstructed, but the tracheostomy is left in place distal to the area of reconstruction with intention to decannulate after a longer time interval and after adequate airway patency has been confirmed. A short-term stent may be secured within the reconstructed area postoperatively. When a stent is placed, endoscopic removal is required, which can be problematic in the event of an airway emergency, such as a broken stent (54). In selected cases, a cartilage graft is placed in the posterior aspect of the cricoid cartilage endoscopically (55). In each of these scenarios, there is anticipation of graft vascularization and graft survival to maintain the expansion of the airway lumen. Laryngotracheal reconstruction can have a number of complications, including pneumothorax from graft harvest, graft resorption, or even graft dislodgement.

A cricotracheal resection may be indicated in select cases when there is a very circumscribed or very severe area of narrowing. In this procedure, rather than expanding the narrowed area, the stenotic portion and the surrounding cartilage is completely removed, and the distal and proximal ends of the gap in the airway are reconnected. Risks include vocal fold paralysis because surgical dissection is carried out in the region of the recurrent laryngeal nerve (53). Children may have a suture placed between the chin and chest to prevent neck extension from causing distraction forces on the anastomosis. Potential postoperative complications include separation of the reconstructed airway, which can be disastrous and may be initially evidenced by subcutaneous air (42). Reintubation must always be completed very cautiously because there is a risk of intubating through an existing false passage or creating a new one.

Alternatively, a tracheostomy may be the most prudent option if there are circumstances that warrant postponing reconstruction until the child's condition or other circumstances can be optimized. A tracheostomy tube is placed in the trachea, distal (inferior) to the subglottis, and bypasses this level of narrowing.

While the factors affecting susceptibility to subglottic stenosis in an individual patient are not completely understood, it seems prudent to always handle the airway gently and to optimize pulmonary function to decrease the need for mechanical support. These additional considerations may be helpful:

1. Minimize trauma by using gentle technique when intubating and avoid repeated attempts (e.g., the more difficult the intubation may be, the greater the expertise required of the person performing the intubation).
2. Use the smallest effective endotracheal tube (ETT), considering the size of patient's airway and the ventilatory requirements. An ETT smaller than predicted may be required in infants and children with known subglottic pathology.
3. Secure the ETT well and minimize the frictional forces caused by motion of the tube and patient relative to each other, such as during patient repositioning. This may require retaping an ETT whenever it is noted to move freely from the lip or cheek so that the distal tip of the tube does not rub against the subglottic airway.
4. Manage suspected GERD or LPR. The reflux may already be exacerbated by the retractions and respiratory effort that create strong negative intrathoracic pressure and pull effluent from the esophagus and stomach to the laryngopharynx (42, 53).

■■ After reintubating with a 3.5 cuffless ETT, the physician contacts BG Walters' parents to discuss the possibility of subglottic stenosis. He recommends an otorhinolaryngology consult, to which they readily agree.

Endoscopy performed by the pediatric ear, nose, and throat (ENT) specialist uncovers a grade II stenosis. The ENT surgeon recommends a tracheostomy tube to allow mechanical ventilation weaning and multisystem stabilization prior to tracheal reconstruction. BG Walters' parents agree to the tracheostomy tube, but request a more specific timeline and goals for her management and plan of care, which the multidisciplinary teams will build over the coming week.

Other Conditions Affecting the Subglottis

Subglottic cysts can also present in the subglottic region. They can be congenital (56), but are more frequently acquired secondary to endotracheal intubation. Interestingly, duration of intubation is not thought to be a key factor in the development of subglottic cysts (57); premature birth and GERD are often seen as associated factors (58). Subglottic cysts tend to occur more frequently on the left side. One theory postulates that because most individuals are right-handed, and most intubation laryngoscopes are designed for right-handed intubation, they may exert more pressure, and subtle trauma, on the left side of the subglottis during intubation (57).

Subglottic cysts may sometimes be apparent radiographically, but definitive diagnosis is achieved endoscopically. Management is through excision or marsupialization (unroofing) of the cyst, which can be completed with microlaryngeal instruments, a microdebrider, or CO_2 laser. Intubation itself can sometimes rupture the cysts. Subglottic cysts can recur, and thus vigilance is warranted. Repeat evaluations with bronchoscopy are often completed. Recent evidence suggests that treatment with the chemotherapeutic agent mitomycin C applied topically to the subglottis can reduce the incidence of recurrence (58).

A subglottic hemangioma is an abnormal buildup of blood vessels in the subglottic tissue, which can cause airway obstruction. Subglottic hemangiomas tend to increase in size for the first 8 to 12 months of life, and then regress spontaneously (59). Traditional management includes steroids; recent evidence suggests that propranolol also may be effective (60). In severe cases, endoscopic or open resection, or a tracheotomy, may be indicated.

Laryngotracheobronchitis (croup) is a condition that occurs in up to 15% of children, typically between 6 months and 3 years of age. This is most often a viral disease that causes airway narrowing involving the subglottis; it presents with a "barky" cough, stridor, and occasionally hoarseness. Mild cases can be managed conservatively; severe cases with significant respiratory distress may require treatment with racemic epinephrine and systemic steroids (61). Intubation is avoided except in severe cases of respiratory failure. In children who develop symptoms of croup before 6 months of age, or who have repeated episodes of croup, additional underlying conditions, such as subglottic stenosis, should be considered.

Airway Abnormalities of the Trachea and Bronchi

The airway below the glottis and vocal cords begins the lower respiratory system. Despite having the vocal cords as a protective mechanism, infection of the airway and foreign bodies are still potential threats to the trachea and bronchi. In addition, the posterior layers of the trachea interface with the anterior tissue layers of the esophagus, so both congenital and acquired conditions affecting the esophagus may also affect the trachea. The congenital malformation most commonly cared for by RTs is esophageal atresia/tracheoesophageal fistula. Other disorders that can cause significant respiratory distress include exudative tracheitis, tracheal masses, and tracheal compression.

Tracheoesophageal Fistula

Esophageal atresia (EA) is a congenital defect in which the esophagus ends in a blind-ended pouch rather than connecting normally to the stomach. A form of EA may also involve a connection between the esophagus and the trachea, known as a **tracheoesophageal fistula (TEF)**. TEF can lead to severe pulmonary complications and requires a multidisciplinary approach to manage both the digestive and respiratory malformations. TEF occurs in about 1 in 3,500 births (62).

Pathophysiology

Esophageal atresia occurs when the embryonic tracheoesophageal septum develops improperly. At around week 4 of gestation, the airway begins to grow out from the foregut, which means that during normal embryological development the trachea and esophagus are connected. The mechanism of how the esophagus and trachea grow and separate is still not fully understood. TEF is a failure of the esophagus and trachea to separate in utero, which normally occurs sometime prior to week 18 of gestation (63). Although isolated esophageal atresia can occur, more than 80% of infants with esophageal atresia have a proximal esophagus that ends in a blind pouch and also have a distal TEF (64), which allows esophageal contents to reflux into the airway. Several other variations of EA are also possible (64) (Fig. 10-11). About half of infants with esophageal atresia will also have an additional congenital anomaly that may be musculoskeletal, gastrointestinal, cardiac, or genitourinary; the additional abnormality is often also one that occurs along the vertical axis (known as a midline defect) (64).

Clinical Manifestations

TEF is normally identified in utero using sonography, and it is one of the key congenital malformations ruled out during the 20-week prenatal anatomy sonography screening. Sonographic evidence includes polyhydramnios, absence of a fluid-filled stomach, small abdomen, lower-than-expected fetal weight, and distended esophageal pouch.

TEF may also be suspected after delivery when a newborn presents with one or more of the following:

- Excessive drooling, with copious, fine white frothy oral secretions, which will recur despite suctioning

- Choking or difficulty managing airway, accompanying cyanosis
- Barking cough
- Respiratory distress, worsening during feeding
- Inability to accept orogastric tube into the stomach

TEF is often associated with anatomic tracheomalacia, which is characterized by a widening of the posterior, membranous component of the trachea and a flattened anterior-posterior diameter of the trachea. (The tracheal "rings" are actually arches, and the common wall between the trachea and the esophagus is membranous.) Functional tracheomalacia is characterized by abnormally increased collapsibility of the trachea, particularly during inspiration. Tracheomalacia can also occur as residual after tracheotomy. Tracheomalacia can cause stridor. Congenital tracheomalacia tends to improve with maturation or with repair of the extrinsic cause, but resolution of symptoms is often very gradual.

After delivery, a chest radiograph will verify the presence of the TEF. Insertion of a nasogastric tube may show coiling in the mediastinal area. Contrast

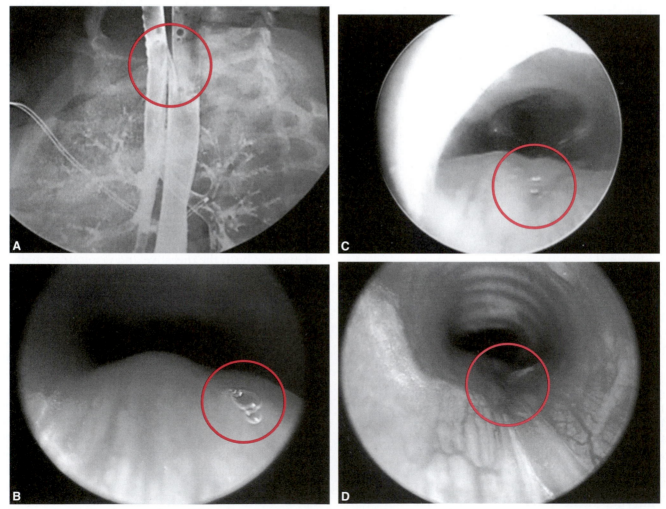

Figure 10-11 Tracheoesophageal Fistula *(Courtesy of Ellen Deutch MD FACS, FAAP)*

studies, where 1 to 2 mL of barium solution is instilled through an 8F suction catheter placed in the esophagus, are rarely needed to confirm a diagnosis of TEF. They significantly increase an infant's risk of aspiration pneumonitis because barium is an irritant if instilled accidentally into the airway. A CT scan of the thorax will also provide important diagnostic information about location of the fistula and assist surgery planning, and it is a less invasive test.

A renal and cardiac ultrasound may also be necessary to rule out other defects such as renal hypoplasia or cardiac anomalies.

Management and Treatment

If diagnosis of TEF is made prenatally, the infant should be delivered at a hospital with a pediatric surgical program, or the infant will need to be transferred there immediately after delivery.

Presurgical management for TEF includes placement of a Replogle tube into the esophageal pouch. This is a large gastric tube that is set to low suction and will remove any oral secretions that may build up to minimize the risk of aspiration. Maintaining infants in a 45-degree sitting position will also help them better manage their own airway. They will not be able to feed normally, so intravenous nutritional support is required. Intubation may be necessary for airway stabilization, and minimal ventilator support is usually necessary because there is no pulmonary dysfunction.

Management is surgical; the details of the procedure depend in part on the configuration of the atresia and fistula. Sometimes a pouch remains in the trachea as a remnant of the TEF despite repair. Depending on the size and the location, this pouch can be problematic in patients who require intubation or tracheotomy because the distal tip of the endotracheal or tracheotomy tube can become malpositioned into this pouch, causing sudden obstruction of ventilation. Management of this complication may include using a longer, or in special circumstances, a shorter tube. The respiratory therapist needs to pay particular care with the endotracheal tube after surgery because the surgeon will strategically place it below the site of the anastomosis. To prevent postoperative complications, it should not be manipulated unless necessary.

Early complications of surgery include leak at the anastomotic site, a recurrence of the TEF, or a stricture or narrowing at the point of anastomosis. Late complications may include GERD, recurrent pneumonias, asthma, esophageal dysmotility, and tracheomalacia.

Course and Prognosis

Survival rates for children with TEF have steadily improved over time, and survival rates for uncomplicated TEF reach close to 100%. More specifically, in one 2006 retrospective study, survival rates were 97% for full-term infants with no other congenital anomalies, but lowered to 50% for infants with a birth weight less than 1,500 g plus major cardiac anomalies (65).

After successful repair, children are relatively healthy. During the first 3 years of life, there is a risk for increased frequency for respiratory infections (63), although this risk tends to decrease over time.

Other Conditions Affecting the Trachea and Bronchi

Exudative tracheitis is a bacterial infection of the trachea that causes edema and oozing of fluid and cellular debris from the airway walls. It is particularly dangerous infection in small children because the tissue edema and exudative debris in the larynx and trachea can cause sudden, complete airway obstruction. Management includes control or vigilant monitoring of the airway as well as antibiotics. Although the most common causative organism is *Staphylococcus aureus*, episodes caused by *Moraxella catarrhalis* tend to be more severe (66).

Tracheal masses and **endobronchial masses** are uncommon in children, but foreign body aspiration should always be considered in a child with tracheal or bronchial symptoms, radiographic findings, or a suggestive history, such as a choking episode. Other tracheal and endobronchial masses that manifest in children include neoplasms such as carcinoid, mucoepidermoid carcinoma and adenoid cystic carcinoma (67, 68), and infections such as atypical mycobacteria (69). Although recurrent respiratory papillomatosis has a predilection for the vocal folds, it may also involve the trachea and bronchi.

Extrinsic compression of the trachea should also be considered. Congenital causes include vascular rings, such as double aortic arch (see Chapter 11). Esophageal foreign bodies can impinge on the trachea, particularly if they remain undiscovered long enough to cause local inflammation and granulation tissue.

As noted previously, ingested button batteries that become lodged in the esophagus constitute a special case and a true medical emergency because the batteries can erode into the trachea with fatal consequences. Aspiration of foreign bodies into the airway is discussed in Chapter 18; it can cause significant airway obstruction and may be a life-threatening event.

Tracheotomies

Rather than a disease or congenital malformation, a **tracheotomy** is a surgical procedure to create an opening in the trachea, below the vocal cord, and placed for long-term airway stabilization. The permanent opening that is created during the surgery is known as a **tracheostomy**. The indications for placement of tracheostomy tubes in children are different from that of adults and are described in Box 10-1.

A tracheotomy creates an opening in the proximal trachea, below the larynx, and therefore below the glottis (vocal folds) and the subglottis. Tracheotomies bypass lesions located above the tracheotomy, including conditions affecting the larynx, pharynx, oral cavity, nose, and face. In children, tracheostomy tubes are most often placed for upper or central airway obstruction, followed in frequency by pulmonary conditions that benefit from mechanical ventilation, and then by conditions associated with neurological impairment (71). Examples of conditions that may require tracheotomy to bypass airway obstruction include subglottic stenosis, subglottic hemangiomas, and craniofacial syndromes such as Robin sequence, Treacher Collins syndrome, CHARGE association, and others. The most common pediatric pulmonary condition that may require tracheotomy for prolonged mechanical ventilation is BPD (72). Examples of neurological conditions for which tracheotomies can be helpful include cerebral palsy and encephalopathy (71–75).

In pediatric patients, tracheotomy stay sutures are placed in the edge of the trachea, on either side of the tracheal incision. If the tracheotomy tube is prematurely dislodged, these ties can be grasped to help pull the incision open, exposing the stoma to facilitate reinsertion of the tube. Care should be taken to keep the right and left ties separated and oriented correctly. It is less common in children to surgically "mature" the stoma by suturing tracheal cartilage to the skin, and emergent cricothyrotomy and "bedside" tracheotomy procedures are uncommon in children.

A tracheotomy stoma is considered unstable until the surgical site has healed sufficiently to decrease the risk of creating a false passage during tracheotomy tube changes. The first tracheotomy tube change is generally performed by the surgeon to confirm adequate healing and can thereafter be delegated to appropriately trained health-care professionals and family members. The first tracheotomy tube change is often accomplished 5 to 7 days after surgery, but it can be safely accomplished as soon as 3 days postoperatively; the decision about this timing is at the discretion of the surgeon (76). Stay sutures are generally removed at the first tracheotomy tube change. Some institutions allow health-care providers to change the tracheotomy tube ties before the first tracheotomy tube change; others do not because of the potential for unintentionally dislodging the tracheotomy tube during manipulation of the ties.

Like adult tracheotomy tubes, pediatric tubes can be cuffed or uncuffed. Pediatric tubes also are available in both pediatric and neonatal sizes; comparably sized tubes have the same inner and outer diameters, but neonatal tubes are shorter. The distance between the chin and the chest in an infant is limited, and the universal adaptor allowing connection to ventilator tubing or other devices may not fit easily into this space. Some tracheotomy tubes have an extension external (anterior) to the neck flange, which allows the universal adaptor to be located further from the child's neck, minimizing local trauma and facilitating normal head position. Unlike adult tracheostomy tubes, most pediatric tracheostomy tubes do not have an inner cannula, so a tracheostomy tube change, whether routine or emergent, requires removing the entire tracheostomy tube. Tracheostomy ties are available in a variety of materials and should be snug but not constricting. To change a pediatric tracheostomy tube, follow the following steps: (77)

- Wash your hands.
- Explain the procedure to the patient and family.
- Suction the airway using sterile technique.
- Prepare a new tracheostomy tube using sterile technique.
- Place ties or holder in the neck plate of new tube.
- Place the obturator (also called introducer) into new tracheostomy tube.
- Lubricate the end of the new tracheostomy tube with water-soluble lubricant.
- Extend the patient's neck.
- Cut tracheostomy ties or release tube securement device.
- If a cuffed tracheostomy tube is in place, completely deflate cuff.
- Gently remove the entire tracheostomy tube.
- Immediately insert the new tube by performing a downward, inward motion.

Box 10-1 Indications for Tracheostomy for Adults and Children

Adults (70)

Prolonged respiratory failure
Decreased level of consciousness
Poor airway protective reflexes
Severe alterations in physiology associated with trauma or medical illness

Children (57)

To bypass upper and central airway obstruction
Provides access for prolonged mechanical ventilation
To facilitate tracheobronchial hygiene
Neurological impairment
Bronchopulmonary dysplasia

- Secure the tracheostomy ties.
- Inflate the cuff using institutional policy, and document cuff pressure (if a cuffed tube is used).

If the new tube cannot be placed, there are several potential options to reestablish an airway:

- Use a tube that is one size smaller than the tube that was removed.
- Use a **Seldinger technique**: Thread the new tracheotomy tube over a small suction catheter, then insert the suction catheter into the stoma to find the pathway into the trachea. Once the suction catheter is in the trachea, use it as a guide over which to slide the tracheotomy tube.
- If the tube still cannot be placed, a small ETT can be placed in the stoma, with care taken not to advance the tube beyond where the tracheostomy tube would have been (measurements for length of tube are provided by the manufacturer).
- If a tube still cannot be placed and the patient is cyanotic, place a gloved finger over the stoma with enough pressure to minimize any air leak, but without pressing hard enough to compress the trachea (which is relatively soft in infants), and use bag-mask ventilation.

Patency of a tracheostomy tube should be evaluated whenever there is question of airway blockage. Positive end-tidal CO_2 (E_TCO_2) measurement is the best method to evaluate airway patency, seen by a positive change in colorimetric $ETCO_2$ or a tidal wave and numerical value in volumetric E_TCO_2. If no E_TCO_2 is available, patency can also be evaluated by passing a suction catheter to the end of the tracheostomy tube, taking care not to pass beyond the end of the cannula to avoid tracheal tissue damage.

■ ■ BG Walters' tracheotomy is performed 2 weeks after her last extubation attempt. Five days after the procedure, she is weaned from mechanical ventilation and maintained on a tracheostomy collar with an FIO$_2$ of 0.30. The surgeon performed the initial tracheostomy tube change on day 6 after surgery and removed the suture stays. You perform the next tube change 5 days later. You bring in a pediatric tracheostomy mannequin for BG Walters' parents to practice tracheostomy tube change procedures, and they perform the third tube change under your supervision.

Two months after Gabrielle's tracheotomy, she has a laryngotracheal reconstruction, which is performed successfully. She is decannulated shortly after she is weaned from mechanical ventilation. She is discharged after her reconstruction on a nasal cannula and home medications to manage her BPD.

■ ■ Critical Thinking Questions: BG Walters

1. What additional considerations should have been made during BG Walters' ETT management after her reintubation?
2. Should BG Walters' parents be allowed to change her airway within the hospital, especially because the plan was to repair her airway and remove the tracheostomy tube prior to hospital discharge?
3. How might BG Walters' chronic lung disease complicate her postoperative care? Would it make it easier or harder to wean her from the ventilator?

▶● Case Studies and Critical Thinking Questions

■ Case 1: BG Chase

BG Chase is 4 hours old and has developed cyanosis that is relieved when she cries. A wisp of cotton held in front of each nare does not move with respiration. You are unable to pass a suction catheter gently through either nare.

- *What can you do to help her immediately in this acute situation?*
- *What is the definitive treatment?*

■ Case 2: Baby Boy (BB) Tompkins

You are called to the bedside of BB Tompkins, a 3-month-old child with Robin sequence who is admitted for failure to thrive. He is sleeping, and you and the nurse notice increased work of breathing with suprasternal retractions and nasal flaring.

- *What can you do to help him at this moment?*

■ Case 3: BG Woodson

BG Woodson, a 4-week-old infant, is admitted to the pediatric floor of a 300-bed suburban hospital where you work as the RT. Olivia was born at full term during a normal delivery, but she has a history of noisy breathing and had an "apparent life-threatening event" that included a cyanotic episode. On the first night of admission, you are called to the bedside to help the medical resident because the infant is having difficulty breathing.

BG Woodson has high-pitched, vibratory, inspiratory stridor with suprasternal retractions and appears to be working hard to breathe. She is lying supine and appears small for her age.

- *What is the most common cause of congenital stridor?*
- *What can you do to alleviate her respiratory distress right now?*
- *Will Olivia need surgical treatment?*

■ Case 4: Jackson Black

You are the RT covering the emergency department (ED) at a 200-bed suburban hospital. Jackson Black's parents have brought him to the ED for respiratory distress. He is 4 years old with hoarseness that is so severe that he has no voice at all, but is able to communicate verbally in a limited fashion using a very hoarse whisper. His parents say that he has been hoarse for as long as they can remember, but it has gotten progressively more severe, and now they notice that his breathing has become noisy and effortful. When you listen, you hear stridor, which is predominantly inspiratory and low-pitched.

- *What initial therapies could help alleviate Jackson's stridor?*

Unfortunately, treatment with steroids and racemic epinephrine are unsuccessful. You review the patient's chart and find a diagnosis of recurrent respiratory papillomatosis.

- *How is this treated?*

■ Case 5: James Brody

You are a neonatal RT in a level III NICU caring for James Brody. He is 6 months old, born at 24 weeks' gestation, and has been successfully weaned to minimal ventilator support. Several attempts to extubate him have been unsuccessful because he develops stridor, which is primarily inspiratory, and work of breathing has significantly increased, requiring reintubation.

- *What can you do to improve his chances of success at the next extubation attempt?*

■ Case 6: BG Hawk

You are the day shift RT at a 75-bed rural community hospital and are called down to the newborn nursery to see BG Hawk, who is just 10 hours old. She was born after a full-term gestation and had Apgar scores of 9 at 1 and 5 minutes. Initial physical examination was remarkable only for a slight increase in white oral secretions, which cleared with suctioning. She reportedly tolerated her first feeding, nursing for about 10 minutes. She is now noted to have crackles on routine auscultation. At the time crackles were noted, she had a normal respiratory rate and increased oral secretions. A 10 French nasogastric tube could not be passed beyond 10 cm.

- *What is the most likely diagnosis?*
- *What temporizing measures would you recommend to manage BG Hawk's airway while awaiting her transfer to a larger pediatric surgery center?*

■ Case 7: BB Turner

BB Turner, a 6-month-old, who had been born prematurely, underwent tracheotomy at 4 months of age for BPD and ventilator dependence. His pulmonary disease has been gradually improving, and his ventilator settings have been stable. When you walk into his room, his oxygen saturation is a bit lower than usual, and he seems to be working harder to breathe.

- *What do you think might be happening? What can you do immediately to assess him?*
- *What would be your next course of action?*
- *You call for assistance to change his tracheostomy tube, obtain the appropriate supplies and equipment, position him with his neck extended, and remove his tracheotomy tube. When you try to insert the new tube, you are unable. What should you do now?*

Multiple-Choice Questions

1. You suspect that a newborn has choanal atresia. What can you do to help her immediately in this acute situation?
   a. Attach a nasal cannula with supplemental oxygen
   b. Place a face mask with supplemental oxygen
   c. Open her mouth
   d. Alert personnel who can place a laryngeal mask airway

2. You are caring for a young child with severe developmental delays who requires bilevel positive airway pressure (BPAP) support. When you adjust his mask, you notice some duskiness at the bridge of his nose under the cuff of the mask. You should:
   a. Notify his care team because this may be evidence of deeper tissue damage
   b. Make sure he is receiving an appropriate antibiotic
   c. Ask the physician to discontinue BPAP therapy and change to another oxygen delivery device
   d. Not worry; this is a common finding with BPAP masks

3. Why should clinicians be concerned about an infant with a large tongue?
   a. A large tongue is likely to cause airway obstruction posterior to it.
   b. A large tongue can cause stridor.
   c. There are no oral airways small enough to fit infants, and therefore it cannot be treated without intubation.
   d. It is not a concern because infants are obligate nose breathers.

4. Masses in the vallecula can cause:
   a. Problems with phonation
   b. Airway obstruction
   c. Death
   d. All of the above

5. Chronic oropharyngeal obstruction frequently causes:
       I. Poor weight gain
       II. Failure to thrive
       III. GERD
       IV. Stridor
       V. Dysphagia
   a. I, II, V
   b. I, II, IV
   c. I, II, III
   d. I, II, III, IV

6. Most cases of laryngomalacia can be managed with:
   a. Surgical reconstruction
   b. Tracheotomy
   c. Body positioning
   d. Endoscopy

7. You are called to assess a 1-month-old baby after her cardiac surgery for patent ductus arteriosus (PDA) ligation. The nursing team notes that her cry has become weaker and breathier compared to previously. What is the most likely cause?
   a. Intraoperative injury to the left recurrent laryngeal nerve
   b. Foreign body left in the airway during intubation for the surgery
   c. Recurrent respiratory papillomatosis
   d. Laryngomalacia

8. A 4-year-old with a history of recurrent respiratory papillomatosis has a tracheostomy. The family and nursing team note that they feel increasing resistance with tracheostomy changes. You examine the tracheostomy site and identify clusters of compressible exophytic red-colored lesions that were not previously noted. Your next step is to:
   a. Recommend that the team consider increasing the size of the tracheostomy tube
   b. Recommend that the team consider evaluation for distal spread of the papilloma
   c. Remove the obstructing lesions at the patient's bedside
   d. Reassure family that this is normal

9. A 3-month-old boy is in the neonatal intensive care unit with stridor, no fever or cough, SpO_2 of 98%, and a history of prematurity. Which of the following is the *least* likely cause of his stridor?
   a. Subglottic stenosis
   b. Laryngotracheobronchitis
   c. Vocal cord paralysis
   d. Subglottic cysts

10. Which of the following methods is the most reliable for confirming that a tracheostomy tube is in place and functioning?
   a. Bilateral equal breath sounds
   b. End-tidal CO_2 reading
   c. Condensation coming from the tracheostomy tube
   d. Hearing airflow at the tip of the tracheostomy tube

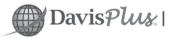 For additional resources login to Davis*Plus* (http://davisplus.fadavis.com/ keyword "Perretta") and click on the Premium tab. (Don't have a *Plus*Code to access Premium Resources? Just click the Purchase Access button on the book's Davis*Plus* page.)

REFERENCES

1. Pirsig W. Surgery of choanal atresia in infants and children: historical notes and updated review. *Int J Pediatr Otorhinolaryngol.* 1986;11(2):153-170.
2. Rothman G, Wood RA, Naclerio RM. Unilateral choanal atresia masquerading as chronic sinusitis. *Pediatrics.* 1994; 94(6, pt 1):941-944.
3. Bergeson PS, Shaw JC. Are infants really obligatory nasal breathers? *Clin Pediatr.* 2001;40(10):567-569.
4. Teissier N, Kaguelidou F, Couloigner V, François M, Van Den Abbeele T. Predictive factors for success after transnasal endoscopic treatment of choanal atresia. *Arch Otolaryngol Head Neck Surg.* 2008;134(1):57-61.
5. Ramsden JD, Campisi P. Choanal atresia and choanal stenosis. *Otolaryngol Clin North Am.* 2009;42:339-352.
6. Benoit MM, Silvera VM, Nichollas R, Jones D, McGill T, Rahbar R. Image guidance systems for minimally invasive sinus and skull base surgery in children. *Int J Pediatr Otorhinolaryngol.* 2009;73(10):1452-1457.

7. Hengerer AS, Brickman TM, Jeyakumar A. Choanal atresia: embryologic analysis and evolution of treatment, a 30-year experience. *Laryngoscope.* 2008;118(5):862-866.
8. Corrales CE, Koltai PJ. Choanal atresia: current concepts and controversies. *Curr Opin Otolaryngol Head Neck Surg.* 2009;17(6):466-470.
9. Durmaz A, Tosun F, Yldrm N, Sahan M, Kvrakdal C, Gerek M. Transnasal endoscopic repair of choanal atresia: results of 13 cases and meta-analysis. *J Craniofac Surg.* 2008;19(5):1270-1274.
10. Belenky WM, Madgy DN, Haupert MS. Nasal obstruction and rhinorrhea. In: Bluestone CH, Stool SE, eds. *Pediatric Otolaryngology.* 4th ed. Philadelphia, PA: Saunders; 2001: 908-923.
11. Elloy MD, Cochrane LA, Albert DM. Refractory choanal atresia: what makes a child susceptible? The Great Ormond Street Hospital experience. *J Otolaryngol Head Neck Surg.* 2008;37(6):813-820.
12. Zuckerman JD, Zapata S, Sobol SE. Single-stage choanal atresia repair in the neonate. *Arch Otolaryngol Head Neck Surg.* 2008;134(10):1090-1093.
13. Allam KA, Wan DC, Kawamoto HK, Bradley JP, Sedano HO, Saied S. The spectrum of median craniofacial dysplasia. *Plast Reconstr Surg.* 2011;127(2):812-821.
14. van Kempen MJ, Rijkers GT, Van Cauwenberge PB. The immune response in adenoids and tonsils. *Int Arch Allergy Immunol.* 2000;122(1):8-19.
15. Brodsky L. Modern assessment of tonsils and adenoids. *Pediatr Clin North Am.* 1989;36(6):1551-1569.
16. Mackay DR. Controversies in the diagnosis and management of the Robin sequence. *J Craniofac Surg.* 2011;22(2): 415-420.
17. Evans AK, Rahbar R, Rogers GF, Mulliken JB, Volk MS. Robin sequence: a retrospective review of 115 patients. *Int J Pediatr Otorhinolaryngol.* 2006;70(6):973-980.
18. Gozu A, Genc B, Palabiyik M, et al. Airway management in neonates with Pierre Robin sequence. *Turk J Pediatr.* 2010;52:167-172.
19. Robison JG, Otteson TD. Increased prevalence of obstructive sleep apnea in patients with cleft palate. *Arch Otolaryngol Head Neck Surg.* 2011;137(3):269-274.
20. John A, Fagondes S, Schwartz I, et al. Sleep abnormalities in untreated patients with mucopolysaccharidosis type VI. *Am J Med Genet A.* 2011;155A(7):1546-1551.
21. Passy V. Pathogenesis of peritonsillar abscess. *Laryngoscope.* 1994;104(2):185-190.
22. Al-Sabah B, Bin Salleen H, Hagr A, Choi-Rosen J, Manoukian JJ, Tewfik TL. Retropharyngeal abscess in children: 10-year study. *J Otolaryngol.* 2004;33(6):352-355.
23. Daniel SJ. The upper airway: congenital malformations. *Paediatr Respir Rev.* 2006;7(suppl 1):S260-S263.
24. Richter GT, Rutter MJ, deAlarcon A, Orvidas LJ, Thompson DM. Late-onset laryngomalacia: a variant of disease. *Arch Otolaryngol Head Neck Surg.* 2008;134(1):75-80.
25. Thompson DM. Abnormal sensorimotor integrative function of the larynx in congenital laryngomalacia: a new theory of etiology. *Laryngoscope.* 2007;117(6, pt 2, suppl 114):1-33.
26. Richter GT, Thompson DM. The surgical management of laryngomalacia. *Otolaryngol Clin North Am.* 2008;41(5): 837-864, vii.
27. Rutter MJ, Cohen AP, de Alarcon A. Endoscopic airway management in children. *Curr Opin Otolaryngol Head Neck Surg.* 2008;16(6):525-529.
28. Woo P. Acquired laryngomalacia: epiglottis prolapse as a cause of airway obstruction. *Ann Otol Rhinol Laryngol.* 1992;101(4):314-320.
29. Mancuso RF, Choi SS, Zalzal GH, Grundfast KM. Laryngomalacia. The search for the second lesion. *Arch Otolaryngol Head Neck Surg.* 1996;122(3):302-306.
30. Cotton RT, Prescott CAJ. Congenital anomalies of the larynx. In: Cotton RT, Myer CM III, eds. *Practical Pediatric Otolaryngology.* Philadelphia. PA: Lippincott-Raven; 1999:497-513.
31. Thompson DM. Laryngomalacia: factors that influence disease severity and outcomes of management. *Curr Opin Otolaryngol Head Neck Surg.* 2010;18(6):564-570.
32. Groblewski JC, Shah RK, Zalzal GH. Microdebrider-assisted supraglottoplasty for laryngomalacia. *Ann Otol Rhinol Laryngol.* 2009;118(8):592-597.
33. Yen K, Flanary V, Estel C, Farber N, Hennes H. Traumatic epiglottitis. *Pediatr Emerg Care.* 2003;19(1):27-28.
34. Gutierrez JP, Berkowitz RG, Robertson CF. Vallecular cysts in newborns and young infants. *Pediatr Pulmonol.* 1999;27(4):282-285.
35. Kumar V, Nagendhar Y, Prakash B, Chattopadhyay A, Vepakomma D. Lingual thyroid gland: clinical evaluation and management. *Indian J Pediatr.* 2004;71(12):e62-e64.
36. Rahbar R, Yoon MJ, Connolly LP, et al. Lingual thyroid in children: a rare clinical entity. *Laryngoscope.* 2008;118(7): 1174-1179.
37. Mussak EN, Kacker A. Surgical and medical management of midline ectopic thyroid. *Otolaryngol Head Neck Surg.* 2007;136(6):870-872.
38. Cavo JW Jr, Lee JC. Laryngocele after childbirth. *Otolaryngol Head Neck Surg.* 1993;109(4):766-768.
39. Wiatrak BJ, Wiatrak DW, Broker TR, Lewis L. Recurrent respiratory papillomatosis: a longitudinal study comparing severity associated with human papilloma viral types 6 and 11 and other risk factors in a large pediatric population. *Laryngoscope.* 2004;114(11, pt 2, suppl 104):1-23.
40. Derkay CS. Task force on recurrent respiratory papillomas. A preliminary report. *Arch Otolaryngol Head Neck Surg.* 1995;121(12):1386-1391.
41. Schraff S, Derkay CS, Burke B, Lawson L. American society of pediatric otolaryngology members' experience with recurrent respiratory papillomatosis and the use of adjuvant therapy. *Arch Otolaryngol Head Neck Surg.* 2004;130(9): 1039-1042.
42. Zur K, Jacobs IN. Management of chronic upper airway obstruction. In: Wetmore R, ed. *Pediatric Otolaryngology: The Requisites in Pediatrics 2007.* Philadelphia, PA: Mosby Elsevier; 2007:173-189.
43. Mudry P, Vavrina M, Mazanek P, Machalova M, Litzman J, Sterba J. Recurrent laryngeal papillomatosis: successful treatment with human papillomavirus vaccination. *Arch Dis Child.* 2011;96(5):476-477.
44. Committee on Infectious Diseases. Recommendations for prevention and control of influenza in children, 2011-2012. *Pediatrics.* 2011;128(4):813-825.
45. Chadra NK, Allegro J, Barton M, Hawkes M, Harlock H, Campisi P. The quality of life and health utility burden of recurrent respiratory papillomatosis in children. *Otolaryngol Head Neck Surg.* 2010;143(5):685-690.
46. Zenk J, Fyrmpas G, Zimmermann T, Koch M, Constantinidis J, Iro H. Tracheostomy in young patients: indications and long-term outcome. *Eur Arch Otorhinolaryngol.* 2009; 266(5):705-711.
47. Marcum KK, Wright SC Jr, Kemp ES, Kitse DJ. A novel modification of the ansa to recurrent laryngeal nerve reinnervation procedure for young children. *Int J Pediatr Otorhinolaryngol.* 2010;74(11):1335-1337.
48. Miyamoto RC, Cotton RT, Rope AF, et al. Association of anterior glottic webs with velocardiofacial syndrome

(chromosome 22q11.2 deletion). *Otolaryngol Head Neck Surg*. 2004;130(4):415-417.

49. Mauritz FA, van Herwaarden-Lindeboom MY, Stomp W, et al. The effects and efficacy of antireflux surgery in children with gastroesophageal reflux disease: a systematic review. *J Gastrointest Surg*. 2011;15(10):1872-1878.

50. Willging JP, Cotton RT. Subglottic stenosis in the pediatric patient. In: Myer CM 3rd, Cotton RT, Shott SR, eds. *The Pediatric Airway: An Interdisciplinary Approach*. Philadelphia, PA: JB Lippincott Co; 1995:111-132.

51. O'Connor DM. Physiology of the airway. In: Myer CM 3rd, Cotton RT, Shott SR, eds. *The Pediatric Airway: An Interdisciplinary Approach*. Philadelphia, PA: JB Lippincott Co; 1995:15-23.

52. Myer CM 3rd, O'Connor DM, Cotton RT. Proposed grading system for subglottic stenosis based on endotracheal tube sizes. *Ann Otol Rhinol Laryngol*. 1994;103(4, pt 1): 319-323.

53. Walner DL, Cotton RT. Acquired anomalies of the larynx and trachea. In: Cotton RT, Myer CM 3rd, eds. *Practical Pediatric Otolaryngology*. Philadelphia, PA: Lippincott-Raven; 1999:515-537.

54. Zalzal GH, Grundfast KM. Broken aboulker stents in the tracheal lumen. *Int J Pediatr Otorhinolaryngol*. 1988;16(2): 125-130.

55. Inglis AF Jr, Perkins JA, Manning SC, Mouzakes J. Endoscopic posterior cricoid split and rib grafting in 10 children. *Laryngoscope*. 2003;113(11):2004-2009.

56. Bruno CJ, Smith LP, Zur KB, Wade KC. Congenital subglottic cyst in a term neonate. *Arch Dis Child Fetal Neonatal Ed*. 2009;94(4):F240.

57. Watson GJ, Malik TH, Khan NA, Sheehan PZ, Rothera MP. Acquired paediatric subglottic cysts: a series from Manchester. *Int J Pediatr Otorhinolaryngol*. 2007;71(4): 533-538.

58. Steehler MK, Groblewski JC, Milmoe GJ, Harley EH. Management of subglottic cysts with mitomycin-C-A case series and literature review. *Int J Pediatr Otorhinolaryngol*. 2011;75(3):360-363.

59. Kazahaya K, Singh DJ. Congenital malformations of the head and neck. In: Wetmore R, ed. *Pediatric Otolaryngology. The Requisites in Pediatrics*. Philadelphia, PA: Mosby Inc; 2007:1-22.

60. Javia LR, Zur KB, Jacobs IN. Evolving treatments in the management of laryngotracheal hemangiomas: will propranolol supplant steroids and surgery? *Int J Pediatr Otorhinolaryngol*. 2011;75(11):1450-1454.

61. Johnson D. Croup. *Clin Evid* (Online). 2009;Mar 10:0321. www.ncbi.nlm.nih.gov/pmc/articles/PMC2907784/.

62. Shaw-Smith C. Oesophageal atresia, tracheo-oesophageal fistula, and the VACTERL association: review of genetics and epidemiology. *J Med Genet*. 2006;43:545-554.

63. Spitz L. Oesophaeal atresia. *Orphanet J Rare Dis*. 2007;2:24.

64. Clark DC. Esophageal atresia and tracheoesophageal fistula. *Am Fam Physician*. 1999;59(4):910-916.

65. Lopez PJ, Keys C, Pierro A, et al. Oesophageal atresia: improved outcome in high-risk groups? *J Pediatr Surg*. 2006;41(2):331-334.

66. Salamone FN, Bobbitt DB, Myer CM, Rutter MJ, Greinwald JH Jr. Bacterial tracheitis reexamined: is there a less severe manifestation? *Otolaryngol Head Neck Surg*. 2004;131(6): 871-876.

67. Deutsch ES, Milmoe G. Stridor in an adolescent: an unusual symptom. *Otolaryngol Head Neck Surg*. 1994;110(3):330-332.

68. Roby BB, Drehner D, Sidman JD. Pediatric tracheal and endobronchial tumors: an institutional experience. *Arch Otolaryngol Head Neck Surg*. 2011;137(9):925-929.

69. Malloy KM, Di Pentima MC, Deutsch ES. Non-tuberculous mycobacteria presenting as an obstructing endobronchial mass in an immunocompetent infant. *Int J Pediatr Otorhinolaryngol*. 2008;3:136-139.

70. Durbin CG. Tracheostomy: why, when and how? *Respir Care*. 2010;55(8):1056-1068.

71. Deutsch ES. Tracheostomy: pediatric considerations. *Respir Care*. 2010;55(8):1082-1090.

72. Carron JD, Derkay CS, Strope GL, Nosonchuk JE, Darrow DH. Pediatric tracheotomies: changing indications and outcomes. *Laryngoscope*. 2000;110(7):1099-1104.

73. Davis GM. Tracheostomy in children. *Paediatr Respir Rev*. 2006;7(suppl 1):S206-S209.

74. Mahadevan M, Barber C, Salkeld L, Douglas G, Mills N. Pediatric trachcotomy: 17-ycar rcview. *Int J Pediatr Otorhinolaryngol*. 2007;71(12):1829-1835.

75. Parrilla C, Scarano E, Guidi ML, Galli J, Paludetti G. Current trends in paediatric tracheostomies. *Int J Pediatr Otorhinolaryngol*. 2007;71(10):1563-1567.

76. Deutsch ES. Early tracheostomy tube change in children. *Arch Otolaryngol Head Neck Surg*. 1998;124(11):1237-1238.

77. Management of a patient with a tracheostomy tube, PAT035, appendix I: tracheostomy tube change procedure. Effective date July 10, 2012. http://www.insidehopkinsmedicine.org/hpo/policies/39/77/appendix_32534.pdf?CFID=100759854&CFTOKEN=af0e8a0db0e06ba3-309F9611-B1B3-88E2-56F8DF7619E494A1. Accessed December 1, 2012.

Chapter 11

Acyanotic Heart Defects

Chapter Outline cont.

Chapter Objectives

After reading this chapter, you will be able to:

1. Identify the common types of acyanotic heart defects diagnosed in children.
2. Identify the two most common acyanotic heart defects.
3. Explain the anatomical variations of different acyanotic heart defects.
4. Discuss the clinical signs and symptoms associated with each heart defect.
5. Explain how the pathophysiology of acyanotic heart defects can mimic pulmonary disease.
6. Differentiate between murmurs found in acyanotic heart defects.
7. Describe the surgical management and treatment strategies for acyanotic heart defects.
8. List the indications for closing a septal wall defect.
9. Describe the respiratory symptoms that may manifest in a patient with a double aortic arch.

■■ Carly Jo Johnson

Carly Jo (CJ) Johnson is a 6-month-old female who presents to the emergency department with "respiratory problems" and a low-grade fever. According to her mother, CJ was a normal baby at birth. She was born at 38 weeks by spontaneous vaginal delivery and weighed 7 lb, 4 oz (3.2 kg). For the past several months, CJ has not seemed to gain weight well despite having a good appetite. Mom has noticed that she seems fatigued after eating and frequently seems to breathe harder and faster while breastfeeding. Over the past 2 days, CJ has been breathing rapidly and not feeding well. She has had some congestion and a cough. This morning she developed a low-grade fever (38°C), which mom treated with acetaminophen.

On clinical examination, the baby appears tachypneic and distressed. Her vital signs are as follows: heart rate 175, respiratory rate 75, blood pressure 85/50, and SpO$_2$ 91% on room air. She looks small for her age, which is confirmed by her weight of 4.8 kg. She is interactive and cries appropriately. However, you notice that she has moderate retractions. On lung auscultation, you can hear fine and coarse rales as well as scattered wheezes. Breath sounds are present throughout. She is warm to touch, although her pulse is rapid and diminished in quality. Her capillary refill time is 4 seconds. The child's liver is 3 to 4 cm below the costal margin.

Approximately 1% of infants suffer from congenital heart disease, which refers to heart diseases or defects present at birth, usually caused by hereditary factors (1). Many different structural abnormalities can lead to the diagnosis of congenital heart disease. Broadly, these abnormalities can be divided into acyanotic or cyanotic defects. This chapter focuses on acyanotic heart defects, and Chapter 12 focuses on cyanotic heart defects.

Acyanotic heart defects refer to any structural abnormality that does not cause right-to-left intracardiac shunting. The term "acyanotic" indicates that the patient should have normal oxygen saturations unlike cyanotic heart disease, which results in lower than normal oxygen saturations. Acyanotic heart defects include the following: septal wall defects, aortic stenosis, pulmonic stenosis, coarctation of the aorta, and double aortic arch.

Diagnosis of congenital heart defects is often made before birth and is frequently observed during fetal ultrasounds performed midway through pregnancy. Early recognition of these defects allows close monitoring as well as counseling by a pediatric cardiologist prior to delivery. Delivery of infants with known cardiac abnormalities is ideally done at a quaternary-care children's hospital with a cardiac surgical team, dedicated cardiac intensive care unit, and an extracorporeal life support (ECLS) program to best support an infant who may have cardiac instability at birth or soon after.

For children who are not diagnosed in utero, a thorough assessment of symptoms and clinical manifestations will allow identification of a cardiac defect. Many diagnostic tools are used to elucidate the type, location, and severity of the defect. These include the following:

- Electrocardiogram (EKG): reading of the electrical activity of the heart
- Chest radiograph
- **Echocardiogram:** using ultrasound to visualize cardiac structures noninvasively

- **Doppler interrogation:** using ultrasound to determine blood flow velocity in different locations in the heart
- **Cardiac auscultation:** listening to heart sounds with a stethoscope and classifying the location and quality of a **cardiac murmur**. A murmur is an abnormal heart sound and is the result of turbulent blood flow across a cardiac structure. Auscultation is an inexpensive bedside assessment that a trained clinician should be able to use to make an accurate diagnosis. A list of abnormal cardiac sounds, their location in the thorax, and associated diagnosis can be found in Table 11-1.

The role of the respiratory therapist in managing hospital patients with congenital cardiac anomalies is mainly supportive, although that should in no way diminish the importance of the therapist's contribution to pre- and postoperative management. Appropriate management of oxygenation and ventilation can have a great impact on the cardiopulmonary system and can help avoid many complications such as hypoxemia and respiratory acidosis. The impact of physiological derangements on a child with congenital heart disease can be significant. Both hypoxemia and acidosis (either respiratory or metabolic) can lead to myocardial dysfunction, inadequate tissue perfusion, and cardiac arrest. Anticipation of potential problems and vigilant clinical reassessment by the multidisciplinary care team can prevent complications in the postoperative period. The bedside respiratory therapist (RT) plays a significant role in early recognition of postoperative issues related to the respiratory system. After undergoing cardiac surgery, pediatric patients may develop extrathoracic upper airway obstruction from postextubation stridor or vocal cord paralysis, pulmonary edema, hypoventilation from residual anesthetic effects, and diffuse atelectasis from splinting. In addition, patients who return from the operating room intubated and mechanically ventilated may need rigorous monitoring of oxygenation/ventilation.

Septal Wall Defects

Septal wall defects are, most literally, holes in the septum of the heart that may occur at various locations. A **septum** is a wall that divides two cavities. In cardiac anatomy, one septum divides the right and left atria (called the intra-atrial septum), and another divides the right and left ventricles (called the intra-ventricular septum). A defect in either of these creates a communication between the two atria or ventricles that allows mixing of blood from the right and left sides of the heart. Mixing of oxygenated and deoxygenated blood can potentially affect cardiac output or oxygenation of tissues in the body.

Atrial Septal Defect

Atrial septal defects represent one of the most common types of congenital heart disease, with a birth prevalence between 13 and 100 out of every 10,000 live births (1). An **atrial septal defect** (ASD) is an opening in the intra-atrial septum, which creates an anatomical connection between the two uppermost chambers of the heart. Approximately 10% to 15% of children with congenital heart disease have a type of ASD (2). ASDs can occur in isolation or as part of more complex congenital heart disease. Because they infrequently cause symptoms during infancy, ASDs may go undiagnosed until childhood or even adulthood.

Table 11-1	Cardiac Auscultation	
Sound/Murmur	**Location**	**Defect**
Soft systolic ejection murmur "Fixed" split S2	Along upper left sternal border	Atrial septal defect
Harsh holosystolic murmur	Loudest at fourth intercostal space, but may be heard throughout the chest	Ventricular septal defect
Harsh, loud systolic ejection murmur Ejection click Paradoxical split		Aortic stenosis
Systolic ejection murmur, with or without click "Fixed" split S2	Left upper sternal border	Pulmonic stenosis
Continuous flow murmur		Coarctation of the aorta

Pathophysiology

The atrial septum is formed by the junction of two important structures: the septum primum and the septum secundum. The **septum primum** is a thin area of tissue connected to the endocardial cushions. The endocardial cushions, found early in embryological development, are segments of tissue in the heart that give rise to the formation of the valves and the septa. The **septum secundum** is a more muscular structure that grows downward from the upper portion of the embryological atria. The fusion of these two structures forms the atrial septum. Any failure in the union of these two structures results in an ASD.

During fetal life, an opening called the foramen ovale is maintained between the left and right atria so that oxygenated blood in the right atrium can bypass the lungs and be diverted into the left atrium and out to the body. After birth, the pressures in the left side of the heart increase and those on the right decrease—resulting in closure of the foramen. If this structure fails to close, the resulting defect is called a patent foramen ovale (PFO). Approximately 15% to 30% of the general population has a PFO that is usually clinically inconsequential (2). In addition to a PFO, there are multiple types of ASDs (Fig. 11-1):

- **Ostium secundum ASD:** the most common type, accounting for two-thirds of all ASDs (2). An **ostium secundum ASD** occurs when the septum primum does not grow to completely cover and fuse with the septum secundum.
- **Sinus venosus type ASD: Sinus venosus** type ASDs (10%) are located directly inferior to the junction of the superior vena cava and the right atrium and are almost always associated with partial anomalous pulmonary venous return (see Chapter 12 for more information on anomalous pulmonary venous return).

- **Coronary sinus type ASD:** occurs in the **coronary sinus**, where the cardiac veins return blood flow to the right atrium. This defect creates a communication between the right and left atrium; it is also referred to as an unroofed coronary sinus.
- **Ostium primum ASD:** a defect in the septum primum that occurs directly superior to the atrioventricular valves. This type of defect almost exclusively occurs as part of an atrioventricular canal defect, where the endocardial cushions fail to form properly.

During fetal circulation, pressure in the right atrium is higher than pressure in the left atrium because of widespread pulmonary vasoconstriction. Therefore, blood flows from the *right* heart to *left* heart across the atrial septum. After delivery, a baby's first breath causes the pulmonary arterial pressure to drop, and right atrial pressure becomes lower than left atrial pressure. Because now left atrial pressure is higher than right atrial pressure, blood flow across an ASD will occur from the *left* heart to the *right* heart, across the defect. Over time, this leads to increased blood volume in the right heart and increased pulmonary blood flow. This has the potential to cause complications such as pulmonary edema and right heart failure; however, even large ASDs with unrestricted flow into the right atrium usually do not cause signs of heart failure.

Clinical Manifestations

Many children, and even adults, are completely asymptomatic from an ASD (Clinical Variation 11-1). If symptoms are evident during childhood, they are usually secondary to a fairly large defect (greater than 6 mm) causing increased workload on the right ventricle and increased blood flow to the lungs. Symptoms may include the following:

- Fatigue
- Exercise intolerance
- Failure to thrive
- Poor weight gain
- Tachypnea
- Congestive heart failure (infrequently)

On clinical examination, a soft systolic ejection murmur can be heard along the upper left sternal border. This murmur reflects the increased flow through the pulmonic valve, rather than flow across the atrial level defect. Increased blood flow through the right ventricular outflow tract (pulmonary arteries) can also cause a "fixed split" of the second heart sound. The second heart sound is caused by the closure of the aortic and pulmonary valves during diastole. During inspiration in a normal heart, the pulmonic valve closes immediately after the aortic valve; however, during expiration, the two close almost at the same

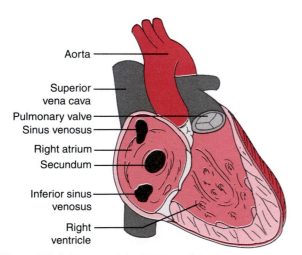

Figure 11-1 Types of Atrial Septal Defects

Aorta

Superior vena cava

Pulmonary valve

Sinus venosus

Right atrium

Secundum

Inferior sinus venosus

Right ventricle

Clinical Variations 11-1

Adult Presentation of ASD

Many patients with ASDs are free of overt symptoms, although most will become symptomatic at some point in their lives. The age at which symptoms appear is highly variable and is not exclusively related to the size of the shunt. Initial symptoms usually present as exercise-induced dyspnea or fatigue. The more common clinical manifestation in later life includes arrhythmias. Atrial fibrillation or flutter is an age-related reflection of atrial dilation and stretch that seldom occurs before 40 years of age.

time—this is a normal "splitting" of the second heart sound (S2). A patient with an ASD has more blood flowing across the pulmonary valve, thus causing the pulmonary valve to close after the aortic valve in inspiration and exhalation—known as a **"fixed" split S2**.

Electrocardiogram (EKG) and chest radiograph findings are usually normal in a patient with an ASD. Over time, a patient can develop evidence of right atrial enlargement and right ventricular **hypertrophy** (increase in size) on the EKG.

An echocardiogram is the diagnostic tool of choice when an ASD is suspected. The two-dimensional images can demonstrate the size and location of the defect, as well as any other associated defects. In addition, Doppler interrogation delineates the direction and velocity of flow across the atrial septum.

Management and Treatment

Many children may have no symptoms associated with an ASD and can be observed by visits to a cardiology clinic for several years. Isolated ASDs that are smaller than 6 mm in diameter will usually spontaneously close on their own by age 2 years (3). An ASD that persists beyond age 2 years or is larger than 6 mm usually requires closure prior to the child starting school. Indications for earlier closure include the following:

- Symptoms of heart failure
- Evidence of pulmonary hypertension
- Risk or history of paradoxical embolus
- History of arrhythmia
- Qp/Qs (see definition and discussion below) greater than 1.5:1 (measurement performed in the cardiac catheterization laboratory)

Symptoms of heart failure result from volume overload of the right ventricle and pulmonary arteries and include tachypnea (caused by pulmonary edema), liver enlargement, and easy fatigability.

Pulmonary hypertension is classically defined as a mean pressure greater than 25 mm Hg in the main pulmonary artery. Over time, excess pulmonary blood flow from a left-to-right intracardiac shunt results in structural changes in the pulmonary arterioles. Specifically, the middle layer of the arteriole undergoes hypertrophy, resulting in an elevated, sometimes fixed pulmonary vascular resistance. This elevation in pulmonary vascular resistance represents an increase in right ventricular afterload—meaning that the right ventricle must generate higher pressures to eject blood into the pulmonary vasculature. Pulmonary hypertension can cause exercise intolerance; syncope (loss of consciousness, accompanied by an inability to maintain upright posture); cyanosis (secondary to reversal of intracardiac shunting from right to left across the ASD); and sudden death. Defects in the atrial septum also pose a risk for paradoxical embolization, where thrombi in the venous system enter the arterial circulation. A paradoxical embolus usually originates in the extremities as a deep venous thrombosis. It can cross the atrial septum, where entry into the cerebral arterial circulation results in an ischemic stroke.

The Qp/Qs measurement is a quantitative way to decide whether a patient meets criteria for early ASD closure. The "Q" refers to *blood flow*, the "p" refers to *pulmonary*, and the "s" refers to *systemic*. This notation compares the ratio of pulmonary blood flow (Qp) to systemic blood flow (Qs). Normally, the ratio of Qp/Qs is 1:1. In most centers, a Qp/Qs greater than 1.5:1, meaning that the pulmonary blood flow is 1.5 times more than systemic blood flow, is an indication for ASD closure. As discussed previously, persistently elevated Qp/Qs can lead to complications such as pulmonary hypertension. These measurements are made in the cardiac catheterization laboratory and can be used as a basis for management recommendations.

ASD closure can occur by cardiac catheterization with an occlusive device known as an Amplatzer Septal Occluder, or in the operating room (OR) using a median sternotomy (cutting through the middle of the sternum). In the OR, the defect can be closed with a primary suture repair or with a patch made of pericardium or Dacron. The method of closure is dependent on the age of the child, the location and size of the defect, and the presence of additional congenital heart defects.

These children usually have a relatively short cardiopulmonary bypass time and are extubated in the immediate postoperative period. The RT should watch for postoperative upper airway obstruction from postextubation stridor, hypoventilation from various anesthetic drugs and narcotics, and atelectasis from splinting. Children may need various forms of respiratory support from supplemental oxygen via nasal cannula to noninvasive ventilation.

Course and Prognosis

If left unrepaired, ASDs result in chronic volume overload of the right side of the heart. After several years, patients are at risk for structural changes in the heart, including right atrial dilation and right ventricular hypertrophy. Atrial dilation can predispose the patient to arrhythmias, including atrial fibrillation and atrial flutter. As pulmonary vascular resistance increases with chronic volume overload, pulmonary hypertension can also develop. In addition, patients are at risk for paradoxical embolization of deep venous thrombi to the brain.

Operative mortality for ASD closure is almost negligible, but does increase if other comorbidities such as chromosomal abnormalities, genetic syndromes, and other organ system failure are present. Most patients have an uncomplicated course after closure in the operating suite or via catheter intervention. Successful ASD closure has excellent long-term outcomes. A recent population-based study from the United Kingdom found a 20-year survival rate of 96.3% for patients with isolated ASD repairs (4). Another study found no significant cardiovascular effects or evidence of pulmonary hypertension in long-term survivors of appropriately timed ASD repair (5). Good long-term outcomes have also been demonstrated in patients following ASD closure with the Amplatzer Septal Occluder device (6).

Ventricular Septal Defect

A **ventricular septal defect (VSD)** is the most common congenital heart lesion, occurring in 1 to 2 per 1,000 live births (2). It is an opening in the interventricular septum, which causes a connection between the right and left ventricles. VSDs can occur as singular lesions but also may occur as part of a constellation of heart defects such as tetralogy of Fallot, pulmonary atresia, complete atrioventricular canal, transposition of the great arteries, patent ductus arteriosus, and others. Some type of VSD is present in 20% of children with congenital heart disease.

Pathophysiology

Three main sections of tissue grow together to form the ventricular septum in the fetus: inlet, trabecular, and conal. A failure of any of these segments of tissue to close results in the various types of VSDs (Fig. 11-2):

- **Perimembranous VSD (80%)**: The most common, the **perimembranous VSD** is located beneath the aortic annulus (the ring of fibrous tissue that anchors the valve leaflets), and if it

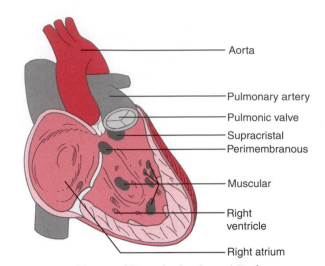

Figure 11-2 Types of Ventricular Septal Defects

Labels: Aorta, Pulmonary artery, Pulmonic valve, Supracristal, Perimembranous, Muscular, Right ventricle, Right atrium

extends into the aortic valve, it can cause aortic regurgitation.
- **Subarterial (or supracristal) VSD (5% to 10%):** This VSD is positioned directly beneath the pulmonic valve
- **Inlet (atrioventricular canal type) VSD (5% to 10%):** The inlet type of VSD occurs posteriorly and runs along the tricuspid valve.
- **Muscular VSD (5% to 10%):** The muscular VSD may be single or multiple and occur anywhere in the muscular septum.

The amount and direction of blood flow through the VSD depends on the size of the defect and the pressure difference between the right and left ventricles. Because pressure in the right ventricle is typically lower than pressure in the left ventricle, blood usually shunts *left* to *right*. Similar to ASDs, left-to-right shunting across a VSD will increase once pulmonary vascular resistance drops during the newborn period.

Small defects with little intracardiac shunting will usually remain asymptomatic. Larger defects can result in increased pulmonary blood flow, increased pulmonary venous return to the left side of the heart, and subsequent left ventricular volume overload. Over time, this overcirculation of the pulmonary vascular bed will cause a fixed increase in pulmonary vascular resistance owing to remodeling of the pulmonary arteries. This is the same mechanism by which any left-to-right intracardiac shunt (including ASDs) causes pulmonary hypertension. After the development of pulmonary hypertension, increased RV pressure can cause reversal in the direction of shunting. This right-to-left shunting of deoxygenated blood across the VSD is called Eisenmenger complex and causes cyanosis in patients who previously had normal oxygen saturations.

Clinical Manifestations

The signs and symptoms of a VSD depend on the size of the defect, the amount of shunting, and the age of the patient. Small defects may be completely asymptomatic. Moderate to large defects, especially those with nonrestrictive left-to-right shunting, can cause the following:

- Tachypnea
- Poor feeding
- Poor growth (failure to thrive)
- Sweating
- Irritability

On clinical examination, patients will have a harsh holosystolic (heard throughout systole) murmur loudest at the fourth intercostal space, but it may be heard throughout the chest. Patients with very large defects will frequently have a softer murmur than will patients with a small defect. A murmur is the result of turbulent blood flow across a cardiac structure. Blood flowing through a small defect produces more turbulence than blood flowing through a larger defect—hence, a louder murmur is heard by the clinician. Some patients with large VSDs may have a palpable thrill (tremor) along the left sternal border. Auscultation of the lungs may reveal rales due to pulmonary edema in a child with symptoms of heart failure.

An EKG may show evidence of left atrial enlargement and left ventricular hypertrophy. In a patient with a symptomatic VSD, the chest radiograph will demonstrate **cardiomegaly** (enlarged heart) and alveolar opacification representing pulmonary edema.

A suspected diagnosis of VSD on clinical examination can be confirmed by an echocardiogram. A two-dimensional image of the ventricular septum can pinpoint the size and location of the VSD. A Doppler interrogation can diagnose the velocity and direction of shunting.

Management and Treatment

Asymptomatic VSDs require no acute treatment. If symptoms of heart failure are present, medical therapy including diuretics, systemic afterload reduction with angiotensin-converting enzyme (ACE) inhibitors, and inotropes (e.g., digoxin) can be initiated. Infants with poor growth may need to be transitioned to a higher calorie formula to accommodate for their increased caloric needs. Definitive therapy is surgical closure using cardiopulmonary bypass. Indications for surgical closure include the following:

- Qp/Qs greater than 1.5:1
- Signs of heart failure despite maximal medical management
- Evidence of pulmonary hypertension
- Subpulmonic or membranous VSD with aortic valve regurgitation

Repair can usually be delayed until the patient is 3 to 6 months of age. However, repair may be required sooner if signs of heart failure or poor growth are present despite medical management. Closure of a VSD is achieved by primary suturing (if the defect is small) or pericardial versus Dacron patch placement. Postoperative complications, although rare, include residual defects and heart block (especially after an inlet-type VSD repair). In addition, children with preoperative elevations of pulmonary vascular resistance are prone to acute pulmonary hypertensive episodes and right ventricular dysfunction in the postoperative period. This subset of patients can be the most challenging to manage. Evidence of elevated pulmonary vascular resistance may require the institution of therapies such as inhaled nitric oxide, intubation with hyperventilation, and intravenous vasodilators. The bedside RT should identify which postoperative patients are at risk for pulmonary hypertension and be prepared to initiate the appropriate therapies, as discussed in Chapter 6.

Course and Prognosis

Some VSDs, especially the muscular type, may close spontaneously. In fact, 75% of small VSDs usually close in the first 2 years of life (6). For those that need to be repaired, operative mortality is quite low at 1%, and patients usually have excellent long-term survival (7). If left untreated, VSDs can result in pulmonary hypertension and left ventricular failure, resulting in a 42% survival at 25 years.

■■ You and the physician discuss a few diagnostic studies to aid in CJ's diagnosis. A chest radiograph shows diffuse alveolar and interstitial opacification. It is unclear if this represents an infiltrate or fluid (pulmonary edema). The cardiac silhouette also looks enlarged. You also decide to perform a bedside blood gas to determine if CJ is oxygenating and ventilating appropriately. The results are as follows: pH, 7.25; $PaCO_2$, 30; PaO_2, 72; HCO_3, 15; base deficit, –8.

A complete blood count shows a normal white cell count and differential and normal hemoglobin. A basic metabolic panel indicates slightly elevated blood urea nitrogen, but no other abnormalities. A rapid respiratory panel is ordered as well.

Atrioventricular Septal Defects

Atrioventricular septal defects (AVSDs) include a spectrum of abnormalities that involve defects in the portion of the atrial and/or ventricular septum directly adjacent to the atrioventricular valves (tricuspid and mitral). AVSDs comprise approximately 5% of people with congenital heart disease (8). This defect is especially common in the subpopulation of children with trisomy 21 (or Down syndrome).

Pathophysiology

The endocardial cushions (as mentioned in the section on ASDs) are segments of tissue that form a platform for the development of the atrial septum, ventricular septum, and atrioventricular valves. Any growth abnormality involving the endocardial cushions can result in defects in the lower portion of the atrial septum (ostium primum ASD), defects in the ventricular septum (inlet VSD), and/or structural abnormalities in the atrioventricular (AV) valves. There are three types of AVSDs:

- **Partial (incomplete):** consists of a defect in the ostium primum (see section on ASDs), as well as an abnormality of the mitral valve
- **Transitional:** involves defects in the ostium primum and in the ventricular septum that is usually restrictive. There are two distinct AVV valves that usually have abnormal leaflets.
- **Complete:** defined by a defect in the ostium primum, a large inlet-type VSD (see section on VSDs), and one common AV valve with multiple leaflets instead of two distinct AV valves

Clinical Manifestations

The clinical manifestations of an AVSD completely depend on the subtype. A partial (incomplete) AVSD may not demonstrate any signs or symptoms and could go undetected until adulthood. The symptoms of an AVSD occur because of unrestricted pulmonary blood flow as a result of significant left-to-right shunting across the VSD component. Patients often present with respiratory distress from pulmonary edema and symptoms of heart failure, which include the following:

- Poor feeding
- Difficulty gaining weight
- Fatigue
- Excessive sweating with feeds or activity

Management and Treatment

Patients with symptomatic AVSDs may be managed with medical therapy, including diuretics, systemic afterload reduction with ACE inhibitors, and intropes (i.e., digoxin). Definitive therapy involves surgical repair. Repair of the partial AVSD includes closure of the defect in the ostium primum with a patch and suture repair of the abnormality in the mitral valve (usually a mitral valve cleft). Surgical repair of a complete AV canal can be quite challenging. The atrial and ventricular septal defects are closed with a single- or double-patch method. The common AV valve leaflets must then be separated into two valve orifices—one for the right AVV and one for the left AVV.

Course and Prognosis

Operative mortality from repair of a complete AV canal, reported at 0% to 8.7%, is usually higher than isolated atrial or ventricular septal defects (9, 10). Recent literature suggests that outcomes are no different in children repaired at less than 3 months of age compared with those greater than 3 months (11). The prognosis depends, in part, on the residual valvar lesions, most commonly left AV valve regurgitation or stenosis. The most common reason for reoperation is left AV valve (mitral valve) regurgitation, which occurs in 6% to 11% of children after AVSD repair (9, 12).

Aortic Stenosis

Aortic stenosis is defined as any discrete narrowing that occurs between the left ventricle and the aorta (Fig. 11-3). It can occur at the level of the aortic valve, above the valve (supravalvar), or below the valve (subvalvar). Obstruction at the level of the aortic valve is by far the most common type of aortic stenosis (70% to 80%) and is the focus of this section. In children, aortic stenosis represents 6% of congenital heart disease (13).

Pathophysiology

The aortic valve consists of three smooth leaflets that open during systole (contraction of the heart chamber muscles) and close during diastole (relaxation of the cardiac muscles) to prevent backflow of blood into the left ventricle. The most common cause of aortic valve stenosis is a **bicuspid** aortic valve, meaning that the aortic valve consists of two functional leaflets instead of three. Because these leaflets have

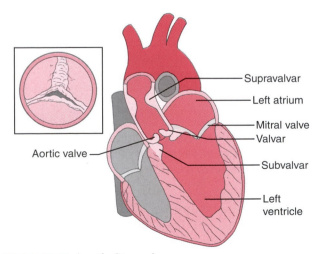

Figure 11-3 Aortic Stenosis

an abnormal shape, symptoms of valve stenosis can either be present at birth or progressively worsen over time as the valves become more stenotic and sometimes calcified. Valve stenosis is classified as mild, moderate, or severe, depending on the degree of obstruction. The severity of obstruction is determined by the difference in pressure across the valve and is calculated from measurements made during the echocardiogram. The gradations of obstruction are as follows:

- Mild (less than 25 mm Hg gradient)
- Moderate (25 to 50 mm Hg gradient)
- Severe (greater than 50 mm Hg gradient)

Even with severe obstruction, cardiac output is usually maintained, but at the expense of increased workload on the left ventricle. Because of this obstruction to blood flow exiting the left ventricle (left ventricular outflow), there is increased afterload, which can eventually cause left ventricular hypertrophy. Over time, **myocardial ischemia** (inadequate supply of blood and oxygen to meet the demands of the heart muscle) can develop because of decreased coronary perfusion and increased myocardial oxygen demand from left ventricular hypertension.

Clinical Manifestations

Symptoms of aortic stenosis depend on the degree of obstruction and vary from an asymptomatic patient with mild disease to a neonate with critical aortic stenosis and cardiovascular collapse. Other symptoms depend on age at presentation. Symptoms in infants can include the following:

- Tachypnea
- Poor feeding
- Growth failure

Symptoms in older children include the following:

- Syncope
- Progressive exercise intolerance
- Fatigue
- Chest pain

On physical examination, patients will have a harsh, loud systolic ejection murmur that may be associated with an ejection click (an abrupt, brief sound). With severe stenosis, an accentuated left ventricular impulse can be palpated on the chest. The first heart sound will be normal, but the second heart sound may have a **paradoxical split**—meaning that the closure of the pulmonary valve is always heard prior to the closure of the aortic valve. This finding occurs because ejection across a stenotic aortic valve during systole takes longer than ejection across a normal pulmonary valve.

The patient's pulse quality may be diminished and rise later than expected (a phenomenon called *pulsus parvus et tardus*). In aortic stenosis, the **pulse pressure** (difference between systolic blood pressure and diastolic blood pressure) is usually narrow, or smaller than expected.

A 12-lead EKG result obtained in the patient with aortic stenosis may be normal, but could also demonstrate left ventricular hypertrophy. Chest radiograph findings may show cardiomegaly if the left ventricle is hypertrophied.

An echocardiogram confirms the diagnosis and is used to delineate the valve morphology and size, severity of obstruction, left ventricular function, and presence of aortic regurgitation.

Management and Treatment

Therapy for patients with aortic stenosis is largely based on the severity of obstruction. Neonates presenting with shock secondary to critical aortic stenosis must be initially stabilized and started on prostaglandin therapy (PGE1). PGE1 will maintain patency of the ductus arteriosus, augmenting systemic perfusion with shunting of blood from the pulmonary artery to the aorta and bypassing the severe obstruction. Patients with mild (less than 25 mm Hg) and usually moderate (25 to 50 mm Hg) aortic stenosis can be followed using serial echocardiograms in the cardiologist's office. Patients with severe aortic stenosis must have a procedure to reduce the obstruction and to create an egress of blood across the left ventricular outflow tract. Usually this involves a balloon **valvuloplasty** in the cardiac catheterization laboratory in which a catheter with a balloon at the tip is passed into the valve orifice and inflated to enlarge the opening. If this procedure is unsuccessful, patients may require a surgical **valvotomy** (division of the valve leaflets) or valve replacement. The Ross procedure involves replacing the diseased aortic valve with the patient's own pulmonary valve. A preserved, cadaveric graft is then used to replace the patient's pulmonary valve. This procedure is indicated when the valve leaflets are not amenable to repair owing to calcification or severe dysplasia (abnormal development or growth).

Any child receiving PGE1 therapy is at risk for developing apnea, which is one of the side effects of PGE1, along with fever and peripheral edema. The incidence of apnea secondary to PGE1 administration has been reported to be between 18% and 23% (14, 15). The bedside RT should be prepared to recognize apnea (defined as the cessation of respiratory effort for greater than 20 seconds) and provide the necessary bedside therapies. Apnea may be associated with desaturation as well as bradycardia. Neonates may require oxygen delivery via nasal cannula or noninvasive continuous positive airway pressure (CPAP) for stimulation and decreased apnea frequency. If apnea continues, the neonate will need to be supported with intubation and mechanical ventilation.

Course and Prognosis

Children with congenital aortic valve stenosis will most likely develop progressive obstruction over time. When left untreated, severe aortic stenosis puts the patient at risk for sudden cardiac death and infective **endocarditis**, or inflammation of the heart valves. It is important that children are followed over time to document worsening obstruction or development of symptoms that necessitate therapy. Outcomes after balloon dilation are usually excellent, with 87% of children experiencing a significant reduction in the severity of obstruction (16). Over time, some children will have recurrence of obstruction and may need a repeat dilation. There are no data to suggest that using balloon dilation on the aortic valve versus surgical valvotomy have different success rates or frequency of restenosis (17).

Pulmonic Stenosis

Pulmonic stenosis, also known as pulmonary valvar stenosis, refers to a narrowing in the right ventricular outflow tract between the right ventricle and the main pulmonary artery (Fig. 11-4), occurring in 7% of all patients with congenital heart disease (1). It can occur as an isolated lesion or along with other cardiac anomalies, including tetralogy of Fallot, VSD, and double-outlet right ventricle.

Pathophysiology

Like the aortic valve, the pulmonic valve consists of three leaflets that open during systole, allowing blood to leave the right ventricle and enter the pulmonary artery. Pulmonic stenosis most commonly occurs at the level of the pulmonary valve but can occur above (supravalvar) or below (subvalvar). Pulmonic stenosis results from abnormally formed valve leaflets that may be dysplastic (as in Noonan syndrome) or form an abnormal dome shape. Obstruction in the right ventricular outflow tract from pulmonic stenosis causes increased workload on the right ventricle and subsequent right ventricular hypertrophy. Like aortic stenosis, pulmonic stenosis can be classified as mild, moderate, or severe, depending on the degree of obstruction.

Clinical Manifestations

Children with mild pulmonic stenosis will usually have no symptoms. However, children with moderate to severe pulmonic stenosis may present with the following symptoms due to increased right ventricular afterload:

- Dyspnea on exertion
- Fatigue
- Cyanosis

Severe pulmonic stenosis can progress to early right ventricular failure. On clinical examination, patients will exhibit a systolic ejection murmur, loudest at the left upper sternal border, with or without an ejection click. Auscultation may also exhibit a "fixed" split S2, due to increased ejection time across the stenotic pulmonic valve. Palpation of the precordium, done by placing a hand over the location of the heart on the thorax, may reveal an increased right ventricular impulse or "heave." Cyanosis occurs if the elevated pressure in the right ventricle is causing deoxygenated blood to shunt right to left across the atrial septum through a patent foramen ovale.

A 12-lead EKG will often demonstrate right axis deviation, right ventricular hypertrophy, and a right bundle branch block in cases of moderate to severe stenosis. Echocardiography is an excellent way to assess the pulmonic valve for anatomy, size, and degree of obstruction.

Management and Treatment

Mild pulmonic stenosis needs no therapy. Moderate to severe pulmonic stenosis often requires therapy because of progressive symptoms of exercise intolerance or right ventricular failure. Interventions can include a transcatheter balloon valvuloplasty, a surgical valvotomy, or valve replacement performed in the OR. The cyanotic neonate with critical pulmonic stenosis is dependent on a patent ductus arteriosus (see Chapter 8) to maintain adequate pulmonary blood flow. Prompt initiation of prostaglandin therapy (PGE1) will maintain a patent ductus arteriosus and is necessary for stabilization of a neonate

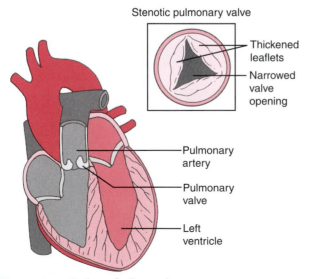

Stenotic pulmonary valve

Thickened leaflets

Narrowed valve opening

Pulmonary artery

Pulmonary valve

Left ventricle

Figure 11-4 Pulmonic Stenosis

with critical pulmonic stenosis until he or she can receive an emergent balloon valvuloplasty in the catheterization laboratory.

Course and Prognosis

The course for mild pulmonic stenosis is generally benign and does not progress over time. Untreated moderate to severe pulmonic stenosis will result in right ventricular failure. Patients with pulmonic stenosis are also predisposed to developing infectious endocarditis and both ventricular and atrial arrhythmias. Balloon valvuloplasty is low risk and successful at reducing stenosis in most patients. Restenosis requiring a repeat procedure has been found to occur in fewer than 5% of patients (18).

■■ CJ receives an albuterol treatment with chest physiotherapy and nasal suctioning to help with her nasal secretions and wheezing. You reexamine her and discover that the wheezing has not changed, but you can now hear a heart murmur. You hear it throughout the chest as a loud, harsh, holosystolic murmur. There is normal splitting of the second heart sound and normal quality of the peripheral pulse.

Coarctation of the Aorta

Coarctation of the aorta is a discrete narrowing of the descending thoracic aorta, usually distal to the takeoff of the left subclavian artery (Fig. 11-5). It occurs in 1 out of every 3,000 live births and represents the sixth most common type of congenital heart disease. Male infants and infants with certain genetic syndromes (e.g., Turner, DiGeorge)

● **Special Populations 11-1**

DiGeorge Syndrome

DiGeorge syndrome is a chromosomal abnormality caused by the deletion of a portion of chromosome 22. The portion deleted will determine the type of errors in fetal development. Chromosome 22 is associated with several different body systems, and may include the following:

- Heart defects, such as VSD, truncus arteriosus, tetralogy of Fallot
- Thymus gland dysfunction
- Hypoparathyroidism
- Cleft palate
- Facial feature abnormalities, such as low-set ears, wide-set eyes, hooded eyes, or a relatively long face
- Learning, behavioral, and mental health problems, which could include attention-deficit-hyperactivity disorder or autism in children and depression, anxiety disorders, or schizophrenia later in life
- Autoimmune disorders such as rheumatoid arthritis and Graves disease, caused by a small or missing thymus

DiGeorge syndrome is most often diagnosed after clinical symptoms manifest, which may include the following:

- Cyanosis
- Failure to thrive
- Weakness or tiring easily
- Hypotonia
- Shortness of breath
- Frequent infections
- Difficulty feeding
- Developmental delays noted by missed infant milestones such as rolling over or sitting up

have an increased prevalence of aortic coarctation (Special Population 11-1). Frequently, aortic coarctation is associated with a bicuspid aortic valve.

Pathophysiology

A coarctation involves the extension of a shelf-like structure into the lumen of the aorta. On a pathology specimen, this "shelf" actually represents thickening of the first two layers of the aortic vessel: the intima (the innermost layer) and the media (a middle layer made mostly of muscle cells). Two theories exist regarding the cause of an aortic coarctation:

- Reduced blood flow through the aortic arch during intrauterine development
- Constriction of ductal tissue that extends into the aortic lumen

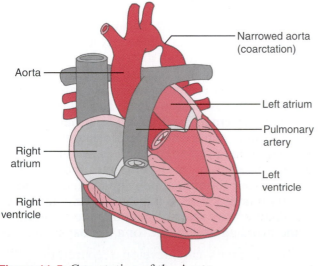

Aorta

Narrowed aorta (coarctation)

Left atrium

Pulmonary artery

Right atrium

Left ventricle

Right ventricle

Figure 11-5 Coarctation of the Aorta

The coarctation is usually located directly opposed to the lumen of the ductus arteriosus and may worsen after ductal closure, which supports the second theory. The area of coarctation in the descending aorta acts as an obstruction to left ventricular outflow causing increased left ventricular afterload.

Clinical Manifestations

This mechanical obstruction to blood in the descending aorta diverts blood flow through the innominate (or brachiocephalic), left carotid, and left subclavian arteries. This results in a difference in systolic blood pressure between the upper and the lower extremities. Blood pressure measured in the upper extremities is at least 10 mm Hg higher than systolic blood pressure in the lower extremities. Older patients may be asymptomatic (which sometimes delays diagnosis) or may present with chest pain with exercise or cool extremities that are painful during physical activity.

On clinical exam, patients may exhibit the following:

• Diminished or absent femoral pulses
• Brachiofemoral delay (a delay occurs between the occurrence of the brachial pulse and the femoral pulse)
• Continuous flow murmur detected from the presence of collateral vessels

Some neonates will have such severe coarctation that their systemic perfusion is dependent on flow through the ductus arteriosus. When the ductus closes, these infants may present with shock (inadequate perfusion as a result of extremely low blood pressure) and cardiovascular collapse.

EKG and chest radiograph findings are usually normal in young children. Over time, children may develop left ventricular hypertrophy visible on EKG results. Rib notching, which appears as concave irregularities on the inferior rib surface from dilated intercostal vessels, may be evident on chest radiograph.

Diagnosis is usually determined through echocardiography and magnetic resonance imaging (MRI).

Management and Treatment

A coarctation of the aorta is repaired surgically by a left thoracotomy incision. The coarctation segment is removed by the surgeon, and the aorta is reconnected in an end-to-end fashion. Alternatively, a homograft segment or Dacron patch may be placed between the two aortic segments if the distance between them is significant. Patients with no other cardiac lesions usually do not need cardiopulmonary bypass for this type of procedure. An alternative to surgical repair is performing a balloon **angioplasty** (dilation and widening

of the narrowed blood vessel) in the catheterization laboratory. Success rates following a balloon angioplasty have been reported at 88% (19).

Course and Prognosis

Depending on the degree of obstruction, patients may go several years before being diagnosed with aortic coarctation. Unrepaired coarctation will result in persistent hypertension and subsequent left ventricular hypertrophy, which could place patients at risk of arrhythmias and left ventricular failure.

The risks of a coarctation operation are somewhat less than those of other heart surgeries because this procedure can be performed without using cardiopulmonary bypass. Operative mortality is less than 1% (20). Patients usually do well postoperatively, but are at risk for the following complications:

• **Persistent hypertension:** Residual hypertension after coarctation repair is thought to be due to an upregulation of the renin-angiotensin-aldosterone system that occurs from reduced blood flow to the kidneys (whose blood supply is distal to the coarctation segment).
• **Vocal cord paresis or paralysis:** Vocal cord paresis can occur secondary to injury to the recurrent laryngeal nerve, which loops around the thoracic aorta near the coarctation site. This is important to remember if the postoperative patient demonstrates evidence of upper airway obstruction (stridor) or hoarseness.
• **Chylothorax:** Injury to the thoracic duct, a thin vessel that empties lymph from the entire body into the internal jugular vein, results in the accumulation of chyle into the pleural space, known as a chylothorax. This can present as respiratory distress with a pleural effusion on chest radiograph.
• **Lower extremity paralysis:** The greater spinal artery, a branch of the descending aorta, supplies the anterior portion of the spinal cord starting at the T10 level. Because the aorta must be cross-clamped during the repair, blood flow to the arterial branches distal to the clamps is halted for the time it takes to perform the repair. This can result in ischemia to the spinal cord if the cross-clamp time is lengthy.
• **Postcoarctectomy syndrome:** This usually occurs in patients who have had coarctation for several years prior to repair. It is caused by reperfusion injury to the intestines and presents with severe abdominal pain, nausea, and sometimes bloody stools. Symptoms usually improve with aggressive management of hypertension and avoiding oral intake for a few days.

Some patients can develop recoarctation that necessitates an intervention (e.g., balloon dilation, stent placement). Recoarctation after surgical repair has been reported at a rate of 5% to 14% (21). Recoarctation rates after balloon angioplasty are slightly higher, at 20% to 33% (19, 22). Long-term survival after coarctation repair was found to be 89% at 20-year follow-up in a large United Kingdom population-based study of children with congenital heart disease (4).

Double Aortic Arch

Aortic arch anomalies occur infrequently (about 1% of congenital heart disease). **Double aortic arch** is one of the more common types of aortic arch abnormality and is the type most likely to cause clinical symptoms. Up to 50% of patients with a vascular ring demonstrate another anomaly, most often cardiac in nature. (15) These may include a VSD, coarctation of the aorta, tetralogy of Fallot, and so forth. Noncardiac anomalies may include genetic syndromes such as DiGeorge syndrome (Special Population 11-2).

Pathophysiology

In the developing fetus, six symmetrical arches undergo remodeling to form the aortic arch and its major branches: the innominate artery, the left common carotid artery, and the left subclavian artery. A double aortic arch occurs when one of these embryological arches fails to remodel correctly and is included in the class of anomalies known as a **complete vascular ring**. Complete vascular rings, including double aortic arch and right aortic arch with aberrant left subclavian artery, encircle and cause compression of both the esophagus and trachea. In double aortic arch, instead of a single left-sided arch, patients have an arch that bifurcates into a right and left aortic arch, which encircle the trachea and esophagus (Fig. 11-6). In a right aortic arch with aberrant left subclavian artery and left ductus arteriosus, the right-sided arch forms the posterior portion of the ring behind the esophagus. The anterior portion of the ring is formed from the takeoff of the left subclavian artery and the connection of the ductus arteriosus to the pulmonary artery overlying the trachea.

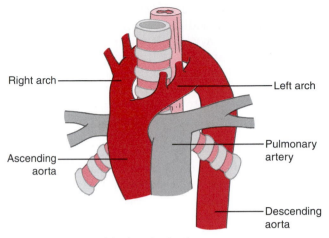

Figure 11-6 Double Aortic Arch

Labels: Right arch, Left arch, Ascending aorta, Pulmonary artery, Descending aorta

Clinical Manifestations

The right aortic arch passes posterior to the esophagus and may cause the following symptoms from compression:

- Feeding difficulty
- Gastroesophageal reflux
- Failure to thrive
- Dysphagia

The left aortic arch abuts the anterior trachea, causing the child to exhibit intrathoracic upper airway obstruction. The following signs and symptoms may be present:

- Cough
- Wheezing
- Stridor
- Persistent infections
- Critical airway obstruction (neonate)

Posterior compression of the esophagus seen on a barium swallow is the classic radiological finding for double aortic arch. The diagnosis can be confirmed by computed tomography angiography or MRI.

Management and Treatment

Once diagnosed, immediate management of double aortic arch depends on how symptomatic the child is. Severe dysphagia or feeding difficulty may need to be mitigated with nasogastric tube feeds. Because of the fixed tracheal obstruction, respiratory symptoms such as wheezing or stridor usually do not respond to conventional therapies such as inhaled bronchodilators or racemic epinephrine. Patients with symptoms of severe upper airway obstruction most often present as neonates and require immediate intubation and mechanical ventilation. Positive pressure ventilation and the use of positive end expiratory pressure (PEEP) can help to stent open airway structures compressed by the anterior

---

● **Special Populations 11-2**

Syndromes Associated with Acyanotic Heart Defects

Down syndrome
Turner syndrome
DiGeorge syndrome
Marfan syndrome
William syndrome
Noonan syndrome

aortic arch. Children diagnosed with double aortic arch should be immediately referred for surgical repair. During surgery, the nondominant left aortic arch is divided and ligated, leaving the dominant right aortic arch intact. This effectively relieves the airway obstruction. However, children may continue to have airway symptoms, such as wheezing or mild stridor, for several months following the operation.

Course and Prognosis

In the neonate, double aortic arch can result in critical upper airway obstruction and death if not managed appropriately. Prognosis is excellent following repair, and intraoperative mortality is almost zero (15). It is important to remember that some patients may continue to have symptoms for several months after surgical repair. Because of compression from the aortic arch, the tracheal cartilage may not develop appropriately (23). This may cause tracheomalacia, a "softening" of the tracheal cartilage that results in collapse during inspiration and manifests as inspiratory stridor or wheezing, depending on the affected site. Children with significant tracheomalacia may require positive pressure ventilation (delivered either noninvasively or by endotracheal tube), especially during a concomitant illness, to overcome airway collapse. There is no specific therapy, except supportive, for tracheomalacia. It will improve as the child grows.

■ ■ CJ's respiratory panel is positive for rhinovirus. An echocardiogram obtained in the emergency department reveals a large, unrestrictive perimembranous VSD with left-to-right shunting. The baby is admitted to the cardiology service where she is treated with oxygen and a dose of furosemide. She is scheduled for a repair in 6 weeks, once her concurrent infection has resolved.

■ ■ Critical Thinking Questions: Carly Jo Johnson

1. What is the cause of the presentation of hypoxemia in CJ Johnson?
2. Why is it important to know this?

▶● Case Studies and Critical Thinking Questions

■ Case 1: Jane Mercer

Jane Mercer is a 5-year-old female recently adopted from China. Her mom noticed that she seemed to tire easily when playing with the other kids, so she took her in for an evaluation at the pediatrician's office. On clinical examination, the pediatrician noted a systolic ejection murmur as well as a fixed split of the second heart sound. An echocardiogram revealed a 5-mm secundum atrial septal defect. Today Jane went to the operating room for patch closure of the ASD. She was just extubated at the bedside in the intensive care unit and is now recovering. Her pulse oximeter is currently reading 87%.

- *You are the RT caring for her; what conditions could cause hypoxemia in the postoperative period?*
- *What therapies should you initiate?*
- *What would you do if the oxygen saturations continued to decrease?*

■ Case 2: Tyrone Dramel

Tyrone Dramel is a 2-month-old male with Down syndrome (trisomy 21) who is presenting to the emergency department with respiratory distress. His mom describes that, since birth, he has had trouble feeding and has not gained very much weight. If he eats for too long, he becomes sweaty, irritable, and sometimes turns blue around the mouth. On examination, Tyrone has no fever, but is breathing very rapidly. You hear scattered wheezing and a few crackles at the bases. You also detect a loud, holosystolic murmur.

- *What types of congenital heart disease could cause this patient's symptoms?*
- *How would you make the diagnosis?*

■ Case 3: Baby Girl (BG) Mack

You are an RT for a transport program, transporting a neonate, BG Mack, with critical aortic stenosis to the nearest children's hospital. BG Mack was born at 38 weeks' gestation earlier today and was noted to have cyanosis and hypotension shortly after birth. Echocardiography revealed critical aortic stenosis and BG Mack was initiated on a PGE1 infusion to keep the ductus arteriosus patent.

- *What is a major side effect of PGE1 that could cause problems during transport?*
- *How is this side effect managed?*

■ Case 4: Martin Gantt

Martin Gantt is an 8-year-old male admitted to the pediatric floor for progressive fatigue and "turning blue" while playing soccer. An echocardiogram revealed moderate pulmonic valve stenosis.

- *What would you expect to hear on clinical examination?*
- *What do you suspect Martin's chest radiograph shows?*

Case 5: Darnell Williams

Darnell Williams is a 6-month-old male infant referred to the cardiac center for repair of coarctation of the aorta. He has no other medical problems and has been growing well at home. He was extubated in the operating room and is now being transitioned to the intensive care unit. You are the RT who will be following him for the day. Darnell seems to initially do well postoperatively and only needs 1/2 L oxygen via nasal cannula to keep his saturations greater than 94%. However, later in the day, you note that he has a very weak cry—in fact, he seems to make no noise at all when he cries.

• What could have caused this?

Case 6: Baby Boy (BB) Tyler

BB Tyler is a 4-day-old full-term male who was intubated shortly after birth for severe cyanosis. Further diagnostic workup revealed evidence of a complete vascular ring caused by a double aortic arch. He is scheduled for surgery at the end of the week. The bedside nurse calls you (the RT) over because the ventilator alarm is sounding for high peak inspiratory pressures. BB Tyler appears agitated and cyanotic on examination, with pulse oximetry readings of 75%. According to the nurse, the quantitative end-tidal CO_2 measurement has increased from 45 to 80 over the last several minutes.

• What could be causing these acute changes?
• How would you immediately manage the infant's current hypoxemia and hypercarbia?
• What steps could be taken to prevent these episodes from occurring in the future?

Multiple-Choice Questions

1. The two most common types of acyanotic heart defects are:
   a. ASD and VSD
   b. VSD and pulmonic stenosis
   c. Aortic stenosis and pulmonic stenosis
   d. Coarctation of the aorta and double aortic arch

2. Which of the following techniques is used as definitive diagnosis of a cardiac defect?
   a. Auscultation
   b. Chest radiograph
   c. Electrocardiogram
   d. Echocardiogram

3. Which of the following acyanotic heart defects usually happens in conjunction with other types of congenital anomalies?
   a. ASD
   b. VSD
   c. Double aortic arch
   d. All of the above

4. Upon auscultation, which of the following acyanotic defects would present with a murmur?
   a. AV septal defect
   b. Aortic stenosis
   c. Coarctation of the aorta
   d. They would all present with a murmur

5. Acyanotic heart defects can often mimic pulmonary disease. Which of the following symptoms would *not* be found associated with acyanotic heart defects?
   a. Pulmonary edema
   b. Stridor
   c. Wheezing
   d. Pneumothorax

6. A 4-month-old baby is admitted to the hospital by her primary pediatrician for poor growth and a heart murmur. Her EKG shows left atrial enlargement and left ventricular hypertrophy, chest radiograph is significant for cardiomegaly and pulmonary edema, and SpO_2 is 95%. When you auscultate, you note a soft holosystolic murmur, loudest at the fourth intercostal space. What acyanotic heart defect do you suspect this infant has?
   a. ASD
   b. VSD
   c. Pulmonic stenosis
   d. Aortic stenosis

7. A baby is diagnosed with a systolic murmur with an ejection click. He is referred to a cardiologist, who diagnoses aortic valve stenosis on echocardiogram. At his 6-week follow-up appointment with the cardiologist, his obstruction is determined to be severe, with some mild hypertrophy of the left ventricle; he also has poor feeding and failure to gain weight effectively since he came home from the hospital. What is a reasonable next step in this baby's management?
   a. Continue to monitor
   b. PGE1 therapy
   c. Valvuloplasty
   d. Valvotomy

8. What are the indications for closing a septal wall defect?
   - I. Qp/Qs greater than 1.5:1
   - II. Signs of heart failure despite maximal medical management
   - III. Evidence of pulmonary hypertension
   - IV. Aortic valve regurgitation
   - a. I, II, IV
   - b. I, II, III
   - c. I, III, IV
   - d. I ,II, III, IV

9. Which of the following respiratory symptoms can manifest in a patient with a double aortic arch?
   - I. Wheezing
   - II. Cough
   - III. Stridor
   - IV. Pulmonary hypertension
   - a. I, III
   - b. I, II, IV
   - c. III, IV
   - d. I, II, III

10. Why are the postoperative risks for coarctation of the aorta less than other acyanotic defects?
    - a. It does not require cardiopulmonary bypass
    - b. It can be performed laparoscopically
    - c. Only mild anesthesia is necessary
    - d. There are no other heart structures implicated in the diseas

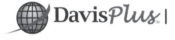 **DavisPlus** | For additional resources login to Davis*Plus* (http://davisplus.fadavis.com/ keyword "Perretta") and click on the Premium tab. (Don't have a *Plus*Code to access Premium Resources? Just click the Purchase Access button on the book's Davis*Plus* page.)

REFERENCES

1. National Birth Defects Prevention Network. *Annual Report.* 2005. www.nbdpn.org. Accessed on April 13, 2013.
2. Nichols DG, Ungerleider RM, Spevak PJ, et al. *Critical Heart Disease in Infants and Children.* 2nd ed. Philadelphia, PA: Mosby; 2006.
3. Hanslik A, Pospisil U, Salzer-Muhar U, et al. Predictors of spontaneous closure of isolated secundum atrial septal defect in children: a longitudinal study. *Pediatrics.* 2006;118(4):1560-1565.
4. Tennant PW, Pearce MS, Bythell M, et al. 20-year survival of children born with congenital anomalies: a population-based study. *Lancet.* 2010;375(9715):649-656.
5. Roos-Hesselink JW, Meijboom FJ, Spitaels SE, et al. Excellent survival and low incidence of arrhythmias, stroke and heart failure long-term after surgical ASD closure at young age. A prospective follow-up study of 21-33 years. *Eur Heart J.* 2003;24(2):190-197.
6. Berger F, Vogel M, Alexi-Meskishvili V, et al. Comparison of results and complications of surgical and Amplatzer device closure of atrial septal defects. *J Thorac Cardiovasc Surg.* 1999;118(4):674-678; discussion 678-680.
7. Scully BB, Morales DL, Zafar F, et al. Current expectations for surgical repair of isolated ventricular septal defects. *Ann Thorac Surg.* 2010;89(2):544-549; discussion 550-541.
8. Hoffman JI. Incidence of congenital heart disease: II. Prenatal incidence. *Pediatr Cardiol.* 1995;16(4):155-165.
9. Bakhtiary F, Takacs J, Cho M, et al. Long-term results after repair of complete atrioventricular septal defect with two-patch technique. *Ann Thorac Surg.* 2010;89(4): 1239-1243.
10. Crawford FA, Stroud MR. Surgical repair of complete atrioventricular septal defect. *Ann Thorac Surg.* 2001;72(5):1621-1628; discussion 1628-1629.
11. Singh R, Warren P, Reece T, et al. Early repair of complete atrioventricular septal defect is safe and effective. *Ann Thorac Surg.* 2006;82(5):1598-1602.
12. Suzuki T, Bove E, Devaney E, et al. Results of definitive repair of complete atrioventricular septal defect in neonates and infants. *Ann Thorac Surg.* 2008;86(2): 596-602.
13. Hoffman JI, Kaplan S. The incidence of congenital heart disease. *J Am Coll Cardiol.* 2002;39(12):1890-1900.
14. Meckler GD, Lowe C. To intubate or not to intubate? Transporting infants on prostaglandin E1. *Pediatrics.* 2009;123(1):e25-e30.
15. Oxenius A, Hug MI, Dodge-Khatami A, et al. Do predictors exist for a successful withdrawal of preoperative prostaglandin E(1) from neonates with d-transposition of the great arteries and intact ventricular septum? *Pediatr Cardiol.* 2010;31(8):1198-1202.
16. Moore P, Egito E, Mowrey H, et al. Midterm results of balloon dilation of congenital aortic stenosis: predictors of success. *J Am Coll Cardiol.* 1996;27(5):1257-1263.
17. McCrindle BW, Blackstone EH, Williams WG, et al. Are outcomes of surgical versus transcatheter balloon valvotomy equivalent in neonatal critical aortic stenosis? *Circulation.* 2001;104(12, suppl 1):I152-I158.
18. Roos-Hesselink JW, Meijboom FJ, Spitaels SE, et al. Long-term outcome after surgery for pulmonary stenosis (a longitudinal study of 22-33 years). *Eur Heart J.* 2006; 27(4):482-488.
19. Yetman AT, Nykanen D, McCrindle BW, et al. Balloon angioplasty of recurrent coarctation: a 12-year review. *J Am Coll Cardiol.* 1997;30(3):811-816.
20. Warnes CA, Williams RG, Bashore TM, et al. ACC/AHA 2008 guidelines for the management of adults with congenital heart disease: a report of the American College of Cardiology/American Heart Association Task Force on

Practice Guidelines (writing committee to develop guidelines on the management of adults with congenital heart disease). *Circulation.* 2008;118(23):e714-e833.

21. Smith Maia MM, Cortês TM, Parga JR, et al. Evolutional aspects of children and adolescents with surgically corrected aortic coarctation: clinical, echocardiographic, and magnetic resonance image analysis of 113 patients. *J Thorac Cardiovasc Surg.* 2004;127(3):712-720.

22. Fletcher SE, Nihill MR, Grifka RG, et al. Balloon angioplasty of native coarctation of the aorta: midterm follow-up and prognostic factors. *J Am Coll Cardiol.* 1995;25(3):730-734.

23. Woods RK, Sharp RJ, Holcomb GW, et al. Vascular anomalies and tracheoesophageal compression: a single institution's 25-year experience. *Ann Thorac Surg.* 2001;72(2):434-438; discussion 438-439.

Chapter 12

Cyanotic Heart Defects

Chapter Objectives

After reading this chapter, you will be able to:

1. Identify the common types of cyanotic heart defects diagnosed in children.
2. Discuss the general evaluation of a neonate suspected of having a cyanotic heart defect.
3. Explain how to perform a hyperoxia test.
4. Define the two components of Ebstein anomaly.
5. List the four types of total anomalous pulmonary venous return and the two broad ways neonates can present.
6. Describe transposition of the great arteries and describe how a neonate will present immediately after birth.
7. Describe an atrial septostomy and in what patient population it is indicated.
8. Define the lesions associated with tetralogy of Fallot and the two ways infants can present.
9. Describe hypoplastic left heart syndrome.
10. Describe the three stages of surgical intervention for hypoplastic left heart syndrome.
11. Describe the benefits and risks of using hypoxic gas mixtures for infants with cyanotic heart defects.
12. State the indications for a prostaglandin E (PGE) infusion for newborns.
13. Define truncus arteriosus and describe how a neonate will present.

■■ Mia Mcnamara

You are working in a 200-bed children's hospital that serves an extensive rural population. You are assisting in the triage area of the emergency department when the nurse asks you to help her look at Mia, a 6-month-old baby brought in by her mom. Her mother tells you and the nurse that at 4 months and 6 months, Mia was seen by her pediatrician who noted a "strong heart murmur." At the 6-month appointment, he recommended consultation with a pediatric cardiologist, and though one is scheduled, it's not for another 6 weeks. Mom has come in today because Mia has had a few episodes of irritability, becoming agitated and inconsolable, and her face and lips turn blue.

As Chapter 11 discussed, the structural abnormalities that lead to the diagnosis of congenital heart disease can be divided broadly into acyanotic or cyanotic congenital heart disease. This chapter focuses on **cyanotic heart defects**, which result from structural abnormalities that lead to significant mixing of oxygenated and deoxygenated blood and cause oxygen saturations of less than 85%. This chapter will discuss several of the more common cyanotic defects, including tetralogy of Fallot, total anomalous pulmonary venous return, transposition of the great arteries, hypoplastic left heart syndrome, Ebstein anomaly, and truncus arteriosus. There are many variations of cyanotic heart defects, and a description of all abnormalities is

beyond the scope of this text. The diseases included in the text are chosen because of the relative frequency with which they are diagnosed, the importance of rapid diagnosis and initial treatment, or the implications of anatomy and presentation of the defect to respiratory management.

In the United States, where children receive very close monitoring and frequent health care in infancy, cyanotic heart disease may present immediately after birth or within the first few months of life. In countries with less-established health-care systems, cyanotic heart disease may not be recognized until later in childhood or early adulthood.

Any neonate who presents with oxygen saturations less than 85% to 90% should be assessed to determine whether the cause of the hypoxemia is lung disease or congenital heart disease. Evaluative measures include chest radiograph, electrocardiograph, hyperoxia test, and echocardiogram; auscultation may often reveal abnormal heart sounds, but normal findings are not conclusive (see Table 12-1). Certain therapeutic measures, such as prostaglandin E_1 (PGE_1) and oxygen delivery, may be warranted while diagnostic procedures are being completed.

A chest radiograph should be taken to assess the lung fields and heart size. An electrocardiograph (ECG) should be obtained, but the results will frequently be normal. A normal result should not rule out the presence of congenital heart defect.

A **hyperoxia test** should also be performed, in which arterial blood gases are obtained on room air and 1.0 fractional concentration of inspired oxygen (FIO_2) and compared to assess a patient's ability to oxygenate. To start, a baseline arterial

Table 12-1 Cardiac Auscultation for Cyanotic Heart Defects

Sound/Murmur	Location	Defect
A harsh crescendo-decrescendo systolic ejection murmur Second heart sound may be single and prominent	Left sternal border	Tetralogy of Fallot
Right ventricular heave Fixed split S2 Loud pulmonary component of S2 S3 gallop (often present) Systolic ejection murmur		Total anomalous pulmonary venous return
No murmur or systolic ejection murmur Possibly a loud second heart sound	Left sternal border	Transposition of the Great Arteries
Little to no murmur detected		Hypoplastic left heart syndrome
Holosystolic murmur Diastolic murmur (possible) Third and fourth heart sounds possible	Left lower sternal border	Ebstein anomaly
Active precordium No murmur, or normal S1, single and loud S2		Truncus arteriosus

blood gas (ABG) is obtained from the right radial artery while the patient is breathing room air. Obtaining the blood gas from the right radial artery is critical to avoid misinterpretation of oxygenation ability because of the neonate's patent ductus arteriosus (PDA), through which shunting of blood occurs. The PDA connects the pulmonary artery to the aorta near the origin of the left subclavian artery. As described in Chapter 2, the PDA is necessary for intrauterine fetal circulation and usually closes over the first few days of life. A right radial ABG will give an accurate measure of the partial pressure of oxygen in the blood (PaO_2), directly from the aorta, before the point at which a PDA may mix deoxygenated blood in aorta and decrease PaO_2. After a baseline ABG is obtained, the patient then should be placed on FIO_2 1.0 using an oxyhood or non-rebreather mask. Ten to 15 minutes later, a repeat ABG is obtained from the right radial artery. If the PaO_2 of the sample on FIO_2 1.0 is higher than 150 mm Hg, the hypoxemia is likely related to lung disease, such as pneumonia or respiratory distress syndrome. If the PaO_2 is lower than 150 mm Hg, a cyanotic heart defect should be suspected because the low PaO_2 likely is due to shunting and mixing of oxygenated and deoxygenated blood. Despite a delivered FIO_2 of 1.0, the complete blood mixing prevents the PaO_2 from rising above an expected level. Once a cyanotic heart defect is suspected, the neonate should be referred to a tertiary care center for further evaluation and management by intensivists and cardiologists.

For any neonate presenting with cyanosis, an intravascular infusion of **prostaglandin E (PGE)** should be started. Prostaglandins are hormone-like substances that perform a variety of functions in the body. PGE_1 will maintain patency of the PDA and allow mixing of oxygenated and deoxygenated blood. Once the specific cardiac lesion has been identified by echocardiogram and the presence of any additional shunts (e.g., patent foramen ovale [PFO], ventricular septal defect [VSD], or atrial septal defect [ASD]) has been verified, PGE may be discontinued.

Echocardiogram is the gold standard for diagnosis and differentiation of congenital cardiac malformations. An echocardiogram uses ultrasound to assess the anatomy of the heart, normal and abnormal patterns of blood flow, and blood pressures at various places within the heart. This test is completed by a cardiologist, usually at the bedside, and the information obtained is important for the respiratory therapist (RT) to understand because it will provide information regarding expected pulmonary blood flow and acceptable SpO_2 ranges, and it may have implications on ideal blood gas values.

■ ■ ■ Mia looks comfortable resting in her mother's lap and does not seem agitated. Her respiratory rate (RR) is 35 breaths/min. You place a pulse oximeter on Mia, and her arterial blood oxygen (SpO_2) is 88%, with a pulse rate of 145 bpm. You place Mia on a nasal cannula and call the pediatrician to the bedside for a consultation.

The pediatrician listens to the heart and notes a harsh systolic ejection murmur along the left sternal border and normal breath sounds. She orders a 12-lead EKG, chest radiograph, hyperoxia test, echocardiogram, and cardiology consultation.

You remove the nasal cannula and return 20 minutes later and obtain a right radial ABG. Results are pH, 7.38; $PaCO_2$, 44 mm Hg; PaO_2, 56 mm Hg; HCO_3, 25.7 mEq/L. You place Mia on a non-rebreather mask at 15 LPM, and her SpO_2 increases to 100%. You return 15 minutes later and draw another ABG. The results are pH, 7.44; $PaCO_2$, 36 mm Hg; PaO_2, 110 mm Hg; HCO_3, 24.1 mEq/L. Based on these results, you are reasonably sure that Mia has some type of cyanotic heart disease.

Tetralogy of Fallot

Tetralogy of Fallot (TOF) (Fig. 12-1) is caused by a combination of four conditions: VSD, an aorta that overrides the VSD, obstruction of the right ventricular outflow tract, and right ventricular hypertrophy (1). It is the most common form of cyanotic congenital heart disease, representing 3.5% of all infants with congenital heart disease and 4.05 per 10,000 live births (2). In addition to this classic intracardiac pathology, other forms of TOF include pulmonary artery or other cardiac abnormalities. TOF may be associated with genetic abnormalities such as trisomy 21, 22q11 deletion, and VACTERL syndrome (vertebral, anal, cardiac, tracheoesophageal, renal and limb abnormalities) (3).

Pathophysiology

The anatomy of TOF centers on four components of intracardiac anatomy:

- A large malaligned, unrestrictive VSD in the membranous portion of the septum that allows flow of blood between the left and right ventricles
- An aorta that straddles or "overrides" the VSD so that blood from both ventricles may enter the systemic outflow tract
- A fixed or variable degree of **right ventricular outflow tract obstruction (RVOTO)** at or adjacent to the pulmonary valve, which causes a decrease in pulmonary blood flow
- Right ventricular hypertrophy as a result of the RVOTO

Other pulmonary artery pathology may be present, leading to variations in pathophysiology and clinical course (Clinical Variation 12-1).

The degree of RVOTO and the relative resistance of the systemic and pulmonary vasculature determine TOF pathophysiology. Cyanosis is directly proportional to the amount of blood being shunted as a result of RVOTO. If there is mild obstruction, patients may have no clinical manifestations. On the opposite end of the spectrum, infants may present in the neonatal period with severe RVOTO and cyanosis due to severe pulmonary stenosis or pulmonary atresia leading to shunting of deoxygenated blood from the right ventricle to left ventricle and aorta. These infants may require early treatment to provide pulmonary blood flow with a PGE_1 infusion

---

Clinical Variations 12-1

Variations of TOF

In addition to the four main components of TOF, there may be additional pulmonary valve abnormalities. These can include an absent or dysplastic pulmonary valve with regurgitation, pulmonary artery stenosis, or pulmonary valve atresia. These can all put additional strain on the right heart and lead to right ventricular hypertrophy, and may also increase blood flow dysfunction to the pulmonary artery, leading to poor oxygenation.

Another variation is known as "pink tet," in which patients may have no cyanotic symptoms because SVR transmitted to the right ventricle via the VSD overcomes the mild RVOTO and provides pulmonary blood flow (4).

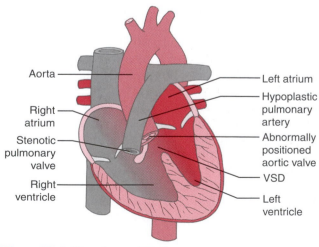

Figure 12-1 Tetralogy of Fallot

to maintain the PDA and early surgical palliation or repair.

RVOTO can also be variable through the course of disease. Infants can initially have little RVOTO and no cyanosis, but over time develop progressive obstruction to pulmonary blood flow with accompanying increase in right-to-left shunt and cyanosis ("blue tetralogy" or "blue tet"). Also, RVOTO can be episodic, with a sudden increase in RVOTO causing a period of hypercyanosis, known as a **tet spell**. Additionally, decreases in systemic vascular resistance (SVR) or systemic blood pressure associated with medications, hypovolemia, or illness can cause shunting of blood from the right to left ventricle. Children with TOF may appear normal between tet spells. Progressive cyanosis or recurrent tet spells are an indication for further medical and surgical treatment.

Clinical Manifestations

The degree of clinical symptoms varies with the degree of RVOTO. Children with mild RVOTO may be asymptomatic, whereas those with significant RVOTO may be cyanotic with an oxygen saturation measurement of less than 85%. The prototypical tet spell is characterized by sudden cyanosis caused by an acute increase in RVOTO and/or decrease in systemic blood pressure, with consequent right-to-left shunting of desaturated blood. Tet spells are usually associated with increased catecholamines, agitation, and/or systemic hypotension.

Most children have no symptoms related to TOF. Even those with significant cyanosis and right-to-left shunt will have few symptoms of feeding intolerance or sweating. Symptoms in older patients in underdeveloped countries may be different (Special Population 12-1). However, patients with "pink tet" (no cyanosis) may have large left-to-right shunting and pulmonary overcirculation that can cause signs and symptoms of heart failure such as tachypnea, feeding difficulties, and poor growth.

On physical examination, cyanosis may or may not be present, depending on the amount of right-to-left shunting. On cardiac auscultation, a harsh crescendo-decrescendo systolic ejection murmur along the left sternal border reflects turbulent flow across the right ventricular outflow tract. The second heart sound may be single and prominent owing to the anterior displaced aorta and lack of pulmonary valve sound. A lung examination will be normal in the majority of patients.

A chest radiograph (Fig. 12-2) may be normal or show a boot-like shape to the cardiac silhouette. Depending on the degree of pulmonary blood flow, the lungs may appear normal or have diminished vascular markings.

An electrocardiogram will show right ventricular hypertrophy and may demonstrate right bundle branch block. Right axis deviation and right atrial enlargement may also be seen.

An echocardiogram is the standard to confirm a TOF diagnosis. The four components of TOF can be seen as well as the degree of RVOTO. The gradient across the right ventricular outflow tract as well as the VSD can be calculated to provide information regarding the degree of obstruction and shunting of blood from the right to left ventricle.

■■ While in a treatment room with Mia and her mom as they wait for Mia to be taken to radiology for her chest radiograph (CXR), you watch Mia, sitting on her mom's lap, become agitated and cyanotic, despite being on 1.0 FIO_2. You call the pediatrician immediately when you see her SpO_2 drop below 92%.

● Special Populations 12-1

TOF in Developing Countries

Older children or adults with unrepaired TOF can be seen in areas of the world without access to surgical repair. These patients experience tet spells associated with exertion and will squat or use Valsalva's maneuver to relieve the cyanosis. This is effective because it increases SVR and will force blood to the pulmonary system. These people may have significant clubbing of hands and feet from cyanosis, similar to that seen in patients with chronic obstructive pulmonary disease (COPD). They will also have poor growth.

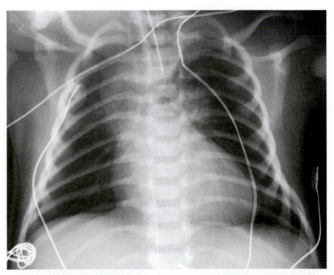

Figure 12-2 Chest Radiograph of a Neonate with TOF
(Courtesy of Jane Benson, MD)

Management and Treatment

Many cases of TOF are diagnosed prenatally. Initial management of the newborn involves assessing the infant using a physical examination and echocardiography. If pulmonary blood flow is critically limited by severe RVOTO or pulmonary atresia, ductal patency may need to be maintained with PGE_1 infusion until palliation or repair can be undertaken in the first days of life.

Infants who have insignificant RVOTO and are not cyanotic may be discharged home for feeding and growing in anticipation of surgical repair in the first few months of life. They may forego surgery until they either have progressive cyanosis or until they have reached appropriate size and weight for primary repair.

Infants who have intermittent tet spells may require initial medical management to decrease cyanosis. Acute spell management includes oxygen, knee-to-chest maneuvers, medications to increase SVR (e.g., phenylephrine), volume administration to increase flow into the pulmonary vasculature, and sedatives such as morphine to decrease catecholamines and perhaps decrease spasm at the opening of the pulmonary valve. In patients who cannot undergo surgical repair, use of propranolol has been found to decrease the frequency of tet spells by decreasing heart rate, hypercontractility, and relaxing the RVOTO.

Surgical repair of TOF involves the following:

• providing relief of RVOTO
• complete separation of atria and ventricles
• preservation of pulmonary valve and tricuspid valve function

This involves closure of the VSD, resecting the obstructions above and below the pulmonary valve, and/or pulmonary valve repair. This surgery is typically performed from the right atrium through the tricuspid valve, although transventricular repair has been used. Full surgical repair can be technically difficult in neonates and small infants who require surgical intervention; therefore, some centers offer initial improvement of symptoms using a systemic-to-pulmonary shunt, such as a modified Blalock-Taussig (BT) shunt (discussed in the management and treatment of hypoplastic left heart syndrome discussion, below), followed by complete repair a few months later. Infants with BT shunts remain cyanotic, with oxygen saturations of 75% to 85%, until repair. Many institutions are moving toward earlier primary repair in infancy, which will decrease morbidity and mortality and the need for further surgical intervention (5).

The advantage of early repair of TOF is the avoidance of prolonged cyanosis, thus avoiding the risks associated with systemic-to-pulmonary shunt.

It also allows for completion of the repair in one operation. However, there are concerns that patients with TOF repaired in infancy may need reoperation later in life for residual RVOTO or pulmonary regurgitation associated with valve incompetency. Proponents of the BT shunt prior to complete repair argue that shunting provides reliable pulmonary blood flow until the child is bigger (typically 3 to 6 months of age). Repair at that time may be more successful and ultimately make reoperation less likely (Evidence in Practice 12-1).

Outcomes from TOF repair are very good, with mortality rates less than 10% in most reports. Data show there is 90% long-term survival even in patients who had the earliest repairs in the 1950s (excluding hospital mortality) (8). In a large retrospective study of a single center's experience with 570 TOF repairs over 50 years, early and late mortality was low at 7%, with no early mortality reported in the last 10 years. Risk of reoperation increased linearly with time in both primary repair and palliation (9).

Late complications are common after TOF repair. RVOTO can recur and cause right ventricular hypertension and need for reoperation. It is common for repaired TOF patients to develop right ventricular dilation and dysfunction that is thought to be due to the accumulated effects of right ventricular hypertension with RVOTO, cardiopulmonary bypass, and perhaps intrinsic myocardial dysfunction. Additionally, techniques for right ventricular outflow tract repair often distort the pulmonary valve, causing pulmonary regurgitation and need for pulmonary valve replacement later in life, often via a right ventricle to pulmonary artery **conduit** or channel. Some patients need repeat operations for conduit stenosis or symptomatic regurgitation. In one review of adult patients who had repair in childhood, half had the

---

● **Evidence in Practice 12-1**

Early Versus Staged Repair for TOF— One Hospital's Experience

In 2000, the Hospital for Sick Children in Toronto, Ontario, reported their experience transitioning from palliation to complete repair in neonates. During the 1990s, the rate of palliation prior to repair fell from 38% to 0%, with a mortality rate of zero during the last 2 years reported. However, children younger than 3 months of age had longer intensive care unit stays and overall hospitalizations, and the authors concluded that repair after 3 months was the optimal time frame (6). Repair in children younger than 28 days of age has been reported not to have increased mortality or hospital length of stay, but may be associated with an increased need for reintervention or reoperation (7).

operation again 30 years after the initial repair (10). Indications for reoperation are variable and include pulmonary regurgitation with enlarging right ventricle, reduced exercise tolerance, and arrhythmias (Evidence in Practice 12-2). Aortic root dilation has also been reported in long-term follow-up studies of patients with TOF (11).

Patients with repaired TOF are at risk for arrhythmias, sinus node dysfunction, and sudden death. This ongoing risk seems to increase with age. Arrhythmia risk 35 years after repair is estimated to be 11% and sudden death to be 8% (13).

Patients with TOF complicated by pulmonary atresia, branch pulmonary stenosis, or multiple aortopulmonary collaterals have more complex treatment schemes and worse outcomes (10). Repair for this class of patients is individualized based on anatomy, but may require palliative shunting to increase pulmonary blood flow, serial stenting of stenotic pulmonary vessels and/or surgical rerouting of pulmonary collaterals to one location, and conduit placement, in addition to standard repair of TOF.

■■ The pediatrician comes in the room, takes Mia from her mother, and lays her on her back on the stretcher, pushing Mia's knees to her chest. The pediatrician explains that this will improve blood flow back to the heart and into the lungs and improve Mia's color and oxygenation. She accompanies you and Mia to radiology and looks at the chest radiograph, noting a "boot-shaped" heart. Mia is then transferred directly to the pediatric intensive care unit (PICU).

The pediatric cardiologist meets Mia in the PICU and performs an echocardiogram, confirming suspicion of tetralogy of Fallot. The echocardiogram notes a VSD, aorta overriding the VSD, mild RVOTO, and mild right ventricular hypertrophy.

● **Evidence in Practice 12-2**

Treatment for Pulmonary Valve Regurgitation

An emerging innovation in treatment of pulmonary regurgitation is percutaneously placed pulmonary valves. A bovine internal jugular vein with a native valve is mounted into a platinum stent and placed into an RV-PA conduit via catheterization, thereby creating a competent pulmonary valve and eliminating regurgitation, all without the need for cardiopulmonary bypass. Early reports demonstrated no mortality and that rates were low for risk of reoperation (12).

Course and Prognosis

Prior to the surgical era, half of all TOF patients died in the first years of life, and survival was not usual past age 30 (14). Surgical intervention has vastly changed prognosis; short- and long-term mortality is now quite low at less than 10% (8). Despite excellent long-term survival, complications and reoperation are common. In addition to pulmonary regurgitation and insufficiency that may cause symptoms and require intervention, right ventricular dysfunction and arrhythmias can impact quality of life. Generally, however, quality-of-life reports of patients with repaired TOF are similar to that of peers and better than children with other chronic diseases. Lower ratings for quality of life in children with TOF are usually related to lower exercise tolerance than that of peers (15). It is promising that outcomes from this common form of congenital heart disease are improving with improved surgical techniques and perioperative care.

Total Anomalous Pulmonary Venous Return

Total anomalous pulmonary venous return (TAPVR) (Fig.12-3) is a type of congenital heart disease that results when there is no connection between the **pulmonary vein confluence** (the location where the pulmonary veins come together) and the left atrium. Rather, the four pulmonary veins connect to one of the systemic veins that drain into the right atrium. This is a life-threatening problem because patients with TAPVR have no blood delivery into the left side of the heart, making it impossible for circulation of oxygenated blood to the body without communication between the right and left sides of the heart, such as with a septal defect. Approximately 1% of all patients with congenital heart disease have TAPVR (9). There is no known pattern of genetic transmission within families. TAPVR usually occurs in isolation, but it may be associated with other cardiac anomalies such as VSDs. TAPVR may be associated with heterotaxy syndrome (an abnormality in which the internal organs of the thorax and abdomen are abnormally arranged within their cavities), in which multiple associated anomalies are almost the rule.

There are four types of TAPVR:

1. *Supracardiac TAPVR* occurs superior to the heart, and the pulmonary vein confluence is posterior to the left atrium. An ascending vertical vein arises from the confluence and drains into the right superior vena cava. More commonly, the ascending vertical vein drains into the left innominate vein, which then drains into the superior vena cava.

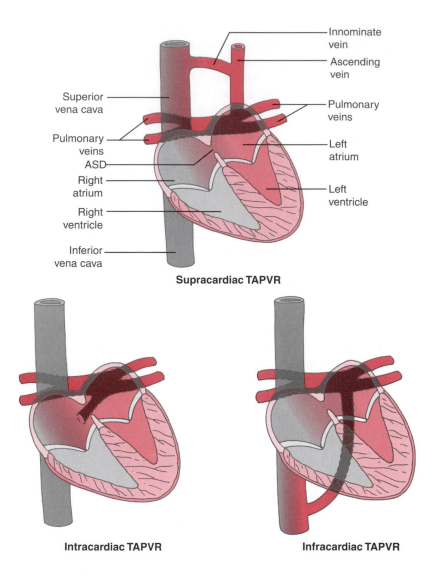

Figure 12-3 Total Anomalous Pulmonary Venous Return. TAPVR results when there is no connection between the pulmonary vein confluence and the left atrium. The connection of pulmonary veins can occur as supracardiac, intracardiac (connected to the coronary sinus), infracardiac, or a combination of the three.

2. *TAPVR to the coronary sinus* (intracardiac) occurs when the pulmonary vein confluence drains directly into the coronary sinus, which is the structure responsible for venous return from the myocardium. The coronary sinus drains into the right atrium.

3. *Infracardiac TAPVR* occurs inferior to the heart, and the pulmonary vein confluence sits posterior to the left atrium. A descending vertical vein drains from the confluence below the diaphragm to the portal vein, hepatic veins, inferior vena cava, or ductus venosus, which then eventually drain into the right atrium.

4. *Mixed-type TAPVR* is a combination of the first three types, in which some pulmonary veins drain to one site and the remainder to another. For example, two veins may drain to the right superior vena cava, whereas the remaining two veins drain to the right atrium.

5. All types of TAPVR have an ASD or PFO as part of the anomaly; otherwise, oxygenated

blood cannot get to the left side of the heart and death would occur.

Key to the understanding of TAPVR and its course is the possibility of obstruction within the pulmonary venous pathways to the right atrium. Obstruction may occur at the level of the atrial septum, the vertical veins, or the ductus venosus. Obstruction is most common in infracardiac TAPVR because the ductus venosus naturally constricts and closes after birth. The clinical implication of obstruction is discussed in more detail in the pathophysiology section.

Pathophysiology

The abnormal anatomy of TAPVR results in left-to-right shunting, requiring that mixed blood shunts again from the right side to the left side of the heart. All oxygenated blood, which normally should fill the left side of the heart, is delivered to the right side of the heart, mixing with deoxygenated blood draining into the right atrium from the inferior and superior vena cavae, and then must cross the atrial septum to provide cardiac output from the left ventricle. Without obstruction, initially after birth, while PVR is still high, saturations may be in the 75% to 85% range as blood mixes in the right atrium and then shunts across the atria. As PVR falls, there will be excessive pulmonary blood flow, and saturations may rise into the 90% range.

With obstruction, oxygenated blood cannot drain from the pulmonary vein confluence into the venous channels that return to the right atrium. This will lead to desaturation, because there is less oxygenated blood being delivered to the right atrium mixing with deoxygenated blood. Additionally, obstruction will cause a backup of blood in the pulmonary vasculature, increasing pulmonary venous pressure that transmits to the pulmonary capillary bed. This increased pressure in the pulmonary capillary bed will cause pulmonary edema and will lead to further desaturation. If the obstruction occurs at the atrial level, there will be an increase in right ventricular volume and pressure overload. This leads to a shift in the ventricular septum as the right heart encroaches into the space of the left heart, causing a decreased left ventricular volume, which leads to decreased cardiac output.

Clinical Manifestations

Patients with TAPVR without obstruction are asymptomatic at birth, and cyanosis is often not apparent. Tachypnea and feeding difficulties develop over the first few weeks of life, with eventual failure to thrive. On physical examination, patients have a right ventricular heave from the increased right ventricular volume, a fixed split S2, and a loud pulmonary component of S2. An S3 gallop is very often present. There may be a systolic ejection murmur from the volume crossing the right ventricular outflow tract. A diastolic murmur from the volume load across the tricuspid valve may be audible, as well as a venous hum in supracardiac TAPVR. Signs of heart failure such as peripheral edema and hepatomegaly may be present. An electrocardiogram shows peaked P waves from right atrial enlargement, right ventricular hypertrophy, and right axis deviation. A chest radiograph shows increased pulmonary vascular markings from excessive pulmonary blood flow, right heart enlargement, and possibly a prominent pulmonary artery. With supracardiac TAPVR to the innominate vein, there may be a characteristic "snowman" appearance of the cardiac silhouette, which is due to the left-sided ascending vertical vein, the prominent left innominate vein, and the right-sided superior vena cava.

With obstructed TAPVR, symptoms are apparent within the first few hours of life. Neonates present with cyanosis, dyspnea, poor oral intake, cardiorespiratory collapse, and metabolic acidosis. The cardiac examination may not be remarkable. There is no right ventricular heave and there is likely no murmur. S2 will be split with an accentuated P2 component. There may be crackles on lung auscultation owing to pulmonary edema, and there will be hepatomegaly.

An electrocardiogram will show right ventricular hypertrophy without right atrial enlargement. A chest radiograph will show a normal heart size but abnormal pulmonary vascular markings. It is important to note that obstruction may not be present upon initial examination; however, all patients should be followed closely until treatment in case obstruction does develop.

An echocardiogram must be done for diagnostic confirmation. All four pulmonary veins should be seen, along with the vertical vein and the pulmonary vein confluence and its relationship to the left atrium. The presence or absence of obstruction needs to be evaluated, and additional cardiac defects must be ruled out. The echocardiogram will show the extent of dilation of the right heart structures, bowing of the atrial septum to the left, and dilation of the pulmonary arteries and small left atrium.

Management and Treatment

All patients with TAPVR, with or without obstruction, require surgical intervention. Surgical repair involves closing the ASD and connecting the pulmonary vein confluence to the left atrium. In TAPVR to the coronary sinus, the common wall of the coronary sinus and left atrium is unroofed, thereby allowing coronary sinus drainage and pulmonary venous blood flow to drain into the left atrium.

Asymptomatic patients without obstruction may be managed conservatively while surgical repair is planned. Even so, obstruction may develop, particularly with infracardiac TAPVR, so patients should be followed closely. For symptomatic patients without obstruction, signs and symptoms of heart failure and overcirculation can be managed with diuretics, but early surgical repair should be planned. Nutrition should also be maximized while surgical planning takes place because these patients often present with failure to thrive. Patients with obstructed TAPVR will be critically ill with cardiovascular collapse. Emergency surgical repair is necessary, and patients should receive supportive care with mechanical ventilation, inotropes, diuresis for pulmonary edema if hemodynamics allow, and correction of metabolic abnormalities. It is important to note that neonates with obstructed TAPVR will initially present with cyanosis and hypoxia despite titration of oxygen and mechanical ventilation.

Nitric oxide is commonly used for newborns with hypoxemia that appears to be the result of pulmonary hypertension. However, inhaled nitric oxide in these patients will worsen cardiac output and cause clinical deterioration; this is because nitric oxide will dilate pulmonary vasculature and there is already pulmonary vascular congestion secondary to pulmonary venous obstruction. This supports the U.S. Food and Drug Administration's (FDA's) recommendation of obtaining an echocardiogram to rule out congenital heart defects prior to initiation of inhaled nitric oxide because the side effects for these patients can be devastating. The diagnosis of TAPVR should be immediately considered in hypoxic patients who deteriorate on nitric oxide so that a cardiologist can be consulted for diagnostic evaluation, and if confirmed, a cardiac surgeon can be notified of the need for emergency surgical repair.

Course and Prognosis

Operative mortality for patients with TAPVR is low at approximately 5% (17). One recent study found higher mortality rates in those with TAPVR associated with single ventricle anatomy and mixed-type TAPVR (18). In this same study, further surgical intervention for recurrent pulmonary vein stenosis was required in approximately 20% of patients, most within 3 months of the initial surgical repair. Long-term mortality rates depend mostly upon the development of pulmonary venous obstruction, which may develop at the surgical connection site itself or within the pulmonary veins. If the pulmonary veins are **hypoplastic** (underdeveloped) or stenotic preoperatively, or if the pulmonary confluence is small, there is an increased risk of having postoperative pulmonary venous obstruction. One large European study found the incidence of postoperative pulmonary venous obstruction to be approximately 20% and that the 1-year survival rate dropped from 86% to 62% if postoperative pulmonary venous obstruction occurred (19). All patients with TAPVR should be followed long-term for the possible development of stenoses in the left atrial-pulmonary vein confluence as well as the pulmonary veins themselves.

Transposition of the Great Arteries

Transposition of the great arteries (TGA) (Fig. 12-4) occurs when the two main arteries leaving the heart have changed places, so that the aorta arises from the right ventricle and the pulmonary artery arises from the left ventricle. There is almost always a PFO, but it may not be large enough to allow sufficient mixing of oxygenated and deoxygenated blood. TGA presents in 3.04 neonates per 10,000 live births (2), with a male predominance. Approximately half of all patients with TGA have no additional cardiac anomalies. The remaining patients may have VSDs, left ventricular outflow tract obstruction, or both. Rarely, there may be aortic abnormalities such as

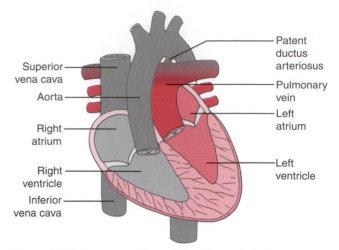

Figure 12-4 Transposition of the Great Arteries

coarctation of the aorta, aortic arch hypoplasia, or interrupted aortic arch. Without treatment or significant intracardiac shunts, TGA is fatal.

Pathophysiology

As described in Chapter 2, in utero the fetus receives oxygenated blood from the placenta. Normally, this blood is carried via the umbilical vein through the ductus venosus to the inferior vena cava, where it enters the right atrium and is directed through the PFO to the left side of the heart and ejected into the aorta so that the fetal brain and heart receive highly saturated blood. Blood from the upper body returns to the right atrium via the superior vena cava and travels across the tricuspid valve into the right ventricle and out the pulmonary artery. The lungs are collapsed in utero and partake in very little oxygen exchange. This causes PVR to be high, and blood is shunted from right to left across the PDA into the descending aorta. This shunting of deoxygenated blood causes lower body organs such as the intestines and kidneys to receive lower saturated blood. There is little blood flow into the lungs in utero because of the PFO and PDA.

Given the abnormal positioning of the aorta and pulmonary artery in TGA, normal fetal circulation is reversed. Oxygenated blood from the placenta travels via the umbilical vein and ductus venosus into the inferior vena cava and right atrium where it is directed across the PFO to the left atrium. It then travels into the left ventricle and out the pulmonary artery. PVR is still high, so the oxygenated blood from the placenta is shunted across the PDA into the descending aorta. Deoxygenated venous return from the superior vena cava drains into the right atrium and travels into the right ventricle and out the aorta. Thus in TGA, the coronary arteries and brain receive poorly saturated blood, and the organs of the lower half of the body receive more highly saturated blood.

Typically after birth, an infant's lungs open and become the primary source of oxygenation. PVR falls quickly in the first 24 hours of life, and the PDA closes within the first few days of life. As PVR falls, blood flow across the PDA becomes bidirectional; it flows from left to right from the aorta into the pulmonary artery during systole, and switches direction during diastole, to flow right to left from the pulmonary artery into the aorta. As the pulmonary vascular resistance continues to fall, PDA flow will become entirely left to right until the PDA fully closes.

In an infant with TGA, oxygenated blood from the pulmonary artery shunts through the PDA into the descending aorta when the PVR is high. As PVR falls, flow across the PDA will become bidirectional. As the PVR continues to fall, deoxygenated blood from the aorta will shunt into the pulmonary artery, and both the upper and lower portions of the body will receive deoxygenated blood, resulting in cyanosis. If PVR remains high, such as from persistent pulmonary hypertension, there will be continued flow of oxygenated blood from the pulmonary artery into the descending aorta; this leads to "reverse cyanosis," with the lower half of the body having higher saturations than the upper half of the body. This is in cotrast to normal infants in whom pulmonary hypertension causes higher saturations in the top half of the body (thus the brain and heart are receiving better oxygenation) and desaturation in the lower half of the body.

Survival of patients with TGA depends upon sufficient mixing of blood for oxygenated blood from the pulmonary veins to get to the body and deoxygenated venous return to get to the lungs. Saturations are dependent upon intracardiac or extracardiac shunts, such as a PFO, ASD, VSD, or PDA.

In the absence of an adequate shunt where mixing of blood can take place, the systemic saturations will be in the 40% to 70% range, and the saturation in the pulmonary vascular bed, if tested, will be 100%. With a PFO, ASD, or moderate VSD, mixing can occur, and saturations will be 75% to 85%. If the VSD is large, pulmonary overcirculation may occur as the PVR falls and deoxygenated blood shunts into the pulmonary circuit. Blood that is more highly saturated may then shunt back to the systemic side and saturations may approach 90%.

Clinical Manifestations

If there is inadequate mixing across an associated intracardiac or extracardiac shunt, a neonate with TGA will present with rapidly progressive cyanosis within the first few hours of life. Rapid diagnosis and emergency intervention are required for survival. The physical examination is usually nonspecific. There is no cardiac murmur. The electrocardiogram is normal, and the chest radiograph is often unremarkable.

If pulmonary hypertension is present, there may be reverse cyanosis (as noted previously) leaving the upper body cyanotic while the lower body will be more normally saturated. Reverse cyanosis may also be present when TGA occurs with an aortic anomaly, such as critical coarctation of the aorta (see Chapter 11); however, aortic obstructions are rare in TGA. An echocardiogram will rule this out.

In neonates with TGA and VSD, cyanosis may not be noticed. These patients develop signs and symptoms of heart failure over the first few weeks of life. They will be tachycardic and tachypneic. They have difficulty with oral feeds, eventually leading to failure to thrive, which may be the presenting symptom. On physical examination, the first heart sound is normal. There may be no murmur, or there may be a systolic ejection murmur at the left sternal border from increased flow across the left ventricular outflow tract. The second heart sound may be loud from the anteriorly placed aorta. The second heart sound may also be loud if the excessive pulmonary blood flow has caused pulmonary hypertension.

An electrocardiogram is usually normal in neonates with TGA. They may develop signs of right axis deviation and right ventricular hypertrophy as the right side of the heart is forced to contract against systemic vascular resistance (SVR). If a large VSD is present, there may be hypertrophy of both ventricles, known as **biventricular hypertrophy**. Arrhythmias are uncommon in TGA, although atrial arrhythmias may occur after atrial septostomy (see the Management and Treatment section that follows) if the arterial supply to the sinoatrial node is injured during the procedure.

The results of a chest radiograph are commonly normal (Fig. 12-5) in patients with TGA. The classic radiographic appearance of TGA with an intact ventricular septum is an "egg on a string" caused by

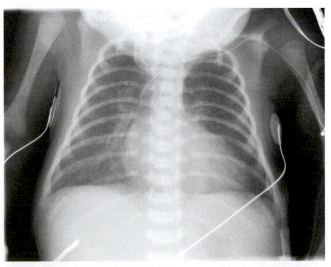

Figure 12-5 Chest Radiograph of Neonate with TGA
(*Courtesy of Jane Benson, MD*)

the cardiac silhouette and the parallel great vessels above; however, this is not universally noted on patients with TGA and intact ventricular septum. There may be prominent pulmonary vascular markings and pulmonary edema if a VSD is present.

An echocardiogram should be done immediately in patients who present with TGA to delineate the exact diagnosis and associated lesions. The relationship of the aorta to the pulmonary artery, the size of the PFO or ASD, the presence of a VSD and PDA, left ventricular outflow tract obstruction, aortic arch, and coronary artery pattern must all be determined.

Management and Treatment

For a neonate with TGA and severe cyanosis from inadequate mixing, an intracardiac shunt must be created immediately so that the infant will survive. An **atrial septostomy** (also known as a Rashkind procedure) is performed, usually at the patient's bedside. The procedure will create a hole in the atrial wall, causing a wide-open atrial-level shunt so that mixing can occur and saturations will stabilize. The procedure is performed by an interventional cardiologist. A balloon catheter is inserted via the umbilical vein or femoral vein and threaded through the inferior vena cava into the right atrium. Using echo guidance, the catheter is manipulated through the atrial septum to cross into the left atrium (Fig. 12-6). The balloon is then inflated and pulled back rapidly across the atrial septum into the right atrium. Saturations should rise immediately after this hole is created and blood from the right and left heart mix. Complications of an atrial septostomy include tearing of the atrial wall, pulmonary veins, or inferior vena cava, as well as atrioventricular valve damage. Emergency surgery may be required if any of these complications occur.

Once the atrial septostomy is performed, the patient can be stabilized prior to surgical repair. The RT's role at this point is usually to support ventilation as needed and provide oxygen

support to maintain a cardiologist-defined SpO_2 range. Because oxygenated and unoxygenated blood will always mix in these patients, normal SpO_2 is not usually expected.

The preferred surgical repair for TGA is the **arterial switch operation**, which was first described in 1975 (20). Prior to the arterial switch operation, TGA was repaired by baffling or tunneling the atria. This would cause systemic venous return to flow to the left side of the heart and out the pulmonary artery, and the pulmonary venous return to course to the right side of the heart and out the aorta. One of the long-term problems with this approach has been that the right ventricle is still the systemic ventricle, being forced to pump against SVR. The right ventricle was not designed to withstand this large amount of pressure, and thus the patient will develop right ventricular failure over time. In the arterial switch operation, the aorta and pulmonary artery are returned to their normal positions. The aorta is connected to the proximal pulmonary artery to form a neo-aorta, and the pulmonary artery is connected to the proximal aorta to form the neo-pulmonary artery. The coronary arteries are excised from the aortic sinus and reimplanted into the neo-aortic root. If a VSD is present, that is closed as well. Studies have shown that outcomes are better if the arterial switch operation is done early in the neonatal period (21, 22). It is important to note that the arterial switch needs to be done before the left ventricle has had time to weaken, when it is still able to tolerate SVR. If surgery is delayed, the left ventricle needs to be retrained to contract against the higher SVR with staged maneuvers such as pulmonary artery banding before surgically attaching the aorta to the left ventricle so that left ventricular failure does not occur after the arterial switch.

Course and Prognosis

Operative mortality for the arterial switch operation is less than 10% (23, 24). Early complications after the operation are usually the result of myocardial ischemia (lack of blood flow to the heart muscle) from abnormalities of the reimplanted coronary arteries. Myocardial ischemia can occur from the following:

- impingement or obstruction of a coronary by surrounding structures
- a tortuous (winding or complex) course caused by repositioning of the coronary artery; this may also include kinking of the coronary artery, which can slow or block blood flow
- stenosis at the connection site of the coronary artery to the neo-aorta

Long-term complications include several progressive abnormal anatomical findings at the surgical sights. One of these is **supravalvar stenosis**, which is

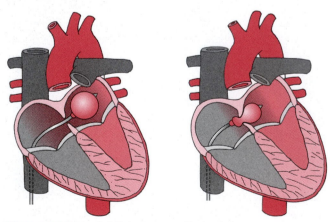

Figure 12-6 Atrial Septostomy Procedure

a narrowing of the vessel above the heart valve, at the suture line of the connection site of the great vessels. This is more commonly seen in the neo-pulmonary artery. Another complication that has been described in long-term follow-up studies is the stretching of the neo-aorta near the connection site, known as neo-aortic root dilation (25). The significance of this finding, however, is still unclear. Patients are also at risk for myocardial ischemia from coronary stenosis. Patients with TGA are followed for life by a pediatric cardiologist and have a regular echo assessment of the neo-pulmonary artery and neo-aorta, as well as assessment of biventricular function, including regional wall motion abnormalities, which would suggest coronary ischemia.

Hypoplastic Left Heart Syndrome

Hypoplastic left heart syndrome (HLHS) (Fig. 12-7) is a cyanotic heart disease in which parts of the left side of the heart do not fully develop. It is the most common of a larger classification of cyanotic heart diseases known as single ventricle syndrome, in which the heart develops with only one functioning ventricle. It occurs in 2.31 per 10,000 live births and accounts for 1% of all patients with congenital heart defects (2). HLHS is more prevalent in boys, with a ratio of 2:1. Many advances have been made in surgical and critical care to improve outcomes of this complex syndrome.

Pathophysiology

In HLHS, the left ventricle is small and unable to support systemic circulation. The mitral and aortic valves may be stenotic or atretic. The left atrium is typically small because of lack of flow, the left ventricle is very small and non-apex forming, and the aorta is small until the location of the PDA, at which point flow from the PDA supplies the normal-size descending aorta. The PDA also supplies the cerebral

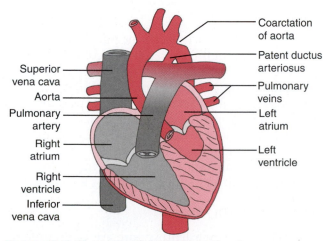

Figure 12-7 Hypoplastic Left Heart Syndrome

Labels: Coarctation of aorta; Patent ductus arteriosus; Pulmonary veins; Left atrium; Left ventricle; Superior vena cava; Aorta; Pulmonary artery; Right atrium; Right ventricle; Inferior vena cava

and coronary blood flow in a retrograde fashion. HLHS also includes an atrial septal defect, supplying oxygenated blood flow to the right heart.

In the postnatal period, blood flow is as follows: Oxygenated blood from the lungs travels through the pulmonary veins and enters the left atrium. When it meets restrictive or absent flow at the mitral valve, the oxygenated blood crosses an atrial connection and enters the right atrium and ventricle, mixing with deoxygenated blood. This mixed blood is ejected via the right ventricular outflow tract into the pulmonary artery where it will enter both the pulmonary vasculature and cross the PDA to supply systemic blood flow. How much blood will flow into the pulmonary vasculature versus how much will cross the PDA depends on the ratio of SVR to PVR. The crossing of blood through the PDA into the descending aorta is necessary to supply blood to the lower body, because of the absence of left ventricular flow into the ascending aorta.

Successful management of patients with HLHS at any age requires an understanding of the delicate balance between pulmonary blood flow and systemic blood flow and the degree of vascular resistance in each system. **Vascular resistance** is the resistance to flow that must be overcome to push blood through the circulatory system. **Pulmonary vascular resistance (PVR)** is the amount of resistance to blood flow through the lungs. **Systemic vascular resistance (SVR)** describes the resistance to blood flow through the peripheral system. PVR in healthy humans is less than one-tenth of SVR. Because of this lower value, the right ventricle does not have to be as large or work as hard to provide adequate blood flow to the lungs when compared with the left ventricle, which pumps against a much larger resistance. Infants with HLHS will have an oxygen saturation that is dependent on the ratio of systemic to pulmonary blood flow and resistance in these two circuits. Because the right ventricle is responsible for providing all blood flow, once the blood leaves the heart it will either travel to the systemic or pulmonary system, rather than travel to the lungs and then the body as in normal circulation. If blood flow between the pulmonary and systemic system is "balanced," then patients will have an SpO_2 of approximately 80% to 85% on FiO_2 of 0.21. An SpO_2 higher than 85% is an indication of higher pulmonary blood flow at the expense of blood flow to the systemic organs, which is critical for survival. Similarly, lower saturations reflect inadequate pulmonary blood flow, which is necessary to properly oxygenate the blood and avoid tissue hypoxia.

Clinical Manifestations

Affected newborns may have few symptoms in the first hours to days of life because the high PVR in the early neonatal period causes pulmonary and systemic blood flow to be nearly balanced. There may be little to no murmur detected, and lung examination will likely be normal. On careful examination, some increased acrocyanosis (blue skin of the hands and feet) may be present and/or liver size may be increased, but these findings may be subtle.

Without prenatal diagnosis, the infant with HLHS may present with shock, hypoperfusion, respiratory distress, and cyanosis associated with PDA closure within the first few days to weeks of life. As the duct naturally closes, systemic blood flow, including cerebral and coronary blood flow, will be diminished. Pulmonary blood flow increases, but oxygenated blood circulates in the pulmonary circuit without systemic delivery. Acidosis and hypoperfusion can be profound, and rescue therapy with PGE infusion to reopen the ductus arteriosus is life-saving.

A chest radiograph (Fig. 12-8) typically will not show diagnostic features particular to HLHS. The heart size may appear small or normal. Depending on the ratio of systemic to pulmonary blood flow, the pulmonary vasculature may be increased or decreased.

An electrocardiogram is less helpful in the diagnosis of HLHS. Right ventricular hypertrophy or lower left ventricular voltages may be seen, but these findings are also normal in the newborn period.

An echocardiogram is the standard to confirm diagnosis. With increasing precision of prenatal ultrasound imaging, many infants are diagnosed before birth and referred for cardiology consultation and prenatal echocardiography. Echocardiography confirms a small left ventricle, stenoses, or atresia of the mitral and/or aortic valves, in addition to a small aorta and aortic arch.

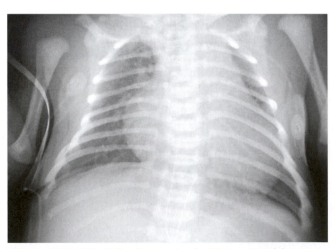

Figure 12-8 Chest Radiograph of a Neonate with HLHS *(Courtesy of Jane Benson, MD)*

Management and Treatment

If there is a prenatal diagnosis of HLHS, then neonates are admitted to the ICU after birth. The PDA is critical to maintaining systemic blood flow in the immediate post-natal period, and a PGE If there has not been a prenatal diagnosis, neonates are commonly discharged from the well-baby nursery as healthy because they are asymptomatic while their PDA is open. With closing of the PDA, usually in the first 2 weeks of life, infants will develop symptoms of poor feeding, lethargy, and cyanosis. They present in cardiovascular collapse with poor perfusion, hypotension, and metabolic acidosis. These patients are admitted to an ICU, where they require stabilization and management of multiorgan failure secondary to hemodynamic collapse. They are often intubated upon presentation for hypoxia. Goal saturations are 75% to 85%. Pressors are required to maintain blood pressure and augment cardiac contractility. Because of inadequate blood flow to critical organs, frequently liver and renal failure occurs, which require supportive care. Surgery should be planned once the patient is stable with improving organ function.

Surgical management of HLHS involves a series of staged procedures that progress toward the ultimate goal of a univentricular circulation that provides the following:

- Systemic blood flow via the right ventricle to a neo-aorta
- Pulmonary blood flow directly into the pulmonary arteries from the vena cava

There are variations in the procedures and timing, but this is most commonly achieved using three staged palliative procedures (Table 12-2):

Stage 1

The classic stage 1 reconstruction, also known as the **Norwood procedure**, is typically performed in the first week of life (26) (Fig. 12-9). This extensive surgery includes the following:

- Creating a neo-aorta using the pulmonary artery and homograft material to reconstruct the aortic arch in continuity with the right ventricle
- Removing the atrial septum (atrial septectomy) to ensure unobstructed blood flow from the pulmonary veins to the right ventricle
- Providing a source of pulmonary blood flow via a systemic-to-pulmonary artery shunt. This is typically via a right subclavian to right pulmonary artery shunt, known as a *modified BT shunt*
- Ligating the PDA

Goals of the stage 1 procedure are to provide reliable systemic blood flow via the right ventricle to a

Table 12-2	Staged Repair for HLHS	
Stage	**Name**	**Description**

1 (Figure 12-9A)	Norwood	1. Design of a neo-aorta to arise from the right ventricle, providing systemic blood flow
		2. Atrial septectomy, to ensure unobstructed blood flow from pulmonary veins to right ventricle
		3. Design of a shunt to provide blood flow directly from systemic circulation to pulmonary artery. This is performed by either:
		  a. Modified BT shunt (connecting the right subclavian vein to the pulmonary artery), or
		  b. Sano modification (connects the right ventricle to the pulmonary artery via a conduit)
		4. PDA ligation

2 (Figure 12-9B)	Bidirectional Glen	1. Connection of superior vena cava to pulmonary artery 2. Removal of pulmonary artery shunt (modified BT shunt or Sano modification)
3 (Figure 12-9C)	Fontan	Connection of inferior vena cava to pulmonary artery (with or without fenestration)

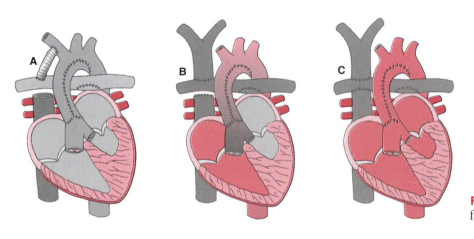

Figure 12-9 Three Stages of Repair for HLHS

neo-aorta and to provide pulmonary blood flow via a systemic-to-pulmonary shunt. This procedure is complex and has significant risk; mortality is reported to be from 10% to 20% (27, 28). In an effort to identify patents most at risk for mortality after stage 1, one study noted risk factors included prematurity, restrictive intra-atrial septum, longer cardiopulmonary bypass time, weight less than 2.8 kg, revision of the systemic-to-pulmonary shunt, and postoperative extracorporeal membrane oxygenation (ECMO) (27).

Modifications of this classic procedure include a right ventricle to pulmonary artery (RV-PA) conduit for pulmonary blood flow rather than the modified BT shunt; this RV-PA conduit was originally proposed by Norwood, but initial attempts were unsuccessful. Sano and colleagues reintroduced a modified version of Norwood's classic RV-PA conduit in 1983 (29), although the benefit of one technique over the other is still unproven

(Evidence in Practice 12-3). This alternative technique is known as a **Sano modification**.

After stage 1 in the neonatal period, infants are managed until stage 2 reconstruction is attempted, typically at 4 to 6 months of life. Mortality between stages 1 and 2 is generally reported to be 10%, making overall mortality before stage 2 for children with HLHS approximately 20% (27, 28).

Stage 2: Bidirectional Glenn Procedure

Stage 2 reconstruction, known as the **bidirectional Glenn (BDG) procedure**, changes pulmonary blood flow to a passive flow or drainage system, which connects the superior vena cava to the pulmonary artery and bypassing the right heart. The systemic-to-pulmonary shunt placed in stage 1 is removed. BDG requires low pulmonary vascular resistance to ensure passive blood flow from the superior vena cava to the pulmonary artery; therefore, a cardiac catheterization is performed before the BDG procedure to

● **Evidence in Practice 12-3**

Stage 1 Procedure: RV-PA Conduit Versus Modified BT Shunt

Theoretical benefit of the RV-PA conduit over the modified BT shunt for pulmonary blood flow after stage 1 is decreased diastolic run off of aortic and coronary blood flow into the pulmonary artery. Despite the plausible physiological benefit, outcomes to date are not distinctively improved with the RV-PA conduit, although studies are ongoing. For example, reviews of two large centers' experiences indicate that the RV-PA conduit does not demonstrate an improved perioperative mortality after stage 1 (27, 28), but may decrease mortality and decrease reoperation risk between stage 1 and stage 2 (27). There is concern that the incision of the right ventricle (ventriculotomy) required for the RV-PA conduit may be associated with RV dysfunction later in life (28). Overall, controversy regarding these two approaches to pulmonary blood flow in stage 1 is ongoing.

document pulmonary pressures. The BDG decreases myocardial work by reducing the amount of blood going through the right heart to prevent overloading the heart (cardiac volume overload). Postoperatively, the right heart has less responsibility for pumping blood to the lungs because the superior vena cava is flowing into the pulmonary artery. The inferior vena cava, however, still provides deoxygenated blood flow to the right atrium, causing some continued mixing of oxygenated and deoxygenated blood; thus the patient will still have some cyanosis.

As opposed to high mortality rates associated with stage 1 and interstage mortality, BDG mortality is quite low. Mortality has been reported to be between 0% and 5% (27).

Stage 3: Fontan Procedure

The final stage of HLHS surgery, the **Fontan procedure**, routes inferior vena cava flow from the right atrium to the pulmonary artery via an intracardiac or extracardiac conduit. This procedure finalizes the separation of pulmonary and systemic blood flow, reducing myocardial work and improving saturations to normal or near-normal range. The Fontan procedure is typically performed when the child is between 2 and 4 years of age and has low mortality, approximately 5%. The conduit from the inferior vena cava to pulmonary artery can include some openings into the right atrium, known as fenestrations, allowing desaturated blood to run off into the right atrium when pulmonary pressures are high and thereby limiting pulmonary blood flow and subsequent cardiac output. Determining which patients will be fenestrated depends on pre-Fontan pulmonary artery pressures, comorbidities, and surgical preference.

Alternatives to Three-Stage Repair

One alternative to the three-staged surgery of HLHS is heart transplantation, but organ availability and long neonatal wait times make this option impractical as a universal approach. Another alternative is a hybrid procedure, which replaces the complex repair of stage 1 with PDA stenting and bilateral pulmonary artery banding. This provides reliable systemic blood flow via the PDA and limits pulmonary blood flow with banding of the pulmonary arteries. This procedure is done by both a cardiac surgeon and an interventional cardiologist in a combined operating room and cardiac catheterization laboratory. The child then undergoes a more comprehensive stage 2 procedure at a few months of age to construct the neo-aorta and attach it to the right ventricle, to repair stenoses of the pulmonary arteries caused by the banding, and to establish an SVC-to-pulmonary artery connection (using the BDG procedure). Theoretic advantage of the hybrid procedure for repair of HLHS is reduction of major surgical procedures and their associated risks. However, early reports do not show decreased mortality over the traditional approach (30). The hybrid approach may be more beneficial in patients who have significant risk factors for mortality with the use of the traditional approach.

Prenatal intervention for HLHS is an emerging practice. Intrauterine, fetal catheter procedures to dilate aortic stenosis or open an intact atrial septum have been performed in a small number of patients, but practice and outcomes are still evolving.

Respiratory Management During HLHS Repair

Respiratory management of HLHS is mainly supportive and is based on appropriate oxygen saturation management and adequate ventilation with avoidance of hypocapnia.

Oxygen Therapy

Oxygen therapy is used as necessary to maintain SpO_2 of 75% to 85% throughout infancy until stage 3 repair. Supplemental oxygen is a potent vasodilator and should only be given when a patient with HLHS is unable to maintain appropriate SpO_2 when breathing room air. Health-care providers must pay close attention to the causes of hypoxemia in this population of patients. An SpO_2 less than 75% or greater than 85% is often an indication of undesired changes in SVR or PVR, which may indicate serious complications of surgical repair such as shunt occlusion.

Hypoxic Gas Delivery

In patients who consistently saturate greater than 85%, hypoxic gas delivery has been used as a means of increasing PVR to maintain appropriate systemic blood flow prior to stage 1 repair. This is done by mixing nitrogen with room air to achieve an FIO_2 of 0.15 to 0.20 (31) delivered via nasal cannula or oxyhood in spontaneously breathing patient or through the ventilator for intubated patients (32). In patients who are intubated, FIO_2 must be evaluated prior to delivery to the patient to ensure FIO_2 does not fall below 0.15, which would put the patient at risk of tissue hypoxia. An external oxygen analyzer should be used on the inspiratory limb of the ventilator circuit and alarms set in a narrow range to alert RTs if the FIO_2 is outside of desired range (32).

Ventilatory Management

Ventilator management is often required before stage 1 repair. This could be due to apnea associated with PGE delivery or respiratory failure associated with cardiac failure. Postoperative mechanical ventilation is also needed after each stage of repair, and close management of $PaCO_2$ is needed to maintain a high PVR and maintain appropriate systemic blood flow. Hypocapnia is also a potent pulmonary vasodilator, so $PaCO_2$ should be maintained in a normal to relatively high range (40 to 50 mm Hg) to maintain an adequate PVR to SVR ratio.

Mechanical ventilation immediately after stage 3 repair should focus more on normal acid base status and normoxemia, and thus techniques similar to other postoperative pediatric patients can be applied. Pressure-controlled ventilation has historically been the method of choice, although alternative techniques such as airway pressure release ventilation have been suggested because it may allow improved pulmonary blood flow and oxygenation (Evidence in Practice 12-4).

Course and Prognosis

Untreated, HLHS is fatal within days to weeks of birth. The three-staged surgery has significant risk, and current combined mortality for the three stages approaches 30%. Mortality for staged surgery prior to about 1995 was much higher, in the range of 50% to 80% (34). As these procedures are still in their relative infancy, the oldest survivors are only in young adulthood at this point. Advances in diagnosis, preoperative and postoperative management, and surgical and anesthetic techniques are advancing the care of these patients, making predictions based on early surgery survivors difficult.

Short-term complications of the staged surgery for HLHS include residual coarctation, atrioventricular valve regurgitation, chylothorax (lymphatic fluid in the pleural space), and partial or complete

● **Evidence in Practice 12-4**

Using Airway Pressure Release Ventilation (APRV) to Improve Pulmonary Blood Flow

Patients with cyanotic heart defects often have low cardiac output in the postoperative period as a consequence of their ventricular dysfunction. Positive-pressure ventilation has been shown to further decrease cardiac output by limiting blood flow into the pulmonary artery during diastole. Fontan operations also make patients very sensitive to the effects of positive-pressure ventilation, further decreasing pulmonary blood flow (17). Spontaneous ventilation normally causes a natural negative pressure that augments venous return, but this is negated when a patient is intubated because of the increased intrathoracic pressure from the ventilator. This increased intrathoracic pressure reduces preload and decreases cardiac output. One study questioned if spontaneous ventilation during airway pressure release ventilation (APRV) would improve pulmonary perfusion compared with pressure control ventilation in children after a Fontan operation or a TOF repair.

After cardiac surgery, patients were placed on APRV on the following settings (see Chapter 15 for more information on APRV): FIO_2, 0.50; P_{high} (pressure maintained in the lungs during the majority of the ventilator cycle), 13 to 20 cm H_2O; P_{low} (pressure to which the ventilator will release at short intervals), 0 cm H_2O; T_{high} (time the ventilator will maintain the P_{high} setting), 2.5 to 3.0 sec; and T_{low} (amount of time the ventilator will allow release of pressure), 0.3 to 0.5 sec. Goal $PaCO_2$ was 40 to 45 mm Hg. If CO_2 trended higher, P_{high} was increased and T_{high} was decreased. The study showed that when patients were spontaneously breathing, pulmonary blood flow and oxygen delivery was significantly increased during APRV compared to PCV, despite having higher mean airway pressures, similar $PaCO_2$, and similar right heart pressures. Patients displayed intermittent reductions in intrathoracic pressure during spontaneous inspiration on APRV. During PCV, however, spontaneous inspiration resulted in only positive deflections. This is a promising result, which shows that even with higher ventilator settings, pulmonary blood flow can be improved and cardiac interference decreased when using APRV (33).

vocal cord paralysis. Systemic hypoperfusion can occur in neonates with unbalanced systemic and pulmonary blood flow, causing necrotizing enterocolitis and/or renal or hepatic dysfunction. These children have prolonged ICU stays and hospitalizations that can increase complications and the complexity of care (34).

Long-term complications of the three-staged HLHS surgery and other variants of single ventricle heart disease are related to cardiac failure of the single ventricle; arrhythmias caused by right atrial dilation and sinus node dysfunction, particularly with earlier versions of the Fontan procedure; and atrioventricular valvular dysfunction.

Despite the complications described, many teens and young adults surviving with Fontan physiology have relatively good quality of life. They are able to go to school, work, and have families. However, close neurodevelopmental examination of survivors of HLHS demonstrates intelligence quotient (IQ) scores lower than those of the general population. One report of 11 children treated in the earliest era found that 7 of 11 (64%) had mental retardation (35). Wernovsky et al. reported that school-aged HLHS patients managed in a similar time period had high utilization of special education (30%), and their median IQ scores were significantly lower than the general population (36). Analysis of neurocognitive testing results from patients treated more recently show improved outcomes, but outcomes that are still different from those of the general population. Goldberg et al. reported that the mean IQ for 26 HLHS patients treated between 1991 and 1996 was 94 compared with other single-ventricle patients, whose mean IQ was 107 (37).

Interestingly, the diagnosis of HLHS is a risk factor for worse neurodevelopmental outcomes when compared with other single-ventricle heart diseases requiring similar palliative surgeries (36, 37). Even children with HLHS who undergo transplantation as treatment versus staged surgery score lower on developmental testing than does the normal population (38). It is postulated that abnormal fetal cerebral blood flow and oxygen delivery may predispose this group of patients to worse developmental outcomes (39). Further study of the etiology of these prenatal insults and improvements in perioperative and operative care will ideally improve these outcomes.

Ebstein Anomaly

Ebstein anomaly is a malformation of the heart in which there are abnormal leaflets of the tricuspid valve, found between the right atrium and ventricle, as well as displacement of the leaflets into the right ventricle. The posterior and septal leaflets are usually abnormal, but the anterior leaflet may be involved as well, and the valve leaflets may be thickened, tethered, and/or redundant. Among patients with congenital heart disease, the prevalence of Ebstein anomaly is less than 1% (Fig. 12-10) (40). Most occurrences are sporadic cases with no family history of Ebstein anomaly or congenital heart disease.

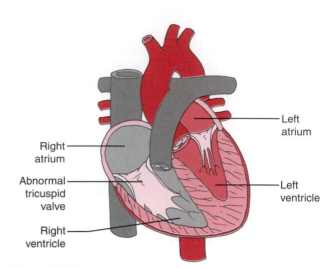

Figure 12-10 Ebstein Anomaly

Older studies have indicated that there may be an association between maternal use of lithium during pregnancy and the occurrence of Ebstein anomaly (41). Ebstein anomaly is usually associated with an atrial septal defect or patent foramen ovale) but may also be associated with other lesions of congenital heart disease, such as a ventricular septal defect. (See Chapter 11 for discussions of each of these defects.)

Pathophysiology

The displacement of the tricuspid valve leaflets in Ebstein anomaly leads to an "atrialized" portion of the right ventricle that is continuous with the right atrium. The abnormalities cause loss of valve integrity and lead to tricuspid **regurgitation**, or backflow into the atrium during diastole. With mild displacement and insufficiency, there may be no clinical symptoms. In more severe cases, significant tricuspid regurgitation leads to an elevated right atrial pressure. When right atrial pressure becomes higher than left atrial pressure, it will cause shunting of deoxygenated blood across the atrial septum to the left atrium. This causes desaturation and cyanosis. Tricuspid regurgitation may be so severe that there is little forward (antegrade) flow of blood out of the right ventricle and into the pulmonary arteries, and these patients will be dependent on the PDA to provide blood flow to the pulmonary arteries.

As described in Chapter 2, with a newborn's first inspiration of oxygen after birth, when the lungs take over for the placenta as the primary organ for gas exchange, PVR begins to fall, but does not reach normal levels for a few weeks. In neonates with Ebstein anomaly, PVR remains high, which may further prevent antegrade flow through the pulmonary valve. This can increase tricuspid regurgitation, leading to increased right-to-left shunting of blood and cyanosis. As PVR decreases, pulmonary blood flow will increase, and saturations will thus increase.

Patients with Ebstein anomaly also have an associated risk of arrhythmias. Approximately 20% to 40% of these patients experience arrhythmias during their lifetime (42, 43). There also may be an accessory electrical conductance pathway between the atria and ventricles that leads to Wolff-Parkinson-White syndrome and associated supraventricular tachycardia (Special Population 12-2). Supraventricular tachycardia may also occur without Wolff-Parkinson-White syndrome. As tricuspid regurgitation increases, the right atrium dilates, which can also lead to atrial fibrillation and atrial flutter.

Clinical Manifestations

As mentioned previously, if the tricuspid valve has little dysfunction and is only mildly displaced, children with Ebstein anomaly may show no clinical symptoms. As displacement and regurgitation increase, symptoms become more prevalent. Cyanosis may present immediately after birth. It may be persistent with severe disease or may improve over the first few weeks of life as pulmonary vascular resistance falls. Cyanosis may recur in adolescence or early adulthood as the tricuspid regurgitation worsens. Older patients may also have dyspnea on exertion and fatigue. On physical examination, cyanosis may be noted and saturations may be less than 85%. In older children and adults, jugular venous distention may be seen along with hepatomegaly (enlarged liver) as the right atrial pressure increases as a result of severe tricuspid regurgitation and/or right ventricular failure. The results of a lung examination will be normal in the majority of patients. On cardiac examination, a holosystolic murmur of tricuspid regurgitation will be present at the left lower sternal border, and a diastolic murmur from tricuspid stenosis may be heard. A third heart sound may be heard, either from right ventricular filling or vibration of the tricuspid valve leaflets. A fourth heart sound may also be heard during atrial systole.

A chest radiograph (Fig. 12-11) may be normal or show cardiomegaly with an enlarged right atrial silhouette. There may also be decreased pulmonary vascular markings if pulmonary blood flow is decreased.

An electrocardiogram will show peaked P waves from right atrial enlargement, possible right bundle branch blocks from delayed conduction of the right ventricle, and possible shortened PR intervals associated with Wolff-Parkinson-White syndrome.

An echocardiogram should be performed to confirm the diagnosis of Ebstein anomaly. The degree of displacement of the valve leaflets can be seen as well as the amount of tricuspid regurgitation, tricuspid stenosis (narrowing), antegrade flow into the pulmonary artery, and shunting of blood between the right and left atria.

Management and Treatment

As with all patients presenting with an unknown cause of cyanosis, a trial of PGE is warranted. If the initial echocardiogram shows antegrade flow into the pulmonary artery, this is evidence of appropriate blood flow through the lungs, and PGE infusion may be discontinued and the baby monitored. Again, as PVR naturally falls in newborns, flow into the pulmonary artery will increase and saturations will increase. If there is minimal antegrade blood flow into the pulmonary artery, PGE infusion should be continued, and the baby should be monitored as PVR decreases. Once antegrade flow into the pulmonary artery occurs, PGE infusion may then be discontinued and saturations monitored.

Anatomical **pulmonary atresia** may also be present, which is abnormal development of the pulmonary valve that sits between the right ventricle

---

● Special Populations 12-2

Wolff-Parkinson-White syndrome

Wolff-Parkinson-White syndrome (WPW) is one of several disorders of the conduction system of the heart that are commonly referred to as pre-excitation syndromes. WPW is caused by the presence of an abnormal accessory electrical conduction pathway between the atria and the ventricles. Electrical signals traveling down this abnormal pathway stimulate the ventricles to contract prematurely, resulting in a supraventricular tachycardia referred to as an atrioventricular reentrant tachycardia.

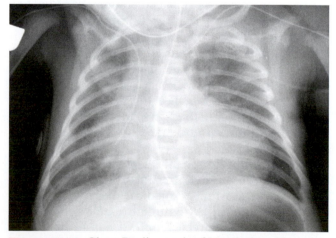

Figure 12-11 Chest Radiograph of Newborn with Ebstein Anomaly *(Courtesy of Jane Benson, MD)*

and the pulmonary artery. If anatomical pulmonary atresia is present, surgical intervention, such as the placement of a **Blalock-Taussig shunt (BT shunt),** is needed. Patients with BT shunts are followed over the first 6 to 12 months until they begin to outgrow the shunt and require more long-term surgical **palliation** (treatment to improve symptoms), which may include Glenn and Fontan procedures, completed over several stages (see Table 12-2). In the Glenn procedure, the superior vena cava is connected directly to the pulmonary artery, and in the Fontan procedure, the inferior vena cava is connected to the pulmonary artery (see Fig. 12-9). These procedures allow venous blood to bypass the right heart and travel to the lungs for oxygenation and allow permanent separation of the pulmonary and systemic circulations.

The decision to repair the tricuspid valve—either with primary repair of the valve or placement of a prosthetic valve, as discussed in Chapter 11—or to proceed with the Glenn or Fontan procedures after a BT shunt depends on the size of the patient, the size of the right ventricle, presence of anatomical pulmonary atresia, and the anatomy of the tricuspid valve. There are specific indications for surgery:

- Increased right heart size
- Right ventricular dysfunction
- Dyspnea
- Exercise intolerance
- Ventricular or atrial tachyarrhythmias not controlled by medical therapy or catheter intervention
- Significant associated cardiac lesions

Neonates who do not need medical intervention will be followed long-term by a pediatric cardiologist. These patients may grow and develop normally until symptoms such as cyanosis and right heart failure develop in adolescence or early adulthood. If tricuspid regurgitation is increasing in severity, tricuspid valve repair or replacement may be indicated. Heart transplantation is also an option for patients with biventricular dysfunction in which repair is thought unlikely to be successful. For patients with heart failure, **inotropes** (medications to improve cardiac contractility) may be necessary to stabilize the patient's blood flow. Once the patient is clinically stable, conversion to long-term heart failure medications (e.g., diuretics and digoxin) is possible.

Arrhythmias may develop in children with Ebstein anomaly at any time. Supraventricular tachycardia (SVT) may be present after birth or it may develop later and be resistant to medical therapy or be well controlled on anti-arrhythmics (e.g., amiodarone). Older patients with recurrent SVT can be treated by an electrophysiologist. Atrial fibrillation and atrial flutter also tend to develop as atrial dilation occurs secondary to significant tricuspid regurgitation. Patients with atrial fibrillation or atrial flutter may need to be treated with cardioversion acutely and then with anti-arrhythmics.

Course and Prognosis

Most patients with Ebstein anomaly survive into adulthood. One study reported that 1-year survival was 67% and 10-year survival was 59% (44). This study showed a shortened life span, with few patients living past 70 years of age. Mortality rates are higher for neonatal patients requiring early intervention (45). Those with a mild form of the disease may live a normal life span. Outcomes are worse with more severe tricuspid valve displacement and regurgitation and right ventricular hypoplasia and dysfunction. For patients who require intervention, one large study reported age at surgery between 2 months and 79 years, with a median age at operation of 20 years (46). Thirty-four percent underwent valve repair, and 66% underwent tricuspid valve replacement. Approximately 5% of all patients who underwent intervention experienced early death, and 7.6% experienced late death over 25 years of follow-up. Another study from the same institution reported that for those who required surgery, 82% required no further intervention at 10 years' follow-up, and 56% required no further intervention at 20 years' follow-up (47). Nearly 80% were reported to have an excellent or good outcome, and more than half of the study group was free of cardiac symptoms, including arrhythmias.

Truncus Arteriosus

Truncus arteriosus (Fig. 12-12) is a condition in which a single great vessel leaves the heart and supplies the systemic and pulmonary circulation. The prevalence of truncus arteriosus is estimated to be 0.74 per 10,000 live births (2).

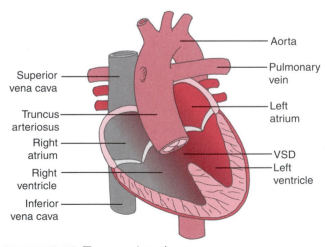

Figure 12-12 Truncus Arteriosus

Pathophysiology

The truncus arteriosus is a large arterial vessel that arises from the developing heart during normal fetal development. By the end of the fifth gestational week, this trunk normally separates into the aorta and main pulmonary artery and their respective valves. Disruption of this embryologic process and persistence of the truncus causes this condition.

The truncus is positioned over the ventricular septum and can be dominant over the right (42%), left (16%), or both (42%) ventricles. The truncus valve is typically abnormal in anatomy and function; stenosis or regurgitation is common. A VSD is present, and coronary artery anomalies can also be present.

There are four types of truncus arteriosus based on the origin of the pulmonary arteries and associated anomalies. The commonly used classification was proposed by Van Praagh in 1965 (42).

- **Type 1:** A main pulmonary artery arises from the truncus.
- **Type 2:** The right and left pulmonary arteries arise separately from the common trunk.
- **Type 3:** One pulmonary artery arises from the ascending aorta, and the other arises from the descending aorta or other vessel such as an aortopulmonary collateral artery.
- **Type 4:** An interrupted aortic arch or coarctation is the origin, rather than pulmonary artery. Type 4 is more commonly associated with DiGeorge syndrome.

As the truncus usually overrides the VSD, blood from both ventricles is ejected into the truncus. The amount of blood that goes to the lungs is dependent on the size of the pulmonary vessels and PVR. After PVR decreases in the first days and weeks of life, if pulmonary vessels are not small enough to restrict blood flow, then pulmonary circulation will be excessive and patients with truncus arteriosus will not be cyanotic. Once excessive pulmonary blood flow develops, congestive heart failure is common in the untreated infant. Abnormal truncal valves will also put an excess volume load on the heart and contribute to congestive heart failure.

One series of 65 patients who underwent primary repair in infancy reported the following associated lesions: interrupted aortic arch (12%), truncal regurgitation (23%), and coronary artery anomalies (18%) (49). Also, association with DiGeorge syndrome, including thymic hypoplasia and hypocalcemia, is well documented.

Clinical Manifestations

Truncus arteriosus may be diagnosed prenatally after routine ultrasound screening for anomalies. Neonates without prenatal diagnosis may present with **asymptomatic cyanosis**, meaning they may be blue with saturations in the 75% to 85% range without respiratory distress. Infants with truncus arteriosus not diagnosed in the neonatal period will present with symptoms associated with congestive heart failure, such as poor feeding, tachypnea, sweating, and hepatomegaly. An active precordium may be appreciated. Murmur may or may not be present depending on the origins and caliber of pulmonary arteries. The first heart sound is normal and second is loud and single. A lung examination may demonstrate rales, and hepatomegaly may be present.

A chest radiograph (Fig. 12-13) may demonstrate abnormal cardiothymic silhouette and increased pulmonary markings caused by excessive pulmonary blood flow. An electrocardiogram is typically nondiagnostic; left ventricular hypertrophy and left atrial enlargement may be seen.

An echocardiogram is diagnostic and will reveal the characteristic truncus vessel arising from the heart. Truncal valve structure and function can be determined with echocardiography. Cardiac catheterization may be required to completely delineate anatomy, although this is rarely needed now that echo techniques have been improved and refined.

Management and Treatment

Successful truncus arteriosus repair was first described by McGoon and colleagues in 1968 in a 5-year-old boy with severe congestive heart failure (50). Their operation was the first to provide pulmonary blood flow via a valved right ventricle to pulmonary artery conduit. Even though perioperative care and operative techniques have improved since their report, the repair they performed

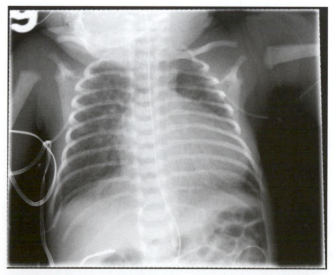

Figure 12-13 Chest Radiograph of Neonate with Truncus Arteriosus (*Courtesy of Jane Benson, MD*)

remains the basis of the treatment of this condition today.

Without surgical intervention, mortality with truncus arteriosus is high. Although earlier techniques involved delayed repair until a few months of life or even palliation of truncus arteriosus with banding of one or more pulmonary arteries, repair of truncus arteriosus in the neonatal period is now the standard. The surgical goals are to achieve the following:

• Isolate pulmonary blood vessels from the truncus
• Provide continuous connection of the pulmonary arteries to the right ventricle, which is typically done by a right ventricle to pulmonary artery (RV-PA) conduit.
• Close the VSD.
• Repair or replace the truncal valve if regurgitant or stenotic.

While awaiting surgery, excessive pulmonary blood flow and congestive heart failure may need to be managed with diuretics. Respiratory management is supportive, and involves pre- and postoperative ventilation support for cardiac and respiratory failure, and oxygen therapy as needed to maintain SpO_2 75% to 85%.

Course and Prognosis

In the early era of truncus arteriosus repair (1980s–1990s), mortality was high at nearly 50% (51). More recently, early postoperative mortality for infants undergoing truncus arteriosus repair has been reported to be 5%. Lower weight at repair (less than 2.5 kg), longer intraoperative cardiopulmonary bypass times, and associated interrupted aortic arch are risk factors for mortality (49, 51).

Early complications of truncus repair include need for early reoperation such as reexploration for bleeding, wound infection, chylothorax, and arrhythmias. Delayed sternal closure is common.

Long-term mortality has been reported to be 5% to 10%, with increased mortality in patients who are small at the time of repair or in those who require truncal valve replacement. Reoperation for replacement of the RV-PA conduit is common, with nearly half requiring this procedure by 3 years of age and 75% needing it by 5 to 8 years (49, 52). Additionally, multiple long-term interventions for complications are common. Procedures such as valve replacements and balloon dilation for conduit obstruction, pulmonary artery obstruction, arch obstruction, or stenosis are common (51).

Advances in perioperative and surgical care have improved outcomes in truncus arteriosus, but need for reoperation and intervention to manage this complex condition is common.

■■ Mia remains in the PICU until surgical repair of her TOF can be scheduled. She remains on oxygen as needed to keep her SpO_2 greater than 80% per the echocardiogram, but she is able to be maintained on room air for most of her presurgical course, requiring supplemental oxygen only during tet spells, along with knee-to-chest maneuvers, which seem to be very successful. Two days later, she is taken to the OR for complete repair, including VSD repair and relief of RVOTO. She returns to the PICU after surgery, where she is on the ventilator postoperatively for 1 day before being successfully extubated to room air.

■■ Critical Thinking Questions: Mia Mcnamara

1. What type of postoperative ventilatory support would you have recommended for Mia?
2. What do you expect Mia's postsurgical respiratory therapy needs will be?
3. If a knee-to-chest maneuver had not been successful at relieving Mia's hypoxemia, what other treatments could have been implemented?

◗● Case Studies and Critical Thinking Questions

■ Case 1: Baby Girl (BG) Kelly

You are working in a level 3C NICU when you are a notified that there is a 40-week female, now 3 hours old, who is being admitted to the NICU from the well-baby nursery. Her mother had an uneventful pregnancy and vaginal delivery. A few hours after birth, the baby was noted to be dusky. When the nurse checked her vitals, her heart rate was 165 bpm, her respiratory rate 60 breaths/min, blood pressure 65/38 mm Hg, and saturations 80% on room air. She was placed on oxygen, and the NICU was contacted for transfer. On arrival, she is visibly cyanotic, with saturations of 70% obtained from a pulse oximeter on her right hand and while breathing 1.0 via a non-rebreather mask. Her vital signs also include a heart rate of 175 bpm, respiratory rate of 80 breaths/min, and blood pressure of 60/35 mm Hg.

• *What could be three causes of BG Kelly's hypoxia?*

BG Kelly's physical examination reveals cyanosis and tachypnea. Her cardiac examination is notable for tachycardia but no murmur. Lungs are clear to auscultation. Abdomen is soft, nontender, and nondistended without organomegaly. Extremities are cyanotic but warm, with normal upper and lower extremity pulses. A chest radiograph is obtained and shows normal cardiac silhouette and normal pulmonary vascular markings. An electrocardiogram is done and shows sinus tachycardia. Laboratory results, including blood culture, are obtained. She is started on antibiotics and a prostaglandin infusion. The physician asks that you remove the oxygen, and a blood gas is drawn from her right radial artery while she is breathing room air. The results are pH 7.28, $PaCO_2$ 30 mm Hg, PaO_2 50 mm Hg, HCO_3 15 mEq/L. The physician now asks for you to place her under an oxyhood and deliver 100% oxygen. After 10 minutes, a repeat blood gas drawn from the right radial artery is pH 7.26, $PaCO_2$ 30 mm Hg, PaO_2 80 mm Hg, HCO_3 14 mEq/L.

- *Based on these results, what is your leading diagnosis for the etiology of BG Kelly's hypoxia?*
- *What should be done to improve oxygenation in BG Kelly at this time?*

■ Case 2: (Baby Boy) BB Adams

You are working in a level 3C NICU when a baby is transferred from an outside hospital. He was born vaginally after an uneventful pregnancy and was noted to be cyanotic a few hours after birth, with saturations of 80% on room air. He was intubated, started on antibiotics and a prostaglandin infusion, and transferred to your hospital. On arrival, his heart rate is 150 mm Hg, respiratory rate is 40 breaths/min (ventilator set at 25 breaths/min), blood pressure is 65/42 mm Hg, and saturations are 88% on 1.0 oxygen. A cardiac examination reveals a regular rate and rhythm and a 2/6 holosystolic murmur heard loudest at the left lower sternal border. His lung examination reveals normal work of breathing and clear lung fields. His abdomen is soft, with his liver palpable 1 cm below the costal margin. His extremities are warm and well perfused, with normal upper and lower extremity pulses. Electrocardiogram shows a sinus rhythm with a shortened PR interval. A chest radiograph shows mild cardiomegaly and clear lungs. An echocardiogram is done and is noteworthy for Ebstein anomaly with moderate tricuspid regurgitation. There is a small amount of flow seen through the pulmonary valve and a large PDA with left-to-right flow and elevated pulmonary artery pressures.

- *What would be your respiratory care recommendations?*

BB Adams is weaned to room air via the ventilator with stable saturations in the 75% to 85% range. He is then extubated. Because there is flow across the pulmonary valve, the prostaglandin infusion is stopped in an attempt to decrease pulmonary artery pressure and encourage antegrade flow across the pulmonary valve.

- *What should you monitor after the prostaglandin infusion is stopped?*

Saturations rise into the 90% to 95% range, and BB Kelly remains stable. He does not have any episodes of supraventricular tachycardia. Follow-up echocardiogram shows a closed ductus arteriosus, mild tricuspid regurgitation, normal antegrade flow into the pulmonary artery across the pulmonary valve, and normal pulmonary artery pressure. He is discharged home a few days later with close follow-up by cardiology.

■ Case 3: BB Moore

You are working in a level 3B NICU when a full-term baby is admitted with hypoxia and poor respiratory effort after an unremarkable vaginal delivery. The mother's pregnancy was normal, and a 20-week prenatal ultrasound showed normal organs, including a four-chamber heart. The baby was noted to be cyanotic in the delivery room and was unresponsive to blow-by oxygen and positive-pressure ventilation, so he was intubated. On admission to the NICU, his saturations are 80% on FIO_2 1.0, heart rate is 175 bpm, and blood pressure is 48/30 mm Hg. He is placed on synchronized intermittent mandatory ventilation (SIMV) with a peak inspiratory pressure of 20 cm H_2O, peak end expiratory pressure of 5 cm H_2O, rate of 30 breaths/min, and FIO_2 1.0 with measured tidal volumes of 8 to 10 cc/kg. The initial chest radiograph shows mild bilateral pulmonary edema, and initial ABG results are pH 7.25, $PaCO_2$ 40 mm Hg, PaO_2 70 mm Hg, HCO_3 17 mEq/L.

- *What type of acid-base abnormality does this blood gas result show? What ventilator adjustments would you recommend?*

His physical examination reveals a nondysmorphic neonate who is sedated. His cardiac examination shows a tachycardic but regular rhythm with no murmurs, and the lung examination is notable for scattered bilateral crackles. His abdomen is soft, nontender, and nondistended, with the liver palpable 1 cm below the right costal margin. His extremities are cyanotic, cool, and mottled, with a capillary refill time of 4 seconds. Blood and urine cultures are sent. He is deemed too unstable for lumbar puncture.

- *What medications should be started immediately?*
- *Does a normal prenatal ultrasound rule out congenital heart disease?*

BB Moore is quickly started on broad-spectrum antibiotics and a prostaglandin infusion. Cardiology is consulted for cyanosis and is on the way to perform an echocardiogram. He is given three 20 cc/kg fluid boluses for hypotension, but continues to be hypotensive with mean arterial pressures of 30 to 35 mm Hg, so he is started on a dopamine infusion. He continues to be hypoxic, now with saturations of 70% on FIO_2 1.0. He is converted to a high-frequency oscillatory ventilator (HFOV) for persistent hypoxia, and nitric oxide is initiated for possible pulmonary hypertension. Within 10 minutes of starting nitric oxide, his saturations are 60% on 1.0 oxygen and a repeat ABG test result is pH 7.20, $PaCO_2$ 38 mm Hg, PaO_2 55 mm Hg, HCO_3 14 mEq/L. Repeat chest radiograph shows severe bilateral pulmonary edema.

- *What is the cause of BB Moore's decompensation after conversion to HFOV and nitric oxide?*

Cardiology arrives and an echocardiogram shows obstructed infra-diaphragmatic TAPVR. His persistent hypotension is treated with further fluids and titration of pressors. He is quickly weaned off of nitric oxide while cardiac surgery is contacted. The baby is taken to the operating room for emergent repair of TAPVR.

■ Case 4: James Smith

You are working in a PICU when a 6-day-old baby boy presents to the emergency room with lethargy, poor feeding, and change in color over the course of the day. The mother had an uneventful pregnancy, with a normal 20-week screening ultrasound. James had an uneventful vaginal delivery and was discharged home after 2 days and an uneventful newborn nursery course. Upon presentation to the ED, James is gray and lethargic. His rectal temperature is 34°C, heart rate is 170 bpm, respiratory rate is 75 breaths/min, and blood pressure is not detectable by noninvasive cuff measurements. His saturations are 70% on room air, so he is intubated and placed on pressure control ventilation. He is given fluid boluses for hypotension, started on a dopamine drip, and admitted to the PICU for further management.

- *What is the differential diagnosis for this patient? Based on this differential, what medications should be started immediately?*

After blood and urine cultures are obtained, antibiotics are given for possible sepsis. Given pulmonary edema on his admission chest radiograph, hepatomegaly on physical examination, and a lactate of 10 mEq/L on admission laboratory results, a PGE infusion is immediately started. An echocardiogram is obtained to evaluate for congenital heart disease.

- *What broad type of congenital heart disease can present like this?*
- *What surgery will James have within the next week?*

Multiple-Choice Questions

1. The most common cyanotic congenital heart disease found in newborns is:
   a. Tetralogy of Fallot.
   b. Ebstein anomaly.
   c. Hypoplastic left heart syndrome.
   d. Transposition of the great arteries.

2. Evaluation of a neonate suspected of having a cyanotic heart defect should include all of the following *except*:
   a. Cardiac catheterization.
   b. Hyperoxia test.
   c. Echocardiogram.
   d. Electrocardiograph.
   e. Chest radiograph.

3. Place in order the steps taken to perform a hyperoxia test.
   I. Obtain an arterial blood gas from the right radial artery
   II. Wait 15 minutes?
   III. Place patient on FIO_2 0.21
   IV. Wait 60 minutes
   V. Place patient on FIO_2 1.0

   a. I, II, V, I
   b. III, I, V, II, I
   c. III, I, V, IV, I
   d. V,I,III,IV,I

4. You are working in the pediatric emergency department (ED) of a community hospital, and a 2-week-old infant comes in with his mother. He was sent to the ED by his primary physician after his 2-week check-up because he has had difficulty feeding and has not been gaining weight appropriately. His SpO_2 on pulse oximetry is 84%. On auscultation you hear a murmur, which the emergency room physician describes as a fixed split S2 with an S3 gallop. The physician orders a 12-lead electrocardiogram and a chest radiograph. The EKG shows peaked P waves, and the chest radiograph shows a normal-sized heart with increased pulmonary vascular markings. Based on these findings, what is the likely diagnosis?
   a. TAPVR
   b. HLHS

c. TOF

d. TGA

5. You are the NICU RT and help admit a new-born, now 1.5 hours old, with worsening cyanosis despite FIO$_2$ delivery via non-rebreather mask. She has no murmur on auscultation and her chest radiograph looks normal. Suspecting either pulmonary hypertension or a cardiac defect, you place a pulse oximeter on her right arm and left leg and note that the SpO$_2$ on her right arm is 72% and her left leg is 87%. Based on these clinical findings, what cardiac abnormality does your patient likely have?

a. TOF

b. TGA

c. HLHS

d. TAPVR

6. In what patient population would an atrial septostomy be indicated?

a. HLHS

b. TOF

c. TGA without a septal defect or shunt

d. TGA with a VSD

e. Ebstein anomaly

7. Tetralogy of Fallot includes which of the following four components (*select the four that apply*)

VI. ASD

VII. VSD

VIII. Aorta that sits over (overrides) the VSD

IX. Right ventricular outflow tract obstruction

X. Small left ventricle

XI. Right ventricular hypertrophy

XII. PDA

a. I, II, III, V

b. II, III, V, VII

c. I, II, III, VII

d. II, III, IV, VI

8. After what stage of surgical treatment for hypoplastic left heart syndrome (HLHS) would you expect a child to have a normal SpO$_2$ on room air?

a. Norwood

b. Bidirectional Glen

c. Fontan

d. I would never expect a patient with HLHS to have a normal SpO$_2$ on room air

9. Which of the following is an appropriate method to deliver a hypoxic gas mixture to an infant with a cyanotic heart defect?

a. Oxyhood delivering only nitrogen gas

b. Bleeding nitrogen into the expiratory limb of a ventilator circuit

c. Replacing room air on a mechanical ventilator with nitrogen

d. Connecting nasal cannula to a blender that mixes nitrogen and room air to a specified FIO$_2$ before delivery

10. The indication for a prostaglandin infusion for newborns is to:

a. Decrease PVR in a neonate with congenital heart disease.

b. Increase systemic blood pressure for neonates with a congenital heart defect.

c. Maintain an atrial or ventricular septal defect in a neonate with congenital heart malformation who requires a shunt.

d. Maintain a patent ductus arteriosus in a neonate with a congenital heart malformation who requires a shunt.

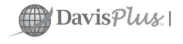 For additional resources login to Davis*Plus* (http://davisplus.fadavis.com/ keyword "Perretta") and click on the Premium tab. (Don't have a *Plus*Code to access Premium Resources? Just click the Purchase Access button on the book's Davis*Plus* page.)

REFERENCES

1. Apitz C, Webb GD, Redington AN. Tetralogy of Fallot. *Lancet.* 2009;374:14621471.

2. Parker SE, Mai CT, Canfield MA, et al. Updated national birth prevalence estimates for selected birth defects in the United States, 2004-2006. *Birth Defects Research (Part A): Clinical and Molecular Teratology.* 2010;88:1008-1016.

3. Michielon G, Marino B, Formigari R, et al. Genetic syndromes and outcome after surgical correction of tetralogy of Fallot. *Ann Thorac Surg.* 2006;8:968-975.

4. Siriapisith T, Wasinrat J, Tresukosol D. Uncorrected pink tetralogy of Fallot in an adult patient: incidental CT findings. *J Cardiovasc Comput Tomogr.* 2010;4(1):58-61.

5. Karl TR. Tetralogy of Fallot: current surgical perspective. *Ann Pediatr Card.* 2008;1:93-100.

6. van Arsedell GS, Maharaj GS, Tom J, et al. What is the optimal age for repair of tetralogy of Fallot? *Circulation.* 2000;102:123-129.

7. Tamesberger MI, Lechner E, Mair R, et al. Early repair of tetralogy of Fallot in neonates and infants less than four months of age. *Ann Thorac Surg.* 2008;86:1928-1936.

8. Nollert G, Fischlein T, Bouterwek S, et al. Long-term outcome in patients undergoing surgical repair of tetralogy of Fallot: 36 year follow-up of 490 survivors of the first year after surgical repair. *J Am Coll Cardiol.* 1997;30: 1374-1383.

9. Lindberg HL, Saatvedt K, Seem E, et al. Single-center 50 years' experience with surgical management of tetralogy of Fallot [published online ahead of print, 2011]. *Eur J Cardiothorac Surg.* doi:10.1016/j.ejcts.2010.12.065.

10. Hickey EJ, Veldtman G, Bradley TJ, et al. Late risk of outcomes for adults with repaired tetralogy of Fallot from an inception cohort spanning four decades. *Eur J Cardiothorac Surg.* 2009;35:156-166.

11. Niwa K, Siu SC, Webb GD, Gatzoulis MA. Progressive aortic root dilation in adults late after repair of tetralogy of Fallot. *Circulation.* 2002;106:1374-1378.

12. Lurz P, Coats L, Khambadkone S, et al. Percutaneous pulmonary valve implantation: impact of evolving technology and learning curve on clinical outcome. *Circulation.* 2008;117:1964-1972.

13. Gatzoulis MA, Balaji S, Webber SA, et al. Risk factors for arrhythmia and sudden death late after repair of tetralogy of Fallot: a multicenter study. *Lancet.* 2000;356:975-981.

14. Bertranou EG, Blackstone EH, Hazelrig JB, et al. Life expectancy without surgery in Tetralogy of Fallot. *Am J Cardiol.* 1978;42:458-466.

15. Kwon EN, Mussatto K, Simpson PM, Brosig C, Nugent M, Samyn MM. Children and adolescents with repaired tetralogy of Fallot report quality of life similar to healthy peers. *Congenit Heart Dis.* 2011;6:18–27.

16. Reller MD, Strickland MJ, Riehle-Colarusso T, et al. Prevalence of congenital heart defects in metropolitan Atlanta, 1998-2005. *J Pediatr.* 2008;153:807-813.

17. Karamlou T, Gurofsky R, Al Sukhni E, et al. Factors associated with mortality and reoperating in 377 children with total anomalous pulmonary venous connection. *Circulation.* 2007;115:1591-1598.

18. Kelle M, Backer CL, Gossett JG, et al. Total anomalous pulmonary venous connection: results of surgical repair of 100 patients at a single institution. *J Thorac Cardiovasc Surg.* 2010;139:1387-1394.

19. Seale AN, Uemura H, Webber SA, et al. Total anomalous pulmonary venous connection: morphology and outcome from and international population-based study. *Circulation.* 2010;122:2718-2726.

20. Jatene AD, Fontes VF, Paulista PP, et al. Anatomic correction of transposition of the great vessels. *J Thorac Cardiovasc Surg.* 1976;72:364-370.

21. Kirklin JW, Blackstone EH, Tchervenkov CI, et al. Clinical outcomes after the arterial switch operation for transposition: patient, support, procedural, and institutional risk factors. *Circulation.* 1992;86:1501-1515.

22. Wernovsky G, Mayer JE, Jonas RA, et al. Factors influencing early and late outcome of the arterial switch operation for transposition of the great arteries. *J Thorac Cardiovasc Surg.* 1995;109:289-302.

23. Emani SM, Beroukhim R, Zurakowski D, et al. Outcomes after anatomic repair for d-transposition of the great arteries with left ventricular outflow tract obstruction. *Circulation.* 2009;120:S53-58.

24. Qamar ZA, Goldberg CS, Devaney EJ, et al. Current risk factors and outcomes for the arterial switch operation. *Ann Thorac Surg.* 2007;84:871-878.

25. Marino BS, Wernovsky G, McElhinney DB, et al. Neoaortic valvar function after the arterial switch. *Cardiol Young.* 2006;16:481-489.

26. Norwood WI, Lang P, Hansen DD. Physiologic repair of aortic atresia-hypoplastic left heart syndrome. *NEJM.* 1983;308:23-26.

27. Pigula FA, Vida V, del Nido P, et al. Contemporary results and current strategies in the management of hypoplastic left heart syndrome. *Sem Thorac Cardiovasc Surg.* 2007;19:238-244.

28. Ballweg JA, Dominguez TE, Ravishankar C, et al. A contemporary comparison of the effect of shunt type in hypoplastic left heart syndrome on the hemodynamics and outcome at stage 2 reconstruction. *J Thorac Cardiovasc Surg.* 2007;134:297-303.

29. Sano S, Ishino K, Kawada M, et al. Right ventricle-pulmonary artery shunt in first-stage palliation of hypoplastic left heart syndrome. *J Thorac Cardiovasc Surg.* 2003;126:504-510.

30. Bacha EA, Daves S, Hardin J, et al. Single-ventricle palliation for high risk neonates: the emergence of an alternative hybrid stage 1 strategy. *J Thorac Cardiovasc Surg.* 2006;131:163-171.

31. Toiyama K, Hamaoka K, Oka T, et al. Changes in cerebral oxygen saturation and blood flow during hypoxic gas ventilation therapy in HLHS and CoA/IAA complex with markedly increased pulmonary blood flow. *Circ J.* 2010;74:2125-2131.

32. Gentile M. Inhaled medical gases: more to breathe than oxygen. *Respir Care.* 2011;56(9):1341-1359.

33. Walsh MA, Merat M, La Rotta, G, et al. Airway pressure release ventilation improves pulmonary blood flow in infants after cardiac surgery. *Crit Care Med.* 2011;39(12):2599-2604.

34. Tibballs J, Kawahira Y, Carter BG, et al. Outcomes of surgical treatment of infants with hypoplastic left heart syndrome: an institutional experience 1983-2004. *J Paediatr Child Health.* 2007;43:746-751.

35. Rogers BT, Msall ME, Buck GM, et al. Neurodevelopmental outcome of infants with hypoplastic left heart syndrome. *J Pediatr.* 1995;126:496-498.

36. Wernovsky G, Stiles KM, Gauvreau K, et al. Cognitive development after the Fontan operation. *Circulation.* 2000;102:883-889.

37. Goldberg CS, Schwartz EM, Brunberg JA, et al. Neurodevelopmental outcome of patients after the Fontan operation: a comparison between children with hypoplastic left heart syndrome and other functional single ventricle lesions. *J Pediatr.* 2000;137:646-652.

38. Ikle L, Hale K, Fashaw L, et al. Developmental outcome of patients with hypoplastic left heart syndrome treated with heart transplantation. *J Pediatr.* 2003;142:20-25.

39. Mahle WT, Wernovsky G. Neurodevelopmental outcomes in hypoplastic left heart syndrome. *Pediatr Cardiac Surg Ann Semin Thorac Cardiovasc Surg.* 2004;7:39-47.

40. Correa-Villasenor A, Ferencz C, Neill CA, et al. Ebstein's malformation of the tricuspid valve: genetic and environmental factors. The Baltimore-Washington infant study group. *Teratology.* 1994;50:137-147.

41. Weinstein MR, Goldfield MD. Cardiovascular malformations and lithium use during pregnancy. *Am J Psych.* 1975;132:529-531.

42. Delhaas T, du Marchie Sarvaas GJ, Rijlaarsdam ME, et al. A multicenter, long-term study on arrhythmias in children with Ebstein anomaly. *Pediatr Cardiol.* 2010;31:229-233.

43. Brown ML, Dearani JA, Danielson GK, et al. Functional status after operation for Ebstein anomaly: the Mayo Clinic experience. *J Am Coll Cardiol.* 2008;52:460-466.

44. Celermajer DS, Bull C, Till JA, et al. Ebstein's anomaly: presentation and outcome from fetus to adult. *J Am Coll Cardiol.* 1994;23:170-176.

45. Shinkawa T, Polimenakos AC, Gomez-Fifer CA, et al. Management and long-term outcome of neonatal Ebstein anomaly. *J Thorac Cardiovasc Surg.* 2010;139:354-358.

46. Jost CH, Connolly HM, Dearani JA, et al. Ebstein's anomaly. *Circulation.* 2007;115:277-285.

47. Brown ML, Dearani JA, Danielson GK, et al. Functional status after operation for Ebstein anomaly: the Mayo Clinic experience. *J Am Coll Cardiol.* 2008;52:460-466.

48. Van Praagh R, Van Praagh S. The anatomy of common aorticopulmonary trunk (truncus arteriosus communis) and its embryologic implications: a study of 57 necropsy cases. *Am J Cardiol.* 1965;16:406-425.

49. Thompson LD, McElhinney DB, Reddy M, et al. Neonatal repair of truncus arteriosus: continuing improvement in outcomes. *Ann Thorac Surg.* 2001;72:391-395.

50. McGoon GC, Rastelli GC, Ongley PA. An operation for the correction of truncus arteriosus. *JAMA.* 1968;205:69-73.

51. Tlaskal T, Chaloupecky V, Hucin B, et al. Long-term results after correction of persistent truncus arteriosus in 83 patients. *Eur J Cardiothorac Surg.* 2010;37:1278-1284.

52. Ullmann MV, Gorenflo M, Sebening C, et al. Long-term results after repair of truncus arteriosus communis in neonates and infants. *J Thorac Cardiovasc Surg.* 2003;51:175-179.

Chapter 13

Asthma

Chapter Outline

Key Terms

Adrenergic
Airway edema
Airway hyperresponsiveness
Airway remodeling
Anticholinergics
Anti-immunoglobulin E (IgE)
  therapy
Antileukotrienes
Asthma
Asthma action plan
Asthma severity
Atopy
Auto-positive end expiratory
  pressure (PEEP)
Biomarkers
Bronchoconstriction
Bronchoprovocation
Cromones
Dyspnea
Exacerbations
Exercise-induced asthma
Exhaled breath condensate
Foreign antigen
Fractional exhaled nitric oxide
  (FeNO)
Heliox
Histamine
Hygiene hypothesis
Immunotherapy
Ketamine
Leukotrienes
Long-acting beta agonists (LABAs)
Magnesium
Mast cells
Methacholine
Mucus
Natural history of asthma
Peak expiratory flow (PEF)

Key Terms cont.

Permissive hypercapnia

Phagocytosis

Phenotypic

Pulmonary function testing (PFT)

Pulsus paradoxus

Short-acting beta agonists (SABAs)

Status asthmaticus

Viscous

Xanthines

Chapter Objectives

After reading this chapter, you will be able to:

1. List the risk factors for the development of asthma.
2. Describe the four key characteristics of asthma.
3. Identify key components of the inflammatory pathway for asthma.
4. Recommend ways to identify triggers for a patient newly diagnosed with asthma.
5. Assist in obtaining a patient history for a child who wheezes and is suspected of having asthma.
6. Classify a patient's asthma severity based on current impairment and anticipated risk.
7. Recommend daily long-term pharmacological therapy for a patient newly diagnosed with asthma.
8. Identify clinical manifestations that would require an increase or decrease in asthma therapy.
9. Diagnose a patient in status asthmaticus.
10. Recommend respiratory support for a patient with asthma and impending respiratory failure and hypoxemia.
11. Recommend initial ventilator settings for an intubated patient in status asthmaticus.
12. Adjust ventilator settings for an intubated patient with asthma to allow adequate time for exhalation.

■■ Derrick Lamb

You are a respiratory therapist who works at a children's hospital in a large urban environment. You volunteer once a month with some of the pediatric pulmonologists providing health-care outreach in the community for children without insurance. The next child in the clinic is a 7-year-old boy named Derrick Lamb; you've met previously in the hospital's emergency department, where his grandmother brought him for wheezing several times in the past year. She has brought him to the clinic today because she says he seems to be wheezing more frequently this winter season.

Asthma

Asthma is a common chronic disorder of the airways with a complex interaction of airflow obstruction, bronchial hyperresponsiveness, and an underlying inflammation. A working definition of asthma has been commissioned by the National Asthma Education and Prevention Program (NAEPP), and is updated as new evidence is uncovered (Box 13-1). The NAEPP's current definition of asthma follows:

Asthma is a chronic inflammatory disorder of the airways in which many cells and cellular elements play a role: in particular, mast cells, eosinophils, T lymphocytes, macrophages, neutrophils, and epithelial cells. In susceptible individuals, this inflammation causes recurrent episodes of wheezing, breathlessness, chest tightness, and coughing, particularly at night or in the early morning. These episodes are usually associated with widespread but variable airflow obstruction that is often reversible either spontaneously or with treatment. The inflammation also causes an associated increase in the existing bronchial hyperresponsiveness to a variety of stimuli. Reversibility of airflow limitation may be incomplete in some patients with asthma (1).

Box 13-1 The National Asthma Education and Prevention Program (1)

The National Asthma Education and Prevention Program (NAEPP) was initiated in March 1989 to address the growing problem of asthma in the United States. The NAEPP is administered and coordinated by the National Heart, Lung, and Blood Institute (NHLBI). The NAEPP works with intermediaries, including major medical associations, voluntary health organizations, and community programs, to educate patients, health professionals, and the public. Every 5 years, an expert panel is commissioned by the NAEPP's Coordinating Committee to summarize current knowledge in asthma epidemiology, pathology, diagnosis, and management. The ultimate goal of the NAEPP is to enhance the quality of life for patients with asthma and decrease asthma-related morbidity and mortality.

One of the defining characteristics of asthma is its heterogeneity, or differing characteristics and symptoms. The interaction of symptoms can vary greatly among patients and within the same patient over time. The interaction of asthma features determines the clinical manifestations, severity of asthma **exacerbations** (increase in symptoms), and success of treatment (2). Many different things can trigger an asthma exacerbation. For many, asthma is an allergic disease, whereas for others, it may be triggered by environmental exposure to things like pollutants or dust mites. Still others have **exercise-induced asthma**, in which symptoms are only present during physical exertion.

Compared to other allergic diseases, asthma has the greatest clinical and economic burden, and most of the epidemiological attention has been focused on improving its treatment strategies above all other allergic diseases. A common cofinding with asthma is **atopy**, the genetic predisposition for hypersensitivity to allergens. Atopy is present in approximately 80% of children with asthma and 60% of adults with asthma (2). It has been difficult to define the relationship between atopy and asthma incidence, however, showing that the pathophysiology of asthma is multifactorial and complicated.

It has been difficult to report the true frequency of asthma, especially with children. Diagnosing asthma in young children is particularly challenging because wheezing in this age group is a common and nonspecific physical finding. Although some 50% of preschool children have wheezing, only 10% to 15% have a diagnosis of "true" asthma by the time they reach school age (3). It is often assumed, for example, that if a diagnosis code for asthma is documented in a medical record, the child has a higher likelihood of asthma, but the lack of a diagnosis does not necessarily indicate lack of disease (4). Many children with asthma are not diagnosed in a timely manner, especially in those without the commonly recognized factors associated with asthma, such as family history or exercise-induced wheezing or coughing (5).

In 2009, approximately 24.6 million Americans had a current asthma diagnosis, including 7.1 million children. The highest prevalence rate was seen in children ages 5 to 17 (109.3 per 1,000 children). Overall, the pediatric rate (all children younger than 18) was 96.1 per 1,000, which was significantly greater than those older than 18 (76.8 per 1,000). More than 10 million U.S. children aged 17 years and under (14%) have been diagnosed with asthma at some point in their life as of 2009 (6).

In addition to an increasing prevalence of pediatric asthma, the number of children seeking medical assistance or treatment for asthma has also increased, as measured by ambulatory visits, emergency department (ED) use, and hospitalizations for asthma. Ambulatory care visits have continued to increase since the year 2000 (7). In 2006, there were 10.6 million physician office visits, 1.2 million hospital outpatient department visits, and almost 1.7 million emergency room visits as a result of asthma (8). In the same year, 444,000 hospital discharges were attributed to asthma (6). Admission rates for asthma in children ages 0 through 4 years and 5 through 14 years are seven times and twice as high, respectively, as those for adults (9). From 2002 to 2007, the annual economic cost of asthma in the United States was $56 billion; direct health-care costs were $50.1 billion, with indirect costs (e.g., lost productivity) contributing an additional $5.9 billion (10). Americans lose approximately 14.41 million work days and 3.68 million school days per year because of asthma, which averages to 0.92 school days lost per student (11).

Tobacco smoke, air pollution, occupations, and diet have all been associated with an increased risk for the onset of asthma. Several other risk factors make asthma more likely in certain populations, including gender, race, family history, prenatal care, birth weight, health history, urban living, and socioeconomic status.

- **Gender:** Boys (16%) are more likely than girls (12%) to have been diagnosed with asthma (6).
- **Race:** In the United States, non-Hispanic black children are more likely to have been diagnosed with asthma (21%) or to still have asthma (16%) than Hispanic children (13% and 8%) or non-Hispanic white children (12% and 8%) (6). Black children in families with incomes less than 50% of the poverty level (approximately $10,000 for a family of four) have twice the risk of asthma as white children in families in the same financial situation (2).
- **Family history:** Asthma has historically been considered a hereditary disorder. A child with a parent with asthma is 1.96 times more likely to have asthma than a child with no parental history of asthma. A child with a parent *and* a grandparent with asthma is more than 4 times more likely to have asthma (12). Given the higher than normal prevalence of asthma in certain populations, it appears that asthma family history in first-degree relatives (parents, siblings) may help in capturing the probability of childhood asthma.
- **Prenatal care:** In utero exposure to environmental tobacco smoke increases the likelihood for wheezing in the infant, although the subsequent development of asthma has not been well defined (2). Diet and nutrition, stress, use of antibiotics, and mode of delivery are currently being studied to assess their effect on the early development of allergies and asthma (3).

- **Birth weight:** There is a strong association between low birth weight and the risk of physician-diagnosed asthma (13).
- **Health history:** The Centers for Disease Control and Prevention have found children in fair or poor health (38%) to be 3.5 times more likely to have ever been diagnosed with asthma and almost 5 times more likely to still have asthma (33%) compared with children in excellent or very good health (11% and 7%) (14). In addition, infants with sensitivity to food allergens early in life are more likely to develop asthma (15). One study also showed that patients who wheezed before age 2 were 4 times more likely to develop asthma later in life (16).
- **Urban living:** Asthma in the United States appears to be more frequent in ethnic minorities and in children growing up in poor urban neighborhoods and is least common in rural areas in combination with farm animal exposure. There are several environmental and lifestyle factors associated with urban living that are suspected to promote the development of asthma, particularly in the first few years of life, including close living quarters, less time spent outdoors, and vehicle exhaust (17). In one study, asthma was consistently reported less frequently among only younger farm-reared children, suggesting that exposures occurring early in life have a significant effect in modifying the incidence or risk of asthma (18). National statistics and differences in state reporting requirements, however, make it difficult to accurately quantify urban versus rural or farm asthma rates. The role of air pollution in the development of asthma remains controversial and may be related to allergic sensitization (19). One epidemiological study showed that heavy exercise (three or more team sports) outdoors in communities with high concentrations of ozone was associated with a higher risk of asthma among school-aged children (20).
- **Socioeconomic status:** Research has found that children in poor families are more likely to have been diagnosed with asthma (17%) or to still have asthma (12%) than children in families that were not poor (12% and 8%) (6).

Despite all these risk factors, there is not a clear picture of asthma or its cause in any age or population. The prevalence of asthma across regional, national, and international populations also varies widely, suggesting that both genetic and environmental exposures may influence the development of asthma. It is hypothesized that environmental factors such as infections and exposure to endotoxins may protect against asthma or may facilitate its development, depending in part on the timing of exposure in infancy and childhood. Our understanding of asthma development and underlying mechanisms includes the concept that gene and environmental interactions are critical factors in the development of airway inflammation and eventual alteration in the pulmonary physiology that is characteristic of clinical asthma.

The diagnosis of asthma usually is based on **phenotypic** (observable) symptoms. Central to the symptom patterns is the presence of airway inflammation, which is variable both from person to person and also in individuals based on the quality of symptom control. The level of symptom control helps determine the amount of medical support needed and is classified by terms such as *intermittent versus persistent* or *acute versus chronic.* Acute symptoms of asthma usually arise from bronchospasm and require and respond to bronchodilator therapy, whereas chronic asthma is thought to be caused by irreversible airway edema, and does not respond to rescue therapies such as bronchodilator.

The most current research findings on the mechanisms of asthma and findings from clinical trials have led to therapeutic approaches that allow most people who have asthma to participate fully in activities they choose. As we learn more about the pathophysiology, phenotypes, and genetics of asthma, treatments will become available to ensure adequate asthma control for all patients and, ideally, to reverse and even prevent asthma processes. The challenge for respiratory therapists remains to help all patients with asthma, particularly those at high risk, receive quality asthma care (2).

Pathophysiology

The airways are in continuous contact with the outside world, which makes them susceptible to contact with allergens as well as potentially harmful physical, chemical, and biological agents. For patients with asthma, this can start a chain reaction that will cause airflow limitation and **dyspnea** (a subjective feeling of shortness of breath). Airflow limitation in asthma is recurrent and caused by a variety of changes in the airway. These include airway edema, bronchoconstriction, airway hyperresponsiveness, and airway remodeling (Fig. 13-1). Mucous plugging is an additional factor that contributes to airflow limitations.

- **Airway edema**: When asthma becomes more persistent, **airway edema** develops as fluid begins to accumulate in the interstitial spaces of the airway, limiting localized air flow.
- **Bronchoconstriction:** The dominant physiological event leading to clinical symptoms of asthma is airway narrowing and a subsequent

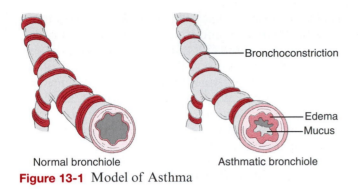

Figure 13-1 Model of Asthma

interference with airflow. In acute exacerbations of asthma, bronchial smooth muscle contraction (**bronchoconstriction**) occurs quickly to narrow the airways in response to exposure to a variety of stimuli, including allergens or irritants.

• **Airway hyperresponsiveness: Airway hyperresponsiveness,** an exaggerated bronchoconstrictor response to a wide variety of stimuli, is a major, but not necessarily unique, feature of asthma. The degree to which airway hyperresponsiveness can be quantified by challenge tests, such as with methacholine, correlates with the clinical severity of asthma. The mechanisms influencing airway hyperresponsiveness are multiple and include inflammation, dysfunctional neuroregulation, and structural changes.

• **Airway remodeling:** Chronic and severe asthma in children and adults is associated with thickening of the airway walls. As a consequence, airflow limitation may be only partially reversible for some people with asthma—they may always have a certain amount of airway narrowing. Permanent structural changes can occur in the airway and are associated with a progressive loss of lung function that is not prevented by or fully reversible by therapy. It is believed that this **airway remodeling** is caused by both the inflammation and repeated and continuous incidences of bronchoconstriction (21, 22), with consequent permanent changes in the airway that increase airflow obstruction and airway responsiveness and can cause a patient to be less responsive to therapy. The structural changes found in airway remodeling can include the following:
• Thickening of the subbasement membrane
• Fibrosis of airway tissues
• Increase in airway smooth muscle tissue
• Blood vessel proliferation and dilation
• Excessive airway wall collagen deposition
• Mucous gland hyperplasia and hypersecretion
Regulation of the repair and remodeling process is not well established, but both the process of

repair and its regulation are likely to be key events in explaining the persistent nature of the disease and limitations to a therapeutic response.

Airway Inflammation

Inflammation is a central part in the pathophysiology of asthma. Airway inflammation involves an interaction of many cell types and multiple mediators with the airways that lead to bronchial inflammation and airflow limitation presenting clinically as coughing, wheezing, and shortness of breath. The process by which this inflammation occurs and leads to clinical asthma is still not well understood. Inflammation is a consistent part of all phenotypes of asthma, although patients may have different triggers, and it is suspected that different inflammatory cells are involved in different types of asthma (Fig.13-2). There are thought to be two possible mechanisms causing airway inflammation during asthma: acute and chronic. All asthma begins as an acute (or type I) response; at some point during the disease, some patients may experience chronic inflammation.

Type I Hypersensitivity Response (Acute Inflammation)

The acute inflammatory cascade in asthma begins with the introduction of a trigger, known as a **foreign antigen,** into the airway. Foreign antigens are chemical or physical irritants that are capable of eliciting an immune response. In asthma, these antigens could be any of the allergic or nonallergic triggers, such as pet dander, dust, pollution, cold air, or cigarette smoke. Antigens come into contact with the airway and are captured by one of three cells:

• **Macrophages:** immune cells found in high numbers in the airway that engulf foreign antigens
• **Dendritic cells:** located beneath the airway epithelium, with sensory nerves projecting into the epithelium to detect physical and chemical irritants
• **Epithelial cells:** cells that capture foreign antigens and send out chemokines (chemical signals) to white blood cells to stimulate an immune response

These cells will present the antigens to T-cell lymphocytes found within the airway mucosa. T cells are a type of white blood cell (WBC) responsible for the body's immune response. T cells will multiply to neutralize and/or eliminate the antigen. The T cells bind to another type of lymphocyte called a B cell, which will release a chemical signal called a cytokine to change the B cell into a plasma cell. The plasma cell releases immunoglobulin E (IgE), which binds to mast cells in the airway to stimulate the

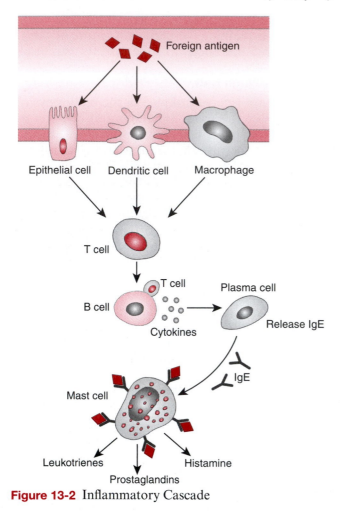

Figure 13-2 Inflammatory Cascade

inflammatory response. **Mast cells** are concentrated beneath the mucous membranes of the respiratory tract. When IgE binds to them, mast cells will release chemical mediators such as **histamine**, **leukotrienes**, and prostaglandins that produce an immediate hypersensitivity response. These mediators will attach to airway smooth muscle cells, triggering muscle contraction and airway narrowing, and they will also mediate inflammatory responses such as tissue swelling, mucus production, and vasodilation. Box 13-2 gives a description of the cells, proteins, and chemical mediators involved in the type I inflammatory response.

Chronic Inflammation

Research has suggested that a different inflammatory process is at work during chronic inflammation, in which there may not be a direct antigen stimulation that begins the inflammatory cascade discussed in the previous section. This process is being studied currently, but two cells seem to be participants in this chronic inflammatory process: eosinophils and neutrophils. Eosinophils are WBCs that contribute to allergic reactions by releasing chemical mediators

such as histamine. They are found in increased numbers in the airway and mucus of most, but not all, people with asthma (23, 24). Neutrophils are the primary cell causing any inflammatory process in the body, are readily attracted to foreign antigens, and are heavily involved in the destruction of antigens. They are found in increased numbers during acute exacerbations, but it is not yet clear what their role is during asthma.

Increased Mucus Production

Mucus is a viscous fluid normally made up of a combination of mucin, leukocytes, inorganic salts, water, and epithelial cells. An important and consistent feature of chronic asthma is the production of excess and **viscous** (sticky, gummy, gelatinous) mucus that blocks peripheral airways and is difficult to expectorate. Evidence in chronic persistent asthma shows goblet cells, which are the mucus-producing cells normally found within the conducting airways, have spread down to more peripheral airways where they do not normally exist. The submucosal glands in the airway of patients with asthma are also larger and contain a greater proportion of mucin as compared to water, contributing to a thicker mucous composition. Bronchoconstriction during an asthma exacerbation can also stimulate excessive production of mucus, which can contribute to further airway occlusion (22).

Natural History of Asthma

The **natural history of asthma** refers to its course over an individual's lifetime, as its progression and symptoms vary throughout an individual's life. It has been proposed that the persistence or increase of asthma symptoms over time is accompanied by a progressive decline in lung function. Recent research suggests that this may not be the case. Rather, the course of asthma may vary markedly among young children, older children and adolescents, and adults, and this variation is probably more dependent on the age of symptom onset than on the symptoms themselves. Asthma at school age is associated with reduced lung function, particularly in patients with severe disease. However, reduced lung function at this age does not necessarily indicate the future path that asthma will take for a particular patient. It is also unclear whether early loss of lung function in asthma is a cause or a consequence of the disease (25). It appears that children whose asthma symptoms were identified before age 3 are more likely to develop loss of lung function than those whose symptoms began later (26, 27).

Much research is currently under way to help clinicians understand this natural history so that an asthma diagnosis can be predicted in very young

Box 13-2   Key Components in the Inflammatory Pathway of Asthma

- **Foreign antigens:** substances from outside the body capable of eliciting an immune response. In asthma, this could be any of the allergic or nonallergic triggers (e.g., pet dander, cold air, pollen, cigarette smoke, dust).
- **Macrophages:** most numerous immune cells in the airway and the major phagocytic cells of the immune system. **Phagocytosis** is the engulfing and destroying of microorganisms, foreign antigens, or cell debris. The major role of the macrophage is to capture foreign antigens and present it to T-cell lymphocytes within the airway mucosa. They can also release cytokines that amplify the inflammatory response.
- **Dendritic cells:** located beneath the airway epithelium. The sensory nerves projecting into the epithelium detect physical and chemical irritants and then present the antigens to T-cell lymphocytes within the airway mucosa.
- **Epithelial cells:** may capture foreign antigens and send out chemokines (chemical signals) to white blood cells to stimulate an immune response; can also produce inflammatory mediators such as histamine.
- **Lymphocytes:** white blood cells (WBCs), making up 20% to 40% of all WBCs in the body; responsible for the body's immune protection. Lymphocytes normally are stored in lymph nodes or spleen (less than 1% circulate in the blood). T-cell lymphocytes (or T cells) originate from the thymus; B cells are formed from stem cells in the bone marrow. Lymphocytes can be stimulated by macrophages or directly by exposure to a specific antigen. Their role is to neutralize or eliminate the antigen. It has been thought recently that an excessive response of T-cell lymphocytes is a contributory factor to asthma persistence and inflammation.
- **Cytokines:** proteins produced by WBCs such as lymphocytes that direct and modify the inflammatory response, and may determine its severity. They provide signals that regulate inflammation and to stimulate lymphocytes to change into different cells to better fight the foreign antigen.
- **Immunoglobulin E (IgE):** excreted by plasma B cells (started out as B lymphocytes) and attach (bind) to mast cells in the respiratory tract. IgE will help stimulate mast cells to fight the foreign antigen and release inflammatory mediators. They can also bind to dendritic cells and lymphocytes and increase the inflammatory response.
- **Mast cells:** concentrated beneath the mucous membranes of the respiratory tract. When covered with IgE molecules, mast cells will bind with foreign antigens and stimulate degranulation, releasing such mediators as histamine, prostaglandin D_2, and leukotrienes. These mediators produce an immediate hypersensitivity reaction within the airway walls. Mast cells may also be activated by osmotic stimuli, such as during exercise-induced bronchospasm, and they may potentially continue to send signals stimulating inflammation even when exposure to allergens is limited.
- **Leukotrienes:** mediate the inflammatory response and are potent bronchoconstrictors derived mainly from mast cells. Inhibition of this mediator has been shown to improve lung function and reduce asthma symptoms.
- **Histamine:** major component of type I (acute) hypersensitivity reactions. Histamine causes dilation of blood vessels, smooth muscle constriction, mucus production, tissue swelling, and itching.
- **Prostaglandins:** hormone within the body that, when secreted by mast cells in the airway, will stimulate bronchoconstriction and inflammation.

Chronic Inflammatory Pathway

- **Eosinophils:** type of WBC, making up 1% to 3% of the total WBC count. Eosinophils contribute to allergic reactions by directly releasing chemical mediators such as histamine and leukotrienes. They are not normally found in large quantities in the airway, but have been seen in increased numbers in most asthma patients.
- **Neutrophils:** most common type of WBC, making up 55% to 70% of all WBC count. Neutrophils are the primary effector cells in inflammation. They are readily attracted to foreign antigens and destroy them by phagocytosis. It is still not clear what their role is in asthma, but they are found in increased numbers in the airways and mucus of patients with asthma during acute exacerbations.

---

patients and prevented in high-risk groups. It is hoped that this will slow or halt airway remodeling and loss of lung function in groups of children who are otherwise suffering from permanent loss of lung function. Another important effect of understanding the natural history of asthma is to offer treatment strategies that will prevent the progression of airway inflammation to airway remodeling and irreversible airway obstruction for children who are in a high-risk category.

Causes and Triggers

The cause of the inflammatory mechanism in asthma varies from person to person. What initiates the inflammatory process and makes some susceptible to its effects is an area not well understood. The expression of asthma is a complex, interactive process that depends on the interplay between two major factors: host factors found within an individual (particularly genetics) and environmental exposures that occur at a crucial time in the development of the immune system. It is important to understand the physiological mechanism that began the development of asthma for individuals and populations in order to control its development and make recommendations for prevention and treatment strategies. It is becoming clear with newer evidence that the cause of asthma may even affect whether certain treatments will be effective and may help guide therapy. One of the most popular trends in allergy and asthma research since the late 1980s has been the "hygiene hypothesis" (discussed later in this chapter), although it is likely that several factors such as innate immunity, genetics, exposure to pathogens at an early age, and other environmental exposures play a varied role in asthma development.

Genetics (Hereditary)

As of 2011, there were 12 genome-wide association studies to look for genetic susceptibility sites for asthma and related traits. Researchers have identified as many as 40 potential chromosomes that may be associated with an increased likelihood of childhood or adult-onset asthma (28). It is well recognized that asthma has an inheritable component to its expression, but the genetics involved in the eventual development of asthma remain a complex and incomplete picture. The relevance of understanding the role that specific genes have in the development of asthma may help focus treatment strategies, but the widespread application of these genetic factors remains to be fully established.

Atopy

Atopy is a hereditary disorder marked by the tendency to develop immediate allergic reactions to substances such as pollen, food, dander, and insect venoms, as manifested by hay fever, asthma, or similar allergic conditions. This genetic hypersensitivity or allergic reaction to specific mechanisms has historically been associated with asthma. However, in reviews during the late 20th century, it appears that the correlation of atopy to asthma is weaker than was previously assumed (21). Defining atopy has also been under scrutiny because testing for atopy by allergen skin prick test does not yet guarantee capturing all affected children (29). Identifying severe allergies as the cause of asthma is important because exposing a sensitized patient to allergens can cause poorly controlled asthma. Furthermore, ongoing allergen exposure is one of the most important factors of asthma that can be controlled, and appropriate interventions can potentially avoid escalation of medical therapy (30). One study that monitored 1,030 children's allergy exposure from birth to age 8 years also found that sensitization to multiple allergens within the first 3 years of life gave the greatest risk for developing asthma at age 8 years, rather than having atopy itself (21).

Environmental Triggers

THE HYGIENE HYPOTHESIS

The **hygiene hypothesis** was first suggested in 1989 by Dr. David Strachan, when he theorized that hay fever prevalence was higher for his young patients because "declining family size, improvements in household amenities, and higher standards of personal cleanliness have reduced the opportunity for cross-infection in young families" (31). The hygiene hypothesis specific for allergic diseases and asthma is that nature may "immunize" against the allergic march by microbial exposures of the respiratory tract, gastrointestinal tract, and possibly the skin, in early life (32). The core of this hypothesis is the complex interaction of the microbial environment and the innate immune system in children. In modern societies, different factors such as small family size, high antibiotics use, and good sanitation contribute to higher living standards and life expectancy. As a result of these societal advances, internal regulatory mechanisms that are activated by interacting with the microbial environment and that are needed to balance the adaptive immune response might be disturbed. (33) Within the first several months, a newborn's innate immunity is learning how to react to various environmental triggers. Without adequate input to boost natural immunity, harmless environmental exposures can become allergens (32). Evidence indicates that the incidence of asthma is reduced in association with certain infections (e.g., *Mycobacterium tuberculosis,* measles, or hepatitis A); exposure to other children (e.g., presence of older siblings and early enrollment in child care); and less frequent use of antibiotics (34–36). It is not suggested, however, that creating a dirtier living environment and exposing young infants to a wide variety of respiratory viruses will improve the rates of asthma. When reviewing the literature on potential causes for asthma, it becomes more likely that there is a complex interaction among the innate immunity proposed by the hygiene hypothesis, environmental or airborne allergens, and early childhood viral infections.

AIRBORNE ALLERGENS

The role of allergens in the development of asthma has yet to be fully defined or resolved, but it is obviously important. Early studies showed that animal danders, particularly dog and cat, were associated with the development of asthma, although exposure early in life may also potentially prevent the incidence of asthma. Sensitization and exposure to house dust mites and household molds and fungi are important factors in the development of asthma in children. Studies to evaluate house dust mite and cockroach exposure have shown that the prevalence of sensitization and subsequent development of asthma are linked (37, 38). In addition, allergen exposure can promote the persistence of airway inflammation and likelihood of an exacerbation.

EARLY VIRAL RESPIRATORY INFECTIONS

Children who have lower respiratory infections caused by respiratory syncytial virus (RSV) are at a threefold to fourfold risk of subsequent wheezing during the early school years (26). A number of long-term prospective studies of children admitted to the hospital with documented RSV have shown that approximately 40% of these infants will continue to wheeze or have asthma in later childhood (39). Most importantly, however, the strongest predictor of subsequent asthma is the occurrence of episodes of wheezing during which rhinovirus infection is found in the upper airway (26). The hypothesis that virus-allergen interactions play a role in the origins of asthma has been supported by experimental studies (40). It is also being investigated whether early antibiotic use may increase the likelihood of asthma. A 2010 study of 1,401 U.S. children found that those with antibiotic use at less than 6 months of age were 1.4 to 1.7 times more likely to develop asthma by age 6 years (41). The adverse effect of antibiotics on asthma risk was particularly strong in children with no parental history of asthma, which should encourage physicians to avoid unnecessary antibiotic use in low-risk children with no genetic predisposition to asthma.

When bringing together all the current knowledge of the causes of asthma, it suggests that asthma in some children might be the result of an initial viral insult, which would enhance local and eventually systemic responses to allergens in children who are predisposed to hypersensitive immune responses. The presence of a virus allergen interactive mechanism at the beginnings of asthma might explain why children with parental history of asthma are more prone to have early sensitization to allergens. Although asthma may be predisposed for some, for many it is probably an interaction between heredity, innate immunity, and a viral insult early in life that begins a chain of events within the airways and starts the progression of asthma.

Triggers for Exacerbation

Asthma, when well controlled, will exhibit few clinical manifestations. A goal in understanding the asthma disease for individuals is to identify what might cause symptoms to worsen and then alleviate opportunities for these items to trigger an asthmatic response. Triggers for children can include exposure to allergens, environmental (nonallergic) exposures to irritants, exercise, and nocturnal mechanisms.

Allergen-Induced Bronchoconstriction

Allergen-induced bronchoconstriction results from an IgE-dependent release of mediators from mast cells that includes histamine, tryptase, leukotrienes, and prostaglandins that directly contract airway smooth muscle (42). U.S. residents as a whole spend up to 60% of their time inside their homes, and a substantial portion of the remaining time in other indoor environments, such as school (43). Long-term exposure to normal and typical indoor allergens can lead to allergic sensitization and stimulate allergic symptoms in children. A study by Sheehan et al. showed an increase in the rate of sensitization to indoor and outdoor aeroallergens throughout childhood and found different aeroallergens to be prominent at different ages (44). The study found that 51.3% of children who underwent skin prick testing were sensitized to at least one indoor aeroallergen and 38.8% were sensitized to at least one outdoor aeroallergen (44).

Indoor allergen triggers, particularly those that occur within the home, are the easiest to control and minimize for children whose allergic symptoms include wheezing and bronchoconstriction. The most common offenders within the home are dust mites, cockroaches, mold, and pets.

- **Dust mites:** The house dust mite is one of the most commonly implicated asthma triggers (45). Numerous well-designed studies have demonstrated that asthma symptoms, pulmonary function, and need for medication in dust mite-sensitive asthma patients correlate with the level of exposure to house dust mites (46).
- **Cockroaches:** Cockroach allergen is a common cause of asthma exacerbations in urban environments. In the National Cooperative Inner-City Asthma Study (NCICAS), children sensitized and exposed to high levels of cockroach allergen showed increasing asthma severity as the level of cockroach allergen exposure increased (47).
- **Mold:** There is a strong link between asthma and mold. The Institute of Medicine's "Report on Damp Indoor Spaces" found sufficient evidence of an association between mold and asthma symptoms in sensitized individuals (48).
- **Pets:** Pet allergens, particularly dog and cat, are well-recognized asthma triggers in sensitized individuals (49). A prospective controlled study of 554 health maintenance organization members with asthma found those with a dog in the home who were sensitized to dog allergen had

a 49% increase in the risk of needing acute asthma care each year, even after adjusting for other risk factors (50).

Nonallergic Triggers

Other, nonallergic triggers within the home and other environments can exacerbate asthma symptoms. These include tobacco smoke, vehicle emissions, nitrogen dioxide, and particulate matter from wood or gas stoves. Common seasonal viruses can also exacerbate asthma.

- **Tobacco smoke:** Environmental tobacco smoke has been linked to an increased risk of developing asthma as well as increased severity and frequency of exacerbations in children with asthma (51).
- **Air pollutants:** Exposure to traffic-related air pollutants has been associated with respiratory symptoms and asthma morbidity, but the effects of chronic air pollution exposures in susceptible populations such as urban children are not well-characterized (52). Data from studies from the last decade support the hypothesis that traffic-related air pollution increases the asthma symptoms and the frequency of health service contacts for asthma, but researchers are still evaluating the proximity to and amount of vehicle emissions exposure required to see a significant increase in symptoms (52–55).
- **Nitrogen dioxide:** The primary source for nitrogen dioxide within the home is a gas cooking appliance. A 2006 study of 728 homes with children diagnosed with asthma found that exposure to indoor NO_2 at levels well below the U.S. Environmental Protection Agency outdoor standard (53 ppb) is associated with increased respiratory symptoms if the children lived in multifamily housing (56).
- **Wood and gas stoves:** Use of gas stoves and wood-burning appliances or fireplaces have been associated with increased wheezing in schoolchildren and increased asthma exacerbations (57).
- **Viral respiratory infections:** In addition to allergen and air pollutants, the asthmatic airway is particularly susceptible to respiratory virus infection as a cause of 40% to 80% of asthma exacerbations both in children and adults (58). Of particular significance is the finding in asthma that the common cold viruses (e.g., rhinovirus), which usually causes only upper respiratory tract symptoms, causes exacerbations, especially in the spring, fall, and winter months.

In summary, a variety of triggers in the home can worsen asthma symptoms. Understanding all the potential environmental and physiological components that contribute to exacerbation will help children and their families to minimize the likelihood for exposure to the triggers and the subsequent need for treatment.

Nocturnal Asthma

Currently, there is no thorough understanding of the causes of nocturnal asthma or the increase in asthma symptoms at night for some people. There have been many suggested mechanisms for the cause of nocturnal asthma, but studies that have isolated each individual suspect have not resulted in any definitive results to either pinpoint the cause or alleviate the symptoms. This leads experts to believe that it is the interaction of several of these physiological and environmental mechanisms that contribute to nocturnal asthma symptoms.

Potential mechanisms are as follows: (59)

- **Sleep state-induced increased airway parasympathetic tone:** This is a potential physiological mechanism that occurs during sleep that may make bronchoconstriction more likely to occur when triggered.
- **Decreased lung volume and subsequent airway smooth muscle unloading:** Typically, bronchial reactivity is greater at lower lung volumes than at higher. Furthermore, when individuals refrain from sighs or deep inspiration, typically increased airway reactivity rapidly ensues. In sleep, fewer deep breaths or sighs are initiated, which will lower lung volume. Theoretically, this can result in unloading of airway smooth muscle, which can contribute to increased bronchoconstriction and may be an important factor leading to nighttime exacerbation of asthma.
- **Circadian modulation of respiratory function:** The mechanisms by which circadian rhythms (physiological phenomena that occur at approximately 24-hour increments, commonly known as the "biological clock") influence pulmonary function in asthma are unknown, although several possibilities have been evaluated. Autonomic tone exhibits circadian variability, meaning that there may be times in the day that bronchial smooth muscle has more or less tone. Airway parasympathetic tone is also increased at night, but changes in state from wakefulness to sleep may be the most important factor modulating parasympathetic flow to the airways rather than circadian rhythms. Circadian variation in the portions of the nervous system that encourage bronchodilation may also contribute to a nighttime decrease in airway function. Airway leukocyte, neutrophil, and eosinophil counts have been shown to be greater in patients with nocturnal asthma during the early morning hours compared with afternoon levels, suggesting that the airways may be more inflamed overnight than during the day.

- **Sleep-related environmental factors:** Allergens in bedding have been suggested as a cause of nocturnal exacerbation of asthma. However, avoidance of these allergens does not abolish nocturnal bronchoconstriction. Breathing cool air at night or reduced nocturnal body temperature has also been suggested to cause nocturnal asthma. However, nocturnal decreases in expiratory airflow persist even when temperature and humidity are maintained at daytime levels.
- **Gastroesophageal reflux disease (GERD):** Asthma guidelines recommend that patients with difficult to control asthma should be evaluated for GERD. Additionally, a cross-sectional study assessing more than 2,600 individuals concluded that those with gastroesophageal reflux (GER) had significantly more nocturnal asthma symptoms (60).
- **Obstructive sleep apnea (OSA):** The mechanical effects of snoring and apneas on the airways might trigger vagal or other neurally mediated reflexes that contribute to bronchoconstriction. GER, a possible trigger for nocturnal asthma, may also link these disorders because GER may be exacerbated by OSA and improves with the use of continuous positive airway pressure. Another potential connection between OSA and asthma is the proinflammatory state induced by OSA, which contributes to both systemic and upper airway inflammation, and it may also augment allergen-induced bronchoconstriction.

Nocturnal asthma has not been as well studied in children as it has been in adults. Nocturnal awakening for asthma exacerbation is not uncommon, even in children with mild-to-moderate asthma (61). Symptoms that may indicate a higher likelihood of nocturnal exacerbations include the following:

- Evening peak flow of less than 80% of personal best the day before
- Albuterol use for symptoms the day before
- A previous night awakening within the last 2 days
- Regular exposure to environmental allergens, particularly high levels of dog or cat allergens (61)

■■ You reintroduce yourself to Derrick and his grandmother, and you and the pediatric pulmonary fellow sit down with them to ask some questions about Derrick's medical history. Derrick tells you that he loves playing basketball and riding his skateboard outside in the summer and hates spending all his time indoors in the winter. He also loves dogs and cats, and Grandma says Derrick is always bringing home stray animals from the neighborhood, even though they are not allowed to have pets in their apartment. They live very close to the interstate highway, but they use public transportation and don't own a car. Derrick seems to have a harder time breathing in the winter when he's cooped up indoors than when he's able to play outside. The grandmother has never noticed that he has had any allergies. He's always been healthy, except for the wheezing that has happened every winter since he was about 3 years old. He wakes up coughing a few times a month during the winter and once or twice in the summer and spring.

Clinical Manifestations

Clinical judgment is needed to assess for asthma. Because there are many different pathophysiological causes and effects in asthma, signs and symptoms can vary widely from patient to patient as well as within each patient over time. Asthma is not a self-contained disease, but occurs and presents in many different forms. Because of the variety of etiologies, asthma is frequently characterized by its heterogeneity, which is a vast array of wheezing phenotypes. Wheezing has been suggested as the most important symptom in identifying asthma in disease population studies. Because of an increased focus on asthma phenotypes, asthma guidelines now recommend phenotype-specific treatment. A 2011 study sought to create a more standardized phenotype classification system, particularly for school children (62), but there is not yet consensus on phenotype categorization (e.g., wheezing with rhinitis, wheezing with rhinoconjunctivitis, atopic wheezing, nonatopic wheezing, and frequent wheezing four wheezing episodes per year).

The current asthma classification system is based on the severity of symptoms and the risk for impairment. Prior to classification, a lengthy diagnostic process is undertaken to gather subjective and objective data regarding that patient's signs and symptoms. These include a patient history; physical examination focusing on the upper respiratory tract, chest, and skin; spirometry to demonstrate obstruction and assess reversibility (in children 5 years of age or older); and the ruling out of other diagnoses. Additional tests that may be warranted include bronchoprovocation testing (BPT), exhaled nitric oxide (FeNO), allergy testing, and biomarkers for inflammation. Once the clinical data is collected, the severity of asthma can be classified.

Signs and symptoms of asthma also include differentiating between control symptoms (those seen every day) and those experienced during an acute exacerbation. Clinicians, patients with asthma, and family members need to be aware of the severity of exacerbation, when to intervene, and when to seek immediate medical attention. This progression should be clearly defined for each person to ensure that safe decisions are made about asthma management.

Diagnosis of Asthma

The first step in controlling asthma is to establish a definitive diagnosis. Clinicians should determine that episodic symptoms of airflow obstruction or airway hyperresponsiveness are present, airflow obstruction is at least partially reversible, and alternative diagnoses are excluded.

Asthma should be suspected when any of the following have occurred (Box 13-3):

In the past 12 months

- A sudden severe episode or recurrent episodes of coughing, wheezing, chest tightness, or shortness of breath
- Colds that seem to "go to the chest" or take more than 10 days to resolve
- Coughing, wheezing, or shortness of breath
  - During a particular season or time of the year
  - In certain places or when exposed to certain things (e.g., animals, tobacco smoke, perfumes)
- Using medications that improve breathing
- Symptom relief when the medications are used

In the past 4 weeks

- Coughing, wheezing, or shortness of breath
  - At night, causing awakenings
  - Upon awakening
  - After running, moderate exercise, or other physical activity (2)

Medical History

The NAEPP recommends taking a detailed medical history of the new patient who is thought to have asthma. The medical history can help identify the symptoms likely to be due to asthma and support the likelihood of asthma. See Box 13-4 for an example patient history form. The history should include items regarding the following:

- Symptoms
- Pattern of symptoms
- Precipitating and/or aggravating factors
- Development of disease and treatment
- Family history
- Social history
- History of exacerbations
- Impact of asthma on patient and family
- Assessment of patient's and family's perceptions of asthma (2)

Physical Examination

The upper respiratory tract, chest, and skin are the focus of the physical examination for asthma. Physical findings that increase the probability of the disease are listed below. The absence of these findings does not rule out asthma because the disease is by definition variable, and signs of airflow obstruction are often absent between attacks.

- Thorax
  - Hyperexpansion of the thorax, especially visible in children
  - Use of accessory muscles
  - Appearance of hunched shoulders
  - Chest deformity
- Auscultation
  - Sounds of wheezing during normal breathing
  - Prolonged phase of forced exhalation (typical of airflow obstruction)

Box 13-3 Key Indicators for Considering an Asthma Diagnosis (2)

Consider a diagnosis of asthma and perform spirometry if any of the indicators noted here are present. The indicators are not diagnostic by themselves, but the presence of multiple key indicators increases the probability of a diagnosis of asthma. Spirometry is needed to establish a diagnosis of asthma.

- Wheezing, especially in children (lack of wheezing and a normal chest examination do not exclude asthma.)
- History of any of the following:
  - Cough, worse at night
  - Recurrent wheeze
  - Recurrent difficulty in breathing
  - Recurrent chest tightness

- Symptoms occur or worsen in the presence of:
  - Exercise
  - Viral infection
  - Animals with fur or hair
  - House dust mites (in mattresses, pillows, upholstered furniture, carpets)
  - Mold
  - Smoke (tobacco, wood)
  - Pollen
  - Changes in weather
  - Strong emotional expression (laughing or crying hard)
  - Airborne chemicals or dusts
  - Menstrual cycles
- Symptoms occur or worsen at night, awakening the patient.

Box 13-4   Items Included in a Patient History Form

A detailed medical history of the new patient who is known or thought to have asthma should address the following items:

- Symptoms
  - Cough
  - Wheezing
  - Shortness of breath
  - Chest tightness
  - Sputum production
- Pattern of symptoms
  - Perennial, seasonal, or both
  - Continual, episodic, or both
  - Onset, duration, frequency (number of days or nights, per week or month)
  - Diurnal variations, especially nocturnal and on awakening in early morning
- Precipitating and/or aggravating factors
  - Viral respiratory infections
  - Environmental allergens, indoor (e.g., mold, house-dust mite, cockroach, animal dander or secretory products) and outdoor (e.g., pollen)
  - Characteristics of home including age, location, cooling and heating system, wood-burning stove, humidifier, carpeting over concrete, presence of molds or mildew, characteristics of rooms where patient spends time (e.g., bedroom and living room with attention to bedding, floor covering, stuffed furniture)
  - Smoking (patient and others in home or day care)
  - Exercise
  - Occupational chemicals or allergens
  - Environmental change (e.g., moving to new home; going on vacation; and/or alterations in workplace, work processes, or materials used)
  - Irritants (e.g., tobacco smoke, strong odors, air pollutants, occupational chemicals, dusts and particulates, vapors, gases, and aerosols)
  - Emotions (e.g., fear, anger, frustration, hard crying or laughing)
  - Stress (e.g., fear, anger, frustration)
  - Drugs (e.g., aspirin and other NSAIDs; beta blockers including eyedrops, others)
  - Food, food additives, and preservatives (e.g., sulfites)
  - Changes in weather, exposure to cold air
  - Endocrine factors (e.g., menses, pregnancy, thyroid disease)
  - Comorbid conditions (e.g. sinusitis, rhinitis, GERD)
- Development of disease and treatment
  - Age of onset and diagnosis
  - History of early-life injury to airways (e.g., bronchopulmonary dysplasia, pneumonia, parental smoking)

- Progression of disease (better or worse)
- Present management and response, including plans for managing exacerbations
- Frequency of using SABA
- Need for oral corticosteroids and frequency of use
- Family history
  - History of asthma, allergy, sinusitis, rhinitis, eczema, or nasal polyps in close relatives
- Social history
  - Day-care, workplace, and school characteristics that may interfere with adherence
  - Social factors that interfere with adherence, such as substance abuse
  - Social support/social networks
  - Level of education completed
  - Employment
- History of exacerbations
  - Usual prodromal signs and symptoms
  - Rapidity of onset
  - Duration
  - Frequency
  - Severity (need for urgent care, hospitalization, ICU admission)
  - Life-threatening exacerbations (e.g., intubation, ICU admission)
  - Number and severity of exacerbations in the past year.
  - Usual patterns and management (what works?)
- Impact of asthma on patient and family
  - Episodes of unscheduled care (ED, urgent care, hospitalization)
  - Number of days missed from school/work
  - Limitation of activity, especially sports and strenuous work
  - History of nocturnal awakening
  - Effect on growth, development, behavior, school or work performance, and lifestyle
  - Impact on family routines, activities, or dynamics
  - Economic impact
- Assessment of patient's and family's perceptions of disease
  - Patient's, parents' knowledge of asthma and belief in the chronicity of asthma and in the efficacy of treatment
  - Patient's or parent's perception and beliefs regarding use and long-term effects of medications
  - Ability of patient and parents, spouse, or partner to cope with disease
  - Level of family support and patient's and parents' capacity to recognize severity of an exacerbation
  - Economic resources
  - Sociocultural beliefs

- Nasopharynx
  - Nasal secretion
  - Mucosal swelling
  - Nasal polyps
- Atopic dermatitis, eczema, or any other manifestation of an allergic skin condition

Pulmonary Function Testing (Spirometry)

Obstructive lung disease is objectively measured using **pulmonary function testing (PFT)**. PFT is a direct measurement of airflow and lung volumes. The specific PFT values of most use for asthma assessment include the following:

- **Forced vital capacity (FVC):** the maximal volume of air forcibly exhaled from the point of maximal inhalation
- **Forced expiratory volume in 1 second (FEV_1):** volume of air exhaled during the first second of an FVC
- **Forced expiratory volume in 6 seconds (FEV_6):** the volume of air exhaled during the first 6 seconds of an FVC
- **FEV_1/FVC:** the percentage of forced vital capacity that is able to be exhaled in the first second of the maneuver

Patients' perception of airflow obstruction varies, and PFT sometimes reveals obstruction that is more severe than would have been estimated from the history and physical examination. One study reports that one-third of the children who had moderate-to-severe asthma were reclassified to a more severe asthma category when PFT reports of FEV_1 were considered in addition to symptom frequency (63). Conversely, a majority of children in another study who had mild-to-moderate asthma classified by symptoms had normal FEV_1 (64).

Abnormalities of lung function are categorized as restrictive and obstructive. Reduced flow measurement values compared to predicted (i.e., a reduced ratio of FEV_1/FVC or FEV_1/FEV_6) indicates obstruction to the flow of air out of the lungs and suggests an obstructive disease. Reduced lung capacity and volumes with normal flow measurements (i.e., a reduced FVC with a normal or FEV_1/FVC ratio) suggests a restrictive disease. The severity of abnormality of PFT measurements is evaluated by comparing a patient's results with reference values based on age, height, sex, and race (65). Up until 2008, however, normal values had not been formally assessed for children less than 8 years old, until a European team reviewed published literature to add valuable data for all age groups (66).

Spirometry should be done both before and after the patient inhales a short-acting bronchodilator, and the two sets of results should be compared to assess for improvement after the bronchodilator is administered as an indicator of the reversibility of the disease. Reversibility of asthma is indicated by American Thoracic Society standards as an increase in FEV_1 of greater than 200 mL and greater than or equal to 12% from the baseline measure after inhalation of a short-acting bronchodilator (67, 68).

Spirometry is recommended in children 5 years old or older, at an age when they are physically able to perform the maneuvers and cognitive development allows them to follow the more complex directions given during the testing. Maximum effort by the patient is necessary when performing the test to avoid important errors in diagnosis and management, so it can sometimes be difficult to assess the quality of the data for young children. Healthy young children complete exhalation of their entire vital capacity in a few seconds, but it can take older patients much longer, especially patients who have airflow obstruction. In these patients, sustaining a maximal expiratory effort for the time necessary for complete exhalation may be more than 12 or 15 seconds—long enough for some patients to find the maneuver uncomfortable or associated with lightheadedness. This accounts for the interest in measurement of the FEV_6 as a substitute for measurement of FVC. In adults, FEV_6 has been shown to be equivalent to FVC in identifying obstructive and restrictive patterns, and to be more reproducible and less physically demanding than FVC (69). Airflow obstruction is indicated by a reduction in the values for both FEV_1 and FEV_1/FVC (or FEV_1/FEV_6) relative to reference or predicted values. See Figure 13-3 for an example flow-volume loop. Predicted values for FEV_1/FVC are based on data from the National Health and Nutrition Examination Survey, the National Center for Health Statistics, and the Centers for Disease Control and Prevention.

Recently, additional PFT results have been identified to assist in improving diagnostic capabilities. A

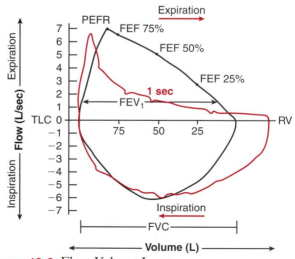

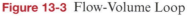

Figure 13-3 Flow-Volume Loop

study of children with asthma with a normal FEV_1 found that forced expiratory flow 25% to 75% (FEF_{25-75}) predicted correlated well with bronchodilator responsiveness (70). FEF_{25-75} percent predicted should be evaluated in clinical studies of asthma in children and might be of use in predicting the presence of clinically relevant reversible airflow obstruction.

The NAEPP recommends that office-based physicians who care for asthma patients have access to spirometry. This will allow for convenient care in one setting and encourage more rapid diagnosis. Clinicians certified in spirometry, such as respiratory therapists (RTs), can assure that the correct technique, calibration methods, and maintenance of equipment will achieve consistently accurate test results. The NAEPP also recommends that when office spirometry shows severe abnormalities, or if questions arise regarding test accuracy or interpretation, further assessment should be performed in a specialized pulmonary function laboratory (2).

Although asthma is typically associated with an obstructive impairment that is reversible, neither spirometry findings nor any other single test or measure alone is adequate to diagnose asthma. Many diseases can be associated with an abnormal spirometry result. The patient's pattern of symptoms (along with other information from the patient's medical history) and exclusion of other possible diagnoses also are needed to establish a diagnosis of asthma.

Bronchoprovocation Testing

Bronchoprovocation is a pulmonary function test that attempts to deliberately stimulate the bronchial smooth muscle to assess airway hyperresponsiveness. After providing a set of baseline spirometry results, the patient uses normal tidal breathing to inhale a substance such as methacholine, histamine, or cold air, and then an FEV_1 measurement is taken again. If the FEV_1 is lower than the baseline measurement, the airways are diagnosed as being hyperresponsive. For patients whose asthma is suspected to be exercise-induced, an exercise challenge rather than an inhaled provocation may be useful. Bronchoprovocation testing is recommended when baseline spirometry is normal or near normal and differential diagnosis is unclear. For safety reasons, bronchoprovocation testing should be carried out by a trained individual in an appropriate facility and is not generally recommended if the FEV_1 is less than 65% predicted. A positive bronchoprovocation test (BPT) is diagnostic for the presence of airway hyperresponsiveness, a characteristic feature of asthma that can also be present in other conditions, such as cystic fibrosis and chronic obstructive pulmonary disease. Thus, although a positive test is consistent with asthma, a negative BPT may be more helpful to rule out asthma.

Once a positive BPT result is seen, a bronchodilator is given, and the patient provides another FEV_1 result to assess for airway responsiveness to treatment. This is important not only for creating an asthma action plan and assessing the effectiveness of chosen treatment techniques, but also it is essential to reverse bronchoconstriction once it has been provoked to decrease the risk of needing emergency resuscitation because of severe bronchospasm.

Traditionally, **methacholine** has been the inhalant of choice when performing BPT. Methacholine chloride is a parasympathomimetic bronchoconsrictor that acts directly on smooth muscle receptors, and it will cause immediate bronchoconstriction. Methacholine is useful to assess whether a particular person's bronchial smooth muscle is hyperresponsive, but it does not stimulate the airways in the same way as they are stimulated by asthma triggers. This has led some asthma researchers to find an inhaled stimulant that will indirectly stimulate the lungs by the release of mediators, similar to the natural process that occurs during an exacerbation (71). A benefit of using indirect stimuli to diagnose the bronchial hyperresponsiveness of asthma is that all the common stimuli that provoke an attack of asthma in daily life (e.g., allergens, cold air, exercise, sulfur dioxide, fog) act indirectly to cause airways to narrow. These same indirect stimuli can also provoke a cough, so this feature has the potential to be used to determine if a patient's cough is associated with airway narrowing during challenge (Clinical Variations 13-1).

BPT can be used later in the management of asthma to evaluate the success of a treatment: How well is it able to protect the patient against attacks from exposure to these common stimuli? For example, well-treated asthma patients will lose their sensitivity to indirect stimuli in response to an appropriate dose of inhaled corticosteroids. Mannitol and adenosine monophosphate are available indirect stimulants for BPT (71). The benefit of direct challenges with methacholine is that they are more sensitive than indirect BPT, but indirect tests are more specific.

Clinical Variations 13-1

Cough Variant Asthma

Although a chronic cough can be a sign of many health problems, it may be the only manifestation of asthma, especially in young children. This has led to the term "cough variant asthma." Monitoring of PEF or methacholine inhalation challenge to clarify whether there is bronchial hyperresponsiveness may be helpful in diagnosis. The diagnosis of cough variant asthma is confirmed by a positive response to asthma medication. Treatment should follow the same stepwise approach to long-term management of asthma.

A positive test for BPT would consist of a reduction in FEV_1 greater than 20%, which indicates the patient as having airway hyperresponsiveness. Likewise, an increase in FEV_1 of at least 20% is considered a positive response to bronchodilator therapy (72).

Allergy Testing

Environmental allergens are a major trigger of asthma, but not all asthmatics have allergies. It can be challenging to determine when allergy skin testing will be useful to help with the diagnosis of asthma. The NAEPP currently recommends that patients be tested only for sensitivity to the allergens to which they may be exposed, followed by an assessment of the clinical relevance of the sensitivity, and that testing be limited to patients who have persistent asthma and are exposed to indoor allergens. Allergy tests are also an essential part of educating patients about the role allergens play in their disease.

In children, the clinical symptoms for allergic and nonallergic asthma are the same. One study attempting to find differences between the two failed to identify any combination of features that could reliably distinguish allergic from nonallergic asthma in children (73). Two-thirds of the children in the study diagnosed with asthma had at least one positive skin test. Thus, the recommendation from this study was that all children with asthma should undergo allergy testing to identify potential allergic triggers and to prevent instituting unnecessary environmental control measures.

The skin test method of allergen evaluation is well known and consists of approximately 50 to 200 tiny scratches, pricks, or needle sticks made on the upper back or arm with small amounts of suspected allergens. After an appropriate time period (10 to 30 minutes), the skin is observed for any reaction. With the discovery of the IgE antibody, in vitro testing has become possible. Using this method, a blood sample is mixed with different allergens and observed for a chemical reaction. The laboratory's equipment and computers analyze the reaction and measure the amount of IgE for each allergen. Results are grouped into classes from 0 (negative) to 6 (high positive).

Biomarkers of Inflammation

Biomarkers are biochemical, genetic, or molecular indicators that can be used to screen for diseases. They are already in use to aid in the diagnosis of cardiovascular disease and cancer. Biomarkers of inflammation can be obtained from sputum, blood, urine, and exhaled air. Their use as aids to the diagnosis and assessment of asthma is currently being evaluated in clinical research trials. Because asthma is a heterogeneous disease, it will require multiple biomarkers for accurate diagnosis.

Fractional Exhaled Nitric Oxide

Fractional exhaled nitric oxide (FeNO) is the most widely used exhaled biomarker of airway inflammation in asthma. Levels of nitric oxide in exhaled breath can be measured relatively quickly in an outpatient clinic, although the gas analyzers required are expensive. FeNO is often increased in patients with atopic asthma and severe asthma and is correlated with airway eosinophilia (74). It has been suggested that FeNO can be most useful to predict the likelihood of response to inhaled steroid therapy. The suggested values of FeNO vary. Low FeNO levels (less than 25 parts per billion) indicate that the patient is unlikely suffering from eosinophilic asthma and is less likely to respond to steroids. A high FeNO level (greater than 50 parts per billion) strongly suggests airway eosinophilia and steroid responsiveness (75). The level of FeNO can also be useful to assess whether the present dose of inhaled corticosteroid is adequate to control airway inflammation. A 2009 Cochrane Review of the research related to FeNO's use for tailoring treatment strategies such as dosage of steroid therapy did not recommend FeNO for this purpose, but did agree regarding its usefulness to monitor eosinophilic asthma (76).

Exhaled Breath Condensate

Exhaled breath condenses when it comes into contact with a cooled collector, allowing the collection of respiratory particles, droplets, and water vapor. The pH of **exhaled breath condensate** has been shown to relate to airway inflammation. Low exhaled breath condensate pH is a biomarker that indicates poorly controlled eosinophilic asthma in a manner similar to high FeNO (77). There is currently no standard type of condenser used to collect exhaled breath condensate. The differing surface properties of each condenser type will cause significant variation in the nature of the particles collected. Variations can also be caused by exercise and environmental conditions (78). This makes it difficult to compare condensate values between sites or studies until standards are better defined.

Sputum Eosinophils

Sputum samples can offer many biomarkers. The percentage of eosinophils in sputum directly measures airway inflammation and is one method of objectively monitoring asthma. Patients with asthma have significantly higher percentages of sputum eosinophils than do patients without asthma. This biomarker has been used specifically for tailoring asthma interventions and has been found to be beneficial in reducing the frequency of asthma exacerbations in adults with frequent exacerbations and severe asthma, although its effectiveness has not been evaluated for children (79).

■■ Derrick's history strongly suggests that he should be worked up for asthma. He is slumped over slightly, and when you listen to his chest you hear mild expiratory wheezing, although Derrick says that he feels "pretty good" today. You place a portable pulse oximeter on his hand. It reads 99%, and his heart rate (HR) is 115 beats per minute (bpm). You perform an FVC with a bedside spirometer, and Derrick's results for FEV_1 are 80% of predicted for his age. Although your current resources do not allow you to do bronchoprovocation or anything else more sophisticated, you give him an albuterol metered dose inhaler (MDI) with a nonelectrostatic holding chamber and show him how to administer it. When he performs another FVC 10 minutes later, his FEV_1 is 93% of predicted.

Differential Diagnosis

The NAEPP recommends consideration of alternative diagnoses when diagnosing asthma. Table 13-1 lists examples of possible alternative diagnoses that may be considered. Additional pulmonary function studies (e.g., measurement of lung volumes and evaluation of inspiratory loops) may be indicated, especially if there are questions about possible coexisting obstructive lung disease, a restrictive defect, vocal cord dysfunction, or possible central airway obstruction. A chest radiograph may be needed to exclude other diagnoses.

It is important to remember that recurrent episodes of cough and wheezing are most often from asthma. Underdiagnosis of asthma is a frequent problem, especially in children who wheeze when they have respiratory infections. These children are often labeled as having bronchitis, bronchiolitis, or pneumonia even though the signs and symptoms are most compatible with a diagnosis of asthma. This is further complicated by the fact that many of the objective diagnostic tests cannot be performed on children younger than 5 years of age (Special Populations 13-1).

● Special Populations 13-1

Diagnosing Asthma in the Very Young (2)

Diagnosis can be difficult in children from birth to age 4 and has important implications. On the one hand, asthma in early childhood is frequently underdiagnosed or misdiagnosed as chronic bronchitis, wheezy bronchitis, reactive airway disease (RAD), recurrent pneumonia, gastroesophageal reflux, and recurrent upper respiratory tract infections. Therefore, many infants and young children do not receive adequate therapy. On the other hand, not all wheezing and coughs in children are caused by asthma, so caution is needed to avoid giving infants and young children inappropriate prolonged asthma therapy. Episodic or chronic wheeze, cough, and breathlessness also may be seen in other conditions, including cystic fibrosis, congenital heart disease, tracheomalacia, and foreign-body aspiration.

Essential elements in the evaluation and diagnosis of children from birth to age 4 include the history, symptoms, physical examination, and assessment of quality of life. A therapeutic trial with medications such as SABAs and inhaled corticosteroids will also aid in the diagnosis. A decrease in symptoms after medication use is consistent with an asthma diagnosis.

Table 13-1	Differential Diagnoses for Asthma	
Infants and Children		**Adults**
Upper Airway Diseases	Allergic rhinitis and sinusitis	• COPD (e.g., chronic bronchitis or emphysema)
Large Airway Obstructions	• Foreign body in trachea or bronchus • Vocal cord dysfunction • Vascular rings or laryngeal webs • Laryngotracheomalacia, tracheal stenosis, or bronchostenosis • Enlarged lymph nodes or tumor	• Congestive heart failure • Pulmonary embolism • Mechanical obstruction of the airways (e.g., benign and malignant tumors) • Pulmonary infiltration with eosinophilia
Small Airway Obstructions	• Viral bronchiolitis or obliterative bronchiolitis • Cystic fibrosis • Bronchopulmonary dysplasia • Heart disease	• Cough secondary to drugs (e.g., angiotensin-converting enzyme inhibitors) • Vocal cord dysfunction
Other	• Recurrent cough not due to asthma • Aspiration from swallowing mechanism dysfunction or gastroesophageal reflux	

Classifying the Severity of Asthma

Once the diagnosis of asthma has been established, information obtained from the diagnostic evaluation, and additional information, if necessary, should be used to characterize the patient's asthma in order to guide decisions for therapy. The NAEPP recommends that clinicians classify asthma severity by using the domains of current impairment and future risk. **Asthma severity** is the intrinsic intensity of disease. Initial assessment of patients who have confirmed asthma begins with a severity classification because the selection of type, amount, and scheduling of therapy should correspond to the level of asthma severity. This initial assessment of asthma severity is made immediately after diagnosis or when the patient is first encountered, before he or she is taking some form of long-term control medication. Assessment is made on the basis of current spirometry results and the patient's recall of symptoms over the previous 2 to 4 weeks. If the assessment is made during a visit in which the patient is treated for an acute exacerbation, then asking the patient to recall symptoms in the period before the onset of the current exacerbation will suffice until a follow-up visit can be made. For individual patient management, the goal is to assess asthma severity prior to initiating therapy and then to assess control for monitoring and adjusting therapy. The severity classification of asthma is shown in Table 13-2 and uses the two domains of current impairment and future risk.

The specific measures used for classifying severity include the following:

- Symptoms
- Use of short-acting beta agonists for quick relief
- Exacerbations
- Pulmonary function

The distinction between impairment and risk emphasizes the need to consider separately asthma's effects on quality of life and functional capacity on an ongoing basis and the risks asthma presents for adverse events in the future, such as exacerbations and progressive loss of pulmonary function.

Assessing Impairment

Classifying asthma severity requires assessing the following components of current impairment:

1. Symptoms
   - Nighttime awakenings
   - Need for short-acting beta agonist for quick relief of symptoms
   - Work/school days missed
   - Ability to engage in normal daily activities or in desired activities
   - Quality-of-life assessments
2. Lung function, measured by spirometry
   - FEV_1
   - FVC (or FEV_6)
   - FEV1/FVC

Table 13-2	Classification of Severity of Asthma by Age (2)			
Components of Severity		**Classification of Asthma Severity (Children 0–4 years of age)**			
		Intermittent	Persistent		
			Mild	Moderate	Severe
Impairment	Symptoms	≤ 2 days/week	>2 days/week but not daily	Daily	Throughout the day
	Nighttime awakenings	0	1–2/month	3–4/month	>1/week
	SABA use for symptom control	≤2 days/week	>2 days/week, but not daily	Daily	Several times per day
	Interference with normal activity	None	Minor limitation	Some limitation	Extremely limited
Risk	Exacerbations requiring oral systemic steroids	0–1/year	≥2 exacerbations in 6 months requiring oral steroids or ≥4 wheezing episodes/1 year lasting >1 day *and* risk factors for persistent asthma		
	Consider severity and interval since last exacerbation. Frequency and severity may fluctuate over time. Exacerbations of any severity may occur in patients in any severity category.				

Table 13-2	Classification of Severity of Asthma by Age (2) —cont'd

Components of Severity		Classification of Asthma Severity (Children 5–11 years of age)			
		Intermittent	Persistent		
			Mild	Moderate	Severe
Impairment	Symptoms	≤2 days/week	>2 days/week but not daily	Daily	Throughout the day
	Nighttime awakenings	≤2/month	3–4x/month	>1/week, but not nightly	Often 7/week
	SABA use for symptom control	≤2 days/week	>2 days/week, but not daily	Daily	Several times per day
	Interference with normal activity	None	Minor limitation	Some limitation	Extremely limited
	Lung function	Normal FEV_1 between exacerbations FEV_1 >80% predicted FEV_1/FVC >85%	FEV_1 > 80% predicted FEV_1/FVC >80%	FEV_1 = 60%–80% predicted FEV_1/FVC = 75%–80%	FEV_1 < 60% predicted FEV_1/FVC <75%
Risk	Exacerbations requiring oral systemic steroids	0–1/year	≥2 exacerbations in 1 year Consider severity and interval since last exacerbation. Frequency and severity may fluctuate over time for patients in any severity category. Relative annual risk of exacerbations may be related to FEV_1.		

Components of Severity		Classification of Asthma Severity (Children ≥12 years of age and adults)			
		Intermittent	Persistent		
			Mild	Moderate	Severe
Impairment Normal FEV1/FVC: 8–19 years 85% 20–39 years 80% 40–59 years 75% 60–80 years 70%	Symptoms	≤2 days/week	>2 days/week but not daily	Daily	Throughout the day
	Nighttime awakenings	≤2/month	3–4/month	>1/week, but not nightly	Often 7/week
	SABA use for symptom control	≤2 days/week	>2 days/week, but not daily	Daily	Several times per day
	Interference with normal activity	None	Minor limitation	Some limitation	Extremely limited
	Lung function	Normal FEV_1 between exacerbations FEV_1 >80% predicted FEV_1/FVC >85%	FEV_1 = >80% predicted FEV_1/FVC >80%	FEV_1 =60%–80% predicted FEV_1/FVC = 75%–80%	FEV_1 <60% predicted FEV_1/FVC <75%
Risk	Exacerbations requiring oral systemic steroids	0–1/year	≥2 exacerbations in 1 year Consider severity and interval since last exacerbation. Frequency and severity may fluctuate over time for patients in any severity category. Relative annual risk of exacerbations may be relatedto FEV_1.		

There is some question about the usefulness of serial PFT results in children. Making treatment decisions for children should be based on frequency and severity of past exacerbations and symptoms, with pulmonary function measures used as an additional guide.

Assessing Risk

A closely related and second dimension of severity is the concept of risk of adverse events, including exacerbations and risk of death. Assessment of the risk of future adverse events requires careful medical history, observation, and clinician judgment. Documentation of warning signs and adverse events will be necessary when a patient is felt to be at increased risk. Patients who are deemed at increased risk of adverse outcomes need close monitoring and frequent assessment by their clinicians.

Although the classification of severity focuses on the frequency of exacerbations, it is important to note that the severity of disease does not necessarily correlate with the intensity of exacerbations, which can vary from mild to very severe and life-threatening. Determination of whether the level of severity is mild, moderate, or severe will depend on consideration of both the frequency and the intensity of the exacerbations. Predictors reported to be associated with increased risk of exacerbations or death include the following:

- Severe airflow obstruction, as detected by spirometry
- Persistent severe airflow obstruction
- Two or more ED visits or hospitalizations for asthma in the past year
- Any history of intubation or intensive care unit (ICU) admission, especially if in the past 5 years
- A patient reporting that he or she feels in danger or frightened by his or her asthma
- Certain demographic or patient characteristics such as female, nonwhite
- Nonuse of inhaled corticosteroid therapy
- Current smoking
- Psychosocial factors such as depression, increased stress, socioeconomic factors
- Attitudes and beliefs about taking medications (2)

Asthma Exacerbations

Exacerbations of asthma are acute or subacute episodes of progressively worsening shortness of breath, cough, wheezing, and/or chest tightness. Exacerbations are characterized by decreases in expiratory airflow that can be documented and quantified by simple measurement of lung function such as spirometry or peak expiratory flow. These objective measures more reliably indicate the severity of an exacerbation than does the severity of symptoms. Milder exacerbations may be managed outside the health-care system, whereas more serious exacerbations may require an urgent office visit, a trip to an emergency department, or a hospital admission. The most severe exacerbations require admission to the ICU for optimal monitoring and treatment. Clinical manifestations of an acute exacerbation are different depending on the age of the patient.

For infants, assessment relies heavily on physical examination and includes the following findings:

- Use of accessory muscles
- Inspiratory and expiratory wheezing
- Paradoxical breathing
- Cyanosis
- SpO_2 less than 90%
- Respiratory rate greater than 60 breaths/min
- Poor feeding

It can also be challenging with preschool-aged children to assess clinical signs and symptoms of exacerbation accurately and make a decision about treatment and hospital admission. More than a dozen clinical scores assessing acute asthma have been published, but few have been validated. The Preschool Respiratory Assessment Measure, for example, is one that has been validated for children ages 3 to 6 years, although it may not be used exclusively (80). Therapists should be aware of the tools used in their institution and be trained in their use.

Markers of severe asthma exacerbation for all patients include the following:

- Difficulty talking in full sentences
- SpO_2 90% to 92%
- PaO_2 less than 60 mm Hg
- Partial pressure of carbon dioxide ($PaCO_2$) greater than 42 to 45 mm Hg
- Use of accessory muscles
- **Pulsus paradoxus** (a greater than 15 mm Hg drop in systolic blood pressure during inspiration)
- Quiet chest (diminished breath sounds, no wheezing)
- Patient unable to lie supine
- Cyanosis
- Sweating
- Confusion
- Decreased level of consciousness
- Hypotension or bradycardia (81)

Arterial blood gas (ABG) presentations in acute exacerbation can vary. In patients who are tachypneic but still effectively ventilating, the ABG results will show respiratory alkalosis with varying degrees of hypoxemia. In severe exacerbations, or when patients begin air trapping and no longer effectively removing CO_2 during exhalation, ABGs will begin to show a pattern of respiratory acidosis and respiratory failure.

The severity of asthma exacerbations is described in Table 13-3. The frequency of asthma exacerbations can vary widely among individuals and within individuals, from very rare to frequent. Although the classification of asthma severity focuses on the frequency of exacerbations, it is important to note that the severity of disease does not necessarily correlate with the intensity of exacerbations.

Patients at any level of severity can have severe and life-threatening exacerbations. Children, in particular, are at a high risk of death or complications from their asthma exacerbations. Severe asthma exacerbations are one of the most common causes of critical illness in children, accounting for approximately 10,000 ICU admissions per year in the United States (82). Although the prevalence of this disease is high in children, the risk factors for the development of severe asthma exacerbations are not well established. One study, conducted to find some predictors of severe exacerbation, observed 188 children admitted to inpatient wards or ICUs with a severe exacerbation. The study found that past exacerbation severity was not a good predictor of the current exacerbation. When comparing the children who were admitted to the ICU compared to the general hospital ward, there were two significant findings: Children admitted to the ICU were significantly more likely to use inhaled corticosteroids than children admitted to the ward, and the strongest predictor of an ICU admission for a severe exacerbation was having an exacerbation triggered by an allergen/irritant (82).

Table 13-3 Severity of Asthma Exacerbations in the Urgent or Emergency Care Setting (2)

	Signs and Symptoms	Initial PEF (or FEV₁)	Clinical Course
Mild	Dyspnea only with activity (assess tachypnea in young children)	PEF ≥70% predicted or personal best	Usually cared for at home Prompt relief with inhaled SABA Possible short course of oral systemic corticosteroids
Moderate	Dyspnea interferes with or limits usual activity	PEF 40%–69% predicted or personal best	Usually requires office or ED visit Relief from frequent inhaled SABA Oral systemic corticosteroids Some symptoms last for 1–2 days after treatment is begun
Severe	Dyspnea at rest; interferes with conversation	PEF <40% predicted or personal best	Usually requires ED visit and likely hospitalization Partial relief from frequent inhaled SABA Oral systemic corticosteroids Some symptoms last for >3 days after treatment is begun Adjunctive therapies are helpful
Status Asthmaticus **Life-Threatening**	Too dyspneic to speak; perspiring	PEF <25% predicted or personal best	Requires ED/hospitalization; possible ICU Minimal or no relief from frequent inhaled SABA Intravenous corticosteroids Adjunctive therapies are helpful

Status asthmaticus refers to severe, persistent, and intractable asthma that does not respond to initial short-acting beta-agonist therapy. Typically, a patient will present following exposure to a potent allergen or irritant, a few days after the onset of a viral respiratory illness, or after exercise in a cold environment. A patient may also have underused or have been underprescribed anti-inflammatory therapy. Patients report chest tightness, rapidly progressive shortness of breath, dry cough, and wheezing. Status asthmaticus is a medical emergency that requires prompt assessment and treatment from the health-care team.

■■ Based on Derrick's symptoms, you and the pulmonologist agree that he has mild persistent asthma. Although he has been sent home with a short-acting beta agonist in the past, you both agree that he should have some form of maintenance therapy to minimize the inflammation present in his airways and to improve his nighttime and winter symptoms.

Management and Treatment

Diagnosing a patient with asthma is only the first step of asthma care. The objectives of patient management are to reduce the symptoms, functional limitations, impairment in quality of life, and risk of adverse events (Box 13-5). The ultimate goal of treatment is to enable a patient to live without manifestations of asthma. Management of asthma includes controlling asthma triggers, making lifestyle and environmental changes, educating the patient and family members, providing a personalized asthma action plan, and initiating pharmacological and nonpharmacological therapies. Of utmost importance is recognition of the signs and symptoms of asthma control and educating families when to seek immediate medical attention. Responsiveness to asthma treatment varies, so follow-up assessment must be made and treatment should be adjusted as frequently as necessary.

Care for an in-patient with an acute asthma exacerbation includes similar pharmacological therapies as offered during chronic management, but additional therapies and monitoring are also available. The health-care team must also make difficult decisions regarding frequency and escalation or reduction of therapy, admission to an intensive care setting, intubation, and mechanical ventilation.

Control of Asthma Triggers

Controlling asthma triggers includes identifying precipitating factors and comorbidities that may aggravate asthma and assessing a patient's knowledge and skills for self-management. Education and control of

| Box 13-5 | Goals of Long-Term Asthma Therapy (2) |

1. Reduce impairment
   • Prevent chronic and troublesome symptoms
   • Require infrequent use (2 or fewer days a week) of inhaled SABA for quick relief of symptoms, not including prevention of exercise-induced bronchospasm
   • Maintain near-normal pulmonary function
   • Maintain normal activity levels, including exercise, other physical activity, and attendance at work or school
   • Meet patients' and families' expectations of and satisfaction with asthma care

2. Reduce risk
   • Prevent recurrent exacerbations of asthma and minimize the need for emergency department visits or hospitalizations
   • Prevent progressive loss of lung function or prevent reduced lung growth (in children)
   • Provide optimal pharmacotherapy with minimal or no adverse effects

environmental asthma triggers should be a part of every patient's asthma management, regardless of severity of symptoms or risk for exacerbation. Exposure to allergens to which one is sensitive has been shown to increase asthma symptoms and exacerbations. For this reason, clinicians should evaluate the potential role that allergens play in each individual's asthma management. Particular focus should be given to indoor inhalant allergens, where the most environmental change is possible. This involves using the patient's medical history to identify allergen exposures that may worsen asthma and to assess sensitivity to seasonal allergies. Skin testing or in vitro testing should also be considered to more effectively determine allergen sensitivity. Patients who have asthma at any level of severity should also do the following:

• Reduce, if possible, exposure to allergens to which the patient is sensitized and exposed
• Avoid exposure to environmental tobacco smoke and other respiratory irritants, including smoke from wood-burning stoves and fireplaces and, if possible, substances with strong odors
• Avoid exertion outdoors when levels of air pollution are high
• Avoid sulfite-containing foods and other foods to which they are sensitive
• Consider allergen immunotherapy when there is clear evidence of a relationship between symptoms and exposure to an allergen to which the patient is sensitive

- Be evaluated for the presence of a chronic comorbid condition when the patient's asthma cannot be well controlled (e.g., allergic bronchopulmonary aspergillosis, GER, obesity, obstructive sleep apnea, rhinitis, sinusitis, chronic stress/depression)
- Consider receiving inactivated influenza vaccination, which is safe for administration to patients older than 6 months of age
- Avoid the use of humidifiers if sensitive to house-dust mites or mold
- Consider possible occupational exposures, particularly in patients who have new-onset disease (2)

Dietary restrictions and food avoidances may also be useful in reducing asthma symptoms.

Education is key to controlling triggers and self-management of asthma. This education should begin at the time of diagnosis and continue at every clinical interaction with the patient. Asthma education should include the following:

- Basic facts about asthma
- What defines well-controlled asthma and the patient's current level of control
- Roles of medications
- Skills (e.g., inhaler technique, use of spacer, self-monitoring)
- When and how to handle signs and symptoms of worsening asthma
- When and where to seek care
- Environmental exposure control measures

Education and reinforcement is particularly important during emergency department visits, when medications are frequently increased or newly prescribed, and when misuse of medications may be a significant instigator of asthma symptoms. Point-of-care pharmacists may also play a role in improving asthma self-management by helping patients understand their mediations and teaching inhaler and self-monitoring techniques.

All patients should also be provided with a written **asthma action plan**. Written asthma action plans should include these two items:

- Daily management
- How to recognize and handle worsening asthma

Patients will be more likely to adhere to their personal asthma action plan and treatment regimen if it achieves well-stated outcomes that both they and health-care providers agree with. If the treatment plan does not fit well in the life and schedule of the patient, or the importance of each aspect of the plan is not understood, it is less likely to be followed. Any deviation from a developed asthma plan will increase the chance of poorly controlled asthma or acute exacerbations.

A 2006 systematic review found that when children's action plans were based on symptoms (rather than peak expiratory flow; discussed in the following paragraph), they required fewer acute care visits, suggesting that symptom-based assessment in children may be more useful than attempting objective pulmonary measurements (83). This focus is not to negate the usefulness of peak expiratory flow measurements, but rather to illustrate that both objective and subjective symptoms are essential components of pediatric asthma action plan development. Action plans should be shared with day-care staff and/or school nurses that care for children with asthma so that they are aware of how to manage acute exacerbations.

In addition to education and an asthma action plan, the NAEPP recommends that daily **peak expiratory flow (PEF)** monitoring be considered for patients who have moderate or severe persistent asthma, poor perception of airflow obstruction or worsening asthma, unexplained response to environmental or occupational exposures, and others at the discretion of the clinician and the patient. A peak flow meter (PFM) is sent home with the patient (Fig. 13-4), and

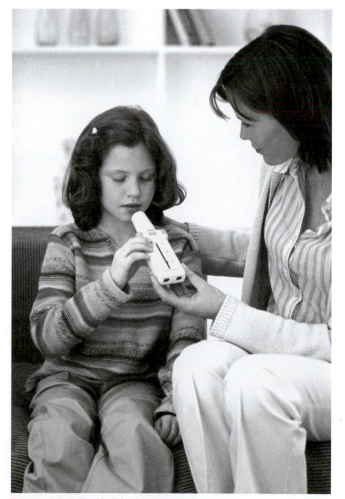

Figure 13-4 Peak Flowmeter *(© Thinkstock)*

he or she will perform a PEF twice daily. A PEF measurement is taken by having the patient stand, take a deep breath to fill the lungs completely, then blow out as hard and as fast as possible in one single exhalation. When this is performed with a mouthpiece PFM, the indicator will tell the maximum, or peak, expiratory flow generated. A personal best is documented as the "goal" PEF, and future measurements will be read as a percentage of this ideal number. This is then used to assess the severity of an exacerbation and used to help guide decisions on when to seek medical assistance. Studies have found that children had low compliance with twice daily PEF (84), the values were less accurate when compared with PFT measurements such as FEV_1 (85), and the values were ineffective in helping with

self-management of school-aged children (86). Even when not completed every day, periodic daily PEF monitoring may be useful when changing treatment strategies or helping teach patients a better understanding of airflow obstruction.

Pharmacological Therapy

Medications for asthma are categorized into two general classes: (1) long-term control medications used to achieve and maintain control of persistent asthma and (2) quick-relief medications used to treat acute symptoms and exacerbations. The mainstay for asthma is an anti-inflammatory for chronic management and a short-acting beta agonist for acute exacerbations. Table 13-4 presents the NAEPP stepwise approach to asthma management based on

Table 13-4	Stages of Asthma and Treatments (2)					
		Step 1	**Step 2**	**Step 3**	**Step 4**	**Step 5**	**Step 6**
Children 0–4 years	Preferred	SABA prn	Low-dose ICS	Medium-dose ICS + LABA or montelukast	Medium-dose ICS + LABA o montelukast	High-dose ICS + LABA or montelukast	High-dose + LABA or montelukast + oral corticosteroids
	Alternative		Cromolyn or montelukast				
		Each step: Patient education and environmental control					
	Quick-relief medication	*SABA as needed for symptoms. Intensity of treatment depends on severity of symptoms. With viral respiratory symptoms: SABA every 4–6 hours, up to 24 hours without physician consult. Consider short course of systemic corticosteroids if exacerbation is severe or patient has history of severe exacerbations*					
		Intermittent	**Persistent Asthma: Daily Medications**				
Children 5–11 years	Preferred	SABA prn	Low-dose ICS	Low-dose ICS + LABA, LTRA, or theophylline or medium-dose ICS	Medium-dose ICS + LABA	High-dose ICS + LABA	High-dose ICS + LABA + oral corticosteroids
	Alternative		Cromolyn, LTRA, nedocromil or theophylline		Medium-dose ICS + LTRA or theophylline	High-dose ICS + LTRA or theophylline	High-dose ICS + LTRA or theophylline + oral corticosteroids
		Each step: Patient education, environmental control, and management of comorbidities. Steps 2–4: consider allergen immunotherapy for patients with persistent, allergic asthma.					
	Quick-relief medication	*SABA as needed for symptoms. Intensity of treatment depends on severity of symptoms: up to three treatments at 20-minute intervals as needed. Short course of oral systemic corticosteroids may be needed.*					

classification. The following sections provide descriptions of each type of medication, its mechanism of action, route of administration, benefits, and potential side effects. Management for exercise-induced bronchospasm does not follow the same step pattern that allergic and nonallergic asthma follow. An overview of exercise induced bronchospasm is found in Clinical Variations 13-2.

Long-Term Control Medications

INHALED CORTICOSTEROIDS

The NAEPP has concluded that corticosteroid therapy improves asthma control more effectively in both children and adults than does any other single long-term control medication. **Corticosteroids** are a group of hormones secreted by the adrenal cortex in the brain, but they can also be manufactured synthetically. The specific types of corticosteroids useful in asthma are the glucocorticoids. They block late-phase reaction to allergens, reduce airway hyperresponsiveness, and inhibit the activation and migration of inflammatory cells. They are the most potent and effective anti-inflammatory medications currently available and are used in the long-term control of asthma. Short courses of oral systemic corticosteroids are often used to gain prompt control of the disease when initiating long-term therapy; long-term oral

systemic corticosteroid is used for severe persistent asthma.

Several systemic corticosteroid preparations are available, such as hydrocortisone, cortisone, prednisone, prednisolone, and methylprednisolone, but they produce undesirable side effects when used to treat asthma, including suppression of the immune system, fluid retention, hypertension, hyperglycemia, diabetes mellitus, osteoporosis, cataract, anxiety, depression, insomnia, colitis, and growth slowing in children. This last side effect is of particular interest regarding corticosteroid maintenance therapy for children with asthma. Even inhaled corticosteroids (ICS) have been tied to a decrease in growth of about 1.5 cm per year, and it is not clear whether children will "catch up" after cessation of steroid therapy (89). Topical application of corticosteroids via inhalation is intended to minimize side effects by directly applying the medication to the lung. There are negative effects unique to ICS:

- Dysphonia (hoarseness or change in voice quality)
- Cough or bronchoconstriction
- Oropharyngeal fungal infections (rinsing mouth after treatment will minimize this risk)
- Inadequate dosing due to misuse of inhalers (using a reservoir device such as a spacer will maximize dosing and correct inhaler use) (Fig.13-5)

Table 13-5 lists the corticosteroids used for oral inhalation. ICS can be given via a metered dose inhaler (MDI), a dry powder inhaler (DPI), or small volume nebulizer (SVN). They can be formulated alone or with a long-acting beta agonist to help better maintain asthma control.

Several database reviews have been done to assess which available corticosteroid is the best choice for different populations. Despite the reviews, there is no

---

Clinical Variations 13-2

Exercise-Induced Asthma

Transient airway narrowing following strenuous physical exercise is referred to as exercise-induced bronchoconstriction (EIB). An episode is generally self-limiting, but it can cause those afflicted to avoid vigorous activity and serious athletes to underperform by limiting endurance and prolonging recovery time. Management of EIB is preventive in nature, and typically involves using a SABA prior to exercise to prevent the symptoms of EIB. Additional pharmacological therapies have been attempted as well to further minimize the risk of exacerbations. Inhaled corticosteroids used for 4 weeks or more before exercise testing significantly attenuated exercise-induced bronchoconstriction (87). Mast cell stabilizers and anticholinergics have also been tested in trials, but they tend not to be as effective as SABAs in preventing the symptoms of exacerbation (88). Interestingly, the results tend to vary across individuals, stressing the importance of having clinicians and patients work together to find the most effective management strategy.

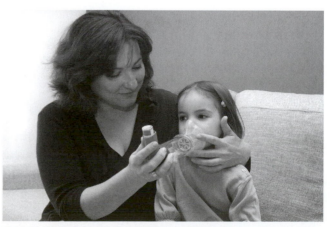

Figure 13-5 Spacer for MDI *(© Thinkstock)*

Table 13-5	Inhaled Steroid Therapy for Asthma			
Generic Name	**Brand Name**	**Formulation/Route of Administration**	**Dosage**	**Recommended Frequency**
Beclomethasone dipropionate HFA	QVAR	MDI (HFA)	40 or 80 mcg/puff	Children ≥5 years: 1–2 puffs twice daily
Budesonide	Pulmicort	Dry powder inhaler (DPI) Nebulized (SVN)	200 mcg/actuation 0.25 mg/2 mL, 0.5 mg/2 mL	Children ≥6 years: 1 actuation twice daily Children 1–8 years old: 0.25 mg twice a day or 0.5 mg given once a day
Ciclesonide	Alvesco	MDI	80 mcg/puff	Adults and children ≥12 years: 80 mcg bid; 320 mcg bid (if previously taking oral corticosteroids)
Flunisolide	Aerobid	MDI	250 mcg/puff	Adults and children ≥6 years: 2 puffs bid. Adults no more than 4 puffs daily, children ≤15 no more than 2 puffs daily
Flunisolide hemihydrate	Aerospan	MDI	80 mcg/puff	Adults ≥12 years: 1 puffs bid, no more than 4 puffs daily Children 6–11 years: 1 puff daily, no more than 2 puffs daily
Fluticasone propionate	Flovent	MDI	44, 110, and 220 mcg/puff	Adults ≥12 years: 88 mcg bid (recommended starting dose), 80–220 mcg bid (if previously taking inhaled corticosteroids), or 880 mcg bid (if previously taking oral corticosteroids) Children 4–11: 88 mcg bid
		DPI (Diskus)	50, 100, and 250 mcg	Adults: 100 mcg bid (recommended starting dose), 100–250 mcg bid (if previously taking inhaled corticosteroids),1,000 mcg bid (if previously taking oral corticosteroids) Children 4–11 years: 50 mcg twice daily
Mometasone furoate	Asmanex Twisthaler	DPI	220 mcg/actuation	Adults and children ≥12 years: 1–2 puffs daily (recommended starting dose if previously taking no corticosteroids or inhaled corticosteroids), 2–4 puffs bid (if previously taking oral corticosteroids)
Triamcinolone acetonide	Azmacort	MDI	100 mcg/puff	Adults ≥12 years: 2 puffs tid or qid Children ≤15 years: no more than 2 puffs daily

Table 13-5	Inhaled Steroid Therapy for Asthma —cont'd			
Generic Name	**Brand Name**	**Formulation/Route of Administration**	**Dosage**	**Recommended Frequency**
Combination Therapies				
Budesonide/ formoterol	Symbicort	MDI (HFA):	80 mcg or 160 mcg budesonide/ 4.5 mcg formoterol	Adults and children ≥12 years old: 2 puffs bid. Daily maximum 640 mcg budesonide/18 mcg formoterol
Fluticasone propionate/ salmeterol	Advair Diskus Advair HFA	DPI	100 mcg, 250 mcg, or 500 mcg fluticasone/50 mcg salmeterol	Adults and children ≥12 years: 1 100-mcg dose inhalation twice daily, about 12 hours apart. Maximal recommended dose: 1 inhalation of 500 mcg dose twice daily. Children ≥4 years: 1 100-mcg dose inhalation twice daily, about 12 hours apart (for those who are symptomatic while taking an inhaled corticosteroid)
		MDI	45 mcg, 115 mcg, or 230 mcg fluticasone/21 mcg salmeterol	Adults and children ≥12 years: 2 inhalations twice daily, about 12 hours apart

compelling evidence to recommend one ICS over others for specific populations (90, 91). There is also no consensus on whether to start with high doses of ICS and taper the dose down or to start with low doses and increase until the patient is asymptomatic. Current trends suggest starting with a moderate dose and decreasing the dosage as able (92). Some corticosteroids are available for delivery as both an inhaler and SVN. There is no evidence that one delivery method is superior (93), though DPI requires coordination of breathing and posture that may not be possible in young children.

CROMONES

Cromones such as cromolyn sodium and nedocromil stabilize mast cells and interfere with chloride channel function, preventing the release of mediators and minimizing airway inflammation. Nedocromil also blocks the activity of eosinophils, airway epithelial cells, and sensory neurons, potentially causing a more potent protective effect. Cromolyn sodium is available in nebulized and MDI forms, and nedocromil is available as an MDI. Recommended dosage is two puffs four times a day or one ampule for nebulization.

Studies have shown that although cromones exhibit fewer side effects, they are not as effective at preventing inflammation or providing symptom-free days as ICS (94–96). Although research has not established whether cromones or ICS are superior in managing persistent asthma, there is still a role for cromones, and they are recommended by the NAEPP as an alternative medication for treatment of mild persistent asthma and as preventive treatment prior to exercise or unavoidable exposure to known allergens.

XANTHINES

Xanthines, such as theophylline, are classified as bronchodilators, although they have much less potency than do beta-2 agonists such as albuterol. They are stimulants, generally stimulating the central nervous system and cardiac muscles, but they may also simulate the respiratory drive or strengthen the diaphragm muscles. The exact mode of action is unclear. Sustained-release theophylline is a mild to moderate bronchodilator that can be used as an alternative, not preferred, adjunctive therapy with ICS for children greater than 5 years old. Theophylline may also have mild anti-inflammatory effects. Excessive amounts of theophylline have been shown to cause headaches, nausea, cardiac arrhythmias, and seizures, thus monitoring of serum theophylline concentration is essential in order to maintain within a therapeutic range of 5 to 15 mcg/mL during asthma management (97). Dosages and dosing schedules should be titrated based on serum theophylline levels to maintain the correct therapeutic range.

Studies have shown that other medications are more effective at managing lung function than theophylline. Long-acting beta agonists, particularly salmeterol, are more effective than theophylline in improving morning and evening PEF, but are not significantly different in their effect on FEV_1 (98). Fewer adverse events occurred in participants using long-acting beta agonists as compared to theophylline. When reviewing the evidence for children, there is not enough research data to make firm conclusions about the effectiveness of xanthines as add-on preventive treatment to ICS, and there are no published pediatric studies comparing xanthines with alternatives in this role (99). The data suggest that xanthines are only suitable as first-line preventive asthma therapy in children when ICS are not available, but they may have a role as add-on therapy in more severe asthma not controlled by ICS.

ANTILEUKOTRIENE

Antileukotrienes, also known as leukotriene modifiers or leukotriene receptor antagonists (LTRA), act by preventing leukotrienes from causing airway inflammation in asthma. They are recommended for the prophylactic and chronic treatment of asthma patients 12 years and older. Antileukotrienes work by inhibiting enzymes that act in the formation of leukotrienes, thus stopping the inflammatory pathway and preventing airway inflammation. There are three different antileukotrienes on the market currently, which are available as oral pills or granules in varying strengths and dosages:

• Zileuton
• Zafirlukast
• Montelukast

Zileuton is available only for patients 12 years and older, whereas zafirlukast is approved for children 5 years and older and montelukast has preparations approved for infants and children 6 months and older. The NAEPP asthma guidelines clearly state that corticosteroids are the most effective anti-inflammatory drug; antileukotrienes are recommended as a secondary and adjunct drug after ICS and long-acting beta agonists have been tried.

IMMUNOTHERAPY

Allergen-specific **immunotherapy** involves having subcutaneous injections of increasing amounts of a known allergen under the skin. It is also known as allergy hyposensitization or desensitization. The injections are formulated based on an individual's allergic sensitivities and provided at a physician's office on a regular basis (e.g., weekly). Side effects of the therapy include a lump at the injection site, rash, wheezing, breathlessness, and very rarely, a fatal allergic reaction known as anaphylaxis. The review of trials found that immunotherapy can reduce asthma symptoms, the need for medications, and the

risk of severe asthma attacks after future exposure to the allergen (100). It is possibly as effective as ICS.

Another form of immunotherapy is known as **anti-IgE therapy**. Omalizumab is a monoclonal antibody that prevents binding of IgE to mast cells, thereby reducing the number of mediators released in allergic reaction and decreasing airway inflammation. It can be used as adjunctive therapy for patients 12 years of age and older who have allergies and severe persistent asthma. Like traditional immunotherapy, anti-IgE therapy involves a subcutaneous injection, and clinicians who administer omalizumab should be prepared and equipped to identify and treat anaphylaxis that may occur. A review of research trials found that anti-IgE therapy led to a reduction, and in some cases, withdrawal, of regular inhaled steroid use and a reduction in asthma exacerbations. The side effects were few and mild to moderate in the short term, but longer-term evaluation is needed. Patient and physician assessments of the effectiveness of therapy were positive. It may be useful in cases of uncontrolled moderate to severe asthma (101).

ANTIHISTAMINES

For children with allergic asthma, antihistamines may assist in managing asthma symptoms. Ketotifen is an oral medication that may be used for maintenance treatment of asthma. It is an oral antihistamine whose mechanism of action is not fully understood, but it may inhibit the release of inflammatory mediators and inhibit bronchospasm by reducing calcium uptake in mast cells and in smooth muscle. As an oral preparation, ketotifen might be useful in managing children with asthma, especially in the preschool age, where independent inhaled therapy can be difficult to perform. Randomized controlled trials indicate that ketotifen alone or in combination with other asthma interventions improves control of asthma and wheezing in children with mild and moderate asthma (102).

LONG-ACTING BETA AGONISTS

Long-acting beta agonists (LABAs) are used in combination with ICS for long-term control and prevention of symptoms in moderate or severe persistent asthma. They work by reversing the narrowing of the airways that occurs during an asthma attack. Available alone as MDI or in combination with different ICS, they are known to improve lung function, symptoms, and quality of life, and to reduce the number of asthma attacks (103, 104). LABAs have been shown to lead to fewer asthma symptoms during the day and the night, less bronchodilator medication required to relieve symptoms, better lung function measurements, and better quality-of-life measurements compared to short-acting beta agonists (105). They have also been shown to be superior to antileukotrienes in reducing oral steroid-treated exacerbations in adults, but this conclusion is not yet evidenced in children (106).

Of the adjunctive therapies available, LABAs are the preferred therapy to combine with ICS for patients 12 years of age and older and patients 5 years of age and older who have severe persistent asthma or asthma inadequately controlled on low- or moderate-dose ICS. The option to increase the ICS dose in children ages 5 to 11 years should be given equal weight to the option of adding LABAs. When added to an established maintenance therapy of ICS, LABAs have allowed many patients to decrease their dosage of ICS (107). Although there are beneficial effects of LABAs in combination with ICS, there is a known increased risk of severe exacerbations and even death with their use (108–110). LABAs should not be taken by people who are not taking regular inhaled steroids because of the increased risk of asthma-related death (108, 111). Although this risk is evident in children, it is unclear whether it is the same, higher, or lower for children than that seen with adults.

Quick-Relief Medications

The mainstay of "rescue" therapy for acute asthma exacerbations is short-acting inhaled bronchodilator therapy. These include **short-acting beta agonists (SABAs)** and anticholinergics, which are both effective in relaxing airway smooth muscles during bronchoconstriction to reverse the signs and symptoms of acute airflow obstruction, namely cough, chest tightness, and wheezing.

SHORT-ACTING BETA AGONISTS
These medications are known as adrenergic bronchodilators. They produce bronchodilation by stimulating beta-2 receptors on airway smooth muscles, thus relaxing the muscle and reversing the airflow obstruction. **SABAs** refer to those medications whose clinical effectiveness range is 2 to 6 hours. SABAs include albuterol, levalbuterol, metaproterenol, and pributerol. They are available for inhalation in nebulized, MDI, and DPI formats, and orally as a tablet or syrup. They can be self-administered and should be available to patients with asthma when symptoms of exacerbation occur, as the onset of action is typically between 1 to 15 minutes. Inhaled dosing is the preferred delivery route because it has a more rapid onset, smaller doses are needed compared with an oral route, side effects such as tremor or tachycardia are reduced, and the drug is delivered directly to the lung. Questions arise as to the efficacy of MDI versus SVN as the method of delivery, and in children in particular, MDI performs as well as nebulizers in delivery of SABAs (112). The side effects most seen with SABAs include tremors, palpitations and tachycardia, headache, insomnia hypertension, nervousness, dizziness, and nausea. Most side effects are due to the adrenaline-like **(adrenergic)** effect that beta agonists have on the systemic system, they and should be minimized when providing SABAs via inhalation. A more serious potential side effect of SABA delivery is a worsening of the ventilation-perfusion ratio (Box 13-6), which is exhibited clinically as hypoxemia.

For home treatment of acute exacerbation, two initial treatments (2 to 6 puffs MDI or 1 SVN) 20 minutes apart are recommended by the NAEPP, followed up with dosing no more frequently than every 3 to 4 hours; more frequent use is a sign of worsening symptoms and requires contact with a clinician.

ANTICHOLINERGICS
Anticholinergics such as ipratropium bromide have been used, with some success, as a quick-relief medication to avoid use of as-needed albuterol in clinical research trials in patients who have mild asthma (113), and they are widely used in the management of both acute and chronic asthma in children (114). Anticholinergics work by blocking parasympathetic nerve fibers such as those seen in airway smooth muscle, thereby allowing relaxation of the muscle and reduction of the intrinsic vagal tone of the airway. Ipratropium bromide can provide additive benefit to SABAs in moderate-to-severe asthma exacerbations and has been used effectively in managing chronic obstructive pulmonary disease. It may be used as an alternative bronchodilator for patients who do not tolerate SABAs. Current guidelines for the management of chronic asthma advise that anticholinergic drugs may be used if children are already on high-dose ICS, but there is not enough data to be sure that they are effective at improving lung function or symptoms. (114)

Box 13-6 SABA Use and Ventilation-Perfusion Mismatch

Regional alveolar hypoxemia has been shown to cause regional pulmonary vasoconstriction. The purpose is to shunt blood flow (perfusion) to areas of the lung with higher oxygen tension in an effort to maximize oxygen delivery to the body. Administration of inhaled beta agonists may reverse the hypoxic pulmonary vasoconstriction by stimulating the smooth muscle of the blood vessel. This will cause increased blood flow to underventilated lung regions and decrease oxygen delivery, causing hypoxemia. There is usually no clinical significance to this hypoxemic event, and PaO_2 usually returns to baseline within 30 minutes; however, a decrease in PaO_2 or SpO_2 during SABA delivery can be a concern for a respiratory therapist.

■ ■ The pulmonologist tells Derrick and his grandmother that he probably has asthma. Although there are many more tests that would help them better understand what triggers his asthma, they are expensive and time consuming and may not offer additional useful information. Though you and the pulmonologist are not sure what causes Derrick's worsening symptoms, the pulmonologist recommends that Derrick no longer bring furry animals inside and avoid having feather pillows and other potential allergic triggers in the house. He provides a list of helpful recommendations for changing the home environment. Additionally, he prescribes Derrick an ICS—Pulmicort, 200 mcg—to be used one actuation, twice a day. The clinic has a free 1-month supply of Pulmicort that you will send home with him to use until they can fill the prescription. He is also prescribed an MDI of albuterol and spacer, which you demonstrate how to use. You also give him a PFM to monitor his symptoms over the next few weeks and encourage him to find his personal best number with which he can compare his breathing when he starts to feel short of breath. He is also sent home with an asthma action plan that describes when to take all of his medications and which symptoms should prompt immediate help. In addition, you provide copies of the action plan for the school nurse and his teacher.

The pulmonologist asks Derrick to come back to the clinic in 2 months so that he can follow up on his symptom control and see how his symptoms were for the remainder of the winter.

Nonpharmacological Therapy

Patients who suffer from asthma frequently search for holistic ways to manage their daily symptoms of asthma and minimize the risk of exacerbation. To date, there is little evidence supporting or refuting the effectiveness of many of these techniques. Although clinicians may not recommend any of these complementary therapies, RTs should be aware of all therapies that patients may be using to control their asthma. Examples of nonpharmacological therapies include herbal therapies, caffeine, dietary changes and vitamin supplementation, acupuncture, manual therapy, breathing exercises, and physical exercise.

Herbal Therapies

Herbal interventions are one complementary therapy sought by patients whose asthma causes a decrease in actual or perceived quality of life. Several studies have shown some promise for different herbal remedies, but the research for such remedies is usually

designed very differently; thus, it is not possible to compare their efficacy with traditional daily control regimens recommended by the NAEPP (Evidence in Practice 13-1).

● **Evidence in Practice 13-1**

Herbal Therapy for Asthma (116)

A 2008 Cochrane Database Review sought to identify which herbal interventions may improve asthma symptoms. The review looked at 21 different herbal preparations, many of which are commonly used in China where they are considered "conventional" treatment. Some of the more promising results are described here.

- Boswellia extract has been used as an anti-inflammatory herbal product. Studies showed an increase in FEV_1, peak expiratory flow rate (PEFR), and FVC in at least one set of subjects reviewed. Side effects included nausea, epigastric pain, and hyperacidity for some.
- Mai-Men-Dong-Tang, also known as Ophiopogon Combination, is a natural Chinese medication used for both stomach and lung dysfunctions to moisten dryness in the digestive and pulmonary tracts. The review found an increase of FEV_1 in a statistically significant number of subjects.
- Propolis is a resin-like material from the buds of poplar and cone-bearing trees. It is used for its anti-inflammatory properties. The review showed positive effects in FEV_1, PEFR, and FEF_{25-75}, as well as a reduction in nocturnal attacks.
- Also known as eucalyptol, 1.8-cineol, is the dominant portion of eucalyptus oil. Its use with patients with asthma showed no differences in PFT results, but did allow for a reduction in oral steroid use and a reduction in dyspnea score.
- Pycnogenol is extracted from a tree called the *Pinus pinaster*, but can also be extracted from peanut or grape seed and witch hazel bark. It has been used for allergies, circulatory problems, high blood pressure, varicose veins, and childhood asthma. In children, it has been shown to increase PEFR, reduce symptom scores, and significantly decrease albuterol use.
- *Tylophora indica* comes from the leaves and roots of a climbing plant. It has been used in India for more than a century to treat bronchial asthma, but has also been suggested for diarrhea and hay fever. In medical studies, patients have experienced an increase in PEFR and reductions in symptom scores and the use of reliever medications such as albuterol. Side effects include loss of salt taste (for those who ingest by chewing on *Tylophora* leaves), sore mouth, nausea, and vomiting.

Caffeine

Caffeine has a variety of pharmacological effects. It is a weak bronchodilator, and it also reduces respiratory muscle fatigue. Studies throughout the 20th century showed that caffeine improves mental performance, elevates oxygen consumption, increases respiratory rates in healthy people, and increases ventilation in patients with chronic obstructive pulmonary disease. It belongs to a group of chemicals called methylxanthines; thus, it is chemically related to the drug theophylline (discussed previously), which lends further credence to its potential use for asthma. A number of studies have explored the effects of caffeine, and it is clear that even small amounts of caffeine can improve lung function for up to 4 hours. What is not clear, however, is whether taking caffeine leads to improvements in symptoms. If taken in too large a dose, caffeine can cause insomnia, nervousness, restlessness, anxiety, agitation, stomach irritation, nausea, vomiting, tachycardia, tachypnea, headache, chest pain, and arrhythmias (115).

Dietary Changes and Vitamin Supplementation

Patients also have a great interest in whether dietary factors may influence the onset or severity of asthma. Asthma as the sole manifestation of a food allergy is rare, and less than 5% of patients experience wheezing without other gastrointestinal or skin symptoms during a food challenge (117). Asthma exacerbations induced by food are rare, since to induce airway hyperresponsiveness, the patient must inhale the food product (such as fish or shellfish being aerosolized while cooking). It is a common misconception by patients and clinicians that food is a frequent cause of wheezing. There are, however, some exceptions when food avoidance may be essential to minimize the risk of severe exacerbations. Sulfites are a food preservative found in processed potatoes, shrimp, dried fruit, and beer and wine. They have been known to cause severe asthma exacerbations, and the incidence of sensitivity in asthma patients has been found to be between 3% and 10% (118). Avoiding foods containing sulfites may decrease asthma incidence in those for whom this is a trigger. Decreasing sodium intake has also been suggested to improve asthma control, but there is no evidence of this being a universal asthma controller, although it may improve lung function in exercise-induced asthma (119). In general, clinicians should promote a healthy diet such as that suggested by the Department of Health and Human Services, including more fruits, vegetables, and whole grains, and eating less saturated and trans fats, salt, and added sugars (2).

Preliminary evidence suggests that antioxidants, such as vitamin C, may reduce asthma severity. Vitamin C is one of the key antioxidants found in the fluid lining of the lung. Low levels have been associated with pulmonary dysfunction (120), and both children and adults with asthma have been found to have lower concentrations of vitamin C than do people with no lung disease (121), although it is not clear whether this is because they have a lower supply or an increased demand. An argument can be made for vitamin C supplementation for patients with asthma, but there is no conclusive evidence that vitamin C or any other antioxidant supplements can prevent or exacerbate the disease. Another supplement that may be useful is vitamin D. Children taking high doses of ICS may benefit from increased intake of calcium and vitamin D because corticosteroid therapy may be associated with adverse growth or reduced bone density (2).

Acupuncture

Acupuncture has traditionally been used to treat asthma in China, and its international use is increasing. It consists of stimulating defined points on the skin, mostly by the insertion of needles. It is thought that needling will reduce local muscle tension or release pain-killing endorphins (122). There are various techniques of acupuncture, and it is usually used as an adjunct, not a sole therapy. There is currently insufficient evidence to make guided recommendations about the effectiveness of acupuncture for treating asthma (123).

Manual Therapy

There are various forms of manual therapy used at home to try and improve asthma quality of life, decrease symptoms, and help manage mucus. Most well-known by respiratory therapists are traditional chest physiotherapy techniques such as percussion, vibration, and postural drainage, although these are not recommended by the NAEPP. Chiropractic techniques aim to increase chest wall and spine movement to try to improve lung function and circulation. A 2011 review of literature on manual therapy found insufficient evidence to support the use of any of these manual therapies to treat asthma (124); however, the risk or side effects are minimal, so there is probably no harm in patients trying or continuing said therapies if they perceive improvement in symptoms or quality of life.

Breathing Exercises

Breathing exercises are frequently taught for numerous conditions, including asthma. They are included in yoga as well as recommended by respiratory and physical therapists, and they are often found in self-help books and other complementary therapies. The physiological mechanism of breath retraining in asthma is to induce mild hypercapnia because hyperventilation (i.e., hypocapnia) often exacerbates asthma symptoms such as air trapping. The ideal primary outcome of this technique would be improvement in quality of life and perceived health, and some studies have suggested that this is achieved (125). It is also a relatively risk-free and inexpensive therapy, so it would be a very desirable option for many patients with asthma. However, there is no consensus as yet on which breathing technique is most effective.

Physical Exercise

Physical exercise and training is recommended for all people who are physically capable, and it has been questionable whether exercise is possible for patients with asthma. There has been no evidence of negative effects of physical training on lung function and wheeze in patients with asthma (126). It can improve cardiopulmonary fitness and improve quality of life, but it does not seem to improve pulmonary function tests.

Assessing Asthma Control

Once an asthma action plan has been developed and a patient is sent home with his or her long-term therapy, part of regular asthma management includes regular assessment of asthma control. Evaluation should be done 2 to 6 weeks after any initiation of or change in an asthma plan. The step system (see Table 13-4) allows clinicians to quickly adjust pharmacological therapies up or down, depending on a patient's level of control. Signs of poorly controlled asthma include the following:

- Symptoms more than 2 days per week
- Symptoms multiple times per day on 2 or more days per week
- Nighttime awakenings more than once a month (0 to 4 years old), or twice a month or more (5 years old and older)
- Some limitation with normal activity
- Use of SABAs for symptom control more than 2 days per week
- FEV_1 60% to 80%
- FEV_1/FVC 75% to 80%
- Exacerbations more than two times per year requiring oral systemic corticosteroids

Signs of very poorly controlled asthma include the following:

- Symptoms throughout the day
- Weekly nighttime awakenings (0 to 4 years old) or more than 2 times per week (5 years and older)
- Extremely limited activity levels
- Use of SABAs for symptom control several times per day
- FEV_1 less than 60%
- FEV_1/FVC less than 75%
- Exacerbations more than 2 (ages 5 years and up) to 3 (0 to 4 years) times per year requiring oral systemic corticosteroids

Any time that asthma is poorly controlled, an increase in the step approach is warranted. Consultation with an asthma specialist should be initiated once step 3 care or higher is needed for children younger than 4 years and should be considered for any patient age 5 and older. Any patient requiring step 4 care or higher should be managed by an asthma specialist.

For children 0 to 4 years old: If a clear and beneficial response to the prescribed asthma treatment is not obvious within 4 to 6 weeks and the patient's and family's medication technique and adherence are satisfactory, treatment should be stopped. Alternative therapies or alternative diagnoses should be considered. Once a clear and beneficial response is sustained for at least 3 months, consider a step down to evaluate the need for continued daily long-term control therapy. Children in this age group have high rates of spontaneous remission of symptoms.

For patients 5 years and older: Declines in lung function or repeated periods of worsening asthma impairment may indicate a progressive worsening of the underlying severity of asthma. Although there is no indication that treatment alters the progression of the underlying disease in children, adjustments in treatment may be necessary to maintain asthma control. Once asthma control is achieved, monitoring and follow-up are essential because asthma often varies over time. A step up in therapy may be needed at any time that asthma is poorly controlled, or a step down may be possible to identify the minimum medication necessary to maintain control.

There is also the possibility of identifying seasonal patterns of asthma. One study found that poorly controlled asthma was present in one-third of children in the summer, compared with close to half the asthma population during spring, autumn, and winter (127).

Acute Exacerbations

An asthma exacerbation is an acute or subacute episode of progressively worsening shortness of breath, coughing, wheezing, and/or chest tightness. It is characterized by decreases in expiratory flow that can be quantified through simple measurements such as PEF. Generally, milder exacerbations can be managed at home using a quick-relief medication (usually a SABA), whereas more serious exacerbations require an unscheduled visit to a doctor's office, urgent care facility, ED, or a hospital admission. The most severe exacerbations, frequently referred to as *status asthmaticus*, are those that do not respond to attempts at bronchodilation with SABAs. They require admission to an ICU for continuous monitoring and advanced treatment.

Early treatment is the best strategy for management of asthma exacerbations. Early treatment includes a written action plan to guide patients in recognizing the signs of an exacerbation and initiating self-management. The key indicator of exacerbation is a decrease in PEF to less than 80% of that predicted or personal best (2). If PEF is 50% to 79%, the patient should monitor response to his or her quick-relief medication. If the response is poor (less than 10% improvement in PEF), then a visit to a clinician is recommended. If PEF is less than 50%, immediate medical attention is required. For infants, physical examination signs of serious distress include accessory muscle use, inspiratory and expiratory wheezing, paradoxical breathing, and a respiratory rate greater than 60.

Patients require careful monitoring and frequent assessment for response to treatment. For patients 5 years and older, PEF may be useful. Pulse oximetry in infants and young children can be useful for assessing exacerbation severity. Saturation of 92% to 94% at 1 hour of exacerbation is a predictor for needing hospitalization, and saturation less than 90% denotes serious distress. Any patient in status asthmaticus requires cardiorespiratory monitoring. A comfortable and supportive environment will also help alleviate some of the patient's anxiety and may improve signs of distress.

Severity assessment scores have been developed and tested in children to help predict the need for hospitalization early in the course of ED treatment (128). Although no one assessment is 100% predictive, they may help determine which patients should be admitted to a hospital in-patient unit and which are more likely to be able to go home after extended ED treatment and observation.

Emergency Department Management

The mainstays of acute exacerbation management within a hospital emergency department are oxygen, beta agonists, and corticosteroids. Adjunct therapies may also be warranted to reverse bronchoconstriction, and these are discussed in this section (2). The goals of treatment are to accomplish the following:

- Correct significant hypoxemia by administering supplemental oxygen. In rare instances, alveolar hypoventilation and hypoxemia will require mechanical ventilation.
- Rapidly reverse airflow obstruction, by repetitive or continuous administration of a SABA *and* early administration of systemic corticosteroids for patients with moderate or severe exacerbations or to those who do not respond immediately and completely to SABA treatment
- Reduce the likelihood of exacerbation relapse or future recurrence by increasing control therapy.

OXYGEN

Children with asthma in severe acute exacerbation have significantly increased oxygen demands and poor respiratory reserve. The potential for rapid desaturation and hypoxemia is great; therefore, oxygen therapy should be administered as needed to reverse hypoxemia and should be delivered via partial or nonrebreather mask (129).

SABA

Despite advances in many other methods of bronchodilation, SABAs are still the mainstay of therapy. They can be administered via nebulizer, MDI, intravenously, subcutaneously, or orally. The most common SABA used in the United States is albuterol, and although as of 2007 no recommendation for children had been made, many clinicians have recently adopted the use of levalbuterol because it has fewer side effects at higher doses.

A nebulized SABA is the most popular route of delivery in the hospital, although higher doses of nebulized SABA may be needed (130), and some evidence suggests that delivery via MDI with a spacer for young children will be more effective than nebulizers during severe exacerbations. Recommended dosages for albuterol include the following:

- Nebulized: 0.15 mg/kg (minimum dose 2.5 mg) every 20 minutes for three doses, then 0.15 to 0.3 mg/kg up to 10 mg every 1 to 4 hours as needed (2)
- MDI: four to eight puffs every 20 minutes, up to 4 hours, then every 4 hours as needed (81)

Dose-ranging techniques have shown that it takes between 4 and 10 puffs of an MDI bronchodilator to provide acute efficacy similar to a single nebulizer treatment (131).

For children presenting with severe acute asthma who are not responding to doses every 20 minutes, current evidence supports the use of continuous nebulized SABAs to increase pulmonary functions and reduce hospitalization (132). It appears to be safe and well tolerated in patients who receive it, and such use may lead to more rapid improvement, improve sleep and be more cost effective (133). Continuous SABA nebulization via a special nebulizer can provide a more consistent delivery of medication and allow deeper tissue penetration, resulting in enhanced bronchodilation. It has been shown to reduce admissions in patients with severe asthmatic exacerbations (134). A reasonable approach to inhaled therapy in severe exacerbations could be the use of continuous nebulized albuterol until PEF is greater than 50% of that predicted, or until serious adverse effects appear (e.g., severe tachycardia, arrhythmias), followed by intermittent SABA every 20 to 60 minutes for hospitalized patients (135). The dosage for continuous nebulized albuterol is 0.5 g/kg/hr (2).

Decreased tidal volume or severe airway obstruction in status asthmaticus may prevent effective aerosolized bronchodilator delivery; thus, intravenous delivery may be necessary. Terbutaline is the current intravenous beta agonist of choice in the United States, whereas other countries also use albuterol. Although most adverse effects of beta agonists are cardiovascular in nature, neither albuterol or terbutaline have been known to cause clinically significant toxicity when used intravenously for pediatric status asthmaticus (136). Oral delivery of albuterol is not an effective way to treat severe, acute asthma (129).

A 2011 Cochrane Review of trials did not find enough evidence to show that inhaled beta-2 agonists work well for patients once they are intubated and mechanically ventilated; thus, the current effect is not established (137). Although more research is needed, SABA therapy is typically continued for patients even after intubation.

CORTICOSTEROIDS

Despite extensive clinical experience with corticosteroids, there remains considerable uncertainty as to the onset of action, dose-response characteristics, duration of treatment, optimal route of administration, and patient populations likely to require or respond best to them during the treatment of acute severe asthma (138). The treatment of acute severe asthma with corticosteroids within 1 hour of presentation to the emergency department has been found to lower hospitalization rates and improve pulmonary function (139). The benefit of systemic corticosteroids appears greatest in patients with more severe asthma, and those not currently receiving steroids (140). Their onset of action may be seen in as little as 2 hours when monitoring PEF, but improvement in FEV_1 may be delayed by as much as 6 hours (135). This is why corticosteroids should be given as quickly as possible, within 1 hour of presentation to the emergency department (2), and aggressive bronchodilator treatment must continue until corticosteroids take effect.

A clear dose response is seen at dosages greater than 40 mg/day of methylprednisolone or the equivalent. Oral and intravenous corticosteroids have similar efficacy in the treatment of acute asthma in adults, and children appear to respond well to oral dosing (139). Systemic corticosteroids produce some improvements for children admitted to the hospital with acute asthma. The benefits may include earlier discharge and fewer relapses, and continuing a course of oral corticosteroids after the exacerbation can also decrease the relapse rate (140).

Inhaled or nebulized corticosteroids are not currently recommended as being equivalent to systemic steroids. Further studies examining differing doses and routes of administration for corticosteroids will clarify the optimal therapy, and the use of corticosteroids within 1 hour of presentation to

an ED significantly reduces the need for hospital admission in patients with acute asthma (141).

Prednisone, methylprednisolone, or prednisolone are the systemic corticosteroids of choice for treating asthma, and are administered in dosages of 1 to 2 mg/kg (maximum 60 mg/day), divided into two doses, delivered until PEF reaches 70% of predicted or personal best (2).

ANTICHOLINERGICS

Anticholinergics have a much slower onset of action (60 to 90 minutes to peak) and produce less bronchodilation at peak effect compared with SABAs. The rationale for implementation of a combination of SABAs and anticholinergic agents in patients with severe asthmatic exacerbations is based on targeting different sites of action (i.e., proximal vs. distal airways) and different pathophysiological mechanisms of airway smooth muscle relaxation (135). Ipratropium bromide is the anticholinergic agent of choice to administer to patients with asthma in the emergency setting because of its selectivity for muscarinic airway smooth muscle receptors through which bronchodilation is mediated and its lack of systemic anticholinergic adverse effects.

A single dose of an anticholinergic agent is not effective for the treatment of mild and moderate exacerbations and is insufficient for the treatment of severe exacerbations. Adding multiple doses of anticholinergics to beta-2 agonists appears safe, improves lung function, and helps prevent hospital admission in some patients. The available evidence only supports their use in school-aged children with severe asthma exacerbation, not for mild or moderate exacerbations (142).

MAGNESIUM

Magnesium is an ion found in abundance in the human body and, when given intravenously, has been shown to have beneficial effects on smooth muscle relaxation and inflammation (143). The use of magnesium sulfate in status asthmaticus has gained support recently, appearing to be of some benefit in the subpopulation of patients with severe airflow limitation, a relative failure to respond to inhaled bronchodilators, and a high risk of hospital admission (144). The addition of intravenous magnesium sulfate to the repetitive administration of inhaled SABAs and systemic corticosteroid treatment among individuals with severe exacerbations is shown to reduce hospitalizations and improve pulmonary function (135). Even a single dose of intravenous magnesium sulfate administered to patients with severe acute asthma has been shown to be effective.

Based on current research, the dose for intravenous magnesium sulfate is 25 to 75 mg/kg/dose up to 2 g in children, over 20 minutes (2, 135). Nebulized inhaled magnesium sulfate in addition to beta-2 agonist in the treatment of an acute asthma exacerbation also appears to improve pulmonary function in patients with severe exacerbations (145).

ANTILEUKOTRIENES

Antileukotrienes could be considered as an adjunct therapy for asthma to avoid intubation by providing another pathway to rapid bronchodilation (2). It is not yet clear whether these agents offer a significant benefit over and above that derived from routine therapy (135). A single dose of intravenous montelukast in moderate and severe exacerbations demonstrated a rapid and significant improvement in pulmonary function within 10 minutes of administration (146). Patients treated with montelukast tended to receive less SABA therapy and had fewer treatment failures than did patients receiving placebo, but oral formulations should not be expected to provide benefit for at least 90 minutes (147–149).

The following therapies that may have been common previously are not currently recommended by the NAEPP for treating acute severe exacerbations in patients admitted to the emergency department:

- Methylxanthines (aminophylline, theophylline)
- Antibiotics (unless there are comorbid conditions such as bacterial infections)
- Aggressive hydration (except for some infants and young children who become dehydrated due to decreased food intake)
- Chest physical therapy
- Mucolytic
- Sedation

DISCHARGE

The decision to discharge from the emergency department can be made once FEV_1 or PEF is greater than or equal to 70% of the value predicted and has been sustained for 60 minutes after the SABA treatment, the patient is in no sign of distress, and physical examination is normal. Patients should receive asthma education at discharge. Asthma education aimed at children and their caregivers who present to the emergency department for acute exacerbations can result in lower risk of future emergency department presentation and hospital admission. There remains uncertainty as to the long-term effect of education on other markers of asthma morbidity such as quality of life, symptoms, and lung function. There is no definitive data as to what type, duration, and intensity of educational packages are the most effective in reducing acute care use (150). Patients and the family should be retrained on the proper delivery method of current medications, and new education should be provided on any new prescriptions. Preventive care at home and avoidance of triggers should also be reviewed.

Home therapy should include the following:

- Continued treatment with inhaled SABAs
- Course of oral corticosteroids: A short course

of corticosteroids following assessment for an asthma exacerbation significantly reduces the number of relapses to additional care, hospitalizations, and use of SABAs without an apparent increase in side effects (151).
- Consideration of initiation of a daily home regimen of ICS: There is some evidence that high-dose ICS therapy alone may be as effective as oral corticosteroid therapy when used in mild asthmatics upon ED discharge (152).
- Magnesium supplementation at home: A current research question is whether chronic magnesium supplementation at home would assist in asthma control, particularly for patients who have a history of acute exacerbations (Evidence in Practice 13-2).

Patients should always follow up with their regular clinician after a visit to the emergency department for acute exacerbation.

■■ Two months later you are working a morning shift in the emergency department when Derrick arrives in obvious distress. His grandmother says that she was unable to fill his prescription for ICS, so instead they had him use his SABA inhaler once a day to keep his symptoms under control. He's been waking up several nights this week and has been up since 0200 with wheezing and coughing. Derrick did a PEF before arriving, and it was 50%. After 4 puffs of his albuterol MDI, there was no improvement in PEF or symptoms, so they came to the ED for help.

He is placed on a monitor, and his vital signs are HR, 134 bpm; RR, 55 breaths/min; SpO_2, 94%; BP, 105/65 mm Hg, with severely diminished breath sounds. You call the physician to the bedside and recommend starting back-to-back albuterol nebulizers at a dosage of 2.5 mg, as well as systemic corticosteroids and potentially a 500 mg dose of IV magnesium. While you are preparing the nebulizer, the grandmother shows you the MDI, whose weight seems very light. When you shake and depress the canister, you note that no spray comes out, and you therefore suspect that Derrick has been taking his inhaler after the medication had been completely used, which may be contributing to his lack of response to therapy. You begin the nebulizer treatment and call the physician to the room to let him know of your findings with the MDI.

Intensive Care Management

If the FEV_1 or PEF continue to be at 40% to 60% of predicted and the patient still displays mild-to-moderate symptoms after 1 to 2 hours of aggressive therapy and observation in the emergency department,

Oral Magnesium (146)

A randomized controlled trial of oral magnesium (300 mg/day) in 37 children ages 7 to 19 years found that oral magnesium supplementation reduced bronchial reactivity to methacholine, diminished allergen-induced skin responses, provided better symptom control, and reduced exacerbations in pediatric patients with moderate persistent asthma. Supplemental oral magnesium, or at least increased dietary intake of magnesium food sources (e.g., whole seeds, grains, nuts, vegetables), may prove an effective adjunctive therapy in asthma. Further research is required in different pediatric populations to confirm this finding, and also larger studies in adults may be needed to determine whether this intervention has any merit.

current therapies should be continued on a general care pediatric floor. Patients will need immediate transfer to an ICU if they display the following symptoms after 60 to 90 minutes of aggressive therapy:

- FEV_1 or PEF of less than 40%
- $PaCO_2$ greater than or equal to 42 mm Hg
- Severe symptoms
- Drowsiness or confusion

One pediatric hospital reviewed their asthmatic admissions and found that 85% of their ICU admissions reported that the child had been previously admitted to the hospital for asthma (153). Additional therapies should be available once a patient is in the ICU. These include noninvasive ventilation, heliox, intubation, mechanical ventilation, and inhaled anesthetics. Patients who fail mechanical ventilation and continue with severe airflow obstruction, hypoxemia, and hypercarbia may also warrant placement on extracorporeal membrane oxygenation (ECMO).

NONINVASIVE POSITIVE-PRESSURE VENTILATION

Noninvasive positive-pressure ventilation (NIPPV) can decrease the work of breathing by offsetting the intrinsic positive end expiratory pressure (PEEP) caused by air trapping when patients are unable to completely exhale during a severe exacerbation. The advantages of NIPPV over intubation include improved comfort, decreased need for sedation, decreased incidence of ventilator-associated pneumonia, and decreased length of ICU and hospital stay (154). On the other hand, NIPPV carries an increased aspiration risk and requires increased monitoring and health-care staff resources. One randomized controlled trial involving adults showed a benefit in the BiPAP group based on improvements in hospitalizations, discharge rates, and

respiratory parameters (155). NIPPV might have a role for pediatric patients with asthma and hypercapnic respiratory failure who do not require immediate intubation, and it is frequently used in children's hospitals with anecdotal success. One retrospective study reviewed the outcomes of pediatric patients placed on NIPPV along with SABAs in the emergency department. Of the patients placed on NIPPV, 88% tolerated the therapy, and it prevented ICU admission in 22% of patients. Clinically, 77% showed an immediate improvement in respiratory rate after initiation of therapy, and 88% showed an increase in SpO_2 (156). Most studies, particularly for severe asthma exacerbations and very young pediatric patients (i.e., weighing less than 20 kg), are small and retrospective, but they have found NIPPV to be safe and that it may improve clinical outcomes (157).

A trial of NIPPV could be implemented in selected patients with acute severe asthma in conjunction with conventional medical treatment such as continuous nebulized SABAs and corticosteroids, but close monitoring is required for the early recognition of respiratory failure, such as decreasing levels of consciousness. RTs should be readily available for these patients, and intubation supplies and personnel should be close at hand to avoid delayed intubation if NIPPV does not improve ventilation (135).

HELIOX

A helium and oxygen mixture, known as **heliox,** has been used to treat airway obstruction since 1934 (158). Heliox has been studied and reported to be effective in a variety of respiratory conditions such as upper-airway obstruction, status asthmaticus, decompression sickness, postextubation stridor, bronchiolitis, and acute respiratory distress syndrome. Because helium is an inert gas that is not known to interact with human metabolism, it can be used on any patient without adverse effects. Heliox is recommended as a useful adjunct in patients with severe asthma, both for spontaneous breathing and mechanical ventilation.

Helium is 86% less dense than room air. The only gas with a lower density is hydrogen, which is highly flammable. As will be discussed in Chapter 15, the lower density of heliox reduces areas of turbulence in the airways and increases laminar flow. Thus, heliox improves the efficiency of gas flow through narrowed orifices. Heliox decreases the work of breathing in patients with increased airway resistance, but it does not treat airway resistance. Rather, it reduces the inspiratory pressure required by the patient or ventilator. When heliox was administered to seven patients with status asthmaticus intubated for respiratory failure, all patients experienced a significant reduction in $PaCO_2$, peak airway pressure, and increased tidal volume within 20 minutes (159).

Heliox has also been used to deliver SABAs during acute exacerbation. It increases the deposition of inhaled particles to the distal airways in patients, and this improved deposition might be even more pronounced in patients with a great degree of airway obstruction (160). Patients with severe asthma may be better served by delivering aerosolized medications with heliox rather than room air or oxygen-enriched air, and improvements in asthma with heliox-propelled nebulized bronchodilators have been seen, especially when it was administered within the first hour of presentation of severe exacerbation (161). No complications or adverse events have been reported.

A review of studies involving pediatric status asthmaticus suggests that heliox may have a beneficial role in the initial treatment of pediatric asthma, especially to serve as a bridge until corticosteroids have a clinical effect (158). A 2010 Cochrane Review concluded that it would not recommend heliox for initial patient management or for all patients presenting to the ED with acute asthma. However, because no large studies have been performed, it is difficult to make blanket statements regarding what patient populations should receive heliox and what a likely protocol should be for its use (162).

ARTERIAL BLOOD GAS

Serial blood gas measurements are useful in severe exacerbations to monitor for signs of respiratory failure. Hypocarbia is found early in clinical presentation, but normalizing CO_2 in the face of persistent respiratory distress should be considered a sign of impending respiratory failure (129). However, ABG values should not be the primary clinical factor for the decision to intubate and place a patient on mechanical ventilation.

INTUBATION

One retrospective study of children admitted to the hospital for acute asthma found the rate of mechanical ventilation to be 10% to 12% (163). Because intubation of a severely ill patient with asthma is difficult and associated with complications, additional treatments such as magnesium or heliox should be attempted to avoid intubation, but intubation should not be delayed once it is deemed necessary. (Clinical Variations 13-3)

Intubation should be avoided unless respiratory failure is impending. Intubation may aggravate bronchospasm, precipitate hypotension and cardiac arrest, and greatly increase the risk of barotrauma, such as pneumothorax and subcutaneous emphysema, through positive-pressure ventilation (166). Absolute indications for intubation are as follows:

- Cardiopulmonary arrest
- Severe hypoxia
- Rapid deterioration of mental status

A relative indication for intubation is progressive respiratory deterioration despite maximal treatment,

---

Clinical Variations 13-3

When Are Patients in Status Asthmaticus Intubated?

The decision of when in a patient's course of treatment to intubate is a challenging one. A 2007 retrospective review found that children with status asthmaticus were three times more likely to be intubated at community hospitals than at a children's hospital. This increased likelihood was despite similar baseline illness, acute asthma severity, and hospital courses (164). Data showed that the children in community hospitals were intubated earlier in the course and had shorter courses than those in children's hospitals, suggesting that the same children might not have been intubated had they been cared for at a children's hospital where they would have received more aggressive noninvasive therapy. It was noted in another review study from London that 85% of children transferred from a community hospital to a PICU needed intubation, suggesting that they are often identified and referred to a higher acuity facility before intubation (165), although the referral and transfer may not be happening early enough to implement higher level therapies that could reverse respiratory failure.

---

including NIPPV. ABG results alone should not determine when to intubate—some patients who are hypercarbic can be managed without invasive support, whereas others with mild hypercarbia may need emergency airway support. Factors associated with the increased likelihood of intubation include exhaustion and fatigue despite maximal therapy, deteriorating mental status, refractory hypoxemia, increasing hypercapnea, hemodynamic instability, and impending coma or apnea (135).

Intubation might cause severe derangement of the cardiopulmonary status of a patient with status asthmaticus. Hypotension can be the result of sedative dosing, preexisting dehydration, or decreased venous return owing to high intrathoracic pressures and overzealous ventilation, or any combination of the three. Arrhythmias, barotrauma, aspiration, laryngeal edema, and seizures are often encountered during the peri-intubation period in ventilated patients with asthma (167), making close monitoring essential.

Most of the complications in patients with asthma receiving mechanical ventilation occur during or immediately after intubation (129), thus it is imperative to determine a plan for airway management and intubation prior to starting the procedure.

To intubate, sedation is indicated to improve comfort, safety, and patient-ventilator synchrony, while at the same time decreasing oxygen consumption and carbon dioxide production. Benzodiazepines can be safely used to sedate a patient with asthma, but time to awakening after discontinuation is prolonged and difficult to predict. The most common alternative is propofol, which is useful in patients with acute severe asthma of rapid onset who may be eligible for extubation within a few hours; the benefit of propofol is that it can be titrated rapidly to a deep sedation level and has rapid reversal after discontinuation. Propofol also possesses bronchodilatory properties. The addition of an opioid (e.g., fentanyl or remifentanil) administered by continuous infusion to benzodiazepines or propofol is often desirable to provide amnesia, sedation, analgesia, and respiratory drive suppression (135). **Ketamine** is another anesthetic agent with strong analgesic action that mediates bronchodilation. Both of these properties make it a popular choice for children with severe asthma requiring mechanical ventilation (168). Once intubated, the use of neuromuscular blockade may be necessary in patients with severe respiratory failure who are difficult to ventilate. Paralytics such as vecuronium and pancuronium decrease chest-wall stiffness, eliminate patient-ventilator dyssynchrony, lower the risk of barotrauma, and decrease oxygen consumption (81).

MECHANICAL VENTILATION STRATEGIES

Acute severe asthma will cause severe pulmonary hyperinflation because of the marked limitation of the expiratory flow. Therefore, the main objective of initial ventilator management is twofold: to ensure adequate gas exchange and to prevent further hyperinflation and ventilator-associated lung injury.

This may require **permissive hypercapnia**, or deliberate hypoventilation and acceptance of higher $PaCO_2$ levels and a more acidic pH. Permissive hypercapnea provides adequate oxygenation and ventilation while minimizing high airway pressures and barotrauma. Specifically, it involves administration of fractional concentration of inspired oxygen (FIO_2) at a value that is as high as necessary to maintain adequate arterial oxygenation, acceptance of hypercapnea, and treatment of combined metabolic and respiratory acidosis with intravenous sodium bicarbonate (2).

No randomized controlled trials have been completed to determine the best ventilation mode in life-threatening asthma. The chosen mode is probably less important than providing settings that minimize dynamic hyperinflation and intrinsic PEEP caused by increased airway resistance. Monitoring lung mechanics is of paramount importance for the safe ventilation of patients with status asthmaticus. Following intubation, controlled modes of ventilation are usually employed. The exhaustion of respiratory muscles after spontaneous breathing against a heavy resistive load of bronchoconstriction makes the assist-controlled mode a reasonable choice in the first 24 hours to

unload respiratory muscles and relieve fatigue (135). If a control mode is used, deep sedation and possibly muscle paralysis is necessary to avoid patient-ventilator asynchrony and to manage controlled hypoventilation.

Traditionally, volume-controlled ventilation has been preferred over pressure controlled. The perceived benefit is that alveolar ventilation may be more consistent than with pressure controlled ventilation, mainly because of fluctuating and rapidly changing airway resistance and intrinsic PEEP. On the other hand, volume-controlled ventilation mandates careful monitoring of inflation pressures. However, no strong clinical data prove the superiority of any type or mode of positive pressure in status asthmaticus, and barotrauma seems to occur regardless of the mode of delivery of positive pressure (169).

Volume ventilation settings would involve low tidal volume, avoiding a high respiratory rate and maintaining an I/E ratio (inspiratory to expiratory time) of at least 1:3 (81). The inspiratory flow rate must be set higher to allow adequate expiration time. A higher inspiratory flow rate will result in higher peak pressures. However, it is not the peak but the plateau pressure that has been associated with barotrauma. Plateau pressure (P_{Plat}) should ideally be kept at less than 30 cm H_2O to reduce regional lung over-stretch injury (170).

Although volume ventilation tends to be the mode of choice, there are some downfalls. As tidal volume is delivered with constant flow in traditional volume-controlled ventilation, relatively less obstructed airways with shorter time constants are likely to receive more volume throughout inspiration compared to more obstructed airways with longer time constants. This would result in uneven ventilation, higher peak inspiratory pressure, and a decrease in dynamic compliance. With pressure control ventilation (PCV), because of a constant inflation pressure, relatively fewer obstructed lung units with shorter time constants would achieve pressure equilibration earlier during inspiration compared with more obstructed areas. Thus, units with shorter time constants would attain their final volume earlier in inspiration, whereas those with longer time constants would continue to receive additional volume later in inspiration. This would result in a more even distribution of inspired gas, delivery of more tidal volume for the same inflation pressure, and improved dynamic compliance. One hospital's study of 40 children admitted for 51 episodes of severe status asthmaticus over 5 years assessed the effectiveness of PCV as the chosen ventilation mode. The studied population had a low incidence of barotrauma, lower duration of ventilation, and blood gas improvement immediately upon initiation (171).

With either pressure or volume ventilation, the recommendations for respiratory rate, I/E ratio, FIO_2, and PEEP are the same.

- Avoid a high respiratory rate to ensure adequate time for exhalation.
- Begin with an I/E ratio of at least 1:2 or 1:3 as an initial setting, and constantly assess flow waveforms and auto-PEEP for adequate exhalation time.
- Begin FiO_2 at 1.0, then wean for a target SpO_2 greater than 90%. Usually, an FIO_2 less than 0.50 is sufficient to achieve this goal, and the need for a high FIO_2 should trigger a search for other causes of hypoxemia, such as pneumothorax and atelectasis.

Intrinsic PEEP or **auto-PEEP** is the gas trapped in the alveoli at the end of expiration, caused by inadequate exhalation time. Auto-PEEP predisposes the patient to increased work of breathing, barotrauma, hemodynamic instability, and difficulty in triggering the ventilator. Auto-PEEP should be assessed frequently to ensure that there is adequate time set for exhalation despite airway obstruction. Auto-PEEP is measured by momentarily occluding the ventilator's expiratory port. Most computer-driven ventilators have a feature or button that can be selected to obtain a one-time measurement of auto-PEEP. The presence of auto-PEEP may also be suspected by observing the flow waveform or the flow volume curve when expiratory flow does not zero before the beginning of the next breath (Fig. 13-6).

ADVANCED THERAPIES

If a patient with severe status asthmaticus is not able to be ventilated despite using intubation, mechanical ventilation using permissive hypercapnea, and paralytics, there are few additional strategies to improve gas exchange while awaiting bronchodilation. Two potential therapies that may be used in large children's hospitals include extracorporeal membrane oxygenation (ECMO) and inhaled anesthetics (Evidence in Practice 13-3).

ECMO could provide adjunctive pulmonary support for intubated patients with asthma who remain severely acidotic and hypercarbic in spite of aggressive conventional therapy and unconventional therapies, including inhaled anesthetics. Although potentially helpful, there has been little experience reported with ECMO in refractory status asthmaticus. Anecdotal case reports have described its use in adults but rarely in children. It is an uncommon use for ECMO, and a review of the Extracorporeal Life Support Organization (ELSO) registry database from 1986 to 2007 identified 64 patients cannulated for status asthmaticus, with a 94% survival rate (172).

● **Evidence in Practice 13-3**

Isoflurane for Status Asthmaticus

Isoflurane, an inhalational anesthetic agent with bronchodilating properties, has been used in patients with severe life-threatening asthma exacerbations that are nonresponsive to conventional therapy. The exact mechanism of its bronchodilatory effect is not clearly established. Some of the proposed mechanisms include stimulation of beta-adrenergic receptors, direct relaxation of bronchial smooth muscles, and antagonism of actions of histamine and acetylcholine (173). Consequently, isoflurane may offer additional bronchodilatation after a maximal therapy with standard bronchodilators, and it is usually immediate and sustained. It is used in patients with the most severe status asthmaticus after intubation but when ventilatory management is unsuccessful and the airways are still not responsive to other therapies. Case study publications on this method began in the 1990s, but no extensive trials have been completed to assess its effectiveness. The most recent case series describes the use of isoflurane in 11 episodes of life-threatening acute asthma in children over a 5-year period in the ICU of a tertiary-care children's hospital (173). All of the patients in this series showed a significant drop in $PaCO_2$ and improvement in pH within 2 hours of administration by mechanical ventilation, suggesting that this is an effective method to improve alveolar ventilation in this population of patients.

Isoflurane for asthma is usually delivered via the inspiratory limb of an ICU ventilator under the direct supervision of the respiratory therapist. Extreme care must be taken when delivering anesthesia via an ICU ventilator because they are not FDA approved for delivery of anesthetic gases. Anesthesia ventilators are designed to safely administer inhaled anesthetics, while ICU ventilators must be modified to deliver it safely. The PICU team of physicians, nurses, and respiratory therapists will also need to be trained by the anesthesiology team on the safe use of this therapeutic modality.

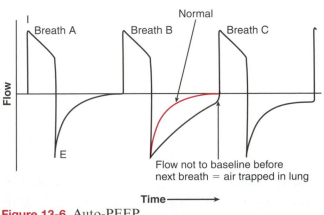

Figure 13-6 Auto-PEEP

Course and Prognosis

Asthma deaths are rare among children and increase with age. In 2007, 152 children younger than 15 years died from asthma (0.2 per 100,000 population) compared to 659 adults older than 85 years (6). A 2012 retrospective review of pediatric intensive care unit (PICU) data from 2004 to 2008 showed that the death rate of children admitted to PICUs with a primary diagnosis of acute asthma was 0.3%, making it a very rare event (163). Children with asthma who live in high-poverty communities have disproportionately high adverse asthma outcomes. There are racial disparities for asthma in ED visits, hospitalizations, and death, which are substantially higher than prevalence disparities alone (2).

Hospitalizations

Asthma is classified as a condition for which hospitalization is preventable, yet it continues to have a high annual rate of hospitalization, particularly for children. The most common reasons for the preventability of asthma hospitalizations cited are usually parent and patient related. Medication-related issues were identified, which included adherence problems, medications not being given soon enough, families running out of medications, and refills not being called in to pharmacies. Inadequate preventive measures was another reason frequently identified; this consisted of failure to avoid known triggers of the child's asthma exacerbations, including exposure to cigarette smoke (the most often cited in this subcategory), household dust, other children with upper respiratory infections, and pet dander, such as allowing a child who is allergic to dogs to play with a puppy (174).

In a 2011 retrospective study of pediatric patients admitted to an ICU for asthma exacerbation, 67% were readmitted to the hospital following discharge from the initial admission and 16.6% were readmitted to the ICU. Of the total children studied, 1.8% of them died from asthma within 10 years of ICU discharge (9).

At times, asthma can be a predictor of additional health-care burden and a coexisting factor for hospitalizations for other respiratory diseases. In a surveillance of 10 states during the 2003 to 2009 influenza seasons, 32% of children hospitalized with influenza had asthma; during the 2009 pandemic, 44% of children had asthma. The median age of the children was 7 years, and 73% had no additional medical conditions (11). This stresses the importance for annual influenza vaccinations and pandemic influenza vaccinations (175). (Special Populations 13-2).

In France, half of all hospitalizations for asthma occurred among children, and their hospitalization rates, contrary to those of adults, have not decreased over the past decade. Despite improvement in asthma management, including treatment and health education, adherence to guidelines remains poor, and

● **Special Populations 13-2**

Intramuscular Versus Intranasal Influenza Vaccinations for Infants With Wheezing/Asthma (175)

Influenza is a highly infectious disease caused by viruses. Influenza has been thought to cause asthma attacks. Few trials have been carried out to test whether asthma attacks following influenza infection (as opposed to following the vaccination) are significantly reduced by having been vaccinated, so uncertainty remains in terms of the difference vaccination makes to people with asthma. The included studies suggest that the vaccine against influenza is unlikely to precipitate asthma attacks immediately after the vaccine is used.

asthma remains a leading cause of hospitalization among children. Two-thirds of children with known asthma were hospitalized for an exacerbation that had been consistently poorly controlled during the previous year, 69% of them had at least one preventable risk factor for hospitalization, and more than 75% had asthma that was not well controlled in the month before hospitalization. These results point out the high proportion of poorly controlled asthma in children without adequate controller therapy (60% of them did not have any controller medication, or they had only low-dose ICS) despite the long-standing nature of this poor control and thus suggest a substantial potential for improvement (176).

The United States has found similar issues with pediatric hospitalizations. One 2009 national study found considerable variation in pediatric asthma hospitalization rates by and within states, suggesting that the use of national hospitalization rates to develop public health intervention policies may not target the populations most at risk (177). The study's findings indicate a significant difference in the overall pediatric asthma hospitalization rates ranging from 51.1 per 100,000 children in Oregon to 185.9 in Kentucky. These rate differences persist even when examining geographic subcategories, and there is no consistent pattern across states when examining rurality. For example, Florida children living in urban areas are most likely to be hospitalized for asthma, whereas in Kentucky and Oregon, children living in rural counties are most likely to be hospitalized (177). These findings support efforts to increase health insurance coverage for children, which may also improve access to prescription drugs that can help manage asthma exacerbations.

Cost of Asthma

From 2002 to 2007, the total incremental cost of asthma for a single patient was estimated to be $3,259 per year. The predicted incremental cost of hospital outpatient visits was $151; for emergency department visits, it was $110, and for in-patient visits, it was $446. The incremental cost of office-based visits for patients with asthma was estimated at $581 per year. Prescription medication expenditures are estimated to cost an additional $1,680 a year for a person with asthma (10).

Lung Function

Pulmonary function testing research has shown differing levels of lung dysfunction among children with asthma. Children with transient forms of preschool wheezing have lower levels of lung function and mildly increased bronchial hyperresponsiveness, but are only at limited, if any, risk of asthma during the school years compared with children who do not wheeze during the preschool years. In contrast, both persistent and late-onset wheezers are at high risk of having asthma bronchial hyperresponsiveness, and the greatest deficits in lung function growth are observed in persistent wheezers and in late-onset wheezers whose symptoms start before age 3 years (26).

"Outgrowing" Asthma

At the onset of puberty, children are frequently "symptom-free" of asthma, and it is said that their asthma is in "remission," or that they have "outgrown" their asthma. In one study, PFT results of such teenagers showed that their results of methacholine challenge were unchanged, but the speed of bronchial constriction was significantly diminished. This has been labeled by one group as "symptom-free but bronchial hyperresponsive" asthma. Of note, the lung function results for the subjects, such as FVC and FEV_1 was similar to that of kids the same age who were still diagnosed with intermittent asthma, suggesting that the lung disease and airway remodeling was not reversed (178).

■■ Derrick was treated with three doses of albuterol and given one oral dose of corticosteroids. When the physician heard that Derrick's albuterol MDI was empty at home during this exacerbation, he decided to hold off on the IV magnesium until you could assess the results of the nebulizer treatments. A PEF 1 hour after the last albuterol treatment was 65% of predicted. You continued two more nebulized treatments over the following 2 hours, and the follow-up PEF was 80%. The physician agrees that Derrick has responded very favorably to treatment, but his risk for exacerbation is much higher than initially anticipated because of his low compliance with control therapy. The physician obtains an additional albuterol MDI and 1-month dosing of ICS for Derrick and contacts the social work office to discuss with Derrick's grandmother ways of obtaining prescription drug coverage.

■■ Critical Thinking Questions: Derrick Lamb

1. What additional diagnostic tests would you have found helpful when Derrick was initially assessed for asthma?
2. How would you classify Derrick's asthma severity if his spirometry was less than 75% of predicted and he had no nocturnal symptoms?
3. If Derrick's PEF hadn't responded to the initial doses of albuterol and corticosteroids, what would be your next recommended therapy?
4. How might you, as the RT, be able to improve Derrick's access to control therapy and long-term care, despite the limitations of the health-care system?

◗● Case Studies and Critical Thinking Questions

■ Case 1: Amanda Peters

You are the evening shift RT working in a 200-bed community hospital and are covering the emergency department's respiratory needs. The triage nurse calls you to assess a 6-year-old girl brought in by her mom for shortness of breath.

You go to the triage area and find Amanda Peters, who is anxious, pale, and diaphoretic, sitting in her mother's lap. You begin your physical assessment while mom tells you some background: She brought Amanda to the emergency room this evening because after her dance class she has been coughing and can't seem to catch her breath. She didn't eat her dinner, and when mom sent her to lie down on the couch she said she couldn't because it was hard to breathe. Mom says Amanda has no history of asthma, and this is the first time she's come to the emergency room for her breathing.

Amanda's vital signs are RR 65 with mild retractions, SpO_2 95%, HR 145, and blood pressure 100/59. When you auscultate, you hear loud inspiratory and expiratory wheezes. When you ask Amanda questions, she answers them in short, two- or three-word sentences. You show her how to do a peak expiratory flow, but each time she tries to take a deep breath it causes her to cough uncontrollably.

• What would you like to do for Amanda?

You find the covering physician and request starting albuterol MDIs for Amanda, to which she agrees. You also discuss oral corticosteroids, to which she also agrees and notifies the nurse to begin that therapy. You arrive back in the triage area and show Amanda how to use the MDI along with a holding chamber. You provide her with six puffs of albuterol, and stay to monitor her for the next 20 minutes before administering additional therapy. While you wait, you ask Amanda's mom for additional history. Amanda has twin 12-year-old brothers, who are very healthy and active, and no one in the family has allergies or asthma. Amanda has always had lots of runny noses and upper respiratory infections, which seem to take longer for her to recover from than the other family members, and they often cause her to cough when no one else has that symptom. She's been to urgent care twice this winter for difficulty breathing and a cough that keeps her up at night. The nurse practitioner at the urgent care center recommended that Amanda be seen by her pediatrician, but Amanda has been so busy with dance classes and other family activities they just haven't had time to go.

- *Based on her symptoms and history, do you think Amanda has asthma?*

Amanda is given eight puffs of albuterol every 20 minutes and is given one dose of oral corticosteroids—she is able to perform a PEF afterward with 60% of predicted value and vital signs are HR, 158 bpm; SpO_2, increased to 97%; BP, 100/60; and she continues to have inspiratory and expiratory wheezes. One hour later her dyspnea and PEF is unchanged, so the on-call pediatrician agrees to admit her overnight for observation and continued bronchodilator therapy.

■ Case 2: Samantha Ocee

You are the RT working in an asthma and allergy clinic in a large town. You are seeing Samantha Ocee, a 16-year-old patient who was diagnosed with asthma at 4 years old. She is here for her annual follow-up examination. Samantha is a healthy-looking teenager who has allergic asthma and up until 6 months ago was receiving immunotherapy twice a week for her outdoor allergy triggers. She was diagnosed at her last visit with moderate persistent asthma, and her control therapy includes a fluticasone/salmeterol diskus twice a day and an albuterol SABA for acute symptoms. You go into the room to discuss her asthma symptoms and quality of life with her. Samantha tells you that she recently got her driver's license and is working after school three evenings a week and on the weekends as a hostess at a local restaurant. She no longer has time to get her allergy

shots, and so she has stopped that part of her therapy. An aunt has been teaching her about herbal therapies for asthma, and so she has been taking propolis, vitamin C, and magnesium supplements daily. She has a PFM at home but only uses it when she experiences symptoms, and she hasn't had an exacerbation or needed her SABA in the last 6 weeks. She also admits to you that often when she's working she does not remember to take her diskus before going to bed at night. You do a PEF with her and she is at 90% of her personal best, and says she's experiencing no symptoms. Her breath sounds are clear bilaterally, and pulse rate is 98 bpm.

- *Based on the information you've gathered, how well do you think Samantha's asthma is controlled? Would you make any recommendations for change in her control therapy?*
- *Would you have any recommendations or comments on her use of alternative therapies?*

■ Case 3: Andy Singh

You are an RT working in a children's hospital in the pediatric ICU. You receive a call from the emergency department that they will be transferring Andy Singh to the PICU. Andy is a 10-year-old who has been in the PICU twice before for status asthmaticus. He is diagnosed with moderate persistent asthma but has a high risk for severe airway limitation during his exacerbations. He has received 2 hours of continuous nebulized albuterol in the ED, along with one dose of IV magnesium and IV corticosteroids. His PEF rate is 40% of his personal best. He was trialed on heliox with his continuous nebulizers, but his SpO_2 had dropped to 88% so he was switched to FIO_2 1.0. The ED RT just placed him on BiPAP with an inspiratory positive airway pressure of 15 cm H_2O and an expiratory positive airway pressure of 5 cm H_2O. His ABG values 30 minutes after BiPAP initiation is 7.10/88/65/24.3. Andy is beginning to become less responsive and sleepy, and though he had audible bilateral wheezes, his breath sounds are becoming diminished. His vital signs are HR, 135 bpm; RR, 35 breaths/min; SpO_2, 89%; and BP, 100/50 mm Hg (dropping to 80/50 mm Hg during inspiration).

- *What should be the next recommended course of action for Andy?*
- *What would you recommend as initial ventilator settings? Would you continue with the same bronchodilator therapy after intubation?*

Multiple-Choice Questions

1. Which of the following would not be a risk factor for developing asthma?
   a. Growing up on a farm
   b. Being a boy
   c. Having a poor health history
   d. Having a grandfather with asthma

2. What are the four main characteristics of asthma?
   I. Airway edema
   II. Bronchoconstriction
   III. Airway hyperresponsiveness
   IV. Atopy
   V. Increased mucus production
   VI. Airway remodeling
   a. I, II, III, IV
   b. I, II, V, VI
   c. II, III, IV, VI
   d. I, II, III, VI

3. Which of the below signs and symptoms should make a clinician suspect a diagnosis of asthma?
   I. Wheezing
   II. Nighttime coughing
   III. Allergic rhinitis
   IV. Symptoms that worsen with viral infections
   V. Symptoms that occur in the presence of pets
   a. I, II
   b. I, II, III
   c. I, II, IV, V
   d. I, II, III, IV, V

4. Classify the asthma severity of the following patient: A 7-year-old with asthma symptoms three to four times a week for which she uses a SABA inhaler. She is awakened a few times a month with coughing and wheezing, occasionally has to sit out at recess for difficulty breathing, and has had two exacerbations this year that required oral corticosteroids.
   a. Intermittent
   b. Mild persistent
   c. Moderate persistent
   d. Severe persistent
   e. Does not have asthma

5. Which of the following are symptoms of poorly controlled asthma?
   a. FEV_1 60 to 80%
   b. FEV_1/FVC 80 to 90%
   c. Nighttime awakenings more than twice per month
   d. Limited activity levels

6. How frequently can patients who are having an acute exacerbation at home take a SABA?
   a. 0 to 15 mg/kg every 20 minutes nebulized for three doses, then 0.15 to 0.3 mg/kg every 1 to 4 hours
   b. 4 to 8 puffs SABA every 20 minutes for up to 4 hours
   c. 10 puffs every 30 minutes for up to 4 hours
   d. 2.5 mg/kg every 4 hours

7. At what point should a patient with an acute exacerbation go for emergency medical care?
   a. PEF less than 50%
   b. PEF 50% to 79%
   c. PEF 40% to 60%
   d. PEF less than 40%

8. Which of the following is/are no longer considered appropriate emergency room treatment(s)?
   a. Magnesium
   b. Mucolytics
   c. Heliox
   d. Continuous SABA

9. You are caring for an intubated patient in status asthmaticus who is sedated and is not taking any spontaneous breaths. You note that the flow waveform is not returning to zero after each breath. Which of the following ventilator changes might offer additional time for exhalation?
   I. Decrease I-time
   II. Increase I-time
   III. Increase RR
   IV. Decrease RR
   V. Inverse I/E ratio
   a. II, III, V
   b. I, IV
   c. II, IV
   d. I, III

10. Which of the following is a recommended method for corticosteroid therapy for a 6-month-old?
    a. Beclomethasone
    b. Budesonide
    c. Fluticasone
    d. Oral prednisone

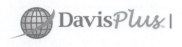 For additional resources login to Davis*Plus* (http://davisplus.fadavis.com/ keyword "Perretta") and click on the Premium tab. (Don't have a *Plus*Code to access Premium Resources? Just click the Purchase Access button on the book's Davis*Plus* page.)

REFERENCES

1. National Institutes of Health. National Asthma Education and Prevention Program (NAEPP). http://www.nhlbi.nih.gov/about/naepp/. Accessed January 1, 2012.
2. U.S. Department of Health and Human Services. National Heart, Lung, and Blood Institute. National Asthma Education and Prevention Program. Expert panel report 3: guidelines for the diagnosis and management of asthma. 2007. http://www.nhlbi.nih.gov/guidelines/asthma/03_sec2_def.pdf.
3. Subbarao P, Mandhane PJ, Sears MR. Asthma: epidemiology, etiology and risk factors. *CMAJ.* 2009;181(9): E181-E190.
4. Jhun Y, Kung A, Voigt R, Johnson S. Characterization of children's asthma status by ICD-9 code and criteria-based medical record review. *Prim Care Resp J.* 2011;20(1):79-83.
5. Molis WE, Bagniewski S, Weaver AL, Jacobson RM, Juhn YJ. Timeliness of diagnosis of asthma in children and its predictors. *Allergy.* 2008;63(3):1529-1535.
6. American Lung Association. Trends in asthma morbidity and mortality. September 2012. http://www.lung.org/finding-cures/our-research/trend-reports/asthma-trend-report.pdf. Accessed July 17, 2013.
7. Myers TR, Tomasio L. Asthma: 2015 and beyond. *Respir Care.* 2011;56(9):1389-1410.
8. Cherry DK, Hing E, Woodwell DA, Rechtsteiner EA. National ambulatory medical care survey: 2006 summary. *Natl Health Stat Report.* 2008;(3):1-39.
9. Triasih R, Duke T, Robertson CF. Outcomes following admission to intensive care for asthma. *Arch Dis Child.* 2011;96:729-734.
10. Barnett SB, Nurmagambetov TA. Costs of asthma in the United States: 2002-2007. *J Allergy Clin Immunol.* 2011; 127(1):145-152.
11. Dawood FS, Kamimoto L, D'Mello TA, et al. Children with asthma hospitalized with seasonal or pandemic influenza, 2003-2009. *Pediatrics.* 2011;128(1):27-32.
12. Valeri MA, Andreski PM, Schoeni RF, McGonagle KA. Examining the association between childhood asthma and parent and grandparent asthma status: implications for practice. *Clin Pediatr.* 2010;49(6):535-541.
13. Bjerg A, Hedman L, Perzanowski M, Lundbäck B, Rönmark E. A strong synergism of low birth weight and prenatal smoking on asthma in schoolchildren. *Pediatrics.* 2011;127(4):905-912.
14. Centers for Disease Control. *Data for Children With Asthma. Summary Health Statistics for US Children: National Health Interview Survey, 2010.* Vital and Health Statistics, series 10, number 250. Publication (PHS)-2012-1576). Atlanta, GA: CDC; 2001.
15. van der Hulst AE, Klip H, Brand PLP. Risk of developing asthma in young children with atopic eczema: a systematic review-atopic eczema. *J Allergy Clin Immunol.* 2007;120: 565-569.
16. Ruotsalainen M, Piippo-Savolainen E, Hyvärinen MK, Korppi M. Adulthood asthma after wheezing in infancy: a questionnaire study at 27 years of age. *Allergy.* 2010;65: 503-509.
17. Gern JE, Lemanske RF Jr, Busse WW. Early life origins of asthma. *J Clin Invest.* 1999;104(7):837-843.
18. Adler A, Tager I, Quintero DR. Decreased prevalence of asthma among farm-reared children compared with those who are rural but not farm-reared. *J Allergy Clin Immunol.* 2005;115(1):67-73.
19. American Thoracic Society. What constitutes an adverse health effect of air pollution? Official statement of the American Thoracic Society. *Am J Respir Crit Care Med.* 2000;161:665-673.
20. McConnell R, Berhane K, Gilland F, et al. Asthma in exercising children exposed to ozone: a cohort study. *Lancet.* 2002;359:386-391.
21. Holgate ST. The sentinel role of the airway epithelium in asthma pathogenesis. *Immunol Rev.* 2011;242:205-219.
22. Grainge CL, Lau LCK, Ward JA, et al. Effect of bronchoconstriction on airway remodeling in asthma. *N Engl J Med.* 2011;364:2006-2015.
23. Chu HW, Martin RJ. Are eosinophils still important in asthma? *Clin Exp Allergy* 2001;31(4):525-528.
24. Williams TJ. The eosinophil enigma. *J Clin Invest.* 2004; 113(4):507-509.
25. Bisgaard H, Bonnelykke K. Long-term studies of the natural history of asthma in childhood. *J Allergy Clin Immunol.* 2010;126(2):187-197.
26. Martinez FD. New insights into the natural history of asthma: Primary prevention on the horizon. *J Allergy Clin Immunol.* 2011;128(5):939-945.
27. Morgan WJ, Stern DA, Sherrill DL, et al. Outcome of asthma and wheezing in the first 6 years of life: follow-up through adolescence. *Am J Respir Crit Care Med.* 2005; 172(10):1253-1258.
28. Akhabir L, Sandford AJ. Genome-wide association studies for discovery of genes involved in asthma. *Respirology.* 2011;16:396-406.
29. Frith J, Fleming L, Bossley C, Ullmann N, Bush A. The complexities of defining atopy in severe childhood asthma. *Clin Exp Allergy.* 2001;41:948-953.
30. Bracken M, Fleming L, Hall P, et al. The importance of nurse-led home visits in the assessment of children with problematic asthma. *Arch Dis Child.* 2009;94:780-784.
31. Strachan DP. Hay fever, hygiene, and household size. *Br Med J.* 1989;299:1259-1260.
32. Liu AH. Hygiene theory and allergy and asthma prevention. *Paediatr Perinat Epidemiol.* 2007;21(suppl 3):2-7.
33. Besswinger C, Bals R. Interaction of allergic airway inflammation and innate immunity: hygiene and beyond. *J Occup Med Toxicol.* 2008;3(suppl 1):S1-S3.
34. Eder W, Ege MJ, von Mutius E. The asthma epidemic. *N Engl J Med.* 2006;355(21):2226-2235.
35. Gern JE, Busse WW. Relationship of viral infections to wheezing illnesses and asthma. *Nat Rev Immunol.* 2002; 2(2):132-138.
36. Sears MR, Greene JM, Willan AR, et al. A longitudinal, population-based, cohort study of childhood asthma followed to adulthood. *N Engl J Med.* 2003;349(15): 1414-1422.
37. Crocker DD, Kinyota S, Dumitru GG, et al. Effectiveness of home-based, multi-trigger, multicomponent interventions with an environmental focus for reducing asthma morbidity. *Am J Prev Med.* 2011;41(2S1):S5-S32.

38. Wahn U, Lau S, Bergmann R, et al. Indoor allergen exposure is a risk factor for sensitization during the first three years of life. *J Allergy Clin Immunol.* 1997;99(6, pt 1):763-769.

39. Sigurs N, Bjarnason R, Sigurbergsson F, Kjellman B. Respiratory syncytial virus bronchiolitis in infancy is an important risk factor for asthma and allergy at age 7. *Am J Respir Crit Care Med.* 2000;161(5):1501-1507.

40. Al-Garawi A, Fattouh R, Botelho F, et al. Influenza A facilitates sensitization to house dust mite in infant mice leading to an asthma phenotype in adulthood. *Mucosal Immunol.* 2011;4(6):682-694.

41. Risnes KR, Belanger K, Murk W, Bracken MB. Antibiotic exposure by 6 months and asthma and allergy at 6 years: findings in a cohort of 1,401 US children. *Am J Epidemiol.* 2011;173:310-318.

42. Busse WW, Lemanske RF Jr. Asthma. *N Engl J Med.* 2001;344(5):350-362.

43. Leickly FE. Children, their school environment, and asthma. *Ann Allergy Asthma Immunol.* 2003;90(1):3-5.

44. Sheehan WJ, Angsithienchai PA, Baxi SN, et al. Age-specific prevalence of outdoor and indoor aeroallergen sensitization in Boston. *Clin Pediatr.* 2010;49(6):579-585.

45. Sporik R, Holgate ST, Platts-Mills TAE, Cogswell JJ. Exposure to house-dust mite allergen (Der p I) and the development of asthma in childhood. *N Engl J Med.* 1990;323(8):502-507.

46. Huss K, Adkinson NF Jr, Eggleston PA, et al. House dust mite and cockroach exposure are strong risk factors for positive allergy skin test responses in the Childhood Asthma Management Program. *J Allergy Clin Immunol.* 2001;107(1):48-54.

47. Rosenstreich D, Eggleston P, Kattan M, et al. The role of cockroach allergy and exposure to cockroach allergen in causing morbidity among inner-city children with asthma. *N Engl J Med.* 1997;336(19):1356-1363.

48. Institute of Medicine (IOM) of the National Academies of Sciences, Board on Health Promotion and Disease Prevention. Damp indoor spaces and health. May 25, 2004. Accessed July 17, 2013. www.iom.edu/Reports/2004/Damp-Indoor-Spaces-and-Health.aspx.

49. Ownby D. Pet dander and difficult-to-control asthma: the burden of illness. *Allergy and Asthma Proc.* 2010;31(5):381-384.

50. Osborne M, Pedula K, O'Hollaren M, et al. Assessing future need for acute care in adult asthmatics: the Profile of Asthma Risk Study: a prospective health maintenance organization-based study. *Chest.* 2007;132(4):1151-1161.

51. Mannino D, Homa DM, Redd SC. Involuntary smoking and asthma severity in children: data from the Third National Health and Nutrition Examination Survey. *Chest.* 2002;122(2):409-415.

52. Patel MM, Quinn JW, Jung KH, et al. Traffic density and stationary sources of air pollution associated with wheeze, asthma, and immunoglobulin E from birth to age 5 years among New York City children. *Environ Res.* 2011;111:1222-1229.

53. Cook AG, deVos A, Pereira G, Jardine A, Weinstein P. Use of a total traffic count metric to investigate the impact of roadways on asthma severity: a case-control study. *Environ Health.* 2011;10:52-59.

54. Chung KF, Zhang J, Zhong N. Outdoor air pollution and respiratory health in Asia. *Respirology.* 2011;16(7):1023-1026.

55. Li S, Batterman S, Wasilevich E, et al. Association of daily asthma emergency department visits and hospital admissions with ambient air pollutants among the pediatric Medicaid population in Detroit: time-series and time-stratified case-crossover analyses with threshold effects. *Environ Res.* 2011;111(8):1137-1147.

56. Belanger K, Gent JF, Triche EW, Bracken MB, Leaderer BP. Association of indoor nitrogen dioxide exposure with respiratory symptoms in children with asthma. *Am J Respir Crit Care Med.* 2006;173:297-303.

57. Garrett MH. Respiratory symptoms in children and indoor exposure to nitrogen dioxide and gas stoves. *Am J Respir Crit Care Med.* 1998;158(3):891-895.

58. Papadopoulos NG, Rhode G, Agache I, et al. Viruses and bacteria in acute asthma exacerbations: a GA(2) LEN-DARE systematic review. *Allergy.* 2011;66(4):458-468.

59. Greenberg H, Cohen RI. Nocturnal asthma. *Curr Opin Pulm Med.* 2012;18(1):57-62.

60. Gislason T, Janson C, Vermeire P, et al. Respiratory symptoms and nocturnal gastroesophageal reflux: a population-based study of young adults in three European countries. *Chest.* 2002;121:158-163.

61. Strunk RC, Sternberg AL, Bacharier LB, Szefler SJ. Nocturnal awakening caused by asthma in children with mild-to-moderate asthma in the Childhood Asthma Management Program. *J Allergy Clin Immunol.* 2002;110(3):395-403.

62. Civelek E, Cakir B, Orhan F, et al. Risk factors for current wheezing and its phenotypes among elementary school children. *Pediatr Pulmon.* 2011;46:166-174.

63. Stout JW, Visness CM, Enright P, et al. Classification of asthma severity in children: the contribution of pulmonary function testing. *Arch Pediatr Adolesc Med.* 2006;160(8):844-850.

64. Bacharier LB, Strunk RC, Mauger D, et al. Classifying asthma severity in children: mismatch between symptoms, medication use, and lung function. *Am J Respir Crit Care Med.* 2004;170(4):426-432.

65. Hankinson JL, Odencrantz JR, Fedan KB. Spirometric reference values from a sample of the general U.S. Population. *Am J Respir Crit Care Med.* 1999;159:179-187.

66. Stanojevic F, Wade A, Stocks J, et al. Reference ranges for spirometry across all ages: a new approach. *Am J Respir Crit Care Med.* 2008;177:253-260.

67. American Thoracic Society and European Respiratory Society Task Force, Pellegrino R, Viegi G, Brusasco V, et al. Standardization of lung function testing. *Eur Respir J.* 2005;26:948-968.

68. Pellegrino R, Viegi G, Brusasco V, et al. Interpretative strategies for lung function tests. *Eur Respir J.* 2005;26(5):948-968.

69. Swanney MP, Beckert LE, Frampton CM, Wallace LA, Jensen RL, Crapo RO. Validity of the American Thoracic Society and other spirometric algorithms using FVC and forced expiratory volume at 6 s for predicting a reduced total lung capacity. *Chest.* 2004;126(6):1861-1866.

70. Simon MR, Chinchilli VM, Phillips BR, et al. Forced expiratory flow between 25% and 75% of vital capacity and FEV1/forced vital capacity ratio in relation to clinical and physiological parameters in asthmatic children with normal FEV1 values. *J Allergy Clin Immunol.* 2010;126(3):527-534.

71. Anderson SD. Provocative challenges to help diagnose and monitor asthma: exercise, methacholine, adenosine, and mannitol. *Curr Opin Pulm Med.* 2008;14:39-45.

72. Cockroft DW. Direct challenge tests: airway hyperresponsiveness in asthma: its measurement and clinical significance. *Chest.* 2010;138:18S-24S.

73. Sinisgalli S, Collins MS, Schramm CM. Clinical features cannot distinguish allergic from non-allergic asthma in children. *J Asthma.* 2012;49(1):51-56.

74. Sethi JM, White AM, Patel SA, et al. Bronchoprovocation testing in asthma: effect on exhaled monoxides. *J. Breath Res.* 2010;4(4):047104.

75. Wadsworth SJ, Sin DD, Dorscheid DR. Clinical update on the use of biomarkers of airway inflammation in the management of asthma. *J Asthma Allergy.* 2011;4:77-86.

76. Petsky HL, Cates CJ, Li A, et al. Tailored interventions based on exhaled nitric oxide versus clinical symptoms for asthma in children and adults. *Cochrane Database Syst Rev.* 2009;4:1-41.

77. Kostikas K, Papaioannou AI, Tanou K, et al. Exhaled NO and exhaled breath condensate pH in the evaluation of asthma control. *Respir Med.* 2011;105(4):526-532.

78. Hoffmeyer F, Raulf-Heimsoth M, Bruning T. Exhaled breath condensate and airway inflammation. *Curr Opin Allergy Clin Immunol.* 2009;9(1):16-22.

79. Petsky HL, Kynaston JA, Turner C, et al. Tailored interventions based on sputum eosinophils versus clinical symptoms for asthma in children and adults. *Cochrane Database Syst Rev.* 2007;2:1-31.

80. Chalut DS, Ducharme FM, Davis GM. The Preschool Respiratory Assessment Measure (PRAM): a responsive index of acute asthma severity. *J Pediatr.* 2000;137(6):762-768.

81. Lugogo NJ, MacIntyre NR. Life-threatening asthma: pathophysiology and management. *Respir Care.* 2008;53(6):726-739.

82. Sala KA, Carroll CL, Tang YS, et al. Factors associated with the development of severe asthma exacerbations in children. *J Asthma.* 2011;48:558-564.

83. Bhogal SK, Zemek RL, Ducharme F. Written action plans for asthma in children. *Cochrane Database Syst Rev.* 2006;3:1-62.

84. Kamps AW, Roorda RJ, Brand PL.Peak flow diaries in childhood asthma are unreliable. *Thorax.* 2001;56(3):180-182.

85. Eid N, Yandell B, Howell L, Eddy M, Sheikh S. Can peak expiratory flow predict airflow obstruction in children with asthma? *Pediatrics.* 2000;105(2):354-358.

86. Wensley D, Silverman M. Peak flow monitoring for guided self-management in childhood asthma: a randomized controlled trial. *Am J Respir Crit Care Med.* 2004;170(6):606-612.

87. Koh MS, Tee A, Lasserson TJ, Irving LB. Inhaled corticosteroids compared to placebo for prevention of exercise induced bronchoconstriction. *Cochrane Database Syst Rev.* 2007;3:CD002739.

88. Spooner C, Spooner GR, Rowe BH. Mast-cell stabilising agents to prevent exercise-induced bronchoconstriction. *Cochrane Database Syst Rev.* 2003;4:CD002307.

89. Sharek PJ, Bergman D, Ducharme FM. Beclomethasone for asthma in children: effects on linear growth. *Cochrane Database Syst Rev.* 1999;3:1-26.

90. Adams NP, Bestall JC, Jones P. Beclomethasone versus budesonide for chronic asthma. *Cochrane Database Syst Rev.* 2000;1:1-209.

91. Manning P, Gibson PG, Lasserson TJ. Ciclesonide versus other inhaled steroids for chronic asthma in children and adults. *Cochrane Database Syst Rev.* 2008;2:1-124.

92. Powell H, Gibson PG. High dose versus low dose inhaled corticosteroid as initial starting dose for asthma in adults and children. *Cochrane Database Syst Rev.* 2003;(4):1-206.

93. Cates CJ, Bestall JC, Adams NP. Holding chambers versus nebulisers for inhaled steroids in chronic asthma. *Cochrane Database Syst Rev.* 2006;(1):1-29.

94. Sridhar AV, McKean MC. Nedocromil sodium for chronic asthma in children. *Cochrane Database Syst Rev.* 2006;(3):1-180.

95. van der Wouden JC, Uijen JHJM, Bernsen RMD, et al. Inhaled sodium cromoglycate for asthma in children. *Cochrane Database Syst Rev.* 2008;(4):1-68.

96. Guevara JP, Ducharme FM, Keren R, Nihtianova S, Zorc J. Inhaled corticosteroids versus sodium cromoglycate in children and adults with asthma. *Cochrane Database Syst Rev.* 2006;(2):1-85.

97. Gardenhire DS. *Rau's Respiratory Care Pharmacology.* St. Louis: Mosby-Elsevier; 2008.

98. Tee A, Koh MS, Gibson PG, et al. Long-acting beta-2-agonists versus theophylline for maintenance treatment of asthma. *Cochrane Database Syst Rev.* 2007;(3):1-40.

99. Seddon P, Bara A, Lasserson TJ, Ducharme FM. Oral xanthines as maintenance treatment for asthma in children. *Cochrane Database Syst Rev.* 2006;(1):1-169.

100. Abramson MJ, Puy RM, Weiner JM. Injection allergen immunotherapy for asthma. *Cochrane Database Syst Rev.* 2010;(8):1-116.

101. Walker S, Monteil M, Phelan K, Lasserson TJ, Walters EH. Anti-IgE for chronic asthma in adults and children. *Cochrane Database Syst Rev.* 2006;(2).

102. Bassler D, Mitra AAD, Ducharme FM, Forster J, Schwarzer G. Ketotifen alone or as additional medication for long-term control of asthma and wheeze in children. *Cochrane Database Syst Rev.* 2004;(1).

103. Cates CJ, Lasserson TJ. Combination formoterol and inhaled steroid versus beta2-agonist as relief medication for chronic asthma in adults and children. *Cochrane Database Syst Rev.* 2009;(1).

104. Ducharme FM, NiChroinin M, Greenstone I, Lasserson TJ. Addition of long-acting beta2-agonists to inhaled corticosteroids versus same dose inhaled corticosteroids for chronic asthma in adults and children. *Cochrane Database Syst Rev.* 2010;(5).

105. Walters EH, Walters JAE, Gibson PG. Regular treatment with long acting beta agonists versus daily regular treatment with short acting beta agonists in adults and children with stable asthma. *Cochrane Database Syst Rev.* 2002;(3).

106. Ducharme FM, Lasserson TJ, Cates CJ. Addition to inhaled corticosteroids of long-acting beta2-agonists versus anti-leukotrienes for chronic asthma. *Cochrane Database Syst Rev.* 2011;(5).

107. Gibson PG, Powell H, Ducharme FM. Long-acting beta2-agonists as an inhaled corticosteroid-sparing agent for chronic asthma in adults and children. *Cochrane Database Syst Rev.* 2005;(4).

108. Cates CJ, Cates MJ. Regular treatment with salmeterol for chronic asthma: serious adverse events. *Cochrane Database Syst Rev.* 2008;(3).

109. Cates CJ, Cates MJ, Lasserson TJ. Regular treatment with formoterol for chronic asthma: serious adverse events. *Cochrane Database Syst Rev.* 2008;(4).

110. Walters EH, Gibson PG, Lasserson TJ, Walters JAE. Long-acting beta2-agonists for chronic asthma in adults and children where background therapy contains varied or no inhaled corticosteroid. *Cochrane Database Syst Rev.* 2007;(1).

111. Ni Chroinin M, Greenstone I, Lasserson TJ, Ducharme FM. Addition of long-acting beta2-agonists to inhaled steroids as first line therapy for persistent asthma in steroid-naive adults and children. *Cochrane Database Syst Rev.* 2009;(4).

112. Cates CJ, Crilly JA, Rowe BH. Holding chambers (spacers) versus nebulisers for beta-agonist treatment of acute asthma. *Cochrane Database.* 2006;(2).

113. Israel E, Chinchilli VM, Ford JG, et al. National Heart, Lung, and Blood Institute's Asthma Clinical Research

Network. Use of regularly scheduled albuterol treatment in asthma: genotype-stratified, randomised, placebo-controlled cross-over trial. *Lancet.* 2004;364(9444):1505-1512.

114. McDonald N, Bara A, McKeanMC. Anticholinergic therapy for chronic asthma in children over two years of age. *Cochrane Database Syst Rev.* 2003;(1).

115. Welsh EJ, Cates CJ. Formoterol versus short-acting beta-agonists as relief medication for adults and children with asthma. *Cochrane Database Syst Rev.* 2010;(9).

116. Arnold E, Clark CE, Lasserson TJ, Wu T. Herbal interventions for chronic asthma in adults and children. *Cochrane Database Syst Rev.* 2008;(1).

117. Beausoleil JL, Fiedler J, Spergel JM. Food intolerance and childhood asthma: what is the link? *Pediatr Drugs.* 2007;9(3):157-163.

118. Vally H, Misso NLA, Madan V. Clinical effects of sulphite additives. *Clin Exp Allergy.* 2009;39:1643-1651.

119. Pogson Z, McKeever T. Dietary sodium manipulation and asthma. *Cochrane Database Syst Rev* 2011,(3).

120. Schwartz J, Weiss ST. Relationship between dietary vitamin C intake and pulmonary function in the First National Health and Nutrition Examination Survey (NHANES I). *Am J Clin Nutr.* 1994;59(1):110-114.

121. Aderele WI, Ette SI, Oduwole O, Ikpeme SJ. Plasma vitamin C (ascorbic acid) levels in asthmatic children. *Afr J Med Med Sci.* 1985;14(3-4):115-120.

122. Green S, Buchbinder R, Barnsley L, et al. Acupuncture for lateral elbow pain. *Cochrane Database Syst Rev.* 2002,(1).

123. McCarney RW, Brinkhaus B, Lasserson TJ, Linde K. Acupuncture for chronic asthma. *Cochrane Database Syst Rev.* 2003;(3).

124. Hondras MA, Linde K, Jones AP. Manual therapy for asthma. *Cochrane Database Syst Rev.* 2005;(2).

125. Holloway EA, Ram FSF. Breathing exercises for asthma. *Cochrane Database Syst Rev.* 2004;(1).

126. Ram FSF, Robinson S, Black PN, Picot J. Physical training for asthma. *Cochrane Database Syst Rev.* 2005;(4).

127. Koster ES, Raaijmakers JA, Vijverberg SJH, van der Ent CK, Maitland-van der Zee A. Asthma symptoms in pediatric patients: differences throughout the seasons. *J Asthma.* 2011;48:694-700.

128. Gorelick M, Scribano PV, Stevens MW, Schultz T, Shuts J. Predicting need for hospitalizations in acute pediatric asthma. *Pediatr Emerg Care.* 2008;24(11):735-742.

129. Mannix R, Bachur R. Status asthmaticus in children. *Curr Opin Pediatr.* 2007;19:281-287.

130. Sabato K, Hanson JH. Mechanical ventilation for children with status asthmaticus. *Respir Care Clin N Am.* 2000;6:171-188.

131. Schramm CM, Carroll CL. Advances in treating acute asthma exacerbations in children. *Curr Opin Pediatr.* 2009;21:326-332.

132. Camargo CA Jr, Spooner C, Rowe BH. Continuous versus intermittent beta-agonists for acute asthma. *Cochrane Database Syst Rev.* 2003;(4).

133. Ackerman AD. Continuous nebulization of inhaled beta-agonists for status asthmaticus in children: a cost-effective therapeutic advance? *Crit Care Med.* 1993;21:1422-1424.

134. Cairns CB. Acute asthma exacerbations: phenotypes and management. *Clin Chest Med.* 2006;27:99-108

135. Papiris SA, Manali ED, Kolilekas L, Triantafillidou C, Tsangaris I. Acute severe asthma: new approaches to assessment and treatment. *Drugs.* 2009;69(17):2363-2391.

136. Chiang VW, Burns JP, Rifai N, et al. Cardiac toxicity of intravenous terbutaline for the treatment of severe asthma in children: a prospective assessment. *J Pediatr.* 2000;137:73-77.

137. Jones AP, Camargo CAJ, Rowe BH. Inhaled beta2-agonists for asthma in mechanically ventilated patients. *Cochrane Database Syst Rev.* 2001;(4).

138. Sherman MS, Verceles AC, Lang D. Systemic steroids for the treatment of acute asthma: where do we stand? *Clin Pulm Med.* 2006;13:315-320.

139. Rowe BH, Spooner C, Ducharme FM, et al. Early emergency department treatment of acute asthma with systemic corticosteroids. *Cochrane Database Syst Rev.* 2001;(1).

140. Rowe BH, Spooner CH, Ducharme FM, Bretzlaff JA, Bota GW. Corticosteroids for preventing relapse following acute exacerbations of asthma. *Cochrane Database Syst Rev.* 2007;(3).

141. Smith M, Iqbal SMSI, Rowe BH, N'Diaye T. Corticosteroids for hospitalised children with acute asthma. *Cochrane Database Syst Rev.* 2003;(1).

142. Plotnick L, Ducharme F. Combined inhaled anticholinergics and beta2-agonists for initial treatment of acute asthma in children. *Cochrane Database Syst Rev.* 2000;(3).

143. Rowe BH, Bretzlaff J, Bourdon C, et al. Magnesium sulfate for treating exacerbations of acute asthma in the emergency department. *Cochrane Database Syst Rev.* 2000;(1).

144. Rowe BH, Camargo CA. The role of magnesium sulfate in the acute and chronic management of asthma. *Curr Opin Pulm Med.* 2008;14:70-76.

145. Blitz M, Blitz S, Beasely R, et al. Inhaled magnesium sulfate in the treatment of acute asthma. *Cochrane Database Syst Rev.* 2005;(4).

146. Gontijo-Amaral C, Ribeiro MA, Gontijo LS, et al. Oral magnesium supplementation in asthmatic children: a double-blind randomized placebo controlled trial. *Eur J Clin Nutr.* 2007;61:54-60.

147. Carmargo CA, Smithline HA, Malice MP, et al. A randomized controlled trial of intravenous montelukast in acute asthma. *Am J Respir Crit Care Med.* 2003;167:528-533.

148. Dockhorn RJ, Baumgartner RA, Leff JA, et al. Comparison of the effects of intravenous and oral montelukast on airway function: a double blind, placebo controlled, three period, crossover study in asthmatic patients. *Thorax.* 2000;55:260-265.

149. Silverman RA, Nowak RM, Korenblat PE, et al. Zafirlukast treatment for acute asthma: evaluation in a randomised, double-blind, multicenter trial. *Chest.* 2004;126:1480-1489.

150. Boyd M, Lasserson TJ, McKean MC, Gibson PG, Ducharme FM, Haby M. Interventions for educating children who are at risk of asthma-related emergency department attendance. *Cochrane Database Syst Rev.* 2009;(2).

151. Rowe BH, Spooner C, Ducharme F, Bretzlaff J, Bota G. Corticosteroids for preventing relapse following acute exacerbations of asthma. *Cochrane Database Syst Rev.* 2007;(3).

152. Edmonds M, Brenner BE, Camargo CA, Rowe BH. Inhaled steroids for acute asthma following emergency department discharge. *Cochrane Database Syst Rev.* 2000;(3).

153. Files DC, Patel N, Gabretsadik T, Moore PE, Sheller J. A retrospective characterization of African and European American asthmatic children in a pediatric critical care unit. *J Natl Med Assoc.* 2009;101(11):1119-1124.

154. American Thoracic Society, European Respiratory Society, the European Society of Intensive Care Medicine,

and the Société de Réanimation de Langue Francaise. International Consensus Conferences in Intensive Care Medicine: noninvasive positive pressure ventilation in acute respiratory failure. *Am J Respir Crit Care Med.* 2001;163:283-291.

155. Soroksky A, Stav D, Shpirer I. A pilot prospective, randomized, placebo controlled trial of bilevel positive airway pressure in acute asthmatic attack. *Chest.* 2003; 123:1018-1025

156. Beers SL, Abramo TJ, Bracken A, Wiebe RA. Bilevel positive airway pressure in the treatment of status asthmaticus in pediatrics. *Am J Emerg Med.* 2007;25:6-9.

157. Williams AM, Abramo TJ, Shah MV, et al. Safety and clinical findings of BiPAP utilization in children 20 kg or less for asthma exacerbations. *Intensive Care Med.* 2011; 37:1338-1343.

158. Frazier MD, Cheifetz IM. The role of heliox in paediatric respiratory disease. *Paediatr Respir Rev.* 2010;11:46-53.

159. Gluck EH, Onoranto DJ, Castriotta R. Helium-oxygen mixtures in intubated patients with status asthmaticus and respiratory acidosis. *Chest.* 1990;98(3):693-698.

160. Anderson M, Svartengren M, Bylin G, Philipson K, Camner P. Deposition in asthmatics of particles inhaled in air or in helium oxygen. *Am Rev Respir Dis.* 1993; 147(3):524-528.

161. Reuben AD, Harris AR. Heliox for asthma in the emergency department: a review of the literature. *Emerg Med J.* 2004;21(2):131-135.

162. Rodrigo GJ, Pollack CV, Rodrigo C, Rowe BH. Heliox for non-intubated acute asthma patients. *Cochrane Database Syst Rev.* 2006;(4).

163. Bratton SL, Newth CJL, Zuppa AF, et al. Critical care for pediatric asthma: wide care variability and challenges for study. *Pediatr Crit Care Med.* 2012;13(4):1-8.

164. Carroll CL, Smith SR, Collins MS, Bhandari A, Schramm CM, Zucker AR. Endotracheal intubation and pediatric status asthmaticus: site of original care affects treatment. *Pediatr Crit Care Med.* 2007;8(2):91-95.

165. Deho A, Lutman D, Montgomery M, Petros A, Ramnarayan P. Emergency management of children with acute severe asthma requires transfer to intensive care. *Emerg Med J.* 2010;27:834-837.

166. Werner HA. Status asthmaticus in children: a review. *Chest.* 2001;(119):1913-1929.

167. Zimmerman JL, Dellinger RP, Shah AN, et al. Endotracheal intubation and mechanical ventilation in severe asthma. *Crit Care Med.* 1993;21:1727-1730.

168. Nehama J, Pass R, Bechtler-Karsch A, Steinberg C. Continuous ketamine infusion for the treatment of refractory asthma in a mechanically ventilated infant: case report and review of the pediatric literature. *Pediatr Emerg Care.* 1996;12:294-297.

169. Carroll CL, Zucker AR. Barotrauma not related to type of positive pressure ventilation during severe asthma exacerbations in children. *J Asthma.* 2008;(5):421-424.

170. Slutsky AS. Mechanical ventilation. *Chest.* 1993;104: 1833-1859.

171. Saranaik AP, Daphtary KM, Meert KL, Lieh-lai MW, Heidemann SM. Pressure-controlled ventilation in children with severe status asthmaticus. *Pediatr Crit Care Med.* 2004;5(2):133-138.

172. Hebbar KB, Petrillo-Albarano T, Coto-Puckett W, Heard M, Rycus PT, Fortenberry JD. Experience with use of extracorporeal life support for severe refractory status asthmaticus in children. *Crit Care.* 2009;13(2).

173. Shankar V, Churchwell KB, Deshpande JK. Isoflurane therapy for severe refractory status asthmaticus in children. *Intensive Care Med.* 2006;32:927-933.

174. Flores G, Abreu M, Tomany-Korman S, Meurer J. Keeping children with asthma out of hospitals: parents' and physicians' perspective on how pediatric asthma hospitalizations can be prevented. *Pediatrics.* 2005;116(4): 957-967.

175. Cates CJ, Jefferson T, Rowe BH. Vaccines for preventing influenza in people with asthma. *Cochrane Database Syst Rev.* 2008;(2):CD000364.

176. Fuhrman C, Dubus J, Marguet C, et al. Hospitalizations for asthma in children are linked to undertreatment and insufficient asthma education. *J Asthma.* 2011;48: 565-571.

177. Knudson A, Casey M, Burlew M, Davidson G. Disparities in pediatric asthma hospitalizations. *J Public Health Manag Pract.* 2009;15(3):232-237.

178. Mochizuki H, Muramatsu R, Hagiwara S, Takami S, Misuno T, Arakawa H. Relationship between bronchial hyperreactivity and asthma remission during adolescence. *Ann Allergy Asthma Immunol.* 2009;103:201-205.

Chapter 14

Cystic Fibrosis

Peter Mogayzel Jr., MD, PhD, MBA
Holly Loosen, PT
Karen Von Berg, PT
Andrea L Honesto, BS, RRT

Key Terms

Active cycle of breathing
Allergic bronchopulmonary
  aspergillosis (ABPA)
Autogenic drainage (AD)
Breath-actuated nebulizer
Breath-enhanced nebulizer
Cystic fibrosis transmembrane
  conductance regulator gene
  (CFTR)
Forced expiratory technique
Hemoptysis
High-frequency chest wall
  oscillation (HFCWO)
Inhaled antibiotics
Intrapulmonary percussive drainage
Lung transplantation
Meconium ileus
Mucolytics
Newborn screening
Pancreatic insufficiency
Percussion
Pilocarpine iontophoresis
Pleurodesis
Positive expiratory pressure (PEP)
Postural drainage
Pulmonary exacerbation
Vibration

Chapter Objectives

After reading this chapter, you will be able to:

1. Identify the two major body systems affected by cystic fibrosis and the subsequent clinical manifestations that affect them.
2. Describe the process for screening and diagnosing cystic fibrosis.
3. Describe six methods of airway clearance available for patients with cystic fibrosis.
4. Recommend inhaled therapies for a patient with cystic fibrosis based on clinical signs and symptoms.
5. Create a daily treatment schedule for a patient with cystic fibrosis.
6. Identify common organisms that contribute to pulmonary exacerbations.
7. List several common complications that manifest during the progression of cystic fibrosis.

■■ Ryan Greb

You are the respiratory therapist working at a pulmonary outpatient clinic associated with a large pediatric hospital. You are preparing for an initial appointment with a new patient. Ryan is a 4-week-old boy who has been diagnosed with cystic fibrosis (CF). The diagnosis was made after Ryan had a "positive" newborn screening test for CF, and he was referred for a sweat test by his pediatrician. The sweat test confirmed the diagnosis of CF.

Cystic Fibrosis

Cystic fibrosis (CF) is a genetic disease characterized by progressive obstructive lung disease resulting from abnormal ion transport in the airway epithelium. The accumulation of viscous secretions leads to obstruction of small airways and chronic infection and inflammation.

Cystic fibrosis is the most common life-shortening genetic disease in Caucasians. It affects approximately 1 in 3,200 Caucasians but is less common in Hispanics and African Americans (1). CF is an autosomal recessive disease caused by mutations in both copies of the **cystic fibrosis transmembrane conductance regulator (CFTR)** gene. Mutations in the *CFTR* gene are classified based on their molecular consequences (Table 14-1). Parents of a child with CF are asymptomatic carriers of a single *CFTR* gene mutation. Approximately 1 in 25 Caucasians carry a *CFTR* gene mutation. The incidence of CF is the same in males and females (1).

Historically, CF has been thought of exclusively as a pediatric disease because individuals with CF typically did not survive into adulthood. However, this is no longer the case. Improvements in therapy have increased the median life expectancy of individuals with CF beyond 38 years (Fig. 14-1) (2). In fact, it is estimated that there will be more adults than

Class	Abnormality	Example
1	CFTR is not synthesized	W1282X*
2	CFTR is synthesized but does not reach the cell surface	F508del
3	CFTR reaches the cell surface but is not activated normally	G551D
4	CFTR reaches the cell surface, but chloride conductance is abnormal	R117H
5	Reduced CFTR synthesis so that less CFTR is at the cell surface	A445E
6	CFTR at the cell surface is less stable	

Table 14-1 Classes of *CFTR* Mutations

Adapted from Zielenski and Tsui (15).

*The number in the mutations designates the location of the change in the protein. The letter before the number is the expected amino acid, and the letter after the number is the mutated amino acid. A similar nomenclature exists for mutations that occur outside of the *CFTR* coding region.

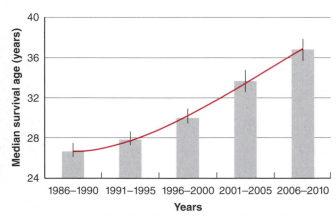

Figure 14-1 Median Predicted Survival for Patients With CF Living in the United States *(From the* 2010 Patient Registry Report, *CF Foundation, Bethesda, MD; with permission)*

children with CF in the United States at the time of publication of this book. This improvement in outcome is thanks to an aggressive approach to pulmonary care and nutritional support provided by multidisciplinary teams at specialized care centers. This strategy has been the cornerstone of CF care that has led to the improvement in survival.

Pathophysiology

Cystic fibrosis is caused by mutations in the *CFTR* gene, which encodes a chloride channel that resides on the surface of airway epithelial cells (3). The lack of chloride secretion into the airway is coupled with excess removal of sodium from the airway lumen (4). The alteration in ion transport leads to dehydration of the liquid layer that coats the lining of the airways. The resulting dehydrated airway surface liquid is thought to impair mucociliary clearance, which is a major airway defense mechanism (5). The accumulation of secretions and loss of airway defenses leads to the colonization of the airways with characteristic bacteria such as *Staphylococcus aureus* and *Pseudomonas aeruginosa*. Approximately 80% of patients eventually become infected with *P. aeruginosa* (Fig. 14-2) (2). The acquisition of certain pathogens such as *P. aeruginosa, Burkholderia cepacia,* and methicillin-resistant *Staphylococcus aureus* (MRSA) are associated with a faster rate of lung function decline and increased mortality (6–8). The airway obstruction and persistent infection present in the CF airway is associated with chronic inflammation. This ongoing inflammation eventually leads to bronchiectasis and parenchymal damage.

Disease-causing mutations in the *CFTR* gene are classified based on the resulting molecular defect (Table 14-1). Although more than 1,900 mutations in the *CFTR* gene have been identified, not all of these mutations cause disease (9). The most common *CFTR* mutation is F508del, which results in production of a protein missing a phenylalanine (abbreviated F) at position 508 of the protein (3). This abnormal protein is misfolded and does not reach the cell surface (10). *CFTR* gene mutations are often described as "mild" or "severe" based on whether they are associated with the absence or presence of pancreatic insufficiency (see the discussion of gastrointestinal manifestations below). Those mutations that have residual chloride transport are associated with milder disease.

Clinical Manifestations

The defective chloride transport that occurs in CF leads to manifestations in many organ systems (Fig.14-3).

Gastrointestinal Manifestations

Gastrointestinal manifestations of CF are common. Approximately 10% to 15% of patients present with bowel obstruction from the failure to pass meconium after birth (2). This condition, known as **meconium ileus**, is a life-threatening complication that often requires surgical intervention.

The vast majority of patients with CF are **pancreatic insufficient**, meaning that the pancreas does not secrete an adequate amount of enzyme to digest food appropriately. Symptoms of this resulting malabsorption include abnormal stools that can be greasy, oily, bulky, or foul smelling; increased bowel gas; and failure to thrive. Treatment with pancreatic enzyme supplements improves absorption and allows for adequate growth. Pancreatic enzyme replacement must be taken with every meal and snack to ensure adequate nutrient and calorie absorption. Even with the use of pancreatic enzyme replacement therapy, patients with CF have increased calorie needs that can be 1.5 to 2 times that of unaffected children (11).

The importance of maintaining adequate nutrition in patients with CF has been reinforced by the observation that children with a higher body mass

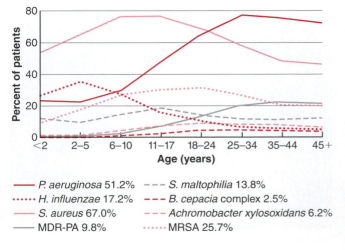

Line	Organism	Prevalence
——	*P. aeruginosa*	51.2%
⋯⋯	*H. influenzae*	17.2%
——	*S. aureus*	67.0%
——	MDR-PA	9.8%
– – –	*S. maltophilia*	13.8%
– – –	*B. cepacia* complex	2.5%
– – –	*Achromobacter xylosoxidans*	6.2%
⋯⋯	MRSA	25.7%

Figure 14-2 Prevalence of Bacteria Cultured From Airway Secretions of Patients With CF *(From the* 2010 Patient Registry Report, *CF Foundation, Bethesda, MD; with permission)*

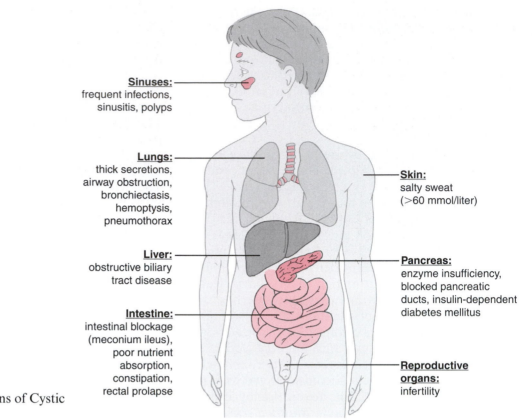

Sinuses:
frequent infections,
sinusitis, polyps

Lungs:
thick secretions,
airway obstruction,
bronchiectasis,
hemoptysis,
pneumothorax

Skin:
salty sweat
(>60 mmol/liter)

Liver:
obstructive biliary
tract disease

Pancreas:
enzyme insufficiency,
blocked pancreatic
ducts, insulin-dependent
diabetes mellitus

Intestine:
intestinal blockage
(meconium ileus),
poor nutrient
absorption,
constipation,
rectal prolapse

**Reproductive
organs:**
infertility

Figure 14-3 Manifestations of Cystic
Fibrosis

index (BMI) have better lung function (Fig.14-4)
(11). Although these data do not demonstrate a
causal relationship, it suggests that patients should
strive to maintain a normal BMI.

Pulmonary Manifestations

Obstruction of the small airways by viscous secretions is associated with infection and inflammation
that eventually lead to bronchiectasis and mucus
plugging (Figs. 14-5 and 14-6). Infants and young
children with CF typically have few, if any, respiratory symptoms when adequately treated. However,
ongoing airway damage eventually leads to chronic
cough and sputum production. The progression to

chronic respiratory symptoms varies and cannot be
easily predicted. The inability to forecast the timing
of the development of future respiratory problems
can be very stressful for families. Although older children with worse lung function tend to have more
cough and sputum production, these symptoms can

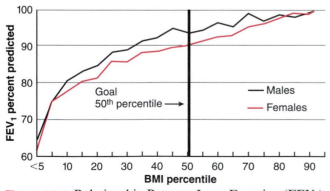

Figure 14-4 Relationship Between Lung Function (FEV$_1$)
and Nutritional Status Measured by Body Mass Index
(BMI) *(From the 2010 Patient Registry Report, CF Foundation,
Bethesda, MD; with permission)*

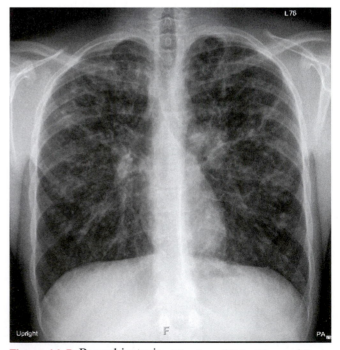

Figure 14-5 Bronchiectasis *(Courtesy of Peter Mogayzel Jr.
MD, PhD, MBA)*

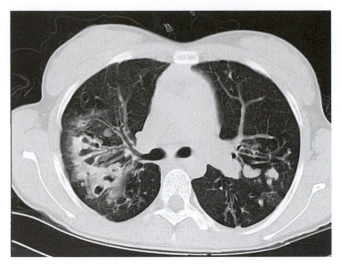

Figure 14-6 Bronchiectasis CT Scan *(Courtesy of Peter Mogayzel Jr. MD, PhD, MBA)*

begin at any age and are not necessarily associated with a significant lung function testing abnormalities.

The widespread use of newborn screening for CF provides the opportunity to begin preventive therapies before respiratory symptoms develop. The goal of therapy is directed toward the prevention of lung damage and maintenance of appropriate weight gain.

As children age, they eventually develop routine cough and sputum production. Physical examination can reveal crackles. A significant proportion of children with CF periodically wheeze because of airway hyperreactivity. This asthma phenotype, which is responsive to albuterol, is quite common in patients with CF. Allergic bronchopulmonary aspergillosis (ABPA) is another source of wheezing in patients with CF (see the section on allergic bronchopulmonary aspergillosis later in this chapter, and Case 3 at the end of the chapter).

Radiology studies can be helpful in monitoring the progression of lung disease. Chest radiographs (Fig. 14-5) or computed tomography (CT) scans (Fig. 14-6) can demonstrate bronchiectasis and mucus plugging. Radiological changes are heterogeneous and are often first observed in the upper lobes. Pulmonary function testing is routinely used to monitor the progression of CF lung disease. Most clinicians focus on the forced expiratory volume in 1 second (FEV_1) because this is the parameter that best correlates with mortality (12).

Other Manifestations

Some degree of sinus disease is universal in children with CF; however, patients can experience a wide range of symptoms. Sinus CT scans will invariably demonstrate some degree of sinus involvement. Therefore, therapy is typically based on symptoms rather than radiological findings. Nasal polyps and hypertrophic mucosa are very common in children with CF. As in the lungs, thick secretions lead to chronic bacterial colonization and recurrent infections. Chronic

therapy with saline irrigation and topical steroids is often successful in managing nasal symptoms. However, surgical intervention may be needed for patients with unremitting symptoms or evidence of bony polyps or other complications.

Alterations in biliary secretions often lead to bile duct obstruction and mild liver function abnormalities. Severe cholestatic liver disease leads to liver cirrhosis and portal hypertension in 3% to 5% of patients with CF (2). Male infertility as a result of congenital bilateral absence of the vas deferens is essentially universal.

Diagnosis

Newborn screening for CF is performed in all 50 states in the United States and in many countries around the world. The newborn screening test identifies infants that *may* have CF; however, not all infants with a positive newborn screen actually have CF. Infants with a positive newborn screening test must have additional testing to definitively make a diagnosis of CF.

Pilocarpine iontophoresis, commonly known as a "sweat test," is the gold standard for diagnosing CF (13). This test measures the amount of chloride in the sweat. The lack of CFTR in the sweat duct prevents the reabsorption of secreted chloride, which leads to increased chloride content in the sweat of patients with CF (14).

The diagnosis of CF can also be made by the detection of two disease-causing *CFTR* gene mutations. Genetic testing is usually performed using panels of common *CFTR* gene mutations. Testing for the most common 23 to 32 mutations in the United States will detect approximately 90% of Caucasians with CF (13). However, the rate of detection is lower for other ethnic groups, in whom less common *CFTR* gene mutations may predominate. Sequencing of the entire *CFTR* gene is commercially available and may be appropriate for diagnosis in some cases. Nasal potential difference (NPD) testing is a technique that measures salt transport in the nasal epithelial cells. This test is very sensitive when detecting abnormalities in chloride transport, and it can be used to diagnose CF (13). However, NPD testing is only available at a limited number of CF research centers.

■■ When Ryan comes to his first CF clinic appointment, he has no respiratory symptoms. However, he has trouble gaining weight and has greasy, foul-smelling stools that suggest malabsorption.

Management and Treatment

Preventive management of CF includes routine care, screening, and prevention through outpatient clinic visits. The current clinical care guidelines recommended by the Cystic Fibrosis Foundation are found in Box 14-1.

Annual Care, Screening, and Prevention Guidelines

- Four or more clinic visits per year
- Four or more respiratory cultures
- Two or more PFTs if 6 years of age or older and physically able
- An influenza vaccine if 6 months of age or older
- Measurement of fat-soluble vitamin levels
- An oral glucose tolerance test if 10 years of age or older
- Measurement of liver enzymes in the blood

Pulmonary management of CF relies on daily prescribed management to improve airway clearance and lung function, as well as early treatment of any pulmonary infections or exacerbations to prevent permanent declines in lung function and quality of life. Daily therapy includes airway clearance techniques, exercise, inhalation therapies, and infection control. Treatment of pulmonary infections and exacerbations includes many of the same techniques, but will require an increase in the timing or mode of therapy to improve symptoms and clear the offending cause.

Airway Clearance

Airway clearance techniques (ACTs) are an essential part of the daily treatment and management for individuals with CF (Table 14-2). Airway clearance is typically performed in conjunction with inhalation therapies (discussed later in this chapter). As noted previously, CF airways produce an excessive amount of thick, sticky mucus that is difficult to mobilize and that impairs mucociliary clearance. The inability to

easily transport mucus up and out of the airways puts patients at higher risk for respiratory infection and airway inflammation.

ACTs enhance secretion mobilization and thereby minimize airway obstruction, infection, and inflammation. Improving ventilation and using expiratory airflow are the keys to a good airway clearance strategy. Many different treatment techniques can be employed, and the decision to use a particular strategy should be based on clinical findings as well as the patient's preference. Systematic reviews have established the short-term effectiveness of various ACTs but have not found conclusive evidence to suggest that one strategy is superior to the others (16, 17). (Evidence in Practice 14-1)

Postural Drainage, Percussion, and Vibration

The most common form of airway clearance for infants in the United States includes **postural drainage**, **percussion**, and **vibration** (2). Postural drainage uses gravity to mobilize mucus from different lung segments. Patients are positioned to anatomically target specific lung segments and drain mucus from the lung periphery into the more central airways. Traditional postural drainage uses 6 to 12 different positions that tip the head and chest downward to drain mucus from the lung fields. This technique can be modified for any patient, regardless of age or disease severity. The *modified technique,* which is more commonly used, employs 4 to 6 positions that don't tip the head and chest downward (Fig. 14-7) (21).

Percussion is performed over the lung segment being drained to loosen mucus from the airway walls. The technique involves cupping the hands and rhythmically clapping over the chest wall. The frequency of clapping transmits an energy wave that

Table 14-2 General Guidelines for Age-Appropriateness of ACT

ACT	Infants	Toddlers	Preschoolers	School-age	Adolescents and Teenagers	Young Adults
Postural drainage, percussion, and vibration	M	M	Y	Y	Y	Y
HFCWO	N	Y	Y	Y	Y	Y
ACBT	N	N	Y	Y	Y	Y
PEP	M	M	Bubble PEP	Y	Y	Y
Oscillating PEP	N	N	As adjunct	Y	Y	Y
Autogenic drainage	M	M	M	Y	Y	Y
Breathing games	N	Y	Y	Y	Y	Y
IPV	N	N	N	Y	Y	Y
Exercise	Y	Y	Y	Y	Y	Y

Y indicates yes; N, no; M, modified technique can be employed.

When to Begin Airway Clearance

The wide availability of newborn screening for CF means that the patients are now often diagnosed prior to the onset of overt pulmonary disease. The question of whether to begin ACT with a newly diagnosed infant is a topic of much discussion in the international CF community. Clinicians favoring the "wait to treat" viewpoint argue that ACT should be delayed until the infant begins to show respiratory symptoms. They would argue that treatment at an early age is an unnecessary burden for the family and that aggressively performed ACT, such as percussion and vibration, may evoke a negative response in the infant. Potential side effects such as gastrointestinal reflux and overstimulation could be detrimental to the infant's overall health.

On the pro side of the early initiation of ACT argument is that preserving lung function in infants with CF is one of the primary goals of disease management. Advocates for commencing airway clearance at diagnosis point to studies demonstrating the presence of lung damage prior to the onset of any clinical symptoms. For example, bronchoalveolar lavage (BAL) studies in infants with CF with stable and or clinically mild lung disease found inflammatory changes in even the first weeks of life (18). The CF clinics in Australia introduced a microbiological surveillance program using bronchoscopy and BAL annually on infants and young children with CF until they are able to expectorate sputum (19). These investigators found that although 84% of the infants were asymptomatic, 21% of infants diagnosed with CF by newborn screening were infected on BAL at diagnosis. Sly et al (19) also demonstrated abnormal radiographic abnormalities indicative of lung disease in 81% of the 57 infants with CF with a median age of 3.6 months. Even more concerning is the fact that these lesions progressed over time (20). Thus, it is clear that the lungs may be undergoing damage before the first clinical symptoms appear. Initiating ACT from the time of diagnosis also enables the family to establish a routine from the start. This builds a solid foundation and establishes the importance of ACT as a therapy that will be part of everyday life for every child with CF.

Advocates of early institution of airway clearance argue that the benefits far outweigh the risks. Overall the evidence supports the argument for earlier intervention because symptoms alone cannot predict the damage occurring in the infant's airways. Infants cannot be traditionally tested for lung function, and specialized tests are not readily available to all patients. Therefore, many feel it is best to aggressively treat and prophylactically assist with airway clearance and infection prevention.

loosens mucus from the airway walls. The action is similar to the effect created when you clap the bottom of a ketchup bottle to get the liquid flowing.

Vibration is generated by gently shaking the chest wall during expiration with your hands or a mechanical device. This helps mobilize secretions by oscillating the airways and increasing expiratory flow rates.

These techniques can be used at any age, and they can focus treatment on the problematic lung segments. The disadvantages of postural drainage, percussion, and vibration are that they cannot be performed independently because they require a caregiver to perform them, and they take a long time to adequately treat all lung segments. Airway clearance in individuals with gastroesophageal reflux (GER), which is common in patients with CF, can potentially cause more harm than good. Evidence suggests that the effects of postural drainage are detrimental for people with GER (21) because airway inflammation can result from aspiration of acidic stomach contents into the airways. This problem has been well studied in young children. For example, a long-term study demonstrated statistically greater lung function decline and radiological changes by age 5 years in children with GER using head-tilted-down postural drainage positions versus children who did not (21). For this reason, modified postural drainage positions that do not tip the child's head down are now the standard of practice when using manual percussion and drainage in all children with CF who are younger than 2 years. Some evidence also suggests that head-down positioning in older children and teenagers with CF can also aggravate GER, but there is no conclusive evidence in adults (22). Based on the current evidence, many clinicians have stopped employing head-down postural drainage positioning in any patient with CF.

Additional airway clearance options for infants include modified autogenic drainage and infant positive expiratory pressure, both of which are discussed later in this chapter.

High-Frequency Chest Wall Oscillation

Maintaining a regular airway clearance program for toddlers can pose a problem for many parents. Toddlers are developing their sense of independence and adventure and often do not like to be contained for ACTs. They may resist the efforts of the caregiver to provide treatment and may not sit still for modified postural drainage and percussion. Families sometimes express concern over not being able to provide adequate treatment to their child. One possible solution to this dilemma is the use of **high-frequency chest wall oscillation (HFCWO)**, which uses an inflatable jacket with an air pulse generator that rapidly fills and deflates the jacket at a set pressure. Both frequency and pressure are adjustable. Examples

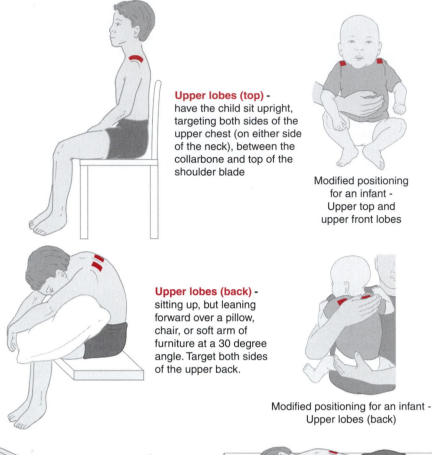

Upper lobes (top) - have the child sit upright, targeting both sides of the upper chest (on either side of the neck), between the collarbone and top of the shoulder blade

Modified positioning for an infant - Upper top and upper front lobes

Upper lobes (back) - sitting up, but leaning forward over a pillow, chair, or soft arm of furniture at a 30 degree angle. Target both sides of the upper back.

Modified positioning for an infant - Upper lobes (back)

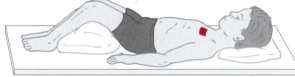

Upper lobes (front) - have child lay on back with arms to side. Standing at child's head, target between the collarbone and nipple.

Lower lobes (back) - have child lay on stomach. Target lower ribs just above lower edge of rib cage on both sides, avoiding the spine.

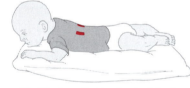

Modified positioning for an infant - Lower lobes (back).

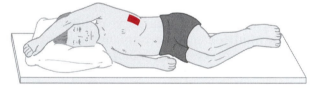

Middle lobes (left and right side front) - have child lie on left side with right arm above head. Target lower ribs, just below nipple area. Repeat on opposite side.

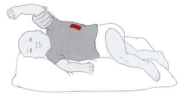

Modified positioning for an infant - Left and right side (front and back, lower and upper).

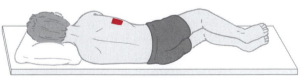

Lower lobes (side) - have child lie on left side, and turn a quarter turn toward his or her stomach. Target lower right side of chest, just above bottom of rib cage. Repeat on opposite side.

Figure 14-7 Postural Drainage for Infants and Children. Positions for modified postural drainage, percussion, and vibration. Note the modified body positioning for infants and toddlers.

of HFCWO include the SmartVest (Electromed, New Prague, MN); The Vest (Hill-Rom, Batesville, IN); and the inCourage System (RespirTech, St. Paul, MN) (Fig. 14-8). The oscillations and increased expiratory flow rate in HFCWO act like mini-huffs or coughs to shear the mucus off the airway wall and move secretions up the airways. The oscillation frequency can be programmed from 6 to 25 times per second to create increased expiratory flow rates in the airways.

HFCWO has also been shown to alter mucus properties by thinning secretions and decreasing spinnability as well as improving the amplitude of the ciliary beat (23). It has been postulated that a resonance phenomenon occurs when the excitatory vibration matches a system's own natural frequency of vibration and amplifies it. Research supports that resonance occurs when the HFCWO frequency matches the patient's own ciliary beat frequency. Improved ciliary beat amplitude can effectively assist the impaired mucociliary transport found in CF.

Settings for HFCWO are selected based on how the individual responds to the therapy. The pressure should be set as high as tolerated for each chosen frequency. There are several approaches to selecting the right frequency for a patient's HFCWO. One approach is to use a constant frequency in an attempt to match the individual's ciliary beat frequency. Another approach is to alter frequencies from low to high to dislodge the mucus at slower speeds before whipping it up and out the airway with the faster oscillations. Patient responses will differ, so it is important to try comfortable settings to determine the best individual outcomes.

HFCWO is a treatment that can be used throughout the life span and fosters independence and consistency with technique delivery. It is also an excellent technique for patients who are too weak, sick, or young to perform other breathing techniques or

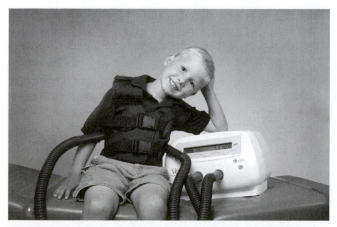

Figure 14-8 High-Frequency Chest Wall Oscillation Device *(From Johns Hopkins University, www.hopkinscf.org; with permission)*

strategies. HFCWO can be introduced as soon as children are large enough to fit into a jacket. Toddlers can sit for their treatment or move around within a limited radius near the machine. Toddlers are at a good age for introducing the unit because they typically enjoy sensory and vestibular stimulation, and their curiosity is piqued with the sensation of HFCWO. Care must be taken to ensure that the heads of young children are stabilized during therapy to avoid any threat of head injury from the vigorous chest wall oscillations.

Another advantage of HFCWO is that it is independent of positioning and technique. Once the correct settings are programmed, the machine will give consistent care every time, whereas other techniques are more dependent on patient or caregiver effort and technique. HFCWO can be a good fit for younger children who are often too distractible to stay on task or to be consistent with technique performance. Once begun, HFCWO can also be used throughout childhood and into adulthood. Settings should be reevaluated periodically to make sure that patients are receiving the maximum benefit as they age.

Forced Expiratory Technique and Active Cycle of Breathing

Preschoolers usually follow the same routine as toddlers, but new therapies such as **forced expiratory technique (FET)** and **active cycle of breathing (ACB)** may be introduced as toddlers develop the patience, attention to instruction, and pulmonary endurance to perform breathing exercises correctly.

FORCED EXPIRATORY TECHNIQUE

A FET, also known as a *huff*, should be incorporated into all ACTs. The huff creates an increased expiratory airflow and thereby mobilizes the mucus from the distal, small airways into the more central airways where it can then be expelled with a cough. Huffing can be incorporated effectively at about 4 years. Children should be taught to hold their mouth in a large O shape while exhaling. A tissue can be held in front of the mouth for visual feedback. Children are encouraged to exhale with enough force to make the tissue fly away. The imagery or practice of fogging up a mirror can also be used to teach huffing. Most babies will begin to mimic the actions of others by about 9 months. Caregivers can incorporate a mock huff or cough into airway clearance sessions to begin to teach this technique.

The effectiveness of a FET (as well as other ACTs) relies on the concepts of *equal pressure point* (EPP) and *collateral ventilation.* The EPP is the region of the airway where the pressure inside the airway (intraluminal pressure) is equal to the pressure exerted eternally from the lung parenchyma (extraluminal pressure) (Fig. 14-9). Extraluminal pressure typically remains constant while intraluminal pressure changes as one inhales and exhales. Airway pressure gradually increases during inhalation and then decreases during exhalation. With a deeper inspiration, the pressure in the distal airways will increase even more. As the pressure decreases during exhalation, there will be a point at which intraluminal and extraluminal pressures are the same, which is the EPP. Just proximal to the EPP (closer to the mouth) there will be a slight compression of the airway. It is this compression, or squeezing, of the airways that helps to move secretions from the distal airways.

ACTs also take advantage of collateral ventilation, which is present throughout the lung. Using interbronchial and bronchoalveolar connections, or channels, air is able to spread throughout the airways, behind any mucus blockages. Many ACTs incorporate an inspiratory hold, lasting 2 to 3 seconds, to use collateral ventilation to open distal airways and alveoli as well as allow air to get behind the mucus to help move it closer to the mouth.

To perform a FET, the patient should take a small breath in, followed by an inspiratory hold to allow for collateral ventilation. The small breath in leads to the EPP being more distal and is thus more likely to mobilize mucus from the small airways. The exhalation should be fast enough to overcome airway resistance, but not so fast as to create airway collapse. A general guideline to teach patients is that they should not hear any harsh or wheezing noises during exhalation. The next huff should be with a medium, or slightly larger than tidal volume, inspiration. The third breath in should be large, approaching inspiratory reserve volume, to mobilize the mucus into the larger, central airways. Each of these breaths should be followed by an inspiratory hold and a forced expiration.

This series of three huffs should be incorporated into most ACTs.

The series of huffs just described is not always necessary. However, many patients may have secretions in the larger airways and would benefit from a FET with large inspiratory volume. As with all ACTs, the huffing portion should be individually tailored to the patient's needs.

Active Cycle of Breathing

The ACB is a basic breathing exercise that is easy to teach and easy for patients to learn. Generally, ACB can be effectively introduced to school-aged children. ACB is adaptable to various treatment settings and can be combined with other ACTs, such as manual postural drainage and HFCWO.

During ACB, patients cycle through three types of breathing (Fig.14-10):

• Breathing control (i.e., normal, ideally diaphragmatic)
• Thoracic expansion
• FET

Patients should always start ACB using their normal breathing pattern. When ready, thoracic expansion breaths are performed. The practitioner can provide a tactile cue to facilitate this deep breathing (e.g., hands on the lower rib cage to facilitate lateral costal expansion). Hand placement provides proprioceptive stimulation to increase ventilation to a certain part of the lung. At most, three to four expansion breaths should be performed. These expansion breaths should always be followed by breathing control, at least three to four breaths, but more can be performed if needed to recover from the deeper breaths. This cycle should be repeated until the patient or therapist hears or feels that mucus has loosened. At this point, a series of huffs should be performed. Coughing should occur if mucus has moved into the central airways. If the patient does not feel the need, the cough should not be forced. The huff and cough should be followed by relaxed breathing. The whole cycle is then repeated.

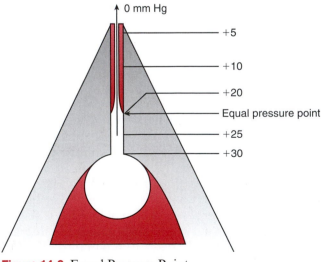

Figure 14-9 Equal Pressure Point

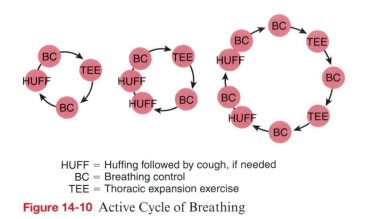

HUFF = Huffing followed by cough, if needed
BC = Breathing control
TEE = Thoracic expansion exercise

Figure 14-10 Active Cycle of Breathing

There is no set number of cycles to be performed during ACB. The number of cycles will vary from patient to patient and treatment to treatment. In general, when ACB is being performed as a sole treatment, patients should spend at least 20 minutes cycling through the breathing pattern (Fig. 14-10). Postural drainage positions may be incorporated with ACB to target specific lung segments.

Positive Expiratory Pressure

Preschoolers can also be introduced to forms of **positive expiratory pressure (PEP)**, which is an airway clearance strategy introduced in the 1970s in Denmark (24). Positive pressure is created in the airways by resisting expiration (25). This positive pressure created in the airways aids airway clearance by the following:

- Stenting airways open to prevent airway collapse
- Facilitating collateral ventilation
- Increasing functional residual capacity (FRC)

Resistance can be created naturally simply by narrowing the opening of the mouth mechanically with an expiratory resistor attached to a one-way valve. Toddlers and preschoolers can be introduced to breathing games that serve as low-level PEP. For example, blowing out through pursed lips as one does to blow bubbles is one way to narrow the exit outlet. Using musical toys, party blow-outs, or games that involve blowing through a straw are other examples. A fun activity for preschoolers and primary school-aged children is "Bubble PEP," which can be performed using common items found in the hospital or home (Box 14-2) (26). The child blows bubbles using respiratory tubing and a bottle containing water and detergent. The depth of water and tubing diameter determine the amount of expiratory resistance and PEP created.

Some preschoolers may be too young to correctly and independently use the PEP and oscillating PEP mechanical devices (discussed below) as their sole mode of airway clearance, but they can be introduced to them as an adjunct to therapy. When the child can incorporate all aspects of device use, including regular huffing and maintenance of a closed system, PEP devices can be considered as a daily treatment option.

PEP devices include the PEP/Rmt (Astra Tech, Mölndal, Sweden); PARI PEP (PARI Respiratory Equipment, Midlothian, VA); and TheraPEP (Smiths Medical, Dublin, OH). The goal with these low-pressure PEP devices is to create between 10 and 20 cm H_2O pressure at midexpiration using either a well-sealed face mask or mouthpiece that attaches to an adjustable resistor. A manometer can be used in conjunction with the device to monitor for target

Box 14-2 Bubble PEP—Underwater PEP

Bubble PEP was developed for use with young children who require help with clearing secretions from their lungs (22). This creative therapy provides positive feedback. It helps the parent to gain the cooperation and interest of the child.

Equipment

- Tubing, 15 to 18 inches long
- Plastic container (e.g., empty milk or juice container, gallon size)
- Dish detergent, few squirts
- Food coloring, few drops (optional)
- Water

Method

1. Fill the gallon container with 4 to 5 inches of water. The depth of the water and the diameter of the tubing will affect the amount of PEP produced.
2. Add detergent and food coloring (optional) to water.
3. Thread tubing through the handle into the base of the water. The end of the tubing should remain at the base of the water.
4. Stand the container in a large basin, tub, or use outside.

Instructions

1. Have patient blow through the end of the tubing with long breaths. Breaths should cause bubbles to rise up into the neck of the container.
2. Older children are asked to perform huffs and cough after a set number of breaths.

expiratory pressures. The technique is relatively simple to use and teach. The child breathes in and out of the device for 10 to 15 breaths. Inhalation should be slightly larger than tidal volume, and expiration should be active enough to overcome the resistance.

The consecutive breaths steadily increase the pressure and air volume in the airways, which results in a temporary increase in FRC. The temporary increase in FRC allows progressive recruitment and re-expansion of previously collapsed alveoli using collateral ventilation between airways and alveoli. However, the increase in FRC will only occur if the series of breaths takes place in a closed system. If air is allowed to escape from any part of the system, then the desired effect will not occur. Therefore, it is important to use a face mask or nose clip with any patient who cannot maintain mouth breathing with a tight seal over the mouthpiece for the series of breaths. As with other ACTs, huffs follow each series of breaths to mobilize and assist with clearing the secretions before the cycle is repeated.

PEP may be a particularly useful ACT for patients who have an asthma component to their respiratory disease because it prevents collapse of narrowed airways (27). In this CF subgroup, the reactive airway collapsibility can trap mucus in the airways. The airway stenting feature of PEP stabilizes the airway and allows air to use collateral ventilation channels to travel down behind the mucus so it can be mobilized.

PEP is also being used for infants at some CF centers. Infants do not have well-developed collateral ventilation channels, but they can still benefit from the temporary increase in FRC through the principle of interdependence. The temporary increase in air volume in the lungs allows healthy alveoli to create an outward pull on deflated alveoli to re-expand obstructed airways. Better aeration throughout the lungs reduces the chances of infection and inflammation by limiting hypoxia in previously collapsed portions of the airways.

The PEP technique is modified for use in infants. The baby is held and a small infant PEP mask is held over the infant's mouth and nose for 10 to 15 breaths. Midexpiratory pressures are expected to be 3 to 5 cm H_2O for infants, as compared to 10 to 20 cm H_2O used with older children and adults. The goal is to optimize lung aeration. The other difference for infants using PEP is that they cannot perform a FET on their own. Therapists can use techniques to stimulate a cough or FET, such as part of the assisted autogenic drainage technique, discussed later.

Oscillating PEP

Oscillating PEP is a subtype of PEP most commonly used by clinicians in the United States (2). These devices, which can be introduced to school-aged children, include the acapella (Smiths Medical, Dublin, OH); Flutter (Aptalis, Birmingham, AL); Quake (Thayer Medical, Tucson, AZ); and RC Cornet (R. Cegla GmbH & Co. Montabaur, Germany). Oscillating PEP devices combine PEP with high frequency expiratory oscillations (25). The flow-dependent oscillations created in addition to the PEP are theorized to act similarly to vibrations created by HFCWO devices. They help decrease sputum viscosity and can improve ciliary beat via resonance if the correct oscillating frequency is established. The vibrations create continuous interruptions of expiratory airflow, allowing waves of positive pressure to mobilize secretions and facilitate their progression up the airway.

The oscillating PEP devices differ slightly in their function and design. The most unique oscillating PEP device is the Flutter. This device uses the benefits of oscillations more than its PEP feature. The frequency of the vibrations depends on the angle that the device is held in the mouth. It is necessary to incorporate an inspiratory hold to allow time for collateral ventilation to get air into previously obstructed airways and alveoli. The Flutter does not provide as much PEP as other devices, so it does not provide the increase in FRC found in the closed system of PEP devices or the acapella device.

The acapella has more PEP features than does the Flutter. The oscillatory frequency of this device is not angle dependent, and it has an expiratory flow option of greater than 15 L/min (Fig. 14-11). The acapella also has an option for lower flows that may be more suitable for younger children and patients with poorer lung function. A dial controls the amount of PEP and frequency of vibrations. Increasing the PEP will decrease the frequency of vibrations. Turning the dial in the other direction increases the oscillatory benefits of the acapella by decreasing the PEP.

The instructions for use of oscillating PEP follow those for its PEP counterpart. Slightly larger than tidal volume breaths are performed in cycles of 10 to 15 breaths with breath holds. This is followed by huffing and coughing, then breathing control, before repeating the cycle. Total treatment time should be 15 to 20 minutes, and it is usually prescribed twice daily; however, as with other ACTs, the program should be individualized to the patient's needs.

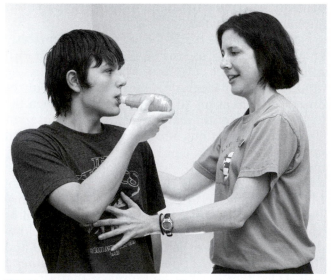

Figure 14-11 Oscillating PEP. Teenage patient with CF using an acapella® oscillating PEP device. *(From Johns Hopkins University, www.hopkinscf.org; with permission)*

Patients with CF who have an asthmatic component or are prone to airway collapse and wheezing may find that the oscillating effect exacerbates these symptoms. Standard PEP may be a gentler option for this subgroup.

High-Pressure PEP

High-pressure PEP (HIPEP) is a technique that is less commonly used in the United States. It employs increased tidal breathing at pressures of 30 to 100 cm H_2O (28). This is followed by a maximal inspiration and huff against the resistor. The patient coughs into the mask, and the technique is repeated until there is no longer any sputum production. The forced expirations into the mask keep the airways open longer. It is a fatiguing treatment for the patient, but it is very time efficient. It is a treatment option for patients with significant secretions and ineffective but excessive coughing. One should be aware that there is a risk of pneumothorax with use of HIPEP, especially for patients with severe airway obstruction.

Autogenic Drainage

Autogenic drainage (AD) is an independent breathing technique in which patients breathe at various lung volumes to mobilize secretions (Fig. 14-12). Older children and young adults can use AD effectively for airway clearance. Autogenic drainage is an individualized technique that aims to enhance linear air velocity over the largest possible area of the bronchial tree in a synchronous and even way. Inspiration should be done with very low airflow with an open glottis. A 2- to 3-second breath hold is performed with every breath. Breathing out is done through open upper airways with high flow. Expiratory pressure needs to be balanced in proportion to the bronchial wall stability to avoid airway collapse. Autogenic drainage is composed of three phases:

• Unstick
• Collect
• Evacuate

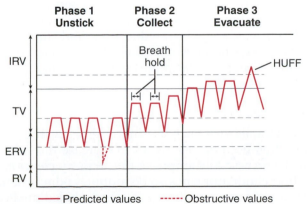

Figure 14-12 Autogenic Drainage

Before starting AD, the upper airways should be cleared (e.g., by blowing nose, coughing). The first phase of AD is "unsticking." In this phase, patients should breathe with low lung volumes, exhaling toward expiratory reserve volume. Once down into the expiratory reserve volume, the patient takes a tidal volume inspiration followed by a 2- to 3-second breath hold. Breathing continues at this level until the secretions are mobilized in the small airways.

The next phase involves "collecting" the mucus in the middle-sized airways. Exhalations are below tidal volume, but not quite as low as in the first phase. Again, breathing stays at this phase until the mucus is gathered in the middle-sized airways. This occurs when there is audible feedback of the mobilized secretions.

The final phase is "evacuation." Breathing changes to large inhalations, toward inspiratory reserve volume, during this phase. The breath hold occurs with every breath at all phases. Exhalations in the evacuation phase are normal, tidal-volume breaths. Once more, secretions will be mobilized into the more central airways. When breath sounds suggest the presence of loose mucus, the final part of AD is to huff and cough. The cough reflex must be controlled until the patient reaches this point.

Assisted autogenic drainage (AAD) may be performed on infants. Assisted autogenic drainage is based on the principles of AD. Optimal expiratory flows are achieved by the caregiver manually changing the lung volume level of tidal breathing. It is recommended that therapists have appropriate training before performing AAD on infants.

Intrapulmonary Percussive Ventilation

Intrapulmonary percussive ventilation (IPV) delivers small bursts of positive pressure (at rates of 100 to 300 cycles/minute) that are superimposed on the patient's own breathing. IPV can be used in cooperative school-aged children. Pressures used typically range from 5 to 35 cm H_2O. Compressed gas (25 to 40 pounds per square inch) generates the oscillations. Patients should breathe normally with a face mask or mouthpiece. The positive pressure reaches the airways and can be effective in treating atelectasis. During the percussive bursts of air into the lungs, a continued pressure is maintained, creating a PEP effect.

Although medications can be delivered with IPV, there are no controlled studies in the CF population using IPV for medication delivery. Certain medications can be broken down when nonapproved devices are used. For this reason, further studies on the clinical efficacy of drug deposition are needed.

■ ■ ■ At the end of Ryan's first appointment, his parents are instructed in the use of modified percussion and postural drainage. The hallmark of CF is the presence of abnormal, viscous secretions within the airways. Airway clearance techniques that promote mobilization of airway secretions are the cornerstone of chronic CF therapies. Although Ryan has no respiratory symptoms, he still has viscous secretions, and his parents are told that airway clearance should be performed twice daily.

Exercise

Exercise is an important adjunct to airway clearance. Physical activity can increase minute ventilation and expiratory air flow. The improved ventilation can open previously collapsed airways and get air behind mucus plugs. The expiratory air flow increase will help shear mucus from the airway walls so it can be moved centrally up the airways for clearance. Exercise as an adjunct to therapy should incorporate huffing and/or coughing to assist with mucus clearance. There is no evidence that supports exercise as a stand-alone ACT, but many studies support the overall improvement in respiratory function.

As infants develop, facilitation of movement and exercise can also be used for airway clearance. Ventilation distribution can also be affected by altering the child's positioning and/or breathing pattern with selected activities. Certain movements or activities can cause a change in breathing pattern that mimics some of the breathing exercises that will be introduced when the child is older. For example, bouncing with a parent or caregiver on a therapy ball or on the caregiver's lap can increase expiratory airflow and simulate huffs.

Challenging the baby to pull up and use shoulder muscles and core abdominal muscles can create breath holds and releases. Additionally, activities and games that promote arm and trunk mobility, such as raising an infant's arms overhead in a "so big" gesture, will optimize lung function through improved chest wall flexibility. Exercise can play a vital role in airway clearance in infants. It is practiced as a staple for CF management in Sweden. In fact, The Lund CF Centre in Sweden has adapted exercise/activity as the infant's primary mode of airway clearance and has not used postural drainage or percussion with any of their patients since 1983 (29)

Games introduced to the infant and toddler can be expanded on with the preschooler. Incorporating hippity-hop balls, trampolines, and riding toys can be fun ways to increase the exercise and activity necessary for the health of a child with CF. Such activities will also promote breathing patterns that can facilitate mucus clearance via increasing

expiratory flow rates. Encouraging climbing activities and upper-body strength with activities such as going across monkey bars and performing wheelbarrows will improve breathing mechanics by optimizing chest/respiratory accessory muscle strength and flexibility.

School-aged children and teens often enjoy participation in more organized individual and team athletics. Activities such as dance, gymnastics, yoga, martial arts, bicycling, hiking, and team sports are great ways to get children active and exercising. Children who are more inclined to video games and computers may benefit from using interactive gaming systems to increase their activity. There are a multitude of games that encourage cardiopulmonary fitness as well as posture and good breathing mechanics (Teamwork 14-1).

Inhalation Therapies

A common part of a patient's everyday routine includes inhaled medications. These treatments are used to prevent the buildup of thick, sticky mucus; manage infection; and help preserve lung function over time. Table 14-3 lists inhaled medications frequently used by patients with CF. It is important to remember that not all patients receive all of the medications available. Individualized treatment plans should be developed based on the patient's age, symptoms, and severity of lung disease. Evidence-based guidelines for the use of these therapies have been published and can aid in treatment decisions (30). These guidelines provide recommendations of effective therapies for children older than 5 years and adults with CF. Unfortunately, they do not provide guidance on when to start a particular therapy or identify the best combinations of therapies. Although these therapies are often used in younger children and may in fact be effective, there is not enough evidence to recommend their use in children younger than 5 years.

The daily treatment routine of inhaled medications and airway clearance can be burdensome to patients and families; however, it is important that patients adhere to these therapies to have the best chance of preserving lung function. Respiratory therapists can provide encouragement, education, and support to patients and families regarding these inhaled treatments and explain the importance of remaining compliant with them.

Bronchodilators

Bronchodilators, such as albuterol or levalbuterol, are often used before ACTs to increase the caliber of the airway and improve mucociliary clearance. A bronchodilator can also be routinely administered before hypertonic saline and other inhaled medications to prevent bronchospasm. Many patients with

Teamwork 14-1 Working Together With Physical Therapy

RESPIRATORY AND PHYSICAL THERAPISTS WORK CLOSELY TOGETHER TO OPTIMIZE DELIVERY OF MEDICATIONS AND SUCCESS OF THERAPY AND EXERCISE. Respiratory therapists delivering medications and airway clearance may be the first to take notice of problems requiring physical therapy attention. Good posture and positioning can greatly enhance the delivery of aerosolized medications. Posture also improves breathing mechanics. The physical therapist can recommend postural interventions that can be applied during respiratory sessions to maximize treatment effectiveness. Simply reminding your patient to sit up straight and/or use a towel roll behind the spine to open up the thoracic cage can greatly improve effectiveness of treatment.

Stress urinary incontinence is a common but treatable secondary impairment that can develop in CF or other chronic respiratory illness. Weakness develops in the pelvic floor muscles from the long-term, repeated stress that coughing and huffing place on the musculature. This results in a leakage of urine with coughing, laughing, or other activities. Because these can be embarrassing complaints, the respiratory therapist should ask if they occur as part of the ACT evaluation. The treating respiratory therapist may be the first to suspect or identify a problem through behaviors observed during airway clearance and nebulizer treatments. Warning behaviors include the following:

- Cough suppression during therapy
- Frequent interruptions of therapy to use the bathroom
- Preventive body posture, such as keeping legs crossed during treatment or coughing

If stress urinary incontinence is identified, a referral to a physical therapist or women's health specialist is recommended.

Physical therapists can also aid in developing an effective exercise program for children with CF at any age. Teaming with the physical therapist and the patient to coordinate airway clearance with exercise and inhalational therapies will optimize the value of these treatments.

Table 14-3	Common Inhaled Medications for Patients with CF	
Bronchodilators	**Mucolytics**	**Antibiotics**
Albuterol	Hypertonic saline	Tobramycin (TOBI)
Levalbuterol	Dornase alfa (rhDNase or Pulmozyme)	Aztreonam (Cayston)
		Colistin

CF administer bronchodilators via nebulizer to also hydrate airway secretions; however, in many cases metered dose inhalers (MDIs) can be used to diminish the overall burden of treatments. Patients who have airway reactivity should use a bronchodilator to treat wheezing and airway obstruction caused by to smooth muscle contraction.

■■ Over the next few years, Ryan continues to gain weight well. Although he is typically healthy, he has had several pulmonary exacerbations requiring oral antibiotic therapy. He has a cough that is present every day. Based on this history, the clinic team discusses and believes that introduction of nebulized therapy to thin the airway secretions would be worthwhile as an addition to Ryan's daily ATCs.

Mucolytics

Although they may not break down the structure of mucus per se, therapies that are designed to thin airway secretions are commonly known as **mucolytics**. Another, and perhaps better term, is mucus modulating agents. Dornase alfa (rhDNase or Pulmozyme) and hypertonic saline are the most commonly used inhaled mucolytics. Based on a systematic review of the published literature, the CF Foundation has strongly recommended the continuing use of these drugs (30).

Mechanism of action

- **Dornase alfa (rhDNase or Pulmozyme)**: This medication digests the excess DNA present within mucus, helping to make it less thick and sticky. This enzyme therapy is effective because CF airway secretions contain a significant amount of bacterial and neutrophil DNA resulting from the presence of chronic infection and the subsequent inflammatory response. The proven efficacy of dornase alfa is limited to CF. Although there are reports of successful of use of dornase alfa in treating atelectasis in patients without CF, there is not enough evidence to recommend it routinely for this use.

- **Hypertonic saline**: Inhaling saline with a high concentration of salt (typically 7%) acts to rehydrate the dehydrated airway secretions by drawing water into the airways to replenish the airway surface liquid. Hypertonic saline also has the benefit of inducing a cough in many patients.

Side effects

- **Dornase alfa:** Sore throat, voice changes, and eye irritation
- **Hypertonic saline:** Bronchospasm, salty taste and burning feeling in mouth/throat

N-acetylcysteine, which breaks disulfide bonds, has been used as a mucolytic for many years, but there is not enough research evidence to recommend its routine use in patients with CF (26). Studies of inhaled mannitol used to hydrate airway secretions in patients with CF suggest that this medication is effective (31, 32). However, this medication is not yet approved for use in the United States.

Inhaled Antibiotics

As noted previously, the airways of patients with CF are often chronically infected with bacteria. The most common bacterium found in the airways of patients with CF is *P. aeruginosa* (Fig. 14-2). It is well known that the presence of *P. aeruginosa* is associated with a more rapid decline in lung function and increased mortality (7). This observation has led to aggressive approaches to eradicate this organism when it is first recovered (33). **Inhaled antibiotics** are a foundation of these eradication strategies. Once the *P. aeruginosa* infection is established, patients often begin chronic inhaled antibiotic therapy to minimize the inflammation from the infection. The use of chronic inhaled antibiotic therapy for suppression is associated with improved lung function and fewer exacerbations (30).

Tobramycin and aztreonam are two inhaled antibiotics approved by the U.S. Food and Drug Administration (FDA) for use in patients with CF. Although not FDA approved for inhalational use, colistin (colistimethate sodium) has been used for many years as treatment for *P. aeruginosa*. The rationale for the use of inhaled antibiotics is that they deliver a high concentration of drug to the airway surface, where it is most needed, while minimizing systemic drug toxicity.

Mechanism of action

- **Tobramycin:** an aminoglycoside antibiotic that blocks bacterial protein synthesis.
- **Aztreonam:** a monobactam antibiotic that inhibits bacterial cell wall formation.

- **Colistin:** a polymyxin antibiotic that disrupts the outer bacteria cell membrane.

Side effects

- **Tobramycin:** Sore throat, voice changes, and redness around eyes
- **Aztreonam:** Cough, nasal congestion, and wheezing
- **Colistin:** Cough, wheezing, and chest tightness

Inhaled antibiotics frequently are used to eradicate *P. aeruginosa* when it is first cultured, even when children are asymptomatic. Recent studies have shown that 28-day course of inhaled antibiotics is very effective at eradicating *P. aeruginosa* (34, 35). The Eradication of Pseudomonas Infection Control (EPIC) trial found that the addition of 14 days of oral ciprofloxacin to 28 days of inhaled tobramycin did not improve the eradication rate of *P. aeruginosa* (35). Ratjen et al (34) demonstrated that 56 days of inhaled tobramycin was no more effective at eradicating the *P. aeruginosa* when compared to 28 days of therapy. Both therapies were able to eradicate the infection in greater than 92% of children. The use of routine administration of inhaled antibiotics with or without oral antibiotics does not appear to decrease the rate of *P. aeruginosa* colonization in children with CF compared to culture-directed therapy (34, 36).

When used to treat chronic *P. aeruginosa* infection, inhaled tobramycin and aztreonam are typically administered in 28-day on/off cycles. This approach is thought to minimize the development of antibiotic resistance. However, patients with more severe lung disease often alternate two antibiotics in monthly cycles so that they are always receiving an inhaled antibiotic. Although inhaled antibiotics are an effective therapy, they do have unintended consequences. The marked increase in the prevalence of fungi recovered from the airways of patients with CF is due in part to the widespread use of inhaled antibiotics (37).

■■ Because he is not yet able to produce sputum, Ryan has a throat culture performed at each clinic visit to monitor his airway microbiology. His most recent culture has grown *Pseudomonas aeruginosa*. Therefore, 1 month of inhaled tobramycin is prescribed as "eradication therapy."

Other Inhaled Therapies

Inhaled steroids are an attractive therapy to treat the inflammation associated with CF lung disease. However, there is not enough evidence to recommend this therapy (26). Inhaled steroids can be considered in patients who wheeze frequently. The same can be said for long-acting bronchodilators. They may be helpful in treating children who have an asthma phenotype, but they should not be prescribed routinely. There is a trial of tiotropium, a long-acting anticholinergic drug, now under way to determine if it has a role in treating patients with CF.

Optimal Delivery of Inhaled Medications

Proper delivery of respiratory medications is essential to ensure that an adequate and effective dose is delivered to the patient (Table 14-4). Therefore, it is important for patients with CF to use the appropriate nebulizer with the proper technique because many of the inhaled medications are dose dependent. Infants, toddlers, and those patients unable to use a mouthpiece treatment should use nebulizers with a mask that provides a tight-fitting seal. Patients who are able to use a mouthpiece should be encouraged to do so for best delivery of medications. Good posture should be encouraged during treatments.

Nebulizers commonly used by patients with CF can be found in Table 14-4. The PARI LC Plus (PARI Respiratory Equipment) is a **breath-actuated nebulizer**, which means it will deliver medication only during inspiration. The Sidestream (Respironics, Murrysville, PA) is a **breath-enhanced nebulizer**, which will increase medication output when it senses an increase in inspiratory flow, then decrease medication delivery when inspiration concludes. Both are approved for use with CF medications. Dornase alfa can be administered with several nebulizer/compressor combinations. However, the only FDA-approved nebulizer for use with inhaled tobramycin (TOBI) is the PARI LC Plus.

Recently, PARI has introduced two electronic vibrating mesh nebulizers, Altera and TRIO, both based on eFlow technology. Portable and more efficient than traditional nebulizers, the eFlow technology can deliver a greater number of respirable particles to the lungs at a faster rate. Inhaled aztreonam (Cayston) is approved by the FDA only for use in the Altera nebulizer. It is administered three times daily in 28-day on/off cycles. The TRIO nebulizer can be used with several medications prescribed for patients with CF; however, this device has not been approved for this specific use with CF medications by the FDA. The vibrating mesh has not been optimized for these medications. Caution must be used when converting from a standard nebulizer to a TRIO device because a greater proportion of the medication will be delivered to the lungs. Typically, a dose reduction of approximately 50% is required for most inhaled therapies.

Although not based on rigorous experimental data, the CF Foundation has recommended a standardized order for the delivery of inhaled medications and airway clearance (26). No medications should be mixed together, with the exception of albuterol (or levalbuterol) and ipratropium bromide, if prescribed. A clean, disinfected nebulizer cup is strongly recommended for each medication.

The recommended order of therapies is as follows:

- Bronchodilator
- Hypertonic saline
- Dornase alfa
- Airway clearance
- Inhaled steroids (including combination drugs)
- Inhaled antibiotics

Disease-Modifying Therapy

Therapies that restore the function of the defective *CFTR* found in CF have the potential to modify the course of CF lung disease to improve lung function

Table 14-4	Which Nebulizer for Which Inhaled Medication?							
	Bronchodilators	**Dornase alfa (Pulmozyme)**	**Hypertonic Saline**	**Budesonide (Pulmicort)**	**TOBI (300 mg)**	**Tobramycin**	**Colistin (150 mg)**	**Cayston**
T Piece Nebulizer	Yes	Yes	Yes	Yes	No	No	No	No
Pari LC Plus	Yes	Yes	Yes	Yes	Yes	No	Yes	No
Sidestream	Yes	Yes	Yes	Yes	No	No	Yes	No
Trio (eFlow)*	No	Maybe	Maybe	No	No	Maybe (170 mg)	Maybe (75 mg)	No
Altera (eFlow)	No	No	No	No	No	No	No	Yes

*eFlow technology allows the faster delivery of drugs with higher respirable fraction; therefore, the dose of several medications can be decreased. However, long-term trials to demonstrate the effectiveness of the reduced dosage of these medications have not been performed. Pulmozyme and hypertonic saline are typically used in Trio/eFlow, with standard dosing. The dose of inhaled antibiotics is typically reduced by 50%. Because of the risk of confusion and potential overdose, bronchodilator use in Trio is not recommended.

and survival. Ivacaftor is the first such therapy approved by the FDA. It is a small-molecule potentiator that activates defective *CFTR* at the cell surface that has been shown to improve sweat chloride, lung function, weight, and quality of life (38). Ivacaftor activates mutated *CFTR* in which glycine has been replaced by aspartic acid at position 551 (G551D). If started early in the course of the disease, this therapy has the potential to alter the progression of CF lung disease for patients with CF as a result of at least one G551D mutation. Therapies directed toward other defective forms of *CFTR* are currently under way.

Infection Control

An important consideration for people with CF is infection control (39). Health-care providers must take precautions to avoid transmitting pathogens from one patient to another in both inpatient and outpatient settings. Many of the bacteria colonizing the airways of children with CF are transmissible to others with the disease. Therefore, it is of vital importance that excellent hand hygiene is practiced. Additional precautions are warranted when individuals are colonized with certain bacteria such as *B. cepacia*. Many CF centers see young patients with CF in clinics separate from individuals colonized with *P. aeruginosa*, *B. cepacia*, MRSA, and other pathogens to prevent early colonization.

Although infection control in the health-care setting is important, most patients acquire colonizing organisms from their everyday environmental exposure, not from CF clinic visits (40). Infection control must become a part of the family's everyday life, especially in the care of their respiratory equipment. Studies have found that many pathogens remain on respiratory equipment after use. Because of these findings, the CF Foundation strongly recommends cleaning and disinfecting nebulizer equipment after each and every treatment (39).

The first step in cleaning any respiratory device is to remove secretions with soap and water. For cleaning, fill a clean basin with warm, soapy water and agitate the equipment pieces in it, removing any debris. Rinse with sterile water and then follow with an appropriate disinfection technique for the device type (Table 14-5). Vinegar is not strong enough to kill *P. aeruginosa* and is therefore not recommended for disinfecting respiratory equipment.

Adherence to Therapy

Improved survival for patients with CF is thanks to the introduction of an aggressive approach to treatment of airway obstruction and infection. A typical therapeutic routine for many patients includes airway clearance twice daily, mucolytic therapy, and inhaled antibiotics. This regimen can take more than 1 hour to administer twice daily. For this reason, CF therapy can be quite burdensome for patients and their families. Adherence to prescribed therapies is vitally important, and the role of the respiratory therapist in encouraging adherence is key to the success of therapy. Studies have shown that children and adults with CF who have better adherence have a slower decline in lung function and fewer exacerbations (41).

There are different challenges to adherence at every age. Adherence to therapy tends to become worse in adolescence and early adulthood as patients gain independence from their parents (41). Caregivers should strive to create an individualized care plan that the patient can realistically complete on a daily basis (Box 14-3). Instilling an understanding of the rationale and importance of therapies will improve adherence in the long run.

Table 14-5	Nebulizer Cleaning After Using Warm, Soapy Water				
	Cold Disinfection[1]	**Boiling[2]**	**Top Rack Dishwasher**	**Electronic Steam Sterilizer[3]**	**Microwave Steam Bags[4]**
Pari LC Plus	Yes	Yes	Yes	Yes	***
Sidestream	Yes	Yes	Yes	Yes	***
Trio (eFlow) ◊	Yes	Yes	NO		NO
Altera (eFlow) ◊	Yes	Yes	Yes	Yes	NO

Adapted from Saiman L, Siegel J (39).

[1]Cold disinfection includes soak in 70% isopropyl alcohol for 5 minutes or 3% hydrogen peroxide for 30 minutes.

[2]Place in boiling distilled water for 5 minutes.

[3] Brand names include Avent Iq24 and Nuk. These are available in the baby supply section of many department stores.

[4] Brand names include Medela, Dr. Brown's, and Munchkin. These are available in the baby supply section of many
   department stores.

[5]For eFlow devices, the aerosol head should always be kept in isopropyl alcohol when not in use. eFlow devices have
   specific cleaning/disinfection requirements. Please refer to manufacturer's care instructions.

***Manufacturer does not recommend this disinfection method; however, it has been advocated by patients and some
   CF centers.

Box 14-3 A Day in the Life of a Teenager with CF

Morning

5:00 a.m.	Wake up
5:30 a.m.	*Morning Therapies*
	Albuterol (5 min)
	Hypertonic saline (15 to 20 min)
	Airway clearance using HFCWO (30 min)
	Inhaled tobramycin (every other month) (15 to 20 min)
6:30 a.m.	Breakfast and off to school

Evening

4:00 p.m.	Homework
6:00 p.m.	Soccer Practice
7:00 p.m.	Dinner
8:00 p.m.	*Evening Therapies*
	Albuterol (5 min)
	Dornase alfa (5 to 10 min)
	Hypertonic saline (15 min)
	Airway clearance using HFCWO (30 min)
	Inhaled tobramycin (every other month) (15 to 20 min)

■ ■ Ryan is now 6 years old. He performs airway clearance twice daily and uses dornase alfa once daily. He does typically cough on a daily basis, but does not produce sputum. *P. aeruginosa* has only been cultured once, and it has not been found again after eradication therapy.

Over the past week Ryan has had an increased amount of coughing and is now producing sputum on a daily basis. He has had one episode of post-tussive emesis. When he is examined in clinic he has crackles on auscultation, and his FEV$_1$ has fallen by 15%.

Pulmonary Exacerbation Therapy

Pulmonary exacerbations can be challenging for patients, families, and care providers (Box 14-4). These episodes are characterized by increased airway secretions, infection, and inflammation. Antibiotics are the mainstay of exacerbation therapy. Antibiotics can be administered either orally or via nebulizer to treat mild exacerbations. Airway clearance should also be increased to at least three to four times daily to mobilize secretions when children are ill. Additional nebulized therapies, such as bronchodilators or mucolytics, can be employed to enhance airway clearance.

More severe exacerbations are treated with intravenous (IV) antibiotics. Generally, patients who require IV antibiotics are admitted to the hospital for at least some portion of their therapy. In addition to IV antibiotics, patients should receive more intensive airway clearance and aggressive nutritional support during the hospital stay (38). From a respiratory standpoint, treatment will vary from patient to patient. Options for inhaled medications include the addition or increased frequency of albuterol, hypertonic saline, or dornase alfa. Airway clearance should be provided at least three to four times daily. There can be an important role for bronchoscopy in exacerbation management. Bronchoscopy can be used therapeutically to treat mucus plugging and atelectasis or diagnostically to obtain cultures from children who do not expectorate sputum.

The role of inhaled antibiotic therapy in patients being treated with IV antibiotics is unclear. Inhaled antibiotics deliver a high concentration of drug directly to the airway during illness, potentially leading to better outcomes. However, there is also the potential for increased toxicity when IV and inhaled aminoglycoside antibiotics are administered together. Unfortunately, there are no studies that clearly define

Box 14-4 Pulmonary Exacerbations

Children with CF experience episodic increases in respiratory symptoms known as *pulmonary exacerbations*. These episodes can be acute or have an insidious onset. Pulmonary exacerbations are thought to be from an overgrowth of bacteria in the airways of patients with CF in combination with increased mucus production and inflammation. Pulmonary exacerbations are characterized by respiratory symptoms including the following:

- Increased cough
- Increased sputum production
- Change in sputum color or composition
- Dyspnea
- Chest pain
- Weight loss
- Hemoptysis

Exacerbations are rarely associated with fever. Physical examination can be deceptive. Although children experiencing a pulmonary exacerbation often have physical findings such as crackles on examination, patients can have a significant increase in symptoms and a fall in lung function yet have a benign examination. Similarly, chest radiographs may not show significant changes during an exacerbation.

an advantage or disadvantage of combined IV and inhaled therapy (42).

The goal of exacerbation therapy is resolution of symptoms and improvement in lung function. The effectiveness of therapy can be monitored by improvement in symptoms, such as cough and sputum production, and physical findings, such as crackles. If the chest radiograph does have significant changes, then a follow-up radiograph should be obtained at the end of therapy. Typically, pulmonary function testing is the most important tool for monitoring the success of therapy. Improvement in FEV_1 can occur after just a few days of therapy and normally peaks within 10 days of IV antibiotics (43).

There are few randomized, controlled trials of exacerbation therapies, making it difficult to make evidence-based recommendations for treatment. Unfortunately, up to one-third of patients do not recover their previous lung function despite aggressive exacerbation therapy (44). Therefore, studies to determine the optimal approach to exacerbation therapy are needed.

■ ■ Based on Ryan's clinical findings, he is diagnosed with a mild pulmonary exacerbation. You and the physical therapist also take this opportunity to reassess Ryan and his family on their adherence to prescribed maintenance therapy and techniques of airway clearance. They deny any problems with performing therapies and maintain that they consistently adhere to the prescribed therapies. After observing their techniques, you and the physical therapist agree that Ryan's exacerbations are not the result of poor adherence to therapy or technique. The team recommends increasing his airway clearance techniques to four times a day and coupling it with a bronchodilator. The pulmonologist also prescribes Ryan a 28-day regimen of inhaled tobramycin and 2 weeks of oral ciprofloxacin.

At a follow-up visit 1 month later, Ryan's PFTs have returned to his baseline predicted values, and he is returned to his standard airway clearance regimen.

Complications

Hemoptysis

Many patients with advanced lung disease will periodically have **hemoptysis**, the expectoration of blood arising from the airway or lungs. Bleeding can range from the expectorating blood-streaked sputum to frank blood. Hemoptysis results from damage to fragile, tortuous bronchial arteries, which often form arteriovenous fistulas with pulmonary vessels. Hemoptysis is more common in patients with severe lung disease.

Acute episodes of bleeding are typically associated with infection. Therefore, treatment with antibiotics should be considered when hemoptysis occurs (45). Evaluation of patients with significant hemoptysis should include hemoglobin count, platelet count, and a prothrombin time to confirm whether the patient is vitamin K deficient. Massive hemoptysis, defined as more than 250 mL of blood, can be life threatening. The definitive treatment of recurrent or massive hemoptysis is bronchial artery embolization.

Pneumothorax

About 3.4% of all patients with CF will experience a pneumothorax in their lifetime (46). The annual incidence of pneumothorax in patients with CF is approximately 1 in 167 patients (47). Pneumothoraces typically present with pleuritic chest pain and dyspnea. Small pneumothoraces, without significant cardiopulmonary compromise, can be treated conservatively with observation and analgesic therapy. Larger pneumothoraces require chest-tube drainage (45). Another optional treatment is **pleurodesis**, which is the creation of adhesions between the two thoracic pleura, to prevent recurrence of pneumothoraces. Careful consideration should be given before performing pleurodesis because the resulting adhesions may influence future transplant decisions. Pneumothorax has traditionally been considered to be a poor prognostic indicator and to be a harbinger of a more rapid decline in lung function.

Allergic Bronchopulmonary Aspergillosis

Allergic bronchopulmonary aspergillosis (ABPA) is an allergic reaction to a fungus commonly found in the environment (48). Allergy to *Aspergillus fumigatus* is the most common form of ABPA. The prevalence of fungi in the airways of patients with CF has increased 10-fold over the past decade to more than 30% in some centers (37). The symptoms of ABPA can overlap those of CF, making the diagnosis difficult in some cases. The classic symptoms include wheezing, loss of lung function, and central bronchiectasis. Criteria have been developed for the diagnosis and treatment of ABPA in patients with CF (48).

- A consensus conference convened by the CF Foundation has suggested minimal criteria for the diagnosis of ABPA in patients with CF (48). These criteria include acute or subacute clinical deterioration (cough, wheeze, exercise intolerance, exercise-induced asthma, change in pulmonary function, or increased sputum production) not attributable to another etiology.
- Total serum immunoglobulin E (IgE) concentration greater than 500 IU/mL (1,200 ng/mL). If ABPA is suspected, and the total IgE level is

200 to 500 IU/mL, repeat testing in 1 to 3 months is recommended

- Immediate cutaneous reactivity to *A. fumigatus* (prick skin test) or in vitro demonstration of IgE antibody to *A. fumigatus.*
- One of the following: (a) precipitins to *A. fumigatus* or in vitro demonstration of IgG antibody to *A. fumigatus;* or (b) new or recent abnormalities on chest radiography (infiltrates or mucus plugging); or (c) chest CT results (bronchiectasis) that have not cleared with antibiotics and standard physiotherapy

The growth of *A. fumigatus* is not required for the diagnosis of ABPA. Serum IgE is typically used both as a screening laboratory test and as a test to follow the progression of disease. Systemic steroids are the mainstay of treatment for ABPA. Inhaled steroids and antifungal therapies are widely employed as adjunctive therapies. However, there is little evidence for the effectiveness of these agents. There have been several case reports of the effective use of omalizumab to treat ABPA (49).

Extrapulmonary Complications

There are several significant extrapulmonary complications of CF, including CF-related diabetes (CFRD), liver cirrhosis, osteoporosis, and depression, all of which occur with increased frequency with age. Up to 50% of adults with CF eventually develop CFRD. The presence of CFRD is associated with an increased rate of pulmonary decline. In fact, rapid pulmonary function decline may be an indicator of occult CFRD (50). Depression has been found to correlate with worse clinical outcomes (51). This finding is most likely owing to less compliance with therapies in depressed patients.

End-Stage Lung Disease

Although survival for patients with CF continues to improve, there comes a point at which patients develop increased respiratory compromise associated with dyspnea and gas exchange abnormalities. Supplemental oxygen can be used to treat hypoxemia, which typically presents first during sleep. Noninvasive positive-pressure ventilation (NIPPV) can be effective in improving nocturnal gas exchange abnormalities, including hypercapnia, and decreasing work of breathing during sleep.

As the lung disease progresses, patients may begin to feel increasingly breathless and air hungry. Their oxygen saturation may begin to drop, and hospital admission may become inevitable. Switching from a nasal cannula to a higher flow, cool aerosol mask may help patients with the feeling of air hunger. As a patient inevitably continues to progress, NIPPV can be used effectively to treat dyspnea, aid in airway clearance, and prevent intubation of patients in respiratory failure. Noninvasive positive-pressure ventilation has been used effectively as a bridge to lung transplantation. However, there is a risk of pneumothorax in patients with severe airway obstruction who use NIPPV.

Finally, intubation does remain an option for respiratory failure. If possible, this option should be discussed and decided on by the patient, family, and care team before a crisis moment. Outcomes for patients with end-stage lung disease who require intubation and mechanical ventilation are poor (52). End-of-life decisions should be discussed before a crisis develops so that patients and families have time to make informed decisions (see Chapter 21). Respiratory therapists may spend a significant amount of time in the room of a patient with end-stage CF lung disease. Therefore, understanding that patients are feeling anxious, breathless, and scared can help the respiratory therapist to provide them much-needed support.

Lung Transplantation

Lung transplantation is an option for some children with respiratory failure. Bilateral lung transplantation is required to treat patients with CF. Lung transplantation is not a cure for CF, but rather a therapy to allow patients to live longer with a better quality of life. Because of improved outcomes, transplantation in childhood is rare. Adolescents are more likely than younger children to require transplantation. Determining the optimal timing for making a referral for transplantation can be challenging. Factors that influence referral include lung function, the presence of hypoxemia and/or hypercapnia, and debility. Allocation of organs is based on a severity score. Transplantation is not appropriate for all individuals with CF. Contraindications to transplantation include history of poor adherence to therapy, colonization with resistant organisms, uncontrolled diabetes, and severe malnutrition. The 5-year survival after transplant for children with CF is approximately 50% (53). However, lung transplantation can provide a significant benefit for carefully selected patients.

Course and Prognosis

The aggressive approach to the care of patients has improved the survival for individuals with CF dramatically (Fig. 14-1). In 1986, the median predicted age of survival with CF in the United States was 27 years. Since that time there has been a steady increase in survival. In 2010, the median predicted age of survival was 38.3 years (2). This is a calculation that describes that age past which half the individuals with CF in the United States will live. However, this is a complicated and imprecise number, and it is not useful in predicting a particular person's chances of living to a particular age. There are many reasons for this increase in survival. Stronger partnerships among people with CF, their families, and CF care center staff are key. Earlier diagnosis because of nationwide newborn screening also plays a critical role. The earlier CF is diagnosed, the sooner treatment can begin.

Despite these promising numbers, 85% of patients with CF die from complications of their lung disease (2). Monitoring lung disease progression is a critical role for health-care providers because it will help patients and their families make timely and informed decisions about care.

Progression of Lung Disease

Airway obstruction, infection, and inflammation leads to progressive damage to the CF lung. The progression of respiratory disease varies and cannot be predicted for individual patients by either the sweat chloride level or genotype. This uncertainty can be frustrating for families and can create a great deal of stress. In general, patients who are pancreatic sufficient tend to have a slower progression of lung disease (54). Several factors have been shown to negatively influence the progression of lung disease, including the following:

- Infection with *P. aeruginosa* (7, 54), *B. cepacia* (55), or MRSA (8, 56)
- Female gender (57, 58)
- Diabetes (54,58)
- Poor nutritional status (11, 54)
- Low socioeconomic status (57)
- Lack of insurance (59)
- Exposure to secondhand smoke (60)
- Presence of polymorphisms in modifier genes such as transforming growth factor-beta (TGF-β) (61) and mannose binding lectin (62)

Pulmonary function tests (PFTs) are the primary mode of following disease progression in patients with CF. The FEV_1 is the test that has traditionally been thought to best relate to mortality in patients with CF (12). However, it is clear that the rate of decline in lung function clearly influences morbidity and mortality (63).

Although CF is a multisystem disease, mortality is due almost exclusively to lung disease. Therefore, it is of vital importance to preserve lung function to enhance survival. The consistent use of airway clearance and inhalational therapies has the potential to continue to improve the lives of children with CF. Patients, families, and caregivers must adopt a unified approach designed to prevent permanent lung damage.

Children with CF can look forward to novel therapies that will treat the basic defect in chloride transport and revolutionize the approach to CF care. Eventually, these disease-modifying therapies will be available for administration to infants with CF diagnosed by newborn screening, thereby preventing or greatly slowing the appearance of the manifestations of CF lung disease. However, none of these therapies will reverse parenchymal lung disease. Therefore, maintaining an aggressive approach to respiratory care and encouraging adherence to the currently available therapies is vitally important.

■ ■ Ryan is now in 10th grade and using many therapies to maximize his lung function. It can be an arduous routine to maintain day in and day out, but Ryan and his parents are committed to maintaining his lung health. He is one of your most pleasant patients, and you often look forward to talking with him at each of his quarterly visits. He used twice-a-day airway clearance using HFCWO, as well as albuterol, hypertonic saline, dornase alfa, and tobramycin (every other month). He is active in soccer and loves to watch scary movies. He is a math tutor for elementary school students and helps maintain the website for his graduating class. He has been hospitalized twice in the last 5 years for pulmonary exacerbations, each in the winter months and associated with upper respiratory infections. In each case he was discharged within 4 days and never admitted to the intensive care unit. He confides to you that the most challenging part of trying to be a "normal kid" is when the clinic team increases his treatment regimen to four times a day during mild pulmonary exacerbations. At those times he's forced to spend his lunchtime in the school nurse's office and has to go home immediately after school to maintain treatment compliance. Based on his PFTs, which remain within 90% of predicted values, his current treatment modalities seem to be effective.

■ ■ Critical Thinking Questions: Ryan Greb

1. If Ryan had presented with more severe pulmonary symptoms in infancy, what would be an effective way for his family to provide airway clearance techniques?
2. What clues would let you or the physical therapist know that Ryan or his parents were not being compliant with his prescribed treatment regimen?
3. What role does infection play in the progression of Ryan's CF lung disease?

▶● Case Studies and Critical Thinking Questions

■ Case 1: Sarah Moses

Sarah Moses is 11 years old and has a baseline FEV_1 of 102% of predicted. She usually has only an intermittent cough. Today she presents in the CF clinic with an increased cough and sputum production, which is not typical for her. Her FEV_1 has also fallen to 88% of predicted. She reports having occasional dyspnea. Her chest examination results are normal.

- *What do you think is going on with Sarah? What clinical information led you to that conclusion?*
- *What should be the recommended course for Sarah, based on her symptoms?*

It is important to realize that pulmonary exacerbations can lead to permanent loss of lung function. Therefore, aggressive therapy should be undertaken for Sarah. Studies have shown that there can be a greater delay in therapy for children with better lung function, as in Sarah's case (64). This is exactly the wrong approach to take because children with good lung function have the most to lose from a delay in care.

■ Case 2: Dylan Warski

Dylan Warski is 14 years old and has CF as a result of two F508del *CFTR* mutations. Airway cultures have repeatedly grown *P. aeruginosa*. His daily pulmonary regimen includes airway clearance twice daily, dornase alfa once daily, albuterol twice daily, and inhaled aztreonam three times daily in 28-day on/off cycles. Over the past 3 months, Dylan has had several episodes of wheezing, and his FEV_1 has fallen by 10%. Dylan's physician is concerned about the increased symptomatology and obtains a serum IgE result, which is 2,600 IU/mL.

- *Based on the above findings, what is the most likely cause for Dylan's pulmonary exacerbation?*

Note that the culture of *A. fumigatus* from the airway is not required for the diagnosis of ABPA. Although the serum IgE measurement can be an effective screening tool for ABPA, it is not adequate for the diagnosis. IgE measurements can also be used to follow the progression of disease and effectiveness of therapy.

- *Once the diagnosis of ABPA is confirmed, what should Dylan's treatments include? How should his daily regimen be adjusted to compensate for this new infection? How would you assess the effectiveness of treatment?*

■ Case 3: Michelle Rivers

Michelle Rivers is 15 years old and has CF. She is a sophomore in high school and maintains a high grade point average while enrolled in college preparatory classes. She is active in varsity soccer. Michelle has had a slow but steady decline in her pulmonary function testing over the past year. Her FEV_1 was 90% of predicted 2 years ago and has steadily declined to her current 80%.

Michelle's prescribed inhaled therapy/airway clearance regimen is as follows:

AM	Afternoon	PM
Nebulized albuterol	Albuterol MDI	Nebulized albuterol
Hypertonic saline	Cayston (every other month)	Hypertonic saline
Dornase alfa		HFCWO (30 minutes)
HFCWO (30 minutes)		TOBI/Cayston
TOBI/Cayston (alternating months)		

The care team is concerned about her progressive decline in lung function, which is excessive for a child with CF, in whom the expected decline in FEV_1 should be approximately 2% per year (65). The clinic physician asks you to work with Michelle to help stop this decline.

- *Given that her subjective symptoms are unchanged, what do you suspect is the reason for Michelle's pulmonary function decline? How can you investigate to determine the cause?*
- *What can you do to halt this decline in adherence to therapy?*
- *If Michelle returned in 3 months and there was no improvement in her pulmonary function results, what do you think the recommendation should be?*

Multiple-Choice Questions

1. Which of the following are manifestations typical in a school-aged child with CF?
   I. Productive cough
   II. Wheeze
   III. Meconium ileus
   IV. Oily stools
   V. Nasal polyps
   a. I, III, IV
   b. I, II, III, IV, V
   c. I, III, IV, V
   d. I, II, IV

2. What test is the "gold standard" for diagnosing CF?
   a. Newborn screening
   b. Sweat test
   c. Nasal potential difference (NPD) test
   d. Genetic testing for *CTFR* gene mutations

3. What is the best method for airway clearance in a 3-year-old child without a history of GER?
   I. Percussion and vibration
   II. HFCWO
   III. ACB
   IV. FET
   V. Oscillating PEP
   a. I, II, III
   b. I
   c. I, II
   d. I, II, III, V

4. Which nebulizer should be used to deliver tobramycin to a 13-year-old with CF?
   a. Small-volume nebulizer
   b. PARI LC Plus
   c. Breath-actuated nebulizer
   d. Altera nebulizer

5. Which ACT can help improve FRC as well as promote clearance of mucus?
   a. HFCWO
   b. Percussion, vibration, and postural drainage
   c. PEP
   d. ACB and FET

6. You are asked to participate in prescription of pulmonary therapies for a 12-year-old who just moved to the area from another state and is new to the clinic. He has not yet had a pulmonary exacerbation, is active in soccer and baseball, and plays the trumpet in the middle school band. His parents both work full time, and he is an only child. There is no other family nearby. What would you recommend as his therapy?
   a. Percussion and vibration, dornase alfa, albuterol SVN, and tobramycin four times a day
   b. HFCWO, albuterol MDI, dornase alfa, and Colistin before school and after soccer practice
   c. HFCWO, albuterol SVN, and *N*-acetylcysteine before and after school
   d. Oscillating PEP, albuterol MDI, dornase alfa, and hypertonic saline before school, during lunch break, and after soccer practice

7. A 9-year-old patient, Jason, had a change to his new daily regimen of CF therapies. His mom has called you because she lost the paper that describes the correct order of therapies, but she still has the list of medications and other therapies. Put in them in the order in which they should be done.
   I. Albuterol (MDI)
   II. Tobramycin
   III. Pulmozyme
   IV. HFCWO
   a. I, II, III, IV
   b. I, II, IV, III
   c. IV, I, II, III
   d. I, III, IV, II

8. Identify common organisms that contribute to pulmonary exacerbations.
   a. *Aspergillosis fumigatus*
   b. *Streptococcus pneumonia*
   c. *Pseudomonas aeruginosa*
   d. *Staphylococcus aureus*

9. Which of the following complications is an adult patient with CF most likely to have had at some point in his or her life?
   a. Pneumothorax
   b. CF-related diabetes
   c. Allergic bronchopulmonary aspergillosis
   d. Liver failure

10. Which of the following is not a strategy that should be employed during any pulmonary exacerbation?
    a. Addition of or increased frequency of bronchodilator
    b. Increase in frequency of ACTs
    c. bronchoscopy
    d. Antibiotic therapy

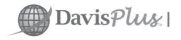 For additional resources login to Davis*Plus* (http://davisplus.fadavis.com/ keyword "Perretta") and click on the Premium tab. (Don't have a *Plus*Code to access Premium Resources? Just click the Purchase Access button on the book's Davis*Plus* page.)

REFERENCES

1. O'Sullivan BP, Freedman SD. Cystic fibrosis. *Lancet.* 2009;373(9678):1891-1904.
2. Cytic Fibrosis Patient Registry. Cystic Fibrosis Foundation, Bethesda, Maryland, 2010.
3. Riordan JR, Rommens JM, Kerem B, et al. Identification of the cystic fibrosis gene: cloning and characterization of complementary DNA. *Science.* 1989;245(4922):1066-1073.
4. Donaldson SH, Boucher RC. Sodium channels and cystic fibrosis. *Chest.* 2007;132(5):1631-1636.
5. Boucher RC. Airway surface dehydration in cystic fibrosis: pathogenesis and therapy. *Annu Rev Med.* 2007;58:157-1570.
6. Jones AM, Dodd ME, Govan JR, et al. Burkholderia cenocepacia and Burkholderia multivorans: influence on survival in cystic fibrosis. *Thorax.* 2004;59(11):948-951.
7. Emerson J, Rosenfeld M, McNamara S, Ramsey B, Gibson RL. Pseudomonas aeruginosa and other predictors of mortality and morbidity in young children with cystic fibrosis. *Pediatr Pulmonol.* 2002;34(2):91-100.
8. Dasenbrook EC, Checkley W, Merlo CA, Konstan MW, Lechtzin N, Boyle MP, et al. Association between respiratory tract methicillin-resistant Staphylococcus aureus and survival in cystic fibrosis. *JAMA.* 2010;303(23):2386-2392.
9. Cystic Fibrosis Mutation Database. http://www.genet.sickkids.on.ca/cftr/app, accessed July 27, 2013.
10. Cheng SH, Gregory RJ, Marshall J, et al. Defective intracellular transport and processing of CFTR is the molecular basis of most cystic fibrosis. *Cell.* 1990;63(4):827-834.
11. Stallings VA, Stark LJ, Robinson KA, Feranchak AP, Quinton H. Evidence-based practice recommendations for nutrition-related management of children and adults with cystic fibrosis and pancreatic insufficiency: results of a systematic review. *J Am Diet Assoc.* 2008;108(5):832-839.
12. Kerem E, Reisman J, Corey M, Canny GJ, Levison H. Prediction of mortality in patients with cystic fibrosis. *N Engl J Med.* 1992;326(18):1187-1191.
13. Farrell PM, Rosenstein BJ, White TB, et al. Guidelines for diagnosis of cystic fibrosis in newborns through older adults: Cystic Fibrosis Foundation consensus report. *J Pediatr.* 2008;153(2):S4-S14.
14. Quinton PM. Missing Cl conductance in cystic fibrosis. *Am J Physiol.* 1986;251(4, pt 1):C649-C652.
15. Zielenski J, Tsui LC. Cystic fibrosis: genotypic and phenotypic variations. *Annu Rev Genet.* 1995;29:777-807.
16. Flume PA, Robinson KA, O'Sullivan BP, et al. Cystic fibrosis pulmonary guidelines: airway clearance therapies. *Respir Care.* 2009;54(4):522-537.
17. Main E, Prasad A, Schans C. Conventional chest physiotherapy compared to other airway clearance techniques for cystic fibrosis. *Cochrane Database Syst Rev.* 2005(1): CD002011.
18. Khan TZ, Wagener JS, Bost T, et al. Early pulmonary inflammation in infants with cystic fibrosis. *Am J Respir Crit Care Med.* 1995;151(4):1075-1082.
19. Sly PD, Brennan S, Gangell C, et al. Lung disease at diagnosis in infants with cystic fibrosis detected by newborn screening. *Am J Respir Crit Care Med.* 2009;180(2): 146-152.
20. Mott LS, Park J, Murray CP, et al. Progression of early structural lung disease in young children with cystic fibrosis assessed using CT. *Thorax.* 2012;67(6):509-516.
21. Button BM, Heine RG, Catto-Smith AG, Olinsky A, Phelan PD, Ditchfield MR, Story I, et al. Chest physiotherapy in infants with cystic fibrosis: to tip or not? A five-year study. *Pediatr Pulmonol.* 2003;35(3):208-213.
22. Elkins MR, Alison JA, Bye PT. Effect of body position on maximal expiratory pressure and flow in adults with cystic fibrosis. *Pediatr Pulmonol.* 2005;40(5):385-391.
23. Dasgupta B, Tomkiewicz RP, Boyd WA, Brown NE, King M. Effects of combined treatment with rhDNase and airflow oscillations on spinnability of cystic fibrosis sputum in vitro. *Pediatr Pulmonol.* 1995;20(2):78-82.
24. Pryor JA. Physiotherapy for airway clearance in adults. *Eur Respir J.* 1999;14(6):1418-1424.
25. Myers TR. Positive expiratory pressure and oscillatory positive expiratory pressure therapies. *Respir Care.* 2007; 52(10):1308-1326, discussion 27.
26. Campbell T, Ferguson N, McKinlay R. The use of a simple self-administered method of positive expiratory pressure in chest physiotherapy after abdominal surgery. *Physiotherapy.* 1986;72(10):498-500.
27. Darbee JC, Ohtake PJ, Grant BJ, Cerny FJ. Physiologic evidence for the efficacy of positive expiratory pressure as an airway clearance technique in patients with cystic fibrosis. *Phys Ther.* 2004;84(6):524-537.
28. Oberwaldner B, Evans JC, Zach MS. Forced expirations against a variable resistance: a new chest physiotherapy method in cystic fibrosis. *Pediatr Pulmonol.* 1986;2(6): 358-367.
29. Lannefors L, Button BM, McIlwaine M. Physiotherapy in infants and young children with cystic fibrosis: current practice and future developments. *J R Soc Med.* 2004; 97(suppl 44):8-25.
30. Flume PA, O'Sullivan BP, Robinson KA, et al. Cystic fibrosis pulmonary guidelines: chronic medications for maintenance of lung health. *Am J Respir Crit Care Med.* 2007;176(10):957-969.
31. Aitken ML, Bellon G, De Boeck K, et al. Long-term inhaled dry powder mannitol in cystic fibrosis: an international randomized study. *Am J Respir Crit Care Med.* 2012;185(6):645-652.
32. Bilton D, Robinson P, Cooper P, et al. Inhaled dry powder mannitol in cystic fibrosis: an efficacy and safety study. *Eur Respir J.* 2011;38(5):1071-1080.
33. Stuart B, Lin JH, Mogayzel PJ, Jr. Early eradication of Pseudomonas aeruginosa in patients with cystic fibrosis. *Paediatr Respir Rev.* 2010;11(3):177-184.
34. Ratjen F, Munck A, Kho P, Angyalosi G. Treatment of early Pseudomonas aeruginosa infection in patients with cystic fibrosis: the ELITE trial. *Thorax.* 2010;65(4): 286-291.
35. Treggiari MM, Retsch-Bogart G, Mayer-Hamblett N, et al. Comparative efficacy and safety of 4 randomized regimens to treat early Pseudomonas aeruginosa infection in children with cystic fibrosis. *Arch Pediatr Adolesc Med.* 2011;165(9):847-856.
36. Tramper-Stranders GA, Wolfs TF, van Haren Noman S, et al. Controlled trial of cycled antibiotic prophylaxis to prevent initial Pseudomonas aeruginosa infection in children with cystic fibrosis. *Thorax.* 2010;65(10):915-920.
37. Sudfeld CR, Dasenbrook EC, Merz WG, Carroll KC, Boyle MP. Prevalence and risk factors for recovery of filamentous fungi in individuals with cystic fibrosis. *J Cyst Fibros.* 2010;9(2):110-116.
38. Ramsey BW, Davies J, McElvaney NG, et al. A CFTR potentiator in patients with cystic fibrosis and the G551D mutation. *N Engl J Med.* 2011;365(18):1663-1672.
39. Saiman L, Siegel J. Infection control recommendations for patients with cystic fibrosis: microbiology, important pathogens, and infection control practices to prevent patient-to-patient transmission. *Am J Infect Control.* 2003;31(suppl 3):S1-S62.
40. Masoud-Landgraf L, Badura A, Eber E, et al. Molecular epidemiology of Pseudomonas aeruginosa in cystic fibrosis patients from Southeast Austria. *Wien Klin Wochenschr.* 2012;124(7-8):262-265.

41. Eakin MN, Bilderback A, Boyle MP, Mogayzel PJ, Riekert KA. Longitudinal association between medication adherence and lung health in people with cystic fibrosis. *J Cyst Fibros.* 2011;10(4):258-264.

42. Flume PA, Mogayzel PJ, Jr., Robinson KA, et al. Cystic fibrosis pulmonary guidelines: treatment of pulmonary exacerbations. *Am J Respir Crit Care Med.* 2009;180(9): 802-808.

43. Collaco JM, Green DM, Cutting GR, Naughton KM, Mogayzel PJ, Jr. Location and duration of treatment of cystic fibrosis respiratory exacerbations do not affect outcomes. *Am J Respir Crit Care Med.* 2010;182(9):1137-1143.

44. Sanders DB, Bittner RC, Rosenfeld M, Hoffman LR, Redding GJ, Goss CH, et al. Failure to recover to baseline pulmonary function after cystic fibrosis pulmonary exacerbation. *Am J Respir Crit Care Med.* 2010;182(5):627-632.

45. Flume PA, Mogayzel PJ, Jr., Robinson KA, Rosenblatt RL, Quittell L, Marshall BC, et al. Cystic fibrosis pulmonary guidelines: pulmonary complications: hemoptysis and pneumothorax. *Am J Respir Crit Care Med.* 2010; 182(3):298-306.

46. Flume PA. Pneumothorax in cystic fibrosis. *Curr Opin Pulm Med.* 2011;17(4):220-225.

47. Flume PA, Strange C, Ye X, Ebeling M, Hulsey T, Clark LL, et al. Pneumothorax in cystic fibrosis. *Chest.* 2005; 128(2):720-728.

48. Stevens DA, Moss RB, Kurup VP, et al. Allergic bronchopulmonary aspergillosis in cystic fibrosis-state of the art: Cystic Fibrosis Foundation Consensus Conference. *Clin Infect Dis.* 2003;37(suppl 3):S225-S264.

49. Lebecque P, Leonard A, Pilette C. Omalizumab for treatment of ABPA exacerbations in CF patients. *Pediatr Pulmonol.* 2009;44(5):516.

50. Moran A, Brunzell C, Cohen RC, et al. Clinical care guidelines for cystic fibrosis-related diabetes: a position statement of the American Diabetes Association and a clinical practice guideline of the Cystic Fibrosis Foundation, endorsed by the Pediatric Endocrine Society. *Diabetes Care.* 2010;33(12):2697-2708.

51. Riekert KA, Bartlett SJ, Boyle MP, Krishnan JA, Rand CS. The association between depression, lung function, and health-related quality of life among adults with cystic fibrosis. *Chest.* 2007;132(1):231-237.

52. Efrati O, Bylin I, Segal E, et al. Outcome of patients with cystic fibrosis admitted to the intensive care unit: is invasive mechanical ventilation a risk factor for death in patients waiting lung transplantation? *Heart Lung.* 2010; 39(2):153-159.

53. Benden C, Aurora P, Edwards LB, et al. The Registry of the International Society for Heart and Lung Transplantation: Fourteenth Pediatric Lung and Heart-Lung Transplantation Report—2011. *J Heart Lung Transplant.* 2011; 30(10):1123-1132.

54. Konstan MW, Morgan WJ, Butler SM, et al. Risk factors for rate of decline in forced expiratory volume in one second in children and adolescents with cystic fibrosis. *J Pediatr.* 2007;151(2):134-139, 9 e1.

55. Courtney JM, Dunbar KE, McDowell A, et al. Clinical outcome of Burkholderia cepacia complex infection in cystic fibrosis adults. *J Cyst Fibros.* 2004;3(2):93-98.

56. Dasenbrook EC, Merlo CA, Diener-West M, Lechtzin N, Boyle MP. Persistent methicillin-resistant Staphylococcus aureus and rate of FEV1 decline in cystic fibrosis. *Am J Respir Crit Care Med.* 2008;178(8):814-821.

57. Barr HL, Britton J, Smyth AR, Fogarty AW. Association between socioeconomic status, sex, and age at death from cystic fibrosis in England and Wales (1959 to 2008): cross sectional study. *BMJ.* 2011;343:d4662.

58. Chamnan P, Shine BS, Haworth CS, Bilton D, Adler AI. Diabetes as a determinant of mortality in cystic fibrosis. *Diabetes Care.* 2010;33(2):311-316.

59. Curtis JR, Burke W, Kassner AW, Aitken ML. Absence of health insurance is associated with decreased life expectancy in patients with cystic fibrosis. *Am J Respir Crit Care Med.* 1997;155(6):1921-1924.

60. Collaco JM, Vanscoy L, Bremer L, et al. Interactions between secondhand smoke and genes that affect cystic fibrosis lung disease. *JAMA.* 2008;299(4):417-424.

61. Drumm ML, Konstan MW, Schluchter MD, et al. Genetic modifiers of lung disease in cystic fibrosis. *N Engl J Med.* 2005;353(14):1443-1453.

62. Buranawuti K, Boyle MP, Cheng S, et al. Variants in mannose-binding lectin and tumour necrosis factor alpha affect survival in cystic fibrosis. *J Med Genet.* 2007;44(3): 209-214.

63. Corey M, Edwards L, Levison H, Knowles M. Longitudinal analysis of pulmonary function decline in patients with cystic fibrosis. *J Pediatr.* 1997;131(6):809-814.

64. Kraynack NC, Gothard MD, Falletta LM, McBride JT. Approach to treating cystic fibrosis pulmonary exacerbations varies widely across US CF care centers. *Pediatr Pulmonol.* 2011;46(9):870-881.

65. Konstan MW, Schluchter MD, Xue W, Davis PB. Clinical use of ibuprofen is associated with slower FEV1 decline in children with cystic fibrosis. *Am J Respir Crit Care Med.* 2007;176(11):1084-1089.

Chapter 15

Pediatric Pulmonary Diseases

Vinay Nadkarni, MD
Roberta Hales, MHA, RRT-NPS, RN
Shawn Colbourn, AS, RRT-NPS

Key Terms

Acute lung injury
Acute respiratory distress
  syndrome (ARDS)
Airway pressure release ventilation
  (APRV)
Antipyretics
Apoptosis
Bronchoalveolar lavage (BAL)
Bronchiolitis
Consolidated
Epinephrine
Exudative stage
Fibrotic stage
Fomites
Nitrogen washout
Pentamidine isethionate
Plateau pressure
Pneumocytes
Proliferative stage
Prone positioning
Refractory hypoxemia
Respiratory syncytial virus (RSV)
Ribavirin
Static compliance
Surfactant
Volume-targeted pressure control
  ventilation

Chapter Objectives

After reading this chapter, you will be able to:

1. Assess the need for hospital admission for a pediatric patient with signs of respiratory distress.
2. Identify the signs and symptoms used when classifying bronchiolitis severity.
3. Select an oxygen-delivery device for a patient with bronchiolitis or pneumonia based on age, required concentration of inspired oxygen, and severity of respiratory distress.
4. List the different pathogens responsible for pediatric pneumonia.
5. Assess the effectiveness of noninvasive ventilation in managing a patient with hypoxemia and alveolar instability associated with pneumonia.
6. Describe the four clinical characteristics of acute respiratory distress syndrome (ARDS).
7. Describe the chest radiograph findings for bronchiolitis, pneumonia, and ARDS.
8. Describe the benefits of advanced modes of ventilation in improving gas exchange in ARDS.
9. Recommend ventilator setting changes for a patient on airway pressure release ventilation with ARDS and respiratory acidosis.

■■ Jacob Smith

You are the respiratory therapist (RT) working in a regional pediatric hospital with a level I PICU and are called to assess an infant in respiratory distress. Jacob Smith is 9 months old and weighs 8 kg—his mother brought him to the emergency department (ED) because of decreased feeding, runny nose, and increased work of breathing (WOB). Jacob's history is unremarkable: He is a term newborn who has had a normal development, with standard immunizations and no prior hospital admissions. Mom states that Jacob has a 2-day history of cold symptoms, including nasal discharge, slight fever, and cough. Today, his respiratory symptoms worsened and include a rapid respiratory rate (RR), wheezing, intercostal retractions, and nasal flaring, along with decreased oral intake and activity level. A nasal swab has been sent to the laboratory for viral testing.

Respiratory disorders account for 27.8% of all pediatric hospital admissions through the ED, and acute respiratory distress is the most common cause of illness requiring hospitalization in infants and children less than 15 years of age (1). These children usually require acute management and frequent assessment of respiratory distress, and a small percentage will need intensive care management to prevent respiratory failure and circulatory collapse. With even mild respiratory impairment, most of these children will require at least one type of respiratory therapy, which could include airway clearance, supplemental oxygen therapy, deep breathing exercises, chest physiotherapy, and inhaled medications. More severe cases will require noninvasive ventilation, specialty gas therapy, and intubation and mechanical ventilation. This chapter will discuss several of those diseases: bronchiolitis, pneumonia, and acute respiratory distress syndrome (ARDS).

Bronchiolitis

Acute viral **bronchiolitis** is an inflammation of the small bronchiolar airways resulting from a viral infection. Bronchiolitis is the most common lower-respiratory tract infection and the leading cause of hospitalizations in children younger than 1 year old in the United States. Approximately 4 million children are infected with bronchiolitis every year, and approximately 1% to 3% (75,000 to 125,000) of full-term infants are hospitalized, with 2% to 5% of those hospitalized requiring mechanical ventilation (2, 3). Bronchiolitis can manifest a full spectrum of severity, from mild tachypnea and expiratory wheezing to profound, acute, life-threatening respiratory failure as a result of near-complete lower respiratory tract obstruction and inflammation. A relatively common life-threatening complication associated with bronchiolitis is apnea, particularly in the premature, low birth weight, or young infant (less than 3 months of age). The natural history of the disease is that severity worsens over the first 72 hours, then plateaus for a few days and resolves over several weeks. Risk factors for more severe symptoms include the following:

- Young age, that is, infants younger than 3 months old
- Low birth weight
- Premature birth less than or equal to 36 weeks
- Congenital heart disease
- Chronic lung disease
- Airway abnormalities (e.g., bronchomalacia)
- Neurological abnormalities with dystonia

Additional risk factors occasionally reported as associated with bronchiolitis include male gender, having older siblings, living in crowded conditions, exposure to tobacco smoke, attending day care, and low socioeconomic status (4, 5). Factors that should lead the health-care provider to consider the need for hospitalization include a history of apnea, difficulty feeding, pronounced respiratory distress (including accessory muscle and/or grunting and respiratory rate greater than 60 breaths per minute), and the need for supplemental oxygen (saturation of arterial blood with oxygen, or SpO_2, less than or equal to 92%) (4, 6).

Acute bronchiolitis is characterized by acute inflammation, increased mucus production, and bronchoconstriction. The initial presentation often begins with nasal congestion followed by lower-respiratory symptoms of cough, tachypnea, wheezing, and coarse crackles. Many viruses cause bronchiolitis. The most common viral pathogen is **respiratory syncytial virus (RSV)**, which accounts for 50% to 80% of all bronchiolitis cases (7, 8). Other contributing viruses include parainfluenza types 1 and 2; adenovirus types 1, 2, and 5; influenza type B; rhinovirus; and human metapneumovirus.

Pathophysiology

Viruses are the most common pathogens that cause bronchiolitis. The virus replication begins in the nasopharyngeal epithelium and spreads downward into the respiratory tract to the bronchial epithelium. After viral replication, inflammation occurs in the bronchial epithelium cells in combination with peribronchial white blood cell infiltration, mostly mononuclear cells, and the resultant submucosal edema, cell sloughing, and necrosis of the bronchial epithelium. Mucus production increases in both quantity and viscosity and mixes with the necrotic epithelium, fibrin, and cellular debris (6). Furthermore, these inspissated (thick) secretions decrease the function of the ciliated epithelium, resulting in extensive mucus plugging, increased airway resistance, and partial or total airway obstruction/trapping of the lower respiratory tract. The degree of obstruction is the foremost contributing factor to ventilation/perfusion (V/Q) mismatch and hypoxemia, along with respiratory failure (9).

RSV infection is particularly problematic because it is extremely virulent and highly infectious, and it is usually transmitted through direct inoculation or contact with infected secretions. The vehicle of transmission is direct contact with secretions rather than airborne mist. Most infants and children acquire the virus from direct contact with infected older children and/or adults. The usual method of RSV transmission is by **fomites**, or secretions that live on inanimate objects. Once an object is contaminated with RSV, the virus can live and remain viable for 2.5 to 8 hours, depending on environmental conditions (10). Additionally, RSV can survive on the hands for a considerable length of time and be transferred back and forth from inanimate and animate objects. This long and variable viability makes it imperative that health-care providers practice good hand hygiene (Teamwork 15-1). The incubation period for RSV is 2 to 8 days, and it can be shed in nasal secretions for up to 3 weeks (average 8 days), and even longer in immune-compromised patients (e.g., cancer patients). Seasonal outbreaks usually occur during the winter months, with a variation in the peak, onset, and duration from year to year. The season typically begins in November, peaks in the winter months, and comes to an end by early spring; however, this time frame can be subject to regional variation. Almost all children are infected with RSV by the age of 2 years, but this does not appear to provide them with immunity from future infections.

Clinical Manifestations

In acute bronchiolitis, a rapid onset of lower-respiratory symptoms usually occurs by days 2 to 5 of the illness. Although fever may be present in the early onset of disease, it is usually low grade or absent in the later stages. Infants usually exhibit decreased physical activity, irritability, and feeding intolerance secondary to tachypnea resulting in decreased fluid intake, which leads to dehydration and contributes to thickened secretions.

Teamwork 15-1 Universal Precautions

HEALTH-CARE PROVIDERS ARE RESPONSIBLE FOR THE SAFETY AND WELFARE OF THEIR PATIENTS. Providing safe, clean environments does not happen by chance. There must be vigilance to prevent the spread of infection to patients, colleagues, and yourself. Health-care workers must presume that every person and inanimate object is a carrier of a pathogen. Therefore, adherence to universal precautions is the responsibility of the entire health-care team. Universal precautions place barriers between providers and the patient. These barriers include wearing personal protective equipment (e.g., gown, gloves), performing hand hygiene, and adhering to isolation/contact precautions to prevent nosocomial spread of the pathogen (viral or bacterial).

Physical assessment focuses on classifying the severity of respiratory distress and hydration and thus the severity of the disease. Clinical signs and symptoms of bronchiolitis include the following:

- Low-grade fever
- Rhinorrhea
- Cough
- Tachypnea, earliest sign of change in status of disease
- Tachycardia
- Retractions, subcostal and intercostal
- Nasal flaring
- Expiratory wheezing, with or without bilateral crackles
- Prolonged expiratory time
- Cyanosis

Respiratory rate, WOB, and hypoxemia are the most clinically significant patient-assessment parameters used to determine the severity of illness, and several patient-assessment tools have been designed to objectively measure respiratory distress (11-13) (Table 15-1, Table 15-2). The most significant consequence of bronchiolitis is hypoxemia. Hypoxemia results from a V/Q mismatch at the alveolar capillary membrane. Specifically, this mismatch occurs because there are alveoli being perfused but not ventilated owing to the collapse of small airways (bronchioles) and microatelectasis. Hypercarbia can occur because of an increase in the dead space-to-tidal volume (V_T) ratio, thus decreasing the amount of functional lung participating in gas exchange. Careful monitoring is necessary to detect periodic breathing, central apnea, and cardiopulmonary instability in the young and premature infant.

Apnea may be attributed to a mix of both central and obstructive apnea. It rarely lasts more than a few days, and fewer than 10% of patients who present with an episode of apnea require intubation and ventilation (5, 6).

Diagnostic Testing

The most common diagnostic testing used for acute bronchiolitis includes viral detection and chest radiographs. The American Academy of Pediatrics (AAP) guidelines (14) do not support the use of these tests in the management of routine cases; however, they are still commonly prescribed clinically to assist in diagnosis of bronchiolitis.

RSV Testing

RSV viral antigen testing has variable sensitivity and specificity, and it is generally good at detecting viruses during the peak viral season. Even so, viral pathophysiology is usually equivalent. The identification of the specific virus has little to no impact on clinical management or outcome of the disease. However, the identification of a specific virus on the hospitalized patient may assist the health-care provider in preventing and reducing the spread of hospital-acquired infections or allow discontinuation of antibiotics or other medication exposures.

Chest Radiographs

Chest radiographs are an important diagnostic tool used in the diagnosis of respiratory distress. In acute bronchiolitis, radiographs may reveal areas of overinflation along with patchy infiltrates attributed to atelectasis. However, the AAP does not

Table 15-1	Respiratory Distress Assessment Instrument (RDAI) (11)					
Symptom	**Points**					
	0	**1**	**2**	**3**	**4**	**Maximum**
Wheezing						
During expiration	None	End	1/2	3/4	All	4
During inspiration	None	Part	All			2
Number of involved lung fields	None	Segmental	Diffuse			2
Retractions						
Supraclavicular	None	Mild	Moderate	Marked		3
Intercostal	None	Mild	Moderate	Marked		3
Subcostal	None	Mild	Moderate	Marked		3
Total						17

The total score on the RDAI is the sum of the scores for each row, with a range of 0 to 17; higher scores indicate more severe respiratory distress.

| Table 15-2 | ED Guidelines for Evaluation/Treatment of Children With Bronchiolitis (13) |

Bronchiolitis Assessment Tool

Respiratory Assessment	Mild	Moderate	Severe
Pulse oximetry in room air	≥95%	92%–94%	<92%
Respiratory rate	<60	60–70	>70
Mental status	Normal	Irritable but active	Lethargic
Feeding	Normal	Less but adequate	Poor
Increased WOB Retractions Accessory muscles	Minimal/none	Intercostal	Substernal Neck or abdominal muscles
Wheeze	Minimal/none	Moderate expiratory	Severe inspiratory/expiratory
Air exchange	Good, equal breath sounds	Localized decreased breath sounds	Multiple areas decreased

Classification of Severity by Using Assessment Tool

Single Severity	
Mild	≥5 factors in the mild category
Moderate	≥5 factors in the moderate category
Severe	≥5 factors in the severe category

Mixed Severity	
Mild/Moderate	Majority of factors are in mild and moderate categories
Moderate/Severe	Majority of factors are in moderate and severe categories

Measuring Response to Albuterol/Racemic Epinephrine Using Assessment Tool

Improvement noted in at least three of seven categories

Zorc J, Florin T, Rodio B (12). Used by permission.

recommend routine radiographic testing because it does not change the clinical management of the disease. Although many infants with bronchiolitis have abnormalities on chest radiographs, the data are insufficient to demonstrate that these findings correlate well with severity of the disease (15). A chest radiograph is warranted when an infant or child does not improve or worsens, exhibits a high fever of unknown origin, and/or another diagnosis is suspected (e.g., pneumonia, ARDS).

■■ In triage, Jacob's physical examination is notable for the following: temperature, 38.3°C; alert and crying; nasal flaring; marked suprasternal and intercostal retractions; RR 54 breaths/min; heart rate (HR), 160 bpm; blood pressure, 92/60 mm Hg; SpO_2, 92% in room air; and capillary refill less than 2 seconds. You note during auscultation that he has a prolonged expiratory phase with expiratory wheezing, scattered coarse crackles, and an occasional grunt. There is minimal to no inspiratory stridor. Based on his clinical findings, Jacob's most likely differential diagnosis is acute viral bronchiolitis.

Management and Treatment

Bronchiolitis is the most frequent cause of hospitalization in the infant population. Management varies widely, and the efficacy of many routinely implemented therapies is not supported by evidence (16). Literature reviews support that the mainstay of bronchiolitis management should be quality supportive care, including adequate hydration, secretion clearance, and comfort measures. The majority of infants and children can be managed at home. A pulse oximetry level of less than 90% or 92% is frequently used as the deciding factor for in-patient admission. Admission should also be considered for patients with symptoms of severe respiratory distress. If hospitalized, there is a wide variety of practice for diagnosis and management of patients with bronchiolitis. The usual therapeutic interventions include oxygen, bronchodilators, glucocorticoids, chest physiotherapy, nasal suctioning, hypertonic saline, continuous airway pressure (CPAP), bi-level positive airway pressure (BiPAP), and antiviral agents. Despite this widespread list, none of these therapies has been shown to have a significant impact on duration of illness and severity of clinical outcomes (9). For these reasons, the AAP has issued evidence-based clinical guidelines focusing on the diagnosis, management, and prevention of bronchiolitis in children up to the age of 2 years (14). These guidelines are not intended to be a substitute for clinical expertise; they are a resource for the health-care provider in the management of acute bronchiolitis. Respiratory care for bronchiolitis should be focused on secretion clearance, frequent monitoring of respiratory status, and escalation of oxygen and ventilatory support as needed by the patient. This section will review all of the current treatments commonly in use for RSV and will address the amount of evidence behind their use, as well as whether they are currently part of the AAP's recommendations for bronchiolitis management.

Suctioning and Mucus Clearance

In acute bronchiolitis, nasal obstruction is the most common problem in young infants. Because infants are classified as obligate nose breathers (Special Population 15-1), nasal congestion and blockage can range from a mild nuisance to a life-threatening respiratory distress. Nasal suctioning and saline drops might help alleviate the nasal congestion, but there is no clear evidence to determine whether it is effective in the overall clinical management. In addition, there is no evidence to support deep suctioning of the pharynx or lower pharynx. Nevertheless, infants may require frequent nasal suctioning to clear their nasal passages. Frequent suctioning has some risks, including inflammation, bleeding, and trauma to the nasal mucosa. Therefore, the selection of the suction device should be geared toward maximum effectiveness with minimal trauma and limited to patients with an SpO_2 less than 90% and/or moderate-to-severe respiratory distress.

The preferred suctioning method uses an acorn nasal aspirator or bulb suction because of the minimal negative pressure; however, in the hospital a suction catheter with a side-control port can be used to nasally suction the patient. At times, a higher negative pressure may be needed to remove the copious

secretions. If higher negative pressure is used, the health-care provider should provide intermittent suction to minimize nasal trauma.

Oxygen Therapy

The delivery of supplemental oxygen therapy is the cornerstone for treatment and prevention of hypoxemia. Oxygen therapy is initiated to maintain a minimum level of SpO_2 at 94%; however, AAP recommends initiating oxygen below an SpO_2 of 90% because it is an acceptable point on the oxyhemoglobin dissociation curve (9, 14). It is important to remember that at the peak of illness a higher level of supplemental oxygen may be needed because several factors may shift the oxyhemoglobin dissociation curve, such as fever, acidosis, and hemoglobinopathies. These shifts cause large decreases in the partial pressure of oxygen (PaO_2) to occur at a SpO_2 greater than 90% (17, 18) (Fig. 15-1). Supplemental oxygen should be titrated based on the complete physical examination because a low oxygen saturation level measured using pulse oximetry is an influential parameter in determining the need for hospital admission. However, the use of continuous pulse oximetry monitoring during an in-patient admission may also contribute to a prolonged hospital course. For this reason, pulse oximetry measurements should be confirmed for accuracy prior to initiating supplemental oxygen and limited to severely ill patients. If the SpO_2 consistently measures below 90% and the infant or child exhibits signs of respiratory distress, then supplemental oxygen is necessary. The selection of an oxygen-delivery device depends on the age and size of the child, patient tolerance, and humidification. (Table 15-3 describes recommended delivery devices.) Oxygen should be discontinued if the infant or child is able to maintain a SpO_2 greater than 90%

Obligate Nose Breathers

Infants prefer to breathe through the nasal passages because of the physical structure of the upper airway. The soft palate is in direct contact with the epiglottis, and the tongue fills most of the oral cavity. These physical structures make it difficult for the infant to effectively breathe through the oral cavity. However, most infants can breathe through their mouths if the nasal passages are blocked.

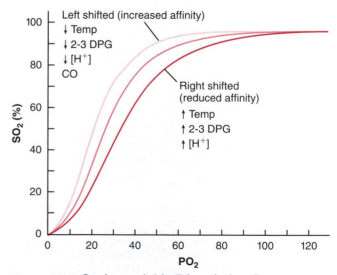

Figure 15-1 Oxyhemoglobin Dissociation Curve

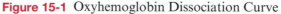

Table 15-3 Oxygen-Delivery Devices

Delivery device	Humidification	Flowrates	User Guidelines
Nasal cannula	no		Prong size is approximately half the diameter of the nares
<2 years of age		up to 2 LPM	Use low-flow meter to deliver accurate flow rates
>2 years of age		up to 4 LPM	Not suitable if nasal passages are congested or blocked
	yes	up to 6 LPM	Secure cannula to face with tape or anchoring device. Check for nasal patency, suction as needed
Simple mask	yes	minimum flow 4 LPM	FiO$_2$ is dependant on: oxygen flow rate, mask size/fit and the patient's ventilation minute volume
Pediatric mask		maximum flow 8–10 LPM	Select a mask that fits snug over child's face. Ensure good mask fit to maximize oxygen concentrations. Mask should be humidified and warmed
Oxyhood	yes		Minimize leaks by closing all open areas. Provide adequate flow, greater than 10–15 LPM (dependent on hood size) to ensure carbon dioxide clearance. Analyze oxygen near patient to ensure consistent delivery of FiO$_2$. Oxygen blender systems allows for precise control of FiO$_2$
Venturi mask	no	Ranges 6–10 LPM	FiO$_2$ ranges from 35%–50% depending on patient's minute ventilation. Minimal flowrate to ensure carbon dioxide clearance
Partial non-rebreather mask	no	Flow is adequate to maintain bag inflation during the entire respiratory cycle.	Prevents exhaled gases mixing with the fresh gas flow. May provide higher concentrations of FiO$_2$ (60%–80%) than is able to be provided by a standard aerosol face mask. Unsuitable if humidification is required
Non-rebreather mask	no	Flow is adequate to maintain bag inflarion during the entire respiratory cycle	Prevents exhaled gases mixing with the fresh gas flow. May provide higher concentration of FiO$_2$ (>80%) than is able to be provided with a standard aerosol face mask. Unsuitable if humidification is required
High-flow nasal cannula	yes	Low-flow cartridge 1–8 LPM. High-flow cartridge 10–40 LPM	Liter flow is dependent on the cartridge in system

while resting and/or feeding with minimal respiratory distress.

High-Flow Nasal Cannula

One of the newest high-flow oxygen-delivery systems being used in patients with impending respiratory failure is the high-flow nasal cannula (HFNC), which provides high-flow gas heated with nearly 100% humidity, allowing higher flows (1 to 8 liters per minute [LPM] pediatric cartridge and 8 to 40 LPM adult cartridge) to be tolerated by patients (19). These flow rates should exceed the patient's inspiratory flow demand at various minute volumes, eliminating the entrainment of room air. To further guarantee FIO$_2$ delivery, the HFNC uses an oxygen/air blender as the main driving gas source. Additionally, the HFNC uses the nasal pharynx as the gas reservoir, reducing the anatomical dead space (upper airway) by flushing the end expiratory gas from the system. This flushing enhances CO_2 clearance and oxygenation, thus improving the patient's respiratory status.

Helium-Oxygen (Heliox) Therapy

Bronchiolitis is an acute inflammatory process of the bronchioles causing increased mucus production and edema. This combination causes airway narrowing, resulting in increased airway resistance and partial or total obstruction. Moreover, the upper-airway tract is narrowed secondary to secretions and inflammation of the nasal passages. This critical narrowing results in turbulent gas flow and increased airway resistance (20). Turbulent flow is a major problem in obstructive lung disease such as acute bronchiolitis. The bronchiole lumens are obstructed and reduced in diameter from mucosal edema, inflammation, and thickened mucus. These dynamic changes result in decreased ventilation in the affected areas causing V/Q mismatch (20). Overall, these changes will affect alveolar gas exchange, resulting in hypoxemia and hypercapnia.

Heliox, a low-density gas mixture of helium and oxygen, has been shown to decrease resistance to gas flow in turbulent flow and obstructive disease conditions such as asthma and croup. In this mixture, helium replaces nitrogen as the carrier gas for oxygen, reducing resistance to air flow within the airways, "allowing increased bulk flow, increased oxygen flow, and decreased WOB" (21). Additionally, CO_2 is four to five times more readily diffusible in helium, assisting with improved ventilation and CO_2 removal. The onset of effects of heliox is rapid, so the clinical benefits will be seen within minutes. For these reasons, patients with acute bronchiolitis, a turbulent flow, and obstructive disease, may benefit from heliox therapy. However, if a patient requires supplemental oxygen greater than 0.40, it is speculated that the benefit of helium will be less likely because the lower the helium, the higher the gas density, resulting in increased turbulent flow in the airways and a decrease in alveolar ventilation. Current evidence suggests that heliox reduces WOB within the first hour of administration (21); however, there is no reduction in the rate of intubation and mechanical ventilation (20).

Commercial-grade heliox is available via H-cylinders in three different mixtures (80:20, 70:30, 60:40). One of the biggest challenges is the heliox delivery system. The lower-density heliox causes inaccurately high readings from flow meters calibrated for air and/or oxygen (22); thus, the liter flow needs to be corrected based on the density of the gas (Table 15-4). For heliox to be effective in spontaneously breathing patients, the optimal delivery system should be closed so that the patient will breathe

Table 15-4	Helium Oxygen Ratio Correction Factor for Oxygen Flowmeters (22)	
Heliox	Helium-Oxygen Mixture
80:20	1.8 times the liter flow
70:30	1.6 times the liter flow
60:40	1.4 times the liter flow

the delivered heliox without entraining room air during inspiration. Additionally, the flow rate of the heliox delivery system must be higher than the peak inspiratory flow rate of the infant or child to avoid titration of room air. The recommended heliox delivery system is through a non-rebreather device, which reduces the risk of air entrainment. Other systems including an oxyhood and nasal cannula are still used but have been deemed suboptimal (22). For example, a study by Stillwell showed that, when delivered via oxyhood, because of its low density, helium tends to separate from the oxygen and concentrate in the top of the hood (23). This minimizes the clinical effectiveness, and thus the study concluded that non-rebreathers and simple masks are satisfactory delivery devices. On the contrary, two studies have shown clinical improvement in children with upper respiratory obstruction in a heliox hood and no difference in oxygen concentrations within a hood (24, 25). When using newer delivery devices such as HFNCs, flow-rate settings should meet the patient's inspiratory flow demand to reduce entrainment of room air.

The administration of heliox with mechanical ventilation can be problematic. Ventilators are calibrated with nitrogen, not helium, as the primary gas source. Helium interferes with the pneumotachometer and ventilator function, causing inaccurate readings of all flow-dependent parameters. These parameters include actual V_T, minute ventilation, inspiratory flow rates, expiratory flow rates, and FIO_2. Because the reading from the ventilator may not be accurate, each of these parameters needs to be directly monitored. Several new-generation ventilators (e.g., Avea ventilator from Viasys Healthcare, Conshohocken, PA; Servo-i from Maquet Critical Care AB, Solna, Sweden) have helium/oxygen administration systems to help circumvent these issues. The delivery of heliox to the infant or child who is breathing spontaneously and mechanically ventilated is challenging. Optimal heliox-delivery systems should prevent or limit entrainment to ensure helium delivery.

Inhaled Bronchodilator Therapy

Bronchodilators are often used in the management of acute bronchiolitis; however, there is no strong evidence that justifies routine use. The

AAP's recommendation is that bronchodilators should not be used routinely in the management of bronchiolitis. However, they do recommend that a carefully monitored trial of B₂-adrenergic and/or alpha-adrenergic bronchodilators is an option and that the use of bronchodilators should be continued only if there is "documented positive clinical response" (14). However, if no clinical benefit occurs, then the bronchodilator should be discontinued because of the potential adverse side effects (e.g., tremors, tachycardia, hypokalemia, hyperglycemia). Some common bronchodilators used to treat bronchoconstriction are albuterol sulfate/salbutamol and racemic epinephrine (Table 15-5).

Epinephrine

Airway edema is a primary component of bronchiolitis. Theoretically, infants and children with bronchiolitis should benefit from inhaled **epinephrine** "because it contains alpha-adrenergic properties in addition to the beta-adrenergic effect" (26). Although trials of inhaled epinephrine have shown temporary clinical improvement, it is probably a result of the alpha-adrenergic effect on the nasal mucosa and bronchiole edema. In general, inhaled epinephrine is not recommended because there is insufficient evidence to determine the clinical significance (27); however, there is evidence to suggest that epinephrine may be favorable to albuterol sulfate (salbutamol) in outpatients (26).

Hypertonic Saline Solution

Airway edema and mucus plugging are the primary pathological constituents of acute bronchiolitis. The cilia that line the airways are responsible for clearing debris out of the lungs. In bronchiolitis, the cilia become dysfunctional from excess mucus and edema. This causes a malfunction of the mucociliary escalator, resulting in viscous mucus and plugging. Hypertonic saline increases the ion concentration in the airway surface liquid and osmotically draws fluid into the airway lumen, thereby replenishing the fluid layer and accelerating mucus clearance (28). Nebulized hypertonic saline is administered with a small-volume nebulizer. Hypertonic saline can cause airway irritation, and coughing may be induced. This coughing aids in the breaking up and clearance of mucus from the lower respiratory tract but can cause further airway irritation. Therefore, if patients experience moderate-to-severe coughing with bronchoconstriction, a prophylactic treatment with a bronchodilator should precede nebulized 3% hypertonic saline.

Nebulized 3% hypertonic saline has been used as a therapeutic treatment for acute bronchiolitis, and several studies suggest a decrease in the length of stay at the hospital and a significant improvement in the clinical severity scores for patients treated with it (29–32). Given these positive results, 3% nebulized hypertonic saline is a reasonable consideration for acute bronchiolitis.

Chest Physiotherapy

Bronchiolitis causes epithelium sloughing, which can cause partial to total airway obstruction. Chest physiotherapy is used to assist in the clearance of secretions and/or obstructions from the tracheobronchial tract. Techniques include vibration, percussion, and postural drainage to help clear the airway obstruction, reduce airway resistance, enhance gas exchange,

Table 15-5 Dosage and Routes for Albuterol and Racemic Epinephrine (26)

Medication	Indication	Concentration	Dosage	Route	Frequency	Diluent
Albuterol sulfate	Bronchospasm	0.5% (5 mg/mL)	1.25–5 mg	Inhaled—SVN	Every 2–6 hours	
		0.5% (5 mg/mL)	0.5 mg/kg/hr up to 10–20 mg/hour	Inhaled—LVN	Continuous	Mix to a total of 25–30 mL per 1 hour of nebulization
		90 mcg	<12 years of age: 4–8 puffs; ≥12 years of age: 4–8 puffs	Inhaled–MDI	Repeat every 1–4 hours as needed with a spacer.	N/A
Racemic epinephrine	Airway inflammation	2.25% solution	0.25–0.5 mL	Inhaled–SVN		Mix with 2–3 mL of normal saline solution

SVN, small-volume nebulizer; LVN, large-volume nebulizer; MDI, metered dose inhaler.

and reduce WOB. The current recommendation on chest physiotherapy for acute bronchiolitis is inconclusive (33), although it may be considered for patients with severe plugging and atelectasis.

Patient Positioning

There is no clear evidence that certain body positions will decrease respiratory distress. Infants and children should be allowed to position themselves in whatever way is comfortable for them. For infants who cannot position themselves, side-lying or supine positions may be used with the head slightly elevated. If prone positioning is used, continuous pulse oximetry monitoring must be used because of the higher risk of sudden infant death syndrome (SIDS) (Special Population 15-2).

Fluid Management

All children with bronchiolitis need hydration and fluid status evaluation. They are very susceptible to dehydration because of high insensible water loss, elevated respiratory rate, fever, copious secretions, and poor feeding (9). In mild respiratory distress, the infant or child may continue to feed but must be observed for changes in respiratory and feeding status. Patients in impending respiratory failure are at risk for aspiration; thus, oral nutrition may need to be held or reduced to decrease the risk of aspiration. If oral feeding becomes inadvisable because of severe respiratory distress, the infant or child should be placed on intravenous fluids to rehydrate. If oral feeding is delayed for more than 2 days, a nasogastric tube should be placed for enteral feeding to provide nutritional support.

Glucocorticoids

Systemic glucocorticoids have been intermittently used for routine treatment of acute viral bronchiolitis for the past 40 years. The rationale is that the anti-inflammatory effects should help in the early stages of bronchiolitis because acute inflammation of the bronchioles is one of the primary components in the disease. However, the evidence shows no benefit in decreasing the in-patient length of stay or clinical outcomes in infants and children treated with systemic glucocorticoids (34). Because the safety of high-dose inhaled corticosteroids for infants is not yet known, the AAP recommends avoiding their use in small children unless there is a clear likelihood of benefit (14).

Antibiotics

The risk for a bacterial infection with bronchiolitis is low, at less than 1% (35–38). Approximately 25% of hospitalized infants with bronchiolitis will have radiographic evidence of atelectasis or infiltrates, often misinterpreted as possible bacterial infection (39). For that reason, antibiotic therapy is still used in the treatment of young infants. Antibiotic therapy is not recommended for routine treatment of viral bronchiolitis, however, and should only be used if there is a suspicion and/or confirmation of a secondary bacterial infection.

Ribavirin (Virazole)

Ribavirin is a broad-spectrum antiviral medication used in the treatment of children with severe RSV. Though it used to be a mainstay of treatment for all patients with RSV bronchiolitis, it is no longer recommended routinely for inpatients with bronchiolitis. This is because of its marginal benefit, if any, for most patients. It should, however, be considered for patients with severe disease or those who have significant underlying risk factors such as congenital immunodeficiency, organ and bone marrow transplants, and chronic lung and congenital heart diseases. Other considerations for not using ribavirin include high cost and lack of demonstrated benefit in decreasing hospitalization or mortality, in addition to the occupational health risk to health-care providers.

● **Special Populations 15-2**

Sudden Infant Death Syndrome

SIDS is defined as the unexplained death of a healthy newborn. It typically occurs in infants 2 to 4 months of age, with a range of 1 to 6 months of age. Risk factors for SIDS include the following:

- Male sex
- Premature or low birth weight
- African American, American Indian, or Native Alaskan
- Sleeping on the stomach
- Being born to mothers who smoke or take drugs
- Exposure to secondhand tobacco smoke
- Overheated homes
- Being born during fall or winter months
- Upper respiratory infection
- Being a sibling of a baby who died from SIDS

  Prevention factors include the following:

- Placing baby on his or her back to sleep
- Not smoking or exposing the baby to secondhand smoke
- Selecting appropriate bedding: firm mattress, fitted sheets, and no lambskin, quilt, pillow, or stuffed animals (to prevent the risk of smothering)
- Caregivers not sleeping with the infant in their bed
- Maintaining a moderate room temperature
- Breastfeeding, which some research has linked to lower incidence of SIDS

In vitro studies have shown that ribavirin has carcinogenic, mutagenic, teratogenic, and embryolethal properties; however, no effects have been reported in humans. Health-care providers, however, should take necessary precautions to protect themselves from prolonged ribavirin exposure. Special precaution should be taken by pregnant women and women attempting to become pregnant because of the potential teratogenic and embryolethal effects.

For those who receive ribavirin treatment, the recommended dosage is 6 g in 300 mL of distilled water administered with a small-particle aerosol generator (SPAG unit) over 12 to 18 hours per day for 3 to 7 days based on clinical response. The most common side effects include irritation of the eye and nasal mucosa (burning and itching) and respiratory distress including wheezing and coughing.

Noninvasive Positive Pressure Ventilation

Noninvasive positive-pressure ventilation (NIPPV) may be used to support the ventilation of an infant or child in impending respiratory failure. The mode of action of NIPPV is likely the result of the splinting of the bronchioles, causing a reduction in airway resistance, functional residual capacity (FRC), and gas trapping in hyperinflated lungs. It also assists in the recruitment of underinflated lung units, resulting in improvement in ventilation-perfusion matching and alveolar gas exchange. These dynamic changes will result in reduced WOB and lower oxygen requirements. A worsening of the cardiorespiratory status (e.g., increased WOB, respiratory rate, heart rate, and oxygen requirement) may indicate that NIPPV is not providing adequate ventilatory support and that invasive mechanical ventilation should be considered.

The modes of noninvasive ventilation include continuous positive airway pressure and BiPAP.

Continuous Positive Airway Pressure

Continuous positive airway pressure (CPAP) is a constant positive airway pressure maintained throughout the respiratory cycle (inspiratory and expiratory phase). CPAP should increase FRC and improve ventilation-perfusion matching, resulting in decreased WOB and respiratory distress. It can be delivered via nasal mask, nasal prongs, or a full-face mask. Care must be taken to inspect and cleanse the bridge of the patient's nose and face to prevent loss of skin integrity. (See Chapter 7 for a discussion of the common side effects of CPAP devices.)

Nasal CPAP delivered via nasal mask or prongs is the most useful method of delivery of CPAP for infants. There are several clinical considerations that may make nasal CPAP delivery less effective. These include the following:

- Loss of pressure in the hypopharynx may result in a variation in the actual CPAP delivered.
- Thickened secretions may impede gas flow from nasal prongs and therefore require adequate humidification and frequent suctioning it is being used.
- Excessive leaks may result in asynchrony between the patient and machine.

Full-face mask CPAP requires an appropriate-sized mask to provide a tight seal and fit. It should encompass the mouth and nose. Care must be taken to avoid placing the mask too high over the eyes or too low on the chin because this creates a leak in the system. Inappropriate mask and headgear may cause potential interface complications and can decrease patient compliance.

Initial CPAP settings for bronchiolitis are similar to those of all pediatric patients, 4 to 5 cm H_2O. The effectiveness of CPAP is determined by evaluating WOB, changes in oxygenation or FIO_2, lung inflation on chest radiograph, and patient comfort:

A. WOB

If there is a decrease in respiratory rate and severity of retractions, grunting, and nasal flaring, maintain current CPAP level and wean FIO_2.

If patient is still in severe respiratory distress, increase CPAP level by 1 to 2 cm H_2O up to a maximum of 10 cm H_2O.

If CPAP 10 cm H_2O does not alleviate severe respiratory distress, consider BiPAP.

B. Stabilization of FIO_2 requirement less than or equal to 0.60

C. Improvement of lung volumes as seen on chest radiograph

D. Improvement of patient comfort, including WOB and vital signs

Patients should be monitored and assessed every 2 to 4 hours for changes in respiratory status. If a patient exhibits increased WOB, reevaluation should be completed immediately, including a chest radiograph and arterial blood gas, assessing for either inadequate or excessive ventilation. Too much CPAP can result in air-leak syndrome, V/Q mismatch, CO_2 retention, increased WOB, and gastric distension.

Bilevel Positive Airway Pressure

Bi-level positive airway pressure, or BiPAP, provides both an expiratory pressure, as with CPAP, and an additional preset inspiratory pressure. It also allows for an optional preset respiratory rate. Like CPAP,

BiPAP is delivered via nasal mask, nasal prongs, or full-face mask, and similar care must be taken to protect the patient's skin integrity. BiPAP should be considered when the infant or child needs extra support for ventilation and/or oxygenation. Initial bilevel settings include selecting a mode, an inspiratory positive airway pressure (IPAP), an expiratory positive airway pressure (EPAP), and FIO_2.

A. Mode of ventilation

1. Spontaneous (pressure support): Patient's spontaneous inspiratory effort triggers the ventilator to deliver IPAP.
2. Spontaneous timed (pressure support with backup rate): Patient's spontaneous inspiratory effort triggers the ventilator to deliver IPAP. If the patient's spontaneous respiratory rate decreases below the preset rate, the ventilator triggers a pressure control breath according to the preset IPAP level.

B. IPAP initial setting: 8 to 10 cm H_2O. Effectiveness of IPAP setting should be assessed by evaluating the following and changing settings as needed:

1. Good chest wall excursion with resolution of tachypnea and hypercapnia
2. Increase IPAP by 2 cm H_2O if there is persistent hypercapnia
3. Increase IPAP by 2 cm H_2O if there is persistent hypoxemia
4. Maximum IPAP varies based on patient size but should be no higher than 20 cm H_2O to avoid gastric distension

C. EPAP initial setting: 4 to 6 cm H_2O

1. Patients with severe hypoxemia or air trapping may require higher levels of EPAP to increase mean airway pressure to improve oxygenation and ventilation matching or to counter elevated levels of intrinsic positive-end expiratory pressure. Increase EPAP by 1 to 2 cm H_2O pressure if hypoxemia is persistent.
2. Maximum EPAP varies based on patient size but should be no higher than 10 to 15 cm H_2O.

Predictors of success for BiPAP include a decrease in $PaCO_2$, improvement in oxygenation, and correction of respiratory acidosis. Predictors of failure for BiPAP ventilation include persistent hypercapnia and acidosis and a decrease in level of consciousness.

Prevention

Because viral infections are transmitted through direct person-to-person contact or contact with fomites, frequent hand hygiene is the first line of protection against infectious viral pathogens.

Health-care providers also should adhere to isolation precautions in the hospital. High-risk infants should have limited exposure to settings where transmission is common, such as day-care settings.

Palivizumab, a humanized monoclonal antibody vaccine, is indicated as a preventive measure against RSV for select infants and children in high-risk groups younger than 24 months. Three groups of children qualify for the vaccine:

1. Infants born before 35 weeks of gestation
2. Infants with chronic lung disease
3. Infants born with hemodynamically significant congenital heart disease (40)

Palivizumab has been shown to reduce hospitalizations in premature infants and children younger than 2 years with hemodynamically significant cardiac disease; however, no studies have yet demonstrated reduced mortality (6). Additionally, it appears the medication is less effective in infants and children with comorbidities, such as very premature infants with chronic lung disease (41).

Additional preventive strategies include the following:

- Avoiding tobacco smoke, which is an independent risk factor in bronchiolitis (42–44)
- Breastfeeding, owing to the fact that human milk contains immune factors that decrease the risk of acquiring viruses such as RSV because it contains immunoglobulin G, immunoglobulin A, and alpha interferon (45).

■■ After donning a gown, gloves, and a mask, you support Jacob's spontaneous respirations by providing blow-by oxygen and positioning him upright to optimize air movement. These maneuvers increase Jacob's SpO_2 above 95%.

Once you've improved Jacob's oxygen, the nurse places an intravenous catheter and starts fluid therapy at maintenance rate. You suggest a trial of inhaled bronchodilator therapy for Jacob because of the bilateral scattered wheezing heard on auscultation. You administer 1.25 mg albuterol sulfate via a small-volume nebulizer with an aerosol mask. After the nebulizer, reassessment reveals no change in breath sounds or current respiratory status. You suggest a trial of racemic epinephrine (0.25 mL of 2.5%) to capitalize on the alpha effect of the medication. There is minimal change in breath sounds, but there may be a slight increase in air entry. The patient care team discusses whether to repeat the racemic epinephrine secondary to the slight improvement in air entry. After much discussion, racemic epinephrine is not repeated. You note that the patient has copious nasal secretions and a consistently low SpO_2 of less than 90%. You recommend nasal suctioning to help alleviate nasal obstruction. The physician and nurse agree. Together, you and the nurse suction the nasal passages at low negative pressure to minimize nasal mucosal trauma. Jacob's SpO_2 increases to 92%, and he exhibits a slight decrease in WOB. You help the nurse transport Jacob to the infant care in-patient unit.

Course and Prognosis

Over the past several decades, a better understanding of the pathophysiology of viral infections has improved outcomes for children hospitalized with acute bronchiolitis. Mortality rates are less than 1% (less than 500 deaths) per year in the United States (46) but can be as high as 600,000 in other parts of the world (47). Most hospitalized infants recover from acute bronchiolitis without sequelae within 3 to 4 days, whereas high-risk infants are hospitalized longer with a higher rate of intensive care admission and mechanical ventilation. One study found that approximately 40% of survivors have subsequent wheezing episodes up to the age of 5 years, and 10% have subsequent wheezing episodes after 5 years (48). It has also been suggested that RSV in infancy is an independent risk factor for recurrent wheezing and asthma (6).

As future researchers investigate the propensity of children with bronchiolitis to develop asthma, present clinical management should focus on preventive measures along with research for developing a valid and reliable severity scoring system that is sensitive to important clinical changes in bronchiolitis.

Pneumonia

Pneumonia is an inflammation of the lung tissue mediated by an immunological response to infectious agents. It is the leading cause of death in children worldwide, killing an estimated 1.6 million children every year (49). In the United States, *Streptococcus pneumoniae* is responsible for 100,000 to 135,000 hospitalizations in children younger than 5 years old each year (50). Although pneumonia is the leading cause of death, it is preventable by immunization, adequate nutrition, and addressing environmental factors. Additionally, it is a largely treatable disease with early and advanced treatment and supportive care. Factors associated with an increased risk of pneumonia include the following:

- Age (very young children with immature immune systems)
- Concomitant immune deficiency diseases (e.g., leukemia) or chronic illnesses (e.g., chronic lung disease, congenital heart disease)
- Smoking or secondhand smoke exposure
- Hospitalization in an intensive care unit (ICU)
- Chronic lung disease requiring long-term inhaled corticosteroids
- Exposure to certain chemicals or pollutants (e.g., chlorine, inhaled pesticides, vomitus, smoke)
- Indoor air pollution
- Living under crowded conditions
- Surgery or traumatic injury
- Ethnicity (Native Alaskans have a 60% greater risk of contracting influenza and pneumonia) (51)

Pneumonia can be caused by bacteria, viruses, fungi, protozoa, chemicals, foreign bodies, or irritants. *S. pneumoniae* is the most common bacterial organism causing pneumonia in children (51).

Other common bacterial causes include the following:

- *Staphylococcus aureus*
- *Streptococcus pyogenes* (group A *Streptococcus*)
- *Klebsiella pneumoniae*
- *Pseudomonas aeruginosa*
- *Haemophilus influenzae*
- *Chlamydia pneumoniae*
- *Mycoplasma pneumoniae*

Viruses more commonly cause pneumonia in younger populations (52). Although measles and RSV are the most common viruses causing pneumonia in children (51), other viral causes include the following:

- Influenza
- Adenovirus
- Metapneumovirus
- Parainfluenza
- Rhinovirus

Other atypical causative agents include mycoplasm tuberculosis, fungal infections, and oral anaerobes.

Pneumonia is often classified into the following four general categories:

- Aspiration pneumonia
- Community-acquired pneumonia
- Hospital-acquired pneumonia
- Immunocompromised (opportunistic) pneumonia

Other types of pneumonia include severe acute respiratory syndrome, bronchiolitis obliterans organizing pneumonia, and eosinophilic pneumonia. Each type of pneumonia is associated with an array of different pathogens and routes of transmission, which helps to dictate the type of "isolation" that is necessary when caring for these patients. The most common routes of transmission are inhalation and aspiration. Transmission via inhalation occurs after a sneeze or cough disperses small respiratory droplets into the air. Transmission via aspiration occurs when oropharyngeal or gastric contents are inhaled into the lungs. Fomites and blood-borne pathogens are other routes of transmission.

Viral infections can impede immunity and secretion clearance and precede bacterial infections that result in co-infection. Although there are distinctive and specific pathogenic causes of pneumonia, the treatment by and large is the same: effective specific antimicrobials combined with meticulous respiratory support and critical care, when needed.

Pathophysiology

The immunological response in pneumonia causes alveoli and lining epithelium of the terminal air spaces to become inflamed (53). The inflammatory cascade (discussed in Chapter 13) activates the release of protein-rich fluid, which aids as a growth medium for pathogens. Edema thickens the alveolar capillary membrane, and transfer of oxygen is impeded, resulting in hypoxemia (Fig. 15-2). Alveoli that are **consolidated** (solidified), fluid filled, or atelectatic cause decreased amounts of oxygen to reach the alveolar capillary membrane, resulting in intrapulmonary shunting and V/Q mismatch. These alterations cause increased pulmonary vascular resistance and impairment in oxygen delivery and carbon dioxide clearance (Fig. 15-3).

Clinical Manifestations

Patients with pneumonia usually present with nonspecific signs and symptoms that widely vary according to age and infectious organism. The most common clinical signs and symptoms are as follows:

* Fever greater than 38.5°C
* Cough with tenacious sputum
* Tachypnea
* Dyspnea
* Chills
* Fatigue

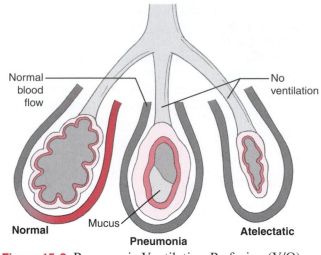

Figure 15-3 Pneumonia Ventilation-Perfusion (V/Q) Mismatch

* Loss of appetite
* Accessory muscle use (intercostal and substernal retractions)
* Nasal flaring
* Crackles sometimes heard over the affected area by auscultation

Respiratory rate, oxygen saturation, and increased WOB are the most clinically significant parameters in characterizing the severity of illness and determining the need for hospitalization (Table 15-6). Additionally, if the family is unable to provide appropriate observation or care in the home, the infant or child should be admitted to the hospital (Special Population 15-3).

Table 15-6	Pneumonia Severity Assessment (54)	
	Mild	**Severe**
Infants	Temperature <38.5°C	Temperature >38.5°C
	RR < 50 breaths/min	RR > 70 breaths/min
		Altered consciousness
	Awake and alert	Nasal flaring
	Taking full feeds	Cyanosis
		Intermittent apnea
		Grunting respiration
		Not feeding
Older Children	Temperature <38.5°C	Temperature >38.5°C
	RR <50 breaths/min	RR >50 breaths/min
		Severe difficulty in breathing
	Mild breathlessness	Nasal flaring
		Cyanosis
	No vomiting	Grunting respiration
		Signs of dehydration

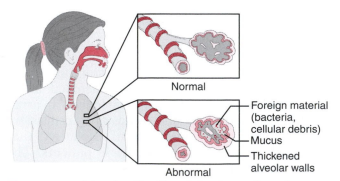

Normal

Foreign material (bacteria, cellular debris)
Mucus
Thickened alveolar walls

Abnormal

Figure 15-2 Alveolar Capillary Membrane Impairment During Pneumonia

Admitting Infants and Children to the Hospital

Clinicians may need to use discretion when assessing the ability of a child to receive adequate care at home before discharging patients from the ED. Some families may not have the resources or the ability to provide the appropriate level of care for their child at that specific time in the child's course of illness. Caution should be used whenever it is suspected that a child may not receive treatments or therapies in a timely manner, if the child may not be monitored 24 hours a day, or if there is any concern that prescriptions will not be filled owing to insurance or economic reasons.

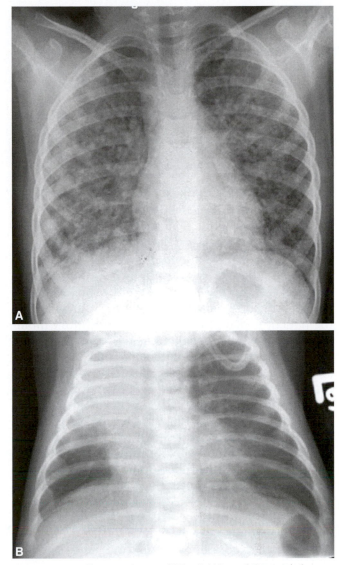

Figure 15-4 Comparison of Viral (A) and Bacterial (B) Pneumonias *(Courtesy of Jane Benson, MD)*

Diagnostic Testing

Diagnostic testing for pneumonia focuses on obtaining a definitive diagnosis of pneumonia and determining the causative agent using sputum cultures, bronchoalveolar lavage, and blood cultures, and then assessing how much of the lung is affected, using chest radiography.

Chest Radiographs

Chest radiographs are very helpful to confirm the diagnosis of pneumonia; however, they can only suggest but cannot confirm the underlying causative agent. Viral and bacterial pneumonias are often similar in clinical presentation, but they present differently radiographically (Table 15-7). Classically, viral pneumonia presents as a diffuse interstitial or peribronchial infiltrate, whereas bacterial pneumonia presents as a lobar or alveolar consolidation (55) (Fig. 15-4). If pleural fluid is present, a lateral decubitus radiograph can help differentiate between a pleural effusion and empyema. If a significant amount of pleural fluid is discovered, a thoracentesis should be performed, and fluid should be sent for culture and sensitivity to determine the pathogen and antibiotic regimen.

Table 15-7	Pneumonia Comparison Table		
Type	**Causative Agent**	**Pharmacological Therapy**	**Radiographic Findings**
Viral	Measles, RSV, influenza, parainfluenza, adenovirus, metapneumovirus	Fluids, oxygen if needed, antiviral medications, ibuprofen, acetaminophen	Diffuse interstitial or peribronchial infiltrates
Bacterial	S. aureus, K. pneumoniae, S. pyogenes, P. aeruginosa, H. influenzae	Amoxicillin, Augmentin, penicillin, clindamycin, erythromycin, vancomycin, second-generation cephalosporin	Lobar or alveolar consolidation
Atypical	M. pneumoniae	Erythromycin	Patchy and segmental or nonsegmental with the presence of airspace opacification

Sputum Cultures

Sputum samples can be used to determine the agent causing the pneumonia. Inducing sputum cultures with nebulized hypertonic saline may be feasible in children who are able to perform the procedure and cooperate. On intubated patients, a simple tracheal aspirate can be performed to obtain sputum into a specimen trap, using a sterile suctioning technique. However, bronchoalveolar lavage may yield a more definitive result.

Bronchoalveolar Lavage

Bronchoalveolar lavage is a diagnostic technique used to determine the pathogenic agent in lung infections, particularly those caused by opportunistic pathogens in an immunocompromised patient. Two techniques are used to obtain a sample: nonbronchoscopic bronchoalveolar lavage (NB-BAL) and bronchoscopic-guided bronchoalveolar lavage. During the NB-BAL, the patient is placed on full cardiorespiratory monitoring and is preoxygenated using 1.0 FIO_2. Using sterile technique, a BAL catheter is placed down the endotracheal tube. Saline is injected and then aspirated into a specimen trap using suction, without withdrawing the catheter. The process of injecting and aspirating saline is repeated until an adequate sample is obtained or the patient shows signs of intolerance (e.g., cardiac instability, hypoxemia, tachypnea). The technique of flexible fiber-optic bronchoscopy is straightforward; however, it is usually limited to diagnose severe acute cases in children because of the invasiveness of the procedure. If a BAL is warranted, it should take place in a setting with a full complement of continuous monitoring and resuscitative equipment.

Blood Cultures

Hospitalized children diagnosed with bacterial pneumonia should have blood cultures done to rule out a blood or multisystem infection. If viral infection is suspected, a nasopharyngeal culture may be indicated.

Management and Treatment

The management and treatment of pneumonia is dependent on the causative agent and severity of the disease (Table 15-7). Most children are treated at home with anti-infectives, **antipyretics** (drugs that reduce body temperature), oral hydration, bronchodilators, and rest. If the pneumonia is severe, then hospitalization may be necessary to provide supplemental oxygen, intravenous fluids, antipyretics, antibiotics, and mechanical ventilatory support. A child is discharged from the hospital when respiratory distress has resolved, the child can maintain an acceptable SpO_2 level, and the child is able to take oral antibiotics without vomiting.

Oxygen Therapy

Oxygen therapy is a life-saving intervention that should be administered when a patient exhibits an SpO_2 that is less than 90% in the absence of cyanotic heart disease. If the patient has underlying congenital heart disease or a chronic condition, SpO_2 levels should be maintained at or slightly above the patient's baseline. In pneumonia, hypoxemia is caused by V/Q mismatch. Oxygen delivery is dependent on adequate alveolar gas exchange and the circulatory system. Failure of these systems can cause tissue hypoxia within 10 to 15 minutes (56). Early recognition and management with oxygen therapy may decrease the likelihood of tissue hypoxia. Maintaining a normal body temperature for pediatric patients is important because fever shifts the oxyhemoglobin dissociation curve to the right, requiring a higher PaO_2 to ensure adequate oxygen delivery. There has been some suggestion, however, that fever may be beneficial in minimizing the inflammatory effects within the lungs (Evidence in Practice 15-1).

Oxygen delivery devices should meet or exceed the patient's inspiratory flow demand to ensure adequate FIO_2 delivery. Nasal cannulas can be used in patients who tolerate low-flow oxygen delivery systems. High-flow delivery systems may be necessary for patients who require an FIO_2 greater than 0.40 or nasal cannula flow rates greater than 6 LPM (Table 15-3). Humidified oxygen delivery systems should be considered to help loosen and mobilize thick secretions.

✚ Anti-infectives

Pneumonia is a treatable disease; however, "less than 20% of children worldwide receive the antibiotics that they need" (49). Antibiotics are prescribed to treat bacterial pneumonia or suspected bacterial co-infection, and rarely, antiviral medications are prescribed to treat viral pneumonia (5). The antibiotic selection should be based on local

---

● Evidence in Practice 15-1

Therapeutic Fevers

Recent animal studies have shown that physiological fever induces a protective stress response by down-regulating the inflammatory cascade (56), which means a fever may reduce the release of inflammatory markers (cytokines, such as tumor necrosis factor and interleukin) and reduce the severity of alveolar inflammation and thus pneumonia symptoms. Ongoing research will determine the utility of a therapeutic fever.

pathogenic patterns and severity of illness. After the initiation of antibiotics, 90% of patients with bacterial etiology will show improvement in signs and symptoms (57). If improvement is not noted, other etiologies or antibiotic-resistant strains of the illness should be suspected.

Antibiotics used to treat pneumonia include the following:

- Amoxicillin (first antibiotic of choice in children younger than 5 years old)
- Augmentin
- Penicillin
- Clindamycin
- Erythromycin
- Vancomycin
- Second-generation cephalosporin

Current treatment for viral pathogens is generally supportive in nature. Specific antiviral medications (e.g., ribavirin for RSV and adenovirus; ganciclovir for cytomegalovirus) are controversial and not widely accepted as effective. The theory is that viral pathogens set up a rich medium for bacterial colonization, which results in a viral/bacterial co-infection. Special cases of pneumonia include *Pneumocystis jiroveci* pneumonia (also known as *Pneumocystis carinii* pneumonia; see Clinical Variation 15-1); cytomegalovirus; and idiopathic, parasitic, and fungal pneumonias. High-risk populations include patients with concomitant diseases such as AIDS, immunocompromised conditions (e.g., leukemia, bone marrow transplants), cystic fibrosis, chronic lung disease, congenital heart disease, and asthma.

Pneumocystis Jiroveci Pneumonia

Pneumocystis carinii pneumonia (PCP) infections were renamed in 2002. It was found that PCP is a rat strain of pneumonia that cannot infect humans, so the new species was named *Pneumocystis jiroveci* pneumonia (PJP). It is named after Dr. Otto Jirovec, who discovered the strain. It is still abbreviated PCP, however, not PJP.

PCP is caused by the fungus *P. jiroveci*. This fungus is common in the environment and does not cause illness in healthy people. PCP is relatively rare in people with normal immune systems, but it is common among people with weakened immune systems, such as premature or severely malnourished children, the elderly, and especially individuals living with HIV/AIDS, in whom it is most commonly observed. PCP can also develop in patients who are taking immunosuppressive medications.

Fluid Management

Hospitalized children with pneumonia should be well hydrated and have their hydration status monitored. Pneumonia predisposes children to dehydration and electrolyte depletion. Fluid-replacement therapy should be titrated to replenish and maintain intravascular volume and electrolytes. Fluid administration needs to be carefully monitored by intake and output measurements, however, to prevent fluid overload, which can cause pulmonary edema. Excessive fluid administration should be avoided because pulmonary edema or leakage of fluid across inflamed lung tissue can contribute to hypoxemia.

Inhaled Bronchodilators

Inhaled bronchodilators are commonly administered to patients with pneumonia who present with wheezing, but their effects are not benign. Bronchodilator use may contribute to hypoxemia by increasing V/Q mismatching; this occurs when bronchodilation overcomes the hypoxic vasoconstriction that is naturally trying to divert pulmonary blood flow away from damaged lung areas. Blood is more evenly redistributed, increasing flow to alveolar capillaries that are not contributing to gas exchange; therefore, deoxygenated blood mixes with oxygenated blood, resulting in lower oxygen saturation (58). Common bronchodilators include albuterol sulfate/salbutamol and racemic epinephrine. If there is no response to bronchodilator therapy, it should be discontinued to limit any potential adverse side effects.

Inhaled Antibiotics

Pentamidine isethionate is an antibiotic administered with a nebulizer or intravenously for *P. jiroveci* pneumonia (Box 15-1). There are important considerations when administering inhaled antimicrobials. The most common method of administration involves using two separate nebulizers: small volume and Respirgard II (Fig. 15-5). Aerosolized pentamidine has been documented as causing conjunctivitis and bronchospasm in health-care workers exposed to the drug during treatments (59). As a result, the patient must be capable of using a mouthpiece so that the health-care provider's exposure to pentamidine is limited. For added protection, the health-care provider should wear an N95 mask to prevent inhalation of the antibiotic. An N95 mask is a specialized face mask that protects against 95% of respirable particles.

Suctioning and Mucous Clearance

The goal of secretion clearance therapy is to mobilize and expel mucus in the respiratory tract. Current secretion-clearance techniques include postural

Box 15-1 Pentamidine Isethionate Procedure

- A negative flow room or laminar flow hood is recommended.
- Examine the prepared solution of pentamidine isethionate for cloudiness. If cloudy, return it to the pharmacy for another dose.
- Use universal precautions, including a particulate respiratory mask.
- Perform basic physical assessment (HR, breath sounds, breathing pattern and frequency, SpO_2, and determination of cognitive ability).
- Administer a bronchodilator in a small-volume nebulizer.
- Coat the mouthpiece of the pentamidine isethionate nebulizer with fruit flavors, or the patient may suck on hard candy to cope with the metallic taste of the medication.
- Administer pentamidine isethionate with the Respirgard II Nebulizer (Figure 15-6).
- Terminate nebulizer flow prior to removal from the patient's mouth.
- Reassess the patient intermittently and at the conclusion of therapy (HR, breath sounds, breathing pattern and frequency, SpO_2, and determination of cognitive ability).
- Discard the nebulizer and other disposable items.

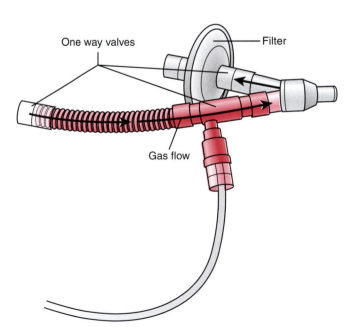

Figure 15-5 Nebulized Pentamidine via Respirgard II Nebulizer System

drainage, percussion and vibration; suctioning, position changes, high frequency chest wall oscillation; forced expiratory technique; positive expiratory pressure (PEP) and oscillating PEP devices; and intrapulmonary percussive ventilation (60, 61). A description of each can be found in Chapter 14. However, current evidence is lacking regarding the effectiveness of these techniques. Poor fluid hydration may lead to inspissated mucus, which hinders adequate secretion clearance. This is another reason for adequate hydration and fluid maintenance.

Glucocorticoids

There is some clinical evidence that corticosteroids can shorten the length of hospitalization and side effects such as sepsis, septic shock, and bacterial meningitis in adults and children (62). It can clearly reduce pulmonary inflammation. One small study of children with severe community-acquired pneumonia showed a mild improvement in outcomes with an early, low-dose, and short-term systemic corticosteroid regimen paired with antimicrobial therapy (62). However, there is not significant evidence that routine use of steroids improves outcomes for pneumonia in either children or adults. Because of their immunosuppressive and other negative effects (discussed in Chapter 13), steroids are not routinely recommended. They may be used for patients with a medical history of severe wheezing or an active component of reactive air disease (5).

Mechanical Ventilation

All patients with pneumonia, regardless of causative agent, are at risk for respiratory failure. Only a small fraction (17%) of children admitted to the ICU in the United States will require assisted mechanical ventilation (63). Mechanical ventilation can be administered noninvasively or invasively. NIPPV may be attempted for patients in impending respiratory failure to reduce the severity of respiratory distress and improve oxygenation and ventilation. Invasive mechanical ventilation is reserved for patients in acute respiratory failure or failure of a trial of NIPPV. Endotracheal intubation should be performed for continued respiratory distress with increasing hypercarbia, acidosis, and hypoxemia. The patient should also be placed on continuous monitoring that consists of cardiorespiratory, pulse oximetry, and capnography. Initial ventilator settings by age can be found in Table 15-8.

Course and Prognosis

In most cases of childhood pneumonia, a full recovery is expected with proper medical treatment, including rest, fluids, antibiotics (when appropriate), and adequate nutrition. In general, the outcome is good for children with pneumonia, and in 2010 the

Age	Rate	VT	T_I	PEEP	FIO₂
6 mo–2 yr	25	6 mL/kg	0.55–0.65 sec	3–5 cm H_2O	1.0*
2–5 yr	20–25	6–8 mL/kg	0.65–0.75 sec	5 cm H_2O	1.0*
5–10 yr	18–20	6–8 mL/kg	0.70–0.80 sec	5 cm H_2O	1.0*
10–15 yr	16–18	6–8 mL/kg	0.–0.90 sec	5 cm H_2O	1.0*
15 yr–adult	14–16	6–8 mL/kg	0.90–1 sec	5 cm H_2O	1.0*

Table 15-8 Suggested Ventilator Settings by Age

VT is based on ideal body weight and corrected for volume loss owing to circuit compliance.

*Please note: starting FIO₂ is based on patients *without* congenital heart disease.

age-adjusted death rate was 2.2% (64). The vast majority of children, 92.5% in one study (65), have no residual disease sequelae. However, children with underlying chronic disease, immune deficiency, or viral/bacterial co-infection tend to have a more severe course and may develop lung problems later in life. Moreover, some studies have followed previously healthy children for 8 to 10 years after they were hospitalized with pneumonia and found little sequelae (66).

Childhood pneumonia remains a global problem. Further research needs to focus on understanding the etiology to aid in the development of vaccines and antimicrobial therapy. Additionally, improvement in living conditions, nutrition, and air quality should help further reduce mortality in developing countries. However, there are still critical gaps that need to be understood—including pathophysiology, etiology, and epidemiology—to reduce mortality in children (67).

■■ Within 1 hour of admission to the inpatient unit, Jacob's RR increases to 75 breaths/min, and he begins to exhibit substernal retractions. SpO₂ is now 90% on a 2 LPM nasal cannula. The pediatrician calls you to initiate HFNC to increase oxygen delivery and obtain an arterial blood gas (ABG) value. You start the HFNC at 6 LPM and an FIO₂ of 1.0. An ABG value 30 minutes later is pH 7.33, PaCO₂ 44 mm Hg, HCO₃ 22.9 mEq/L, PaO₂ 68 mm Hg. You and the physician are both concerned about respiratory failure, and you agree to begin CPAP at +5 cm H_2O. Within 20 minutes, Jacob's SpO₂ has increased to 98%, and FIO₂ is weaned to 0.70. His RR has decreased to 50 breaths/min, and he has no noticeable retractions.

Acute Respiratory Distress Syndrome

Acute respiratory distress syndrome is an acute heterogeneous disease that causes an "overwhelming pulmonary inflammation leading to severe hypoxemia and respiratory failure" (68). ARDS is reported in both adults and children; however, many clinicians believe that children are underdiagnosed because they are classified according to the underlying disease (69). Additionally, the majority of children meeting the criteria for ARDS first meet the criteria for **acute lung injury (ALI)**. ALI is an umbrella term used for lung damage displaying hypoxemic respiratory failure characterized by bilateral pulmonary infiltrates rich in neutrophils and the absence of clinical heart failure. For these reasons, efforts to understand pediatric ARDS can be challenging. The estimated incidence of ALI in the United States is 50,000 to 190,000 cases, with 40% of these patients having ARDS (70). Despite scientific evidence and modern medical interventions, mortality rates remain high, at 22% to 35% in children (71). Furthermore, survival rate varies according to the patient's age and underlying lung injury.

Many conditions or factors cause direct or indirect lung insults and lead to ARDS. Direct lung injuries include the following:

- Near drowning
- Pneumonia
- Inhalational injuries
- Aspiration of gastric contents

Indirect lung injuries include:

- Sepsis
- Trauma
- Pancreatitis
- Severe bleeding
- Fat embolism (68)

The most common etiology of ARDS in children is a lower respiratory tract infection. In addition, the severity of hypoxia has been shown to be a strong predictor of mortality along with multisystem organ failure. There is no specific cure for ARDS, so supportive measures that encourage resting the lung and ensuring optimal oxygen delivery to the end organs remain the primary focus.

Pathophysiology

ARDS is classified as a restrictive lung disease with reduced lung compliance secondary to loss of **surfactant** function, atelectatic regions, and accumulation of interstitial/alveolar plasma leakage (72). ARDS has been defined using the following four characteristics:

1. Acute onset of symptoms
2. Bilateral infiltrates on chest radiograph (Fig. 15-6)
3. No evidence of left atrial hypertension (suggesting a cardiac cause for the infiltrates)
4. A defined degree of hypoxia

The pathogenesis of ARDS is characterized into the following three phases (Table 15-9):

1. The **exudative stage** begins when the inflammatory cascade is triggered from a direct or indirect lung injury, resulting in damage to the cellular lung structure. Outpourings of inflammatory mediators increase the permeability of the alveolar capillary membrane. Protein-rich fluid leaking into the alveoli (pulmonary edema) causes injury to type I **pneumocytes** (lung cells), resulting in loss of epithelial integrity and fluid extravasation (leakage). Damage to type II pneumocytes impedes the removal of the edema fluid and decreases surfactant reproduction, resulting in a further decrease in pulmonary compliance. Alveolar gas exchange is obstructed and results in hypoxemia, hypercarbia, and acidosis (respiratory failure).

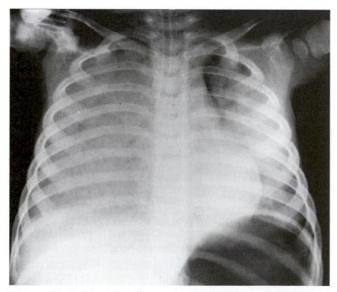

Figure 15-6 Chest Radiograph of ARDS in a 3-Year-Old
(Courtesy of Jane Benson, MD)

Table 15-9	Stages of ARDS (68)	
Stage	**Time Frame**	**Histological Appearance**
Exudative stage	Days 1–7 from the initial injury	Diffuse hemorrhage, edema, leukocyte infiltration, cellular apoptosis
Fibroproliferative stage	Begins on day 7 of illness	Fibroblast proliferation, hyperplasia of type II pneumocytes, inflammation
Fibrolytic stage	Approximately 3 weeks after the onset of illness	Fibrosis, honeycombing, bronchiectasis

From: Tomashefski JF, Jr. (72).

2. The **proliferative stage** is characterized by the proliferation (rapid increase) of type II pneumocytes and fibroblasts (cells that play a role in wound healing). Type II pneumocytes transform into type I pneumocytes, and surfactant production further decreases. Damage to the type I pneumocytes is irreversible, and the denuded (bare) space is replaced by the deposition of proteins, fibers, and cellular debris, resulting in hyaline membranes (the fibrous layer of the alveoli) (73). In this phase, the patient is susceptible to ventilator-induced lung injury (VILI) and secondary infection (lung and blood borne). Additionally, many patients die in this phase from multisystem organ failure.
3. The **fibrotic stage**, also called the chronic or late phase, results in total lung remodeling. It leads to widespread fibrosis and scarring. In this phase, alveolar gas exchange improves, and patients may be extubated from mechanical ventilation. Lung recovery may take 6 to 12 months. Depending on the severity of the initial insult, patients who survive may be left with chronic lung disease.

Clinical Manifestations

The evolution of clinical signs and symptoms of ARDS depends on the mechanism of direct or indirect injury, and ARDS is often defined as a "constellation of clinical, radiological, and physiological abnormalities" (74). Patients exhibit subtle symptoms that evolve over a period of 24 to 72 hours; however, these symptoms are unlikely to meet ARDS criteria.

Additionally, underlying medical conditions may mask the presence of ARDS and delay appropriate early interventions.

Clinical signs and symptoms of ARDS include the following:

- Tachypnea (earliest sign of pulmonary edema)
- Coughing
- Dyspnea
- Cyanosis refractory to oxygen therapy
- Fever
- Rales
- WOB (accessory muscle use, retractions, grunting)
- Hypotension (later symptom)

The final consequence of lung injury is the inability to maintain adequate gas exchange, which leads to respiratory failure and tissue hypoxia.

Patient-Assessment Tools

Several patient assessment tools have been developed to help diagnose ARDS:

- The Murray Lung Injury Score (Table 15-10), which includes radiographic evidence, hypoxemia, ventilatory support, and lung compliance (75)
- The American-European Consensus ARDS Diagnosis Criterion, an internationally agreed-upon definition and set of diagnostic criteria based on timing of onset, patient oxygenation status, radiographic evidence, and pulmonary artery wedge pressure (76)
- The Oxygen Saturation Index (Evidence in Practice 15-2), designed in an attempt to create a noninvasive scoring system that would minimize the need for ABG sampling in children (77)

It is important to recognize the transition from ALI to ARDS. The PaO_2/FIO_2 ratio is one diagnostic indicator that can be monitored to differentiate ALI from ARDS:

- ALI PaO_2/FIO_2 ratio is less than 300
- ARDS $PaO_2/FIO2$ ratio is less than 200

Early identification of ARDS is the key to early intervention. However, comorbid pathologies, iatrogenic complications (complications caused by a medical procedure), and multiorgan system failure may complicate the clinical picture and/or diagnosis.

Diagnostic Tests

Patients who are suspected of having ARDS should undergo a variety of diagnostic tests. The results of a chest radiograph and ABG testing are necessary to meet the characteristic definition of ARDS. Also

Table 15-10 Murray Lung Injury Score (75)

Parameter	Finding	Value
Chest Radiograph	No alveolar consolidation	0
	Alveolar consolidation in one quadrant	1
	Alveolar consolidation in two quadrants	2
	Alveolar consolidation in three quadrants	3
	Alveolar consolidation in four quadrants	4
Hypoxemia	PaO_2/FIO_2 >300	0
	PaO_2/FIO_2 225–299	1
	PaO_2/FIO_2 175–224	2
	PaO_2/FIO_2 100–174	3
PEEP	PaO_2/FIO_2 <100	4
	PEEP ≤5 cm H_2O	0
	PEEP 6–8 cm H_2O	1
	PEEP 9–11 cm H_2O	2
	PEEP 12–14 cm H_2O	3
	PEEP ≥15 cm H_2O	4
Pulmonary Compliance	Compliance ≥80 mL/cm H_2O	0
	Compliance 60–79 mL/cm H_2O	1
	Compliance 40–59 mL/cm H_2O	2
	Compliance 20–39 mL/cm H_2O	3
	Compliance ≤19 mL/cm H_2O	4

Score 0: No lung injury
Score 0.1–2.5: Mild-to-moderate lung injury
Score >2.5: Severe lung injury (ARDS)

To calculate the score, add the numerical value assigned to the finding and divide the answer by 4.
From: Murray JF, Matthay MA, Luce JM, et al. (75).

included in typical ARDS diagnostics are laboratory test values, which will help the health-care team with holistic patient management.

Chest Radiograph

Radiography is the primary tool used to diagnose ARDS. Initial radiographs after the triggering event may be normal or slightly abnormal. Subsequent radiographs may show progressive bilateral interstitial and alveolar infiltrates without cardiomegaly. CT scans, although not routinely used, reveal infiltrates in the posterior regions of the lung.

Oxygen Saturation Index (OSI) (77)

In a 2010 article by Thomas and colleagues, the PaO_2 in the PaO_2/FIO_2 ratio and in the oxygen index $(OI = \frac{(Paw)(FIO_2)(100)}{PaO_2})$ was replaced with SpO_2 in an attempt to validate a noninvasive scoring system and to minimize the need for ABG sampling in children.

$$OSI = [(FIO_2 \times Mean\ Airway\ Pressure)/SpO_2]$$

An OSI of 6.5 would be the equivalent of the ALI criteria, and 7.8 would be the equivalent of ARDS criteria. Study results showed this to be a reasonable substitution for the traditional oxygen index. It also has two clinical advantages: It may make for easier enrollment in ARDS research studies, and it may also assist with more accurately diagnosing children with ALI/ARDS.

Arterial Blood Gases

ABGs are measured to monitor for hypoxemia, hyperoxemia, and hypocarbia/hypercarbia. In addition, the information from a pH and base deficit is useful in management. The ABG results are necessary to calculate the PaO_2/FIO_2 ratio to determine if the criteria are met for the diagnosis of ARDS. SpO_2 has been suggested as a substitute for PaO_2 in the oxygen index calculation (see Evidence in Practice 15-2), and there has been some promising results that will minimize the need for ABG measurements during the diagnosis of ARDS.

Laboratory Studies

A complete blood cell count is used to evaluate indicators of infection (white blood cells) and anemia (hemoglobin). Significant anemia, less than 10 g/dL, can compromise oxygen-carrying capacity. Electrolyte analysis (using the results of a metabolic panel) assists with the evaluation of intravascular volume and metabolic acidosis.

Management and Treatment

There is no definitive treatment for ARDS. The cornerstone of management is early detection and treatment of the primary cause to avoid complications and poor outcomes. Strategies for managing respiratory symptoms include minimizing iatrogenic lung injury and avoiding hypoxemia. Because ARDS is a complex physiological process, it is often challenging to find a balance between providing adequate ventilation and avoiding lung injury, and advanced and novel mechanical ventilation techniques are often used to achieve it.

Oxygen Therapy

Oxygen therapy should be initiated at the first sign of hypoxemia. The goal of oxygen therapy is to maintain SpO_2 at 92% to 98% to avoid free radicals and **nitrogen washout**. It is important to remember that oxygen is a medication, and prolonged exposure of FIO_2 greater than or equal to 60% over an extended time (longer than 24 hours) at normal barometric pressure (1 atmosphere) causes oxygen toxicity (78). Oxygen free radicals lead to an inflammatory response, resulting in tissue damage and/or **apoptosis** (programmed cell death). A result of alveolar cell damage is fibrotic lung remodeling. Delivery of 1.0 FIO_2 will cause nitrogen washout. Nitrogen constitutes about 79% of room air and does not participate in gas exchange at the alveolar level. It acts as an alveolar-stabilizing gas, preventing alveolar collapse or atelectasis during gas exchange. When FIO_2 is increased, the amount of nitrogen within the alveoli decreases (i.e., is "washed out" of the alveoli), and it is no longer available for alveolar stabilization. This can cause microatelectasis. Additionally, the tracheobronchial tree and alveoli are susceptible to increased mucus plugging, atelectasis, and secondary infection because of impairment of the mucociliary epithelial blanket.

High-flow delivery systems are the optimal choice for delivering oxygen to patients with ARDS. It may be difficult to maintain the balance of meeting the patient's oxygen demand while avoiding oxygen toxicity. ABG measurements should be obtained if the patient shows signs of altered mental status or continued hypoxemia with increasing oxygen demands, known as **refractory hypoxemia**. Mechanical ventilation should be considered if the patient's oxygen saturation cannot be maintained at greater than 90% on high-flow oxygen concentrations of 0.70 to 0.90.

Mechanical Ventilation

Mechanical ventilation is a life-saving intervention in the management of ARDS. The goals of mechanical ventilation are to do the following:

- Reverse hypoxemia and hypercarbia
- Increase alveolar recruitment
- Minimize the risk of lung injury (barotraumas and volutrauma)
- Reduce WOB
- Reduce metabolic demand

There are numerous mechanical ventilation strategies being used for the treatment of ARDS. The lung-protective strategies include the following:

1. Minimizing atelectrauma
   - Titration of optimal peak end expiratory pressure (PEEP) to maintain alveolar recruitment

2. Minimizing volutrauma
  - Maintain plateau pressures less than 30 cm H_2O
  - The use of low V->T values—6 mL/kg of ideal body weight
3. Minimizing oxygen toxicity
  - Maintain FIO_2 less than 0.60
4. Accepting physiological markers outside the normal range
  - Permissive hypercapnia
  - Permissive hypoxemia

The mode of ventilation is not as important as the strategy and approach to the disease process. All current modes of mechanical ventilation use nonphysiological positive pressure, in contrast to normophysiological negative pressure. The goal of the strategies just described is to help minimize further injury to the lung. It is important to remember that trying to correct for normal physiological markers such as normocarbia ($PaCO_2$ 35 to 45 mm Hg) and normoxemia (PaO_2 80 to 100 mm Hg) can be detrimental to the lung. For this reason, permissive hypercapnia and hypoxemia are used in the management of ARDS. Hypercapnia may be tolerated if a pH of more than 7.25 can be maintained. A PaO_2 of less than 60 mm Hg may also be tolerated; however, serum lactate concentration and central venous saturation (65% to 75%) must be closely monitored to detect anaerobic metabolism. Trying to correct the blood gases to a normal state may result in exposing the lung to higher than necessary ventilatory pressures, resulting in further VILI. While ARDS requires supportive treatment and careful approaches to ventilation, at the same time, treatment of the underlying triggering mechanism cannot be overlooked.

Several different modes of ventilation may be useful in treating ARDS, and the advantages and disadvantages of each are discussed in the following sections. Table 15-11 summarizes the features of each of the different modes of ventilation.

Patient Monitoring

Physiological monitors essential to managing ARDS patients during mechanical ventilation include cardiorespiratory monitors, pulse oximeters, and capnography or transcutaneous CO_2 monitors. These devices should be available at the bedside prior to the initiation of endotracheal intubation.

Noninvasive Positive-Pressure Ventilation

NIPPV may be the first intervention for patients presenting with ventilatory failure. If FIO_2 requirements cannot be kept at 0.60 or less, or continued respiratory distress is observed, then NIPPV should be initiated in an attempt to avoid endotracheal intubation. The goals of NIPPV are the same as mechanical ventilation, with the primary goal being to increase FRC. Critical care ventilators with NIPPV modes should be used to ensure adequate flow and precise FIO_2 delivery.

CPAP may be the first mode of choice, but BiPAP should be considered if the patient does not improve after 2 hours of therapy (79). ARDS is a restrictive lung disease, and the addition of inspiratory assistance may be needed to augment spontaneous subnormal V_T and decrease physiological dead space ventilation. If the patient continues to display signs of hypoxemia and has increasing hypercarbia after 2 hours, intubation may be necessary to ensure adequate oxygenation and ventilation (79).

Invasive Mechanical Ventilation

Endotracheal intubation should be performed if the patient does not improve with BIPAP or presents in acute respiratory failure. At the initiation of mechanical ventilation, V_T values should be reduced to 6 mL/kg of ideal body weight. The ventilator should initially be set to deliver an FIO_2 of 1.0. Attempts to rapidly wean the FIO_2 to less than or equal to 0.60 should promptly be made, while maintaining a SpO_2 of 92% to 98%. Early observation studies showed PEEP greatly improves oxygenation in patients with ARDS, leading to its widespread use, but the level

Table 15-11 Ventilator Mode Descriptions

Modes	Target	Flow Wave Form	Pressure Wave Form	Cycle
A/C volume control	Volume	Square	Accelerating	Time
A/C pressure control	Pressure	Decelerating	Square	Time
SIMV volume control	Volume	Square	Accelerating	Time
SIMV pressure control	Pressure	Decelerating	Square	Time
Volume-targeted pressure control	Volume	Decelerating	Square	Time

of PEEP needed to achieve maximum benefit with minimum complications has not been established (80). It is not unusual to start with a PEEP of 10 cm H_2O for cases of ARDS. If the FIO_2 cannot be reduced to below toxic levels (less than or equal to 0.60), PEEP should be increased by 2 cm H_2O every 10 to 20 minutes until an SpO_2 of 88% to 95% can be maintained or oxygen weaning can be achieved. An SpO_2 of 88% to 95% may be tolerated, and ABG values should be frequently monitored. The health-care practitioner should pay close attention to the mean airway pressure (Paw) reading on the ventilator. Paw and oxygenation are directly related, so by increasing the PEEP, you are directly increasing the Paw. Other ways to increase Paw, listed from the most to the least effective, follow:

- Increase positive end expiratory pressure
- Increase inspiratory time (T_I)
- Increase peak inspiratory pressure (PIP)
- Increase V_T
- Increase RR

Whereas PEEP and low V_T values play a role in lung-protective ventilation, the choice of the ventilatory mode may provide some added benefit. Ventilator manufacturers have proprietary names for their modes and change frequently, thus clinicians must maintain proficiency with the modes in use within their own institution and understand how each functions. Modes that provide decelerating flow patterns may deliver desired V_T values while requiring lower PIP. Ventilator adjustments based on the desired physiological outcomes are described in Box 15-2.

Regardless of the mode of ventilation, plateau pressures should be monitored regularly for patients with ARDS. **Plateau pressure** is the amount of pressure applied to the alveoli and is measured by creating a short inspiratory pause during a mechanical breath. Plateau pressure is indirectly related to alveolar compliance; a higher plateau pressure is indicative of a lower or worsening compliance, whereas a lower plateau pressure reflects a higher or improving compliance.

Plateau pressure can then be used to calculate static compliance. **Static compliance** is a measurement of lung distensibility, taken under conditions of no airflow. Compliance is calculated as:

$$\text{Compliance } (\Delta \text{ volume}/\Delta \text{ pressure}$$
$$\text{Where } \Delta \text{ volume} = \text{measured } V_T, \text{ and (pressure} =$$
$$\text{plateau pressure} - \text{PEEP}$$

Pressure Control Modes of Ventilation

Pressure control ventilation modes can be used in assist control (A/C) or synchronized intermittent mandatory ventilation (SIMV). The RT sets a PIP, and the delivered V_T will vary depending on the patient's lung compliance and airway resistance. Pressure control uses a decelerating flow pattern and may deliver the desired targeted V_T at a low PIP (Fig. 15-7). If a pressure control mode is chosen, the health-care provider must closely monitor exhaled tidal volumes and minute ventilation. Changes in lung compliance or airway resistance will increase or reduce minute ventilation, resulting in undesired physiological outcomes. This may include hyperventilation or pneumothorax for rapid increases in compliance and hypoventilation for decreases in compliance. Pressure control modes give health-care providers greater control over Paw. Because Paw is directly related to oxygenation, ventilator changes in these modes can produce predictable changes in oxygenation.

Inverse-ratio pressure control ventilation (IRPCV) may be used to increase Paw when increases in PEEP are no longer desirable. Increasing the inspiratory time will result in increased Paw and oxygenation. Note that this ventilator strategy is uncomfortable for the patient, so adequate sedation is necessary.

Volume-Controlled Modes of Ventilation

A/C and SIMV may be used to achieve a volume target (VT), known as volume-controlled ventilation. The health-care practitioner sets a VT, and the PIP will vary depending on compliance and resistance of the lungs. The benefit of using the volume-controlled mode is that there is a guaranteed set minute ventilation (RR $\times$ V_T), which makes CO_2 management more predictable. Changes in compliance and resistance will result in an increase or decrease in airway pressures. The minute ventilation will not change under these conditions. PIPs may be higher in volume-controlled modes than in pressure-control modes while achieving the same VT. This is due to the accelerating flow pattern use to deliver the breath (Fig. 15-7).

Volume-Targeted Pressure Controlled Modes of Ventilation

In an attempt to provide the benefits of pressure ventilation along with the consistent VT delivery of volume ventilation, a hybrid mode of ventilation was

---

Box 15-2 Mechanical Ventilator Adjustments

To decrease CO_2:	To increase O_2:
↑ Tidal volume	↑ FIO_2
↑ Respiratory rate	↑ PEEP
To increase CO_2:	To decrease O_2:
↓ Tidal volume	↓ FIO_2
↓ Respiratory rate	↓ PEEP

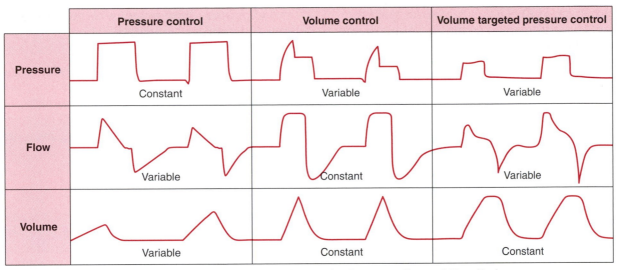

	Pressure control	Volume control	Volume targeted pressure control
Pressure	Constant	Variable	Variable
Flow	Variable	Constant	Variable
Volume	Variable	Constant	Constant

Figure 15-7 A Comparison of Pressure and Flow Curves for Pressure Control Ventilation, Volume Control Ventilation, and Volume Targeted Pressure-Control Ventilation

designed. **Volume-targeted pressure-control ventilation** uses an adaptive pressure delivery algorithm to meet a VT set by the end user. This is also described as a dual-control mode of ventilation. Depending on the ventilator manufacturer, the mode may be called PRVC or AutoFlow on the ventilator and can be used as an A/C or SIMV mode. After a series of quick test breaths, the ventilator determines the appropriate pressure to use to deliver the targeted VT based on the current calculated compliance and resistance of the lungs. The ventilator will adjust the pressure by plus or minus 3 cm H_2O as lung compliance and resistance change until the volume is met or the clinician determines that high- and low-pressure alarm limits are met. There are two benefits to using this mode for ARDS: It provides the benefit of a lower PIP by using the decelerating flow pattern of pressure control ventilation, and it assures a set minute volume (Fig. 15-7).

If plateau pressures, in any mode, cannot be maintained below 30 cm H_2O, alternative modes of ventilation must be considered. Early intervention with airway pressure release ventilation or high-frequency oscillatory ventilation should be considered under these conditions.

Airway Pressure Release Ventilation

Airway pressure release ventilation (APRV), or biphasic positive airway pressure, is an alternative mode of ventilation that provides a continuous airway pressure to promote alveolar recruitment (oxygenation) and ventilation/perfusion matching, as well as an intermittent time-cycled release to augment the patient's spontaneous ventilation, hence CO_2 clearance. Depending on the ventilator, there are several other names, including Biphasic (Avea CareFusion,

San Diego, CA), Bilevel (Dräger-Europe, Germany), Bi-vent (Siemens, Washington, DC), and DuoPAP (Hamilton, Switzerland). A benefit of this mode of ventilation is the encouragement of spontaneous breathing. Spontaneous respirations are independent of the ventilator cycle, similar to a CPAP mode, resulting in gas distribution that is more dependent on the active respiratory system drawing gas into the lungs (81). Spontaneous respirations may allow recruitment of these dependent lung regions without increasing airway pressure. Additional benefits of spontaneous respirations include improved hemodynamic stability, as seen by higher cardiac output and reduced ventricular load, and better patient-ventilator synchronization, exhibited by decreased WOB and increased patient comfort. In contrast, historically advanced modes of ventilation such as high-frequency ventilation and IRPCV have required the administration of sedation and neuromuscular blockades, which inhibit spontaneous respirations and cause uneven gas distribution, causing an increase in V/Q mismatch.

The goals of APRV are to do the following:

• Increase FRC
• Increase surface area for gas exchange
• Maximize oxygenation and ventilation
• Minimize VILI

The initial settings are determined by the patient's age, Paw during conventional ventilation, and pulmonary dynamics determined by the flow/time curves. The settings manipulated in APRV are P_{high}, P_{low}, T_{high}, T_{low}, and FIO_2 (82):

• P_{high} is the pressure the ventilator will maintain in the lungs during the majority of the ventilator cycle, with ranges typically from

20 to 35 cm H_2O. This setting is designed for alveolar recruitment. The initial setting should be equal to plateau pressure when on conventional ventilation.

- P_{low} is the pressure the ventilator will release to at short intervals, usually a fraction of a second, typically set at 0 cm H_2O. The move from P_{high} to P_{low} is designed to allow for a bulk exhalation and CO_2 clearance from the large airways.
- T_{high} is the amount of time the ventilator will maintain the P_{high} setting, which typically ranges from 3 to 5 seconds. A longer T_{high} allows more time for alveolar recruitment.
- T_{low} is the amount of time the ventilator will allow release of pressure from the airways and alveoli. It is typically restricted to between 0.2 and 0.6 seconds. The T_{low} will be adjusted to allow enough time for approximately 50% to 75% of the gas in the lungs to be exhaled. This is assessed by observing the expiratory flow patterns on the ventilator (Fig. 15-8). If more than 75% of the gas in the lungs is exhaled during T_{low}, then alveolar collapse and microatelectasis is possible.

As a guideline, to maximize alveolar recruitment and gas exchange, the bulk of time (80% to 95%) should occur at P_{high}, while limiting the time at P_{low}. The T_{low} is adjusted and continuously reassessed by using the peak expiratory flow pattern (PEFR). Full exhalation of all alveolar contents should be avoided and is evaluated by visualizing the end of exhalation occurring at a flow rate between 25% and 75% of PEFR. A short T_{low} is used to prevent alveolar derecruitment and maintain adequate end-expiratory lung volume (EELV). Ventilator-adjustment strategies focus on manipulating the end-inspiratory and end-expiratory lung volumes to increase oxygenation and improve ventilation.

Oxygenation:

- Assess PEFR greater than 50% and less than or equal to 75%.
- Increase P_{high} and/or T_{high} simultaneously. This will increase Paw, which in turn will increase alveolar volume, surface area, and gas exchange.
- Assess hemodynamics and assure adequate cardiac output.

Ventilation:

- Assess PEFR greater than 50% and less than or equal to 75%.
  - If T_{low} allows for PEFR of greater than or equal to 75%, then increase T_{low} to achieve 50% PEFR.
  - If PEFR is less than or equal to 50%, then decrease T_{low} to optimize alveolar ventilation.
- Increase P (difference between P_{high} and P_{low}) by increasing P_{high} and decreasing T_{low} to increase EELV.
- Assess sedation to assure spontaneous ventilation.
- Attempt weaning when FIO_2 less than or equal to 40% with SpO_2 greater than or equal to 95%, or when hypocarbia is evidenced by ABG or capnography results.
- Decrease P_{high} and increase T_{high} to decrease ventilator minute ventilation and increase the patient's spontaneous minute ventilation.
- Allow APRV to more closely mimic traditional CPAP settings. This will manifest as a low P_{high} and long T_{high}, with fewer drops to P_{low}.

Multiple benefits are attributed to APRV, including improved alveolar recruitment and oxygenation and decreased VILI because of lower inflating pressures. In addition, APRV facilitates spontaneous breathing and may improve patient tolerance to mechanical ventilation by decreasing patient-ventilator dyssynchrony (82). Although APRV is used as a lung-protective strategy, there is no conclusive evidence for whether it is superior to optimal lung-protective conventional ventilation.

High-Frequency Oscillatory Ventilation

High-frequency oscillatory ventilation (HFOV) is used in the pediatric ARDS population as a lung-protective mode of ventilation if plateau pressures cannot be kept at less than or equal to 30 cm H_2O during conventional ventilation. HFOV is not indicated for oxygenation failure secondary to cardiac and circulatory failure because of the high continuous distending pressures used. The benefit of HFOV includes providing effective oxygenation and

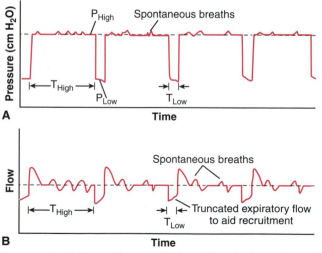
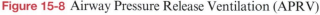

Figure 15-8 Airway Pressure Release Ventilation (APRV)

ventilation through very small VT delivered at high rates, increasing lung surface area for gas exchange.

HFOV works on six basic principles of physics (83):

1. **Bulk flow ventilation:** Fresh gas flow to the alveoli closest to the primary airways causing tidal ventilation with volumes less than or equal to anatomical dead space
2. **Taylor dispersion:** Radial diffusion of gas molecules across a concentration gradient between the center and periphery of the airways
3. **Pendelluft:** Movement of gas across adjacent alveolar units that occurs because of inequalities of time constants and pressure gradients
4. **Asymmetric velocity profiles:** Flow of fresh gas particles centrally down the length of the airway while the returning alveolar peripheral gas particles diffuse toward the outer airway wall
5. **Cardiogenic mixing:** Cardiac contractions that enhance peripheral airway mixing
6. **Molecular diffusion:** Diffusion of O_2 and CO_2 molecules across the alveolar-capillary membrane

Settings for pediatric HFOV are identical to those used for HFOV in the neonatal population. Adjustable settings include Paw, amplitude or P, hertz, and FIO_2. See Table 15-12 for specifics on adjusting HFOV settings to improve ventilation or oxygenation.

- The Paw can be compared with PEEP. It is a continuous distending pressure used to keep the lung "open" and is the primary setting for oxygenation, besides FIO_2. ARDS patients should be initiated on HFOV using a Paw of 3 to 5 cmH_2O above the Paw reading on the conventional ventilator.
- The P is the change in pressure fluctuating above and below the Paw. This is the pressure

Table 15-12	Blood Gas Management High-Frequency Oscillatory Ventilation Oxygenation and Ventilation Adjustments

Desired Result

HFOV Setting	↑PaO₂	↑PaCO₂	↓PaO₂	↓PaCO₂
FIO₂	↑	—	↓	—
Paw	↑	—	↓	—
Amplitude (P)	—	↓	—	↑
Hz	—	↑	—	↓

Oxygenation and ventilation during HFOV are decoupled. This means that adjusting a parameter that affects CO_2 clearance will not affect oxygenation and vice versa.

used to clear CO_2. After the transition is made to HFOV, chest wiggle factor (equal and continuous vibrations of portions of the skin and body, visible to the naked eye) should be evaluated. The P should be increased until chest wiggle is seen in the appropriate area. Definition of adequate "chest wiggle" for patients is as follows:

- Infants: from the umbilicus to the nipple line
- Prepubescent patients: from the groin to the nipple line
- Pubescent through adult patients: from the midthighs to the nipple line
- The frequency, measured in hertz (Hz), is the rate at which the HFOV delivers the change in pressure. This is accomplished using a bellows oscillating at a high frequency (rate) with an active exhalation. The active expiratory component is unique to the oscillator and enables it to use rates as high as 15 Hz (900 breaths per minute). The frequency is initially set at 6 to 15 Hz, depending on the age of the patient. Frequency for younger patients is set at higher hertz (10 to 15 Hz), whereas that for older patients is set at lower hertz (6 to 10 Hz) because the frequency is indirectly related to the small volume displacement in the system (i.e., faster rates = smaller volume per breath). Thus, older patients may need more volume to ventilate (and thus, more time per breath to inhale and exhale), and younger patients may need less.
- The inspiratory time during HFOV is determined as a percentage of total time. The I-time (inspiratory time) percentage should be left at 33%, giving a 1:2 I/E ratio. In older patients, the I-time percentage may be increased to 50% as a last resort to improve CO_2 clearance. By increasing the I-time percentage, you increase volume displacement. The I-time percentage should not exceed 50% because of potential air trapping as a result of the 1:1 I/E ratio.
- The starting FIO_2 should always be set at 1.0. During the conversion from conventional to HFOV, there will be some derecruitment of the lung, and a higher FIO_2 will be needed to compensate for the ventilator change.

If transcutaneous CO_2 monitoring is available, it should be placed on the patient 1 hour before the transition. Correlation between the transcutaneous CO_2 monitor and an ABG value should also be done. Transcutaneous CO_2 can serve as a trend/guide even if the values do not match. If the transcutaneous monitor CO_2 value rises after conversion, the $PaCO_2$ values should also be rising (84).

Even though current theory is that HFOV is lung protective because of the lower distending pressures, there is no evidence that HFOV reduces mortality in ARDS patients (82).

Glucocorticoids

Steroids are still controversial in the literature, and there is no real consensus on their role in ARDS. There is no benefit regarding survival, and use of steroids may increase mortality. Great caution must be used if treating ARDS patients with steroids (85).

Surfactant

There may be efficacy in the delivery of exogenous surfactant for ARDS since there is evidence of type II pneumocyte damage and surfactant deactivation. BAL studies in patients with ARDS have shown decreased levels of surfactant protein A (SP-A) and surfactant protein B (SP-B) (86). One prevalent pathway of surfactant dysfunction in lung injury is through biophysical or chemical interactions with substances present in the alveoli as a result of permeability edema or inflammation (86). The goal of surfactant replacement in patients with ARDS is to decrease surface tension in the alveoli and increase surface area for gas exchange. If this can be accomplished, plateau pressures should be able to be maintained below 30 cm H_2O. Most research has concentrated on increased oxygenation and decreased mortality as their primary outcomes. The dose of surfactant for ARDS is still controversial, but in a recent study by Wilson and colleagues, Calfactant was delivered at 10 mL/kg for patients less than or equal to 10 kg and 80 mL/m^2 for patients greater than 10 kg (86). A meta-analysis of surfactant therapy in children with acute respiratory failure including bronchiolitis and acute lung injury showed decreased mortality, improved oxygenation, increased ventilator-free days, and decreased duration of mechanical ventilation (68, 86). Surfactant replacement may hold promise in the future treatment of ARDS. During delivery, the patient should be monitored for adverse effects, including:

• Hypoxemia
• Decreased ventilation
• Bradycardia
• Pulmonary hemorrhage
• Pneumothorax

The route of administration is direct instillation via the endotracheal tube. Delivery of the ordered dose may take 20 to 60 minutes. Regurgitation up the endotracheal tube is a sign that the dose is being administered too quickly, and the practitioner should halt administration until the endotracheal tube clears. The dose should be split into two syringes, one for the right lung and the other for the left. The patient is positioned laterally on the right

or left side depending on which side the surfactant will be administered. Patients should be preoxygenated with 100% oxygen for 20 to 60 minutes until a SpO_2 of 100% or a plateau is reached. Vital signs, including HR, RR, SpO_2, blood pressure, end-tidal CO_2, V_T exhaled, and PIP, should be monitored, and intra-administration interventions should be performed based on their results. In the event of oxygen desaturation with bradycardia, the patient should be suctioned and administration held until the patient recovers. The patient should not be suctioned for 60 minutes after administration to allow dispersion of the surfactant to the alveoli. Patients in pressure-controlled modes of ventilation need to be monitored for increasing exhaled V_T. Rapid increase in pulmonary compliance may cause the lung to overdistend, resulting in pneumothorax.

Nitric Oxide

Nitric oxide (NO) is an inhaled selective pulmonary vasodilator that alters levels of cyclic guanosine monophosphate (cGMP) in the pulmonary vasculature creating vasodilatation. This increases blood flow to the ventilated regions of the lung and increases oxygenation. The half-life of NO is extremely short (approximately 5 seconds), and it rapidly binds with hemoglobin, deactivating it; thus, the effects are limited to the pulmonary vasculature (86). Doses used to treat ARDS are usually between 10 and 20 ppm, although doses as low as 1 ppm improve oxygenation (68). Current literature reports increased oxygenation; however, there is no reported decrease in mortality (68).

Some of the toxic effects of NO delivery that need to be monitored during delivery are methemoglobin (MetHb) formation and nitrogen dioxide (NO_2). MetHb is formed when NO binds with it, thus cooximetry must be performed when therapy is initiated and then daily during therapy. Therapy should be discontinued when MetHb levels are greater than 5%. NO_2 is a toxic by-product formed when NO combines with oxygen. When NO_2 mixes with oxygen and water, nitric acid is formed (HNO_3). To minimize this reaction and reduce the patient's risk of exposure, the delivery system must be purged before use. Ventilator flow rates should be high enough to keep a fresh gas flow and decrease the reaction between O_2 and NO molecules. Other factors that increase risk of exposure to NO_2 include high FIO_2 and high doses of NO (above 80 ppm). Monitor alarm limits should be set to warn of NO_2 levels 3 ppm or greater. Current delivery systems can deliver precise concentrations of NO and reduce the risk of exposure to NO_2. The delivery systems ensure a consistent concentration of NO in parts per million regardless of minute ventilation.

Prone Positioning

Prone positioning, or the placement of a patient facedown, may be considered if the patient continues to have difficulty oxygenating or ventilating. Although there are improvements in oxygenation associated with prone positioning, the effects are short-lived, and there is no association with a reduction in mortality (88)

Placing patients in a prone position needs to be done with great care and observation. The airway needs to be monitored by one person, and all of the monitoring lines and IV lines must be watched during the turn. Planning must be done in advance to ensure the procedure is accomplished without complications. There are kinetic beds designed to turn patients onto their right and left side throughout the hour. The practitioner programs the frequency of and duration of positioning. This may be an option for patients who are difficult to move.

Extracorporeal Membrane Oxygenation

Extracorporeal membrane oxygenation (ECMO) is indicated if the patient continues to deteriorate despite maximal ventilation and oxygenation attempts. It is recommended that ECMO support be started within 7 days of the initiation of mechanical ventilation (89). While there are no known absolute indications, relative and specific contraindications, such as bleeding risk and genetic abnormalities, need to be considered (see Chapter 6 for more information on inclusion and exclusion criteria for ECMO) (89).

ECMO permits rest of the lung by removing deoxygenated blood from the body and circulating it through a membrane oxygenator. A membrane oxygenator performs the entire process of respiration. Oxygen-rich blood is then pumped back into the body and circulated by the heart or augmented by the ECMO pump to the end organs.

There are two types of ECMO: venovenous (VV) and veno-arterial (VA). VV is the method of choice for treating patients in respiratory failure. Blood is withdrawn from the internal jugular vein and returned to the patient through another lumen of the same cannula, distal to the withdraw port. The patient's native heart function circulates the blood throughout the body.

VA is required if the patient has combined circulatory and respiratory failure. During VA ECMO, blood is pulled from the internal jugular vein and returned via the carotid artery. Survival in one study among adults with severe respiratory failure supported with ECMO was 50% (90). Pediatric data have mostly been limited to small sample size, but survival data are even more promising at 58.3% (91) to 77% (92). ECMO is considered a rescue therapy and is reserved as a last resort for acute respiratory failure and ARDS. Considerations should be made for ventilation strategies while on ECMO. Usually, patients are placed on minimal ventilator settings with a FIO_2 of less than 0.40 and a plateau pressure of less than 20 cm H_2O (87). However, newer approaches use higher PEEP levels (12 to 15 cmH_2O) to prevent lung opacification and/or atelectasis. This strategy may assist with shortening ECMO bypass time and expediting earlier decannulation. In addition, pulmonary hygiene is imperative on ECMO. At a minimum, suctioning should occur every 4 hours, along with a daily chest radiograph.

Course and Prognosis

Although the overall mortality rate from ARDS has been reduced with advancements in modern medical interventions, it still remains high. Research has found that patients who die within the first 72 hours of ARDS onset usually die because of the presenting injury or illness; patients who die after 72 hours usually die from complications (93). The most common cause of death after 72 hours was sepsis/multiorgan failure followed by central nervous system complications (93). Other causes include respiratory, cardiac, hepatic, gastrointestinal, and renal failure. Patients who do survive ARDS often have neurocognitive disorders. Depression and anxiety are the main morbidities among survivors (94). In addition, 18% to 43% have been found to develop post-traumatic stress disorder (94). Development of neurocognitive impairment is not related to the severity of disease or age; however, studies show that hypotension (MAP less than 50 mm Hg) and hypoxemia (prolonged SpO_2 less than 90%) may be contributing factors (94). The incidence of neurocognitive disorders associated with ARDS may remain underreported (94). This may be related to the perceived underreporting of the disease process itself.

The impact of ARDS is broad. Survivors face health-related quality of life and functional disabilities. Survivors and caregivers often are not prepared to deal with the newfound disabilities and impairments (95). This tremendous burden on their lives remains an issue that needs further study to improve long-term outcomes. Additionally, future research should focus on gaining insight into ARDS epidemiology and identifying risk factors to decrease the incidence of emotional and neurocognitive sequelae.

■■ Jacob remained on CPAP for about 24 hours to stabilize his FRC and maintain oxygenation. He was weaned back to an NC and was maintained on it until SpO_2 was greater than 95% on room air. Feeds were reinitiated as his RR returned to baseline. Jacob was discharged home 5 days after admission.

■ ■ Critical Thinking Questions: Jacob Smith

1. What would you have suggested as the next step in therapy if CPAP had not improved Jacob's respiratory distress?
2. Would you expect Jacob to have any long-term sequelae from his bronchiolitis? Is there anything his family should be aware of regarding his respiratory care for the next several years?
3. If Jacob's SpO$_2$ had remained greater than 92% throughout his ED visit, do you think that would have changed the course of his care? Should he have still been admitted to the hospital?

▶● Case Studies and Critical Thinking Questions

■ Case 1: Jennifer Dodson

Jennifer Dodson is 5 years old and weighs 20 kg. Her mother brought her to the ED after visiting Jennifer's pediatrician. Jennifer is exhibiting increased WOB, decreased breath sounds with crackles in the right-middle and right-lower lobes, and general malaise. In triage, her physical examination is notable for temperature 39.0°C, altered mental status, nasal flaring, marked substernal and intercostal retractions, respiratory rate greater than 40 breaths/min, HR of 130 bpm, blood pressure of 115/85 mm Hg, SpO$_2$ of 88% in room air, and capillary refill of less than 2 seconds. Using appropriate universal precautions (e.g., gown, gloves, and mask), you initiate a nasal cannula at 3 LPM and sit her upright. These maneuvers increase her SpO$_2$ to greater than 95%.

The physician assesses the past medical history and history of present illness. The history is unremarkable: Jennifer was a term newborn and has no prior admissions, no prematurity, and normal development and immunizations. Her mother states that Jennifer has a 2-week history of cold symptoms, including nasal discharge, slight fever, and cough. Today, she had worsening of respiratory symptoms, including a rapid respiratory rate, wheezing, and increased respiratory effort (e.g., intercostal retractions and nasal flaring), along with decreased oral intake and activity level.

• *Based on these clinical findings, what is Jennifer's most likely differential diagnosis?*

After the physician has completed his assessment, a chest radiograph is ordered, along with an intravenous catheter and routine blood culture. Jennifer is given a sterile sputum culture sample cup and asked to spit mucus in the cup if possible. Her mom is encouraged to help her obtain the sample while keeping the cup as sterile as possible.

• *If Jennifer is unable to provide a sputum sample spontaneously, what would you recommend as the next step to obtain a specimen?*

Jennifer is moved to the school-aged inpatient unit and maintained at with a 3L NC. You encourage Jennifer to cough for you, and you hear a loose, uncontrollable, and nonproductive cough. Auscultation still reveals crackles in the right-middle and lower lobes. Chest radiograph is returned and confirms the diagnosis of pneumonia.

• *What additional therapies might you suggest for Jennifer?*

■ Case 2: Megan Knox

Megan is 10 years old and weighs 45 kg. She has been transported by helicopter to the ICU for management of respiratory failure with refractory hypoxemia. Upon arrival, she is being hand-ventilated with a 6.0 cuffed endotracheal tube with FIO$_2$ of 1.0 at a rate of 25 breaths/min. Vital signs are HR, 130 bpm; SpO$_2$, 85% to 87%; blood pressure, 85/55 with vasopressor therapy, and capillary refill time of 5 to 6 seconds. Her breath sounds reveal bilateral course crackles via auscultation and no WOB. She is heavily sedated with fentanyl and midazolam. Megan is moved to the ICU bed and placed on mechanical ventilation.

• *What initial ventilator settings would you recommend for Megan?*

After Megan is placed on mechanical ventilation, the physician orders ventilator parameters of volume control, VT 350 mL, rate 25; PEEP, 10 cm H$_2$O; and FIO$_2$, 100%. She orders a chest radiograph and laboratory studies including blood cultures, complete blood count with differential, metabolic panel, and ABG test. After the ABG test and chest radiograph are completed, the physician asks you to perform PaO$_2$/ FIO$_2$ ratio and Murray score to determine the degree of severity of Megan's respiratory illness. The chest radiograph reveals bilateral interstitial and alveolar infiltrates without cardiomegaly. ABG values are 7.27/58/26.3/150.

• *What is Megan's PaO$_2$/ FIO$_2$ ratio?*
• *What is her Murray score?*

Based on these findings, Megan meets the criteria for the diagnosis of ARDS. Arterial and central venous catheters are placed without complications. She is started on IV isotonic crystalloid fluid therapy at maintenance rate. Megan remains on vasopressor therapy with normotensive blood pressure. A follow-up ABG test reveals worsening acidosis with hypercarbia and persistent hypoxemia.

- *What additional therapies can you suggest to improve oxygenation and ventilation?*

Multiple-Choice Questions

1. A 6-month-old girl is brought to the pediatric ED by her grandmother. She has had a low-grade fever, runny nose, and a cough for 3 days. She has refused finger foods since the start of the fever and has refused bottles for the last 6 hours. Vital signs are HR, 158 bpm; SpO_2, 91%; and RR, 65 breaths/min. On physical examination, you note substernal retractions and decreased breath sounds with inspiratory and expiratory wheezing. The baby seems sleepy and difficult to arouse. The ED physician is caring for a patient in a critical care room but asks for your impressions and recommendation regarding admitting the baby. What should you suggest?
   a. Observe for 1 to 2 hours in the ED, assessing for signs of improvement
   b. Admit to the pediatric in-patient unit
   c. Discharge home
   d. Admit to the ICU

2. Which of the following signs are indicative of severe bronchiolitis?
   I. SpO_2 less than 92%
   II. RR 60 to 70 breaths/min
   III. Inspiratory and expiratory wheezing
   IV. Intercostal retractions
   a. I, III
   b. II, IV
   c. I, II, III
   d. I, III, IV

3. A 4-year-old with pneumonia has an SpO_2 of 90% on room air and thick nasal and airway secretions that are difficult to clear. What would be the best oxygen delivery device to increase SpO_2 greater than 95%?
   a. NC at 1 LPM
   b. Simple face mask at 3 LPM
   c. Non-rebreather at 15 LPM
   d. HFNC at 8 LPM

4. What is the most common bacterial pathogen causing pediatric pneumonia?
   a. *Staphylococcus aureus*
   b. *Streptococcus* pneumonia
   c. Respiratory syncytial virus
   d. *Haemophilus influenzae*

5. An 8-year-old boy has been transferred to the PICU for pneumonia and impending respiratory failure. You start him on CPAP plus 5 cm H_2O and an FIO_2 of 0.75. Which of the following would be evidence of improved respiratory status?
   a. Improved SpO_2
   b. Decreased RR
   c. Decreased FIO_2 to less than 0.60
   d. Decreased WOB
   e. All of the above

6. Which of the following are clinical characteristics necessary for a diagnosis of ARDS?
   I. Bilateral infiltrates on chest radiograph
   II. Unilateral infiltrates on chest radiograph
   III. Evidence of left atrial hypertension
   IV. Normal left atrial pressures
   V. Acute onset of symptoms
   VI. Hypoxia
   a. I, III, V, VI
   b. II, III, VI
   c. I, IV, V, VI
   d. II, IV, V, VI

7. Chest radiograph findings for pneumonia include all of the following except:
   a. Patchy and segmental or nonsegmental with the presence of airspace opacification.
   b. Diffuse interstitial or peribronchial infiltrates.
   c. Patchy infiltrates attributed to atelectasis.
   d. Lobar or alveolar consolidation.

8. The benefit of pressure-controlled over volume-controlled modes of ventilation is:
   a. Breath-to-breath VT variations.
   b. Decelerating flow patterns during mandatory breaths.
   c. Consistent PIPs despite changes in lung compliance and airway resistance.
   d. All of the above.

9. The benefit of volume-control over pressure-control modes of ventilation is:
   a. Consistent minute ventilation despite changes in lung compliance and airway resistance.
   b. Accelerating flow patterns during mandatory breaths.
   c. Breath-to-breath variation in PIPs.
   d. All of the above.

10. A 12-year-old patient with ARDS caused by near drowning has been on APRV for 4 days. Goal blood gas values are pH greater than 7.25, $PaCO_2$ less than 55 mm Hg, and PaO_2 greater than 60 mm Hg. A routine ABG result provides the following: pH, 7.23; $PaCO_2$, 62 mm Hg; PaO_2, 55 mm Hg. Which of the following would be the best ventilator setting changes to improve acid-base status and oxygenation?
   I. Increase P_{high}
   II. Decrease T_{high}
   III. Increase T_{high}
   IV. Increase FIO_2
   V. Increase T_{low}
   a. I, II, IV
   b. I, IV, V
   c. I, II, IV, V
   d. I, III, IV

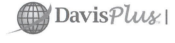 **DavisPlus** | For additional resources login to DavisPlus (http://davisplus.fadavis.com/ keyword "Perretta") and click on the Premium tab. (Don't have a *Plus*Code to access Premium Resources? Just click the Purchase Access button on the book's DavisPlus page.)

REFERENCES

1. Merrill C, Owens PL, for the Healthcare Cost and Utilization Project. Reasons for being admitted to the hospital through the emergency department for children and adolescents, 2004. HCUP Statistical Brief no. 33. Rockville, MD: Agency for Healthcare Research and Quality; June, 2007. Available at: http://www.hcup-us.ahrq.gov/reports/statbriefs/sb33.pdf. Accessed July 18, 2012.
2. Leader S, Kohlhase K. Respiratory syncytial virus-coded pediatric hospitalizations, 1997 to 1999. *Pediatr Infect Dis.* 2002;21(7):629-632.
3. Centers for Disease Control and Prevention. Respiratory syncytial virus activity—United States, July 2008–December 2009. *MMWR Morb Mortal Wkly Rep.* 2010;59(8):230-233.
4. Wainwright C. Acute viral bronchiolitis in children—a very common condition with few therapeutic options. *Paediatr Respir Rev.* 2010;11(1):39-45.
5. Teague WG. Bronchiolitis/viral lower respiratory tract infections. In: *ACCP/AAP Pediatric Pulmonary Medicine Board Review.* lst ed. Northbrook, IL: American College of Chest Physicians; 2010;113-126. http://publications.chestnet.org/data/Books/PPMBREV/ppmbrev-10-113.pdf. Accessed July 18, 2012.
6. Wright M, Piedimonte G. Respiratory syncytial virus prevention and therapy: past, present, and future. *Pediatr Pulmonol.* 2010;46(4):324-347.
7. Shay DK, Holman RC, Newman RD, et al. Bronchiolitis-associated hospitalizations among US children, 1980-1996. *JAMA.* 1999;282(15):1440-1446.
8. Centers for Disease Control and Prevention. Respiratory syncytial virus activity—United States, 2003-2004. *MMWR Morb Mortal Wkly Rep.* 2004;53(49):1159-1160.
9. Wagner T. Bronchiolitis. *Pediatr Rev.* 2009;30(10):386-395.
10. Boone SA, Gerba CP. Significance of fomites in the spread of respiratory and enteric viral disease. *Appl Environ Microbiol.* 2007;73(6):1687-1696.
11. Lowell DI, Lister G, Von Kloss H, et al. Wheezing in infants: the response to epinephrine. *Pediatrics.* 1987;87:939-945.
12. Liu LL, Gallaher MM, Davis RL, et al. Use of a respiratory clinical score among different providers. *Pediatr Pulmonol.* 2004;37(3):243-248.
13. Zorc J, Florin T, Rodio B, for the Children's Hospital of Philadelphia. ED pathway for evaluation guidelines/treatment of children with bronchiolitis. January 2011. http://intranet.chop.edu/emergency_dept/nursing/clin_pathway/bronchiolitis/. Accessed May 7, 2011.
14. American Academy of Pediatrics, Subcommittee on Diagnosis and Management of Bronchiolitis. Diagnosis and management of bronchiolitis. *Pediatrics.* 2006;118(4):1774-1793.
15. American Academy of Pediatrics, Steering Committee on Quality Improvement and Management. Classifying recommendations for clinical practice guidelines. *Pediatrics.* 2004;114(3):874-877.
16. Zentz SE. Care of infants and children with bronchiolitis: a systematic review. *J Pediatr Nurs.* 2011;26(6):519-529.
17. Forster RE II, Dubois AB, Briscoe WA, et al. *The Lung: Physiologic Basis of Pulmonary Function Tests.* Chicago, IL: Year Book Medical Publishers; 1986.
18. Chernick V, Boat TF, Wilmot RW, et al. *Kendig's Disorders of the Respiratory Tract in Children.* 6th ed. Philadelphia, PA: W. B. Saunders; 1998.
19. Gilmore MM. Preterm VLBW infants: post-extubation respiratory support. *J Perinatol.* 2006;26:449-451.
20. Liet JM, Ducruet T, Gupta V, et al. Heliox inhalation therapy for bronchiolitis in infants. *Cochrane Database Syst Rev.* 2010;14(4):CD006915.
21. Wolfson MR, Bhutani VK, Shaffer TH, et al. Mechanics and energetics of breathing helium in infants with bronchopulmonary dysplasia. *J Pediatr.* 1984;104(5):752-757.
22. Myers T. Use of heliox in children. *Respir Care.* 2006;51(6):619-631.
23. Stillwell PC, Quick JD, Munro PR, et al. Effectiveness of open-circuit and oxyhood delivery of helium-oxygen. *Chest.* 1989;95(6):1222-1224.
24. Cambonie G, Milesi C, Fournier-Favre S, et al. Clinical effects of heliox administration for acute bronchiolitis in young infants. *Chest.* 2006;129(3):676-682.

25. Weber JE, Chudnofsky CR, Younger JG, et al. A randomized comparison of helium-oxygen mixture (Heliox) and racemic epinephrine for the treatment of moderate to severe croup. *Pediatrics.* 2001;107(6):E96.

26. Hartling L, Russell KF, Patel H, et al. Epinephrine for bronchiolitis. *Cochrane Database Syst Rev.* 2004;1: CD003123.

27. Wainwright CE, Altamirano L, Cheney M, et al. A multicenter, randomized, double-blind, controlled trial of nebulized epinephrine in infants with acute bronchiolitis. *N Engl J Med.* 2003;349:27-35.

28. Robinson M, Hemming AL, Regnis JA, et al. Effect of increasing doses of hypertonic saline on mucociliary clearance in patients with cystic fibrosis. *Thorax.* 1997;52: 900-903.

29. Kuzik BA, Al Qaghi SA, Kent S, et al. Nebulized hypertonic saline in the treatment of viral bronchiolitis in infants. *J Pediatr.* 2007;151(3):266-270.

30. Mandelberg A, Tal G, Witzling M, et al. Nebulized 3% hypertonic saline solution treatment in hospitalized infants with viral bronchiolitis. *Chest.* 2003;123(2):481-487.

31. Sarrell EM, Tal G, Witzling M, et al. Nebulized 3% hypertonic saline solution treatment in ambulatory children with viral bronchiolitis decreases symptoms. *Chest.* 2002; 122(6):2015-2020.

32. Tal G, Cesar K, Oron A, et al. Hypertonic saline/epinephrine treatment in hospitalized infants with viral bronchiolitis reduces hospitalization stay: 2 years experience. *Israel Med Assoc J.* 2006;8(3):169-173.

33. Perrotta C, Ortiz Z, Roqué i Figuls M. Chest physiotherapy for acute bronchiolitis in paediatric patients between 0 and 24 months old. *Cochrane Database Syst Rev.* 2007;1: CD004873.

34. Patel H, Platt R, Lozano JM, et al. Glucocorticoids for acute viral bronchiolitis in infants and young children. *Cochrane Database Syst Rev.* 2004;3:CD004878.

35. Antonow JA, Hansen K, McKinstry CA, et al. Sepsis evaluation in hospitalized infants with bronchiolitis. *Pediatr Infect Dis J.* 1998;17(3):231-236.

36. Purcell K, Fergie J. Concurrent serious bacterial infections in 2396 infants and children hospitalized with respiratory syncytial virus lower respiratory tract infections. *Arch Pediatr Adolesc Med.* 2002;156(4):322-324.

37. Greenes DS, Harper MB. Low risk of bacteremia in febrile children with recognizable viral syndromes. *Pediatr Infect Dis J.* 1999;18(3):258-261.

38. Levine DA, Platt SL, Dayan PS, et al. Risk of serious bacterial infection in young febrile infants with respiratory syncytial virus infections. *Pediatrics.* 2004;113(6): 1728-1734.

39. Hall CB. Respiratory syncytial virus: a continuing culprit and conundrum. *J Pediatr.* 1999;135(2, pt 2):2-7.

40. Dawson-Caswell M, Muncie HL Jr. Respiratory syncytial virus in children. *Am Fam Physician.* 2011;83(2):141-146.

41. The IMpact-RSV Study Group. Palivizumab, a humanized respiratory syncytial virus monoclonal antibody, reduces hospitalization from respiratory syncytial virus infection in high risk infants. *Pediatrics.* 1998;102(3, pt 1):531-537.

42. Simões EA. Maternal smoking, asthma, and bronchiolits: clear-cut association or equivocal evidence? *Pediatrics.* 2007;119(6):1210-1212.

43. Carbonell-Estrany X, Quero J, Bustos G, et al. Rehospitalization because of respiratory syncytial virus infection in premature infants younger than 33 weeks of gestation: a prospective study. *Pediatr Infect Dis J.* 2000;19(7):592-597.

44. Law BJ, Langley JM, Allen U, et al. The Pediatric Investigators Collaborative Network on Infections in Canada study of predictors of hospitalization for respiratory syncytial virus infection or infants born at 33 through 35 completed weeks of gestation. *Pediatr Infect Dis J.* 2004;23(9):806-814.

45. Tsutsumi H, Honjo T, Nagai K, et al. Immunoglobulin A antibody response to respiratory syncytial virus structural proteins in colostrum and milk. *J Clin Microbiol.* 1989;27(9):1949-1951.

46. Shay DK, Holman RC, Roosevelt GE, et al. Bronchiolitis-associated mortality and estimates of respiratory syncytial virus-associated deaths among US children, 1979-1997. *J Infect Dis.* 2001;183(1):16-22.

47. Krilov LR. Respiratory syncytial virus disease: update on treatment and prevention. *Expert Rev Anti Infect Ther.* 2011;9(1): 27-32.

48. van Woensel JB, Kimpen JL, Sprikkelman AB, et al. Long-term effects of prednisolone in the acute phase of bronchiolitis caused by respiratory syncytial virus. *Pediatr Pulmonol.* 2000;30(2):92-99.

49. World Health Organization. Pneumonia. http://www.who.int/mediacentre/factsheets/fs331/en/index.html#. Accessed July 18, 2012.

50. Centers for Disease Control and Prevention. Vaccines & preventable diseases: pneumococcal vaccination. http://www.cdc.gov/vaccines/vpd-vac/pneumo/default.htm. Accessed July 18, 2012.

51. British Thoracic Society of Standards of Care Committee. BTS guidelines for the management of community acquired pneumonia in childhood. *Thorax.* 2002;57 (suppl 1):i1-i24.

52. Day G, Provost EM, Lanier AP; the Office of Alaska Native Health Research. *Alaska Native Mortality Update 1999-2003.* Anchorage, AK: Alaska Native Epidemiology Center; 2006.Bennett NJ, Domachowske J. Pediatric pneumonia. http://emedicine.medscape.com/article/967822. Updated June 21, 2012. Accessed July 18, 2012.

53. Scott JA, Wonodi C, Moïsi JC et al. The definition of pneumonia, the assessment of severity, and clinical standardization in the Pneumonia Etiology Research for Child Health study. Clin Infect Dis. 2012 April 1; 54(Suppl 2): S109–S116.

54. The Merck Manual. Pneumonia in immunocompromised patients. http://www.merckmanuals.com/professional/sec05/ch052/ch052e.html?qt=pneumonia&alt=sh. Updated May, 2008. Accessed July 18, 2012.

55. Busl KM, Greer DM. Hypoxic-ischemic brain injury: pathophysiology, neuropathology and mechanisms. *NeuroRehablilitation.* 2010;26(1):5-13.

56. The Merck Manual. Community-acquired pneumonia. http://www.merckmanuals.com/professional/sec05/ch052/ch052b.html. Updated May, 2008. Accessed July 18, 2012.

57. Burggraaf J, Westendorp RGJ, in't Veen JCCM, et al. Cardiovascular side effects of inhaled salbutamol in hypoxic asthmatic patients. *Thorax.* 2001;56:567-569.

58. Waskin H. Toxicology of antimicrobial aerosols: a review of aerosolized ribavirin and pentamidine. *Respir Care.* 1991;36:1026-1036.

59. Percussionaire® Corporation. IPV® Impulsator® for home care. www.ipvhome.com/impulsator.asp. Accessed July 18, 2012.

60. Fink JB. Forced expiratory technique, directed cough, and autogenic drainage. *Respir Care.* 2007;52(9):1210-1221.

61. Nagy B, Gaspar I, Papp A, et al. Efficacy of methylprednisolone in children with severe community acquired pneumonia [published online ahead of print May 15, 2012]. *Pediatr Pulmonol.* doi: 10.1002/ppul.22574.

62. Turner DA, Cheifetz IM. Pediatric acute respiratory failure: areas of debate in the pediatric critical care setting. *Expert Rev Respir Med.* 2011;5(1):65-73.

63. Xu JQ, Kochanek KD, Murphy SL, et al, for the Division of Vital Statistics. Deaths: final data for 2007. *National Vital Statistics Reports.* 2010;58(19). http://www.cdc.gov/nchs/data/nvsr/nvsr58/nvsr58_19.pdf. Accessed July 18, 2012.

64. Lee GE, Lorch SA, Sheffler-Collins S, et al. National hospitalization trends for pediatric pneumonia and associated complications. *Pediatrics.* 2010;126(2):204-213.

65. Don M, Canciani M, Korppi M. Community-acquired pneumonia in children: what's old? What's new? *Acta Paediatr.* 2010;99(11):1602-1608.

66. Scott JAG, Abdulla Brooks W, Malik Peiris JS, et al. Pneumonia research to reduce childhood mortality in the developing world. *J Clin Invest.* 2008;118(4):1291-1300.

67. Randolph AG. Management of acute lung injury and acute respiratory distress syndrome in children. *Crit Care Med.* 2009;37(8):2448-2454.

68. Kneyber MCJ, Brouwers AGA, Caris JA, et al. Acute respiratory distress syndrome: is it underrecognized in the pediatric intensive care unit? *Intensive Care Med.* 2008;34(4):751-754.

69. Willson DF, Chess PR, Notter RH. Surfactant for pediatric acute lung injury. *Pediatr Clin North Am.* 2008;55(3):545-575, ix.

70. Chiefetz IR. Pediatric acute respiratory distress syndrome. *Respir Care.* 2011;56(10):1589-1599.

71. Petty TL, Ashbaugh DG. The adult respiratory distress syndrome: clinical features, factors influencing prognosis and principles of management. *Chest.* 1971;60(3):233-239.

72. Tomashefski JF, Jr. Acute respiratory distress syndrome. *Clin Chest Med.* 2000;21(3):1-34.

73. Dahlem P, van Aalderen WMC, Bos AP. Pediatric acute lung injury. *Paediatr Respir Rev.* 2007; 8(4):348-362.

74. Murray JF, Matthay MA, Luce JM, et al. An expanded definition of the adult respiratory distress syndrome. *Am Rev Respir Dis.* 1988;138(3):720-723.

75. Bernard GR, Artigas A, Brigham KL, et al. The American-European Consensus Conference on ARDS: definitions, mechanisms, relevant outcomes, and clinical trial coordination. *Am J Respir Crit Care Med.* 1994;149(3):818-824.

76. Thomas NJ, Shaffer ML, Willson DF, et al. Defining acute lung disease in children with the oxygenation saturation index. *Pediatr Crit Care Med.* 2010;11(1):12-17.

77. Mach WJ, Thimmesh AR, Pierce JT, et al. Consequences of hyperoxia and the toxicity of oxygen in the lung. *Nurs Res Pract.* 2011;2011:260482.doi: 10.1155/2011/260482.

78. Muñoz-Bonet JI, Flor-Macián EM, Roselló PM, et al. Noninvasive ventilation in pediatric acute respiratory failure by means of a conventional volumetric ventilator. *World J Pediatr.* 2010;6(4):323-330.

79. Girard TD, Bernard GR. Mechanical ventilation in ARDS: a state-of-the-art review. *Chest.* 2007;131(3):921-929.

80. Habashi NM. Other approaches to open-lung ventilation: airway pressure release ventilation. *Crit Care Med.* 2005;33(3, suppl):S228-S240.

81. Wunsch H, Mapstone J. High-frequency ventilation versus conventional ventilation for treatment of acute lung injury and acute respiratory distress syndrome. *Cochrane Database Syst Rev.* 2004;(1): CD004085.

82. Krishnan JA, Brower RG. High-frequency ventilation for acute lung injury and ARDS. *Chest.* 2000;118(3):795-807.

83. Berkenbosch JW, Tobias JD. Transcutaneous carbon dioxide monitoring during high-frequency oscillatory ventilation in infants and children. *Crit Care Med.* 2002;30(5):1024-1027.

84. National Heart, Lung, and Blood Institute. Steroids do not prolong survival in intensive care patients with ARDS on life support, finds NHLBI study. NIH News website. http://www.nih.gov/news/pr/apr2006/nhlbi-19.htm. Published April 19, 2006. Accessed July 18, 2012.

85. Willson DF, Thomas NJ, Markovitz BP, et al. Effect of exogenous surfactant (calfactant) in pediatric acute lung injury: a randomized controlled trial. *JAMA.* 2005;293(4):470-474.

86. Afshari A, Brok J, Moller AM, et al. Inhaled nitric oxide for acute respiratory distress syndrome (ARDS) and acute lung injury in children and adults. *Cochrane Database Syst Rev.* 2010;(7):CD002787.

87. Curley MAQ, Hibberd PL, Fineman FD, et al. Effect of prone positioning on clinical outcomes in children with acute lung injury: a randomized controlled trial. *JAMA.* 2005;294(2):229-237.

88. Extracorporeal Life Support Organization (ELSO). *Patient Specific Guidelines: A Supplement to the ELSO General Guidelines (April 2009).* Ann Arbor, MI: ELSO; April, 2009. http://www.elso.med.umich.edu/Guidelines.html . Accessed July 18, 2012.

89. Brogan TV, Thiagarajan RR, Rycus PT, et al. Extracorporal membrane oxygenation in adults with severe respiratory failure: a multi-center database. *Intensive Care Med.* 2009;35(12):2105-2114.

90. Peng CC, Wu SJ, Chen MR, et al. Clinical experience of extracorporeal membrane oxygenation for acute respiratory distress syndrome associated with pneumonia in children. *J Formos Med Assoc.* 2012;111(3):147-152.

91. Pettignano R, Fortenberry JD, Heard ML, et al. Primary use of the venovenous approach for extracorporeal membrane oxygenation in pediatric acute respiratory failure. *Pediatr Crit Care Med.* 2003;4(3):291-298.

92. Stapleton RD, Wang BM, Hudson LD, et al. Causes and timing of death in patients with ARDS. *Chest.* 2005;128(2):525-532.

93. Hopkins RO, Miller RR III. Neurocognitive and psychiatric sequelae among survivors of acute respiratory distress syndrome. *Clin Pulm Med.* 2008;15(5):258-266.

94. Hough CL, Herridge MS. Long-term outcome after acute lung injury. *Curr Opin Crit Care.* 2012;18(1):8-15.

Chapter 16

Pediatric Infectious Airway Diseases

Stacey Mann, BS, RRT

Key Terms

Angioedema
Aryepiglottic folds
Bacterial tracheitis
Cricothyroidotomy
Drooling
Dysphagia
Dysphonia
Endoscopy
Epiglottitis
Immunocompromised
Laryngotracheobronchitis
Leukocytosis
Mucopurulent exudates
Respiratory distress
Subglottic airway
Supraglottic larynx
Westley croup score

Chapter Objectives

After reading this chapter, you will be able to:

1. Identify the "4 Ds" referred to in the clinical presentation of epiglottitis.
2. Identify similarities and differences in the clinical presentation of epiglottitis, croup, and bacterial tracheitis.
3. Identify the most definitive way to diagnose both epiglottitis and bacterial tracheitis.
4. Differentiate between the radiographic findings of epiglottis, croup, and bacterial tracheitis.
5. Identify the most common organism associated with epiglottitis and discuss why there has been a decline in outbreak of the disease over the last several years.
6. List four common viruses that cause croup in the pediatric patient population.
7. Use the Westley croup score to assess a patient's symptoms of croup.
8. List three possible treatments for croup that respiratory therapists can administer.
9. Identify one microorganism found today that may contribute to the changing epidemiology and virulence of bacterial tracheitis.

■■ Timmy Jones

You begin working your dayshift in a level I pediatric trauma center emergency department (ED) where you are the only respiratory therapist (RT) working this 12-hour shift. Two hours into your relatively quiet shift, Timmy, a 4-year-old boy, presents to the ED with obvious respiratory distress. He is having difficulty talking and is only able to put two to three words together at a time. He is immediately triaged by a nurse, and his vital signs are heart rate (HR), 140 bpm; blood pressure (BP), 100/65 mm Hg; respiratory rate (RR) 40 breaths/minute; temperature 103.9°F; and oxygen saturation (SpO_2), 89% on room air. He is taken into an examination room where he waits to be seen by a resident. The triage nurse tells you about this patient, and you immediately go into his room to do an assessment. Upon entering the room, you notice his pronounced respiratory distress.

Acute infections of the respiratory tract are common in pediatric patients. Upper and lower airway infections are commonly encountered in the ED. Visits for respiratory disease account for 10% of all pediatric ED visits and 20% of all pediatric hospital admissions (1). The severity of upper respiratory tract infections can range from a mild, self-limited disease to potentially life-threatening airway obstruction. The various upper airway infections can pose significant diagnostic and therapeutic challenges because they present with similar symptoms but require vastly different medical management. As with many infections, the primary challenge with pediatric upper airway infections lies in identifying the causative pathogen and determining the extent of disease progression. Because of these challenges, a working diagnosis is frequently used when making treatment decisions until a definitive diagnosis is made. Clinical teams caring for children need to be aware of the clinical presentation of the various pediatric upper respiratory infections (Box 16-1) because prompt recognition and early and appropriate treatment save lives (2). The involvement of RTs is typically not necessary for retropharyngeal and peritonsillar abscesses; infectious mononucleosis does not typically require hospitalization and respiratory stabilization; and diphtheria is rarely found in developed countries. Therefore, this chapter will focus on epiglottitis, croup, and bacterial tracheitis.

A well-trained clinician can frequently make an upper airway diagnosis based solely on history and physical examination, using radiographs and laboratory examinations to aid in diagnosis when the clinical picture is unclear. In some cases, airway collapse is imminent, and clinicians must bypass these noninvasive diagnostic techniques and proceed directly to **endoscopy**, a procedure in which a camera is used on the end of a flexible tube inserted into the body for definitive diagnosis and airway protection (3). A summary of important clinical distinguishing features between croup, epiglottitis, and bacterial tracheitis can be found in Table 16-1.

Box 16-1   Infectious Causes of Acute Upper Airway Obstruction in Children

Epiglottitis (supraglottitis)
Croup (laryngotracheobronchitis)
Bacterial tracheitis
Retropharyngeal abscess
Peritonsillar abscess
Laryngeal diphtheria
Infectious mononucleosis

Table 16-2	Clinical Features of Acute Infectious Upper Airway Obstruction		
Clinical Features	**Croup**	**Epiglottitis**	**Bacterial Tracheitis**
Onset	Gradual viral symptoms 1–7 days	Rapid onset 6–12 hours	Viral symptoms followed by rapid deterioration
Typical age at onset	6 months to 3 years	2–7 years	6 months to 8 years
Seasonal occurrence	Late fall to winter	Throughout the year	Fall to winter
Causative agents	Parainfluenza RSV Adenovirus Influenza A & B	Hib (typically) S. pneumoniae S. aureus K. pneumoniae H. parainfluenzae Beta-hemolytic streptococci (groups A, B, C, and F)	S. aureus H. influenzae M. catarrhalis S. pneumoniae
Pathology	Subglottic edema	Inflammatory edema of supraglottis	Thick, mucopurulent membranous tracheal secretions
Radiographic findings	Subglottic narrowing on AP view; steeple sign	Thickening, rounding of epiglottis; thumb sign	Subglottic narrowing on AP view; hazy irregular soft tissue densities; pneumonia
Fever	Low grade	High fever	High fever
Cough	Barking or seal-like	None	Present
Sore throat	None	Severe	None
Drooling	None	Frequent	None
Posture	Any position	Sitting forward, mouth open, neck extended (tripod position)	Any position
Voice	Normal or hoarse	Muffled	Normal or hoarse
Appearance	Nontoxic	Toxic	Toxic

Epiglottitis

■■ During your examination of Timmy's chest, you discover moderate intercostal retractions and occasional use of accessory muscles during respiration. You listen to breath sounds and hear poor aeration throughout the lungs, which sound mostly clear with the occasional rhonchi. Timmy is anxious and prefers sitting upright, in a forward position with his mouth open. He complains of a bad sore throat. You place him on a 100% non-rebreather mask and go to find the physician.

Epiglottitis, also known as supraglottitis, is a bacterial infection of the epiglottis and the surrounding tissues, including the entire **supraglottic larynx** (the portion of the larynx above the vocal cords), which can progress rapidly to life-threatening airway obstruction (4). This includes the **aryepiglottic folds**, which are prominent folds of mucous membranes stretching between the lateral margin of the epiglottis and the arytenoid cartilage, which are also

affected (Fig. 16-1). The tightly bound epithelium at the level of the vocal cords greatly limits the inflammatory edema, such that the vocal cords and **subglottic airway** (the lower part of the larynx just below the vocal cords down to the top of the trachea) are usually normal in appearance. This is why the term *supraglottitis* is often interchanged with *epiglottitis*, because the supraglottic structures are mostly affected (4). As the supraglottic edema increases, the epiglottis is forced posteriorly, causing progressive airway obstruction (3) (Evidence in Practice 16-1).

Epiglottitis typically affects children between 2 and 5 years old, although a recent 10-year retrospective review suggests that older children are now more commonly affected (2). The study found that the mean age of affected children was 5.8 years from 1992 to 1997, whereas the mean age was 11.6 years from 1998 to 2002 (2).

Pathophysiology

Historically, *Haemophilus influenzae* **type b (Hib)** was the most common cause of epiglottitis. Despite the widespread use of Hib vaccination (given in

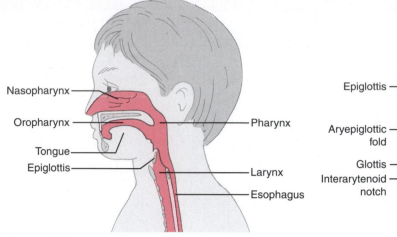

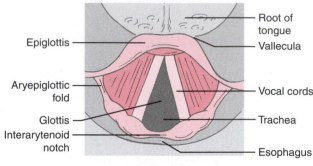

Figure 16-1 Upper Airway Anatomical Structures

● **Evidence in Practice 16-1**

George Washington—Epiglottitis

Perhaps the most famous case of epiglottitis involved the first president of the United States. George Washington is widely believed to have died of epiglottitis during the influenza epidemic of 1799. One early December morning, George Washington awoke with a severe sore throat. Throughout the day, his condition rapidly deteriorated as he developed difficulty in swallowing, a muffled voice, and persistent restlessness. Although a tracheotomy was suggested by one of his physicians, the procedure was not well practiced at the time, and a series of bloodlettings was performed instead. He died less than 24 hours from the onset of his symptoms (5). If tracheotomy had been more common during this time, perhaps George Washington's life could have been saved.

---

infancy through 18 months), a number of cases of Hib-related epiglottitis are still reported in both immunized and nonimmunized children. For these reasons, an up-to-date immunization history should not exclude the possibility of epiglottitis in a child with a clinically consistent presentation (4). Infectious pathogens associated with epiglottitis in the postvaccination era include the following:

- Group A *Streptococcus pneumoniae*
- *Staphylococcus aureus*
- *Klebsiella pneumoniae*
- *Haemophilus parainfluenzae*
- Beta-hemolytic streptococci (groups A, B, C, and F).

Candidal and viral infections (herpes simplex type 1, varicella-zoster, and parainfluenza) have also

been implicated, particularly in **immunocompromised** patients (such as patients with cancer or who have had an organ transplant) (6).

Noninfectious causes such as direct trauma and thermal injury may also lead to swelling of the epiglottis. Injury to the epiglottis secondary to ingestion of hot foods or liquids, caustic agents like the chemical sulfuric acid, foreign bodies, smoke inhalation, **angiodema** (an allergic reaction that causes rapid swelling just below the skin, typically found around the lips and eyes), and sidestream exposure to "crack" cocaine have been reported in children and adults. All of these clinical entities often present with symptoms and radiographic findings similar to those of acute infectious epiglottitis (6).

Clinical Manifestations

In light of the now-infrequent nature of childhood epiglottitis and the potential for rapid clinical deterioration, the diagnosis of this condition requires a high index of suspicion and careful attention to the subtle clues in the patient's history and physical examination.

Subjective Clinical Signs

Affected children typically present with rapidly progressive signs and symptoms (Box 16-2). Characteristically, the children appear toxic, assuming an upright sitting position with the chin up and mouth open, bracing themselves on their hands. This classic position is known as the tripod position and allows for maximal air entry (3). Patients often have difficulty in managing their secretions because of painful and difficult swallowing, also known as **dysphagia**. Due to the dysphagia, **drooling** occurs, which is a classic sign of epiglottitis. Dysphagia and drooling are just two of the "4 Ds" that can be associated with epiglottitis (Box 16-3). Dyspnea, or difficulty

- Severe throat pain
- Fever
- Irritability
- Drooling

breathing, is a chief complaint of patients with epiglottis. Speech is limited because it is painful, and **dysphonia** or disorders of the voice can occur. The voice tends to be muffled rather than hoarse (as in children with croup; discussed later in this chapter). Stridor is a late finding and signals near-complete airway obstruction.

Children with epiglottitis are usually anxious, which is a strong indication that their airway is significantly compromised and may, in fact, worsen the degree of upper airway obstruction.

Past and Recent Medical History

Secondary sites of infection are present 50% of the time, including meningitis (inflammation of the spinal cord and brain), otitis media (middle-ear infection), pneumonia, and cellulitis (infection of the skin) (3).

Laboratory Test Results

Patients with epiglottitis have elevated leukocyte white blood cell (WBCs) counts and frequently have positive blood cultures for the bacterial pathogen (4).

Airway and Respiratory Symptoms

The definitive diagnosis of epiglottitis requires direct visualization of a red swollen epiglottis under laryngoscopy (4). Because of the higher likelihood of airway obstruction in children, in patients who exhibit a significantly compromised airway, direct examination of the epiglottis should be attempted only in an interdisciplinary collaboration with an anesthesiologist and an otolaryngologist in a controlled setting, such as an operating room (OR), which allows for the establishment of an artificial airway (4). The child should be attended at all times by someone

capable of obtaining an airway, and any anxiety-provoking maneuvers such as phlebotomy and radiographs should be avoided until an airway has been established. Also, in patients who have mild-to-moderate respiratory distress or in older, cooperative patients, the classic cherry red epiglottis may be visualized with gentle compression of the anterior portion of the tongue with a tongue depressor (Fig. 16-2A). In these patients, radiological examination can confirm the diagnosis and rule out foreign body, retropharyngeal abscess (the collection of pus in the back of the throat), or croup. Lateral neck radiographs taken with hyperextension of the neck are the single most-useful study and may demonstrate the classic thumb sign, indicative of the thickening and rounding of the epiglottis (Fig.16-2B). It should be noted, however, that with this practice, rapid respiratory compromise may develop in a delayed manner, necessitating emergency airway intervention (6).

Drooling
Dysphagia
Dyspnea
Dysphonia

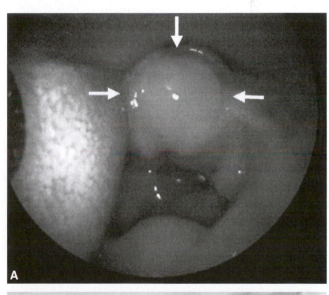

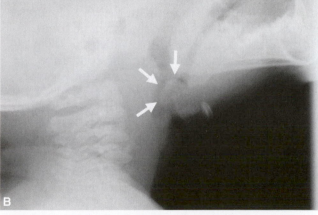

Figure 16-2 Neck Radiograph (A) and Endoscopic View (B) of Epiglottis *(Source: International Journal of Pediatric Otorhinolaryngology,* with permission*)*

■■ Upon the resident taking the history and completing the physical examination, you learn that Timmy was seen by his pediatrician 3 days ago and is currently being treated for an otitis media with amoxicillin. The physician asks Timmy's mom if he is up to date with his immunizations, and she says he has not gotten all of his Hib vaccines owing to a national shortage. Timmy begins to drool and is starting to have stridor on inspiration. You pull the physician aside and say, "I am worried about being able to maintain Timmy's airway, and I think we should get the attending physician involved in his care. Now that he is drooling, I am concerned about epiglottitis, which is an airway emergency" (Teamwork 16-1). Based on what you both have just learned in Timmy's history and physical examination, the resident agrees, and you get the attending physician while he stays with the Timmy to monitor his airway.

Management and Treatment

The typical management of epiglottitis includes rapid airway stabilization, treatment of hypoxemia, and the administration of pharmacological interventions aimed at minimizing airway edema.

Oxygen Therapy

Oxygen is a supportive therapy used to treat hypoxemia in these patients while assessing and stabilizing the patient's airway.

Airway Stabilization and Management

When epiglottitis is suspected, immediate coordinated care should be arranged between otolaryngology, anesthesiology, critical care intensivists, and RTs to protect the patient from complete airway obstruction. It is important for RTs to aid in looking for the early warning signs of **respiratory distress** and airway obstruction. A good therapist can aid the physicians in their diagnosis by recognizing the clinical signs and symptoms of epiglottitis and voicing their concerns regarding proper airway management to the physician.

Patients for whom epiglottitis is suspected should be expeditiously transported to the OR to secure an airway. In the OR, all emergency airway equipment should be available and set up in advance, including the following:

- Oral airways
- Laryngoscopes
- Rigid bronchoscope (a hollow stainless steel scope used to visualize the airway and typically remove foreign bodies or dilate the airway and place stents)
- Flexible bronchoscope (a longer and thinner scope than the rigid bronchoscope that tends to be preferred because of its smaller size and ability to navigate into individual lobes or bronchi of the lung, and because it causes less discomfort to the patient)
- Instruments for **cricothyroidotomy/tracheotomy**

 Teamwork 16-1 Hint and Hope

As an RT, it is important to use your airway and respiratory assessment skills and be able to communicate your thoughts on management and treatment to the rest of the healthcare team. For example, in the case of Timmy Jones, the RT continually assessed and monitored Timmy's airway status. When the RT was concerned, she voiced her specific concern to the physician who was focused on obtaining the history and physical information from Timmy's mom. Often, when team members feel they need to challenge the patient assessment or decisions of clinicians in authority, rather than clearly voicing their concerns they drop hints in the hope that the leader will arrive at a similar conclusion. Nonspecific responses such as "Timmy doesn't look very good" or "I don't think that's right," are not useful when timely care is necessary. In this case, it was the prioritization of the physician in the face of rapidly declining airway stability that the RT felt needed to improve. The RT gained the attention of the resident by saying "I am worried about being able to maintain Timmy's airway, and I think we should get the attending physician involved his care. Now that he is drooling, I am concerned about epiglottitis, which is an airway emergency."

It is important to remember that physicians and nurses, as well as other health-care providers, have many different things they are assessing and monitoring, whereas the RT's primary responsibility is airway stability and respiratory status. The RT is the ideal person to focus on assessing and managing the patient's airway. When RTs are concerned, they need to clearly voice their concerns in an appropriate way to the other members of the health-care team to ensure the best possible care and outcomes for their patients.

It is preferable for the patient to maintain spontaneous ventilation if possible.

Once the patient is anesthetized, the supraglottic structures are visualized. The typical examination reveals redness and edema of the supraglottis, including the epiglottis, aryepiglottic folds, and arytenoids (3). An abscess is sometimes present, and landmarks are frequently obscured. Oral intubation should be attempted at this time. After oral intubation, specimens should be obtained from the epiglottis and sent for identification and sensitivity. Before concluding the procedure, the oral tube should be changed to a nasotracheal tube. Historically, patients underwent tracheotomy when diagnosed with epiglottitis; nasotracheal intubation is now preferred (3).

If oral intubation is not successful, a surgical airway with cricothyroidotomy or tracheotomy is performed.

In older children and adults who do not have respiratory distress and have at least a 50% laryngeal lumen as seen with flexible laryngoscopy, it is reasonable to forgo intubation and monitor the patient closely (5). All patients who have epiglottitis should be admitted to the intensive care unit (ICU) for observation and definitive treatment. Emergency intubation equipment should be kept at the bedside in the ICU, and personnel trained in difficult airways should be on standby in case artificial airway management is necessary.

Intensive Care Unit Management

Once the artificial airway is secure, the patient is transferred to the ICU for observation and definitive treatment. Typically, these patients do not have lung disease and therefore do not need high ventilator settings to maintain normal blood gases. The role of the RT is to place the patient on normal rest settings on the ventilator, assess blood gases periodically per physician order, and assess for a leak around the airway, at minimum twice per 12-hour shift. Generally, symptomatic improvement and the development of an audible air leak around the tracheal tube occur within 24 to 48 hours (4).

Antimicrobial Therapy

Blood may be drawn and sent for a complete blood cell (CBC) count and blood cultures. Elevated WBC counts are frequently present, but positive blood culture results are extremely variable (6). Broad-spectrum antibiotic coverage is started in the ICU; ceftriaxone, cefuroxime, and ampicillin-sulbactam are the preferred antibiotics. Adjustments in antibiotic coverage are made as necessary for culture and sensitivity results. The duration of drug therapy is determined by the clinical response.

Corticosteroids

Steroids are also commonly used to decrease the mucosal edema of the epiglottis, but no data exist in the literature to prove any benefit from their use (6).

Extubation

Generally, an audible air leak around the tracheal tube usually occurs within 24 to 48 hours, and the patient can be extubated (2). Once extubated, the patient should be placed on standard oxygen therapy, the airway should still be monitored closely, and all emergency airway equipment should remain at the bedside so that health-care providers are prepared for emergent reintubation if necessary (2). Patients with epiglottitis have a significant chance of decompensation after extubation owing to the inflammation and edema that may still be present in the airway, so being prepared for reintubation is an important management strategy.

■ ■ The attending physician agrees with you and the resident in regard to Timmy's deteriorating condition and marked respiratory distress. He suspects Timmy may have epiglottitis and pages the ear, nose, throat (ENT) specialist and anesthesia provider. Timmy is rushed to the OR where he is nasally intubated using a fiber-optic bronchoscope. After establishing an artificial airway, Timmy is admitted to the pediatric intensive care unit (PICU) for intravenous (IV) antibiotics, corticosteroids, and monitoring.

Course and Prognosis

Historically, Hib was once a major cause of morbidity and mortality in children aged 2 to 7 years (2). The overall incidence of epiglottitis has decreased significantly since the introduction of the conjugated Hib vaccine in 1988 and its widespread use by 1995 (6). The Hib vaccine is recommended at age 2 months, 4 months, 6 months (depending on the brand), and 12 to 15 months. By 1996, the incidence of invasive Hib disease among children younger than 5 years declined by more than 99% (6).

A 2010 study looking specifically at an 8-year (1998 to 2006) retrospective review of epiglottitis admissions in the United States revealed the absolute number of cases has decreased. In this study, looking at pediatric patients (less than 18 years of age), Shah and Stocks found there was a trend toward more children less than 1 year of age being admitted with epiglottitis. In 1998, 26.8% were less than 1 year of age compared with 41.1% of patients found in 2006 (7). Among pediatric patients, for the entire study period, 34.4% of this group was less than 1 year of age. Across all ages, this study showed that there are

Adult Epiglottitis

The clinical presentation of childhood epiglottitis differs from that of adults. Adults tend to have a more gradual course, are less likely to present with airway compromise, and frequently have symptoms that are limited to sore throat and painful swallowing (3).

less-frequent admissions in the less than 18-year-old cohort, with an increase in the age groups of 45- to 64-year-old patients and patients greater than 85 years of age (7) (Clinical Variations 16-1). The findings of this study suggest patients less than 1 year of age are still plagued by this illness more than other pediatric patients owing to the small anatomy of the infant airway. As a result of the Hib vaccine, there has been an epidemiological shift in epiglottitis in that there are fewer cases of pediatric epiglottitis but an increase in adult epiglottitis. Studies from other countries have correlated a decrease in the spectrum of Hib infections, which has led to the emergence of other causative organisms (7).

Because epiglottitis usually has an acute onset and is not seen with the frequency it once was, it is possible that pediatric teams have minimal real-life experience with this disorder. For that reason, a high index of suspicion needs to occur in patients presenting with the rapid onset of signs and symptoms consistent with epiglottitis. Patients who are admitted to the ICU for close observation and/or intubated quickly to protect the airway and treated with IV antibiotics and steroids have an excellent prognosis with no long-term complications and are typically discharged within a week of onset.

Croup

Laryngotracheobronchitis (commonly known as **croup**) is a viral-mediated inflammatory condition of the subglottic airway, which corresponds to the area between the true vocal folds and the trachea. This is the narrowest point of the pediatric airway and the most common site of inflammatory conditions causing clinically significant airway obstruction in children (6). Croup is the most common childhood upper airway disorder and typically affects children between the ages of 6 months and 3 years, with a peak incidence of 60 cases per 1,000 children aged 1 to 2 years (8). Croup has a peak incidence in early fall and winter but can be seen throughout the year. The incidence of croup is 1.4 to 2 times higher in boys than in girls (9). This inflammatory disorder is characterized by a distinctive barking cough that is usually accompanied by stridor, hoarse voice, and respiratory distress (10).

Pathophysiology

The narrowest portion of the pediatric airway is at the level of the cricoid cartilage, termed the subglottis, just below the vocal cords. This anatomical feature makes children more susceptible than adults to airway obstruction from infectious diseases such as croup. Poiseuille's law tells us that airway resistance is inversely proportional to the fourth power of the radius of the airway. The equation is:

$$V \text{ (Flow)} = (\Delta P \, \pi \, r^4)/(8 \, n \, L),$$

in which V is flow, ΔP is the pressure gradient between the two ends of a tube (airway), r is the radius, n is the viscosity of the medium, and L is the length. Considering that the change in airway flow is directly proportional to the airway radius elevated to the fourth power, an airway with a diameter of 7 mm that develops a 0.5-mm edema will have a flow of 54% of baseline, assuming pressure remains unchanged (11). This means that even small reductions in the radius of the airway because of inflammation or edema can exponentially increase airway resistance and work of breathing (WOB) (9).

The most-frequent etiological agents associated with croup are as follows:

• Parainfluenza viruses (types I, II, III)
• Respiratory syncytial virus (RSV)
• Influenza viruses A and B
• Adenovirus

Parainfluenza I, II, and III account for up to 80% of all croup cases. Parainfluenza I is the etiological agent in 50% to 75% of patients who are hospitalized for croup (6). Influenza-mediated croup is associated with a more severe disease compared with parainfluenza. Other reported etiologies include *Mycoplasma pneumoniae*, herpes simplex type I, measles, and varicella (9). Human metapneumovirus and human coronavirus NL63 are two newly described pathogens that are strongly associated with croup in children (12).

Clinical Manifestations

Patients with croup typically present with a hoarse voice, a harsh barking cough often described as sounding similar to a seal, a low-grade fever, and variable degrees of stridor and respiratory distress. These symptoms tend to be worse at night and with agitation (Clinical Variations 16-2).

Past Medical History

In contrast to epiglottitis, children with croup usually present with a 1- to 3-day history of upper respiratory symptoms that may or may not include a fever. These patients do not typically present with the same life-threatening appearance characteristic of epiglottitis.

Spasmodic Croup

Spasmodic croup is a term that describes a condition clinically similar to croup. Patients with spasmodic croup typically have a barking cough with stridor, but lack a fever and a history of viral illness. Onset tends to be sudden and usually occurs at night. Episodes are frequently recurrent and resolve within hours, either spontaneously or with cool, humidified air. The precise pathogenesis of spasmodic croup is unknown, although it is thought to be allergic as opposed to infectious (11). Treatment for severe forms of spasmodic croup is the same as for viral croup (11).

Respiratory Distress

Depending on the degree of inflammation and subglottic narrowing, each child will develop varying degrees of respiratory distress (13).

The symptoms of croup can be classified as mild, moderate, or severe. The **Westley croup score** is a tool commonly used to characterize the severity of respiratory impairment in children with croup (Table 16-2). It takes into consideration the more common symptoms of the following:

- Stridor
- Chest retractions
- Air entry
- Cyanosis
- Level of consciousness (13)

Children with Westley croup scores of 1 to 3 are considered to have mild respiratory distress and croup. Those with scores of 3 to 8 are in moderate respiratory distress and therefore are considered to have moderated croup. Children with scores greater than 8 are considered to have severe croup (13).

Children with mild croup tend to have inflammation limited to the larynx and upon examination are found to have symptoms of hoarseness, intermittent barky cough, and inspiratory stridor that may be noticeable only with agitation. More severe cases of croup are associated with the extension of the inflammation to the trachea and bronchi and present with inspiratory stridor that is audible at rest and possibly biphasic (inspiratory and expiratory) stridor, suggesting a more severe fixed airway obstruction. Tachypnea, nasal flaring and intercostal retractions, hypoxia, or desaturation are often ominous signs associated with croup and indicate worsening obstruction and impending respiratory failure (9).

The subtle onset and clinical presentation of croup readily distinguish it from epiglottitis, and, in most instances, little confusion exists between them. In fact, only 2% of patients initially diagnosed with croup are given an incorrect diagnosis (11).

Laboratory and Diagnostic Procedures

Radiographic examination of the soft tissues of the neck may help establish the diagnosis of croup, while ruling out other important conditions such as epiglottitis, congenital abnormalities, foreign body, or retropharyngeal abscess. The anterior to posterior (AP) soft tissue neck film typically shows narrowing of the subglottic area or the steeple sign (3) (Fig. 16-3). Lateral neck films may show haziness in the subglottis and normal supraglottic structures in contrast to the findings present with epiglottitis. Radiographic findings may be absent in as many as 50% of the patients with croup, and the diagnosis is made frequently based on the history and physical examination alone (3).

Table 16-2	The Westley Croup Scoring Tool (5)	
Symptom	**Score**	
Stridor	None	0
	When agitated	1
	At rest with stethoscope	2
	At rest without stethoscope	3
Retractions	None	0
	Mild	1
	Moderate	2
	Severe	3
Air entry	Normal	0
	Decreased	1
	Markedly decreased	2
Cyanosis in room air	None	0
	With agitation	4
	At rest	5
Level of consciousness	Normal	0
	Disoriented	5
Total Score	**0–17**	

Management and Treatment

Less than 10% of croup patients require hospitalization, and management is largely dependent on the severity of symptoms (11). Croup is usually self-limited and frequently requires only supportive care. Oxygen therapy is typically the first treatment option, followed by inhaled racemic epinephrine and possibly corticosteroid administration. In some cases of severe croup in which stridor is still present, heliox therapy may be used, and in some rare cases for which supportive therapy is not successful, intubation is required to stabilize the patient's airway.

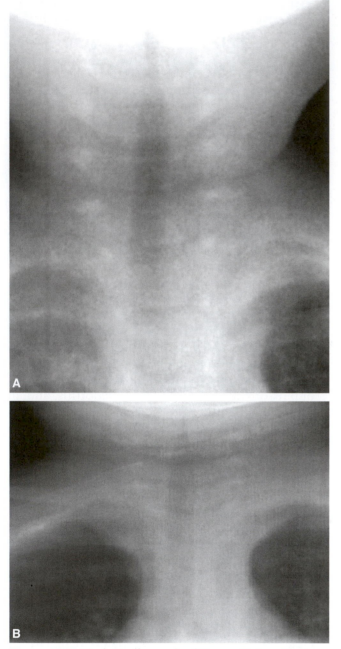

Figure 16-3 Neck Radiograph of Croup Taken During Inspiration (A) and Exhalation (B) *(Courtesy of Jane Benson, MD)*

Oxygen Therapy

Traditionally, croup has been treated with humidified air, as either heated or cool mist. The presumed effect is to soothe the inflamed mucosa, decrease coughing due to irritation, and liquefy secretions, making them easier to expectorate. Unfortunately, no scientific evidence exists to support the theory that humidified air has any effect on subglottic mucosa or that it positively influences patient outcome. Furthermore, mist tents can increase respiratory distress by provoking anxiety because of separation from the parents and may lessen the ability to effectively monitor the patient because of the thick mist; blow-by humidification and oxygen (when the patient is hypoxemic) is thus preferred (3).

Inhaled Medications

The use of nebulized racemic epinephrine has been well established as an effective, albeit temporary, means of relieving upper airway obstruction by local vasoconstriction and decreasing the mucosal edema (4). Racemic epinephrine has been available in the United States since 1971. The alpha-adrenergic effect on mucosal vasculature is highly effective in reducing airway edema (3). Due to the potential for side effects, including agitation, tachycardia, and hypertension, the use of racemic epinephrine is commonly reserved for patients who have moderate-to-severe respiratory distress per their Westley croup score (6). The most common pediatric dosage of nebulized racemic epinephrine is 2.25% (0.25 to 0.75 mL in 2 mL normal saline), with clinical effect lasting up to 1 to 2 hours (9).

Treatment with racemic epinephrine causes rapid improvement in clinical status (within 10 to 30 minutes) and appears to decrease the need for intubation (9). The effect, however, is transient because epinephrine has a short half-life and disappears within 2 hours of administration. A single dose may relieve the symptoms of some children in considerable distress, but others may need repeat doses.

In the past, children treated with racemic epinephrine have been hospitalized for observation because of the potential for rebound edema, which refers to tracheal edema that returns to baseline after 1 to 2 hours of administration of racemic epinephrine (9). Recent studies, however, suggest that these patients may be safely discharged after a 3- to 4-hour observation period, provided that they are stridor free and show no signs of respiratory distress and that the parents can provide reliable monitoring and return to the hospital if necessary (11).

Corticosteroids

Because of their significant anti-inflammatory effects, corticosteroids are commonly prescribed for the treatment of croup. They can be administered by way of nebulization or via oral or IV routes. Although the exact mechanism of action for corticosteroids is unclear, they have been shown to reduce submucosal edema and decrease the inflammatory reaction (3). In general, because the result of steroid administration will not be appreciated for at least 3 hours, they are usually administered with racemic epinephrine (3).

There has been much debate over the past several years about the efficacy of corticosteroids in the treatment of croup. Several studies have shown substantial improvement in children with severe croup treated with corticosteroids regardless of their route of administration (14). For example, a recent review by the Cochrane Collaboration looked at 38 studies in which glucocorticoids were administered for croup. The review showed that patients who received glucocorticoids had a significantly improved Westley croup score at 6 hours and at 12 hours. It also showed a decrease in return visits and/or readmission, a reduced length of time in the ED or hospital, and a decrease in the use of racemic epinephrine. These benefits occurred in children with mild-to-moderate and moderate-to-severe croup. There was a fivefold decrease in the rate of intubation in children with severe croup, and children already intubated spent one-third less time on the ventilator (14). Dexamethasone is the most commonly used corticosteroid for the treatment of croup (9). Both oral and intramuscular dexamethasone are effective if comparable drug dosages are used.

When the routes of administration of steroids are compared, oral dosing has some advantages. It is easy to administer, is inexpensive, does not carry risks such as infection at the injection site, and does not cause pain and anxiety that may occur during intramuscular administration. The major disadvantage of oral use is the unpleasant taste of the drug. Unfortunately, it is often not tolerated well by younger children and can cause vomiting.

Over the years, studies have compared the effectiveness of nebulized budesonide and intramuscular dexamethasone. Budesonide is a synthetic corticosteroid with strong topical anti-inflammatory effects and low systemic activity and is commonly used for the treatment of croup in children (15). The onset of action of inhaled budesonide is more rapid than that of oral or IV dexamethasone. This may be attributed to the more direct delivery of nebulized budesonide to the inflamed, edematous subglottic area. The majority of recent studies found no statistically significant difference between oral dexamethasone and nebulized budesonide (10, 15).

Heliox Therapy

The administration of a mixture of helium and oxygen (heliox) can be of benefit in the treatment of selected patients with severe forms of croup. Heliox is a particularly attractive therapy in children with upper airway obstruction, where age and size-related differences in airway diameter can lead to more turbulent airflow than in adults with larger airways. When turbulent airflow is combined with narrowed airways, inefficient gas exchange may occur.

Helium has a density approximately one-seventh that of air (16). By using helium in patients with upper airway obstructions, this turbulent airflow is converted to a more laminar flow, therefore bypassing any obstructions and decreasing airway resistance. It is important for RTs and other clinicians to understand that, in patients with narrowed airways owing to inflammation and edema, the lower density of heliox acts as a carrier gas through the airways that allows increased delivery of oxygen and medication while potentially decreasing WOB and improving gas exchange.

When used medically, helium is delivered in a mixture containing between 20% and 40% oxygen. This replicates the nitrogen-oxygen ratio in room air but substitutes nitrogen with helium. It is important to note that for heliox to be effective, the mixture should contain only oxygen and helium. Helium is manufactured in H cylinders and can be mixed as 80:20, 70:30, or 75:25 helium-to-oxygen mixtures. To ensure there is no room air/nitrogen entrained into the heliox mixture, heliox is delivered with a high-concentration oxygen device such as a non-rebreather mask or with high-flow devices such as an aerosol mask, but it can also be used with noninvasive bi-level positive airway pressure and in patients who are intubated and receiving mechanical ventilation (MV). To significantly lower the density of the inhaled gas, helium needs to comprise 60% to 80% of the mixture, which limits its usefulness in patients with a high oxygen requirement (fractional concentration of inspired oxygen [FIO_2] less than 0.40). Patients requiring less than 0.40 oxygen will not see the full benefit of heliox therapy.

Other limiting factors to delivering heliox are the expense and the complexity of the delivery setup. One H cylinder of heliox costs approximately $54, whereas an H cylinder of oxygen costs $18. Delivery of heliox requires a helium-oxygen regulator and an oxygen analyzer as well. When comparing cost, delivering heliox is three times as expensive as oxygen.

In a 2010 Cochrane review of heliox administration for croup in children, 45 trial reports were identified, with only two randomized controlled trials meeting eligibility criteria (17). One study compared heliox with 30% humidified oxygen, whereas the other study compared heliox with 100% oxygen with additional racemic epinephrine nebulization. Both trials found a greater improvement in croup score in the helium-oxygen group, although this change was not statistically significant (17). As a management strategy for patients with croup, heliox serves as more of a therapeutic bridge because it does not decrease airway inflammation or edema. Heliox can reduce WOB enough to prevent intubation and allow steroids and other medications to reach therapeutic peak (16).

Airway Management

In patients with severe forms of croup that do not respond to supportive treatment such as nebulized epinephrine, corticosteroids, and heliox, endotracheal intubation and MV may be necessary. In these cases, it is recommended that a smaller than normal endotracheal tube (ETT) be used. Extubation can usually be accomplished within 2 to 3 days, when an air leak around the ETT can be detected.

Course and Prognosis

Since the early 1900s, advances in management of croup have transformed this condition from a deadly upper airway disease to a relatively benign self-limited condition (6). Most patients with croup can be treated in the primary care or ED setting using supportive treatment. For patients in an outpatient setting who have severe symptoms that do not resolve over 2 to 4 hours with corticosteroids and racemic epinephrine, admission to the ICU and treatment with heliox, it may be necessary to use IV antibiotics and intubation. Mortality from croup in intubated patients is rare, with rates reported as low as 0.5% (13).

It is common for a child with a croup diagnosis to have recurring croup after the initial bout. Up to 5% of children may have more than one episode. Patients who are younger than 6 months when they first present with croup, those who have an unusually long duration of symptoms (greater than 1 week), those who have unusually severe symptoms, and those who have recurrent croup should be evaluated for congenital or acquired airway narrowing (6). For patients with recurring symptoms, airway examination with endoscopy is indicated. Ideally, the examination is delayed for 3 to 4 weeks so that persistent inflammatory changes do not mask any anatomical abnormalities, such as subglottic stenosis.

Bacterial Tracheitis

Bacterial tracheitis, also known as bacterial laryngotracheobronchitis, **pseudomembranous croup**, or bacterial croup, was first described in detail by Jones and colleagues in 1979 (19). Although it is a rare disease, clinicians should consider the diagnosis in any child with respiratory distress. The peak incidence is in the fall and winter, affecting children from age 6 months to 8 years, with the average age of 5 years (3). Furthermore, in a study by Gallagher and Meyer, males were diagnosed with two times more frequency than females (20). Bacterial tracheitis is characterized by marked subglottic edema and thick mucus or pus-containing secretions (11).

Pathophysiology

In bacterial tracheitis, bacteria invade the trachea and stimulate both local and systemic inflammatory responses. This results in production of thick, **mucopurulent exudates** (secretions with a high concentration of mucus and pus), ulceration, and sloughing of the tracheal mucosa (21). This can result in a variable degree of upper airway obstruction. The severity of the upper airway obstruction depends on the location

Box 16-4	Common Pathogens Causing Bacterial Tracheitis (7,12)

- *Staphylococcus aureus*
- *Haemophilus influenzae*
- Alpha-hemolytic streptococcus
- *Streptococcus pneumonia*
- *Moraxella catarrhalis*
- *Streptococcus pneumoniae*

and extent of the damage to the tracheal mucosa, the patient's age and underlying medical condition, and the size of the airway (21).

The most common pathogen associated with bacterial tracheitis is *S. aureus,* although several others have been implicated (Box 16-4).

In one of the largest recent multicenter studies out of the United Kingdom and Australia, 34 pediatric patients with bacterial tracheitis were evaluated. In this series, *S. aureus* was the most common bacteria present, infecting 62% of the patients studied in the UK and 55% of the patients studied in Australia (22). Two patients were isolated for Hib. Eighty-five percent of the patients studied also had viral testing performed. Thirty-one percent of these patients had positive viral results, with 13.8% with influenza A, 6.9% with parainfluenza type I, 6.9% with parainfluenza type III, and 3.5% with adenovirus (22). This study illustrates that bacterial tracheitis often presents as a secondary illness following an acute respiratory viral infection. The viral illness is believed to cause transient alterations in the immune response that predisposes the patient to bacterial infection (21). This theory is strongly supported by the observation that bacterial tracheitis cases occur most often during the winter months when viral upper respiratory tract infections are more prevalent (21).

Clinical Manifestations

The clinical presentation of bacterial tracheitis has features of both epiglottitis and viral croup.

Patient History

Children with bacterial tracheitis typically present with a several-day history of upper respiratory symptoms such as a low-grade fever, cough, and stridor (similar to patients with croup) (10). Presentation for medical attention is often precipitated by an acute deterioration, when a patient develops a high fever, toxic appearance, and evidence of airway obstruction. These patients' infections are generally more toxic than those with croup.

Physical Examination

Other findings on physical examination include stridor, hoarseness, cough, and tachypnea (21). Unlike the classic description of children with epiglottitis, those with bacterial tracheitis have a substantial cough, appear comfortable when lying flat, and are usually able to swallow their oral secretions and therefore do not present with drooling (11, 21). Another important distinction between bacterial tracheitis and viral croup, the more commonly seen clinical presentation, is that there is poor response to the conventional medical therapy of croup, including the administration of racemic epinephrine and systemic corticosteroids (21).

Radiography

Radiographically, bacterial tracheitis may be indistinguishable from croup, with the AP chest radiograph frequently showing marked subglottic narrowing (steeple sign) (11). In some cases on lateral radiograph, the tracheal air column may appear diffusely hazy, with multiple luminal soft tissue irregularities indicative of pseudomembrane detachment from soft tissue (3). Many patients with bacterial tracheitis also present with pulmonary infiltrates on radiograph, suggesting a concurrent pneumonia-like illness. These patients typically have a more severe course of illness. Because radiological findings vary so much with bacterial tracheitis, there is no one clinical or radiographic feature capable of firmly making the diagnosis (3).

Laboratory Data

Results of laboratory investigations, including a CBC with differential counts and blood cultures, are generally nonspecific. **Leukocytosis** (increase in the number of white blood cells) may or may not be present; however, most cases do report an increase in immature cells on differential blood count (21). Blood cultures infrequently show positive identification of the responsible bacteria.

Bronchoscopy

Direct visualization and bronchoscopy are the most definitive ways to diagnose bacterial tracheitis. The typical bronchoscopic findings of bacterial tracheitis include a normal or only slightly inflamed epiglottis, prominent subglottic edema, ulcerations, and copious purulent secretions (8). These thick secretions can partially obstruct the trachea and main bronchi and should be removed with suction and sent for Gram stain, culture, and sensitivity to allow for targeted antibiotic therapy.

The diagnosis of bacterial tracheitis is most often made on the basis of the patient's history and results of the physical examination, combined with findings from laboratory and bronchoscopic examination (21).

Management and Treatment

Management and treatment of the patient with bacterial tracheitis aim to maintain a patent airway and also include administration of IV antibiotics and removal of secretions by endoscopy or ETT as necessary.

Antibiotics

Once a definitive diagnosis of bacterial tracheitis has been made, broad-spectrum IV antibiotics should be initiated. Antimicrobial agents should be targeted to the most frequent isolated organisms including

- *S. aureus*
- *Moraxella catarrhalis*
- *Streptococcus pneumoniae*
- *Haemophilus influenzae* (21)

Appropriate regimens include a semisynthetic penicillin such as nafcillin, with a third-generation cephalosporin agent such as ceftriaxone or cefotaxime for coverage of Gram-negative organisms as a first line of therapy. Cefuroxime and ampicillin-sulbactam have been used for initial therapy as well (3). If methicillin-resistant *S. aureus* (MRSA) is a concern at the admitting institution, coverage should be extended to cover this organism using vancomycin (21). Ultimately, antibiotic therapy should be dictated by the Gram stain, culture, and sensitivity results and should cover a 10- to 14-day course.

Corticosteroids

Traditionally, the management of bacterial tracheitis has included treatment with corticosteroids, based on the rationale that this reduces airway inflammation and edema. In the multicenter study out of the UK and Australia, 30 patients received systemic corticosteroids. There was no statistically significant difference in the duration of intubation or hospital stay between the group of patients who received corticosteroids and the group that did not (22). Unlike viral croup, there are currently no data to suggest that inhaled or systemic steroids provide any clinical benefit in the treatment of bacterial tracheitis (21).

Airway Management

Endotracheal intubation is frequently required for patients with bacterial tracheitis for stabilization of the airway, management of acute respiratory failure, or pulmonary toilet. The decision to intubate should be individualized and will depend on the severity of the upper airway obstruction as well as the likelihood of further deterioration while awaiting a clinical response to antibiotic therapy. If intubation is not successful, a tracheostomy may be necessary. In the acute setting, a needle cricothyrotomy (which involves passing a percutaneous over-the-needle catheter in the cricothyroid membrane to provide ventilation when conventional means have failed) would be the next emergency intervention. Clearance of airway secretions is more effective with an ETT in place because suctioning can be done frequently and aggressively, preventing occlusion of the airway by thick exudates (21). When intubation is indicated, the ETT selected needs to be a smaller size than normally chosen for the age to account for the airway inflammation present (21). Younger children are more likely to require intubation owing to the small size of their airway. The level of comfort of the attending physician and the availability of a skilled bronchoscopist also play a major role in the decision regarding intubation (21). Children managed without endotracheal intubation need close observation in a hospital with expertise in pediatric airway management (21).

Intubation is often required for 3 to 7 days, until the patient is afebrile, there is an air leak present around the ETT, and there is a decrease in the quantity and viscosity of secretions (3). Occasionally, additional endoscopy or bronchoscopy may be needed to remove pseudomembranous material. While patients are intubated, they will require basic rest settings on the mechanical ventilator to maintain adequate arterial blood gas results.

Children managed with bacterial tracheitis without endotracheal intubation need close observation in a tertiary care center and generally get admitted to the PICU for 48 to 72 hours for close monitoring. During their ICU admission, these children are typically maintained on IV antibiotics and basic oxygen therapy, if indicated. In a 2010 retrospective chart review out of Boston Children's Hospital, six patients ranging in age from 10 months to 16 years were admitted to the PICU and treated for bacterial tracheitis between January 2009 and March 2009 (23). All patients underwent urgent laryngoscopy and bronchoscopy for removal of mucopurulent secretions. All patients were treated with broad-spectrum IV antibiotics. None of the patients required urgent intubation, although one was kept on a ventilator for 48 hours until disease resolution was confirmed with laryngoscopy and bronchoscopy (23). No patients required tracheotomy, and there were no cardiopulmonary arrests. The mean hospital stay was 4.8 days, and all patients were transitioned to oral antibiotics for 10 to 14 days after discharge. This study showed that, although bacterial tracheitis is a potentially fatal illness, early identification and consistent, proactive treatment and management in a controlled operative environment might be able to decrease the rate of complications and the need for intubation in pediatric patients.

Course and Prognosis

The mortality rate due to bacterial tracheitis has decreased dramatically since the 1900s. In the early 20th century, the mortality rate was as high as 10% to 40% (21). This rate has declined slowly over time, and the most recent and largest case studies reported from 2004 to present show no mortality associated with the illness. The improvement in mortality rate likely is due to the early recognition and improved treatment of the infection with aggressive airway-clearance techniques and early initiation of broad-spectrum antibiotics (21). Full recovery with no long-term morbidity is expected in the vast majority of children with bacterial tracheitis, especially if there are no complications during the acute illness.

The most frequent complication associated with bacterial tracheitis is pneumonia. Other less common complications include acute respiratory distress syndrome (ARDS), septic shock, toxic shock syndrome, pulmonary edema, pneumothorax, and, rarely, cardiopulmonary arrest (21).

In a retrospective study out of Vermont Children's Hospital, between 1997 and 2006 there were 35 patients with potentially life-threatening upper airway infections admitted to the PICU with the diagnosis of epiglottitis (n = 2), viral croup (n = 16), and bacterial tracheitis (n = 17) (24). Twenty of these patients developed respiratory failure. Fifteen of these patients (75%) had bacterial tracheitis, three patients (15%) had viral croup, and two patients (10%) had epiglottitis (24). As shown by these data, bacterial tracheitis was the most common potentially life-threatening upper airway infection in children. Four patients developed ARDS, with two requiring high-frequency oscillatory ventilation. All four patients with ARDS developed multiple-organ dysfunction syndrome, but all patients in this study survived.

The increasing burden of serious MRSA infections and other bacterial "superbugs" may contribute to the changing epidemiology and degree of severity of this disease. Bacterial tracheitis should be considered as part of the differential diagnosis in all children who present with acute life-threatening upper respiratory infection. With early intervention and treatment, prognosis is good, with low rates of long-term morbidity.

■ ■ Timmy is monitored closely in the PICU, and within 48 hours of being intubated, he is responding to the antibiotics and steroids. He no longer has a fever and has developed an air leak around his nasal tracheal tube. Timmy is awake and anxious to be extubated. You speak with the PICU team, and they agree to extubate him. You gather all of the emergency airway equipment at the bedside just in case he needs to be reintubated. Timmy is extubated without difficulty and placed on 0.40 FIO_2 via aerosol face mask, and his SpO_2 is 99%. Within 2 hours, you are able to wean Timmy to room air. He is discharged from the hospital the following day.

■■ Critical Thinking Questions: Timmy Jones

1. If Timmy had presented to the ED with mild symptoms of upper airway obstruction and you were unsure of the diagnosis being epiglottitis, what could you have recommended to the physician instead of immediate airway protection?
2. If the ENT doctor and anesthesiologist were unable to intubate Timmy in the OR because of swelling and edema in the airway, what else could be done to protect his airway?
3. If Timmy did not show a quick response to the antibiotics and steroids, what would you expect to be true of his airway?
4. How do you think Timmy would have presented differently if he had viral croup instead of epiglottitis?
5. If Timmy had presented with a high fever and slight cough, but had no drooling and was comfortable lying down, what would you suspect his diagnosis to be?

▶● Case Studies and Critical Thinking Questions

Case 1: Ryan Smith

You are working as the floating RT in a small 250-bed community hospital. You are called to the ED to assess an 8-year-old boy, Ryan Smith. Ryan is a previously healthy little boy who is up-to-date with all of his immunizations. He presents today with a chief complaint of sore throat and fever of 103°F, which came about abruptly in the last 4 hours.

While taking the history and performing the physical examination, you learn that Ryan has had a history of runny nose and nasal congestion for the past 3 days. He has pharyngeal redness, and a rapid strep test is performed and comes back negative. A soft tissue neck radiograph is obtained that shows mild thickening of the epiglottis and aryepiglottic folds.

After 2 hours of observation in the ED, Ryan begins to have difficulty swallowing and develops drooling. He now has stridor, wheezing, and a muffled voice.

• What do you think is Ryan's primary diagnosis?
• What should the caregivers in the ED do to help treat Ryan?
• When the PICU transport team arrives, what should they do prior to transporting Ryan back to their facility?

Case 2: Jacob Davis

You are working as a pediatric RT in a large, 800-bed tertiary medical center and are assigned to the pediatric ED for your 12-hour shift. At approximately 0900, Jacob, a 3-year-old boy, presents to the ED with difficulty breathing. He has had a fever and runny nose for the past 2 days. Overnight he has had worsening respiratory distress and now has inspiratory stridor at rest.

Physical examination of Jacob reveals that he is alert, with stridor at rest. He is not drooling. His vital signs are as follows:

• RR of 60 breaths per minute
• SpO$_2$ 92% on room air
• HR of 140 bpm
• Temperature of 39.2°C (102.6°F)

His oropharyngeal examination is normal. His chest examination reveals mild intercostal and supraclavicular retractions with decreased air exchange. He is noted to have some cyanosis with agitation. The remainder of his examination is unremarkable.

• What do you suspect is Jacob's primary diagnosis?
• What is Jacob's Westley croup score?
• What treatment would you recommend for this patient?
• Is Jacob ready to be discharged to home?

Case 3: Stephanie Johnson

You are an RT in a 400-bed hospital covering the ED and part of the 12-bed ICU. You receive a page to the ED and respond to find a 9-year-old girl, Stephanie, who has presented to the ED in respiratory distress. Stephanie's vital signs are as follows:

• RR of 30 breaths/minute
• SpO$_2$ of 89% on room air
• HR of 120 bpm
• Temperature of 38.1°C (101.5°F)

On taking her history and performing a physical examination, you learn that Stephanie has had upper respiratory tract symptoms, a sore throat, a low-grade fever, and mild hoarseness for the past 3 days. Stephanie has mild-to-moderate respiratory distress and has inspiratory stridor and a nonproductive cough. She is found laying flat on the stretcher and has moderate substernal retractions. Over the next few hours, Stephanie's breathing becomes more labored, and her temperature rises to 39.4°C (103°F).

• What do you think is Stephanie's primary diagnosis?
• What do you think would be an appropriate way to diagnose Stephanie's illness?
• What would you recommend to treat Stephanie?

Multiple-Choice Questions

1. Which of the following is a classic radiographic finding of epiglottitis?
   a. Steeple sign
   b. Pneumonia
   c. Thumb sign
   d. Subglottic narrowing

2. Which two types of treatment listed below are appropriate for patients with croup?
   I. Antibiotics
   II. Corticosteroids
   III. Racemic epinephrine
   IV. Vasopressors
   a. I, II
   b. II, III
   c. III, IV
   d. II, IV

3. Which of the following clinical signs and symptoms is specific only to epiglottitis?
   a. Fever
   b. Barking cough
   c. Drooling
   d. Inspiratory stridor

4. Which of the three upper respiratory infections listed below presents with a history of upper respiratory symptoms for multiple days?
   a. Epiglottitis
   b. Croup
   c. Bacterial tracheitis
   d. Both b & c

5. Which of the following is not a microorganism that commonly causes bacterial tracheitis?
   a. *S. aureus*
   b. *M. catarrhalis*
   c. *S. pneumoniae*
   d. Respiratory syncytial virus

6. Which of the following is the tool used to make a definitive diagnosis for both epiglottitis and bacterial tracheitis?
   a. Endoscopy
   b. Radiography
   c. Blood culture
   d. Sputum culture

7. A pediatric patient presents to the ED with the following symptoms of croup: stridor at rest with auscultation, mild retractions, decreased air entry, no cyanosis, and a normal level of consciousness. What is the patient's Westley croup score?
   a. 6
   b. 4
   c. 2
   d. None of the above

8. Which of the following is not a clinical sign of croup on presentation?
   a. Severe toxicity
   b. Hoarseness
   c. Barking cough
   d. Inspiratory stridor

9. Which of the following is the most common complication found in patients with bacterial tracheitis?
   a. Cardiopulmonary arrest
   b. Pneumonia
   c. Toxic shock syndrome
   d. ARDS

10. Which of the following initiatives are most important in treatment and management of patients suspected of having epiglottitis?
    I. Minimize anxiety-producing procedures
    II. Endoscopy
    III. Blood cultures
    IV. Radiography
    a. I, II
    b. II, III
    c. II, IV
    d. All of the above

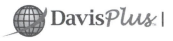

For additional resources login to Davis*Plus* (http://davisplus.fadavis.com/ keyword "Perretta") and click on the Premium tab. (Don't have a *Plus*Code to access Premium Resources? Just click the Purchase Access button on the book's Davis*Plus* page.)

REFERENCES

1. Baker MD, Ruddy RM. Pulmonary emergencies. In: Ludwig S, ed. *Textbook of Pediatric Emergency Medicine.* Philadelphia, PA: Lippincott Williams & Wilkins; 2000:1067-1086.
2. Wheeler DS, Dauplaise DJ, Giuliano JS Jr. An infant with fever and stridor. *Pediatr Emerg Care.* 2008;24(1):46-49.
3. Stroud RH, Friedman NR. An update on inflammatory disorders of the pediatric airway: epiglottitis, croup and tracheitis. *Am J Otolaryngol.* 2001;22(4):268-275.
4. Rafei K, Lichenstein R. Airway infectious disease emergencies. *Pediatr Clin North Am.* 2006;53:215-242.
5. Guardiani E, Bliss M, Harley E. Supraglottitis in the era following widespread immunization against *Haemophilus influenzae* type B: evolving principles in diagnosis and management. *Laryngoscope.* 2010;120(11):2183-2188.
6. Sobol SE, Zapata S. Epiglottitis and croup. *Otolaryngol Clin North Am.* 2008;41:551-566.
7. Shah R, Stocks C. Epiglottitis in the United States: national trends, variances, prognosis, and management. Laryngoscope. 2010;120(6):1256-1262.
8. Shah S, Sharieff GQ. Pediatric respiratory infections. *Emerg Med Clin North Am.* 2007;25:961-979.
9. Wald E. Croup: common syndromes and therapy. *Pediatr Ann.* 2010;39(1):15-21.
10. Rajapaksa S. Starr M. Croup—assessment and management. *Aust Fam Physician.* 2010;39(5):280-282.
11. Rotta AT, Wiryawan B. Respiratory emergencies in children. *Respir Care.* 2003;48(3):248-260.
12. van der Hoek L, Sure K, Ihorst G, et al. Human coronavirus NL63 infection is associated with croup. *Adv Exp Med Biol.* 2006;581:485-491.
13. Wright RB, Rowe BH, Arent RJ, Klassen TP. Current pharmacological options in the treatment of croup. *Expert Opin Pharmacother.* 2005;6(2):255-261.
14. Cetinkaya F, Tüfekci B, Kutluk G. A comparison of nebulized budesonide, and intramuscular, and oral dexamethasone for treatment of croup. *Int J Pediatr Otorhinolaryngol.* 2004;68(4):453-456.
15. Frazier MD, Cheifetz IM. The role of heliox in paediatric respiratory disease. *Paediatr Respir Rev.* 2010;11(1):46-53.
16. Vorwerk C, Coats T. Heliox for croup in children. *Cochrane Database Syst Rev.* 2010;(2):CD006822.
17. Russell KF, Liang Y, O'Gorman K, Johnson DW, Klassen TP. Glucocorticoids for croup. *Cochrane Database Syst Rev.* 2011;(1):CD001955.
18. Jones R, Santos JI, Overall JC Jr. Bacterial tracheitis. *JAMA.* 1979;242(8):721-726.
19. Gallagher PG, Myer CM III. An approach to the diagnosis and treatment of membranous laryngotracheobronchitis in infants and children. *Pediatr Emerg Care.* 1991;7(6): 337-342.
20. Al-Mutairi B, Kirk V. Bacterial tracheitis in children: approach to diagnosis and treatment. *Paediatr Child Health.* 2004;9(1):25-30.
21. Tebruegge M, Pantazidou A, Thorburn K, et al. Bacterial tracheitis: a multi-centre perspective. *Scand J Infect Dis.* 2009;41(8):548-557.
22. Shargorodsky J, Whittemore KR, Lee GS. Bacterial tracheitis: a therapeutic approach. *Laryngoscope.* 2010; 120(12):2498-2501.
23. Hopkins A, Lahiri T, Salerno R, Heath B. Changing epidemiology of life-threatening upper airway infections: the reemergence of bacterial tracheitis. *Pediatrics.* 2006;118(4):1418-1421.

Chapter 17

Neuromuscular Disorders

Sharon McGrath-Morrow, MD
Suzanne Preswitch, MD

Key Terms

Areflexia
Botulism
Demyelination
Duchenne's muscular dystrophy (DMD)
Flaccid paralysis
Gangliosides
Guillain-Barré syndrome (GBS)
Insufflation-exsufflation device
Limb-girdle muscular dystrophy (LGMD)
Maximum expiratory pressure (MEP)
Maximum inspiratory pressure (MIP)
Myasthenia gravis (MG)
Neuropathy
Paresis
Ptosis
Scoliosis
Spinal muscular atrophy (SMA)
Spirometry
Tetanus
Trismus

Chapter Outline cont.

Chapter Objectives

After reading this chapter, you will be able to:

1. Discuss the indications for noninvasive ventilation in a patient with a neuromuscular disorder.
2. Identify at least two common genetic diseases that cause neuromuscular weakness.
3. Identify the cause of hypoxia in a patient with an underlying neuromuscular disorder without underlying lung disease.
4. Determine when to use an insufflation-exsufflation device in a patient with a neuromuscular disorder.
5. Describe how spirometry, maximum inspiratory pressure, and maximum expiratory pressure can help predict risk of respiratory failure in a patient with a neuromuscular disorder.
6. Describe the significance of a bell-shaped chest radiograph in an infant who presents with hypotonia and hypoxia.
7. Explain the utility of an overnight sleep study in detecting early chronic respiratory failure in a patient with a neuromuscular disorder.
8. Describe different mucociliary clearance techniques and their importance in preventing the development of atelectasis and pneumonia in patients with neuromuscular weakness.

■■ William Stubbs

You are working in a small rural community hospital and covering the emergency department (ED), which is packed with children at the height of flu season. You are sent to assess a 15-year-old boy, William Stubbs. William came to the ED the previous evening, reporting that his hands and feet felt "weird." When questioned further, he reported that they felt numb and tingly. He reported no problems with swallowing. Yesterday, he had no cough, wheezing, or respiratory distress. His oxygen saturations were 98% on room air. He was seen by the ED physician and sent home with the diagnosis of "viral syndrome."

William's parents brought him back to the ED today because he is having difficulty walking, with persistent tingling. He has no significant past medical history. He has never had any operations nor been hospitalized. His only medications are multivitamins and occasional diphenhydramine for allergies. William's parents report that he had diarrhea about 1 week ago but was otherwise doing well.

William is anxious, and his respiratory rate (RR) is 35 breaths/min. His oxygen saturations are in the low 90s on room air. He is noted to have a frequent throat clearing. He has a weak cough. Arterial blood gas (ABG) test results show a pH of 7.40, with a $PaCO_2$ of 35 mm Hg and PaO_2 of 75 mm Hg. He is admitted to the inpatient unit for further observation and diagnostic workup.

Neuromuscular disorders are a diverse group of conditions that affect the function of voluntary skeletal muscles. Often, the presentation of acute illness can be mild. However, medical providers need to be aware that these conditions can often deteriorate, many times very quickly, and require immediate and definitive treatment.

Respiratory complications and ventilatory failure are frequently the major cause of morbidity and mortality in patients with a neuromuscular disorder. There are many different types of neuromuscular diseases that afflict the pediatric population. Some conditions are genetic (e.g., spinal muscular atrophy [SMA]), whereas others are acquired (e.g., tetanus). Some conditions are progressive with age (e.g., Duchenne's muscular dystrophy [DMD], limb-girdle muscular dystrophy [LGMD]), whereas others can be episodic (e.g., myasthenia gravis [MG]) or static (e.g., SMA). And some neuromuscular diseases can have an infectious or immune etiology (e.g., botulism, Guillain-Barré syndrome [GBS]). See Table 17-1 for an overview of the disorders discussed in this chapter.

Identification of respiratory abnormalities and the initiation of preventative therapies may help stabilize lung function or help slow lung decline in this vulnerable group of individuals. A decline in respiratory muscle function can lead to decreased tidal volume (V_T) values and ineffective cough (1). Therefore, objective measurements of lung function can be helpful in guiding the initiation of

Table 17-1	Overview of Neuromuscular Diseases			
Disorder	**Cause**	**Presentation**	**Treatment**	**Course**
Guillain-Barré syndrome	Atypical immune response after an infection (*C. jejuni*, cytomegalovirus, *M. pneumonia*, *H. influenzae*, and Epstein-Barr virus) Antiganglioside antibodies bind to peripheral nerves, causing impaired function.	Presents with weakness in both arms and legs, progressing to partial paralysis No previous significant history	Support ventilation Plasmapharesis Intravenous immunoglobulin (IVIG)	4 weeks
Myasthenia gravis	Autoimmune disorder - Congenital = genetic mutations - Neonatal = transplacental exchange of immunoglobulins - Juvenile = chronically produced serum antibodies	Fluctuating muscle weakness and fatigue; begins with ocular and facial weakness	Monitor respiratory failure; anticholinesterase therapy	May be chronic Neonatal resolves in 2-4 weeks
Tetanus	Neurotoxin from *C. tetani* spores that enter the body through a wound; incubation 3-21 days; tetanus toxin prevents inhibitory motor neurons	Trismus Hands clenched Feet dorsiflexed Full-body spasms Body rigidity	Support ventilation Pain management Cardiovascular support Intramuscular (IM) TIG Antibiotic	Low mortality Resolution Few long-term sequelae
Botulism	Bacterial—*C. botulinum*; progressive neuroparalytic disease; block acetylcholine transmission across neuromuscular junction Food-borne, wound, infant	Descending flaccid paralysis over hours or days Starts with constipation and difficulty swallowing, ptosis, loss of head control	Support ventilation Infant = BabyBIG Others = antitoxin Antibiotics	Low mortality No recurrence
Muscular dystrophy	Genetic disorder (males); progressive breakdown of muscle fibers	Gradual loss of skeletal and cardiac muscle strength; heart failure	Aggressive respiratory support - NIV during acute illness - Support respiratory failure - Treat sleep apnea	Survival to 18–21 years, longer with aggressive preventive strategies
Spinal muscular atrophy	- Genetic disorder - Lower motor neuron degeneration, caused by programmed cell death - Three types in childhood	Proximal bilateral muscle weakness, tongue fasciculations	Support respiratory failure (tracheostomy, mechanical ventilation)	Types I and II - die in childhood Type III lives to adulthood

adjuvant therapy in patients with neuromuscular disease.

The role of the respiratory therapist (RT) is of central importance in performing diagnostic testing, such as pulmonary function tests, and providing maintenance therapies, including airway clearance and respiratory support. Furthermore, the RT must be able to recognize acute changes in respiratory status and to quickly address respiratory decompensation when it occurs. The RT's responsibilities include the following:

- Spirometry
- Overnight sleep studies

- Pulmonary clearance techniques
- Noninvasive positive pressure ventilation (NIPPV)
- Acute and chronic mechanical ventilation (MV)

Standard **spirometry** may be used in the evaluation of lung volumes and ventilation in children and adolescents (Fig. 17-1) (Table 17-2). The inability to expire fully to residual volume (RV) because of respiratory muscle weakness may result in a decreased forced vital capacity (FVC) and a functional restrictive lung disease. These children have decreased pulmonary reserve and may be at increased risk for pulmonary decompensation, especially during respiratory illnesses. Minimally, an annual assessment of pulmonary function should be performed in children with neuromuscular disorders who are old enough to complete the maneuvers because these tests can provide valuable information about subtle progression of respiratory muscle weakness and episodic changes, even in the absence of clinical symptoms. Establishing baseline spirometry values by 6 years of age can allow for longitudinal assessment and early interventions when indicated. Measurements of **maximal inspiratory pressure (MIP)** and **maximal expiratory pressure (MEP)** are easily performed and can help assess respiratory muscle strength in children with a neuromuscular disorder. To perform MIP and MEP, the clinician uses a handheld device and has the patient breathe in quickly and out quickly and forcefully to residual volume.

With increasing age, respiratory failure is more common in individuals with progressive neuromuscular diseases (e.g., DMD). Individuals with DMD, for example, often develop compromised airway

Table 17-2	Select Lung Volumes and Spirometry Values
Lung Value	**Definition**
Total lung capacity	The maximum amount of gas able to be contained in the lungs
Tidal volume	The amount of gas inhaled and exhaled during normal resting breathing
Residual volume	The amount of gas remaining in the lungs after a complete exhalation
Forced vital capacity	The amount of air that can be forcefully exhaled after a maximum inspiration
Maximum inspiratory pressure	The pressure obtained when a patient quickly breathes in fully to total lung capacity
Maximum expiratory pressure	The pressure obtained when a patient breathes out quickly and forcefully to residual volume

tone, which can be associated with obstructive apneas and hypopneas during sleep (2, 3). Because symptoms of early respiratory failure can often be detected during sleep, an overnight polysomnography (sleep study) can be useful in diagnosing early signs of respiratory failure in patients with a neuromuscular disorder. Overnight polysomnography should be considered in any child with moderate-to-severe restrictive lung disease; however, the frequency at which sleep studies are needed depends on each patient's clinical condition.

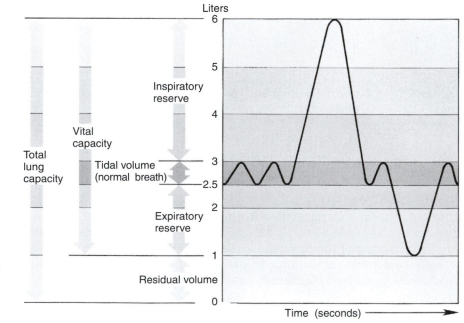

Figure 17-1 Pulmonary Volumes
(Taber's Cyclopedic Medical Dictionary. F.A. Davis, Philadelphia, 2009, p. 1937; with permission)

Individuals with neuromuscular disease should also be monitored for the development of **scoliosis**. Scoliosis is a lateral curvature of the spine and may accelerate decline in lung function by worsening lung restriction. Scoliosis should be followed and treated with appropriate therapies that may include the use of scoliosis vests, braces, or surgery. Therapies are usually determined by an orthopedic or rehabilitation physician. Treatments and interventions often depend on the severity and progression of the scoliosis.

Measures to improve pulmonary clearance and prevent atelectasis may be beneficial in patients with weak respiratory muscle strength. Such interventions may include the routine use of chest physiotherapy, flutter valve therapy, and insufflation-exsufflation devices (Table 17-3). **Insufflation-exsufflation devices** can help with airway clearance and prevent mucus accumulation in the lung and airways. These therapies help prevent the development of atelectasis in the lung. Manual or device-driven chest physiotherapy can help move secretions from distal to more proximal airways, allowing secretions to be easily removed by a patient's natural cough or by the cough-assist device.

In patients with symptoms of early respiratory failure, nighttime noninvasive positive pressure ventilation may improve long-term survival and increase quality of life. Patients with neuromuscular diseases can become sick quickly, so regimens should be increased during episodes of acute illness (4). Also, individuals with neuromuscular disorders should be properly immunized to common respiratory pathogens. Influenza vaccines should be given on a yearly basis, and household members should be immunized as well. Patients should also receive the pneumococcal vaccine.

Swallowing dysfunction as a result of face and muscle weakness is common in patients with neuromuscular diseases. Cough or congestion with meals may suggest dysfunctional swallowing and aspiration. Poor weight gain may be an indicator of excessive caloric expenditure caused by increased work of breathing (WOB) or difficulty taking in adequate calories. Dietary changes or nutrition via gastrostomy tube may be used in patients at risk for pulmonary aspiration as a result of swallowing abnormalities or in individuals who fatigue during meals.

Stresses for patients with neuromuscular disorders can occur with perioperative, postoperative, or intensive care management and should be anticipated. Recommendations have been made in the postoperative and intensive care management of individuals with DMD, for example, and may be generalizable to patients with other neuromuscular disorders (4).

During severe neuromuscular impairment, patients may need to be mechanically ventilated. Despite flat faces and paralysis, children will still be fully aware of their situation; clinicians must remember that discussions around the patient can

Table 17-3	Mucociliary-Clearance Techniques	
Technique	**Description**	**To Use**
Chest physiotherapy	Method of manual clearance of mucus, including percussion, vibration, and postural drainage	*Percussion*: A trained person uses a cupped hand to rhythmically clap over the chest wall. *Vibration*: Gently shaking the chest wall during expiration with your hands or a mechanical device *Postural drainage*: Positioning the patient to allow mucus to drain automatically from small airways to large conducting airways, to facilitate clearance
Oscillating positive expiratory pressure therapy (e.g., flutter valve)	Combines positive expiratory pressure with high-frequency expiratory oscillations to help decrease sputum thickness and improve mobilization of mucus	Patient sits upright and breathes out slowly through device, causing oscillations within the lungs
Insufflation-exsufflation device	Inflating the lungs with a positive pressure, followed by an active negative pressure exsufflation that creates a peak and sustained flow high enough to provide adequate shear and velocity to loosen and move secretions toward the mouth for suctioning or expectoration	Cycles (3–5) cycles of insufflation-exsufflation, followed by about 30 seconds of rest; repeated until secretions have been sufficiently expelled

be fully understood. Special care should be given to the patient to provide appropriate emotional support.

Guillain-Barré Syndrome

Guillain-Barré syndrome (GBS) is a neurological condition that affects peripheral nerves and presents as progressive ascending weakness in both arms and legs and **areflexia**, or absence of reflexes. Symptoms move upward from the arms and legs toward the head. It mostly affects motor function, but can also impair sensation. GBS is the most common cause of acute **flaccid paralysis** (relaxed or absent muscular tone) in children.

The annual incidence in children is between 0.4 and 1.4 cases per 100,000 children younger than 16 years of age. Incidence in adults is significantly higher, with rates of 1.1 to 2.8 per 100,000 annually. There is a bimodal peak in incidence in young adults and in the elderly. Overall rates range from 1.1 to 1.8 per 100,000 (5).

GBS typically presents in previously healthy individuals and often following acute illness with a variety of infectious disease agents. It is thought that most cases of GBS are caused by an atypical peripheral nerve immune response to an infection. It has been documented following infection with *Campylobacter jejuni*, cytomegalovirus, *Mycoplasma pneumonia*, *Haemophilus influenzae*, and Epstein-Barr virus. There have also been documented cases following immunizations, but this risk is considered to be very low (6).

Pathophysiology

The exact cause of GBS is not clear, but several factors have been identified that may play a role. One of the most likely causes is related to the development of antiganglioside antibodies. **Gangliosides** are complex molecules that are in nerve cell membranes and are instrumental in recognition of cells and cell-to-cell communication. In GBS, antiganglioside antibodies bind to peripheral nerves, causing their impaired functioning. In patients who develop GBS following infection with *C. jejuni*, the bacteria has been shown to express lipo-oligosaccharides that mimic the carbohydrate structure of gangliosides on the cell. This can produce antiganglioside antibodies that cause **neuropathy**, a disease or malfunction of the nerves. Additional factors that lead to GBS include local complement activation, which causes nerve cell damage, and an individual patient's genetic predisposition to developing the disorder. These factors combine to impair nerve conduction and can result in weakness, sensory loss, and loss of deep tendon reflexes, such as when you hit your knee or ankle tendons and your ankle or knee jerks automatically (6).

There are multiple variants of GBS. The "classic" disorder is known as acute inflammatory demyelinating polyradiculoneuropathy. **Demyelination** refers to loss of the myelin sheath on the nerve axon (Box 17-1). The myelin sheath is essential in the rapid conduction of nerve impulses through the neuron (Fig. 17-2). Patients present with weakness in both arms and legs, progressing to partial or incomplete paralysis, known as **paresis**. Loss of deep tendon reflexes also occurs. Progression of symptoms can be over the course of several days or can have a rapid and severe onset, causing respiratory failure in 24 to 48 hours. Lumbar puncture shows no signs of infection.

Another variant of GBS, acute motor axonal neuropathy, was first recognized in China and is strongly associated with *C. jejuni* infection. Axons are the part of the nerve cell that transmits electrical impulses away from the body of a nerve. Acute motor sensory axonal neuropathy is a variant more commonly found in adults and is seen throughout the world. This variant tends to be more severe, and recovery time can be prolonged. Finally, Miller-Fisher syndrome is also a demyelinating form of GBS that presents with descending (starting at the head and moving toward the arms and legs) paralysis, ataxia (lack of coordination of the limbs), loss of reflexes, and external ophthalmoplegia. Ophthalmoplegia is the paralysis of any of the muscles involved in the external movement of the eye (7).

Clinical Manifestations

Children with GBS typically have no significant history of neurological issues. They often have a respiratory or gastrointestinal illness prior to developing

---

Box 17-1 Neuron Basics

The basic cell that makes up all nerves is called the neuron (see Fig. 17-2). Neurons have a large central body called the *soma*. The nucleus of the cell is in the soma. Fingerlike projections from the cell body are called *dendrites*. Information is conducted away from the soma along a lengthy projection called the *axon*. The insulation on the axon is called *myelin*. Myelin helps the signal conduct down the axon more efficiently and functions as insulation. Ranvier nodes break up the conduction down the axon. In GBS, the myelin is attacked, causing disease. Neurons transmit signals between other neurons by releasing chemicals called neurotransmitters. This exchange occurs at the junction between nerve cells called the *synapse*. Diseases such as myasthenia gravis, botulism, and tetanus attack the cell at the synaptic junction.

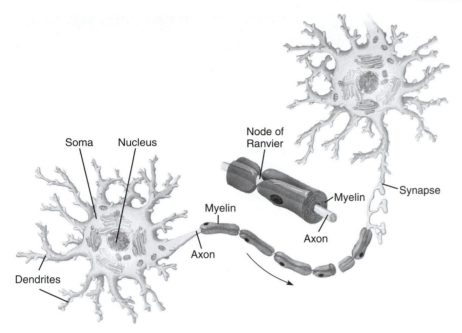

Figure 17-2 Motor Neuron *(Taber's Cyclopedic Medical Dictionary. F.A. Davis, Philadelphia, 2009, p. 1574; with permission)*

GBS. They may complain of numbness, tingling, or weakness in the arms and legs. Younger children may not be able to walk. This typically precedes respiratory compromise. Occasionally, presentation is more consistent with upper airway obstruction or illness. As weakness and paralysis progress, children will develop the following:

- Tachypnea
- Retractions
- Nasal flaring
- Decreased aeration
- Hypoxia

If cranial nerves are affected, swallowing can become impaired. This can lead initially to hoarseness, drooling, and ultimately dehydration. Patients often have difficulty clearing upper airway secretions. As GBS progresses to respiratory failure, chest radiograph would possibly show basal atelectasis and decreased lung volumes. Blood gas findings would be consistent with respiratory failure. Decline in respiratory function from GBS can be tracked by measuring MIP, MEP, and FVC measurements at the bedside using handheld devices. Progressive decreases in these measurements may indicate impending respiratory failure and can help the health-care provider determine when to escalate care for these patients.

A lumbar puncture, which provides a sample of the fluid surrounding the brain and spinal cord, known as cerebrospinal fluid (CSF), is the key to confirming the diagnosis of GBS. If onset of disease is rapid, the CSF might not show any changes. However, it is diagnostic of GBS to have an elevated CSF protein without any evidence of acute inflammation or infection, such as increased white blood cells or bacteria.

Electromyography (EMG) and nerve conduction studies are part of the routine workup for GBS. In an EMG, an electrode is used to assess if muscles are functioning properly based on electrical activity of a given muscle. A nerve conduction study tests if there is nerve damage by stimulating the nerve with small amounts of electricity. These tests can help differentiate between axonal and demyelinating variants of GBS and are part of the routine workup for children presenting with acute onset of weakness (8–10).

■ ■ The next morning, the pediatric neurology service is consulted on William's case. They recommend a lumbar puncture, magnetic resonance imaging of the brain and spinal cord, and EMGs. Tests were normal except for his EMGs, which were consistent with GBS. Stool studies were positive for *C. jejuni*.

Later on that day, William has difficulty swallowing his lunch and starts drooling. His hands and arms get progressively weaker. MIPs and MEPs are obtained. His MIP and MEP were –60 cm H_2O and 50 cm H_2O. His FVC was 1.2 L. Based on his declining status, plasmapheresis treatments were initiated. At 11:30 p.m., William's parents call his nurse to the room because his color doesn't look right. Pulse oximetry on room air is 75%. The nurse immediately puts him on supplemental oxygen and pages you, the RT on call. You notice that William is tachypneic to 45 breaths per minute and is drooling profusely. MIPs and MEPs at this point are –20 cm H_2O and 35 cm H_2O. William's FVC is 0.6 L. The rapid-response team is called to the room.

Management and Treatment

Medical management of GBS involves supportive care of the patient along with treatments such as plasmapheresis and intravenous immunoglobulin infusions (IVIG). Plasmapheresis is a procedure in which blood is removed from the body and unwanted antibodies are removed. The "pheresed" blood is then returned to the patient. IVIG is a blood product that replaces antibodies in certain diseases, including GBS, immunodeficiencies, and some infections.

If needed because of dysphagia (difficulty swallowing), enteral or parenteral nutrition may be required. Care must be taken to prevent development of decubitus ulcers by changing the patient's position frequently and good nursing care. Patients with GBS are also at increased risk for deep-vein thrombosis owing to immobility.

Patients with GBS may also have acute and chronic nerve pain, which may require treatment. Due to weakness of the eyelids, patients need monitoring and treatment of corneal abrasions. In addition, close monitoring is needed for early identification of autonomic dysfunction, preferably in a pediatric intensive care (PICU) setting (6). Patients may have high heart rates (HRs), increased temperatures, and unstable blood pressure (BP) owing to autonomic dysfunction. From a respiratory perspective, vigilant observation is needed for patients with GBS. It is recommended that vital capacity (using a handheld bedside device) and RR be monitored every 2 to 4 hours initially during the acute phase and every 6 to 12 hours in the recovery phase. Patients may rapidly and unexpectedly deteriorate and require MV. Intubation and MV may be required if vital capacity drops below 20 mL/kg. Patients may also benefit from tracheostomy because duration of ventilatory support can be variable (see Special Populations 17-1). Modes of ventilation vary with the individual need of the patient, but typically synchronized intermittent mandatory ventilation pressure control/pressure support or volume ventilation are used.

> ■■ The PICU fellow on call arrives and decides to intubate William using rapid sequence intubation. Following intubation, William remains cyanotic, requiring bagging with high pressures. He is then suctioned for a large mucous plug. His oxygen saturations improve, and he is easily ventilated using lower pressures. He is transferred to the PICU for further management.

Course and Prognosis

The typical course of GBS is about 4 weeks, with peak of symptoms at about 2 weeks. Overall mortality rate for children is less than 5%. Death is frequently

---

● Special Populations 17-1

Tracheostomy Patients

The decision about performing a tracheotomy on a patient with a neuromuscular condition is never made lightly. It is an emotional decision for both the family and the medical team.

In the more acute onset disorders, such as GBS or botulism, the PICU team and the family would work together to decide if a tracheotomy is needed. Patients with GBS get a tracheotomy when their course is severe and prolonged MV is anticipated. In infants with botulism, a tracheotomy is often not indicated because of the size of the patient and the risks.

For children with chronic and progressive neuromuscular diseases such as Duchenne's muscular dystrophy or some forms of spinal muscle atrophy, the decision to perform a tracheotomy is usually made later in life. Often, as neuromuscular weakness progresses, the decision is made in concert with a pediatric pulmonologist to implement chronic ventilator support. If possible, NIPPV should be tried initially because this mode of ventilation is associated with fewer complications when effective. However, tracheostomy and positive-pressure ventilation may be necessary in some patients. Complications from tracheostomy placement, such as airway obstruction and granulomas, or infections, such as tracheitis, can occur and can be life threatening.

---

associated with respiratory failure, arrhythmias, dysautonomia, and pulmonary embolism. Approximately 90% to 95% of children make a full recovery without any neurological impairment. However, 5% to 10% will have long-term permanent disability such as weakness, pain, or continued dependence on ventilator support. Most patients with GBS benefit from rehabilitation services, including physical therapy, occupational therapy, and speech and language therapy to maximize recovery. Speech and language pathologists often work with RTs in the acute rehabilitation setting. These therapists help patients improve their breath support and swallowing. Patients also work with RTs during their recovery. Tracheostomy patients especially benefit because they may need coaching regarding use of speaking valves on tracheostomy tubes and increasing the vocal volumes (11).

> ■■ William continues to receive plasmapheresis for the next week. A nasogastric tube is placed for nutrition. After 1 week of MV, he appears ready to tolerate weaning of pressures. He is weaned to pressure support and is extubated on day 12 of his hospitalization.

Myasthenia Gravis

Myasthenia gravis (MG) is an autoimmune disorder characterized by fluctuating muscle weakness and fatigue. Respiratory failure can occur during an MG crisis. Unlike some muscular dystrophies, the cardiac muscle is not involved in MG. There are three different types of MG: congenital, neonatal, and juvenile. Congenital MG is caused by mutations in different pre- and postsynaptic proteins. The prevalence of congenital MG is 25 to 125 per 1,000,000 live births (12). Neonatal MG is caused by the passive transfer of maternal acetylcholine receptor (AChR) antibodies to the newborn. Neonatal MG is transient but can cause severe muscle weakness, and respiratory support may be needed until symptoms resolve. Juvenile MG is most similar to adult MG and is often caused by the production of AChR antibodies. Episodic symptoms of juvenile MG can be chronic or lifelong.

Asian populations tend to have a higher incidence of juvenile MG than do Caucasian populations. The majority of Asian children with juvenile MG present between the ages of 2 and 4, with equal occurrence between males and females (13). In contrast, post-pubertal juvenile MG in the Caucasian population occurs primarily in females.

Pathophysiology

Congenital MG syndromes are caused by several different genetic mutations that are primarily transmitted in an autosomal recessive manner. Patients with congenital MG have a decreased EMG response and negative serum antibodies to AChR and muscle-specific kinase antibodies. Patients with congenital MG can respond to anticholinesterase therapy. Several genes involved in the expression of proteins at the neuromuscular junction have been shown to be associated with congenital MG (12).

Neonatal MG occurs in infants born to mothers with MG and is due to the transplacental exchange of pathogenic immunoglobulins, with or without AChR antibodies, from mother to infant.

In contrast, juvenile MG is an autoimmune disease. Many patients with juvenile MG make antibodies to the acetylcholine receptor. Some patients with juvenile MG have muscle-specific kinase antibodies, whereas a small group of patients are seronegative. The serum antibodies to AChR are chronically produced by affected individuals and lead to disruption or alterations in the postsynaptic membrane, resulting in the episodic nature and clinical features of MG (13).

Clinical Manifestations

Clinical symptoms of congenital MG syndromes are usually detected at birth but are highly variable. Symptoms can include ocular, bulbar, and limb muscle fatigability that can manifest as poor feeding, choking spells, and muscle weakness (14). MG exacerbations can lead to respiratory failure and are often triggered by infections, fever, and stress. Symptoms may include a poor cry and suck, facial muscle weakness, and **ptosis** (drooping of the eyelid).

In mothers with MG, transmission of anti-cholinesterase receptor antibodies can cross the placenta and cause transient neonatal MG. Neonatal MG does not occur in all infants of mothers who have MG; however, all infants of MG mothers should be delivered in tertiary care centers to treat potentially life-threatening complications because neonatal MG cannot be predicted (15). An infant with neonatal MG may be hypotonic and have facial weakness and poor sucking. More severe cases can present with profound respiratory failure at birth and hypotonia. Symptoms of neonatal MG usually occur by day 2 of life and resolve by 2 to 4 weeks of age.

Juvenile MG may have different clinical presentations. Interestingly, ocular development without respiratory complications is the primary clinical symptom in 70% of Asian patients aged 2 to 4 (13). Although Caucasian female patients with juvenile MG often have ocular symptoms such as ptosis (drooping eyelids), they are more likely to have facial and bulbar weakness and respiratory crises associated with their MG. An MG respiratory crisis can manifest as acute respiratory failure caused by sudden respiratory muscle weakness and plugging of the lower airways with mucus (13).

Management and Treatment

The role of the RT in managing MG patients includes recognizing and managing respiratory symptoms caused by impaired respiratory muscle strength and avoiding tracheal aspiration. Because MG can manifest as rapid and intermittent episodes of respiratory decompensation, the RT must be able to recognize and manage impending respiratory failure. This includes measuring lung function when appropriate and providing aggressive bronchial hygiene. This may include suctioning, maintaining airway patency, and initiating and managing noninvasive or positive-pressure ventilation when required.

Neonatal MG can be mild or severe, but because it is caused by maternal antibody transmission to the newborn, it is transient. Severely affected infants may require MV, supportive care, and anticholinesterase medications until recovery (15).

In patients with congenital MG, the use of prophylactic anticholinesterase therapy may help with preventing sudden respiratory failure or apnea triggered by stress or infection. This is often determined by the treating neurologist. Parents should also be trained in the use of apnea monitors and cardiopulmonary resuscitation because of the risk of sudden respiratory failure and episodic apneas (13).

Juvenile MG can be chronic and lifelong, and clinical symptoms can be episodic. As with congenital MG, respiratory involvement can occur suddenly and be life threatening, even in patients who may normally have only mild symptoms. Respiratory support and airway management during these episodes can be lifesaving. Anticholinesterase therapy such as pyridostigmine may help control symptoms. With more severe and chronic symptoms, some patients will undergo thymectomy, or removal of the thymus gland, when a thymus tumor (thymoma) is present. Steroids and other immunosuppressive agents are used in patients with severe and unrelenting symptoms of MG. These often cause side effects when used for long periods of time. With exacerbations, some patients benefit from plasma exchange and the administration of intravenous immunoglobulin.

Some pharmacological agents have been shown to be useful with certain underlying gene defects. Agents that have been used include the following:

- Acetylcholinesterase inhibitor
- 3,4-diaminopyridine
- Quinidine sulfate
- Fluoxetine
- Acetazolamide
- Ephedrine (16)

Course and Prognosis

Prognosis in congenital MG is variable and is generally worse in those children with disease progression and life-threatening exacerbations. Neonatal MG usually resolves within 2 to 4 weeks of onset of symptoms. Some patients with juvenile MG will undergo remission, whereas others will require lifelong therapy. Optimal outcomes can be better achieved when patients are treated by neuromuscular specialists (17).

Tetanus

Tetanus is a neurological disease caused by a neurotoxin that is produced by the anaerobic bacterium *Clostridium tetani*. Tetanus can affect neonates, children, and adults. There is no increased risk based on gender. Because of the widespread use of immunizations, tetanus rarely occurs in developed countries, with only 40 or fewer cases reported in the United States per year since 1999. However, tetanus remains a major cause of illness and death in the developing world (18). According to the World Health Organization, in 2009 there were 9,836 cases of tetanus in children younger than 5 years old worldwide, with an estimated 61,000 deaths in that population in 2008. There were 4,712 reported cases of neonatal tetanus in 2009, with 59,000 estimated deaths in 2008 (19, 20).

Pathophysiology

Tetanus occurs when *C. tetani* spores enter the body through a wound or other damaged tissue. These spores are found throughout the environment, including in soil; in animal and human feces; and on wood, nails, and other objects. For illness to occur, the spores need to germinate in an environment with reduced oxygen content, such as a wound. Incubation time is typically between 3 and 21 days, with a median of 8 days. The spores produce tetanus toxin, which ultimately prevents inhibitory motor neurons from functioning normally. This causes unopposed stimulation of excitatory motor neurons, resulting in muscle spasms and rigidity, which are characteristic of the disease (21).

Clinical Manifestations

In neonates, infection can occur during or shortly after delivery if unhygienic practices are used. For example, in some developing countries, local customs can increase the risk of tetanus spores being introduced to a neonate, such as using nonsterile instruments for cutting the umbilical cord or coating the cord with unpasteurized cow's milk butter. Neonates typically demonstrate symptoms in the first 3 to 14 days of life, usually on days 6 to 8. Newborns with tetanus typically do not have difficulty with feeding initially. However, over time, babies often are unable to open their mouths to feed due to facial muscle spasms and rigidity, which progresses to the inability to suck. The facial rigidity often starts with the facial muscles related to chewing and smiling. This is called **trismus** or lockjaw. Unique to tetanus is the finding of risus sardonicus, which is a flat-lipped grimace caused by facial muscle tightness (Fig. 17-3). This is seen in older children, but can be difficult to appreciate in babies. Babies keep their hands clenched and feet dorsiflexed, or pointed downward. They continue

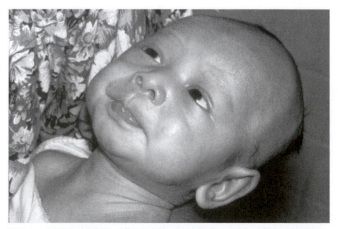

Figure 17-3 Infant With Neonatal Tetanus Displaying Risus Sardonicus *(Courtesy of World Health Organization)*

to develop full-body spasms and rigidity, which are characterized by opisthotonic posturing. Opisthotonic posturing is quite dramatic, with the patient appearing board-like with rigidity (22).

In older children, infection is typically caused by introduction of the spores into a wound. Contaminated wounds, especially deep puncture wounds and traumatic wounds with devitalized tissue, are common sites that introduce the *C. tetani* spores into a host. As with infants, typical presentation for older children begins in the facial muscles. Trismus and risus sardonicus are seen. Muscle spasms and rigidity can occur throughout the body. Respiratory symptoms can include chest wall muscle rigidity and diaphragmatic dysfunction. Laryngeal or glottic spasm can result in upper airway obstruction. Aspiration pneumonia is often seen in the setting of dysphagia and increased airway secretions. Patients can become cyanotic and apneic as a result of the spasms of the airway causing respiratory arrest (22). In any age group, a chest radiograph would show possible aspiration pneumonia or atelectasis as a result of increased secretions. Blood gas findings would be consistent with respiratory failure.

Additional symptoms of tetanus are related to autonomic dysfunction. Hemodynamic instability may result in hypertension, hypotension, tachycardia, bradycardia, and other arrhythmias. These arrhythmias can result in fatal cardiac arrest (23).

Management and Treatment

Treatment of tetanus is supportive and typically involves MV until symptoms of muscle rigidity and spasms improve. Patients may need a tracheotomy to ensure a stable airway for long-term ventilator support. Medically induced paralysis is often needed for comfort. Additional treatment may include cardiovascular system support with fluids, antiarrhythmics, and pressors. Pain management and medications (e.g., benzodiazepines) to help with spasms are essential. If the patient requires MV, vecuronium may be used because it is less likely to contribute to autonomic instability. Nutrition may need to be provided via enteral tube owing to dysphagia and the risk for aspiration (23).

Additional treatment involves the causative agent of tetanus. Human tetanus immune globulin (TIG) is given intramuscularly following diagnosis. Metronidazole provides antibiotic treatment. Wounds should be cleaned and débrided (24).

Prevention of tetanus is provided by routine immunizations. The routine childhood immunization series includes four doses of tetanus toxoid, which can help prevent tetanus. All patients who have a wound that may be at high risk for contamination with *C. tetani* spores should have their immunization history reviewed. Additional doses of tetanus toxoid

and a dose of human TIG may be required to prevent tetanus (24).

Course and Prognosis

The number of fatalities from tetanus in the United States and other industrialized countries that provide the routine immunization series have dropped significantly since the 1940s when this series began to be implemented. In 1947, there were 0.4 cases of tetanus per 100,000 people in the United States. By the 1990s, the rate had dropped to 0.02 cases per 100,000 people. Case fatality rates dropped from 91% prior to immunization to 11% by the 1990s. Adults older than 60 years of age are at highest risk for death. No deaths have been reported in patients who have received their entire primary vaccination series against tetanus (25).

Most cases of tetanus occur in developing countries, where access to appropriate medical care is not available. If tetanus is treated aggressively and appropriately in a PICU setting, mortality is low. Long-term sequelae are minimal in children treated appropriately in the PICU setting. Often, prolonged stays in the PICU are required, along with tracheotomy and MV so that the effects of the tetanus toxin resolve. Prevention of tetanus by appropriate immunizations is paramount in developing countries to decrease morbidity and mortality because access to advanced medical care is often unavailable.

Botulism

Caused by the toxin produced by the bacteria *Clostridium botulinum*, **botulism** is a progressive neuroparalytic disease that has several distinct clinic presentations. Botulism results in acute symmetric descending flaccid paralysis. Paralysis occurs because toxins produced by *C. botulinum* block acetylcholine transmission across the neuromuscular junction at the presynaptic motor neuron terminal. This results in neuromuscular blockade and flaccid paralysis (26).

There are three botulism types, based on how it is contracted: food-borne botulism, wound botulism, and infant botulism. All forms of botulism are rare in the general population. In the United States, there are approximately 145 cases reported each year. The most common form seen is infant botulism, which represents about 65% of all cases. In 2007, there were only 91 reported cases of infant botulism in the United States, with ages ranging from 1 to 44 weeks. The median age for infant botulism was 15 weeks. In a typical year, 15% of cases are food related. In 2007, there were 28 reported cases of food-borne botulism, with an age range of 13 to 74 years. Wound botulism usually represents 20% of all cases reported annually in the United States. Only 22 cases were reported in 2006, with ages of those contracting the disease ranging from 23 to 58 years (18, 27).

Pathophysiology

In infant botulism, affected babies absorb toxin produced in their intestines when the gut is colonized with *C. botulinum*. It is thought that colonization with the toxin-producing bacteria occurs because normal gut flora has not been well established because of infant age. Unprocessed honey is the most frequently cited food associated with infant botulism, but only accounts for 20% of the cases (26). The remainder of botulism cases are caused by contaminated soil or dust or other contaminated foods.

In food-borne botulism, illness develops following ingestion of food containing botulinum toxin. The toxin is produced in food when *C. botulinum* thrives in appropriate conditions, including an anaerobic environment, low pH, low-salt and -sugar content, and in temperatures between 4° and 121°C. Food-borne botulism is frequently associated with ingestion of home-canned foods that were not appropriately processed (26).

In wound botulism, wounds are contaminated by *C. botulinum* spores that germinate and produce toxin in the anaerobic environment of an abscess. This form of botulism is uncommon in children and is associated strongly with intradermal use of black tar heroin (18).

Clinical Manifestations

Symptoms of botulism can evolve over the course of several days or can have an abrupt onset over the course of a few hours. In infants, the first symptom is typically constipation, followed by symptoms that represent impaired function of the cranial nerves. Babies have difficulty feeding and present with a weak suck and swallow. They will often lose their gag reflex. The infant will develop a weak cry and will have decreased movements, loss of head control, and loss of facial expression. In addition, infants with botulism will have impaired movement of their extraocular muscles. This can result in ocular palsies, where the eye cannot move in all directions, and it is often associated with ptosis (drooping eyelid). This progresses to generalized hypotonia and weakness. Respiratory failure can occur when the diaphragm is affected and becomes paralyzed or when there is weakness in respiratory musculature (18, 26).

In older children, symptoms start with cranial nerve involvement as well. Frequent initial complaints include diplopia (double vision), dysphagia (difficulty swallowing), dysphonia (difficulty making sounds), and dysarthria (difficulty speaking clearly). Paralysis then progresses downward to affect voluntary muscles, which can result in respiratory failure (18, 26).

In all types of botulism, signs of progressive weakness and paralysis start in the face and progress downward. Signs of respiratory distress typically seen in babies, such as grunting, nasal flaring, or retractions, are not seen with botulism because of facial muscle paralysis. Instead of appearing anxious owing to impending respiratory failure, patients will present with emotionless expressions. Airway obstruction can occur as a result of pharyngeal muscle paralysis. The patient will have inadequate V_T values owing to weakness and paralysis of chest wall muscles, including the intercostal muscles. Diaphragmatic paralysis can occur. A chest radiograph would show flattened diaphragms, decreased lung volumes, atelectasis, and possible evidence of aspiration caused by dysphagia, which occurs early in the disease. Blood gases values would initially show hypercarbia, and as respiratory status decompensates, blood gas values would be indicative of respiratory failure (26).

Clinical history is very important in making the diagnosis of botulism. For example, history of eating unprocessed honey or foods preserved by home-canning methods can help lead the physician to a diagnosis. To confirm the diagnosis, *C. botulinum* should be identified in a patient's stool sample. In addition, other causes of paralysis should be ruled out, including GBS, tick-borne infections, and myasthenia gravis (25).

Management and Treatment

The management and treatment of botulism will vary depending on the form.

BabyBIG

Treatment of infant botulism includes providing the human-derived antitoxin botulism immune globulin (BabyBIG) as soon as possible. Use of BabyBIG has significantly shortened hospital stays, decreased time on MV, and decreased length of tube feeding time in babies with botulism (25, 28, 29).

Antitoxin

In older children, teens, and young adults, treatment includes use of antitoxin as well. The antitoxin can arrest the progression of paralysis but cannot reverse it. However, because the antitoxin is equine in origin, hypersensitivity reactions can occur, but they are rare.

Antibiotics

If needed, medications such as penicillin or metronidazole should be given to treat wound botulism, after administration of antitoxin (18, 26).

Nutritional Support

In all age groups, botulism may impair safe swallowing. Long-term provision of nutritional support via enteral tube may be necessary.

Mechanical Ventilation

From a pulmonary perspective, long-term MV is often needed to give the patient time to recover from the effects of botulism toxin. Appropriate techniques that help with mucociliary clearance can help prevent the development of atelectasis from mucous plugging. Also important is the prevention of aspiration events by using enteral tube feeds and maintenance of nothing by mouth status. MV modes would be dependent on the age and condition of each patient. For smaller children, pressure ventilation is often used. Larger children can often use volume ventilation. Because the patient's lungs typically are healthy, the goal of ventilator support is to maintain the condition of the lungs to avoid additional complications such as atelectasis or ventilator-associated pneumonia.

For infants, treatment with certain antibiotics, including erythromycin or gentamicin, can increase risk for MV and prolong neuromuscular blockade and paralysis. They are never indicated in patients with botulism.

Course and Prognosis

The mortality rate for botulism prior to the 1940s was 60% to 70%. With current medical practices, overall mortality is now 3% to 5%, with excellent prognosis for full recovery, provided no complications occur (26). To improve outcomes, medical care should be provided in an appropriate setting to avoid complications of long-term immobilization and ventilator dependence. Following weaning off ventilator support, rehabilitation will be needed to help the patient regain strength that was lost during the illness. Many patients will have full recovery, but the disease may leave some patients debilitated. Physical and occupational therapy are often needed. Speech and language pathologists can help with swallowing rehabilitation and recovery of speech (26) (Teamwork 17-1).

Muscular Dystrophies

Duchenne's muscular dystrophy (DMD) is the most common, lethal, X-linked genetic disease, resulting in rapidly worsening muscle weakness and a decrease in muscle mass over time. It occurs almost exclusively in males who are born of mothers who are asymptomatic carriers of the gene mutation. DMD affects 1 in 3,500 newborn males (30). The disease is caused by mutations in the DMD gene that produces the protein dystrophin. Although the gene was identified 20 years ago, there is no cure for the disease. There are other forms of muscular dystrophy, such as limb-girdle, Becker, congenital, facioscapulohumeral, myotonic, oculopharyngeal, distal, and Emery-Dreifuss muscular dystrophy (Clinical Variations 17-1).

Teamwork 17-1 Multidisciplinary Rehabilitation Teams

IT IS COMMON FOR PATIENTS RECOVERING FROM NEUROMUSCULAR DISEASES SUCH AS GBS TO REQUIRE INPATIENT REHABILITATION FOLLOWING AN ACUTE-CARE HOSPITALIZATION. In the rehabilitation environment, the RT works in conjunction with the medical team, speech therapists, occupational therapists, and physical therapists to help the patient return to the functional status he or she had prior to illness. RTs work with speech therapists to strengthen swallow and vocalization using speaking valves in patients with tracheostomies. Occupational therapists and physical therapists work to increase core strength to support recovery of breathing muscles—key to improving and maintaining the respiratory status of the patient. RTs provide invaluable services to the medical team regarding a patient's tolerance for bronchial hygiene using insufflation-exsufflation devices and chest physiotherapy, ventilator support, and optimal timing for weaning off chronic MV. The RT also is instrumental in educating families about long-term respiratory therapies that may be needed for children after discharge from inpatient rehabilitation.

Pathophysiology

With age, patients with DMD gradually lose both skeletal and cardiac muscle strength and function. Children with DMD appear normal at birth and are often not diagnosed before 3 or 4 years of age, when gait abnormalities become noticeable and calf muscles may appear to be overdeveloped. Mutations in the gene that produces dystrophin lead to the breakdown of muscle fibers that is progressive with time (33). In addition to skeletal muscle breakdown, patients with DMD develop heart disease associated with dilation of all four chambers of the heart and impairment of left ventricular function. In DMD, loss of muscle function in the heart may not occur at the same time as skeletal muscle declines (33). For instance, patients with DMD may lose their ability to walk long distances before they exhibit cardiac abnormalities. Swallowing abnormalities and scoliosis or curvature of the spine can also develop in patients with DMD (34). Early mortality in DMD is usually the result of respiratory and/or cardiac failure.

Clinical Manifestations

Most patients with DMD become wheelchair bound by approximately 10 years of age (35). As they age, patients with DMD are often not aware of the severity of their respiratory muscle weakness because of its gradual progression. It has been recommended that ambulatory patients with DMD have their FVC measured annually, and more often if they are having respiratory symptoms (36). Nonambulatory patients with DMD should be followed more closely. They should have their pulmonary status assessed biannually, and these tests should include FVC, room air pulse oximetry, peak cough flow, and MIP/MEP measurements. In addition, patients who have FVCs less than 50% predicted require NIPPV, and patients with suspected hypoventilation should have an awake end-tidal carbon dioxide ($E_T CO_2$) measurement performed using capnography.

Management and Treatment

During acute illnesses and postoperatively, patients with DMD are at increased risk for respiratory decompensation and lung atelectasis caused by respiratory muscle weakness and weak cough.

The use of NIPPV and an insufflation-exsufflation device (Fig. 17-4) to prevent mucous plugging and atelectasis should be strongly considered following any surgical procedure or with respiratory illnesses when indicated. During surgical procedures, depolarizing muscle relaxants such as succinylcholine can lead to fatal reactions and should never be used in patients with DMD. The 23-valent pneumococcal polysaccharide and influenza vaccines are recommended for DMD patients.

Chronic Respiratory Therapies

As the respiratory muscles weaken with age, patients with DMD will develop a weak cough, and they will eventually develop chronic respiratory failure. To prevent atelectasis, an insufflation-exsufflation device should be initiated as part of daily maintenance therapy when the following occurs:

- FVCs are less than 40% of that predicted
- Cough flows are less than 270 L per minute
- MEPs are less than 40 cm H_2O or if patients have difficulty clearing upper and/or lower respiratory secretions (36)

The initiation of NIPPV should be considered in any patient who has any of the following:

- FVCs less than 30% of that predicted
- Decreased oxygen saturations (less than 95%) while awake
- Abnormal polysomnography (or sleep studies) that suggests hypoventilation and hypercarbia ($E_T CO_2$ values greater than 45 mm Hg) (36)

Routine longitudinal follow-up and testing of these patients is essential because timely initiation of chronic therapies has been shown to increase quality of life and longevity.

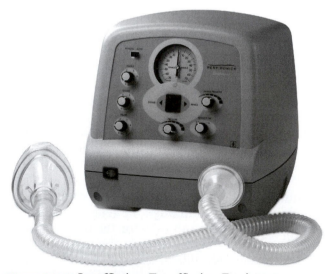

Figure 17-4 Insufflation-Exsufflation Device *(Courtesy of Respironics Media Resource Library, http://www.mrl.respironics.com)*

Patients who have LGMDs develop progressive limb-girdle weakness with upper- and lower-limb wasting. Similar pulmonary function testing and initiation of chronic respiratory therapies as used in DMD patients may also be effective in patients with LGMD.

Currently, respiratory management and care for DMD and LGMDs is supportive and based primarily on respiratory symptoms and pulmonary function tests (31, 37).

Sleep-Related Disordered Breathing

The majority of DMD patients develop sleep-related hypoxemia and upper airway obstruction prior to daytime symptoms (38). Overnight sleep studies have proven to be very useful in identifying patients with early chronic respiratory failure. In patients with evidence of chronic respiratory failure, nighttime NIPPV should be considered and initiated. NIPPV at night can improve daytime symptoms and help prevent acute respiratory failure with lower respiratory illnesses. When initiating NIPPV, it is important to have a properly fitted nasal mask. Full face masks that cover the mouth should not be chosen for home use because aspiration can occur from upper airway secretions or gastric contents. Nasal pillows may be useful for mild chronic respiratory failure but may not be as effective as the nasal mask in treating hypoventilation. Because NIPPV is being used for chronic respiratory failure, bi-level positive airway pressure (BiPAP) should be used with a backup rate. Side effects of the nasal mask may include pressure sores on the bridge of the nose with improperly fitted masks, drying of the nasal mucosa from high flows, and midfacial changes with prolonged chronic use starting in childhood. Humidified air will prevent nasal passage drying, and proper fitting of the mask can help prevent pressure sores and midfacial changes. Caregivers need to be trained carefully in using NIPPV. If the mask is not properly fitted or placed on the patient, hypoventilation will occur, and the patient may become hypoxic. Patients with DMD do not usually have underlying parenchymal lung disease. If they are hypoxic, it is most often due to hypoventilation from weak respiratory muscles or mucous plugging and atelectasis. Patients with DMD who are receiving NIPPV should not require supplemental oxygen unless they are acutely ill with a respiratory illness. If they require supplemental oxygen, this may suggest that they are being underventilated and require increased pressures or mask adjustment or that they have mucous plugging owing to poor mucociliary clearance.

Acute Respiratory Illnesses

Aggressive management of respiratory symptoms during a pulmonary illness can help prevent acute respiratory failure. The insufflation-exsufflation device should be used frequently during respiratory illnesses to help prevent mucous plugging and atelectasis. Chest physiotherapy (CPT) should always be used in conjunction with an insufflation-exsufflation device because CPT alone may move mucus, but patients are often too weak to cough it up. Adequate cough has been shown to correlate with MEPs of 60 or greater, whereas cough was ineffective with MEPs below 45 (39).

Maintenance Pharmaceuticals

Pharmaceutical agents have been used in the treatment of DMD. The use of glucocorticoids may prolong ambulation and reduce the development of scoliosis in DMD; however, side effects are frequent and include the development of osteoporosis and fractures (40). Steroids are usually given orally once a day. Clinical trials are ongoing to investigate other therapeutic options such as nonsense mutation suppression with aminoglycosides, which may help 13% to 15% of DMD patients who have gene mutations that cause a truncated dystrophin protein (41). There is also much interest in gene therapy trials, in particular delivery of the dystrophin gene by an adeno-associated virus-based vector. Animal studies have been encouraging, and there is interest in developing this mode of therapy for human trials (42).

Course and Prognosis

It has been reported that an FVC of less than 1 L is the best predictor of poor survival in a patient with DMD (43). One study reported that patients who had FVCs less than 1 L went on to have a 5-year survival rate of 8% (44). The average lifespan of patients with DMD who do not receive NIPPV or tracheostomy and ventilator support is approximately 18 to 21 years (44, 45). With aggressive cardiopulmonary interventions, including NIPPV, insufflation-exsufflation therapy, and cardioprotective medications, survival may be substantially increased (45). With aggressive preventative therapies and intervention, a median survival of 35 years has been reported in a group of DMD patients (35). Survival for individuals with LGMDs is extremely variable and may partially depend on the specific genetic mutation.

Spinal Muscular Atrophies

Spinal muscular atrophy (SMA) is characterized by lower motor neuron degeneration, and respiratory muscle strength is disproportionately weaker than the diaphragm muscle. SMA is a leading cause of death in children younger than 2 years of age. It is an autosomal recessive disease with a carrier frequency of 1:35, affecting 1 in 6,000 to 1 in 10,000 live births (46). It is a group of disorders caused by deletions or mutations in the survival of the motor neuron 1 (*SMN1*) gene. There are three types of SMA in children: SMA types I, II, and III, with type I being the most severe and type III the least (46) (Table 17-4). There is no cure for SMA at this time, and care is primarily supportive.

Pathophysiology

The severity of SMA is determined by the copy number of the *SMN2* gene (47). This gene is normally inactive during the fetal period and allows normal programmed cell death (apoptosis) in the developing fetus. This gene becomes active in the healthy mature fetus to stabilize the number of neurons. In its absence, programmed cell death persists. This impairs muscle maturation and degeneration and death of lower motor neurons in the spinal cord.

Clinical Manifestations

Disease severity varies based on the type. The most severe form of the disease is SMA type I, or Werdnig-Hoffman disease. Most children with SMA type I will die before 2 years of age owing to respiratory failure if respiratory support interventions are not implemented. These patients develop tongue fasciculations, characterized by involuntary fine tongue movements; bilateral muscle weakness, with proximal muscles (arms and legs) weaker than distal muscles (hands and feet); and profound hypotonia. These symptoms usually present before 6 months of age. Infants with SMA type I have a classic bell-shaped chest wall seen on chest radiograph caused by severe respiratory muscle weakness (Fig. 17-5).

Children with SMA type II have symptoms that are less severe than those of SMA type I. These children usually develop muscle weakness between 6 and 18 months of age. Children with SMA type II can usually sit but not stand. They are at risk for respiratory failure because of respiratory muscle weakness, particularly with lower respiratory tract illnesses, and they often develop scoliosis.

SMA type III is the least severe form of SMA. These children are usually diagnosed after 18 months and frequently not until after 3 years of age. They will

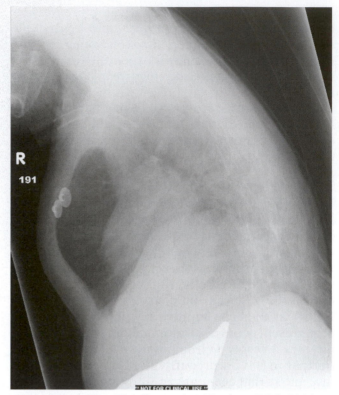

Figure 17-5 Chest Radiograph of Patient With SMA Type I. Note the typical bell-shape. *(Courtesy of Jane Benson, MD)*

exhibit gait abnormalities caused by proximal muscle weakness and easy fatigability with walking, but may have normal life expectancies (46). Prolonged independent ambulation in SMA type III is associated with later disease onset (48).

Management and Treatment

Noninvasive or positive-pressure ventilator support is essential to increase survival in patients with SMA type I because these children will develop respiratory failure by 2 years of life. If possible, the use of ventilator support versus palliative care should be discussed with the family of patients with SMA type I prior to the development of acute respiratory failure (49). Generally, the use of NIPPV to support longer survival or palliative care in children with SMA type I is considered an appropriate option. However, decisions for care should be made in conjunction with family members and the healthcare team on a case-by-case basis. SMA type I patients also require insufflation-exsufflation devices to prevent mucous plugging and atelectasis. Because of respiratory muscle weakness and ineffective coughs, children with SMA type I will develop atelectasis and lobar collapse without frequent suctioning and use of the insufflation-exsufflation device. Nasogastric or gastric tube feedings are needed to support nutrition in these children. Oxygen desaturations can occur rapidly in these individuals as a result of poor

Table 17-4	Spinal Muscular Atrophy		
Type	**Best Function**	**Age of Onset**	**Life Expectancy**
I	Never sits	0–6 months	<2 years
II	Never stands	7–18 months	>2 years
III	Stands and walks	>18 months	Adult

respiratory effort, hypoventilation, and mucous plugging of the airways.

Onset of respiratory symptoms in children with SMA type II is later than with SMA type I, and severity is variable; however, many children with SMA type II are at risk for developing respiratory failure and may require chronic NIPPV and aggressive bronchial hygiene. These children may also need enteral tube feedings owing to impaired swallowing and risk of aspiration. Scoliosis is also common in these children, and they often require treatment. Parents will need to be trained in the use of airway suctioning techniques, insufflation-exsufflation devices, chest physiotherapy, and NIPPV. Home pulse oximetry to assess oxygen saturations should be considered. Children who require NIPPV or tracheostomy with positive-pressure ventilation should be followed closely by a pediatric pulmonologist, and families should be educated on how to identify worsening respiratory distress. As with other muscular dystrophies and chronic diseases, a multidisciplinary approach that involves the pediatrician, neurologist, nutritionist, pulmonologist, cardiologist, speech-language therapist, RT, and others may help to optimize long-term outcomes in these patients.

Patients with SMA types II and III should undergo pulmonary function testing on an annual or biannual basis, as described with the DMD patients. Because of significant respiratory weakness, patients with SMA type II with more severe respiratory involvement may not be able to perform maneuvers required for pulmonary function tests. Although patients with SMA type III are less likely to have respiratory symptoms compared with patients with SMA types I or II, they are at increased risk for pulmonary complications, and their pulmonary function should be assessed on a regular basis and with respiratory illnesses.

Active research is ongoing in the development of therapies that may improve or correct symptoms in SMA. These include drug trials that will target neuroprotection and increasing *SMN2* transcripts (47). Gene therapy is also another potential therapy for SMA.

Course and Prognosis

Most children with SMA type I will die by age 2 years if ventilator support is not initiated. NIPPV and airway-clearance techniques, such as chest physiotherapy, postural drainage, and insufflation-exsufflation devices, have been used successfully in children with SMA type I and may extend life, allow for vocalization, and facilitate return to a home environment (40). Longer survival has also been achieved with tracheostomy and positive-pressure ventilation in some children with SMA type I.

In SMA type II, hypoventilation is common, particularly during sleep, and NIPPV may be necessary. Children with SMA type III seldom require respiratory support but may benefit from NIPPV and airway-clearance techniques during periods of respiratory illnesses or in the postoperative period. SMA type II children typically live into adulthood, and SMA type III children have a normal life expectancy.

■■ William's chest radiograph following extubation showed bilateral basilar atelectasis. A cough-assist device and intensive chest physiotherapy were initiated. William's MIPs and MEPs the following day were 70 and -80 with FVC of 2.2 L. He is transferred to a rehabilitation hospital to work on strengthening his extremities and to improve his oromotor skills. He does well in rehabilitation. A swallow study is performed at 4 weeks into his hospital course. It showed some penetration but no frank aspiration. After the swallow study, William's nasogastric tube was removed, and he was placed on a diet of thickened liquids and solids. A follow-up chest radiograph at week 6 showed resolution of atelectasis. Spirometry is normal at discharge. William will continue to receive outpatient occupational, physical, and speech therapies.

■■ Critical Thinking Questions: William Stubbs

1. Do you think the team made a mistake when they discharged William from the ED during his first visit? Were there any clinical signs that were significant enough to warrant admission at that point?
2. When William was intubated, what ventilator settings would you expect to use?
3. Do you suspect that William's symptoms will manifest again? If so, how should he be educated to identify his symptoms?

▶● Case Studies and Critical Thinking Questions

■ Case 1: Thomas Ming

Thomas Ming is 12 weeks old and was brought by his parents to the ED for evaluation of his constipation and "funny-looking" face for the last 12 hours. Thomas was born at home at 42 weeks. His birth weight was 8 pounds, 7 ounces. His parents do not believe in routine immunizations. They grow all of their own vegetables and do home canning. Mom started introducing solids a week ago, but Thomas is primarily breastfed. On examination, Thomas is an appropriately sized baby for his age. You notice immediately that his eyelids appear droopy. Although many health-care providers are examining him, he does not cry. In fact, his face looks flat. During his time in the ED, you notice that Thomas's respiratory effort is becoming weaker, and you note shallow breathing. You place him on an oxygen saturation monitor, and his oxygen saturation is 90%.

- *What is the likely cause of Thomas's symptoms?*
- *What tests would you do next to assess his pulmonary status?*
- *What would be indications for MV?*
- *What would you expect the prognosis to be for recovery from this illness for Thomas?*

■ Case 2: Tiffany Bradley

Tiffany Bradley is 3 months old and presents to the ED with mild cyanosis, a weak cry, and poor oral intake. Tiffany was born full term, and her mother has noticed that she has been a poor feeder since coming home from the hospital, with each feeding taking up to 45 minutes. Recently, her oral intake has decreased. Her mother also has noticed that Tiffany is floppier than her previous child, who was born 2 years ago. On examination, Tiffany has poor muscle tone, but she will smile and follow her mother with her eyes. She cannot reach to the midline. Her tongue appears to have mild fasciculations. She also has poor head control and a pectus excavatum but does not appear to be in significant respiratory distress. She is tachycardic but not

tachypneic. Her oxygen saturation is 82% on room air but increases to 95% on a simple face mask. Her chest radiograph is significant for a bell-shaped chest wall and bilateral lower-lobe atelectasis.

- *What is in the most likely diagnosis for Tiffany? What specialist(s) do you think should be called?*
- *What further tests would be helpful to guide Tiffany's respiratory management?*
- *Is she at risk for respiratory failure, and what would you do if she is?*
- *What should Tiffany's parents be told about MV?*

■ Case 3: John Barnes

John Barnes is 18 years old and has Duchenne's muscular dystrophy. He started college in the fall and has been feeling acutely short of breath for the past few days, which precipitates his visit to the ED. He has a motorized wheelchair and an assistant who helps him with his day-to-day activities. He uses a cough-assist device on occasion, but not on a regular basis. In the ED, he is slightly cyanotic and short of breath, with an oxygen saturation of 75%. His chest examination is remarkable for fine crackles throughout, and he has a gallop on heart examination. His chest radiograph shows an enlarged heart, pulmonary edema, and bibasilar atelectasis.

- *Why do you think John is hypoxic?*
- *Will oxygen alone treat his hypoxia?*
- *What else would you initiate to help with John's respiratory distress?*
- *Are there any cardiovascular tests that may be useful?*

Multiple-Choice Questions

1. John is a 7-year-old with DMD who is at the pulmonary clinic for a routine visit. He has complained of being more tired lately, even without additional exertion. He is not complaining of any acute symptoms of respiratory distress, and his parents say that he has been taking naps as soon as he comes home from school most weekdays. What evaluations would you recommend to help understand the reason for John's tiredness?
   a. MIP and MEP
   b. Full pulmonary function test (PFT) evaluation
   c. Chest radiograph
   d. Polysomnography

2. Which of the following neuromuscular diseases can be genetically linked?
      I. Guillain-Barré syndrome
      II. Myasthenia gravis
      III. Tetanus
      IV. Botulism
      V. Muscular dystrophy
      VI. Spinal muscular atrophy
   a. I, II, V, VI
   b. V, VI
   c. II, V, VI
   d. IV, V, VI

3. You are caring for a 12-year-old who is experiencing an exacerbation of MG. You come in

to do her bedside full pulmonary function test and note that her SpO_2 is measuring 92%, whereas yesterday when you saw her, her SpO_2 was 100%. What do you suspect is the cause?

   a. She has just exerted herself by moving around the room.

   b. Her respiratory symptoms are worsening, and she should be evaluated for impending respiratory failure.

   c. She was sleeping before you came in and is experiencing sleep apnea.

   d. She aspirated her breakfast.

4. Which patient would benefit most from an insufflation-exsufflation device?

   a. A 6-year-old with SMA type III, for home therapy

   b. A 14-year-old with DMD, admitted to the hospital for pneumonia, on NCPAP at night

   c. A newborn with tetanus, intubated and on MV

   d. A 1-year-old with SMA type I with tracheostomy tube on MV at night

5. Which pulmonary function study would be best to evaluate progressive muscle weakness in a teenager with GBS?

   a. MIP and MEP

   b. Peak expiratory flow rate

   c. Minute ventilation

   d. Negative inspiratory force (NIF)

6. What are the causes of botulism in the pediatric population?

   a. School-aged children eating honey contaminated with *C. botulinum*

   b. Infant gut colonization of *C. botulinum*

   c. Eating home-canned foods

   d. Abscess infection with *C. botulinum*

7. You have a patient who presents to the ED with no previous history of neuromuscular abnormalities. She has been tripping frequently over the last few days and notes weakness in her arms and legs. What is the most likely cause for her neuromuscular symptoms?

   a. Botulism

   b. Tetanus

   c. Myasthenia gravis

   d. Guillain-Barré syndrome

8. What would be the recommended routine pulmonary evaluation for a school-aged child with DMD who has no current respiratory support?

   I. FVC annually

   II. Biannual room air SpO_2

   III. Annual polysomnography

   IV. Awake E_TCO_2 measurement

   a. I, II, III, IV

   b. I, II

   c. III, IV

   d. I, III, IV

9. Mucociliary treatment for a 6-year-old with a neuromuscular disorder can include all of the following except:

   a. Insufflation-exsufflation device.

   b. Percussion and vibration.

   c. High-frequency chest wall oscillation.

   d. Oscillating positive expiratory pressure.

10. Which neuromuscular disorders are rare in developed countries, such as the United States?

   I. Guillain-Barré syndrome

   II. Myasthenia gravis

   III. Tetanus

   IV. Botulism

   V. Muscular dystrophy

   VI. Spinal muscular atrophy

   a. I, II, III, IV

   b. III, IV, V, VI

   c. II, III, IV

   d. III, IV

DavisPlus | For additional resources login to Davis*Plus* (http://davisplus.fadavis.com/ keyword "Perretta") and click on the Premium tab. (Don't have a *Plus*Code to access Premium Resources? Just click the Purchase Access button on the book's Davis*Plus* page.)

REFERENCES

1. McGrath-Morrow S, Lefton-Greif M, Rosquist K, et al. Pulmonary function in adolescents with ataxia telangiectasia. *Pediatr Pulmonol.* 2008;43:59-66.

2. Testa MB, Pavone M, Bertini E, Petrone A, Pagani M, Cutrera R. Sleep-disordered breathing in spinal muscular atrophy types 1 and 2. *Am J Phys Med Rehabil.* 2005;84(9):666-670.

3. Suresh S, Wales P, Dakin C, Harris MA, Cooper DG. Sleep-related breathing disorder in Duchenne muscular dystrophy: disease spectrum in the paediatric population. *J Paediatr Child Health.* 2005;41:500-503.

4. Finder JD. A 2009 perspective on the 2004 American Thoracic Society statement, Respiratory Care of the Patient With Duchenne Muscular Dystrophy. *Pediatrics.* 2009;123(suppl 4):S239-S241.

5. McGrogan A, Madle GC, Seaman HE, de Vries CS. The epidemiology of Guillain-Barré syndrome worldwide: a systematic literature review. *Neuroepidemiology.* 2009;32:150-163.

6. van Doorn PA, Ruts L, Jacobs BA. Clinical features, pathogenesis, and treatment of Guillain-Barré syndrome. *Lancet Neurol.* 2008;7(10):939-950.

7. Asbury AK. New concepts of Guillain-Barré syndrome. *J Child Neurol.* 2000;15(3):183-191.

8. Faloona J, Walsh-Kelley CM. Upper airway dysfunction—an unusual presentation of Guillain-Barré syndrome. *Ann Emerg Med.* 1992;21(4):125-127.

9. Lacroix LE, Galleto AH, Gervais A. Delayed recognition of Guillain-Barré syndrome in a child: a misleading respiratory distress. *J Emerg Med.* 2010;38(5):e59-e61.

10. Roodbol J, de Wit M, Walgaard C, de Hoog M, Catsman-Derrevoets C, Jacobs B. Recognizing Guillain-Barre syndrome in preschool children. *Neurology.* 2011;76(9):807-810.

11. Agrawal S, Peake DW. Management of children with Guillain-Barré syndrome. *Arch Dis Child Educ Pract Ed.* 2007;92:ep161-ep168.

12. Abicht A, Müller J, Lochmüller H. Congenital myasthenic syndromes. In: Pagon RA, Bird TD, Dolan CR, Stephens K, Adam MP, eds. *GeneReviews.* Seattle, WA: University of Washington, Seattle; 1993.

13. Evoli A. Acquired myasthenia gravis in childhood. *Curr Opin Neurol.* 2010;23(5):536-540.

14. Liewluck T, Shen XM, Milone M, Engel AG. Endplate structure and parameters of neuromuscular transmission in sporadic centronuclear myopathy associated with myasthenia. *Neuromuscul Disord.* 2011;21(6):387-395.

15. Gveric-Ahmetasevic S, Colic A, Elvedji-Gasparovic V, Gveric T, Vukelic V. Can neonatal myasthenia gravis be predicted? *J Perinat Med.* 2008;36(6):503-506.

16. Schara U, Lochmüller H. Therapeutic strategies in congenital myasthenic syndromes. *Neurotherapeutics.* 2008;5(4):542-547.

17. Dunand M, Botez SA, Borruat FX, Roux-Lombard P, Spertini F, Kuntzer T. Unsatisfactory outcomes in myasthenia gravis: influence by care providers. *J Neurol.* 2010;257(3):338-343.

18. American Academy of Pediatrics. *The Red Book: 2009 Report of the Committee on Infectious Diseases.* 28th ed. Elk Grove Village, IL: American Academy of Pediatrics; 2009.

19. World Health Organization. Neonatal tetanus. http://www.who.int/immunization_monitoring/diseases/neonatal_tetanus/en/index.html. Updated September 27, 2012. Accessed January 10, 2013.

20. World Health Organization. Tetanus. http://www.who.int/immunization_monitoring/diseases/tetanus/en/index.html. Updated September 27, 2012. Accessed January 10, 2013.

21. Roper MH, Vandelaer JH, Gasse FL. Maternal and neonatal tetanus. *Lancet.* 2007;370(9603):1947-1959.

22. Thayaparan B, Nicoll A. Prevention and control of tetanus in children. *Curr Opin Pediatr.* 1998;10(1):4-8.

23. Bunch TJ, Thalji MK, Pellikka PA, Aksamit TR. Respiratory failure in tetanus: case report and review of a 25-year experience. *Chest.* 2002;122(4):1488-1492.

24. Centers for Disease Control and Prevention. Tetanus—Puerto Rico, 2002. *Morb Mortal Wkly Rep.* 2002;51(28):614-615.

25. Underwood K, Rubin S, Deakers T, Newth C. Infant botulism: a 30-year experience spanning the introduction of botulism immune globulin intravenous in the intensive care unit at Children's Hospital Los Angeles. *Pediatrics.* 2007;120(6):e1380-e1385.

26. Sobel J. Botulism. *Clin Infect Dis.* 2005;41:1167-1173.

27. Centers for Disease Control and Prevention. Botulism: General information. National Center for Zoonotic, Vector Borne and Enteric Diseases. http://www.cdc.gov/nczved/divisions/dfbmd/diseases/botulism. Updated November 11, 2010. Accessed January 10, 2013.

28. Fox CK, Keet CA, Strober JB. Recent advances in infant botulism. *Pediatr Neurol.* 2005;32(3):149-154.

29. Anderson T, Shah U, Schriener M, Jacobs I. Airway complications of infant botulism: ten-year experience with 60 cases. *Otolaryngol Head Neck Surg.* 2002;126(3):234-239.

30. Manzur AY, Kinali M, Muntoni F. Update on the management of Duchenne muscular dystrophy. *Arch Dis Child.* 2008;93(11):986-990.

31. Pegoraro E, Hoffman EP. Limb-girdle muscular dystrophy overview. In: Pagon RA, Bird TD, Dolan CR, Stephens K, Adam MP, eds. *GeneReviews.* Seattle, WA: University of Washington; 1993:32.

32. Broglio L, Tentorio M, Cotelli MS, et al. Limb-girdle muscular dystrophy-associated protein diseases. *Neurologist.* 2010;16:340-352.

33. Romfh A, McNally EM. Cardiac assessment in Duchenne and Becker muscular dystrophies. *Curr Heart Fail Rep.* 2010;7(4):212-218.

34. Nozaki S, Umaki Y, Sugishita S, Tatara K, Adachi K, Shinno S. Videofluorographic assessment of swallowing function in patients with Duchenne muscular dystrophy. *Rinsho Shinkeigaku.* 2007;47:407-412.

35. Kohler M, Clarenbach CF, Bahler C, Brack T, Russi EW, Bloch KE. Disability and survival in Duchenne muscular dystrophy. *J Neurol Neurosurg Psychiatry.* 2009;80(3):320-325.

36. Birnkrant DJ, Ashwath ML, Noritz GH, et al. Cardiac and pulmonary function variability in Duchenne/Becker muscular dystrophy: an initial report. *J Child Neurol.* 2010;25(9):1110-1115.

37. Finder JD, Birnkrant D, Carl J, et al. Respiratory care of the patient with Duchenne muscular dystrophy: ATS consensus statement. *Am J Respir Crit Care Med.* 2004;170(4):456-465.

38. Barbé F, Quera-Salva MA, McCann C, et al. Sleep-related respiratory disturbances in patients with Duchenne muscular dystrophy. *Eur Respir J.* 1994;7(8):1403-1408.

39. Szeinberg A, Tabachnik E, Rashed N, et al. Cough capacity in patients with muscular dystrophy. *Chest.* 1988;94(6):1232-1235.

40. Iannitti T, Capone S, Feder D, Palmieri B. Clinical use of immunosuppressants in Duchenne muscular dystrophy. *J Clin Neuromuscul Dis.* 2010;12(1):1-21.

41. Malik V, Rodino-Klapac LR, Viollet L, Mendell JR. Aminoglycoside-induced mutation suppression (stop codon readthrough) as a therapeutic strategy for Duchenne muscular dystrophy. *Ther Adv Neurol Disord.* 2010;3(6):379-389.

42. Wang Z, Kuhr CS, Allen JM, et al. Sustained AAV-mediated dystrophin expression in a canine model of Duchenne muscular dystrophy with a brief course of immunosuppression. *Mol Ther.* 2007;15(6):1160-1166.

43. Hukins CA, Hillman DR. Daytime predictors of sleep hypoventilation in Duchenne muscular dystrophy. *Am J Respir Crit Care Med.* 2000;161(1):166-170.

44. Phillips MF, Quinlivan RC, Edwards RH, Calverley PM. Changes in spirometry over time as a prognostic marker in patients with Duchenne muscular dystrophy. *Am J Respir Crit Care Med.* 2001;164(12):2191-2194.

45. Ishikawa Y, Miura T, Ishikawa Y, et al. Duchenne muscular dystrophy: survival by cardio-respiratory interventions. *Neuromuscul Disord.* 2011;21(1):47-51.

46. Schroth MK. Special considerations in the respiratory management of spinal muscular atrophy. *Pediatrics.* 2009;123(suppl 4):S245-S249.

47. Zanoteli E, Maximino JR, Conti RU, Chadi G. Spinal muscular atrophy: from animal model to clinical trial. *Funct Neurol.* 2010;25(2):73-79.

48. Montes J, Gordon AM, Pandya S, De Vivo DC, Kaufmann P. Clinical outcome measures in spinal muscular atrophy. *J Child Neurol.* 2009;24(8):968-978.

49. Mitchell I. Spinal muscular atrophy type 1: what are the ethics and practicality of respiratory support? *Paediatr Respir Rev.* 2006;7(suppl 1):S210-S211

Chapter 18

Pediatric Accidents With Pulmonary Involvement

Elizabeth A. Hunt, MD, MPH, PhD
Deeraj Goswami, MD

Key Terms

Aspiration
Carboxyhemoglobin
Cytochrome oxidase
Dry drowning
Dysfunctional swallowing
Escharotomies
Eschars
Hydrocarbons
Hydroxycobalamin
Hyperbaric chambers
Laryngospasm
Lipoids
Methemoglobin
Negative pressure pulmonary
  edema
Rule of nines
Secondary drowning
Serosanguineous
Silent aspiration
Sodium thiosulfate
Wet drowning

Chapter Outline cont.

Chapter Objectives

After reading this chapter, you will be able to:

1. Differentiate between wet and dry drowning and how they present.
2. List the three major therapies for negative pressure pulmonary edema.
3. Understand how to initiate and titrate positive end expiratory pressure when concerned about pulmonary edema.
4. Discuss the differences in therapy between routine acute respiratory distress syndrome (ARDS) and near-drowning–induced ARDS
5. Discuss the symptoms that would make an elective intubation indicated, even in a seemingly stable burn patient.
6. List the factors that make inhalation injury more likely in burn patients.
7. Determine when a hyperbaric chamber should be considered after carbon monoxide poisoning.
8. Know the treatment of the two major systemic complications of inhalation injury: carbon monoxide and cyanide poisoning.
9. Discuss how behavior and development are important for aspiration risk.
10. Discuss the difference between a partial and complete foreign body obstruction and how to treat each.
11. Discuss the differences and similarities between a hydrocarbon and lipoid aspiration.
12. List the therapies and effects for the treatment of gastric and oropharyngeal secretion aspiration.

■■ John Smith

You are working in the pediatric intensive care unit (PICU) during the summer when one of your colleagues calls and gives you an update about John Smith, an 8-year-old patient being transferred from the general pediatric floor to the PICU. John suffered a near-drowning in a local pool. It was estimated that he was submerged underwater for 2 to 3 minutes. He required rescue breaths but no chest compressions, and he coughed up large amounts of water in the field. John was brought into the pediatric emergency department (ED) looking well and actively trying to explain what happened.

Unintentional injuries are the leading cause of death in children aged 1 to 15 years (1). They can also be a major source of pulmonary morbidity and long-term sequelae if there are direct effects to the airway or lung tissues. Accidents with pulmonary involvement include near-drowning, burn injuries, and aspiration. Each of these injuries has subcategories that affect the pathological severity and clinical manifestations and determine the method and extent of treatment.

Near-Drowning

Drowning is the leading cause of unintentional injury deaths for children aged 1 to 4 years and the third most common cause in children aged 5 to 9 years. Males are almost four times more likely to die from drowning than are females, and African Americans are 1.2 times more likely to die than Caucasian children of the same age (1). Furthermore, for every fatal drowning, four children have to visit an emergency room for medical therapy as a result of near-drownings. Lack of supervision and lack of education (regarding water safety and swimming lessons) are thought to be the primary factors leading to near-drownings, but medical conditions such as seizures and prolonged QT syndrome (associated with an increased risk of arrhythmias and loss of consciousness) can also increase the likelihood for drowning.

The term *near-drowning* refers to a person who has been submerged or partially submerged in water and has had a life-threatening experience but has not died in the period of time immediately surrounding the event. The person may still, however, be at high risk of dying in the days or weeks following the event. Alternatively, the term *drowning* refers to a person who has died, usually at the scene of the event. Near-drownings are not only complicated by the factors that lead to them, but also by the body of water in which they occur because salt water, freshwater, and chlorinated water each have different effects on alveolar tissue and surfactant stability. Most near-drownings occur at the child's home or at the local pool, and education on pool fencing has led to a decrease in the frequency over the last few years (2). Respiratory therapists (RTs) need to recognize the factors that led to a drowning or near-drowning and the environment in which it occurred because the optimal therapy may change significantly based on the details of the event.

The events in drownings have been studied in animals and humans for years and begin with breath holding, panic, and an attempt to struggle to the surface (3, 4). Inhaling tiny amounts of water or other foreign materials (e.g., sand) can cause **laryngospasm**, an involuntary muscle contraction of the laryngeal cords, and this helps to prevent fluid or other materials from entering the lungs. When the laryngeal cords no longer contract, typically after a person loses consciousness, and fluid is aspirated into the lungs, this is called a **wet drowning**. There are times, however, when laryngospasm will persist after the individual loses consciousness so that no fluid enters the lungs, and this is referred to as a **dry drowning**. In cases of dry drownings, the individuals typically die from asphyxia leading to cardiac arrest. Of note, as described in the next section, the majority of the pathophysiology related to near-drownings is independent of whether or not *any* water is aspirated.

Acute decompensations can occur in near-drowning patients, and some medical practitioners advocate intensive care unit (ICU) admissions for all near-drowning patients admitted to the hospital (5). Regardless, a period of observation is warranted; the location could be at the discretion of the medical provider.

Pathophysiology

The pathophysiological mechanisms that occur within the lungs after a near-drowning will determine the clinical path that the patient may take and the subsequent pulmonary complications that may develop. This can include pulmonary edema, secondary drowning, surfactant dysfunction and atelectasis, aspiration pneumonia, and acute respiratory distress syndrome (ARDS).

Laryngospasm is the first physiological mechanism to occur when a person is submerged in water for an extended length of time. This glottic closure exists in an attempt to prevent aspiration of contents from the airway into the lungs. This protective mechanism will quickly cause problems if the inciting factor is not removed and air is not able to enter the lungs. Paradoxically, another of the primitive reflexes that is retained until the brain is severely damaged is for the body to continue to attempt to breathe, so these attempts will occur even when the glottis is closed. To clarify, the body is attempting to (1) take a breath (by drawing air into the lungs to oxygenate its tissues) at the same time it is trying to (2) prevent a breath from being taken (by keeping the glottis closed to prevent any contents being aspirated into the lungs). This causes significant physiological changes and acute lung damage.

Negative Pressure Pulmonary Edema

The first physiological change is an increase in the negative pressure in the thorax. The pressure generated can be very high, even in small children, and can damage the alveolar and capillary bed. This leads to fluid being pulled into the lung parenchyma as if in a vacuum. The first cases were described in 1977 and soon called **negative pressure pulmonary edema** or postobstructive pulmonary edema (Fig.18-1) (6, 7).

Secondary Drowning

In normal cardiorespiratory dynamics, blood flow to the right heart and the lung are increased during inspiration. Drowning victims have a high sympathetic

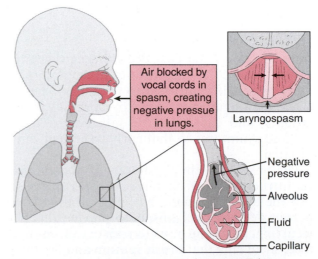

Figure 18-1 Negative Pressure Pulmonary Edema

release increasing heart rate and raising systemic vascular pressure, thus increasing oxygen demand of the left ventricle. Simultaneously, pulmonary vascular resistance increases, thus increasing the oxygen demand of the right ventricle. In this setting, oxygen delivery is minimal because no air is entering the lung, and heart work is increased because the systemic pressure and pulmonary resistance are higher. Overall, more blood flow enters the lung, but there is very high resistance to that blood exiting the heart and lung.

The resistance of blood leaving the lungs essentially causes a backup and significantly increases the hydrostatic pressure in the vessel. The blood in the lung is under such high hydrostatic pressure that fluid can begin to leak into the pulmonary parenchyma and cause cardiac-induced pulmonary edema. Clinicians should be aware that the effects of both types of edema can either be seen immediately or have a temporal delay. This delay is called **secondary drowning**, and it can occur up to 24 hours after the initial event and be seen in 5% to 10% of near-drowning cases (8, 9).

Surfactant Dysfunction and Atelectasis

Surfactant is a chemically complex agent whose main function is to stabilize the air-liquid interface of the alveoli and bronchioles and to lower surface tension. Lower alveolar surface tension improves lung compliance, prevents alveolar collapse, and reduces work of breathing (WOB).

The severity of a near-drowning does not always correlate with the potential for atelectasis. The type of water and a wet drowning can affect surfactant deactivation, thereby increasing the likelihood of respiratory complications. Intubation can also affect the symptoms that are seen. Aspiration of freshwater, pool water with chlorine included, or salt water will cause surfactant dysfunction. Freshwater can inactivate surfactant on contact, and both salt water and freshwater can cause fluid shifts that further cause surfactant breakdown (10).

Aspiration Pneumonia

Lung infections after near-drowning can occur primarily because of aspiration of contaminated water or gastric contents into the lungs. Pneumonia can be a significant source of morbidity in these patients, and care must be taken to recognize risk and symptoms so that early treatment can be initiated.

The primary pathophysiology of pneumonia is the introduction of bacteria or other organisms into the lung. The body has evolved to have numerous defense mechanisms to prevent this from occurring, including hairs to trap organisms in the nose, small cilia that brush sputum and organisms out of the respiratory track, and a large number of immunological cells living along the respiratory track. The aspiration that occurs in many near-drownings overcomes these defenses and infects the lung with organisms from the water or the gastrointestinal (GI) track.

The published incidence of aspiration pneumonia in near-drowning victims has varied in studies from 0% to more than 50% (11–13). Therefore, it is difficult to know the extent of this problem in this patient population. Anecdotally, the severity of the drowning and the amount aspirated (infectious load) is thought to lead to a higher risk of pneumonia, but no studies have proven this. The symptoms of pneumonia can be subtle and similar to numerous other pathological problems and may cause the lack of these studies.

Acute Respiratory Distress Syndrome

Discussed in detail in Chapter 15, ARDS is a primary definition that allows the medical community to categorize patients. Near-drowning is one of the many causes of ARDS. The definition of ARDS is as follows:

- Acute onset of symptoms
- Bilateral infiltrates on chest radiograph
- No evidence of left atrial hypertension, such as a pulmonary capillary wedge pressure less than 18 mm Hg, which would suggest a cardiac cause for the infiltrates
- A defined degree of hypoxia

Near-drowning primarily causes direct lung injury either by infection or disruption of the alveolar-capillary membrane. This type of ARDS may have worse outcomes and is a major cause of morbidity in pediatric near-drowning patients (14).

The disruption of the alveolar capillary membrane induces proinflammatory events that start the cycle and is called the *exudative phase* of ARDS. Inflammatory cells invade the alveolar space, and fluid and proteins migrate across the barrier and further pull fluid in by osmosis (Fig. 18-2). This leads to poor compliance and poor oxygen exchange and the need for increased respiratory support. Positive-pressure ventilation and lung stretch can further encourage the release of inflammatory cytokines, and mechanical ventilation (MV) on its own can cause lung injury, even in a healthy patient.

The fibroproliferative stage of ARDS follows the exudative phase after the acute inflammation has stopped. Chronic inflammation can increase lung dead space, cause pulmonary hypertension, and scar the alveolar capillary membrane. The recovery phase begins when that membrane begins to heal and once again allows no movement of proteins across it (15).

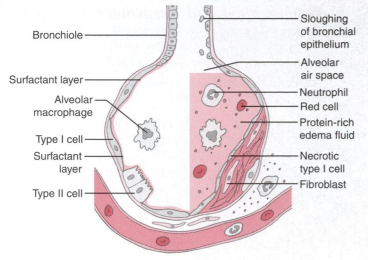

Bronchiole

Surfactant layer

Alveolar macrophage

Type I cell

Surfactant layer

Type II cell

Sloughing of bronchial epithelium

Alveolar air space

Neutrophil

Red cell

Protein-rich edema fluid

Necrotic type I cell

Fibroblast

Figure 18-2 Phases of ARDS

Clinical Manifestations

Fluid filling the lung can cause poor gas exchange and hypoxia. This will lead to children showings signs of respiratory distress, including the following:

- Tachypnea
- Cyanosis
- Retractions
- Nasal flaring
- Rales
- Hypoxia/hypoxemia
- Cough
- Poor oxygenation despite increased oxygen and ventilatory settings (see Chapter 15 for additional information on the physiological mechanisms causing hypoxemia during ARDS)
- Frothy fluid, sometimes pink in color, coughed or coming up an endotracheal tube (ETT)
- **Serosanguineous** fluids (consisting of blood and serum) from the airway
- Chest radiograph ranging from normal to increased vascular marking (mild) to complete whiteout of the lungs bilaterally (severe)
- Atelectasis commonly seen in intubated and nonintubated patients. Areas of the lung are collapsed and have no air for gas exchange. Atelectasis from drowning is primarily caused by the destruction of surfactant by the aspiration of water. It will also cause similar clinical manifestations, which typically include the following:
- Grunting (younger children)
- Fever
- Chest pain
- Asymmetric breath sounds
- Consolidation on film with slight mediastinal shift toward the area of collapse
- "Roving" atelectasis—lungs collapse, moving from one area of the lung to another

- Change in lung compliance, noted during pressure ventilation as a change in tidal volume (V_T) achieved at similar inspiratory pressures

Clinical signs specific to aspiration pneumonia include the following:

- Fever
- Consolidation on chest radiograph (CXR)
- Thick secretions with polymorphonuclear cells and organisms from sputum or endotracheal sample

ARDS and pulmonary edema are very similar in their clinical presentation. The primary factor is fluid crossing the alveolar membrane. In pulmonary edema, and particularly in negative pressure or "flash" pulmonary edema, the fluid crossing the disruption of the membrane is extremely acute, whereas in ARDS, the disruption is more a subacute process. Clinical signs of pulmonary edema include the following:

- Rales
- Poor air entry
- Hypercarbia
- Poor lung compliance
- Bilateral infiltrates on CXR

■■ John continued to look healthy in the ED, with no abnormalities on the laboratory results, including a room air arterial blood gas (ABG) with pH 7.32, $PaCO_2$ 44 mm Hg, PaO_2 71 mm Hg, HCO_3 20 mEq/L. He has a mild cough, and his vital signs were as follows: heart rate (HR) of 104 bpm, blood pressure of 104/58 mm Hg, temperature of 98.6, pulse oximetry of 97% on room air, and respiratory rate (RR) of 34 breaths per minute. A CXR was obtained, and only mild interstitial markings were seen. John was about to be discharged when it was decided by a more senior clinician that the HR and RR were elevated beyond normal, and despite looking otherwise healthy, John warranted admission to the ward for further observation. Just prior to transfer, 3 hours after presentation, John started to have occasional desaturations to 92% and was placed on 1-L nasal cannula and transferred to the floor. On the floor, over a several-hour period, John had worsening and persistent desaturations requiring progressive escalation of support to 60% oxygen by face mask. The PICU response team (you are a team member) was called to the floor to evaluate the patient. You review the ABG values for the patient from when he was in the ED and notice that the numbers individually are relatively unremarkable. However, you have a concern that the CO_2 was slightly elevated despite there being a significant amount of tachypnea (i.e., you would have been expecting a respiratory alkalosis). You suspect he was already showing signs of lung impairment at that time. You are very happy he was admitted and that you now have been called to transition him to a higher level of care. You note that John now is frequently coughing and has tachypnea and nasal flaring, in addition to the increasing oxygen requirement, all of which is consistent with possible aspiration or pulmonary edema (i.e., delayed symptoms related to the near-drowning event).

You assist in transporting John to the PICU immediately to manage his respiratory failure with the goal of starting noninvasive positive-pressure ventilation (NIPPV) to assist with oxygenation, most likely continuous positive airway pressure (CPAP). Upon arrival in the PICU, he is now in worsening respiratory distress with oxygen saturations in the high 80s on the 100% non-rebreather used for transport, with moderate-to-severe retractions. The decision is made to intubate John immediately. He requires bag-mask ventilation (BMV) to maintain saturations while medications and supplies are prepared for intubation. The saturations are approximately 88% with BMV, so you discuss a plan with the physician and agree to increase the positive end expiratory pressure (PEEP) on the resuscitation bag to 10 cm H_2O and use a slightly longer inspiratory time. The saturations subsequently increase to 95%. Because there is good chest movement with BMV, the sedation and paralysis medications are administered, and the RT notices improved compliance of the lung, with further improvement in the saturations as they increase to 99%. The intubation is completed with only a mild desaturation to 92%, likely secondary to excellent preoxygenation. Once the tube is in place, frothy serosanguineous fluid begins to come out of the tube.

Management and Treatment

The lung damage from pulmonary edema in a near-drowning victim occurs well before a medical provider can begin therapy. There are a few key strategies that will help reduce and stop the damage that has already occurred:

- Early initiation of positive pressure
- PEEP
- Overall fluid balance

The earlier these therapies are started, the more likely a patient will have a full recovery.

Early Initiation of Positive Pressure

Intubation is the most common way to initiate positive pressure in near-drowning patients. A possible alternative is NIPPV. This supports respiratory effort while avoiding the possible complications of intubation. Adult data suggest that this may reduce mortality and morbidity and length of hospital stay, but its use in children is still questioned by some, despite a potential benefit in a significant reduction in sedation needs (16, 17). One of the major downfalls is that the airway is not secure, leading to increased gastric distention as well as increased risk of gastric secretion aspiration and continued decompensation. Furthermore, it can be difficult to achieve pressure high enough to adequately ventilate and oxygenate a patient with this disease process. Of note, teams may tend to escalate the settings on NIPPV when it initially works, but it becomes less effective over time with worsening lung disease. Whereas some titration of pressure may be warranted, it needs to be watched closely so that a child isn't on both very high NIPPV settings as well as high concentrations of oxygen, such that the child is at a high risk of rapidly desaturating during intubation attempts. This is even more dangerous when the child is also hemodynamically unstable. Clinicians may do well to remember the mantra that "things are likely to get worse before they get better," and opt for early intubation in a child who requires escalating support.

PEEP

PEEP is used to stent airways open and can also be used to increase the pressure of the alveoli in an attempt to keep fluid from leaking out of the capillary bed. Essentially, the gradient that is causing the fluid leakage is either reduced or overcome. Fluid could potentially be "pushed" back into the capillary bed if the gradient is overcome, which may further improve lung function (18). The starting PEEP is usually 5 but can reach up to 12 and beyond in severe lung disease. The concern is usually overdistension of the lungs, and this can be checked by CXR. Lung expansion in excess of 10 ribs is abnormal, and a decrease in PEEP should be considered at that time.

PEEP increases intrathoracic pressure and decreases blood flow into the heart, which can cause hemodynamic instability such as lower systemic blood pressures, higher central venous pressure, and decreased blood flow and oxygen to vital organs. The RT should continually assess the potential effect that positive pressure may have on other organ systems and suggest alternative settings or therapies if the current treatment has decreased cardiac function.

Overall Fluid Balance/Diuretic Therapy

The severity of the drowning can impact many organs in the body. This can often lead to fluid overload after initial resuscitation. Fluid overload is an independent factor of morbidity and mortality in the PICU, and use of early diuretics or continuous renal-replacement therapy (dialysis essentially) is of benefit (19). There is also widespread use of diuretics in patients with negative pressure pulmonary edema and no other organ involvement; however, data suggest this may not be needed (20).

■ ■ John was initially placed on ventilator settings of peak inspiratory pressure (PIP) of 26, PEEP of 6, and RR of 24 breaths per minute with 100% oxygen, but there were still copious secretions from the ETT and his saturations were consistently in the high 80s. The PEEP was increased to 8, and the frothy material stopped coming from the ETT. The saturations stabilized in the mid-90s over 15 minutes, and then over the next 30 minutes the oxygen was able to be weaned to 60% with no decrease in saturations. Initial CXR showed a complete whiteout of the lungs, which had significantly improved by the following day. The patient's lung compliance progressively improved over the next 24 hours, and the ventilator settings were weaned down to PIP, 1; PEEP, 5; and RR, 10, to prepare for extubation. However, on your daily rounds, you notice that the V_T values are half what they were overnight, breath sounds are poor on the right, and John has some increasing tachypnea. An ABG test and a CXR are ordered after discussion with the physician.

As the patient moves past the acute-management phase, there is potential for many pulmonary complications. These are described in the following sections, along with the reasons they occur in near-drowning patients and their treatment.

Treatments for Atelectasis

The general management and treatment of atelectasis in near-drowning is similar to that for any other cause, but some of these therapies are controversial.

This is often due to lack of evidence on efficacy of therapy. Strategies include chest physiotherapy, PEEP, DNase, and exogenous surfactant.

Chest Physiotherapy

Chest physiotherapy (CPT) is the best-described and best-studied therapy for persistent atelectasis. It is a mainstay for the treatment of atelectasis, although the data on its efficacy are not clear. The mobilization of secretions from small airways allows air reentry and expansion of terminal bronchioles and alveoli. The simultaneous use of humidified saline has been shown to increase sputum clearance better than CPT alone (21). However, the addition of bronchodilator therapy has yet to be proven helpful.

PEEP

Increased PEEP is also used to expand previously collapsed areas of lung. This is thought to be especially helpful in near-drowning patients because of their surfactant loss that potentiates airway collapse. The expansion of collapsed bronchioles and alveoli with higher-end expiratory pressures allows surfactant production and decreased surface tension. This keeps these alveoli expanded when the PEEP is lowered and finally taken away (22).

DNase

DNase is an aerosolized medication that hydrolyzes bacterial DNA often found in the sputum plugs that cause atelectasis. This medication is a mainstay for patients with cystic fibrosis. However, it has also been used in patients with atelectasis and no chronic respiratory disease, but it is usually for patients with thick secretions and plugs. It is often used in conjunction with CPT, with improved sputum clearance and improved air entry as the mechanism for expansion of the atelectatic areas. There are pediatric data supporting its use in patients who have persistent atelectasis despite CPT and bronchodilator therapy (23).

Exogenous Surfactant

As noted previously, the primary mechanism for atelectasis in near-drowning patients is surfactant destruction. Theoretically, it would make sense that giving surfactant to these patients should resolve this issue. However, there are only a few case reports of surfactant being used in near-drowning patients, and their purpose was the treatment of ARDS (discussed later in this chapter) and not primary atelectasis (24, 25). Surfactant is very expensive, and large volumes (3 mL/kg) are used even in the smallest children. These issues, in combination with the fact that the other therapies discussed usually effectively resolve atelectasis, are probably why surfactant is not used regularly.

■■ John's CXR showed right lower lobe and right middle lobe collapse. CPT and humidified saline therapy were initiated. The ventilator settings were increased to a PIP of 20 and PEEP of 7, with improvement on subsequent CXR. You notice on your next shift that John began to have increased thick yellow secretions, and the nurse stated the he now had a new-onset fever. A CXR and an endotracheal culture were obtained; they showed a new right-sided consolidation, an endotracheal culture with many polymorphic nuclear cells (neutrophils), and a Gram stain showing gram–positive cocci.

Treatments for Aspiration Pneumonia

Treatment for aspiration pneumonia includes alveolar stabilization and bronchial hygiene (discussed in the previous section), as well as treating the infectious causes and managing consolidation.

Antibiotics

Antibiotics are a mainstay for the treatment of any type of pneumonia. However, the variability of the organisms that can potentially cause pneumonia in near-drowning victims can make it challenging to determine which antibiotic to use. The fluid that is aspirated could be gastric contents or polluted freshwater, salt water, pond scum, and so forth, all of which vary in terms of the organisms growing in them. Therefore, when a near-drowning patient develops a clinical picture suggesting pneumonia, it is important to initiate broad-spectrum antibiotics that will cover anaerobes and aerobes as well as gram-negative and gram-positive organisms. There are no data on which antibiotic is best, but those commonly used include piperacillin/tazobactam, meropenem, cefepime, vancomycin, ceftriaxone, and clindamycin, among others.

Prophylactic antibiotics were widely used until concern about resistant infections grew in the late 1990s. Multiple studies have shown that prophylactic antibiotics neither prevent infections nor improve morbidity or mortality (5, 26). Some clinicians will still advocate the use of antibiotics if the body of water is considered heavily polluted. However, in the case of empirical coverage, if no bacterial growth is noted at 48 hours, it would be prudent to consider stopping antibiotics at that time.

DNase

The consolidation seen in pneumonia is a combination of dividing and dead bacteria and attacking and dead inflammatory cells. These cells can cause plugging of small airways, especially in patients who are intubated and unable to cough on their own. The breaking up of the plugs allows for the improvement in symptoms; thus, DNase might theoretically improve

the course of a patient with aspiration pneumonia after a near-drowning event. However, there are no apparent studies directly looking at DNase and its use in pneumonias in near-drowning patients.

■■ John was started on antibiotics, his fever abated, and he showed an improvement in respiratory symptoms over the next 12 hours. The endotracheal culture grew out streptococcus pneumonia, and ceftriaxone was continued for a 7-day course. John had a deteriorating course the following 12 hours, including tachypnea, increased oxygen demands, increased ventilator settings, and decreased exhaled V_T values on the ventilator. CXR in the morning showed bilateral infiltrates. John's ventilator settings were PIP of 30 cm H_2O, PEEP of 8 cm H_2O, RR of 24 breaths per minute, fractional concentration of inspired oxygen (FIO_2) of 0.90 because of recurrent desaturations, and his ABG values were pH 7.21, partial pressure of oxygen (PaO_2) of 62 mm Hg, partial pressure of carbon dioxide ($PaCO_2$) of 60 mm Hg.

Treatments for ARDS

The incidence of ARDS in near-drowning victims is difficult to ascertain from studies. Most near-drowning victims do not come to the ED, and the reported data are mostly from the subset of patients admitted to the ICU. Drowning is a relatively rare cause of ARDS in the ICU, but the percentage of near-drowning patients admitted to the ICU who are ultimately diagnosed with ARDS varies from less than 5% to as high as 50% (27–29).

Chapter 15 presented a full discussion of ARDS; thus, this section specifically discusses the therapies in relation to near-drowning.

Ventilator Strategy

There are no specific data on the use of ventilator strategies for ARDS induced by near-drowning. High PEEP and low V_T ventilation of 6 mL/kg are considered optimal for treatment of ARDS patients. Permissive hypercapnia and hypoxia to decrease lung injury from lung overdistension are also advocated. High-frequency oscillator ventilation and airway pressure release ventilation have been discussed as possible treatments, but neither has been proven to be better for ARDS than the conventional ventilator. The mechanism of action is thought to be decreased stretch leading to less inflammation and less chronic lung damage.

Corticosteroids

There are some specific data on steroid use in near-drowning patients. As with ARDS from any cause, there is also similar controversy about its use.

Steroids were heavily used in near-drowning patients until studies demonstrated no improvement in morbidity and mortality. There is also a concern about increased risk of infections with their use (5, 30). There are some animal data that dexamethasone may prevent the lung injury from saltwater aspiration (31). Generally, the use of steroids in near-drowning patients is not advocated. The mechanism of action is thought to be a decrease in the inflammation during the exudative phase, thereby causing less scarring during the fibroproliferative phase. This would argue for its early use, if a decision is made to use it at all.

Nitric Oxide

There is one case report of the use of nitric oxide in a near-drowning patient (32). The use of inhaled nitric oxide (iNO) in these patients may be a hot topic based on animal research that shows iNO abnormalities in animals that drown (33). Nitric oxide causes pulmonary arterial dilatation and improves blood flow to the pulmonary parenchyma. Improved oxygen exchange is thought to be the mechanism of action.

Patient Positioning

Patient positioning has not been proven to be helpful in ARDS. There are no specific data in near-drowning patients.

Surfactant

There is no consensus on the use of surfactant for ARDS. The data are no better than for those in near-drowning patients. There are numerous case reports of its use in this population, but the numbers do not support a definitive answer on its benefits (24, 25, 34, 35). The mechanism of action is the replacement of surfactant that is broken down by fluid entering the alveolar space (Evidence in Practice 18-1).

● **Evidence in Practice 18-1**

Give Back What Is Not Working (35)

A 2010 case report looked at giving back surfactant that is inactivated during drowning. The case was a 2 ½-year-old girl who was found in a pool, apneic and pulseless. Last known visual contact was 20 minutes before retrieval, and core temperature was 27.3°C at the ED. The child had a return of spontaneous circulation after 30 minutes and three doses of epinephrine. She had poor oxygen saturations after stabilization; saturations were 65% on FIO_2 1.0, with PaO_2 of 35 mm Hg. She was given calfactant (80 mL/m^2) administered through an ETT in the supine and decubitus positions. The child had a rapid resolution of her hypoxia and was extubated 8 days later with no known neurological complications.

Extracorporeal Membrane Oxygenation

Respiratory failure from near-drowning is uncommon, but there are cases of severe respiratory failure resistant to standard medical care. The last "treatment" modality available is extracorporeal membrane oxygenation (ECMO), which gives the lung rest and allows it to heal. The Extracorporeal Life Support Organization (ELSO), which has ECMO registry, indicates the overall survival in this cohort of patients is approximately 50%. There are no specific data on near-drowning patients, but there are case reports of its use (36, 37). There are also case reports of its use to actively rewarm patients after drowning (38–40). The most difficult part of making a decision about whether a patient with ARDS secondary to near-drowning is an ECMO candidate is determining whether that patient received severe anoxic injury to the brain, which would mean the disease process is no longer clearly reversible. To help determine the potential reversibility of the disease process, it is essential to ascertain the history regarding the amount of time submerged and details related to any chest compressions before making a decision about ECMO in a near-drowning patient.

Course and Prognosis

Unfortunately, near-drowning events are common in children. The majority of these events are minor, and the children are never even seen in the ED. The studies for outcome measures in drowning typically focus on neurological outcomes. There are two studies that discuss pulmonary function tests for the survivors of near-drowning events; one found there was no increased risk of reactive airway disease, and the other had trends for an increase in airway hyperactivity (41, 42).

The studies of neurological outcomes have been conducted based on a series of key locations—at the location of the drowning event (Emergency Medical System data), in the ED (initial resuscitation), and in the PICU (continued resuscitation). See Table 18-1 for variables associated with death or poor neurological outcomes (43). There is one exception to the prolonged submersion variable associated with poor neurological outcomes: Survivors have been reported for prolonged submersions in very cold water, but even then there are only a handful of case reports that describe these survivors (40, 44–46).

Multisystem organ failure is a significant cause of morbidity and mortality, but it is an uncommon complication that, when seen, is usually limited to severe near-drowning cases. The heart, brain, liver, and kidneys may be affected primarily because of hypoxic injury, and lung-specific care can potentially be harmful for these organs. For example, the acidosis allowed in permissive hypercapnia for

Table 18-1   Variables Associated With Death or Poor Neurological Outcomes in Near-Drowning

Location of Drowning	ED	PICU
• Submersion >25 minutes • CPR >25 minutes • Epinephrine or other vasoactive medication given at scene	• CPR (any) • Fixed and dilated pupils • Initial pH <7	• Apnea • Glasgow Coma Scale = 3 • Intracranial pressure >20 and cerebral perfusion pressure <50 • Abnormal head CT at 36 hours

lung function can be harmful for a heart that has been damaged and whose function is poor. These complicated factors have to be considered individually, and often a compromise is made depending on the patient's overall medical condition (Special Populations 18-1).

Inhalation Injuries

Inhalation injuries are not a common burn finding in children. Burns from hot water and liquids are the most common types of burns seen in children, and these are the least likely to cause inhalation injuries. Steam from these substances is the only exception, and inhalation injuries from steam can be very severe. Thirty percent of children with burns will have concomitant inhalation injuries. The likelihood increases if the victims are exposed to an actual fire and if this fire is in an enclosed space (47).

There are several major concerns with inhalation injury. The first two are upper airway injury and lung damage from the heat and the burning chemicals and gases that are inhaled. The third is the systemic complications that occur from the absorption of these chemicals and gases. Upper airway injury is correlated with the intensity of the heat; lung damage and systemic complications are dependent on the substances ignited during the fire (48).

The pathology and clinical signs and symptoms vary based on the cause of injury, but the course of healing and prognosis are similar. Each type of inhalational injury is described separately, but course and prognosis are compiled together at the end of the section.

Upper Airway Injury

Upper airway burns can be very subtle in their presentation. A child can be talking and looking well; however, the development of respiratory distress can be insidious and life threatening. It is important for RTs to recognize these subtle signs because early therapy could be lifesaving.

Pathophysiology

The pathophysiology of upper airway damage is direct thermal injury. The heat in enclosed spaces can reach up to 1,000°F (49). The upper airway has adapted and become very efficient at heat transfer. This prevents injuries to the lung but can cause severe injuries to the nasopharynx and oropharynx. Heat transfer causes tissue damage and resulting inflammation and edema. This could potentially cause airway obstruction and death.

Clinical Manifestations

The airway obstruction in burn victims is similar to that from any other cause. The obstruction in this case is from airway edema and can occur very quickly. Actual symptoms are very late findings, and advanced airway management must occur quickly to prevent potential respiratory arrest. Clinical signs include the following:

• Singed nares
• Soot along mouth or nose
• Facial burns
• Stridor
• Dyspnea
• Increased WOB/retractions
• Cyanosis

● **Special Populations 18-1**

Permissive Hypercapnia or Not?

Prolonged hypoxia from a near-drowning event can cause pulmonary and systemic pathology. The most severe of these would be a cardiac arrest in a child, which is causing multisystem organ failure. The heart function can initially be poor, and the potential for recurrent cardiac arrest would be high. It would be likely that lung damage would be severe in this type of patient as well, and the use of lower pressures could prevent further lung injury. ARDS ventilation strategies, such as permissive hypercapnia, would be beneficial for the lung but could potentiate rearrest in the child. Acidosis in a poorly functioning heart may be the added factor that causes rearrest. This may be a case where the medical team will not allow permissive hypercapnia and acidosis.

Management and Treatment

Airway and respiratory management of patients with smoke inhalation is a mainstay of therapy. Assessment of respiratory distress and airway stabilization, followed by management of upper airway edema, is essential within the first several hours of therapy.

Intubation

Early intubation is essential for children who have a smoke-inhalation injury. There is support in the literature that delaying intubation can lead to increased difficulty with a later attempt (50). Therefore, it is essential that intubation occur quickly in patients with any of the clinical signs noted for upper airway injury. The ETT should be cuffed and age appropriate. The risk of airway complications is increased with cuffed ETTs, but this does not outweigh the potential risks of respiratory compromise secondary to leaks or the need for a tube exchange (51, 52). The most severe complication of a cuffed tube is tracheal stenosis, and this can require further surgical care to correct in the future. The intubation should be performed by the most experienced airway technician because it can be technically difficult and may require the use of advanced equipment (e.g., video laryngoscope, fiber-optic laryngoscope). Lower-airway injury also is likely in these cases, and the patient may need significant amounts of ventilatory support.

A full evaluation of the airway should be completed early, either after the intubation or before, depending on the risks of the patient. This could include a nasopharyngeal scope and/or bronchoscopy if there is concern about vocal cord or lower airway injury. Intubation allows for adequate ventilation and oxygenation despite swelling that would inhibit air exchange.

Racemic Epinephrine

Racemic epinephrine is an aerosolized version of epinephrine that is typically used in patients with croup, but it has also been used in patients suffering burns, postextubation obstruction, and bronchiolitis. The primary mechanism of action is an alpha effect and mucosal vasoconstriction that decreases edema and a beta effect of muscle relaxation that further increases airway diameter. This allows better airflow through swollen areas and improved respiratory symptoms. There are no primary studies looking at its use in burn patients, but multiple small studies discuss and advocate its use in patients with mild respiratory symptoms from inhalation injuries (53, 54).

Dexamethasone

Dexamethasone is a steroid whose anti-inflammatory effects are helpful with airway edema. It is also primarily used for croup and postextubation obstruction but is not as fast acting as racemic epinephrine. The half-life (how long until half the drug is metabolized by the body) is very long (36 to 48 hours), and the onset of action is thought to be around 4 to 6 hours. Whereas racemic epinephrine is used to acutely improve mild symptoms of airway edema, dexamethasone is used to decrease any further edema formation. There are also no primary studies of its use for airway burns, but some experts advocate its use under certain conditions (55).

Direct Lung Injury

Thermal injuries do not typically affect parenchymal tissue because of the excellent heat dissipation by the upper airway. Any particle larger than 10 μm will get trapped in the upper airway; particles between 3 μm and 10 μm will be deposited in the proximal bronchioles; and particles smaller than 3 μm will find themselves in the distal airway and alveoli (Fig.18-3) (56). The burning of plastics and other compounds, however, can lead to multiple products that can cause severe damage to all parts of the airway, including the lungs (48, 57). The extent of damage can be correlated with the components in the smoke, the length of exposure, and the patient's minute ventilation (57).

Pathophysiology

The pathophysiology of lung injury from smoke inhalation is multifactorial but is initiated by mucosal and cell injury. Other important components include surfactant destruction, alveolar capillary membrane damage, and increased blood flow (58, 59). The presence of body burns and concomitant fluid management potentiates further lung damage and increases the likelihood of pulmonary edema and ARDS. This requires increased respiratory support and further damages the lung parenchyma.

Mucosal and cell injury will lead to edema formation within the first 24 hours. The initial injury will cause an immediate release of inflammatory cytokines, which will increase blood flow and weaken the already-damaged alveolar capillary membrane.

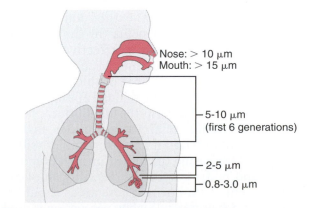

Figure 18-3 Particle Deposition in the Airway

Infectious fighting cells will cross the barrier along with fluid in an attempt to clear the dead cells and protect the body from secondary infections. The epithelial layer will shed and hemorrhage, leading to clumps of debris sitting in the tracheobronchial tree. These areas are filled with inflammatory cells and cytokines and are also prime breeding areas for bacteria (60). These clumps of debris can continue to evolve and form fibrin-like casts that can severely affect gas exchange and make it very difficult to oxygenate and ventilate a patient, even on the highest settings (61).

Clinical Manifestations

The manifestations of direct lung injury are very similar to those of upper airway injury. The assumption is anyone with upper airway inhalation injury will also have direct lung injury. Clinical signs include the following:

- Singed nares
- Soot along mouth or nose
- Carbonaceous secretions
- Dyspnea
- Hypoxia
- Retractions/respiratory distress

The primary means of diagnosis is bronchoscopy and it is advocated by the majority of burn centers. Fiber-optic bronchoscopes are available in diameters as small as 2.8 mm, allowing endoscopic inspection of patients with ETTs as small as 3.5 cm.

Management and Treatment

Respiratory care for inhalation injury focuses on bronchial hygiene and minimizing the effects of airway edema on oxygenation and ventilation. Although none of these therapies will reverse airway damage or speed healing of airway cells, they will stabilize the respiratory system to allow the time necessary for pulmonary recovery.

Chest Physiotherapy

CPT is probably the most-used treatment for patients with lung inhalation injury. Pain, MV, and the extreme hazard of accidental extubation can make its use difficult, but the benefits far outweigh the risks. CPT has been shown to effectively remove secretions in a variety of patients. Victims of inhalation injury have a large number of thick secretions, especially after the sloughing of dead epithelial cells. CPT is thought to increase the likelihood of self-removal or suctioning of airway secretions, making it less likely that distal airway bronchioles will be plugged and decreasing the nidus for infections.

Grafts and body-surface injuries can complicate CPT in patients with burns. These areas should be avoided as much as possible when percussion is used,

and other modes of physiotherapy may take precedence. Early ambulation and allowing the patient to sit in a chair are possibilities. These decrease the likelihood of muscle underuse and improve pulmonary physiotherapy by ventilating areas of the lung that are partially collapsed (62).

Bronchodilators

The primary bronchodilator used in patients with smoke inhalation is albuterol. Albuterol is a β_2-agonist and is often used for asthma to dilate constricted areas of the bronchial tree to allow for better airflow out of the lung. The effect it has on airway resistance can be substantial and potentially can allow for a significant decrease in the MV required for a burn patient. The second major effect is a decrease in inflammation. There are animal models that show that albuterol decreases the production of certain cytokines from the body, many of which initiate the process of alveolar-capillary leak, including TNF-α and leukotrienes (63, 64).

There are currently no prospective trials on albuterol or any β_2-agonist in humans with inhalation injuries. There are some animal data that showed an improvement in peak and plateau airway pressures as well as the PaO_2/FIO_2 ratio, and a similar study was completed with tiotropium, a muscarinic antagonist, which showed similar results (65, 66). A pilot study is under way at Shriners Hospitals for Children at the University of California at Davis to test the efficacy of albuterol in children with inhalation injuries (67).

Inhaled Nitric Oxide

The primary clinical use of iNO is as a pulmonary vasodilator for neonates with persistent pulmonary hypertension. The vasodilatation of the pulmonary artery allows better blood flow and improved oxygenation of the blood. The pathophysiology of inhalation injury can severely affect gas exchange at the alveolar level. Inhaled nitric oxide has been used in burn patients to attempt to improve the gas exchange and shunting that can frequently occur in these patients. There has been one small retrospective study in children with inhalation injury and iNO (68). The study showed improvement in the oxygenation of children but was not large enough to show an effect on morbidity or mortality.

Nebulized Heparin and Other Anticoagulants

Heparin's primary use is as a systemic anticoagulant to inhibit clot formation. Clots and fibrin casts are major inhibitors of ventilation and oxygen exchange, and they are a primary component of the lung injury in smoke inhalation. These casts can be extremely difficult to treat because they are unlikely to be removed by suctioning, CPT, and other forms of bronchial hygiene.

There are multiple animal studies advocating for nebulized heparin use in inhalation-induced lung injury. These benefits were further supported by a single-center study of burn patients in New York (69). These patients were all adults, but the study showed that mortality was significantly improved with heparin use. Nebulized heparin is a very promising treatment for inhalation injury and is starting to be widely used in major burn centers.

Heparin prevents clots, but the casts that form in inhalation injury need to be broken and removed. New animal data suggest that nebulized tissue plasminogen activator may be extremely helpful in removing these casts and resolving the obstruction in air exchange (70). However, there are no human studies that discuss its use.

Corticosteroids

The primary effect of steroids is to reduce inflammation after acute injury or infection. Because corticosteroids inhibit the immune system, the concern is the potential for increased risk of infections with its use. Inhalation injury has significant secondary immune and inflammatory responses that cause further lung damage. Steroids are also used as adjunctive therapy for albuterol in asthmatics. The physiological effects are similar despite the differences in the disease processes of inhalation injury and asthma. However, there have been no clinical data supporting the use of corticosteroids in patients with burns. In fact, the clinical data that are available seem to say steroid use is of no benefit (71).

Escharotomy

Eschars are areas of dead tissue that occur after severe burns. The integument of the skin can become very stiff, and the surrounding tissue can become very edematous and/or ischemic if the eschars inhibit the flow of oxygenated blood to vital tissues. Eschars can threaten both limbs and lives. Any eschar that is circumferential causes the highest risk (e.g., if encircling the arm, the distal extremity is at risk).

The most life-threatening eschars are those that encircle the chest wall and act as a tight band, with the potential to have severely detrimental effects on respiratory mechanics. If an RT notes that compliance is changing and much higher pressures are required to reach the same V_T values, it is essential to investigate whether the problem may be worsening chest wall compliance caused by a chest-encircling eschar rather than (or in addition to) worsening lung compliance. In severe cases, this affects not only respiratory mechanics but also hemodynamics because the use of increased mean airway pressures will ultimately impede venous return and negatively affect cardiac output. **Escharotomies** are incisions in the skin that can release the pressure from the eschars and cause changes in surrounding tissues (Fig. 18-4). The effects in patients' lung compliance can be drastic and lifesaving (72). The V_T values increase significantly at the same inspiratory pressures, chest expansion should return to normal, and hemodynamics may normalize within minutes.

Systemic Complications

The combustion of chemicals and formation of toxic gas is the primary cause of direct lung injury. The absorption of some of the chemicals and gases is the primary cause of systemic injury from smoke inhalation. The alveolar capillary membrane is highly vascularized. This is needed to allow for adequate gas exchange but means that the membrane will absorb noxious chemicals.

Carbon Monoxide Poisoning

Carbon monoxide is produced in high quantities during any fire. Inhalation injuries are more common in an enclosed space, making it even more likely that a victim of an inhalation injury will have carbon monoxide poisoning. The gas itself is odorless, and symptoms can be subtle. It is important to remember this possible complication because quick therapy could potentially reverse its deleterious effects.

Pathophysiology

Carbon monoxide is a competitor of oxygen for the heme-containing proteins. The most important of these is hemoglobin because it carries oxygen to the entire body for energy production. Carbon monoxide affinity for hemoglobin is 200 times that of oxygen and is called **carboxyhemoglobin** when attached (73). Hemoglobin will carry carbon monoxide to the rest of the body, but it cannot be used for energy production; thus, organs become oxygen starved. Furthermore, the oxygen on hemoglobin is more tightly bound, decreasing its availability for tissues even further. The lack of oxygen delivery can cause a significant number of systemic issues depending on the carboxyhemoglobin levels in the body.

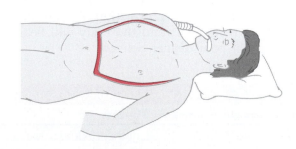

Figure 18-4 Chest Wall Escharotomy

Clinical Manifestations

The clinical manifestations of carbon monoxide poisoning are directly dependent on the amount of carboxyhemoglobin measured (Table 18-2). The light analysis of pulse oximetry reads carboxyhemoglobin the same as oxyhemoglobin. Therefore, pulse oximetry will show normal oxygen saturations despite poor oxygen delivery to the tissues. There are pulse oximeters that can quantify carboxyhemoglobin, but they are not in widespread use at this time.

Management and Treatment

The treatment for carbon monoxide poisoning must occur quickly and be started even before definitive diagnosis. Treatment focuses on overcoming the affinity hemoglobin has for carbon monoxide. The first and easiest of these is 100% oxygen via a non-rebreather mask. The half-life of carboxyhemoglobin at room air is approximately 5 hours; at 100% oxygen, it is decreased to 1 hour. Hyperbaric chambers have also been used on children with carbon monoxide poisoning, but their benefits are questionable. **Hyperbaric chambers** are pressure chambers that allow the delivery of FIO_2 of 1.0 at higher-than-atmospheric pressure. This will decrease the half-life of carboxyhemoglobin and increase the partial pressure of oxygen and the amount that is dissolved in the blood (not attached to hemoglobin). This increases the oxygen delivery to systemic tissues and decreases the half-life of carboxyhemoglobin. It should be considered for a hemodynamically stable child who is showing signs of poor oxygen delivery, altered mental status, and acidosis.

Cyanide Poisoning

Cyanide is produced in fires from the combustion of plastics and certain glues that are used in homes and vehicles. Cyanide toxicity can also be deadly, especially if treatment is not started immediately (74).

Pathophysiology

Cyanide is absorbed into the bloodstream and binds to cytochrome oxidase. **Cytochrome oxidase** is a component of the electron transport chain that turns oxygen into energy for the body. Aerobic metabolism is then prevented, and the body needs to use anaerobic metabolism for energy production. Anaerobic metabolism is inefficient, and the body will begin to show signs of poor oxygen delivery.

Cyanide poisoning also will not be picked up on pulse oximetry. The amount of oxyhemoglobin does not change, but the body's ability to use the bound oxygen is the problem.

Clinical Manifestations

Cyanide poisoning can be very difficult to diagnose and so is assumed until proven otherwise in most inhalation injuries. The deciding factor for the diagnosis should be persistent metabolic acidosis despite adequate oxygenation as seen by ABG values. The reasoning is that lung injury affects oxygen exchange, but acidosis should not occur with a PaO_2 greater than 60 mm Hg in a hemodynamically stable patient. Cyanide bioassays have not been proven to be helpful, and treatment should be started if the diagnosis is possible (75).

Management and Treatment

The two major treatments for cyanide toxicity are sodium thiosulfate and hydroxocobalamin. **Sodium thiosulfate** helps increase the conversion of cyanide to specific nitrates. This prevents the binding with cytochrome oxidase so that aerobic metabolism will continue. The concern is that the nitrates combine with the heme groups on red cells to create **methemoglobin**. Methemoglobin will hold onto oxygen, but delivery of oxygen to the body is decreased. Infants are extremely sensitive to this process because fetal hemoglobin readily converts to methemoglobin. Oxygen delivery can be compromised, especially if the amount of carboxyhemoglobin is elevated as well (Clinical Variation 18-1) (76).

Hydroxocobalamin is the precursor to vitamin B_{12}. It binds cyanide and forms cyanocobalamin, and it is excreted without any toxic effects. This therapy is most often used in children because of the concerns for use of methemoglobinemia (77, 78).

Course and Prognosis

The course and prognosis for burn injuries are variable. First, it is difficult to know the severity of the inhalation injury until days after the incident. Second, morbidity and mortality are greatly influenced by the concomitant body surface area burns. What we do know is inhalation injury is now the leading cause of death in burn patients.

There is a delay in the effects of tissue injury in smoke inhalation. The epithelial layer can slough off, but this can take 3 to 4 days. Bronchoscopy at

Table 18-2 Carboxyhemoglobin Signs and Symptoms (73)

Carboxyhemoglobin levels	3%–20%	20%–40%	>60%–70%
Systemic effects	Lightheadedness, nausea, headache	Confusion, disorientation	Ataxia, seizures, coma, cardiopulmonary collapse

Clinical Variations 18-1

Cyanide Poisoning

It is common that burn patients will be taken to the closest ED for stabilization. It is important to know the subtle signs of cyanide poisoning because it is easily treated but just as easily missed. Clinical signs include the following:

- Unusually red or pink skin (oxygen not being removed from hemoglobin)
- Headache, nausea, altered mental status (early signs of hypoxia)
- Lactic acidosis despite adequate oxygenation

Quick therapy is lifesaving, and patients die because of delayed diagnosis.

---

this time is better able to evaluate the extent of injury and the morbidity and mortality risks for the victim.

Thirty percent of burn patients will also have smoke-inhalation injuries. The morbidity and mortality rate is between 3% and 10% for all burns and increases to 20% to 30% with concomitant smoke inhalation. Pediatric mortality is directly dependent on total body surface area (TBSA) burned. Patients with a 73% TBSA burn have a 10% burn-associated predicted mortality, but the mortality rate increases dramatically to 50% at the same TBSA when the victim has a smoke-inhalation injury as well (47, 78). Calculating the percentage of burns is based on patient age and thickness of the burns. A common formula used to calculate the percentage of skin burned is the **rule of nines**. When using this calculation for adults, the head represents 9%, each upper extremity 9%, the back of the trunk 18%, the front of the trunk 18%, each lower extremity 18%, and the perineum the last 1%. In children, percentage of burn calculation should take into consideration the age of the child because body proportions are different from those of adults. The rule of nines has been adapted for children to include the head as 18% and each lower extremity as 13.5%, with the rest of the calculations the same as adults. The Berkow formula was designed as a way to more accurately calculate TBSA burns in children and has percentages based on age (79).

Multisystem organ failure is a common finding in severe burns. The cause can be from the primary burn and lung injury leading to ARDS, rhabdomyolysis (skeletal muscle destruction, causing acute renal failure), and sepsis, among many others. Carbon monoxide and cyanide poisoning can also cause multisystem organ failure. When the end organs are starved for oxygen, the body begins anaerobic metabolism. The acids that are made during this process further damage these organs, leading to their failure. The more organs affected, the higher the morbidity and mortality rate for the patient (Teamwork 18-1).

Chronic complications are rare in child victims of inhalation injury. There is concern, however, for possible decreased exercise endurance and cardiac limitation during maximal exercise (54, 80). The severity of the complications correlate with the severity of inhalation injury. Overall, most children do well with minimal, if any, noticeable effects.

Aspiration

The study of aspiration in children is complicated by the different causes and variability in treatment. Simply, **aspiration** is defined as material passing the vocal cords and into the tracheobronchial tree. The material can be volatile, solids, or oral secretions. Because the epidemiology, pathophysiology, management, and prognosis are so different for the various causes of aspiration, they will be discussed in separate sections below.

Lung injury is the common component for any type of aspiration and leads to respiratory distress and decompensation. RTs must be able to identify different types of aspiration since treatment for one could potentially harm a patient that is affected by another.

Teamwork 18-1 Sometimes You Have to Be a Mediator

PATIENTS WITH MULTIPLE INJURIES AND MEDICAL CONCERNS CAN HAVE A NUMBER OF DIFFERENT SURGICAL AND MEDICAL TEAMS TAKING CARE OF THEM. For instance, our burn patient is a trauma patient and a PICU patient. The two teams are helping take care of the child, and sometimes the goals of therapy can contradict each other. The patient may have a small pneumothorax that would benefit from 100% oxygen, but this could be harmful to the lungs and the rest of the body. The teams may express their ideas to you because you are at the bedside and the one making ventilator changes. It is important to bring the team together rather than becoming frustrated with contradicting orders. There are strategies that may help:

- Stating the objective reasons why you believe making changes could be harmful
- Calling other members of your team to the bedside to have a group discussion and then make a decision together

Foreign Body Aspiration

Potential foreign body aspiration is a common phenomenon in children. The peak age for aspiration is between 1 and 2 years, and the majority of aspiration events occur before the age of 4 years (81). Food and other organic material is the most frequently aspirated material in younger children, whereas plastics and produced goods are more commonly aspirated in older children (Fig. 18-5) (82). The National Safety Council and other product safety commissions have increased their scrutiny of toys and other materials approved for children, but one-fifth of fatally aspirated objects have passed this inspection (83). Foreign body aspiration will continue to be a problem despite improved safety by companies and monitoring by parents.

Pathophysiology

The pathophysiology of foreign body aspiration in children is split into two separate aspects. The first is a behavior/anatomy component of why it occurs, and the second is the body's response to the aspiration.

Behavior

It is no coincidence that the "terrible twos" is a peak time of aspiration for children. Children ages 1 to 2 years are inquisitive, prone to put objects in their mouths, and will routinely test the limits of their caregivers and their own bodies. They are also easily distracted and are often not focused on eating. Children are often just beginning to ambulate; supervision is then more difficult, thereby increasing the chance of accidents. Older children are affected by many of the same traits. Often, children will place objects in their mouths, pen caps being common, and get distracted or bump into something and aspirate rather than swallow the object.

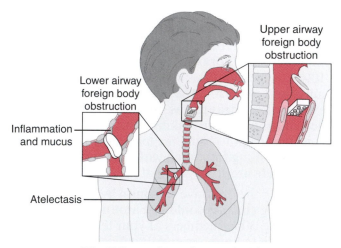

Figure 18-5 The Effects of Foreign Body Airway Obstruction on the Airway

Anatomy and Physiology

Children have a number of anatomical and physiological qualities that increase their likelihood of aspiration. The process of chewing food is a complicated neuromuscular process that is initiated by the tearing of food with incisors. The first of these incisors usually come in around age 1 year. The molars used to grind food do not come in until around 2 years of age. The food that is swallowed before age 2 years is often still in chunks, whereas the food swallowed after the molar eruption is typically chewed completely prior to swallowing (81).

Swallowing involves the control of numerous cranial nerves and coordination of at least 20 muscles. Some of these muscles and nerves are not fully developed until the age of 8 years, thereby leading to poor muscle coordination and possible aspiration.

Upper Airway Foreign Body

The upper airway is defined as the nasopharynx and oropharynx—essentially the area above the vocal cord. To aspirate a foreign body in the upper airway, the foreign body must be small enough to enter the upper airway but large enough to become trapped above the vocal cords. The body's response is dependent on the area that is being obstructed by the object. An object that is completely blocking the vocal cords can cause minimal to no airflow into the lungs. This can lead to a negative pressure pulmonary edema and, if the obstruction is not removed, a hypoxic cardiac arrest.

A partial foreign body airway obstruction (FBAO) has its own concerns. Airflow may be enough to allow for adequate oxygenation, but there may be significant amounts of localized inflammation and edema that could turn a partial obstruction into a complete one. It is for these reasons that medical personnel must work quickly when a patient shows signs of an upper-airway foreign body.

Lower Airway Foreign Body

The majority of foreign body aspirations are found and removed shortly after the initial incident. There are times, however, when there is no history of aspiration and the symptoms are subtle, so that the diagnosis is not made for weeks and sometimes months. The pathophysiology of these events is significantly different from that of an upper airway foreign body.

The initial response to a lower airway foreign body is inflammation and swelling. This decreases the diameter of the bronchial tree, and a plug is formed around the foreign body by secretions, inflammatory cells, and mucus. The plug does not allow airflow to the distal bronchioles and alveoli, and this area becomes atelectatic. The plug can become a nidus of infection, and a partial lobar pneumonia can occur (84). The chronic inflammation can cause bronchiole hyperreactivity similar to that seen in asthma.

Clinical Manifestations

The clinical manifestations of upper versus lower FBAO may differ and may help clinicians distinguish which portion of the airway is affected. Quick assessment is necessary depending on the size of the object aspirated and the degree of airway obstruction to reverse symptoms and prevent complete airway obstruction.

Upper Airway Foreign Body

The symptoms of upper airway obstructions vary dependent on the type of obstruction and the timing of presentation. Upper airway obstructions usually present quickly after inhalation, and the symptoms are rarely subtle. They include, in increasing level of severity, the following:

- Coughing
- Change in phonation (different voice)
- Wheezing
- Stridor
- Retractions
- Hypoxia/cyanosis

Drooling and difficulty swallowing can also be seen, but this is more common with esophageal foreign bodies and with inflammation and swelling of the glottis in epiglottitis.

Lower Airway Foreign Body

The difficulty with lower airway foreign body aspirations is the variability in their symptoms. The initial symptoms involve the irritation of the airway, including coughing and respiratory distress. Once in the lower airway, these acute symptoms disappear until the chronic wheezing and recurrent pneumonias occur. Anywhere from 10% to 50% of foreign bodies are removed without the child having any symptoms, making the history key in the diagnosis.

Clinical symptoms can include the following:

- Wheezing
- Decreased breath sounds
- Crackles
- Dullness to percussion, secondary to pneumonia
- Fever, secondary to pneumonia
- On CXR, hyperinflation of ipsilateral (same) side (Fig. 18-6)

Management and Treatment

The management and treatment of an upper airway foreign body is simple: immediate removal of the foreign body. The algorithm divides, depending on whether the child is coughing. If the patient

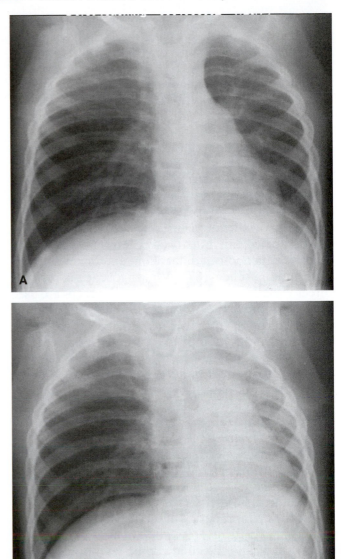

Figure 18-6 Chest Radiograph of a 20-Month-Old Who Aspirated a Peanut Into the Right Bronchus Intermedius *(Courtesy of Jane Benson, MD)*

is coughing, provide no medical care until the object is removed from the airway or the child's medical status deteriorates.

There are some maneuvers that can allow delay until the definitive procedure can be completed if the child is stable but still shows sign of a foreign body. The first of these is prone positioning (85). This increases the diameter of the airway and allows for spontaneous respiration and improved airflow. Racemic epinephrine can be used to decrease the swelling around a foreign body, potentially improving airflow; however, it can also cause a partial obstruction to become a complete obstruction.

A complete airway obstruction requires immediate attempts to remove the foreign body. One of these maneuvers that anyone can perform is abdominal thrusting, typically called the Heimlich maneuver (86). Back thrusts are the treatment of choice in children younger than 1 year because of concerns that the Heimlich maneuver can cause liver injury. The best scenario is that the foreign body is ejected completely out of the airway, but the object may need to be removed under direct visualization.

The removal under direct visualization is complicated in children, potentially requiring sedation (in a partial obstruction) or the need for urgent removal (in a complete obstruction). With a partial obstruction, it is important to keep the child spontaneously breathing. Medications used for sedation that have been reported individually or in combination include ketamine, propofol, midazolam, and dexmedetomidine, among others (87). A laryngoscope is used for direct visualization, and then Magill forceps are used to either remove the object or, if unable, to push the object through the trachea and past the main bronchus in an attempt to oxygenate and ventilate through one lung. A balloon catheter is another unique way of potentially removing a foreign body. The catheter is passed beyond the area of obstruction, the bulb is expanded, and then the object and the catheter are removed (88).

The most invasive therapy for an upper airway foreign body is an emergency cricothyroidotomy. This is usually a last resort, but it is lifesaving in certain situations. A scalpel is used to make a small incision along the cricothyroid membrane. This incision is used to pierce the membrane and enter the trachea. An endotracheal or tracheostomy tube can be placed through the incision, and the child can be temporarily ventilated until a stable airway is placed (89).

Removal of the foreign body in the lower airway is essential to the resolution of symptoms. This is done by rigid bronchoscopy and allows diagnosis and removal. It is the recommendation of many experts that bronchoscopy be completed on all children with a history of choking, even in the absence of any radiological signs (90). A short course of antibiotic therapy and steroids is suggested after a long impaction (91).

There have been three reported cases of using ECMO for delayed presentation of a foreign body. ECMO was used to stabilize an extremely ill patient either to allow for foreign body removal or immediately after the removal (92–94).

Course and Prognosis

The general prognosis of foreign body aspiration is complete recovery and resolution of all symptoms. The only exception is for children who had a complete obstruction and asphyxiation. Mortality in these cases is up to 45%, and survivors have a 30% risk of neurological devastation caused by prolonged hypoxia (95).

Chemical Pneumonitis

Chemical pneumonitis is the inhalation or ingestion and then aspiration of certain chemicals that cause inflammation and damage to the lung. Many chemicals can cause chemical pneumonitis, but this section focuses on the two most common and damaging causes: hydrocarbons and lipoid products.

Hydrocarbons

Hydrocarbons are chemical compounds made only of hydrogen and carbon. The majority of hydrocarbons are found in crude oil and made into gasoline and certain oils. Methane, butane, and propane are commonly used hydrocarbons that are found in fuels, lighters, and cleaning products.

Injuries usually occur after ingestion of hydrocarbons and their subsequent aspiration. Hydrocarbons have a very low viscosity, and the poor development of swallowing in children leads to the high likelihood of aspiration. Aspiration of hydrocarbons accounts for approximately 2% of the accidental poisonings seen in children, but some studies suggest they are 7% of cases that actually seek medical attention (96, 97).

Pathophysiology

As discussed, the majority of hydrocarbons are of low viscosity, increasing the probability of aspiration. They also have very low surface tension, which allows the hydrocarbon to spread diffusely and evenly over the affected area. Hydrocarbons are very volatile and can be absorbed by the alveoli instead of oxygen, leading to cyanosis and acute respiratory distress.

Ventilation/perfusion mismatch is the subacute pathology caused by hydrocarbon aspiration, primarily through bronchospasm, atelectasis from surfactant breakdown, and destruction of the alveolar-capillary membrane.

- Bronchospasm causes airway constriction and poor airflow and oxygen exchange. This leads to poor systemic oxygenation and end-organ dysfunction.
- Atelectasis occurs after the direct interaction of hydrocarbons with surfactant and continued damage after the breakdown of the alveolar-capillary membrane (98, 99).
- The breakdown of the alveolar-capillary membrane induces inflammatory cells and hemorrhaging, causing an ARDS-like situation for affected children. Areas of lung that were not affected by hydrocarbons can still have induced injury from the systemic inflammatory response, which further complicates therapy.

Systemic effects are rare but can be severe. They include the following:

- Central nervous system: Tremors, coma
- Cardiac: Cardiomyopathy
- Gastroenterology: Vomiting, nausea

Clinical Manifestations

The respiratory distress seen in hydrocarbon aspiration can be severe and can occur immediately. Clinical signs are as follows:

- Tachypnea
- Coughing
- Cyanosis/hypoxia
- Retractions
- Atelectasis seen on CXR
- Pneumatoceles, which is a late finding during resolution of acute disease

Management and Treatment

The therapy for hydrocarbon aspiration is dependent on the severity of symptoms. The majority of potential aspiration events require no major medical interventions or even hospital admission (100). The primary morbidity and mortality comes from ARDS-like symptoms, and it is no surprise that treatment is very similar to that used for any cause of ARDS. Surfactant therapy, inhaled and systemic steroids, and nitric oxide are the only therapies that are distinctly discussed for consideration in this section (Table 18-3).

Exogenous Surfactant

Studies of surfactant use in ARDS include hydrocarbon aspiration, but there are no prospective studies looking at its use in this subpopulation. There are animal data that suggest an improvement in compliance, blood gas measurements, and survival (101). There is only one case report that showed a significant improvement in respiratory status of a 17-month-old boy after two doses of surfactant (102). The pathophysiology of direct surfactant damage gives reason

to believe it may be beneficial despite equivocal results in ARDS caused by other conditions. Prospective large studies would need to be undertaken before widespread surfactant use in hydrocarbon-induced lung injury could be advised.

Corticosteroids

There are some data on the use of inhaled and systemic steroids for hydrocarbon aspiration. The benefits are decreased inflammation and secondary injury from the localized and systemic inflammatory response. Inhaled steroids have few if any major side effects, but the concern about systemic steroids has always been increased infection risk. There are a handful of case reports advocating the use of steroids in this subpopulation of ARDS, but there are no prospective data on its use (103–105).

Nitric Oxide

There is only one case report discussing the benefit of nitric oxide in hydrocarbon aspiration. This one patient had an improvement in oxygenation and pulmonary hypertension (106).

Course and Prognosis

The clinical course of hydrocarbon aspiration is usually complete recovery. The major cause of morbidity is lung injury. However, lung injury only occurs in about 12% of cases, and the extent of injury is variable. The mortality for all cases was only 2% in the largest retrospective study completed (107).

There are conflicting data on the long-term effects in patients with hydrocarbon-induced lung injury. The largest of these studies showed pulmonary function abnormalities in children 8 to 14 years after the inciting event (108). These were all asymptomatic children, and it is important to know that these children were all studied well before ARDS guidelines were established. In two small studies, there were no significant changes in pulmonary function after these events (99, 109).

Lipoids

The aspiration of **lipoids**—oils and animal fats—is an uncommon cause of respiratory distress in children. However, many of these substances, such as mineral oil or petroleum jelly, are used as home remedies for a number of minor medical conditions, including chronic constipation, dry lips, and GI upset. There can be a delay in the respiratory symptoms after lipoid aspiration, and medical personnel must be vigilant in recognizing home therapies that could potentially cause severe lung injury.

Pathophysiology

The pathophysiology of lipoid aspiration is similar to that seen in hydrocarbon aspiration. There is a behavioral aspect to lipoid aspiration in that children

Table 18-3	Clinical Decision-Making for Aspiration (99)	
Symptoms of Respiratory Distress	**CXR Findings Consistent With Aspiration**	**Admit/ Discharge**
Yes	Yes	Admit
No	Yes	Admit
Yes	No	Monitor for 6 hours and repeat CXR if normal and symptoms improved: Discharge
No	No	Discharge

attempt to swallow material they shouldn't swallow, and anatomical and physiological development make aspiration likely. There are important differences, however, and these can affect clinical manifestations and therapy.

The first of these differences is the taste and acidity of the chemicals. Oils and fats either have no taste or taste good to children. Hydrocarbons are usually fairly noxious, and there will be an immediate negative response from the child who ingests them. Therefore, with lipoids, it can be more difficult to obtain a history of aspiration, and more of the substance could be aspirated. Oils can diminish or inhibit the gag reflex, again making the determination of aspiration difficult (110). Parents give the lipoid product for therapy and may not associate a medication as a possible cause for respiratory failure. This increases the probability of subsequent events and might not be discussed as a potential cause of respiratory distress by the parent.

The primary cause of lung injury in lipoid aspiration is direct inflammation. The oils cause a cytokine release, and macrophages and other inflammatory cells are released into the lung parenchyma. The subsequent inflammatory response is similar to that seen with hydrocarbons. The difference is the inflammatory response can be blunted, and symptoms can be acute or occur years after initial exposure. Lipoids also stay in the alveolar space, which can further delay and prolong symptoms. Lipoid aspiration does have an effect on the mucociliary response of the tracheobronchial tree. This inhibits the expectoration of the lipoid and allows persistent inflammation (111).

Clinical Manifestations

There can be repeated lipoid aspirations before a child shows any respiratory symptoms. History is extremely important and is usually the key component in the diagnosis of a lipoid aspiration. There are no clinical symptoms or radiological studies that suggest a lipoid aspiration, and the symptoms are similar to many of the other pathological conditions that cause respiratory distress:

- Tachypnea
- Persistent cough
- Cyanosis/hypoxia
- Recurrent pneumonias
- Lipid-laden macrophages on bronchoalveolar lavage constitute a definitive diagnosis

Management and Treatment

Medical personnel must have patience when treating lipoid aspiration. The majority of cases have an indolent (inactive or slow) course as explained in the pathophysiology section above. Therefore, the treatment focuses on decreasing the acute and chronic inflammation and decreasing secondary injury from

pneumonia. The two mainstays for treating lipoid pneumonia are antibiotics and steroids (112–115). There is a case report of using intravenous immunoglobulin, but its use is not as widely reported as steroids and antibiotics (115). This treatment is used primarily during the initial presentation; there is no evidence that early treatment or any treatment improves the course of the disease.

Course and Prognosis

The outcome and prognosis of lipoid aspiration are favorable, and patients are likely to make a complete recovery. However, there are cases of acute decompensation and death. The course is indolent, and it can take years for patients to make a full recovery. Some data indicate that the chronic inflammation from the indolent course can cause fibrosis and lung insufficiency (116). This has led to right heart failure in some adult patients, but no long-term outcome studies have been completed with children (117).

Oral Secretions

Secretions can include both oral and gastric secretions. The section on oral secretions includes the aspiration of formula and other material in children with oral motor pathology. The section on gastric secretions will focus on reflux and the effect of gastric contents on the lung parenchyma.

The aspiration of oropharyngeal secretions has become an increasing problem in the pediatric population. **Dysfunctional swallowing** is a broad term that describes abnormalities in swallowing or managing oropharyngeal secretions; it is a well-recognized cause of aspiration in children and can be caused by prematurity, CNS abnormalities, and craniofacial syndromes (118, 119). Aspiration of oropharyngeal secretions causes lung damage and increases the likelihood of pneumonias. Furthermore, the major causes of dysfunctional swallowing are not temporary in nature, thus leading to recurrent aspiration, lung damage, and pneumonias (Special Populations 18-2).

Data suggest that oropharyngeal aspiration is the most common cause of recurrent pneumonias in children and the cause of 8% of all pneumonias seen in the hospital (120). This number is likely to increase because there is a link between neurologically impaired children and pneumonias. The number of neurologically disabled patients is increasing, primarily as a result of improvement in neonatal intensive care unit and PICU survival. However, it is important to note that there are children with recurrent aspiration who have no apparent risks of dysfunctional swallowing. These children are often misdiagnosed and can go months to years without being adequately treated (121).

● **Special Populations 18-2**

Temporary Versus Permanent Enteral Feeding

Children with cerebral palsy (CP) or neuromuscular disorders are more likely to have dysfunctional swallowing than healthy children. Children with CP are different from patients who are neurocognitively normal or who have anatomical abnormalities. Children with CP and neuromuscular disorders are unlikely to show improvement in their dysfunctional swallowing. In fact, they are more likely to get worse and aspirate more over time. Temporary therapy for children with CP is probably not the best option, and surgical intervention is probably warranted. By contrast, children who may benefit from temporary enteral feeding include the following:

- Burn patients: High caloric needs and pain control may increase aspiration risk.
- Patients with head trauma: It is useful if full recovery is thought to be likely.
- Infants with recent surgery: It may take time for infants to relearn how to feed orally.

Pathophysiology

The pathophysiology of oropharyngeal aspiration is similar to that of the aspiration of hydrocarbons and lipoids. The muscles and cranial nerves required to swallow involve a significant amount of coordination. This is developed over time but can be significantly delayed in patients with the risk factors for dysfunctional swallowing. Prematurity can cause a developmental delay, and oral and motor tone may be decreased. CNS abnormalities can cause cranial nerve dysfunction, making it impossible to completely coordinate swallowing. Craniofacial syndromes may make coordinated swallowing impossible secondary to anatomical concerns. Many of these issues are temporary and require surgical or medical management to decrease aspiration risk.

The aspiration of oral secretions, even without any foreign liquids, can cause damage to the lungs. It becomes a major issue when it occurs repeatedly, since the recurrent damage can cause a significant amount of long-term damage. Aspiration usually causes an immediate reaction from the child. Normal chemoreceptors and reflexes cause coughing in an attempt to remove the material from the airway. There are times when patients who aspirate don't elicit any of these reflexes. This is termed **silent aspiration** and can occur in as many as 80% of all patients who aspirate (122).

The oropharyngeal secretions and liquids that are aspirated are mostly made of water. The components that cause lung damage are the enzymes that are found in saliva and the acidity of foreign liquids. The primary function of saliva is to moisten food and begin the digestion of proteins and sugars contained in it. These enzymes will also break down proteins of the lung parenchyma, causing local inflammation and further lung damage. The acidity of saliva is usually around pH 7.0 (normal), but it can vary and cause cell damage as well. Liquids do not usually break down lung proteins, but they cause localized inflammation and can cause cellular damage due to acidity. Both vehicles of aspiration can bring oral bacteria with them and infect the lung, causing pneumonias (119, 120).

Clinical Manifestations

Children affected by aspiration of oropharyngeal secretions can be healthy or have a number of medical conditions. Symptoms, then, will vary based on a particular child's health. The most common clinical signs of oral secretion aspiration include the following:

- Cough
- Tachypnea
- Hypoxia/cyanosis
- Recurrent pneumonia

There are two specific gold-standard diagnostic tests for the aspiration of food and secretions. Placing dye in the oropharyngeal space and then subsequently checking the airway will prove that secretions are being aspirated. Simple endotracheal suction will show this in an intubated patient. Radioactive dye could be used in a patient who is not intubated, followed by sequential CXRs (121). The gold standard to diagnose the aspiration of food is the videofluoroscopic study (VFSS) (122). A VFSS allows a trained practitioner to look at the dynamic changes that are required for swallowing and can actively show food traveling past the vocal cords. The food is also radioactive and will show up as radiopaque on any image.

Management and Treatment

The therapy for aspiration is dependent on its cause. A temporary solution may be required if a child is premature and developmentally delayed. A more long-term option may be needed for a child who has a craniofacial abnormality. It may be impossible to prevent aspiration of oral secretions in some neurologically impaired patients, and treatment is only partially beneficial.

Enteral Feeding

Enteral feeding is one of the primary therapies for oral motor dysfunction. This can be done using a nasogastric tube or a nasoduodenal tube. These tubes are placed at the bedside and involve minimal risks. Unfortunately, these tubes are temporary, can easily be removed, can be misplaced and cause aspiration, and potentially increase the risk of upper airway infections. Gastric tubes and gastrojejunal tubes are more permanent types of enteral feeding. These require surgical procedures, increasing the risk of complications, but they are relatively routine procedures in the surgical world (123). There is some evidence of fewer respiratory complications when placing the distal end of the tube past the stomach (124).

Glycopyrrolate

Glycopyrrolate is an anticholinergic medication that inhibits the muscarinic receptors. These receptors allow salivation, and studies show that drooling and secretions are significantly decreased with its use. There are no data that suggest it improves respiratory status or decreases the likelihood of pneumonias (125).

Tracheostomy

Tracheostomy is surgical procedure to place a tube through the trachea cutaneously to bypass the upper airway. It is used in children for a number of reasons, one of which is persistent aspiration from oral secretions. The tracheostomy tube allows the suctioning of these secretions in children who have a weak cough from neuromuscular disorders. Theoretically, this should decrease lung damage from continued aspiration, but no studies were found that have explored this potential benefit. If a cuffed tracheostomy tube is used, it will further protect from aspiration.

Course and Prognosis

Chronic aspiration rarely occurs in healthy children. However, it can cause persistent respiratory symptoms, including wheezing, cough, chronic congestion, and pneumonias (121). Chronic aspiration is an even bigger problem in patients with other medical conditions. This is most commonly seen in former premature infants who have chronic lung disease. Their reserve is poor, and even the mildest of aspirations can cause respiratory failure and more lung damage. Persistent lung damage can cause pulmonary hypertension and lead to heart failure. Children with neurological and developmental abnormalities can have a number of these events before receiving medical or surgical therapy, and their lung function could be limited, at best, by then. Aggressive and early treatment of aspiration is extremely important in reducing the morbidities associated with chronic aspiration (126).

Gastric Secretions

The reflux of gastric contents is one of the most common symptoms seen in healthy infants and in infants with numerous medical conditions. Gastroesophageal reflux disease (GERD) rarely has any major complications in infants. GERD in infants can cause discomfort, and the major treatment is to increase the pH of the gastric contents to cause less pain. Complications can arise when the gastric secretions are aspirated, which can cause significant lung injury and morbidity.

Pathophysiology

The pathophysiology of gastric and oral secretion aspiration is closely linked. Reflux can occur and can cause damage to the esophagus and upper airway, but damage will not occur to the trachea and lower airway unless swallowing dysfunction is also present. Prematurity and neurological disorders predispose children to both swallowing dysfunction and reflux. Muscle tone of the lower esophageal sphincter is fundamental to keeping gastric contents out of the esophagus and can be poor in both conditions. Reflux and swallowing dysfunction can be seen in completely normal infants, too, and can be silent as in the aspiration of oral secretions (127).

Gastric contents are acidic and full of enzymes that continue the breakdown of food for digestion. During digestion, the pH of the stomach can reach 1 to 2 and when empty is 4 to 5. Acidity alone can cause an inflammatory response and cytokine release that will damage the lung parenchyma. Repeated events will cause continued damage to the lung, as can recurrent pneumonias from bacteria aspirated from the mouth. Pepsin is the unique enzyme in the stomach that breaks down dietary proteins. Pepsin can hydrolyze lung parenchymal proteins and can be a major cause of fibrosis in chronic aspiration of gastric contents. Pepsin has been used as a marker of chronic aspiration, but the prevalence of respiratory symptoms developing from gastric aspiration is still unknown (128).

Clinical Manifestations

Clinical signs of gastric aspiration include the following:

- Cough
- Tachypnea
- Wheezing
- Hypoxia/cyanosis
- Recurrent pneumonias

There are a number of studies used to diagnose reflux. It is important to note that the child must have a swallowing dysfunction in order to aspirate. A pH probe is the study of choice for reflux. There are multiple ways the test can be done, but in general a probe is placed down the esophagus with multiple ports that test for pH and/or fluid. The ports can tell how high the reflux events are rising, as well as the pH of the contents. The data are reported as reflux index or the percentage of time esophageal pH is less than 4 (129).

There are some studies that report the testing of pepsin in airway secretions. This would show that the protein is entering the lung and would be a direct evaluation of gastric aspiration. This test has yet to be validated against other routine studies (130).

Management and Treatment

Medical management is only partially successful if a patient continues reflux and aspiration. The focus of management is to decrease the pH that is being refluxed using H_2 blockers or proton pump inhibitors (PPIs) and to decrease the transit time through the digestive track. H_2 blockers and PPIs increase the pH of gastric contents but do not prevent aspiration. There is also a concern that the decrease in pH may actually increase the likelihood of a secondary pneumonia from aspiration, although this has only been shown in adults (131). Medications such as metoclopramide and erythromycin have been used to decrease transit time in the stomach because they are promotility agents, thereby decreasing the chance of reflux.

Surgical management is the only definitive treatment for aspiration of gastric contents. The primary surgery is called a Nissen fundoplication, which decreases the chance of reflux by tightening the lower esophageal sphincter. The top portion of the stomach is wrapped around the esophagus and sutured. This keeps the sphincter tight and prevents flow of gastric contents into the esophagus. This can be done with or without a gastric tube if there is concern for aspiration of oral secretions (132).

The simplest therapy for gastric aspiration is positioning. The best position to decrease the likelihood of aspiration is supine with the head at approximately 30 degrees to use gravity to help prevent secretions from rising up the esophagus.

Course and Prognosis

The outcome from gastric aspiration is similar to that of oropharyngeal aspiration. The comorbidities are very important when looking at the effects of aspiration. Many premature infants have chronic lung disease; neuromuscular patients have poor respiratory effort at baseline; cerebral palsy patients have lower lung volumes from scoliosis; and all of these patients are at risk for reflux and aspiration. The more aspiration events patients have, the more likely they are to develop lung inflammation and recurrent pneumonias. Inflammation leads to chronic fibrosis and poor pulmonary function and is the major morbidity of aspiration.

■ ■ John was maintained on MV for a total of 8 days while his pulmonary status was uncertain. During that time, you and the team of ICU nurses, physicians, and RTs continuously struggled to manage the hypoxemia and tachypnea from his pulmonary edema and atelectasis, as well as the pneumonia he had been diagnosed with early on. On day 8, John was extubated to bi-level positive airway pressure and continued on that for 3 additional days before being weaned to a 2-L nasal cannula. Two weeks after his near-drowning in the pool, he was transferred out of the ICU to the school-age pulmonary inpatient unit. He was sent home 6 days later without respiratory support.

■ ■ Critical Thinking Questions: John Smith

1. When John was decompensating shortly after his arrival and required bag-mask ventilation, what interventions would you have suggested to the physician if you were unable to see chest movement during ventilation attempts?
2. When John presented with atelectasis and PEEP was increased, why was the PIP also increased? What would be some additional ventilator strategies that might have improved John's lung inflation?
3. Do you think at any point that John was developing ARDS? What evidence helped you come to that conclusion?

▶● Case Studies and Critical Thinking Questions

■ Case 1: Jamie Lynn

Jamie Lynn is a 6-year-old girl who was found on the floor of her room by firefighters at 2 a.m. The firefighters were called when a neighbor noticed flames coming from the basement of the house. All the other residents were removed from the house before the firefighters arrived. The flames were spreading to the main floor, and the firefighters were able to remove Jamie Lynn after about 15 minutes. She was unconscious when removed but woke up in the ambulance on the way to the hospital. She was coughing heavily upon entering the ED, and her face was covered with soot. Jamie Lynn begins to develop very quiet stridor after the initial triage.

- *What should the initial management decision be for Jamie Lynn?*
- *What are some of the most important laboratory results to obtain when concerned*

about inhalation injury and possible systemic complications?

Jamie Lynn was doing well after intubation with these vital signs: heart rate (HR), 104 bpm; blood pressure (BP), 104/72; RR, 24 breaths per minute; pulse oximetry, 100% on 100% oxygen; and temperature, 99.4°F. The ABG values were 7.34/42/480, but the lactate was 4. The lactate test was repeated and came back at 5.4. The carboxyhemoglobin came back at 24%.

- *What is the potential concern?*
- *How do you treat it and what by-product should be monitored?*

■ Case 2: Stephan Hyde

Stephan Hyde is a 2-year-old boy who comes into the ED because his mother states he has been wheezing for the last 2 days. The mother says he has no history of wheezing and has not been sick recently. When you listen to him, you hear normal breath sounds on the right but poor breath sounds and wheezing on the left.

- *What are your concerns? What is the best way to further investigate your diagnosis?*
- *What should we do next for Stephan?*

■ Case 3: TJ Johnson

TJ Johnson is an 18-month-old boy who was watching his dad in the family garage. The dad was using an ethanol-based cleaner to remove grease from one of his tools. He heard his son coughing and noticed TJ was holding the cleaner in his hand. There were drips of the fluid on TJ's shirt, and the dad was concerned he may have swallowed some of the cleaner and brought him into the ED.

- What are the keys to deciding what TJ needs?
- What should you do next?
- Should TJ be admitted or discharged?

Multiple-Choice Questions

1. What is the best ventilator change for a patient showing signs of worsening pulmonary edema?
   a. Decrease PEEP
   b. Increase PIP
   c. Increase PEEP
   d. Decrease FIO_2
   e. Increase respiratory rate

2. Which of the following is *not* a poor prognostic sign for a drowning patient in the ED?
   a. CPR in the field
   b. CPR upon entering the ED
   c. Initial pH of 7.3 on ABG laboratory test
   d. Fixed and dilated pupils

3. Inhalation risk is at its highest in a patient who has
   a. High minute ventilation.
   b. Been exposed to a fire in an enclosed space.
   c. Been exposed to a fire in which numerous chemicals and plastics were found burned in the house.
   d. All of the above

4. Which patient below is best suited to undergo treatment in a hyperbaric chamber?
   a. A 10-year-old boy who had a flash burn from a gasoline tank explosion with facial burns and a carboxyhemoglobin of less than 0.9%
   b. A 17-year-old girl who was found in a fire of a chemical plant, has altered mental status, a BP of 70/45, and a carboxyhemoglobin of 58%
   c. A 6-year-old boy who was found in a house fire, has no respiratory symptoms, has vital signs including a BP of 98/44, a RR of 34, and carboxyhemoglobin of 48%
   d. A 2-year-old girl who was found in a house fire and was treated at an outside facility and transferred to you after 6 hours with normal vital signs and mental status and a carboxyhemoglobin level obtained 5 hours ago of 48%.

5. What is the first line of treatment for a patient who is thought to have carbon monoxide poisoning?
   a. Call to see if there is a hyperbaric chamber available anywhere near your facility
   b. Intubate the patient
   c. Place the patient on 100% non-rebreather mask
   d. Start sodium thiosulfate

6. A child has a known hydrocarbon aspiration at home. The child has no initial symptoms, but the chest radiograph shows bilateral interstitial infiltrates. How should this patient be triaged?
   a. Admit
   b. Wait 6 hours and repeat the CXR
   c. Discharge
   d. Check ABG values and if normal, discharge

7. A 6-week-old infant born at 34 weeks has had three recurrent pneumonias. A VFSS showed aspiration of thin liquids past the vocal cords

but a toleration of thickened feeds. The patient is breastfed. What should be done for this child's nutrition?

a. Place a surgical gastric tube
b. Feed through a nasogastric tube for 2 to 3 weeks and repeat the test
c. Allow the infant to feed normally
d. Have the mother pump and thicken the breast milk and repeat the swallow study in the future

8. A 2-year-old boy was seen chewing on a candy wrapper and then choking. The child is brought to the ED not talking, coughing occasionally, and in severe respiratory distress. The ED physician uses a laryngoscope but is unable to remove the wrapper with Magill forceps. The physician says the wrapper is completely obstructing the airway. What should you suggest he do?

a. Immediate tracheostomy
b. Attempt to use the Magill forceps and push the wrapper past the vocal cords to relieve the obstruction

c. Intubate the patient
d. Sedate the patient to make him more comfortable

9. What is the best way to initially attempt to remove a complete obstruction in a 9-month-old infant?

a. The Heimlich maneuver
b. Surgical removal
c. Blind finger sweep
d. Back thrusts

10. Which patient population would benefit from exogenous surfactant therapy?

 I. Near-drowning
 II. ARDS
 III. Aspiration
 IV. FBAO

a. I, II, III
b. I, III, IV
c. I, II, IV
d. II, III, IV

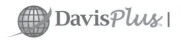 For additional resources login to Davis*Plus* (http://davisplus.fadavis.com/ keyword "Perretta") and click on the Premium tab. (Don't have a *Plus*Code to access Premium Resources? Just click the Purchase Access button on the book's Davis*Plus* page.)

REFERENCES

1. Centers for Disease Control and Prevention, National Center for Injury Prevention and Control. Web-based Injury Statistics Query and Reporting System (WISQARS). http://www.cdc.gov/injury/wisqars. Published November 24, 2009. Accessed January 15, 2013.
2. Thompson DC, Rivara FP. Pool fencing for preventing drowning in children. *Cochrane Database Syst Rev.* 2000;2: CD001047.
3. Karpovich PV. Water in the lungs of drowned animals. *Arch Pathol.* 1933;15:828-833.
4. Orlowski JP. Drowning, near-drowning, and ice-water submersions. *Pediatr Clin North Am.* 1987:34(1):75-92.
5. van Berkel M, Bierens JJ, Lie RL, et al. Pulmonary oedema, pneumonia and mortality in submersion victims; a retrospective study in 125 patients. *Intensive Care Med.* 1996;22(2):101-107.
6. Oswalt CE, Gates GA, Holmstrom MG. Pulmonary edema as a complication of acute airway obstruction. *JAMA.* 1977; 238(17):1833-1835.
7. Willms D, Shure D. Pulmonary edema due to upper airway obstruction in adults. *Chest.* 1988;94(5):1090-1092.
8. Pearn JH. Secondary drowning in children. *Br Med J.* 1980;281(6248):1103-1105.
9. Pratt FD, Haynes BE. Incidence of "secondary drowning" after saltwater submersion. *Ann Emerg Med.* 1986;15(9) 1084-1087.
10. Giammona ST, Modell JH. Drowning by total immersion: effects on pulmonary surfactant of distilled water, isotonic saline, and seawater. *Am J Dis Child.* 1967;114(6):612-616.

11. Modell JH, Graves SA, Ketover A. Clinical course of 91 consecutive near-drowning victims. *Chest.* 1976;70(2): 231-238.
12. Kennedy GA, Kanter RK, Weiner LB, Tompkins JM. Can early bacterial complications of aspiration with respiratory failure be predicted? *Pediatr Emerg Care.* 1992;8(3): 123-125.
13. Lee KH. A retrospective study of near-drowning victims admitted to the intensive care unit. *Ann Acad Med Singapore.* 1998;27(3):344-346.
14. Nichols D. *Rogers' Textbook of Pediatric Intensive Care.* Philadelphia, PA: Lippincott Williams & Wilkins; 2008.
15. Ware LB, Matthay MA. The acute respiratory distress syndrome. *New Engl J Med.* 2000;342:1334-1349.
16. Pelosi P, Jaber S. Noninvasive respiratory support in the perioperative period. *Curr Opin Anesthesiol.* 2010;23(2): 233-238.
17. Ruza F. Noninvasive ventilation in pediatric acute respiratory failure: a challenge in pediatric intensive care units. *Pediatr Crit Care Med.* 2010;11(6):750-751.
18. Kredel M, Muellenbach RM, Schlegel N, et al. Pulmonary effects of positive end-expiratory pressure and fluid therapy in experimental lung injury. *Exp Lung Res.* 2011;37(1): 35-43.
19. Lubrano R, Cecchetti C, Elli M, et al. Prognostic value of extravascular lung water index in critically ill children with acute respiratory failure. *Intensive Care Med.* 2011;37(1): 124-131.
20. Koh MS, Hsu AA, Eng P. Negative pressure pulmonary oedema in the medical intensive care unit. *Intensive Care Med.* 2003;29(9):1601-1604.

21. Peroni DG, Boner AL. Atelectasis: mechanisms, diagnosis and management. *Paediatr Respir Rev.* 2000;1(3):274-278.
22. Fowler AA 3rd, Scoggins WG, O'Donohue WJ Jr. Positive end-expiratory pressure in the management of lobar atelectasis. *Chest.* 1978;74(5):497-500.
23. Hendriks T, de Hoog M, Lequin MH, Devos AS, Merkus PJFM. DNase and atelectasis in non-cystic fibrosis pediatric patients. *Crit Care.* 2005;9(4):R351-R356.
24. McBrien M, Katumba JJ, Mukhtar AI. Artificial surfactant in the treatment of near drowning. *Lancet.* 1993;342(8885):1485-1486.
25. Cubattoli L, Franchi F, Coratti G. Surfactant therapy for acute respiratory failure after drowning: two children victim of cardiac arrest. *Resuscitation.* 2009;80(9):1088-1089.
26. Fields AI. Near-drowning in the pediatric population. *Crit Care Clin.* 1992;8(1):113-129.
27. Dahlem P, Van Aalderen WM, Bos AP. Pediatric acute lung injury. *Pediatr Respir Rev.* 2007;8(4):348-362.
28. Gregorakos L, Markou N, Psalida V, et al. Near-drowning: clinical course of lung injury. *Lung.* 2009;187(2):93-97.
29. Forler J, Carsin A, Arlaud K, et al. Respiratory complications of accidental drowning in children. *Arch Pediatr.* 2010;17(1):14-18.
30. Munt P, Fleetham J. Corticosteroids and near-drowning. *Lancet.* 1978;311(8065):665-666.
31. Xinmin D, Yunyou D, Qinzhi X, et al. Dexamethasone treatment attenuates early seawater instillation-induced acute lung injury in rabbits. *Pharmacol Res.* 2006;53(4):372-379.
32. Taknoa Y, Hirosako S, Yamaguchi T, et al. Nitric oxide inhalation as an effective therapy for acute respiratory distress syndrome due to near-drowning: a case report. *Nihon Kokyuki Gakkai Zasshi.* 1999;37(12):997-1002.
33. Pence HH, Pence S, Jurtul N, Kocuglu H, Bakau E, Kok AN. Changes in nitric oxide levels in striated muscles of rats following different types of death. *Soud Lek.* 2005;50(1):2-6.
34. Suzuki H, Ohta T, Iwata K, et al. Surfactant therapy for respiratory failure due to near-drowning. *Eur J Pediatr.* 1996;155:383-384.
35. Varisco BM, Palmatier CM, Alten JA. Reversal of intractable hypoxemia with exogenous surfactant (calfactant) facilitating complete neurological recovery in a pediatric drowning victim. *Pediatr Emerg Care.* 2010;26(8):571-573.
36. Eich C, Bräuer A, Kettler D. Recovery of a hypothermic drowned child after resuscitation with cardiopulmonary bypass followed by prolonged extracorporeal membrane oxygenation. *Resuscitation.* 2005;67(1):145-148.
37. Guenther U, Varelmann D, Putensen C, Wrigge H. Extended therapeutic hypothermia for several days during extracorporeal membrane-oxygenation after drowning and cardiac arrest: two cases of survival with no neurological sequelae. *Resuscitation.* 2009;80(3):379-381.
38. Wollenek G, Honarwar N, Golej J, Marx M. Cold water submersion and cardiac arrest in treatment of severe hypothermia with cardiopulmonary bypass. *Resuscitation.* 2002;52(3):255-263.
39. Coskun KO, Popov AF, Schmitto JD, et al. Extracorporeal circulation for rewarming in drowning and near-drowning pediatric patients. *Artific Organs.* 2010;34(11):1026-1030.
40. Bolte RG, Black PG, Bowers RS, et al. The use of extracorporeal rewarming in a child submerged for 66 minutes. *JAMA.* 1988;260(3):377-379.
41. Butt MP, Jalowayski A, Modell JH, Giammona ST. Pulmonary function after resuscitation from near-drowning. *Anesthesiology.* 1970;32(3):275-277.
42. Laughlin JJ, Eigen H. Pulmonary function abnormalities in survivors of near-drowning. *J Pediatr.* 1982;100(1):26-30.
43. Buford A, Ryan LM, Klein BL, et al. Drowning and near-drowning in children and adolescents. *Pediatr Emerg Care.* 2005;21(9):610-618.
44. Young RSK, Zaineraitis EL, Dooling EC. Neurological outcome in cold water drowning. *JAMA.* 1980;244(11):1233-1235.
45. Sekar TS, MacDonnel KF, Namsirikul P, Herman RS. Survival after prolonged submersion in cold water without neurologic sequelae: report of two cases. *Arch Intern Med.* 1980;140(6):775-779.
46. Siebke H, Rød T, Breivik H, Lind B. Survival after 40 minutes' submersion without cerebral sequelae. *Lancet.* 1975;305(7919):1275-1277.
47. Barrow RE, Spies M, Barrow LN, Herndon DN. Influence of demographics and inhalation injury on burn mortality in children. *Burns.* 2004;30(1):72-77.
48. Einhorn IN. Physiological and toxicological aspects of smoke produced during the combustion of polymeric materials. *Environ Health Perspect.* 1975;11:163-189.
49. Fein A, Leff A, Hopewell PC. Pathophysiology and management of the complications resulting from fire and the inhaled products of combustion: review of the literature. *Crit Care Med.* 1980;8(2):94-98.
50. Madnani DD, Steele NP, de Vries E. Factors that predict the need for intubation in patients with smoke inhalation injury. *Ear Nose Throat J.* 2006;85(4):278-280.
51. Haponik EF, Meyers DA, Munster AM, et al. Acute upper airway injury in burn patients: serial changes of flow-volume curves and nasopharyngoscopy. *Am Rev Respir Dis.* 1987;135(2):360-366.
52. Dorsey DP, Bowman SM, Klein MB, et al. Perioperative use of cuffed endotracheal tubes is advantageous in young pediatric burn patients. *Burns.* 2010;36(6):856-860.
53. Hudson DA, Jones L, Rode H. Respiratory distress secondary to scalds in children. *Burns.* 1994;20(5):434-437.
54. Fidkowski C, Fuzaylov G, Sheridan R, Coté C. Inhalation burn injury in children. *Paediatr Anaesth.* 2009;19(suppl 1):147-154.
55. Miller K, Chang A. Acute inhalation injury. *Emerg Med Clin North Am.* 2003;21(2):533-557.
56. Demling R, Lalonde C, Youn YK, Picard L. Effect of graded increases in smoke inhalation injury on the early systemic response to a body burn. *Crit Care Med.* 1995;23(1):171-178.
57. Enkhbaatar P, Traber DL. Pathophysiology of acute lung injury in combined burn and smoke inhalation injury. *Clin Sci (Lond).* 2004;107(2):137-143.
58. Murakami K, Traber DL. Pathophysiological basis of smoke injury. *News Physiol Sci.* 2003;18:125-129.
59. Head JM. Inhalation injury in burns. *Am J Surg.* 1980;139(4):508-512.
60. Walker HL, McLeod CG, McManus WF. Experimental inhalation injury in the goat. *J Trauma.* 1981;21(11):962-964.
61. Herndon DN. Inhalation injury. In: Herndon DN, ed. *Total Burn Care.* 2nd ed. Philadelphia, PA: Elsevier; 2002:242-253.
62. Mlcak RP, Suman OE, Herndon DN. Respiratory management of inhalation injury. *Burns.* 2007;33(1):2-13.
63. Zhang H, Kim YK, Govindarajan A, et al. Effect of adrenoreceptors on endotoxin-induced cytokines and lipid peroxidation in lung explants. *Am J Respir Crit Care Med.* 1999;160(5, pt 1):1703-1710.
64. Gauglitz GG, Finnerty CC, Herndon DN, Micak RP, Jeschke MG. Are serum cytokines early predictors for the outcome of burn patients with inhalation injuries who do not survive? *Crit Care.* 2008;12(3):R81.
65. Palmieri T, Enkhbaatar P, Bayliss R, et al. Continuous nebulized albuterol attenuates acute lung injury in an

ovine model of combined burn and smoke inhalation. *Crit Care Med.* 2006;34(6):1719-1724.

66. Muscarinic receptor antagonist therapy improves acute pulmonary dysfunction after smoke inhalation in sheep. *Crit Care Med.* 2010;38(12):2399-2344.

67. Palmieri T. Use of B-agonists in inhalation injury. *J Burn Care Res.* 2009; 30(1):141-142.

68. Sheridan RL, Zapol WM, Ritz RH, Tompkins RG. Low-dose inhaled nitric oxide in acutely burned children with profound respiratory failure. *Surgery.* 1999;126(5):856-862.

69. Miller AC, Rivero A, Ziad S, Smith DJ, Elamin EM. Influence of nebulized unfractionated heparin and N-acetylcysteine in acute lung injury after smoke inhalation injury. *J Burn Care Res.* 2009;30(2):249-256.

70. Enkhbaatar P, Murakami K, Cox R, et al. Aerosolized tissue plasminogen activator improves pulmonary function in sheep with burn and smoke inhalation. *Shock.* 2004;22(1):70-75.

71. Robinson NB, Hudson LD, Riem M, et al. Steroid therapy following isolated smoke inhalation injury. *J Trauma.* 1982;22(10):876-879.

72. Orgill DP, Piccolo N. Escharotomy and decompressive therapies in burns. *J Burn Care Res.* 2009;30(5):759-768.

73. Kao LW, Nañagas KA. Carbon monoxide poisoning. *Med Clin North Am.* 2005;89(6):1161-1194.

74. Barillo DJ, Goode R, Esch V. Cyanide poisoning in victims of fire: analysis of 364 cases and review of the literature. *J Burn Care Rehabil.* 1994;15(1):46-57.

75. Geller RJ, Barthold C, Saiers JA, Hall AH. Pediatric cyanide poisoning: causes, manifestations, management, and unmet needs. *Pediatrics.* 2006;118(5):2146-2158.

76. Tung A, Lynch J, McDade WA, Moss J. A new biological assay for measuring cyanide in blood. *Anesthes Analg.* 1997;85(5):1045-1051.

77. Berlin CM. The treatment of cyanide poisoning. *Pediatrics.* 1970;46(5):793-796.

78. Shepherd G, Velez LI. Role of hydroxocobalamin in acute cyanide poisoning. *Ann Pharmacother.* 2008;42(5):661-669.

79. Gómez R, Cancio LC. Management of burn wounds in the emergency department. *Emerg Med Clin North Am.* 2007;25(1):135-146.

80. Desai MH, Mlcak RP, Robinson E, et al. Does inhalation injury limit exercise endurance in children convalescing from thermal injury? *J Burn Care Rehabil.* 1993;14(1):12-16.

81. Altkorn R, Chen X, Milkovich S, et al. Fatal and non-fatal food injuries among children (aged 0-14 years). *Int J Pedatr Otorhinolaryngol.* 2008;72(7):1041-1046.

82. Rimell FL, Thome A, Stool S, et al. Characteristics of objects that cause choking in children. *JAMA.* 1995; 274(22):1763-1766.

83. Milkovich SM, Altkorn R, Chen X, et al. Development of the small parts cylinder: lessons learned. *Laryngoscope.* 2008;118(11):2082-2086.

84. Zur KB, Litman RS. Pediatric airway foreign body retrieval: surgical and anesthetic perspectives. *Pediatr Anesthes.* 2009; 19(1):109-117.

85. Gomez-Acevedo HH. Maneuver for the recovery of a foreign body causing a complete airway obstruction: illustrative case. *Pediatr Emerg Care.* 2010;26(1):39-40.

86. Heimlich HJ. A life-saving maneuver to prevent food-choking. *JAMA.* 1975;234(4):398-401.

87. Bullock SM, Rabar S, Demott K; Guideline Development Group. Sedation for diagnostic and therapeutic procedures in children and young people: summary of NICE guidance. *BMJ.* 2010;341:c6819.

88. McAfee SJ, Vashisht R. Removal of an impacted distal airway foreign body using a guidewire and a balloon angioplasty catheter. *Anaesth Intensive Care.* 2011;39(2):303-304.

89. Toye FJ, Weinstein JD. Clinical experience with percutaneous tracheostomy and cricothyroidotomy in 100 patients. *J Trauma.* 1986;26(11):1034-1040.

90. Even L, Heno N, Talmon Y, Samet E, Zonis Z, Kugelman A. Diagnostic evaluation of foreign body aspiration in children: a prospective study. *J Pediatr Surg.* 2005;40(7): 1122-1227.

91. Daines CL, Wood RE, Boesch RP. Foreign body aspiration: an important etiology of respiratory symptoms in children. *J Allergy Clin Immunol.* 2008;121(5):1297-1298.

92. Brown KL, Shefler A, Cohen G, DeMunter C, Pigott N, Goldman AP. Near-fatal grape aspiration with complicating acute lung injury successfully treated with extracorporeal membrane oxygenation. *Pediatr Crit Care Med.* 2003;4(2):243-245.

93. Ignaco RC Jr, Falcone RA Jr, Brown RL. A case report of severe tracheal obstruction requiring extracorporeal membrane oxygenation. *J Pediatr Surg.* 2006;41(10):E1-E4.

94. Isherwood J, Firmin R. Late presentation of foreign body aspiration requiring extracorporeal membrane oxygenation support for surgical management. *Interact Cardiovasc Thorac Surg.* 2011;12(4):631-632.

95. Lima JA. Laryngeal foreign bodies in children: a persistent life-threatening problem. *Laryngoscope.* 1989; 99(4):415-420.

96. Bronstein AC, Spyker DA, Cantilena LR Jr, Green JL, Rumack BH, Giffin SL. 2008 Annual Report of the American Association of Poison Control Centers' National Poison Data System (NPDS): 26th Annual Report. *Clin Toxicol (Phila).* 2009;47(10):911-1084.

97. Press E, Adams WC, Chittenden RF, et al. Co-operative kerosene poisoning study: evaluation of gastric lavage and other factors in the treatment of accidental ingestions of petroleum distillate products. *Pediatrics.* 1962; 29(4):648-674.

98. Giammona ST. Effects of furniture polish on pulmonary surfactant. *Am J Dis Child.* 1967;113(6):658-663.

99. Eade NR, Taussig LM, Marks MI. Hydrocarbon pneumonitis. *Pediatrics.* 1974;54(3):351-357.

100. Anas N, Namasonthi V, Ginsburg CM. Criteria for hospitalizing children who have ingested products containing hydrocarbons. *JAMA.* 1981;246(8):840-843.

101. Widner LR, Goodwin SR, Berman LS, Banner MJ, Freid EB, McKee TW. Artificial surfactant for therapy in hydrocarbon-induced lung injury in sheep. *Crit Care Med.* 1996;24(9):1524-1529.

102. Horoz OO, Yildizdas D, Yilmaz HL. Surfactant therapy in acute respiratory distress syndrome due to hydrocarbon aspiration. *Singapore Med J.* 2009;50(4):e130-e132.

103. Kamijo Y, Soma K, Yasushi A, Ohwada T. Pulse steroid therapy in adult respiratory distress syndrome following petroleum naphtha ingestion. *J Toxicol Clin Toxicol.* 2000;38(1):59-62.

104. Steele RW, Conklin RH, Mark HM. Corticosteroids and antibiotics for the treatment of fulminant hydrocarbon aspiration. *JAMA.* 1972;219(11):1434-1437.

105. Gurkan F, Bosnak M. Use of nebulized budesonide in two critical patients with hydrocarbon intoxication. *Am J Ther.* 2005;12(4):366-367.

106. Patwari PP, Michelson K. Use of inhaled nitric oxide for hydrocarbon aspiration. *Chest.* 2005;128:445S.

107. Beamon RF, Siegel CJ, Landers G, Green V. Hydrocarbon ingestion in children: a six-year retrospective study. *JACEP.* 1976;5(10):771-775.

108. Gurwitz D, Kattan M, Levison H, Culham JA. Pulmonary function abnormalities in asymptomatic children after hydrocarbon pneumonitis. *Pediatrics.* 1978; 62(5):789-794.

109. Olstad RB, Lord RM. Kerosene intoxication. *Am J Dis Child.* 1952;83(4):446-453.

110. Franquet T, Giménez A, Rosón N, Torrubia S, Sabaté JM, Pérez C. Aspiration diseases: findings, pitfalls, and differential diagnosis. *Radiographics.* 2000;20(3): 673-685.

111. Proetz AW. The effects of certain drugs on living nasal ciliated epithelium. *Ann Otol Rhinol Laryngol.* 1934;43: 450-463.

112. Marchiori E, Glaucia Z, Mano C, Hochhegger B. Exogenous lipoid pneumonia: clinical and radiological manifestations. *Respir Med.* 2011;105(5):659-666.

113. Furuya M, Martinez I, Zúñiga-Vásquez G, Hernández-Contreras I. Lipoid pneumonia in children: clinical and imagenological manifestations. *Arch Med Res.* 2000; 31(1):42-47.

114. Ayvazian LF, Steward DS, Merkel CG, Frederick WW. Diffuse lipoid pneumonitis successfully treated with prednisone. *Am J Med.* 1967;43(6):930-934.

115. Amato GM, Novara V, Amato G. Lipid pneumonia: favorable outcome after treatment with intravenous immunoglobulins, steroids, cephalosporins. *Minerva Pediatr.* 1997;49(4):163-169.

116. Chin NK, Hui KP, Sinnah R, Chan TB. Idiopathic lipoid pneumonia in an adult treated with prednisolone. *Chest.* 1994;105(3):956-957.

117. Casey JF. Chronic cor pulmonale associated with lipoid pneumonia. *JAMA.* 1961;177:896-898.

118. Newman LA, Keckley C, Peterson MC, Hamner A. Swallowing function and medical diagnoses in infants suspected of dysphagia. *Pediatrics.* 2001;108(6):E106.

119. Morton RE, Wheately R, Minford J. Respiratory tract infections due to direct and reflux aspiration in children with severe neurodisability. *Dev Med Child Neurol.* 1999; 41(5):329-334.

120. Owayed AF, Campbell DM, Wang EEL. Underlying causes of recurrent pneumonia in children. *Arc Pediatr Adolesc Med.* 2000;154(2):190-194.

121. Lefton-Greif M, Carroll JL, Loughlin G. Long-term follow-up of oropharyngeal dysphagia in children without apparent risk factors. *Pediatr Pulmonol.* 2006;41(11):1040-1048.

122. Weir K, McMahon S, Taylor S, Chang AB. Oropharyngeal aspiration and silent aspiration in children. *Chest.* 2011;140(3):589-597.

123. Sleigh G, Sullivan PB, Thomas AG. Gastrostomy feeding versus oral feeding alone for children with cerebral palsy. *Cochrane Database Syst Rev.* 2004;(2):CD003943.

124. Metheny NA, Stewart BJ, McClave SA. Relationship between feeding tube site and respiratory outcomes. *J Parenter Enteral Nutr.* 2011;35(3):346-355.

125. Bachrach SJ, Walter RS, Trzcinski K. Use of glycopyrrolate and other anticholinergic medications for sialorrhea in children with cerebral palsy. *Clin Pediatr.* 1998;37(8): 485-490.

126. Khoshoo V, Edell D. Previously healthy infants may have increased risk of aspiration during respiratory syncytial viral bronchiolitis. *Pediatrics.* 1999;104:1389-1390.

127. Sheikh S, Allen E, Shell R, et al. Chronic aspiration without gastroesophageal reflux as a cause of chronic respiratory symptoms in neurologically normal infants. *Chest.* 2001;120(4):1190-1195.

128. Beck-Schimmer B, Bonvini JM. Bronchoaspiration: incidence, consequences and management. *Eur J Anesthesiol.* 2011;28(2):78-84.

129. Vandenplas Y, Sacré-Smits L. Continuous 24-hour esophageal pH monitoring in 285 asymptomatic infants 0-15 months old. *J Pediatr Gastroenterol Nutr.* 1987;6(2):220-224.

130. Farhath S, He Z, Nakhla T, et al. Pepsin, a marker of gastric contents, is increased in tracheal aspirates from preterm infants who develop bronchopulmonary dysplasia. *Pediatrics.* 2008;121(2):253-259.

131. Sarkar M, Hennessy S, Yan YX. Proton-pump inhibitors use and the risk for community-acquired pneumonia. *Ann Intern Med.* 2008;149(6):391-398.

132. Srivastava R, Berry JG, Hall M, et al. Reflux related hospital admissions after fundoplication in children with neurological impairment: retrospective cohort study. *BMJ.* 2009;339:b4411.

Chapter 19

Pediatric Neurological Accidents

Jennifer Schuette, MD

Key Terms

Capnometry
Cerebral perfusion pressure (CCP)
Cranial vault
Cushing's triad
Diffuse axonal injury
Glasgow Coma Scale (GCS)
Intracranial pressure (ICP)
Monro-Kellie doctrine
Neurogenic pulmonary edema (NPE)
Penumbra
Rapid sequence intubation (RSI)
Spinal cord injury (SCI)
Traumatic brain injury (TBI)
Ventilator-associated pneumonia
  (VAP)

Chapter Objectives

After reading this chapter, you will be able to:

1. Summarize the epidemiology of traumatic brain injury and spinal cord injury in the pediatric population.
2. Describe the pathophysiology of spinal cord injury and its potential effects on spontaneous respiration.
3. List the indications for endotracheal intubation in pediatric patients who have suffered a neurological injury.
4. Describe the best practices for intubating a pediatric patient with a neurological injury, including protecting the cervical spine and minimizing the effect of the procedure on intracranial pressure in the patient with known or suspected traumatic brain injury.
5. Describe the relationship between ventilator settings, intrathoracic pressure, and intracranial pressure.
6. Identify the risks of pulmonary complications in pediatric patients who have suffered a neurological injury, as well as the possible thoracic comorbidities in the pediatric patient who has suffered multisystem trauma.
7. Discuss various approaches to ventilator management in the pediatric patient who has suffered a traumatic brain injury.
8. Define extubation readiness for a pediatric patient with a neurological injury.

■■ Johnny Taylor

You are the pediatric respiratory therapist (RT) carrying the trauma beeper when you are called to prepare for the arrival of a 5-year-old boy who was struck by a motor vehicle after running into the street in his neighborhood. When emergency medical services (EMS) providers arrived at the scene, bystanders reported that the boy, Johnny Taylor, was hit by a sport utility vehicle traveling at approximately 30 mph and that he was struck head on, thrown into the air, and then landed in the roadway approximately 15 feet away. The EMS providers said Johnny had a decreased level of consciousness but was making adequate respiratory effort. He opened his eyes when people spoke to him, and he withdrew from painful stimuli. He was crying, and his speech was understandable but confused (i.e., he said he was hungry and asked if he could eat his baseball); he was occasionally consolable when neighbors whom he knew spoke to him in a comforting manner. Intravenous access was obtained, Johnny was immobilized with a cervical collar and backboard, and he is en route to the pediatric emergency department (ED) of your hospital.

For RTs, managing ventilation in a patient with a TBI can be challenging. For some patients, it requires supporting spontaneous efforts, whereas for others it requires completely overriding their physiological breathing patterns to maintain appropriate carbon dioxide levels in the blood. Ventilation can have a profound effect on brain injury and healing, and proper respiratory management is a key component of intensive-care brain-injury management.

Traumatic Brain Injury

A **traumatic brain injury (TBI)** is caused by a bump, blow, or jolt to the head or a penetrating head injury that disrupts the normal function of the brain (1). TBI is one of the leading causes of death and morbidity in the pediatric population; recent estimates suggest that nearly half a million ED visits are made each year as the result of TBIs in patients aged 0 to 14 years in the United States, resulting in 35,000 hospitalizations and more than 2,000 deaths. Children aged 0 to 4 years and adolescents aged 15 to 19 years represent two of the three largest demographic groups who suffer TBIs (with those older than 65 being the third overrepresented group). Males aged 0 to 4 years have the highest rates for TBI-related ED visits, hospitalizations, and deaths (1). TBIs in children resulting from a motor vehicle accident, either as a vehicle occupant or as a pedestrian/cyclist struck by a motor vehicle, account for approximately 50% of pediatric TBI hospitalizations. Falls account for another 10%, with slightly over 7% of pediatric TBIs occurring as the result of firearm injuries. Pediatric TBIs are unintentional in 86% of cases and are the result of assault 10% of the time; a very small percentage (under 2%) are self-inflicted (2).

Pathophysiology

Anatomically, the brain sits within the bony calvarium, wrapped in three layers of tissue (the dura mater, the arachnoid mater, and the pia mater), which provide a protective covering (Fig. 19-1). Injury to the brain in pediatric patients most commonly occurs as the result of blunt force trauma. Primary injury is the direct result of the translation of kinetic force to the skull and the brain (Fig. 19-2). Injury can occur on the same side of the brain where the trauma

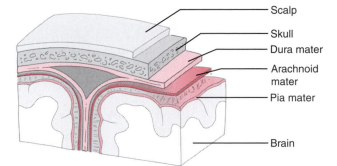

Figure 19-1 The Brain's Protective Barrier

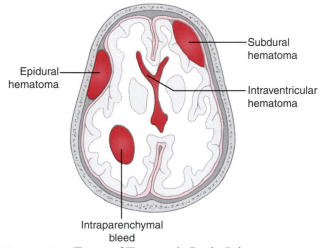

Figure 19-2 Types of Traumatic Brain Injury

is sustained or on the opposite side of the brain as the neural tissue accelerates, decelerates, and makes contact with the skull (a "contrecoup" injury).

The most common patterns of primary injury are as follows:

- Skull fracture
- Contusion ("brain bruise"): focal injury to the brain that results when there is forceful contact between the brain and any bony skull surface or protuberance
- Epidural hematoma: a collection of blood between the skull and the dura, most commonly the result of damage to an arterial vessel and thus resulting in a more-rapid deterioration. Adults who suffer an epidural bleed are often described as having a "lucid interval" before suffering a diminishing level of consciousness; this is less common in younger patients.
- Subdural hematoma: a collection of blood between the dural covering and the brain, usually the result of damage to bridging veins between the skull and the brain
- Intraparenchymal hemorrhage: blood that collects within the substance of the brain itself

- Intraventricular hemorrhage: bleeding into the central cerebrospinal fluid-filled spaces of the brain

Secondary injury occurs when, in response to the primary event, there is a cascade of biochemical responses, which can lead to brain edema and further loss of functional brain tissue if not rapidly addressed. Types of secondary injury include **diffuse axonal injury** (shearing injury to the deeper brain structures), ischemic and hypoxic injury, and vascular compromise brought about by increased pressure within the skull or brain herniation from one skull compartment into another. The focus of patient care after TBI is to minimize the amount of secondary injury that occurs, and appropriate airway management and respiratory support are crucial elements of this strategy (3).

In a patient who has suffered a TBI, there can be direct, neurologically mediated effects on the patient's ability to breathe, as well as additional noncranial injuries that can greatly affect the respiratory system (4, 5). It is important to keep these possible injuries and their effects in mind when assessing the adequacy of ventilation in patients who have sustained a TBI.

Direct TBI effects on the respiratory system are as follows:

- Hemispheric injury and brainstem injury, which can directly affect the level of consciousness and the patient's ability to protect the airway
- Cerebral edema
- Spinal cord injury, which potentially results in loss of control to the muscles of respiration
- Loss of airway patency secondary to foreign objects, secretions, facial fractures, or soft tissue edema
- Altered oropharyngeal muscle tone secondary to a decreased level of consciousness or as a direct result of the anatomical site of injury
- Release of proinflammatory mediators as a direct effect of TBI that affects the lungs

The following are noncranial injuries that affect the respiratory system:

- **Aspiration pneumonitis:** inflammation of the lung tissue, caused by aspiration.
- **Pulmonary contusion:** bruising of the lung tissue as a result of blunt injury, which damages the pulmonary capillaries, causing blood and other fluids to leak into the lung tissue. This damage can interfere with gas exchange, causing hypoxemia.
- **Pneumothorax:** a collection of air between the lung and thoracic wall that can be caused by a blunt or puncture injury to the thoracic cavity or by an airway injury.

- **Pulmonary edema:** increased fluid in the lung parenchyma, which has two main causes in the trauma patient. Postobstructive pulmonary edema, also known as negative pressure pulmonary edema, is discussed in Chapter 18. In this patient population, it is caused by upper airway obstruction secondary to facial or airway trauma. Neurogenic pulmonary edema, which develops within a few hours after a neurological insult, is discussed later in this chapter.
- **Rib fracture:** bony injury that can cause flail chest, pneumothorax, puncture trauma to the lung, or pulmonary contusions.
- **Airway, esophageal, or diaphragm rupture:** these soft tissue injuries can cause a mechanical interference with breathing.

Clinical Manifestations

Patients with TBI can present along a wide spectrum depending upon the specific area of the brain or spinal cord that has been injured, the extent of that injury, as well as other nonneurological injuries that can affect the patient's hemodynamic stability. It is vital to assess the adequacy of the airway, the effectiveness of respirations, and the level of perfusion in the rapid initial assessment of the patient with a traumatic injury. Patients with significant neurological injury may have lost the ability to protect the airway, may have ineffective respirations to support oxygenation and ventilation, or may have neurological or nonneurological injuries that result in hemodynamic compromise. Any of these clinical sequelae can result in worsening of the secondary brain injury; thus, evaluation of the respiratory and neurological systems is essential.

Respiratory Patterns

Observing a trauma patient's respiratory pattern can provide clues to the presence of an intracranial injury (Fig. 19-3). Although tachypnea is the most common respiratory pattern exhibited in a patient with brain injury, the following respiratory alterations should alert the provider to a possible intracranial injury (6):

- Cheyne-Stokes respirations: alternating between hyperventilation and hypoventilation in a cyclical pattern
- Apneustic breathing: deep inspirations with a long inspiratory pause, followed by a short exhalation
- Ataxic breathing: complete loss of breathing rhythmicity. Breaths are irregularly timed and have varying tidal volume (V_T) values.
- Cluster breathing: group of quick breaths in an irregular sequence, regularly separated by long pauses

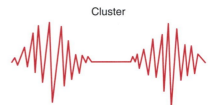

Normal

Regular rate and rhythm, consistent tidal volumes

Tachypnea

Regular rhythm, increased rate, consistent tidal volumes

Cheyne-Stokes

Cyclical pattern alternating between hyperventilation and hypoventilation

Apneustic

Deep inspirations with an inspiratory pause, followed by a short exhalation

Ataxic

Complete loss of breathing rhythmicity; breaths are irregularly timed and have varying tidal volumes

Cluster

Group of quick breaths in an irregular sequence, regularly separated by long pauses

Figure 19-3 Respiratory Patterns Associated With Brain Injury

Glasgow Coma Scale

The **Glasgow Coma Scale (GCS)** (Table 19-1) is a clinical tool often used to quickly assess consciousness and neurological status during the acute assessment of a patient who has suffered intracranial injury. First described in 1974, it is still in widespread use today to guide acute therapy as well as to predict future recovery. Pediatric modifications have been made to the GCS, as shown in Table 19-1; however, this scale has never been statistically validated in a pediatric population. GCS relies on the assessment of three functions: eye opening (on a scale of 1 to 4), verbal response (1 to 5), and motor abilities (1 to 6). A maximum score that indicates good neurological function is thus 15; a score of 3 is the minimum and generally corresponds with a grim overall prognosis.

Table 19-1	Glasgow Coma Scale		
Score	**Response**		
Eye opening	**0–1 year**	**>1 year**	
4	Spontaneous	Spontaneous	
3	To shout	To voice	
2	To pain	To pain	
1	None	None	
Verbal	**0–23 months**	**2–5 years**	**>5 years**
5	Cries appropriately	Uses appropriate words	Oriented and able to converse
4	Cries	Uses inappropriate words	Disoriented and able to converse
3	Cries/screams inappropriately	Cries or screams	Inappropriate words
2	Grunts	Grunts	Incomprehensible sounds
1	None	None	None
Motor	**0–1 year**	**>1 year**	
6	Spontaneous	Obeys commands	
5	Localizes pain	Localizes pain	
4	Flexion response to pain	Flexion response to pain	
3	Abnormal flexion (decorticate)	Abnormal flexion (decorticate)	
2	Abnormal extension (decerebrate)	Abnormal extension (decerebrate)	
1	None	None	

■■ Upon Johnny's arrival at the hospital, the trauma team begins a rapid assessment. His airway is intact, his lungs are clear to auscultation, and he exhibits strong central and distal pulses. He does not open his eyes to painful stimuli, is making incomprehensible sounds, and withdraws from painful stimuli. Although the paramedic who assessed Johnny at the scene gave him a Glasgow Coma Score of 10, based on these findings his score is a 7, and the emergency room physician asks you to prepare for an endotracheal intubation.

Intracranial Pressure

Intracranial pressure (ICP) is the pressure within the **cranial vault** (the portion of the skull where the brain is encased), and it is guided by the **Monro-Kellie doctrine**, which states that the total volume within the cranial vault is strictly limited by the fixed walls of the skull. This volume is composed of the brain, blood, and cerebrospinal fluid (CSF). If the volume of one of these three components changes, ICP can be maintained at a steady level only if one of the other components makes a compensatory change in the opposite direction. For example, an intracranial hemorrhage that results from a TBI causes an increase in the volume of blood in the cranial vault. To prevent an increase in ICP, the health-care team must find a way to reduce the volume of intravascular blood, brain tissue, or CSF. (This can be accomplished by evacuating [removing] the hematoma in the operating room, for example.) This basic principle guides many of the therapeutic interventions used in treating TBI (7).

Monitoring ICP requires placing a catheter in the brain, an invasive procedure that can be done at the bedside by the neurosurgical team (Fig. 19-4). During the initial management period of TBI in the ED and early in the ICU course, it is not feasible to directly monitor ICP. Therefore, other mechanisms are used to estimate ICP and help guide therapy. ICP levels in healthy individuals fluctuate widely but are normally less than 10 mm Hg; in the setting of illness or injury, most providers will intervene if ICP is greater than 20 mm Hg.

In infants who still have an open fontanel (the "soft spot" on the top of the skull, where the plates

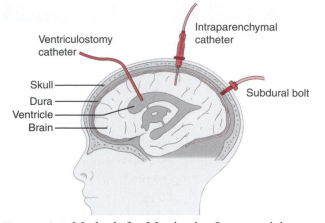

Figure 19-4 Methods for Monitoring Intracranial Pressure

of bone that make up the skull have not yet fused), one can palpate this area as a crude means of assessing ICP; a bulging and taut fontanel is a concern for (but by no means diagnostic of) increased ICP in an infant with an altered level of consciousness. By 1 year of age, the fontanel has usually closed.

One of the hallmarks of increased ICP in a patient with a brain injury is a clinical picture known as **Cushing's triad**, in which bradycardia, hypertension, and irregular respirations are all present. A unilateral change in the pupillary examination is also highly suggestive of a degree of increased ICP that is causing the brain to herniate, or bulge, into another area of the cranial vault or downward into the spinal canal (Fig. 19-5). Any one of these signs is extremely ominous, and often the most effective initial strategy to acutely decrease ICP is to manipulate the degree of ventilation to create a respiratory alkalosis. This strategy of hyperventilation has long been used both as an initial approach to treat increased ICP and, historically, as a long-term therapy as well. The effectiveness of this strategy is based on the fact that hyperventilation and the low partial pressure of

carbon dioxide (PCO_2) that it produces result in a vasoconstriction of the cerebral vascular system. In keeping with the Monro-Kellie doctrine, this vasoconstriction leads to a decrease in the cerebral blood volume and thus a decrease in ICP (8). Although very effective for the acute control of elevated ICP, hyperventilation is no longer used as a mainstay of longer-term ICP management because data have shown that such a strategy can result in ischemic injury to the brain, including those areas not affected by the initial injury (9).

The interaction of ICP and the partial pressure of carbon dioxide in the arteries ($PaCO_2$), partial pressure of oxygen in the arteries (PaO_2), and mean arterial blood pressure has long been studied but is still not fully understood. In the normal brain, there are multiple mechanisms in place to ensure that ICP is maintained at a steady level, even in the face of changes in blood pressure. This system, known as autoregulation, is depicted in Figure 19-6. This figure also demonstrates the effect that alterations in ventilation and oxygenation have on cerebral blood flow, and thus ICP. As demonstrated, hyperventilation results in vasoconstriction and a decrease in cerebral blood flow, whereas only severe hypoxemia (PaO_2 less than 50 mm Hg) results in an increase in cerebral blood flow. Of note, the cerebral vasculature seems to be particularly sensitive to changes in $PaCO_2$ within the physiological range (20 to 60 mm Hg), thus making alteration in patient ventilation a viable strategy for controlling increased ICP.

> ■■ You arrive at the bedside to assist with Johnny's intubation; he is placed on a non-rebreather mask at a fractional concentration of inspired oxygen (FIO_2) of 1.0, and the medications and equipment required for intubation are gathered. The anesthesiologist is considering the safest approach to intubating a patient with suspected TBI and unknown condition of the cervical spine.

Management and Treatment

Management and treatment of patients with TBI involve many different body systems. Initial management includes airway protection and rapid assessment and control of ICP. Continued management will include management of cerebral perfusion pressure, which incorporates mechanical ventilation (MV) and pharmacological therapies.

Intubation

Performing an endotracheal intubation to protect the airway is widely practiced for patients who present with a GCS score of 8 or lower (10). The treating physician may also choose to gain control of the

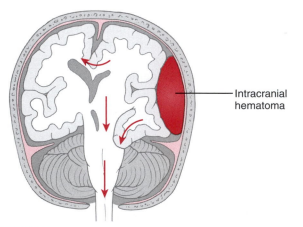

Figure 19-5 Types of Brain Herniation

Intracranial hematoma

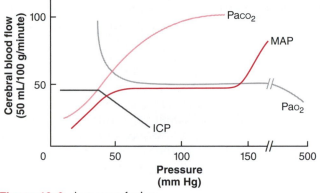

Figure 19-6 Autoregulation

airway for those patients whose GCS score is greater than 8 but steadily declining over time.

Once the decision is made to intubate, it is crucial to do the following:

- Minimize the likelihood of exacerbating a cervical spine injury should one exist
- Guard against the possibility of aspiration
- Limit the effect of the noxious stimulus of intubation on ICP

Minimizing Cervical Spine Injury

The condition of the cervical spine is usually unknown when performing the intubation of a patient with presumed traumatic neurological injury in the acute setting. Therefore, it is essential that inline stabilization of the cervical spine be maintained throughout the procedure. This is most easily achieved by having an additional care provider positioned at the head of the bed and slightly to the patient's left so that one hand can be placed on either side of the patient's head throughout the intubation. This provider is responsible for maintaining the patient's head in a neutral and midline position and for notifying the provider who is intubating the patient if significant head motion is occurring and if control of head position is being threatened. This provider should have no other additional patient care responsibilities and so should be separate from the care provider who completes the intubation and the RT assisting the intubating provider, both of whom are also positioned at the head of the bed. The data in the literature are conflicting regarding the effectiveness of this approach on limiting cervical spine motion, as well as whether or not it hinders intubation unnecessarily (11, 12). Although airway adjuncts such as video laryngoscopes and intubating laryngeal mask airways are available in some centers to assist in maximizing cervical spine protection during intubation by allowing airway control with minimum extension of the cervical spine, neither the equipment nor the staff proficient in its use are universally available.

Guarding Against Aspiration

Aspiration, the inhalation of either oropharyngeal or gastric contents into the lower airways, is another significant concern when managing the airway of a child with TBI. Patients who have suffered a TBI are at risk for aspiration as a result of any combination of the following (12):

- Recent food ingestion
- Delayed gastric emptying associated with the stress of trauma
- Vomiting
- Decreased protective upper airway reflexes
- Facial or oropharyngeal trauma resulting in blood or other foreign material in the oral cavity

In 1961, Brian Arthur Sellick introduced the use of cricoid pressure to minimize the risk of aspiration in patients during the induction of anesthesia (13). This maneuver (also known as Sellick's maneuver) is based on the theory that applying pressure externally over the cricoid membrane will effectively seal off the esophageal opening and inhibit gastric contents from entering the airway (Fig. 19-7). Since its introduction, some have questioned the utility of this technique, voicing concern regarding appropriate technique and effectiveness in preventing aspiration (14–16). In its 2010 Emergency Cardiac Care update, the American Heart Association no longer recommends cricoid pressure in the setting of cardiac arrest, suggesting that the risk of delaying intubation outweighs the potential benefits (17).

In all likelihood, the most effective way to decrease the risk of aspiration in a patient with TBI is to secure the airway by performing a **rapid sequence intubation (RSI)** (Box 19-1). RSI is the introduction of an endotracheal tube (ETT) with minimal passage of time between anesthetic drug delivery and the onset of ideal intubating conditions. Additional components of RSI include preoxygenation with 100% oxygen, minimizing positive-pressure ventilation prior to intubation to avoid filling the stomach with air (and thus increasing the risk of vomiting

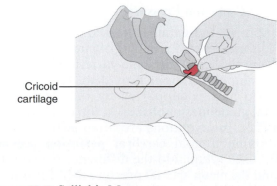

Cricoid cartilage

Figure 19-7 Sellick's Maneuver

Components of a Rapid Sequence Intubation

- Preoxygenation with FIO_2 1.0
- Minimization of positive pressure mask ventilation
- Administration of rapidly acting medications
- Cricoid pressure (Sellick's maneuver)

and aspiration), and the use of cricoid pressure. Medications should be selected that provide adequate sedation, analgesia, and paralysis in a reliable and fast-acting fashion, with special attention to avoiding any medications that might cause an increase in ICP. Specifically, ketamine is a drug that has historically been avoided in patients with TBI secondary to animal data that it is associated with an increase in ICP; more recently, the avoidance of ketamine use in this patient population has been called into question (18). Drugs that have a high risk for causing hypotension and a resultant decrease in brain perfusion (such as the combination of a narcotic and a benzodiazepine) must be avoided. One approach is to anesthetize with etomidate and then paralyze with rocuronium for intubation.

Limiting the Effects of Intubation on ICP

Intubation is a noxious stimulus that can result in increased ICP, leading some providers to seek interventions that would blunt this response. One approach has been to administer intravenous IV lidocaine prior to intubation in the hopes of anesthetizing the airway. However, it is unclear if this practice has a significant protective effect (19, 20). The most crucial elements of airway management in patients with TBI are appropriate recognition of inadequate ventilation and/or oxygenation, avoidance of both prolonged hypercapnia and aspiration, and efficient insertion of an artificial airway after achieving appropriate levels of sedation and muscle relaxation.

Cerebral Perfusion Pressure

The approach to treating increased ICP in a patient with TBI uses a tiered grouping of interventions (21). Although there may be some variations in this approach among different providers, the approach described here is supported by the most recent national guidelines published in the pediatric literature (22). Interventions are often geared toward maintaining a goal **cerebral perfusion pressure (CPP).** CPP is equal to the difference between the ICP and the mean arterial pressure (MAP), approximated by multiplying the diastolic blood pressure

by two-thirds and adding that to one-third of the systolic pressure:

$$CPP = MAP - ICP$$

The precise goals for CPP in pediatric TBI patients have yet to be established by a prospective randomized trial. A goal of 60 to 70 mm Hg is often used based on adult studies, but CPPs as low as 50 may be sufficient in younger patients (23). Adjunctive monitoring devices looking at cerebral oxygen usage are sometimes used to more precisely assess the adequacy of oxygen delivery to the brain in any given patient.

The tiered management strategies described in the following sections are suggested for all patients with a severe TBI, defined as having a GCS score of 8 or less. This approach is based on expert consensus, with the top-tier therapies having a stronger base of support within the scientific literature than those in the second tier (24). The physiological rationale for each therapy is described with each intervention (summary in Table 19-2).

First-Tier Therapy

- Appropriate positioning: Head of the bed at 30 degrees with the head positioned in the midline. This maximizes venous drainage from the head back into the systemic circulation.
- Adequate sedation and analgesia: Unaddressed pain or agitation can increase the brain's metabolic demand, which results in increased blood flow to meet that demand.
- Normoventilation ($PaCO_2$ of 35 to 40 mm Hg): Unless there is clinical evidence of acute herniation (Cushing's triad, unilateral fixed and dilated pupils), the $PaCO_2$ should be maintained in the normal range. *Hypoventilation must be avoided* (Teamwork 19-1).
- CSF drainage: Pressure monitors can be placed in the space between the brain and the skull, within the brain parenchyma itself, or within

Table 19-2	Management of CPP	
First Tier	**Second Tier**
Head of bed elevated 30 degrees	Moderate hyperventilation
Head midline	Barbiturate coma
Adequate sedation and analgesia	Moderate hypothermia
Normoventilation	Decompressive craniectomy
CSF drainage with ventriculostomy	
Neuromuscular blockade	
Hyperosmolar therapy	

Teamwork 19-1 Therapist-Driven Protocols

THE PURPOSE OF THERAPIST-DRIVEN PRO-TOCOLS IS TO ALLOW HEALTH-CARE WORK-ERS TO ADJUST THE SETTINGS OF MEDICAL DEVICES OR THE DOSAGE OF MEDICATIONS TO MAINTAIN PATIENT PARAMETERS (E.G., BLOOD GAS RESULTS, HEART RATE) WITHIN A TARGET THERAPEUTIC RANGE. A complex disease process such as TBI requires physicians to make multiple therapeutic interventions to keep ICP within a theoretically safe range. Having a therapist make changes in MV without requiring physician input for each adjustment frees the physician to focus on other pressing patient decisions. It is the physician's responsibility to be precise in both what the therapeutic goals are and what reportable conditions are. An example would be, "Adjust respiratory rate to maintain E_TCO_2 at 35 to 40 mm Hg. Notify physician if respiratory rate greater than 30 breaths per minute." It is the RT's responsibility to monitor the noted parameters and immediately notify the physician if parameters migrate outside of the desired values.

the ventricle (CSF-containing space) of the brain (Fig. 19-4); if the monitoring device is located in the ventricle (known as a ventriculostomy), CSF can be removed through the catheter to offset a sudden increase in ICP.

- Neuromuscular blockade: If sedation and analgesia alone do not adequately limit the metabolic demands of the brain, neuromuscular blockade can be used as the next step. Neuromuscular blocking agents act as chemical paralytics, inhibiting all activity of the body's voluntary muscles. Theoretically, this decreases ICP by lessening the metabolic demand on the brain, improving venous return from the head by relaxing the thoracic cage, and eliminating shivering (25). Because the neurological examination is not possible when the patient is muscle relaxed, continuous electroencephalogram (EEG) monitoring should be considered to ensure that electrical seizure activity does not go unrecognized and untreated, which would further exacerbate ICP.
- Hyperosmolar therapies (e.g., mannitol, hypertonic saline): The goal of hyperosmolar therapies is to decrease the amount of extravascular fluid in the brain; this is accomplished by increasing the osmolality of the blood, which then pulls fluid into the vascular space. This

fluid is then delivered to the kidneys, where it is removed.

Second-Tier Therapy

- Moderate hyperventilation ($PaCO_2$ of 30 to 35 mm Hg): As previously described, hyperventilation results in cerebral vasoconstriction, and this limitation to blood flow can decrease ICP by lowering the cerebral blood volume. The concern, however, is that cerebral vasoconstriction will result in ischemia (inadequate blood flow to certain areas of the brain).
- Barbiturate coma: The physiological goal of this therapy is to achieve burst suppression by EEG, a bedside test that measures the electrical activity in the brain. Burst suppression translates into slowing the brain's activity to its lowest level and thus limiting the amount of blood flow required to deliver adequate oxygen and glucose to the brain.
- Moderate hypothermia (core temperature 32° to 34° C): This therapy is also aimed at limiting the brain's metabolic needs, but it remains controversial because of the potential side effects, such as increased risk of bleeding and infection.
- Decompressive craniectomy: Removal of a bone flap from the skull to effectively increase the size of the cranial vault can be attempted when other interventions fail to control ICP adequately; studies have also looked at this intervention earlier in the course of therapy (26).

Mechanical Ventilation Strategies

The most effective initial MV strategy for patients with a TBI should focus on normoventilation. Acute hyperventilation in the setting of a sudden increase in ICP has been shown to alleviate the acute clinical findings of cerebral herniation caused by the cerebral vasoconstriction that results from alkalosis (27–30). In this setting, hyperventilation would be used as a temporizing measure while other, longer-term and more-effective therapies (such as hyperosmolar therapies or barbiturates) can be administered. In the 1980s, hyperventilation was used aggressively beyond the acute stage as a means to control ICP. However, evidence has accumulated to suggest that prolonged hyperventilation may not be an effective long-term strategy and may even have a potentially detrimental effect:

- The initial positive alkalotic effect that hyperventilation has on the cerebral vasculature declines over time. This is because the pH of the perivascular space normalizes over approximately 24 hours (31).
- The **penumbra**, which is the at-risk area of the brain that surrounds the injured tissue, may actually be hypersensitive to changes in $PaCO_2$

after the injury has occurred (32). This, along with the low cerebral blood flow that generally occurs regionally after a traumatic injury, could result in ischemic injury to areas of the brain that are potentially salvageable.

• Prolonged hyperventilation can result in a rebound effect on cerebral blood flow when normoventilation is restored such that there is actually supranormal flow in some areas as the $PaCO_2$ returns to normal; thus, any period of hyperventilation must be followed by a weaning phase to normalize the pH and $PaCO_2$ (33).

Therefore, current recommendations for the management of patients with TBI are to use ventilator strategies that maintain a normal $PaCO_2$ except in the case of impending or actual brain herniation. In that scenario, acute hyperventilation ($PaCO_2$ of 30 to 35 mm Hg) can be used until pharmacological agents described in the first-tier therapies are available, with P_aCO_2 being allowed to normalize as soon as clinically feasible. Prophylactic hyperventilation is not recommended because of the risk of ischemia described above (34, 35). Box 19-2 summarizes the respiratory-based TBI management strategies.

With close management of $PaCO_2$ necessary for TBI, **capnometry** or end-tidal CO_2 (E_TCO_2) monitoring is a preferred method for serial trending of CO_2 levels. The American Association for Respiratory Care's clinical practice guidelines offer guidance on the use and management of E_TCO_2 monitoring (36). Care must be taken to correlate E_TCO_2 with $PaCO_2$ regularly to ensure accuracy of measurement, as well as to assess the reliability of E_TCO_2 readings. The common causes for inaccurate E_TCO_2 readings are listed in Box 19-3.

Extubation

Little research has been done to determine the safety and appropriate timing of extubation and/or the use of a surgical tracheostomy for children with severe TBI. Research with adult patients suggests that there

are delays in extubating patients with TBI even after they meet normal extubation criteria (i.e., adequate respiratory effort, intact protective airway reflexes as demonstrated by a cough and gag, and the ability to maintain oxygenation and ventilation with minimal positive-pressure support) (37). There is no reason to think that the pediatric experience is any different. Overall, there is a perception among pediatric intensivists that tracheostomies in pediatric patients are underutilized for a variety of reasons (38), and further work is required in this area to maximize the rehabilitation potential of these high-risk patients.

Box 19-3 Common Causes for Inaccurate E_TCO_2 Reading (63)

Inaccurate Numbers
• High V_D/V_T ratios (dead space to tidal volume ratios)
• Alterations in breathing patterns
• Large changes in V_T
• Delivery of helium through E_TCO_2 device
• High respiratory rate
• High airway resistance (sidestream capnographs)
• High inspiration-to-expiration (I/E) ratios (sidestream capnographs)
• Contamination of monitor or sampling system with secretions or condensate
• Leaks in ventilator circuit
• Leaks around ETT cuff (or presence of an uncuffed tube)
• Bronchopleural fistula
• Dialysis or extracorporeal membrane oxygenation (ECMO)

False Negatives
• Low cardiac output
• Severe airway obstruction
• Pulmonary edema

Box 19-2 RT Goals for TBI Management

1. Keep head of bed (HOB) at 30 or more degrees, even during mask ventilation.
2. Incorporate E_TCO_2 as soon as it is available; this includes its use during mask ventilation.
3. Use acute mild hyperventilation (CO_2 30 to 35 mm Hg) until other first-tier therapies are available
4. Use continuous E_TCO_2 to drive ventilation.
5. Use normoventilation (CO_2 35 to 40 mm Hg) for duration of TBI care, with exceptions listed above in item 3.

■■ After Johnny is safely intubated, ongoing clinical assessment reveals the following: afebrile, heart rate of 52, and blood pressure of 164/98 while he is being bagged at a rate of 12. Pulse oximetry reveals a saturation of 98% on an FIO_2 of 1.0. The surgical resident reexamines Johnny and notes that the right pupil is large and does not respond to light, whereas the left pupil is a normal size and responds briskly to light. The remainder of the physical examination is limited because of the sedation and muscle-relaxant medications given for intubation. The trauma attending physician requests that you increase the rate at which you are bagging to 20 to 25 times per minute.

After a brief period of hyperventilation with manual bagging, Johnny's blood pressure and heart rate return to age-appropriate values, and the pupillary examination normalizes. He is transported to the computed tomography (CT) scanner, where a head CT reveals intracranial blood and concern for early herniation. He is then transported to the ICU for further care and management, at which time an ICP pressure monitor is placed, which reveals an ICP of 32 mm Hg. (Normal ICP is under 10 mm Hg; in a patient with TBI, the goal of therapy is usually to maintain an ICP under 20 mm Hg.) The medical team is considering the most appropriate medical therapy, including ventilator strategy, for Johnny.

Course and Prognosis

The physical, behavioral, and cognitive sequelae after a moderate-to-severe TBI can be significant and profound. It was once thought that infants and younger children had a more favorable chance for good recovery than do older children as a result of the "plasticity" of the still-maturing brain; this is the ability of one part of the brain to take over the function of another area of the brain that has been injured. More recent evidence, however, suggests that younger patients may actually fare worse. Specifically, the continued recovery seen in school-aged and older children over the course of 1 to 2 years after their injury seems to plateau in the younger age groups (39, 40).

Several predictors have been studied to better describe a patient's prospects for functional recovery. The GCS, for example, has some predictive value in categorizing those patients at higher risk for dying prior to discharge. In one study, 20% of children with a GCS score less than 8 died prior to hospital discharge, whereas no children with scores greater than 8 died. Furthermore, the combination of a lower GCS score; a higher Pediatric Risk of Mortality (PRISM) score (a grouping of physiological parameters assessed over the first 24 hours of hospitalization, such as heart rate, blood pressure, and pH); and younger age at the time of injury were most predictive of mortality (41).

Additional predictors of less-favorable outcomes, particularly in the areas of behavior and cognition, have also been described (41, 42):

- Consciousness: Longer duration of impaired consciousness
- Amnesia: Longer duration of posttraumatic amnesia
- Etiology of the injury: Infants sustaining nonaccidental trauma in particular have worse outcomes (Special Population 19-1).

● Special Populations 19-1

Shaken Baby Syndrome

Shaken baby syndrome is a nonaccidental neurological trauma occurring when a baby has been subjected to violent, whiplash-type shaking injuries inflicted by an abuser. This shaking causes tearing of the cerebral veins and bleeding into the subdural space. The reported incidence of severe or fatal shaken baby syndrome in the United States is 1,300 cases per year, but it can be assumed that it is underreported because medical providers do not always include this in their differential diagnosis of the fussy infant (62). The most common significant clinical finding that is not seen in other types of brain trauma is retinal hemorrhage, as well as bruising on the arms or trunk where the baby was forcefully grabbed. In addition to patient management of TBI, other children living in the home should be examined for signs of physical abuse.

- The specific region of the brain affected: Injury to the brainstem can result in impaired respiratory control, whereas frontal lobe injury often leaves a patient with behavioral issues.
- The presence of diffuse axonal injury: This is a pattern of multiple punctuate areas of hemorrhage, which is associated with disruption of neural pathways. Essentially, this causes a severing of the connections between neurons, usually from an extreme acceleration/deceleration injury, and often results in severe functional losses as a result of the global nature of this injury.
- Medical markers
  - Elevated ICP
  - Fever
  - Persistent seizures beyond 24 hours of injury
  - Fluctuations in blood pressure

■■ Sedation, paralysis, and hyperosmolar therapy are initiated for Johnny with good effect, and his ICP decreases below 20 mm Hg. At this point, the medical team receives a call from the neuroradiologist who is reviewing the CT scans that were completed in the ED. In addition to the intracranial injuries described previously, the cervical spine CT is showing fractures of cervical vertebrae 3 and 4, with concern for impingement on the spinal cord at that level. With Johnny now paralyzed and sedated to control the ICP, the team is not able to perform a physical examination. As the RT, you are asked to recommend an appropriate ventilator strategy given this new injury finding and to formulate a plan going forward that takes the cervical spine injury and its potential effects and sequelae into account.

Spinal Cord Injury

Spinal cord injury (SCI) is a relatively rare event in children, accounting for only 1% to 2% of traumatic injuries. Only 3% to 5% of all new SCIs each year occur in children younger than 15 years. Between 60% and 80% of pediatric spinal cord injuries occur at the level of the cervical spine—in adults, this number is significantly lower at 30% to 40%. This difference is thought to be due to the proportionally larger mass of the child's head relative to the rest of the body, such that the fulcrum of force is located higher in the spine. Injuries to the pediatric cervical spine are more likely to occur at a higher anatomical level up to the age of 8 years; beyond that time, the injury pattern takes on that of the adult population, with more injuries affecting the lower cervical spine. These younger age groups are also more likely to suffer a ligamentous (SCI without radiological abnormality [SCIWORA]) rather than bony injury. This is likely related to the anatomical difference in younger age groups: different configuration of the vertebrae, incomplete ossification of the spinal bones, and ligaments that are more easily able to deviate from their initial position when a force is applied to them (44, 45). When fractures do occur in children, they are more commonly the result of motor vehicle accidents than any other cause (46), although sports-related injuries player a larger role in the adolescent group.

Pathophysiology

Injury to the spinal cord from trauma can occur owing to bleeding around the cord resulting in external compression, bony fracture with impingement on the cord from the vertebral body, or extreme stretching of the cord in the setting of hyperextension or hyperflexion that leads to tissue disruption. The injury to the cord can be temporary or permanent and can be partial (where some spinal cord pathways remain intact) or complete (where all neurological function is lost distal to the site of injury). It is important to understand the anatomy involved to better predict the result of an injury at a given spinal level, in addition to the subsequent requirements for respiratory support and the risks of pulmonary complications.

Clinical Manifestations

The level at which the injury occurs will be the driving factor of patient clinical manifestations. The cervical spine is composed of seven vertebral bodies and the ligaments that attach them to each other (Fig. 19-8). Injuries to the first and second cervical vertebrae (C1 and C2) are often fatal because the mechanics of breathing and hemodynamic control are often acutely lost. Injuries to C3 to C5 result in

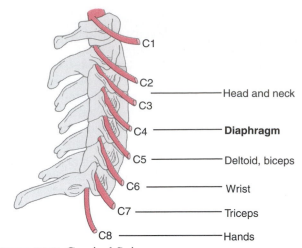

Figure 19-8 Cervical Spine

compromise of the phrenic nerve, which innervates the diaphragm; a common mnemonic taught in medical school is, "C3-4-5 keeps the diaphragm alive." Injuries at this level can also compromise the intercostal and abdominal muscles; these latter muscle groups are innervated by the thoracic nerve roots, which also lose function if the cervical injury is a complete one. The diaphragm is the most important muscle for inspiration, providing 65% of the V_T in normal breathing; the intercostal muscles are innervated by the thoracic nerve roots, and these muscles assist in inspiration by elevating the rib cage. It is important to note that additional muscles of respiration (the scalene, the sternocleidomastoid, the trapezius, and the pectoralis major) also participate in respiration, and their function is often preserved in all but the highest levels of SCI (47–49).

Injuries to the lower cervical cord (C5 to C8) usually spare the diaphragm but can result in a loss of strength in the secondary muscles of respiration. In particular, injuries at this level can compromise the patient's ability to take deep breaths and to cough effectively, placing the patient at risk for atelectasis and pneumonia (49) (see Chapters 7 and 15). The primary muscles of expiration are the pectoralis major in the chest, the rectus abdominus, the transverses abdominus, and the internal and external obliques. Generally speaking, patients with injuries that occur above the level of C5 are likely to need long-term ventilation, whereas patients with injuries at or below the level of C5 can often be weaned from mechanical support over time (45). Keep in mind, however, that even patients who suffer injuries in the thoracic spine are at risk for respiratory complications as a result of the effect of this type of injury on the secondary muscles of respiration (49).

In the acute setting, especially when patients have additional injuries to the head or thorax that require

MV, the cervical spine injury may not be the primary driver for ventilator management. Instead, adjustments of ventilator settings may be more focused on maintaining normal ventilation and providing adequate oxygenation in the days to weeks following injury to minimize secondary cerebral injury. However, over the course of time and throughout the recovery phase, longer-term issues related to the SCI may become prominent in the management strategy. Both the level of the injury and whether there is complete or partial cord injury will affect the long-term prognosis from a respiratory standpoint.

Partial or complete injury to the spinal cord can cause respiratory failure and also hinder the ability to wean and liberate a patient from MV. The specific etiologies for both can be grouped as follows (49):

- Impaired inspiratory ability
  - Decreased respiratory muscle strength with the development of fatigue
  - Paradoxical chest wall movement that increases the work of breathing (WOB)
  - Decreased inspiratory capacity as measured at the bedside by the maximal negative inspiratory force
  - Atelectasis
- Impaired expiratory ability
  - Increased secretions
  - Decreased cough effectiveness
- Autonomic nervous system dysfunction
  - Increased secretions
  - Bronchospasm
  - Pulmonary edema

Management and Treatment

Appropriate management of the pulmonary system should begin as soon as possible after the injury occurs to minimize respiratory complications, which have been shown to increase over the first 5 days after injury. In adult patients with SCI, respiratory failure occurs, on average, 3 to 4.5 days after injury (50). It is likely that most pediatric patients with significant SCI, especially in the younger age ranges, will be intubated early in the course of management for airway protection and to allow for the needed radiological evaluation. As described previously for the TBI patient with unknown cervical spine status, it is crucial to maintain inline spine immobilization during the intubation of patients with an SCI.

Acute Respiratory Management

Atelectasis represents the most common acute respiratory complication of SCI and can result in pneumonia and respiratory failure; thus, interventions to avoid atelectasis are a primary focus of early pulmonary care. Potential interventions include aggressive bronchial hygiene with frequent suctioning and the use of recruitment maneuvers (sigh breaths, inspiratory holds), as well as the use of bronchodilators. Larger V_T values (12 to 15 cc/kg) can also decrease the likelihood of atelectasis developing.

The management of secretions in the acute phase can be aided by the use of warm moist air, bronchodilators, and mucolytics. Suctioning is a double-edged sword because it can result in hypoxia, hypotension, infection if sterile technique is not maintained, tracheal mucosal damage, vagal nerve stimulation with resultant bradycardia, patient anxiety and fear, and, paradoxically, stimulation of more secretions (49).

Subacute Respiratory Management

During the subacute management phase, there are a number of evaluation tools that can be used to assess any given patient's ability to breathe adequately and to protect the airway. The following are all important facets in planning for a long-term pulmonary strategy for patients with SCIs (45):

- **Pulse oximetry:** The goal for oxygen saturations in the acute phase of therapy should be greater than 95%; when feasible (based on the patient's overall physical condition, which may occur beyond the acute phase), the saturations should be carefully assessed during wakefulness, sleep, and with and without activity; cervical SCI patients are at risk for sleep-disordered breathing, with the potential for both cerebral and obstructive origins. Sleep-disordered breathing may result in periods of hypoxia, as well as poor cognitive function and endurance when awake.
- **Capnography:** Respiratory effort is primarily driven by the serum CO_2 levels. It is important not to overventilate patients with SCI because this can blunt their respiratory drive and prevent spontaneous ventilation. It is equally vital not to allow them to remain underventilated, which increases the risk of atelectasis, infection, and airway collapse. Maintaining E_TCO_2 at 35 to 45 mm Hg will minimize the risk of both.
- **Pulmonary function testing (PFTs):** Although potentially of limited use in younger children who are unable to cooperate or patients with comorbid conditions that limit the ability to follow commands, PFTs can still provide important information regarding the respiratory strength in a patient with an SCI (45, 51):
  - **Forced vital capacity (FVC):** the maximal amount of air that can be exhaled following a maximal inhaled breath. Both an inability to forcefully inflate the lungs and chest wall dysfunction that hinders forced exhalation can

result in limitations in FVC. FVC has been shown to have predictive value regarding the ability to maintain adequate gas exchange over a prolonged period of time without an unacceptable increase in WOB, as well as documenting early respiratory compromise in the setting of an acute illness during the chronic management phase.

- **Maximum inspiratory pressure (MIP) and maximum expiratory pressure (MEP):** assess the degree of inspiratory and expiratory muscle weakness, respectively; the procedure for obtaining MIP and MEP is described in Chapter 17.
- **Peak expiratory flow rate (PEFR):** describes the maximum expiratory flow that can be generated during a forced expiration and is commonly used in the assessment of a patient suffering an acute asthma exacerbation (and described in Chapter 13); a decline in this measurement may suggest progressive airway obstruction as a result of plugging or infection.
- **Diaphragm fluoroscopy:** This procedure provides a radiological observation of diaphragm movement during inspiration. As well as being useful in the acute phase of support to assess the degree of function of the diaphragm in a patient able to take spontaneous breaths, this study is also useful in the subacute period. Approximately one-fifth of patients with loss of diaphragm function after SCI will have some recovery of movement, and this study can be used to follow that progress over time as well as to assess the response of the diaphragm to phrenic nerve pacing (52).
- **Video fluoroscopy/modified barium swallow:** This study, which assesses a patient's ability to complete a coordinated process of chewing and swallowing without evidence of aspiration, becomes the longer-term assessment for a patient with SCI. Because patients with SCI often have an impaired cough and gag reflex, it becomes important to identify the "silent aspirator" (described in Chapter 18) to prevent the long-term pulmonary damage that this can cause. Additionally, patients who will require a more-definitive feeding device, such as a gastrostomy tube, can be identified.
- **Sleep studies:** These studies measure the EEG, respiratory movement, and airflow throughout the phases of sleep. These studies are particularly useful in identifying those patients suffering from the sleep-disordered breathing issues described previously; a useful clinical sign of such disruptions in normal sleep include failure to gain weight despite the delivery of adequate calories.

There are a number of devices and therapeutic interventions that can be used in the subacute phase of recovery to assist the patient with respiratory muscle weakness (45). Some can be used prior to the patient being extubated, and others are measures to support the patient after extubation. It should be noted that some have limited use in the pediatric population because they require a degree of cooperation that the youngest patients cannot provide.

- **Respiratory muscle training:** daily exercises aimed at improving muscle strength
- **Abdominal binders:** prevent positional loss of lung volumes that can result from decreased abdominal tone; adult studies have shown that an abdominal binder can increase spontaneous V_T by as much as 16%, and it is therefore recommended early in care (53).
- **Noninvasive positive-pressure ventilation:** administered via face or nasal mask, provides continuous positive airway pressure (CPAP) or inspiratory and expiratory airway pressure (bi-level support, or BiPAP) to decrease the likelihood of hypoventilation and atelectasis in a patient with respiratory muscle weakness; these devices have a good track record in other chronic respiratory diseases in childhood, such as cystic fibrosis and cerebral palsy.
- **Diaphragm pacing:** allows for electrical stimulation of a poorly functioning diaphragm through electrodes placed on the muscle or the phrenic nerve that controls it (phrenic nerve pacing); this relatively new technology offers the possibility of freedom from equipment and technology, at least for some portion of the day (52).
- Airway clearance devices/techniques (discussed in detail in Chapter 14)
- Chest percussion and postural drainage
- Positive expiratory pressure (PEP) device: oscillating handheld apparatus that delivers vibrations to the airways during exhalation via a mouthpiece or mask, facilitating secretion clearance
- Insufflator-exsufflator device (described in Chapter 17): provides rapid cycling between positive inspiratory pressure and negative expiratory pressure to simulate the effect of coughing; should not be used for longer than 5 minutes, and assistance may be needed to suction produced secretions.
- High-frequency chest wall oscillation: vest that oscillates the chest wall through rapid inflation and deflation of the device, which increases airflow into the lungs and moves secretions into the larger airways for easier mobilization

- Intrapulmonary percussive ventilation: delivers high-flow bursts of air into the airways via a face mask or mouthpiece interspersed with periods of exhalation; acts to loosen secretions and relax spasm in the smaller airways. Nebulized medications can also be delivered with this device.

Course and Prognosis

In one of the largest published series to date that addressed the outcome in pediatric cervical SCI, 45% of patients required ICU management, with an average length of stay of 24 days (33). Twenty-seven percent of the patients died prior to hospital discharge, but only just more than a quarter of the deaths were directly related to the SCI; the other mortalities were the result of injuries to other organ systems, most commonly the brain. In this group of pediatric cervical SCI patients, 66% demonstrated initial neurological deficits, with a quarter of these patients exhibiting a complete injury (i.e., loss of all neurological function below the level of the injury). The mortality rate in the group with complete injury was 75%. Sixty-eight percent of the patients who had neurological findings had complete recovery of function. The authors of this series did not comment on the need for short-term or prolonged respiratory support (44).

In another retrospective review of pediatric cervical SCI (35), there was believed to be an increased opportunity for weaning from respiratory support over a period of weeks to months. This was felt to be due in part to the transition from flaccid (no muscle tone) to spastic (increased muscle tone) paralysis of intra-abdominal musculature, allowing less paradoxical motion of the rib cage over time and thus improved respiratory mechanics. In this study, "weaning readiness" was defined as a patient meeting the following criteria:

- Hemodynamic stability
- Free of infection
- In metabolic balance and positive nutritional balance (i.e., demonstrating appropriate weight gain with standard caloric intake)
- Able to generate a negative inspiratory force of –3 to –5 cm H_2O and a V_T of at least 1 to 3 cc/kg
- Stable gas exchange on room air (saturation greater than 95% and E_TCO_2 of under 45 mm Hg)
- Nonparadoxical spontaneous diaphragm motion either unilaterally or bilaterally

As with many adult studies, weaning was accomplished by ever-increasing lengths of "sprints," or time off of the ventilator. This was different from the typical in-patient weaning method, in which there is a gradual but relatively permanent reduction

in respiratory rate over time. When weaning was attempted, 63% of the patients were successfully weaned from support, with injury level being the best predictor of success (46). Although the adult literature suggests that the decision for tracheostomy should not be delayed for longer than 1 to 2 weeks after injury (49), there is very little data in the pediatric literature to form a conclusion regarding the timing of this procedure.

In terms of survival and long-term outcome, a 2007 study of cervical spine injury in pediatric patients over the course of 25 years at a level I trauma center showed the overall mortality rate was 28%, and two-thirds of the patients had neurological deficits (44).

> ■■ You return to take care of Johnny the following day, and the bedside nurse informs you that the secretions have markedly increased very acutely and are frothy-pink in character. As you suction him, you are struck by the volume of the secretions and also that the lung compliance with hand bagging seems to have gotten worse from the previous day. You call for the physician so that this new finding can be discussed and a ventilator strategy can be developed.

Neurogenic Pulmonary Edema

Neurogenic pulmonary edema (NPE) is a sudden increase in pulmonary interstitial fluid associated with numerous central nervous system (CNS) insults, including each of the following (54):

- Intracranial hemorrhage
- TBI
- Cervical spine injury
- Cerebral vascular accidents (strokes)
- Intracranial tumors
- Epilepsy
- Infection
- Multiple sclerosis

The estimated incidence of NPE varies widely; it seems to be most commonly seen in patients who have subarachnoid hemorrhage, and some estimate the incidence in severe TBI to be as high as 20% (55).

Pathophysiology

The mechanisms underlying the development of sudden pulmonary edema in the setting of CNS injury with no underlying cardiac or pulmonary pathology are poorly understood. Two different pathways seem to be at play: a hemodynamic mechanism and an inflammatory mechanism.

The proposed hemodynamic etiology has also been referred to as the "blast injury" theory, which proposes that a sudden increase in ICP causes a dramatic α-adrenergic catecholaminergic response. This then results in a rapid increase in the systemic and pulmonary vascular resistance—making it much harder for blood to move through the vascular beds. In the pulmonary circulation, this damages all three of the anatomical components that separate the vascular space from the alveoli: the pulmonary capillary endothelium, the basement membrane of the alveolar capillaries, and the alveolar endothelium. Once all three of these layers are compromised, there is leakage of red blood cells and proteins into the alveolar space, resulting in the pink, frothy secretions classically seen in pulmonary edema (56).

Also likely playing a role in the development of NPE is the systemic inflammatory response that develops in the setting of a significant neurological insult. A number of specific inflammatory mediators have been implicated, and many of these substances have the direct effect of increasing permeability of the capillary endothelium. This leads to the escape of red cells and plasma from the blood vessels (known as *extravasation*) into the pulmonary interstitium, and from there into the air spaces in severe cases. Interestingly, the catecholamine release described previously can itself result in upregulation, or hyperresponsiveness, of the inflammatory system (54).

Clinical Manifestations

The clinical signs in NPE are similar to those seen in patients with pulmonary edema caused by other etiologies: hypoxia, tachypnea (if spontaneously breathing), tachycardia, and pulmonary crackles noted especially at the bases are the most common findings. Unlike pulmonary edema seen secondary to left ventricular (LV) failure, an abnormal cardiac examination with extra heart sounds, like a gallop rhythm, is usually not present in patients with NPE.

The chest radiograph will most commonly demonstrate bilateral pulmonary infiltrates, although NPE has been reported to occur unilaterally. Cardiac studies (electrocardiogram, echocardiogram, and central venous pressure) will be normal unless there is associated cardiac pathology such as a cardiac contusion or decreased function secondary to hypoxic or ischemic damage suffered at the time of the initial injury.

The differential diagnosis should include aspiration pneumonia and, if the patient has been intubated for more than 48 hours, **ventilator-associated pneumonia (VAP)** (see Table 19-3). Aspiration pneumonia is certainly a risk for patients with an impaired level of consciousness, especially if the airway was left unprotected for a prolonged period of time prior to hospitalization. NPE usually develops more quickly, whereas the signs and symptoms of aspiration pneumonia and VAP tend to develop over a longer period of time. In both types of pneumonia, one could also expect to see thickened, purulent secretions as well as fever (although fever in patients with brain injuries is common, making this sign somewhat less reliable).

Management and Treatment

The primary ventilator strategy to address NPE is increased positive end expiratory pressure (PEEP), which acts to decrease the transmural pressure gradient and minimize the amount of fluid moving from the vascular space into the alveolar space. One must keep in mind the theoretical effect that PEEP could have on the patient's ICP; an increase in PEEP, if transmitted from the intrathoracic space to the intracranial vault, could result in a higher ICP. Similarly, if the increase in PEEP leads to a fall in the venous return from the intracranial space, the cerebral blood volume could increase and also result in increased ICP. Studies suggest, though,

Table 19-3	Differential Diagnosis of Edema and Pneumonia			
	Neurogenic Pulmonary Edema	**Cardiogenic Pulmonary Edema**	**Ventilator-Associated Pneumonia**	**Aspiration Pneumonia**
Cause	Neurological injury	LV failure	Introduction of microorganisms into pulmonary system via artificial airway or ventilation	Introduction of gastric or oropharyngeal secretion, food, or fluids into pulmonary system via unprotected airway
Timing of Signs and Symptoms	Rapid; several hours after a neurological event	Gradual; a result of LV failure	Gradual; after >48 hours of MV	Gradual; after suspected aspiration incidence
Secretions	Pink, frothy	Pink, frothy	Yellow/green, thick, purulent	Yellow/green, thick, purulent
Fever	No	No	Yes	Yes

that a PEEP value of less than 15 is unlikely to adversely affect cerebral hemodynamics (57, 58).

A change from conventional ventilation to a high-frequency ventilation (HFV) mode can also be considered in patients with NPE when hypoxia is not adequately addressed by increasing the PEEP. Some studies have found that the use of HFV may actually lead to a fall in ICP while improving oxygenation; the primary theoretical explanation for this is an increase in venous return resulting in a fall in intracranial blood volume (59, 60).

An additional strategy that can be employed is prone positioning (61). Studies performed in various populations with acute lung injury (ALI) or acute respiratory distress syndrome (ARDS), while not definitively showing a survival benefit for those patients in whom prone positioning is used, have suggested that, in certain subpopulations of patients, prone positioning may be of benefit (62). In the TBI population, where hypoxia could certainly exacerbate the neurological injury by endangering functional brain that surrounds the original insult, this strategy could be considered. The ICP must be carefully monitored, however, because some studies have suggested that being prone may result in an increase in ICP (63). Because of this, attempts should be made to keep the head of the bed elevated, even in the prone position.

Although hypoxia is the primary respiratory concern in NPE, inadequate ventilation can also become an issue. In this clinical scenario, permissive hypercapnia is not a viable option given the effect such a strategy would have on the ICP. Maintaining the ICP in the normal range is the primary objective for patients with NPE; therefore, normal CO_2 levels should be the goal.

■ ■ You and the physician decide to increase Johnny's PEEP from 5 cm H_2O to 10 cm H_2O. You will continue to suction and will monitor for changes in volume of secretions and increasing lung compliance. You ask the nurse to inform you if the MAP trends downward because that may give you a clue that the increase in PEEP may be impeding venous return. At the end of your shift, Johnny is still maintained on a PEEP of 10 cm H_2O, and you have been able to wean his FIO_2 to 0.40 and still maintain a saturation of arterial blood with oxygen (SpO_2) greater than 97%. There has been no change in MAP.

Course and Prognosis

If managed aggressively, NPE is usually a reversible process. The key goals of therapy are maintaining normal oxygenation, avoiding hypercarbia, and using ventilator strategies that do not exacerbate

ICP. The patient's overall prognosis is much more dependent on the underlying brain injury.

■ ■ Johnny is maintained on MV for the next 2 weeks while his neurological injuries heal. When he meets extubation criteria on day 17, he is given a spontaneous breathing trial on CPAP +5 cm H_2O and tolerates this level of support for more than 2 hours. He is extubated to a 2-L nasal cannula (NC) and is started on deep-breathing exercises and PEP therapy to mobilize secretions. When Johnny leaves the ICU 3 days later, he is breathing room air and mobilizing secretions well on his own. He will be continuing deep-breathing exercises and respiratory muscle training with the physical therapist in the hospital and at the rehabilitation facility to which he will be discharged.

■ ■ Critical Thinking Questions: Johnny Taylor

1. What would be included on your differential diagnosis if, after intubating Johnny, he was somewhat hard to bag and decreased breath sounds were noticed on his left side?
2. If Johnny developed worsening hypoxia 3 to 4 days into his ventilator course, what would be included on your differential diagnosis?
3. What would be your initial intervention if Johnny had a sudden spike in ICP to 35?
4. After 2 weeks on the ventilator, Johnny has successfully maintained normal oxygenation and ventilation on pressure support of 10 cm H_2O and CPAP of 5 cm H_2O. What additional clinical information should the medical team consider in assessing Johnny's readiness for extubation?

▶● Case Studies and Critical Thinking Questions

■ Case 1: Carlos Durez

You are working in the pediatric ICU when an 8-year-old boy is admitted after suffering a TBI sustained in a crash of an all-terrain vehicle. You are told he has a significant epidural hemorrhage and will be taken to the operating room for evacuation of the blood as quickly as possible. He was intubated in the ED for a GCS score of 8. No ICP monitor is in place, and the boy remains sedated and paralyzed after the intubation. His initial vital signs on admission to the ICU are as follows:

• Temp 35.0°C
• HR 136

- *RR 20 (ventilator rate)*
- *BP 110/65*
- *SpO_2 98% on FIO_2 of 1.0*
- *E_TCO_2 65*

Additional ventilator settings are peak inspiratory pressure (PIP) of 22 and PEEP of 5. The chest radiograph done in the ED after intubation showed a well-positioned ETT and clear lung fields.

- *What ventilator adjustment(s) would you recommend based on the current information?*
- *If your initial attempts to improve ventilation were not successful, what should the next step in patient management be?*

■ Case 2: Sarah Collins

You receive sign-out on a 10-year-old, 40-kg PICU patient who has been hospitalized for 5 days following a TBI suffered when she was struck by a motor vehicle while riding her bike. The patient has a significant head injury and was intubated in the field for a GCS score of 5. Her ICP has been reasonably well controlled with sedation, paralysis, and hyperosmolar therapy, and the medical team is hoping to start weaning these therapies in the next 24 hours. The patient's bedside nurse reports that she has been running a fever of 39°C for most of the past 24 hours and that the ETT secretions have become thick, yellow, and foul smelling. Her current ventilator settings are pressure-regulated and volume-controlled, with a TV of 350 cc, intermittent mandatory ventilation (IMV) of 20, PEEP of 5, FIO_2 of 0.40, and inspiratory time of 1 second. She is hitting PIPs of 28 to 30 with each ventilated breath. Her most recent arterial blood gas (ABG) values are:

- *pH 7.32*
- *$PaCO_2$ 55*
- *PaO_2 60*
- *Saturation 90%*

These findings are a significant change from her last ABG values, for which the PaO_2 was in the 90s.

- *What ventilator adjustments would be appropriate at this time to address the hypoxia?*
- *What changes would be effective in dealing with the hypercarbia?*

■ Case 3: DaJuan Rodriguez

A 15-year-old, 70-kg patient was admitted to the hospital yesterday after being ejected from a vehicle during a motor vehicle accident. His initial GCS score in the trauma bay was 5, and he

was intubated and admitted to the pediatric ICU. From the start, he required high ventilator settings to maintain adequate oxygenation and ventilation; a chest CT done shortly after admission revealed bilateral pulmonary contusions but no pneumothorax or hemothorax. His head CT showed diffuse axonal injury, a finding with multiple small punctuate hemorrhages that often corresponds to significant shearing injury in the brain and a very guarded prognosis. An ICP monitor was placed, and the readings have been less than 20 throughout the night. Over the course of the last 24 hours, the ventilator settings have been increased to maintain normocarbia and adequate ventilation; the patient currently is being ventilated in a volume-control mode with settings of TV of 700, IMV of 24, PEEP of 12, and FIO_2 of 0.90 to maintain oxygen saturations greater than 92%. You are called to the bedside when the patient has a sudden fall in saturation as measured by the pulse oximeter; this is accompanied by a significant drop in blood pressure and an increase in ICP to more than 30.

- *What would be the most likely cause of this patient's sudden deterioration?*
- *What would be the most appropriate intervention?*
- *If these hemodynamic and respiratory changes occurred in a more subacute fashion, what should be included on the differential diagnosis?*

■ Case 4: Bobby Patton

A 12-year-old, 50-kg patient has been in the hospital for 6 weeks following a cervical spine injury suffered when he dove into a shallow body of water. He did not suffer a head injury. He remained intubated and in the ICU for the first 4 weeks after his injury. He was extubated 2 weeks ago and then slowly weaned from high-flow NC oxygen to a conventional NC. Neurologically, he has no function in his lower extremities and limited movement in his upper extremities. He intermittently has developed areas of atelectasis on his chest radiograph, which has responded to more aggressive chest physiotherapy. He was transferred out to the inpatient floor 48 hours ago. As you are assessing him, you note decreased breath sounds at the bases bilaterally.

- *What respiratory support modalities might be used in this patient to decrease the likelihood of continued problems with atelectasis?*

• *If noninvasive ventilation is unsuccessful in providing adequate support for this patient, what additional intervention is available for long-term support of the respiratory system other than MV?*

■ Case 5: Janey Quinlan

Janey is a 6-month-old infant brought in by her babysitter for multiple episodes of vomiting after falling from a changing table 6 hours previously. There is no history of fever or diarrhea, and the baby has no known significant past medical history. The initial assessment reveals a lethargic infant with a piercing cry who opens her eyes and withdraws her arm when her nail bed is pinched. The anterior fontanel is noted to be bulging and taut.

• *What is this patient's GCS score?*

Janey's GCS score falls acutely to 7 during the evaluation, and she is intubated.

• *How would you best assess the adequacy of the rate at which the child is being ventilated immediately after extubation?*
• *If a CT scan of the head is consistent with significant cerebral edema, what first-tier therapies would you select to begin managing the ICP?*

Multiple-Choice Questions

1. What is the initial goal $PaCO_2$ when ventilating a patient with a significant TBI?
   a. Less than 25 mm Hg
   b. 25 to 30 mm Hg
   c. 30 to 35 mm Hg
   d. 35 to 40 mm Hg
   e. 40 to 50 mm Hg

2. Which of the following is unlikely to be the cause of respiratory compromise in a patient who was intubated 24 hours ago for a GCS score of 6 after suffering a TBI when he was struck by a car at a high rate of speed?
   a. Atelectasis
   b. Pneumothorax
   c. Hemothorax
   d. VAP
   e. Aspiration pneumonitis

3. Which spinal nerves are responsible for enervating the diaphragm?
   a. C1 to C5
   b. C3 to C5
   c. C5 to C8
   d. T1 to T3
   e. T1 to T5

4. What should be the first intervention for an intubated TBI patient who has a sudden and marked elevation in ICP?
   a. Needle decompression of the thoracic cavity
   b. Bolus dose of sedation
   c. Bolus dose of paralytic medication
   d. Manual ventilation to lower $PaCO_2$
   e. Increase PIP on the ventilator

5. A sudden increase in pink-tinged secretions being suctioned from the ETT in a patient with TBI and cervical SCI is most likely caused by:
   a. Pulmonary contusion.
   b. Hemothorax.
   c. NPE.
   d. Tracheal injury.
   e. VAP.

6. All of the following are appropriate therapies to reverse atelectasis in a ventilated patient with TBI except:
   a. Increase PEEP.
   b. Increase PIP.
   c. Decrease rate.
   d. Institute chest PT.
   e. Recruitment maneuvers such as inspiratory hold.

7. Which of the following increases a TBI patient's risk for an aspiration event?
       I. Delayed gastric emptying
       II. Loss of cough and/or gag
       III. Facial trauma
   a. I, II
   b. II, III
   c. I, III
   d. I, II, III
   e. None of the listed choices increase the risk of aspiration.

8. Long-term respiratory support for a patient with a cervical SCI at the level of C2 to C3 is *most* likely to include which of the following?
   a. Tracheostomy and MV
   b. Tracheostomy without MV
   c. Intermittent BiPAP
   d. Supplemental oxygen
   e. Respiratory support is unlikely to be required.

9. All of the following are consistent with the clinical presentation of a tension pneumothorax in a multiple trauma patient whose injuries include a TBI except:
a. Sudden drop in blood pressure.
b. Sudden drop in oxygen saturation.
c. Sudden drop in ICP.
d. Decreased breath sounds on one side.
e. Tracheal deviation.

10. Patients presenting with TBI should have an artificial airway placed if their GCS score is equal to or less than:
a. 12.
b. 11.
c. 10.
d. 9.
e. 8.

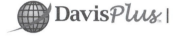 **DavisPlus** | For additional resources login to DavisPlus (http://davisplus.fadavis.com/ keyword "Perretta") and click on the Premium tab. (Don't have a PlusCode to access Premium Resources? Just click the Purchase Access button on the book's DavisPlus page.)

REFERENCES

1. Faul M, Xu L, Wale MM, Coronado VG. *Traumatic Brain Injury in the United States: Emergency Department Visits, Hospitalizations and Deaths 2002–2006.* Atlanta, GA: Centers for Disease Control and Prevention; 2010.
2. Tilford JM, Aitken ME, Anand KJ, et al. Hospitalizations for critically ill children with traumatic brain injuries: a longitudinal analysis. *Crit Care Med.* 2005;33(9):2074-2081.
3. Granacher RP Jr. *Traumatic Brain Injury: Methods for Clinical and Forensic Neuropsychiatric Assessment.* 2nd ed. Boca Raton, FL: CRC Press; 2008.
4. Baigelman W, O'Brien JC. Pulmonary effects of head trauma. *Neurosurgery.* 1981;9(6):729-740.
5. Stevens RD, Lazaridis C, Chalela JA. The role of mechanical ventilation in acute brain injury. *Neurol Clin.* 2008;26(2):543-563.
6. Nyquist P, Stevens RD, Mirski MA. Neurologic injury and mechanical ventilation. *Neurocrit Care.* 2008;9(3):400-408.
7. Gruen JP, Weiss M. Management of complicated neurologic injuries. *Surg Clin North Am.* 1996;76(4):905-922.
8. Stocchetti N, Maas AI, Chieregsato A, van der Plas AA. Hyperventilation in head injury: a review. *Chest.* 2005;127(5):1812-1827.
9. Bullock R. Hyperventilation. *J Neurosurg.* 2002;96(1):157-159.
10. Adelson PD, Bratton SL, Carney NA, et al. Guidelines for the acute medical management of severe traumatic brain injury in infants, children, and adolescents. Resuscitation of blood pressure and oxygenation and prehospital brain-specific therapies for the severe pediatric traumatic brain injury patient. *Pediatr Crit Care Med.* 2003;4(suppl 3):S12-S18.
11. Hastings RH, Wood PR. Head extension and laryngeal view during laryngoscopy with cervical spine stabilization maneuvers. *Anesthesiology.* 1994;80(4):825-831.
12. Dupanovic M, Fox H, Kovac A. Management of the airway in multitrauma. *Curr Opin Anaesthesiol.* 2010;23(2):276-282.
13. Sellick BA. Cricoid pressure to control regurgitation of stomach contents during induction of anaesthesia. *Lancet.* 1961;2(7199):404-406.
14. Brisson P, Brisson M. Variable application and misapplication of cricoid pressure. *J Trauma.* 2010;69(5):1182-1184.
15. Landsman I. Cricoid pressure: indications and complications. *Paediatr Anaesth.* 2004;14(1):43-47.
16. Smith G, Ng A. Gastric reflux and pulmonary aspiration in anaesthesia. *Minerva Anesthesiol.* 2003;69(5):402-406.
17. Field JM. Part 1: executive summary: 2010 American Heart Association guidelines for cardiopulmonary resuscitation and emergency cardiovascular care. *Circulation.* 2010;122(18, suppl 3):S640-S656.
18. Filanovsky Y, Miller P, Kao J. Myth: ketamine should not be used as an induction agent for intubation in patients with head injury. *CJEM.* 2010;12(2):154-157.
19. Vaillancourt C, Kapur AK. Opposition to the use of lidocaine in rapid sequence intubation. *Ann Emerg Med.* 2007;49(1):86-87.
20. Salhi B, Stettner E. In defense of the use of lidocaine in rapid sequence intubation. *Ann Emerg Med.* 2007;49(1):84-86.
21. Madikians A, Giza CC. Treatment of traumatic brain injury in pediatrics. *Curr Treat Options Neurol.* 2009;11(6):393-404.
22. Kochanek PM, Carney N, Adelson PD, et al. Guidelines for the acute medical management of severe traumatic brain injury in infants, children, and adolescents. *Pediatr Crit Care Med.* 13(suppl 1):S1-S82.
23. Hutchison JS, Frndova H, Lo TY, Guerguerian AM. Impact of hypotension and low cerebral perfusion pressure on outcomes in children treated with hypothermia therapy following severe traumatic brain injury: a post hoc analysis of the Hypothermia Pediatric Head Injury Trial. *Dev Neurosci.* 2010;32(5-6):406-412.
24. Adelson PD, Bratton SL, Carney NA, et al. Guidelines for the acute medical management of severe traumatic brain injury in infants, children, and adolescents. *Pediatr Crit Care Med.* 2003;4(suppl 3):S2-S4.
25. Hsiang JK, Chesnut RM, Crisp CB, Klauber MR, Blunt BA, Marshall LF. Early, routine paralysis for intracranial pressure control in severe head injury: is it necessary? *Crit Care Med.* 1994;22(9):1471-1476.
26. Bell MJ, Kochanek PM. Traumatic brain injury in children: recent advances in management. *Indian J Pediatr.* 2008;75(11):1159-1165.
27. Lassen NA. Brain extracellular pH: the main factor controlling cerebral blood flow. *Scand J Clin Lab Invest.* 1968;22(4):247-251.
28. Lassen NA. Control of cerebral circulation in health and disease. *Circ Res.* 1974;34(6):749-760.
29. Lundberg N, Kjällquist A, Bien C. Reduction of increased intracranial pressure by hyperventilation: a therapeutic aid in neurological surgery. *Acta Psychiatr Scand Suppl.* 1959;34(139):1-64.
30. Raichle ME, Posner JB, Plum F. Cerebral blood flow during and after hyperventilation. *Arch Neurol.* 1970;23(5):394-403.

31. Muizelaar JP, Marmarou A, Ward JD, et al. Adverse effects of prolonged hyperventilation in patients with severe head injury: a randomized clinical trial. *J Neurosurg.* 1991;75(5):731-739.

32. McLaughlin MR, Marion DW. Cerebral blood flow and vasoresponsivity within and around cerebral contusions. *J Neurosurg.* 1996;85(5):871-876.

33. Muizelaar JP, van der Poel HG, Li ZC, Kontos HA, Levasseur JE. Pial arteriolar vessel diameter and CO_2 reactivity during prolonged hyperventilation in the rabbit. *J Neurosurg.* 1988;69(6):923-927.

34. Adelson PD, Bratton SL, Carney NA, et al. Guidelines for the acute medical management of severe traumatic brain injury in infants, children, and adolescents. *Pediatr Crit Care Med.* 2003;4(3 suppl):S1-S75.

35. Curley G, Kavanagh BP, Laffey JG. Hypocapnia and the injured brain: more harm than benefit. *Crit Care Med.* 38(5):1348-1359.

36. Keenan HT, Runyan DK, Marshall SW, Nocera MA, Merten DF, Sinal SH. A population-based study of inflicted traumatic brain injury in young children. *JAMA.* 2003;290(5):621-626.

37. Coplin WM, Pierson DJ, Cooley KD, Newell DW, Rubenfeld GD. Implications of extubation delay in brain-injured patients meeting standard weaning criteria. *Am J Respir Crit Care Med.* 2000;161(5):1530-1536.

38. Principi T, Morrison GC, Matsui DM, et al. Elective tracheostomy in mechanically ventilated children in Canada. *Intensive Care Med.* 2008;34(8):1498-1502.

39. Taylor HG, Alden J. Age-related differences in outcomes following childhood brain insults: an introduction and overview. *J Int Neuropsychol Soc.* 1997;3(6):555-567.

40. Anderson V, Catroppa C, Morse S, Haritou F, Rosenfeld J. Functional plasticity or vulnerability after early brain injury? *Pediatrics.* 2005;116(6):1374-1382.

41. Campbell CG, Kuehn SM, Richards PM, Ventureyra E, Hutchison JS. Medical and cognitive outcome in children with traumatic brain injury. *Can J Neurol Sci.* 2004;31(2):213-219.

42. Johnson AR, DeMatt E, Salorio CF. Predictors of outcome following acquired brain injury in children. *Dev Disabil Res Rev.* 2009;15(2):124-132.

43. Keenan HT, Runyan DK, Marshall SW, Nocera MA, Merten DF, Sinal SH. A population-based study of inflicted traumatic brain injury in young children. *JAMA.* 2003;290(5):621-626.

44. Platzer P, Jaindl M, Thalhammer G, et al. Cervical spine injuries in pediatric patients. *J Trauma.* 2007;62(2):389-396; discussion 394-396.

45. Porth SC. Recognition and management of respiratory dysfunction in children with tetraplegia. *J Spinal Cord Med.* 2004;27(suppl 1):S75-S79.

46. Padman R, Alexander M, Thorogood C, Porth S. Respiratory management of pediatric patients with spinal cord injuries: retrospective review of the duPont experience. *Neurorehabil Neural Repair.* 2003;17(1):32-36.

47. Lanig IS, Peterson WP. The respiratory system in spinal cord injury. *Phys Med Rehabil Clin North Am.* 2000;11(1):29-43, vii.

48. Winslow C, Rozovsky J. Effect of spinal cord injury on the respiratory system. *Am J Phys Med Rehabil.* 2003;82(10):803-814.

49. Berlly M, Shem K. Respiratory management during the first five days after spinal cord injury. *J Spinal Cord Med.* 2007;30(4):309-318.

50. Claxton AR, Wong DT, Chung F, Fehlings MG. Predictors of hospital mortality and mechanical ventilation in patients with cervical spinal cord injury. *Can J Anaesth.* 1998;45(2):144-149.

51. Birnkrant DJ. The assessment and management of the respiratory complications of pediatric neuromuscular diseases. *Clin Pediatr (Phila).* 2002;41(5):301-308.

52. Shaul DB, Danielson PD, McComb JG, Keens TG. Thoracoscopic placement of phrenic nerve electrodes for diaphragmatic pacing in children. *J Pediatr Surg.* 2002;37(7):974-978.

53. Gilbert J. Critical care management of the patient with acute spinal cord injury. *Crit Care Clin.* 1987;3(3):549-567.

54. Baumann A, Audibert G, McDonnell J, Mertes PM. Neurogenic pulmonary edema. *Acta Anaesthesiol Scand.* 2007;51(4):447-455.

55. Bratton SL, Davis RL. Acute lung injury in isolated traumatic brain injury. *Neurosurgery.* 1997;40(4):707-712; discussion 712.

56. Hachenberg T, Rettig R. Stress failure of the blood-gas barrier. *Curr Opin Anaesthesiol.* 1998;11(1):37-44.

57. Huynh T, Messer M, Sing RF, Miles W, Jacobs DG, Thomason MH. Positive end-expiratory pressure alters intracranial and cerebral perfusion pressure in severe traumatic brain injury. *J Trauma.* 2002;53(3):488-492; discussion 492-493.

58. McGuire G, Crossley D, Richards J, Wong D. Effects of varying levels of positive end-expiratory pressure on intracranial pressure and cerebral perfusion pressure. *Crit Care Med.* 1997;25(6):1059-1062.

59. Salim A, Miller K, Dangleben D, Cipolle M, Pasquale M. High-frequency percussive ventilation: an alternative mode of ventilation for head-injured patients with adult respiratory distress syndrome. *J Trauma.* 2004;57(3):542-546.

60. Barrette RR, Hurst JM, Branson RD. A comparison of conventional mechanical ventilation with two forms of high-frequency ventilation for the control of intracranial pressure in closed head injury. *Respir Care.* 1987;32:733-740.

61. Fletcher SJ, Atkinson JD. Use of prone ventilation in neurogenic pulmonary oedema. *Br J Anaesth.* 2003;90(2):238-240.

62. Slutsky AS. The acute respiratory distress syndrome, mechanical ventilation, and the prone position. *N Engl J Med.* 2001;345(8):610-612.

63. Lee ST. Intracranial pressure changes during positioning of patients with severe head injury. *Heart Lung.* 1989;18(4):411-414.

Chapter 20

Ethics in Perinatal and Pediatric Respiratory Care

Renee Boss, MD, MHS
Megan McCabe, MD, FAAP

Chapter Outline cont.

Chapter Objectives

After reading this chapter, you will be able to:

1. Identify four ethical principles that underpin modern bioethics.
2. Understand the obligations of professional competence.
3. Discuss the clinician's duty when a medical error occurs.
4. Define professional ethics in the setting of a pandemic or public health emergency.
5. Describe how the best-interest standard is applied to medical decision-making in pediatrics.
6. Understand the differences between informed consent and assent for clinical care and research in pediatrics.
7. Understand the role of hospital ethics committees.
8. Describe moral distress in relation to caring for critically ill and dying children.
9. Explain the ethical issues and arguments around resuscitation of high-risk newborns.
10. Describe and apply the rule of double effect to symptom management at the end of life.
11. Discuss why non–heart-beating organ donation is currently controversial.

■■ Daniel Rogers

Daniel Rogers is a 12-year-old boy who was diagnosed with Duchenne's muscular dystrophy at the age of 6 years. Since that time, he has become progressively weaker, moving from being able to walk independently to requiring leg braces and to now using a wheelchair. Due to his muscular weakness, he has developed scoliosis and is now admitted to the pediatric intensive care unit (PICU) after a posterior spinal fusion. He is intubated postoperatively and is moderately sedated.

Bioethics is the discipline dedicated to the ethical and moral complexities that arise during the course of biomedical research and clinical patient care. The field of bioethics draws from knowledge and expertise in philosophy, law, history, theology, public health, and medicine. Bioethics integrates these approaches in the formulation of guiding principles for the ethical practice of medical research and patient care. This chapter reviews essential elements of both clinical and professional ethics in medicine, providing an overview of how societies, health-care systems, individual clinicians, and researchers share ethical responsibilities and duties in providing health care for patients and families. Specific attention is given to the unique bioethical concerns that may arise during the care of children and their families (1).

Historically, several different philosophical frameworks for thinking about medical research and patient care have evolved (2). Each framework offers a different lens for moral decision-making and for understanding the ethical duties and responsibilities of clinicians, health-care systems, and societies. There are five common philosophical frameworks for moral decision-making: utilitarian, justice, rights, virtue, and the common good. A complete review of these philosophies is beyond the scope of this chapter, but Table 20-1 provides a brief overview of how benefits and burdens might be weighed differently by each approach to decision-making.

This chapter begins with a discussion of basic ethical principles as they apply to patient care and clinical research. It then describes the essential elements of professional ethics, including issues related to professional competence, medical errors, and duty to practice in a public health emergency. It also reviews topics related to clinical ethics, including confidentiality, informed consent and assent, goals of care, futility, and conscientious objection. Finally, it examines how bioethical principles, professional ethics, and clinical ethics interact in the care of pediatric patients with complex diseases (e.g., extreme prematurity, spinal muscle atrophy type 1), as well as issues related to end-of-life care and organ donation.

Principles of Bioethics

In practice, four ethical principles have guided much of patient care and research since the 1970s: autonomy, justice, beneficence, and nonmaleficence (3).

Table 20-1	Five Philosophical Frameworks for Moral Decision-Making
Philosophical Framework	**Approach to Moral Issues**
Utilitarian	The decision should generate the greatest good for the greatest number of people.
Justice	The decision must treat everyone fairly.
Rights	The decision must respect moral rights (e.g., to privacy, to not be injured).
Virtue	The decision should promote the individual reaching his or her highest potential (e.g., for honesty, compassion, courage).
The Common Good	The decision must enhance the common good of a group/community/society.

These principles should guide all patient care interventions (Fig.20-1).

Autonomy

The term **autonomy** represents a person's right to make decisions that are based on his or her personal values, without undue influence from others, including family members or clinicians. This means, for instance, that patients have a right to decide to forgo chemotherapy for advanced cancer if they believe that the length of their life is less valuable than the ability to live their days without the burden of medications and hospitalization. Patients' right to autonomy confers a duty on clinicians to provide enough information about diagnosis and treatment—the

risks, benefits, and predicted outcomes—so that patients can make educated decisions. It also confers a duty for clinicians to elicit, respect, and incorporate patients' goals, values, and wishes into their treatment plans.

Autonomy is generally a right given to adults who have the capacity to make independent decisions about their medical care. When the patient is a child, however, the principle of autonomy typically refers to the rights of parents to make decisions for their child. Parents' rights to make decisions for their child's medical care must be respected as long as they do not endanger, abuse, or neglect the child (4). For children who are in the custody of the state as a result of abuse or neglect, state-appointed social workers and lawyers will act as decision-makers regarding medical care. When patients are very young, they are not generally allowed any substantive voice about their medical care. A 1-year-old child, for instance, is not permitted to refuse a vaccination that the parent requests. Distraction, deception, manipulation, and limited physical or chemical restraints may be permissible in some settings in which a young child's noncompliance interferes with a medical treatment felt to be in the child's best interest (Box 20-1).

Children's right to and capacity for autonomy increases with their emotional and cognitive development. Adolescents can often contribute in an educated and thoughtful way to decisions about their own medical care or participation in research. Preadolescents may be able to understand enough about a particular medical decision that it is appropriate to engage them in expressing their wishes about care. As discussed later in this chapter, respecting autonomy for older children often entails ensuring informed consent from parents and informed assent from the pediatric patient (Special Populations 20-1).

Box 20-1	Enhancing Compliance With Pediatric Patients

Medical treatments and interventions may make children frightened and anxious. When such treatments or interventions are deemed necessary, clinicians and parents often need to collaborate in using the least-coercive, developmentally appropriate means for enhancing patient compliance.

Distraction: using a toy or game to draw a child's attention away from a nebulizer
Deception: telling a child that a medicine will taste good
Manipulation: offering a present to a child if he or she will accept a medicine
Physical restraint: wrapping a child in a papoose to give him or her a nebulizer

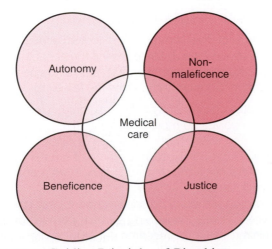

Figure 20-1 Guiding Principles of Bioethics

● Special Populations 20-1

Emancipated Minors and Medical Decision-Making

Emancipated minors are children younger than 18 who live independently of their parents. Emancipated minors may consent to or refuse medical care as if they were adults. The criteria and process for emancipation vary by state and courts, but generally include the following:

- Live separately from their parents
- Are financially independent or self-supporting
- Have parents who surrendered their rights and responsibilities
- Are married
- Have entered into active military service

Justice

The principle of **justice** requires health care to be delivered fairly, so that no one patient group unduly suffers the burden of scarce resources. Justice means that all individuals have a right to equal access to medical care and to a minimum standard of health care. It means, for instance, that children living in the poorest areas of a city should have the same access to a minimum standard of skilled medical care as those living in the richest areas of a city. The ideal of equal access to medical care is obviously constrained by the resources that are readily available in a particular setting. Governments, health-care systems, and individual clinicians often have to set priorities about the medical care that can be delivered within those constraints. Justice does confer a level of responsibility for health-care providers to improve the health status of community members who might be fundamentally harmed by poverty, racism, or inequality. Justice also confers upon clinicians and health-care systems a duty to demonstrate cultural competence so that medical care can be delivered effectively and compassionately to diverse populations.

In clinical research, respecting the principle of justice requires that all people have an equal opportunity to become participants in human subjects research. Particular protections for vulnerable populations, such as pregnant women and children, have evolved because there has been greater realization of the injustice of denying novel medical therapies to these populations (6). In the past 15 years, there has been a move away from the historical prohibition against research in children. Since 1998, the National Institutes of Health have required that children be included in human subjects research protocols, absent a compelling reason to exclude them (7). The ethical principles that govern research in children are

not different from those that govern research in adults: respect for persons, justice, and beneficence. Applying these principles to research in children is made even more complex by children's developmental variability and ability to give assent, additional concerns about risk in a vulnerable population, and the intricacies of family decision-making. It is the role of an institutional review board to evaluate the risks and benefits involved in research protocols (Special Populations 20-2).

Beneficence and Nonmaleficence

The principle of **beneficence** obligates clinicians to provide care that will be beneficial to the well-being of the patient and will serve the best interests of the patient. Care provided in this context may include cure of disease, relief from pain, or enhancing health and quality of life. Social and spiritual support of patients and families are important.

The principle of **nonmaleficence** obligates clinicians to care for patients in a way that causes no harm. Protecting a patient from harm may include adequate pain and symptom management, avoiding burdensome therapies that have minimal chance of improving the patient's well-being, and treating the patient with compassion and honesty. Medical treatments frequently entail some level of harm or risk to the patient; the principles of beneficence and nonmaleficence often have to be weighed against each other when determining what is in the patient's best interest.

Professional Ethics

Professional ethics address the interactions among professionals, individuals, and society. Professional governing bodies develop standards of behavior for their members. The American Association for

● Special Populations 20-2

Research in Infants and Children (53)

Subpart D of The Common Rule is often used by institutional review boards to determine the acceptability of risk posed by research participation in the pediatric population. Subpart D stipulates the following:

- Healthy children may only participate in research that involves no more than minimal risk.
- Children with a particular illness or disease may be eligible to participate in research of greater than minimal risk if the research offers them a potential direct benefit.
- Children without a particular disease may participate in research involving a minor increase over minimal risk if the research will provide vital information about a particular disorder.

Respiratory Care, for example, has issued a statement of professional conduct that defines the professional ethical standards for respiratory therapists (RTs) (Box 20-2) (9). These principles of professional conduct are based on the foundational principles of medical ethics described previously. This code of conduct blends theoretical principles and medicolegal restrictions on professional behavior to create a guide for practitioners. They address RTs' duties

Box 20-2 American Association for Respiratory Care's Position Statement on Professional Conduct (9)

In the conduct of professional activities, the RT shall be bound by ethical and professional principles. RTs shall do the following:

• Demonstrate behavior that reflects integrity, supports objectivity, and fosters trust in the profession and its professionals
• Seek educational opportunities to improve and maintain their professional competence and document their participation accurately
• Perform only those procedures or functions in which they are individually competent and that are within their scope of accepted and responsible practice
• Respect and protect the legal and personal rights of patients, including the right to privacy, informed consent, and refusal of treatment
• Divulge no protected information regarding any patient or family unless disclosure is required for the responsible performance of duty authorized by the patient and/or family or is required by law
• Provide care without discrimination on any basis, with respect for the rights and dignity of all individuals
• Promote disease prevention and wellness
• Refuse to participate in illegal or unethical acts
• Refuse to conceal, and will report, the illegal, unethical, fraudulent, or incompetent acts of others
• Follow sound scientific procedures and ethical principles in research
• Comply with state or federal laws that govern and relate to their practice
• Avoid any form of conduct that is fraudulent or creates a conflict of interest and follow the principles of ethical business behavior
• Promote health-care delivery through improvement of the access, efficacy, and cost of patient care
• Encourage and promote appropriate stewardship of resources

and rights with regard to patients, colleagues, and the larger society. This section explores how professional ethics are applied to some common issues that RTs face.

Professional Competence

■■ Daniel remains intubated in the PICU after his posterior spinal fusion. His parents are at the bedside when you and your preceptor come in to do a ventilator check and suction him. Mrs. Rogers asks you to introduce yourselves.

A fundamental duty of professional ethics requires that clinicians attain **professional competency** through an appropriate level of training relevant to their area of expertise. Health-care providers are often obligated to complete both classroom training and practical training in patient care before assuming responsibilities as an independent practitioner. Health-care providers are required to maintain ongoing continuing education in their areas of expertise to remain knowledgeable about relevant medical advances and evolving standards of care.

Although teaching hospitals and training programs necessarily incorporate patient care by trainees, this care should always be performed under the close supervision of experienced clinicians. Practical training programs have social utility because future patients benefit from the experiences that learners have during their supervised training. When a patient agrees to receive medical care at a training facility, this constitutes a broad type of consent to allow trainees to participate in that care (10). Nevertheless, individual trainees have a duty to disclose their level of experience to patients and families. Patients have a right to request more information about the trainees' level of participation in clinical care and the details of their supervision. These duties and rights are regulated in many states via a patient bill of rights (11).

Clinicians also have a duty to notify supervisors when there are concerns about the professional competency of peers. In addition, clinicians have a duty to notify supervisors of any concerns regarding system-based problems that have the potential to compromise patient safety. This may include concerns about faulty equipment, nonstandard use of therapies, or unsafe staffing levels (Teamwork 20-1).

Medical Errors

■■ Three days after his posterior spinal fusion, Daniel has been extubated and is on the in-patient floor recovering from surgery. He is on bi-level positive airway pressure at night. When you look at the orders, you see that he is ordered for a backup rate of 12, inspiratory positive airway pressure (IPAP) of 20, expiratory positive airway pressure (EPAP) of 6, and fractional concentration of inspired oxygen (FIO₂) of 21%. While you look over the settings on the machine, you see that it has been set for a backup rate of 20 and an IPAP of 12. The EPAP is 6, and the FIO₂ is 21%.

A **medical error** implies a preventable adverse event—a threat to patient safety that could have been avoided. A medical error may cause a patient to experience an avoidable infection, injury, medication overdose or underdose, misdiagnosis, or even death. Medical errors may or may not result in actual patient harm; errors that do not cause patient harm are often called "near misses."

The Institute of Medicine's 2000 report *To Err is Human* estimated that at least 44,000 and as many as 98,000 people die from medical errors yearly in the United States (12). Since that report's publication, many health-care systems have put large-scale quality and safety initiatives into place to help identify and prevent medical errors. In addition to this effort, most institutions have developed guidelines for disclosing errors to patients and their families. To many people in health care, this has been a significant cultural change. In the past, although errors did occur, they were rarely addressed openly with patients and families. However, on multiple levels, there are ethical reasons to disclose errors to patients.

Patient safety can be compromised both as the result of an inherent risk of medical treatment or as the result of an error. Inherent risks include those unavoidable harms that are known to occur in a defined population as a consequence of a medical treatment. For instance, a certain number of patients will suffer from laryngeal edema following extubation, and some of those patients may require reintubation to protect their airway. In this case, patient safety is not compromised due to a mistake on the part of the health-care provider but as a known adverse effect of translaryngeal intubation. Another example of inherent risks associated with medical care includes medication side effects, such as tachycardia following a nebulized bronchodilator. Clinicians have an obligation to anticipate and disclose these foreseeable events and the likelihood of their occurrence to patients before providing the medical treatment or intervention. When the inherent risk is potentially severe, such disclosure may take the form of a formalized written informed consent.

Medical errors can occur in any health-care setting, although they are most common in settings where highly technical care is delivered, such as intensive care units. In 2007, the Joint Commission found that as many as half of all serious adverse medical events were due to poor communication—between clinicians and patients and between clinicians and other clinicians (13).

Although individual clinicians may make errors during the care of patients, it is the duty of a medical system to have in place multiple routine checks and balances to prevent, detect, and ameliorate mistakes made by individuals. Some of the interventions aimed at decreasing medical errors include computerized documentation and order-entry systems that eliminate problems from poor handwriting, automated allergy notifications, work hour limits, standardized methods for handoffs of patient information, and certified hospital translators. Increasingly, efforts are being made to educate patients about the steps they can take to minimize the chance of a medical error, such as asking clinicians to wash their hands, asking surgeons to initial the targeted

Teamwork 20-1 Unsafe Staffing Levels

MOST HOSPITAL DEPARTMENTS HAVE A MINIMUM STAFFING LEVEL, OR THE NUMBER OF RTs NECESSARY TO PROVIDE SAFE PATIENT CARE DURING AVERAGE ACUITY. Patient care acuity, however, can increase rapidly, and staff members have to feel confident enough to speak up to front-line supervisors if they are unable to complete their assigned patient care for any reason. There are several techniques you can use as a front-line RT to ensure that you or one of your coworkers are not sacrificing the care of one patient while working with another:

- Check in at regular intervals with coworkers. This is particularly important for RTs, who frequently work in multiple units or may not always see or hear what other RTs are doing.
- Know how to contact your coworkers when you need help. Do they have a pager number? Is there a lead or floating therapist assigned to help others?
- At the beginning of the shift, identify a therapist with a lighter assignment or one who may be able to help when other assignments increase.
- At the beginning of the shift, identify the RT who is most likely to experience a rapid increase in acuity in his or her patients. This could be someone with the largest number of patients or the one with the highest number of open beds in the unit. It could also be the therapist in a surgical unit who will be receiving many postoperative patients throughout the shift.

body site prior to surgery, and following up with clinicians about the results of medical tests.

When a medical error does occur, clinicians have a duty to carefully analyze what occurred, why it occurred, what has happened because of the error, and what could yet occur. This process of analysis should involve the senior clinicians caring for the patient; some institutions have formal disclosure policies that require hospital administrators be involved. Clinicians should also seek support for the emotional stress that can accompany medical mistakes. The process of error analysis should be thorough and systematic but should also be expedited. Respect for persons means that patients have a right to prompt, complete, and transparent disclosure of the harm to the patient that has resulted from, or could result from, the medical error. When an error causes severe patient harm, or even death, a sentinel event analysis can help avert recurrent events. Despite fear of litigation following disclosure of medical mistakes, there is significant evidence to suggest actual litigation is rare (14).

Pandemics and Public Health Emergencies

Professional codes of ethics often address the rights and obligations of health-care providers in the event of public health emergencies or other types of disasters. Hospitals, as well as local, state, and federal governments, may compel personnel to be available to work in public health emergencies. After September 11, 2001, the Model State Emergency Health Powers Act gave state medical licensers the authority to require health-care providers to work in such scenarios (15). This limit on medical personnel's personal autonomy has been justified by the need on the part of the greater population for the special skills possessed by health-care providers. RTs are likely to be key care providers in public health emergencies, based on recent experience with both the severe acute respiratory syndrome (SARS) and H1N1 pandemics and mass-casualty events worldwide (16).

In the setting of a public health emergency, clinicians may have competing obligations. As noted previously, clinicians have a duty to stabilize and treat patients by drawing from their relevant experience and training and the available resources. Clinicians have a simultaneous duty to protect themselves and their own health so that they might continue caring for patients, will not become patients themselves, and can meet their obligations to their own families. Because of this, some health-care systems require personnel to be vaccinated against certain diseases, such as influenza. Proponents of this **mandatory vaccination** raise several ethical claims. The first is that unvaccinated health-care workers are a source of nosocomial infection for patients, particularly the most vulnerable patients such as those receiving intensive care. Nosocomial infections are the cause of significant patient morbidity and mortality and hospital costs; at least 80% of health-care providers must be vaccinated to decrease nosocomial infections (17). Mandatory vaccination may also prevent workforce disruption during the height of an epidemic. It may prevent health-care providers from becoming additional burdens on a strained health system and requiring medical treatment themselves. Some health-care providers refute a professional duty to receive vaccination, citing concerns about adverse effects, vaccine shortages, and inconvenience. This has been seen as a conflict between personal and professional ethics (18).

There are a number of considerations and obligations for health-care systems and local and national governments in scenarios of public health emergencies. There are several ways to minimize the risk to populations, including efforts to educate, vaccinate, quarantine, or provide postexposure medical and psychological support. Increasingly, hospitals and governments are collaborating in disaster planning and engaging in mass disaster simulations. Health-care systems and governments have important roles to play in determining the need for medical equipment and developing objective criteria to allocate resources in the event that patients need more medication, equipment, or medical personnel than is available. In the recent H1N1 epidemic, standard respiratory therapies—both mechanical ventilators and modes of noninvasive ventilation—were at the center of ethical debates about rationing of health care.

Disaster ethics may require that patients' personal autonomy be limited and decisions about allocation of resources be made at a public health level. Ideally, decision-making about resources should be a transparent and publicly debated process. This will promote just allocation and ongoing public trust that decision makers are acting in their best interests. Allocation policies must be objective, must be consistently applied, and must work to maximize benefit to most people in need. Clinicians must accept a suspension of their own personal professional autonomy because they are required to protect the integrity of the triage process.

Clinical Ethics

Clinical ethics refers to the application of bioethical principles to patient care, research, and health policy. Clinical ethics can assist individual clinicians in analyzing and settling complex clinical cases involving conflict about what should be done for a particular patient. These ethically complex cases may raise issues of confidentiality, best interests, veracity, informed consent, goals of care, and futility. Clinicians involved in these situations may experience moral distress or compassion fatigue.

Confidentiality

Several professions have an obligation to respect confidentiality, including health-care providers and lawyers. Medical **confidentiality** refers to clinicians' duty to not reveal information disclosed to them by a patient or about a patient. This duty reflects the ethic of respect for persons. Legal protection for medical confidentiality is not absolute; clinicians do have an obligation to breech patients' confidentiality if they disclose that they have, or they plan to, harm themselves or others. This means, for instance, that a clinician must make a legal report if a mother reveals that she is physically abusing her toddler.

In pediatrics, conflicts regarding confidentiality can arise when parents ask clinicians to refrain from telling children about their medical condition, treatments, or prognosis. For example, a father may request that a child not be told that she has cancer. Conflicts about confidentiality can also arise when children ask clinicians not to reveal information to their parents, such as the results of a pregnancy test. In each case, the clinician's role is to understand why the patient or parent wishes to withhold the truth. Through discussion of the risks and benefits both of disclosing and of withholding the information, the clinician can often assist in creating a safe and respectful space where the information can be shared.

The rise in the use of social media by health-care providers has posed new concerns about patient confidentiality. Using the internet to share information about patients, whether in the form of photographs or text, violates confidentiality. Increasingly, hospital medical training programs are developing strict staff policies about the use of cameras and social media (19).

Best-Interest Standard

Because children possess, at best, a limited degree of autonomy, they are never considered legally competent to make medical decisions. Morally and legally, it is the parents' right to make decisions for their child. The goal of these decisions is that they are in the child's best interest. The **best-interest standard** holds that decisions should ideally maximize the child's welfare. In fact, parents are only held to a standard of making a decision for their child that is reasonable. That is to say, families do not have to make the best decision for their child as judged by doctors or by the court as long as their decision does not diverge too far from what clinicians and societies define to be reasonable.

Determining what is in a child's best interest can sometimes be ambiguous and conflicted. For instance, if an extremely premature infant has no more than a 5% chance of surviving the neonatal period, some would argue that it is unclear whether aggressive intensive care is in that infant's best interest (20). In such a scenario, the clinicians may believe that it is in the infant's best interest to provide only palliative care, while the parents may believe it is in the infant's best interest to pursue all intensive therapies that have any chance of prolonging life. When faced with conflicts like this, clinicians should strive to reach understanding and compromise through the process of consistent, compassionate, and truthful communication. In addition, careful consideration should be given to the ways in which a family's culture, religion, and beliefs shape their values and decisions. It is important to involve individuals whom the family identifies as important counselors to them, such as extended family members or community religious leaders. For those cases in which clinicians feel that families are not making reasonable decisions for their child, it may be necessary to involve the hospital ethics committee and/or legal counsel. In extreme cases, the legal system may take over responsibility for guardianship and decision-making.

Informed Consent

■ ■ Six months after Daniel's surgery, he is back in the hospital. You are working on the pediatric inpatient floor again and go into Daniel's room to help with his chest physiotherapy regimen. He continues to weaken from his muscular dystrophy. He tells you he is back in the hospital to be part of "an experiment." You ask him what kind of experiment, and he tells you "I don't really know, but my parents signed me up, and they hope it will help me get better."

The concept of **informed consent** is based on a duty to honor patient autonomy. It requires clinicians and researchers to provide the facts and information that a patient needs to make a reasoned decision; it requires patients to have the ability to exercise reasoned judgment (21). Obtaining informed consent from a patient or research participant involves much more than acquiring a signature; true informed consent is a process that requires clear communication about risks and benefits, adequate time for questioning and understanding, protection from undue influences, and transparency about the right to revoke consent at any point. Informed consent requires veracity, or truthfulness, on the part of the clinician.

Informed consent can only be provided by a legal adult 18 years or older. In pediatric medicine and pediatric clinical research, usually one or both parents must provide informed consent for their child's treatment or participation. Although the legal standing of adolescent parents younger than 18 years old varies from state to state, most states recognize some degree of emancipation for adolescent parents and permit them to provide informed consent for their own children.

As noted previously in this chapter, when making medical decisions for their child, parents are not obligated to make the best possible decision or to take the recommendations of the health-care team, as long as the decision they make is reasonable and free from abuse, neglect, or harm. Clinicians are obligated to provide adequate information and guidance to parents to enhance their ability to provide truly informed consent.

Assent

Assent is a concept unique to pediatrics. **Assent** refers to the agreement by a child who cannot legally give informed consent but who parents and providers believe has some capacity for understanding the decision at hand and for expressing preferences. Children as young as 11 years can have the capacity to weigh hypothetical outcomes of different treatment options. In uncomplicated situations, children as young as 7 or 8 years old might be able to participate in decision-making about their treatment and to provide assent.

The American Academy of Pediatrics (AAP) has outlined the steps necessary for pediatric assent (4). Similar to obtaining informed consent from adults, when clinicians and researchers assure assent, they provide children with adequate information about their condition and the predicted risks and benefits from the treatment or intervention, and they answer all questions to the children's satisfaction. The most important aspect of these conversations is that they must be tailored to the child's developmental abilities to reason and make decisions. Clinicians and researchers should also explore the degree of autonomy that characterizes the child's decision. For example, a child may agree to experimental chemotherapy despite advanced cancer because she knows it is what her mother wants, even though the child herself would prefer to never return to the hospital. The clinician may still honor the child's assent to the experimental chemotherapy, but should assess how best to help the child talk with her mother about her goals and expectations.

There are times when parents and children disagree about medical decisions. There are clinical situations in which children may assent to a treatment, but their parents will not, or vice versa. Such conflicts demand ongoing and honest communication between members of the health-care team and the family about what is in the child's best interest to determine the best course of action. Because a child's assent does not have the legal weight of the adult parent's consent, clinicians may proceed based on a parent's consent even without a child's assent if the treatment or intervention has clear therapeutic benefit.

Goals of Care

When participating in the delivery of medical care for a patient, it is important that clinicians and families communicate about what are desirable and undesirable patient outcomes. For children with a life-limiting illness with no known cure, a variety of treatment options may be considered. There is often no clinical indication for choosing one treatment over the others. Some treatments may extend the lifespan, but with considerable burdens of side effects; other treatments may maximize a child's quality of life but may result in fewer days or weeks of life. Because the clinical and ethical value of one treatment over another is not clear, these decisions should be made together with families. Families should be encouraged to reflect upon and articulate what is important to them as their children undergo treatment for their condition. Often, young parents have not had other opportunities to think about their values related to medical care, particularly life-sustaining therapies, and may need considerable support from clinicians to clarify their goals (22). Involving leaders from the family's social network as well as religious and cultural communities is critical.

Establishing these **goals of care** early in the treatment process can assist clinicians in determining which interventions make sense given the priorities for that patient. Many hospitals have policies regarding who is responsible for eliciting a patient or family's goals of care and clarifying procedures for these discussions. A family's goals of care should be documented clearly and be available across health-care settings so that all clinicians who might care for the child (e.g., emergency room clinicians) will have access to the details. A variety of standardized tools exist for documenting a family's goals and values, such as *My Wishes* (23). A family's goals of care are often not static; clinicians should be prepared to adjust their medical management as the family's priorities evolve. As a child's illness worsens, it is particularly important to clarify the goals related to location of care, such as home hospice, as well as resuscitation goals.

Futility

Medical **futility** is a concept that describes medical treatments that are not expected to result in any benefit to the patient. Interventions may be considered futile or medically ineffective either because they will not prolong life or because the quality of life that they will lead to is unacceptably poor. Clinicians are not obligated to provide futile care, and in fact they have an ethical obligation *not* to provide futile care that will cause undue suffering for the patient. Futile care violates the principle of nonmaleficence.

Determining which interventions are unequivocally futile is fraught with some ambivalence. There is no national or international agreement about how small the chance of therapeutic benefit must be for a treatment to be considered futile or medically ineffective. Interventions that clearly fall out of the standard of care for similar patients with similar diseases are most clearly defined as futile. For instance, extracorporeal membrane oxygenation (ECMO) is considered medically futile in infants who have pulmonary hypoplasia caused by lethal osteogenesis imperfecta; not only does this treatment not cure the pulmonary hypoplasia, but it also poses a risk of significant additional harm to the patient. On the other hand, many interventions are believed to have a small or uncertain chance of benefit to the patient. There may be disagreement among professional medical societies, individual clinicians, and families about which of these interventions might be futile (24). In these cases, clinicians should look for guidance from their institution's policies, the hospital ethics committee, and state law regarding medically ineffective care.

Moral Distress

Moral distress describes the dilemma clinicians experience when they are prevented from doing what they feel is best for their patients or when they feel obligated to do something they believe is not in their patients' best interest. A clinician, for instance, might experience moral distress when asked to perform cardiopulmonary resuscitation (CPR) for a 5-year-old who is dying from end-stage cancer. Clinicians treating children with HIV in Africa might feel moral distress when they cannot obtain the antiretroviral treatments for their patients that they know are available in other countries. Clinicians may feel moral distress about perceived unsafe staffing levels in their intensive care unit (25). Moral distress commonly occurs when families request, or deny, therapies that clinicians feel strongly about. Given the ethical and legal deference given to the right of parents to make decisions for their children, clinicians may often feel they do not have a right to deny that autonomy (26).

Because of the different roles and responsibilities that multidisciplinary members of a health-care team have when caring for patients, members of that team often experience moral distress in ways that reflect their roles. Physicians, for example, often feel the greatest moral responsibility for denying requests for medically ineffective care; nurses may experience the greatest moral distress around issues of quality of care or breakdowns in team collaboration (27).

RTs may feel moral distress about performing terminal extubations during withdrawal of mechanical ventilation (MV), particularly if they feel inadequately prepared to participate in end-of-life care (28, 29). The differing roles and experiences of multidisciplinary team members can result in conflict; families often perceive this conflict and find that it undermines their trust in medical care. Clinicians can best manage these conflicts when the environment makes it safe for them to communicate honestly with each other (30).

When clinicians do not have an opportunity to directly address their moral distress and receive support from colleagues, compassion fatigue and burnout can occur. **Compassion fatigue** results from ongoing stress in health-care providers who do not have adequate ability or time to engage in self-care practices. Symptoms of compassion fatigue can include apathy, anger, anxiety, self-doubt, difficulty focusing, work absences, and substance abuse. Unaddressed compassion fatigue may lead to burnout and cause clinicians to experience difficulties in their job or to consider leaving the health-care field (31, 32).

When clinicians' moral objection to the care for a particular patient or group of patients is strong, they are permitted to withdraw their participation in that care. The terms *conscientious objection* and **conscientious refusal** refer to clinicians' moral and legal right to not provide care that they find ethically objectionable (33). The legitimacy of clinicians' personal moral beliefs is permitted to exceed their professional responsibilities in this setting, with the goal of protecting their integrity and self-respect. Medical institutions generally have a written policy for conscientious refusal, which describes the steps clinicians must take in order to decline care of a patient. Conscientious refusal, while protecting the rights of clinicians, does have the potential to infringe on patients' rights. If, for example, a neonatologist refuses to intubate a newborn with Trisomy 18 as a matter of conscientious objection, this may obstruct the infant's right to medical care (34). When terminating their participation in a patient's care because of conscientious refusal, clinicians have a duty to transfer that care to a qualified health-care provider and to continue providing that care if the patient's health is at significant risk.

■■ You don't see Daniel again until 3 years later, when he has been admitted to the PICU. This time, he has been admitted after developing ventricular tachycardia related to cardiomyopathy. He is intubated and needs to have a defibrillator placed. One of the residents on the case is wondering if this constitutes futile care because Daniel is likely to die from muscular dystrophy. An ethics consult is requested. After discussion with Daniel (although he is intubated, he is able to use his computer for communication), his family, and the treating medical team, the hospital ethics committee supports the decision to pursue a defibrillator. The defibrillator is placed, and Daniel is able to be extubated after a long period of intubation. During this hospitalization, there are several meetings with his family and both out-patient and in-patient medical teams. They agree that, when Daniel is better able to speak for himself, they will discuss with him the possibility of tracheotomy and long-term MV and develop a plan for decision-making. Daniel goes home and returns to school.

The Joint Commission mandates that all hospitals formalize a procedure for addressing ethical conflicts that arise during the care of patients. Most hospitals satisfy this requirement by maintaining one or more **hospital ethics committees**, comprising multidisciplinary members from both the medical and lay communities. The chair of the hospital ethics committee generally has some level of advanced training in bioethics. Although committee members are not required to have extensive ethics training, they should have enhanced skills and interests that increase their expertise beyond that of the average clinician (Fig. 20-2). The role of hospital ethics committee members is to act as advisors, arbitrators, and ethical experts to the health-care team. Hospital ethics committees do not have the authority to make medical decisions; this authority remains with the patient's medical team. Hospital ethics committees also are not acting in the capacity of legal counsel, even though questions posed to the committee sometimes overlap with concerns about legal permissibility.

In some hospitals, separate ethics committees are established to specifically address pediatric issues; in other settings, representatives knowledgeable about pediatric medicine participate in the larger hospital ethics committee that reviews both adult and pediatric cases. Hospital ethics committees should be consulted whenever there is uncertainty or disagreement about the ethical permissibility of a particular area of clinical care. For instance, hospital ethics committees are commonly consulted to comment on conflicts between clinicians and families about what is in the patient's best interest. Many hospitals also require that an ethics consultation occur routinely as part of certain clinical protocols, such as during a determination of medically ineffective treatment.

An ethics consultation may be requested by any member of the medical team, any hospital staff member, or any family member. The hospital ethics committee may provide consultation either by individual committee members, by subgroups of the committee, or by the committee as a whole. Committees generally invite involved multidisciplinary clinicians, family members, and if appropriate, the patient to participate in the consultation and present their perspectives about the issue at hand. The ethics committee then proceeds with careful deliberation of the clinical scenario in light of normative ethical principles. The documented findings of the hospital ethics committee are generally included in the patient's medical record.

In addition to providing consultation for individual clinical cases, many hospital ethics committees play integral roles in the development of hospital protocols to address ethically complex clinical scenarios, such as organ donation, establishing goals of care, and do-not-resuscitate orders. Hospital ethics committees also often participate in organizational policies and business ethics for which they may contribute to administrative guidelines, such as receiving gifts from pharmaceutical companies. Most hospital ethics committees engage in education of the wider medical community about ethical issues related to patient care.

Health Policy Ethics

Clinical ethics also inform health policy on a national and international level. Health policy ethics focus on broad issues that have an impact on the way health care is delivered across a variety of settings. Questions about human rights, access to essential medicines, stem cell research, responsible biotechnology, and national health care are just some of the concerns of health policy ethics. In the United States, the Presidential Commission for the Study of Bioethical Issues works with the president to establish policies that promote ethically responsible clinical medicine and medical research. Historically, the commission has published statements concerning such topics as caring for the aged, human cloning, and biotechnology.

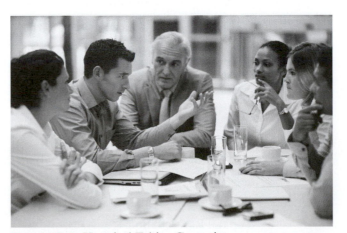

Figure 20-2 Hospital Ethics Committee *(© Thinkstock)*

Clinical Scenarios With Ethical Implications for Pediatric Respiratory Care

There are many scenarios in a pediatric RT's daily responsibilities that have the potential to cause ethical dilemmas. This section describes several of the more common scenarios, the ethical implications, and some strategies to employ to address them.

Newborn Resuscitation in Cases of Extreme Prematurity or Severe Congenital Anomalies

Newborn resuscitation is an extremely common procedure. The goal is to support infants during the transition from fetal life to independent respiration and circulation. For most newborns, this is the simple act of drying and stimulating the infant, assessing for good perfusion and respiratory effort, and subsequently passing them over to proud and excited parents. For the preterm infant or the infant with congenital anomalies, neonatal resuscitation can go far beyond these routine maneuvers. Intubation, vascular access, CPR, or other invasive procedures may be required within the first minutes after birth. These children need the support of a newborn intensive care unit for days to months as their bodies adjust to extrauterine life. As advances in both respiratory technology and medical care have allowed the immediate survival of many infants who would otherwise not survive, the ethical dilemmas faced by care providers have become stark and frequent. This is true both for infants at the threshold of viability and those with severe congenital anomalies. Although technology can save lives, it can also serve to sustain bodily function at times when recovery or future development is impossible, thereby prolonging suffering and delaying but not preventing death. This section reviews the ethical challenges created by the question of when and how to best support these ill and fragile infants and their families.

Ethical questions may arise even before an infant is born. Prenatal screening with ultrasound and maternal blood work has allowed the earlier identification of some severe congenital anomalies. This provides families and health-care providers the opportunity to make decisions regarding maintenance versus termination of a pregnancy. If the pregnancy is maintained, a plan for the delivery and the support provided to the infant after birth becomes the central question. This same decision-making process may need to occur in an abbreviated time frame when a woman develops preterm labor at 23 weeks' gestational age.

The decision regarding which infants to resuscitate and how to resuscitate has both ethical and legal implications. The legal implications require an understanding of both federal and state law, and hospital policies drafted with the participation of hospital counsel will reflect both federal and local regulations. Professional societies such as the AAP have published guidelines for decision-making regarding high-risk newborns (35). These guidelines do not provide specific algorithms but rather create a framework for practitioners (Fig. 20-3). The ethical framework used by these guidelines is interest based, meaning that decisions should be made based on what is perceived to be in the patient's best interests. Ethicists use this approach in part because principle-based approaches (e.g., beneficence, autonomy) are often difficult to integrate with real-world decision-making because often the principles will conflict. In cases of adults who cannot make decisions for themselves, an interest-based approach (i.e., "What is in the best interest of the patient?") is well accepted. Using this approach for infants rests on the fundamental assumption that infants are individuals with rights and interests equal to all other individuals, regardless of chronological age. Because infants are developmentally incapable of expressing and advocating for their interests, clinicians rely on surrogate decision-makers to answer the question "What is in the best interest of the patient?"

Determining the best interest of an individual patient requires an examination of rights. In the case of high-risk newborns, there are several individuals and groups to consider. First is the newborn, followed by the family (parents and siblings), and finally the medical team and larger society. The rights of the infant are primary in this discussion, although not solely important. The infant first has the right to life and therefore medical treatment that sustains life. This right is fundamental but not inviolable, meaning that in certain situations other rights may take precedence (36). The infant also has a right to justice, or equal treatment, unless there is a moral reason for

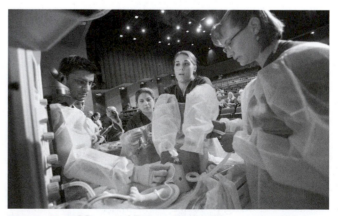

Figure 20-3 Neonatal Resuscitation Team *(Courtesy of Keith Weller)*

not honoring this right. This right is particularly important when evaluating decisions around resuscitation. Characteristics such as gender, race, and socioeconomic status are broadly thought to be morally irrelevant and therefore cannot be used to drive decision-making. It is a matter of justice to ensure that the infant has a competent surrogate decision-maker. Typically, this is a parent, but in circumstances in which the parent is incapacitated or incapable, there is a justice obligation to provide the infant with a capable advocate. This can be another family member or someone appointed by the courts to represent the child. Finally, the infant also has a right to avoid suffering that is without benefit. Adults are entitled to decline medical treatment that they perceive to be excessively burdensome or unlikely to be beneficial. Children and infants have this same right.

When making decisions with clinicians about newborn resuscitation, parents have both rights and obligations. Our society holds that parents have the primary right to make decisions for their children, and this includes medical decisions. This right incorporates several others. The parents' rights include the right to clear, accurate information regarding diagnosis, treatment options, and risks and benefits; the right to incorporate their own values or religious beliefs into decision-making for their children; and the right to choose or refuse treatments. These parental rights, however, are not unlimited. The rights of the infant or child, as described previously, take precedence (36). A common example is the right of Jehovah's Witnesses to refuse transfusion. Parents who are Jehovah's Witnesses may not refuse transfusion on behalf of their child if the refusal would lead to serious harm, suffering, or death. In this case, the right of the child to life supersedes the right of the parents to make decisions based on their religious beliefs. Parents also do not have the right to demand treatments for their children that are nonbeneficial or harmful. For example, parents do not have the right to demand delivery room resuscitation for an infant born at 21 weeks' gestation. In this situation as well, the infant's right to avoid suffering supersedes the decision-making right of the parents.

The rights of the medical team can also come into play during decisions about newborn resuscitation. The medical team has the right to avoid provision of futile or harmful interventions. Medical teams can be harmed when obligated to provide care that is morally distressing. Medical teams have the obligation to provide the family with complete and accurate information and support them through the decision-making process. They also have the obligation to be clinically competent and properly trained to provide the care they offer.

Some argue that the larger society also has rights and interests that should be incorporated into the decision-making regarding resuscitation of high-risk newborns. For example, the significant investment of money and medical resources required to care for these infants might otherwise be used to provide medicines or food to hundreds of people. Some argue for distributive justice, or the idea that societal resources should be allocated equally to all of its members. At this time, there are no frameworks for equitable application of these decisions, so they rarely come into play in daily practice.

Given all of these potentially competing rights and obligations, how does interest-based decision-making about neonatal resuscitation occur? The first step is to ensure that all relevant parties (parents, medical team) are informed of the known facts. In the case of a high-risk newborn, this would include what is known regarding prognosis. For extremely premature infants, this would include mortality rates based on their estimated weight and gestational age, as well as the types of disabilities likely to occur should they survive. Similarly, for the child with congenital anomalies, the expected length and likelihood of survival, known need for surgical or technological interventions, and expected functional outcomes are important facts to review. It is also essential that areas of uncertainty are clear to both the medical team and the infant's family. Other important facts include what interventions are available and their expected likelihood of success.

The next step is to identify the values and views of the parents and medical team. This includes jointly determining what quality of life is believed to be acceptable for the infant and what burden of suffering is acceptable in the hope of survival.

Decisions will generally fall into three distinct groups (Table 20-2). The first group is one in which survival is extremely unlikely and would be

Table 20-2	Guided Decision-Making for Resuscitation
Outcome	**Decision**
Survival is extremely unlikely, accompanied by unacceptable suffering and poor quality of life.	Noninitiation of resuscitation
Survival is likely, with good quality of life a likely result.	Initiate resuscitation
Survival is unclear but likely to be poor; patient may have low quality of life.	Interest-based decision-making should occur prior to determining the need to resuscitate.

accompanied by unacceptable suffering or poor quality of life. In this group, noninitiation of resuscitation is appropriate because the infant will not benefit. The second group is one in which survival is likely and resuscitation is likely to result in good quality of life. The third group is one in which chance of survival is unclear but likely to be poor, and survivors may have a low quality of life. In this third group, interest-based decision-making should occur (35). The parents, with the support of the medical team, should carefully weigh the rights and interests of the infant in order to make a decision. Regardless of the outcome of the decision to resuscitate, ethical medical practice demands that all patients, including newborns, be provided compassionate care to ensure comfort.

Despite the best efforts of the medical team, there are times when resuscitation is pursued, and yet the patient only worsens or does not respond. When medical technology is serving only to delay death, without a hope for recovery, this would be considered medically futile care. The next step may be a discussion of withdrawal of life-sustaining therapy.

In Western ethics, withdrawal of life-sustaining therapy is considered to be morally equivalent to the noninitiation or withholding of life-sustaining therapies (37). This is a difficult concept for many people because the act of removing something creates the appearance of causation or producing the subsequent effect. For example, withdrawal of MV in patients with intractable respiratory failure will be followed by their death. Many providers are uncomfortable in this situation because they feel that they have "caused the patient to die." The same providers are often more comfortable with having never intubated and ventilated a patient with known intractable respiratory failure, even though this patient will die as well. Although the emotional experience of these two approaches is different, the ethical implications are the same. In the case of high-risk newborns where prognosis may be uncertain and the involved parties agree that initial attempts at resuscitation and supportive care are appropriate, the moral equivalence of withholding and withdrawing treatments becomes particularly important. Ethical decision-making requires significant certainty of outcome when withholding treatment will lead to death. As described previously, many cases do not allow this certainty. In those situations, a trial of therapy may allow for clarity. The patient may respond well and therefore benefit from further interventions. Alternatively, the patient may not respond or decline, in which case the burdens and benefits of continued intervention must be reevaluated. If care providers and the patient's parents determine that ongoing treatment is likely to result in suffering and little benefit, withdrawal of life-sustaining treatment is ethically appropriate (35).

Spinal Muscular Atrophy Type 1

Spinal muscular atrophy (SMA) is an inherited neuromuscular disease that causes degeneration of the spinal cord motor neurons. It occurs at a rate of 1 in 6,000 to 10,000 live births (38–41). The gene that causes SMA is located on chromosome 5 and is called *SMN*, for *survival motor neuron*. Affected patients develop progressive muscle atrophy and weakness. There is a wide range of clinical presentations, ranging from infants who are symptomatic at birth or soon after to adults with only mild weakness and normal function. SMA is divided into four types based on functional ability (Table 20-3) (42).

SMA is progressive, such that children with SMA type 1 will ultimately lose all voluntary and involuntary skeletal muscle function, including the ability to communicate. The respiratory muscle weakness leads to poor airway clearance as a result of a weak cough, hypoventilation with sleep, chest wall and lung developmental abnormalities, and therefore, increased susceptibility to pulmonary infections and impaired lung parenchymal function. Bulbar dysfunction leads to difficulty with swallowing and airway protection. As a result, respiratory dysfunction and disease are the major causes of morbidity and mortality in children with SMA types 2 and 3. Despite their neurological impairment, children with SMA do not have cognitive disabilities.

The Child Neurology Society published a Consensus Statement for Standard of Care in Spinal Muscular Atrophy in 2007 (42). In this document, the recommendations for diagnosis, acute care, respiratory support, nutritional care, orthopedic care, rehabilitation, and palliative care are outlined. There are strong recommendations for early initiation of airway clearance therapies, nutritional support, and noninvasive ventilation because these have been shown to improve both functionality and survival for children with SMA. Far more controversial is the question of tracheotomy and MV for children with SMA type 1.

Table 20-3	Types of Spinal Muscular Atrophy		
Type	Best Function	Age of Onset	Approximate Life Expectancy
1	Never sits	0–6 months	<2 years
2	Never stands	7–18 months	>2 years
3	Stands and walks	>18 months	Adult
4	Walks into adulthood	10–30 years	Adult

From a strictly physiological point of view, tracheotomy and MV will prolong the survival of children with SMA type 1, although not indefinitely. In medical practice, however, there is wide variation in terms of offering and/or recommending invasive ventilatory support. This variability in practice reflects the ethical complexity of medical care for these patients. For many practitioners, the fundamental conflict is that tracheotomy and MV will prolong survival for a child with SMA type 1, but that child will lose his ability to talk and eventually will become "locked in," unable to communicate, even by eye blinking.

The ethical analysis of this problem has focused on delineating an acceptable quality-of-life threshold for children with SMA type 1 and on weighing the benefits and burdens of the treatment (best-interest standard). Overall, there has been a movement away from quality-of-life arguments. This has happened for two reasons. One, multiple studies have shown that medical-care providers routinely perceive the quality of life of chronically ventilated patients to be far lower than the patients themselves perceive it to be (43). Additionally, there are no specific published studies on quality of life as assessed by mechanically ventilated SMA type 1 patients. Therefore, medical providers' judgments on the quality of life of any individual patient remain pure speculation.

By applying a best-interest standard, medical providers hope to balance the benefits and burdens of a given treatment to help a patient or family decide whether or not to pursue that intervention. The survival benefit of tracheotomy and MV is present for children with SMA type 1. In some countries, such as Japan, and for some religious groups, this benefit trumps all others. To live, regardless of the circumstances, is better than dying. Others see that tracheotomy itself comes with burdens. By the nature of the device, it impairs phonation and verbal communication. This is of particular note in SMA type 1 because the patients who do undergo tracheotomy are most often between 6 and 18 months of age. They have not yet developed alternative means of communicating their needs. Additionally, tracheotomies require frequent tracheal suctioning for airway clearance, a procedure that is known to be uncomfortable. Finally, many view a tracheotomy and MV as serving to prolong the dying process unacceptably. As one author notes, "Such children can see, until weakness of the ciliary muscles limits accommodation and facial weakness causes complete ptosis. Until that time, they can take pleasure in looking at their caregivers, toys, and movies. . . . The burdens of these children's lives include their inability to communicate their feelings, desires, discomfort, suffering, or pain, other than by tears or an elevation in heart rate." (44)

The struggle to define who ultimately determines best interest for a given patient remains a challenge. As in the previous example of a high-risk newborn, the most ethical and practical approach to decision-making relies on a combination of medical facts and identification of values by the deciding parties. The rights and interests of the child must be identified. A process of shared decision-making will need to occur. This is also known as **deliberative decision-making** (45). When physicians or other medical providers make a decision alone, subsequently informing the patient or family of their actions, this is known as **paternalism**. When the physician or medical provider simply performs whatever action the parent or family requests, this is known as **consumerism**. Neither paternalism nor consumerism will produce decisions that are medically appropriate and mutually acceptable (Box 20-3).

For shared decision-making to occur, there must be a true choice at hand. In addition, the choices must be value sensitive. In the case of children with SMA type 1, there are three viable alternatives: tracheotomy and MV; respiratory support with airway clearance and noninvasive ventilation, but a specific agreement not to proceed beyond this level of support; and exclusive comfort care (46). Each of these options is medically and ethically acceptable in certain circumstances, and therefore the choice should be made on the basis of the recommendations of the medical team and the values of the family functioning as surrogates for their child. This process has inherent obligations for the participants. The medical team must share their knowledge and experience with the patient or family. The patient or family must share their values and priorities with the medical team. Once this exchange of information has occurred, a plan of action can be identified. Both parties must then evaluate, agree upon, and initiate the plan.

Box 20-3 Decision-Making Models

Deliberative: Decisions about care are determined through a discussion with care providers and family members.

Paternalism: Medical providers make a decision alone, later informing the patient or family of their actions.

Consumerism: The physician or medical provider performs any action the parent or family requests.

End-of-Life Care

■ ■ Eighteen months after his last hospital stay, Daniel returns to the hospital with respiratory failure that is a result of his muscular dystrophy. This time he cannot be weaned from the ventilator. His parents and primary care team report that, during his time at home, Daniel repeatedly informed them that he did not wish to live with a tracheotomy or chronic ventilation. The clinical psychologist who has worked with Daniel spends a long time reviewing the issue with him. He continues to refuse a tracheotomy, and all who interact with him believe that this is a reasoned decision. He and his parents determine a time for him to be extubated after other family members and friends can be present for a life celebration. They request that all comfort measures be provided but that he not undergo CPR, reintubation, or noninvasive ventilation. The cardiology team turns off his defibrillator prior to extubation.

RTs often participate in end-of-life care when newborn or pediatric patients die. As discussed in the section on resuscitation of high-risk newborns, patients may die when life-sustaining interventions are not performed, when they are not successful, or when they are withheld. The most common end-of-life scenario involving RTs is terminal extubation. **Terminal extubation** is the removal of MV and the endotracheal tube (ETT) from a patient who is expected to die.

Although the management of patients during the process of withdrawing life-sustaining therapies is a medical procedure, there are some ethical issues that are important for all participants to understand. Withdrawal of life-sustaining therapy does not mean that the patient is no longer receiving care. Care at the end of life is medical, psychosocial, and spiritual. Aggressive symptom management is a key part of end-of-life care. The goal of symptom management is to provide comfort; it does not seek to extend life or hasten death.

In patients who have respiratory failure, one very common symptom is dyspnea, also called air hunger. It is a subjective experience that patients describe as uncomfortable. It can be unusual awareness of breathing or breathlessness. Narcotic medications such as morphine can be effective in treating the sensation of dyspnea, although they provide no improvement in lung function. The fact that narcotics relieve dyspnea in patients is well known, but many medical providers express reluctance or anxiety about prescribing them at the end of life. They hesitate because they also know that narcotics can suppress a patient's respiratory drive and even

lead to apnea, and therefore they fear that by treating the patient's dyspnea, they will in fact hasten or cause the patient's death. Medical providers and ethicists agree, however, that the provision of narcotics to a dyspneic patient is ethically permissible under what is known as the rule of double effect.

The **rule of double effect** states that an action that is known to have two possible effects, where the intended one is beneficial and the unintended one is not beneficial, can be morally permissible under specific circumstances. These circumstances are as follows:

• The act itself must be either good or morally neutral.
• The person must be acting with good intent.
• The bad effect is necessary to achieve the good effect.
• The good effect must be more significant than the bad effect (3).

How does this affect the patient with dyspnea at the end of life? The intended effect of the morphine is relief from air hunger. The unintended effect is the potential of narcotic medications, including morphine, to decrease a patient's drive to breathe, which can result in an ineffective respiratory rate or even apnea. If we examine the provision of morphine to a dyspneic patient, what do we find?

• **Is it a good or morally neutral act?**
Providing the patient with relief is a good act. To meet this criterion, the medication given must be known to provide relief of the symptom being treated. Other sedative medications, which can also decrease respiration, are not known to provide relief of dyspnea, and therefore administering them for this purpose would not be a good act.
• **Is the provider acting with good intent?**
By using morphine, the medical provider is attempting to relieve a distressing symptom and therefore is acting with good intent. If the intention is to cause apnea leading to death, this would not be an action with good intent. It is important to distinguish the difference between actions that may allow death to come faster (hastening death) and actions that directly lead to death (killing).
• **Is the bad effect necessary to achieve the good effect?**
Finding the appropriate balance in dosing does require careful titration of the medication, but the bad effect of morphine (respiratory depression) is not required to relieve dyspnea.
• **Is the good effect more significant than the bad?**
Given that the patient is receiving palliative care and the primary goal is relief of suffering and provision of comfort, improving the distress

from dyspnea is more significant than the risk of slowing down the breathing or causing apnea.

If the intention and practice of the provider meets the conditions of the rule of double effect, then giving morphine to a terminal patient with dyspnea is in fact ethically permissible, even if it suppresses the patient's respiratory effort. In the United States, the Supreme Court has made it clear that terminally ill patients have a right to adequate pain medication, even if that medication hastens death (47).

Many patients who undergo terminal extubation show signs of respiratory distress postextubation. This can be very disturbing to both families and medical providers who witness this, particularly if they are unprepared for it. One approach has been the use of neuromuscular blocking agents to suppress the physical evidence of respiratory distress or dyspnea. Neuromuscular blocking agents are drugs such as succinylcholine, vecuronium, and pancuronium. They act at the neuromuscular junction to block muscle contraction, resulting in paralysis. They are commonly used during anesthesia and intubation to keep patients immobile and relax the muscles. At times, they are also used in the intensive care unit to allow full MV without competition from the patient's respiratory effort. Neuromuscular blocking agents have no ability to relieve symptoms such as pain or shortness of breath.

Medical providers and ethicists agree that neuromuscular blocking agents have no role in managing patients during terminal extubation. We can apply the rule of double effect to understand why. The intended effect is to decrease external signs of distress in the patients. The unintended effects are twofold. First, the medications cause apnea through paralysis of the respiratory muscles. Second, a fully paralyzed patient cannot express any distressing symptoms, such as pain or nausea, or engage in verbal or nonverbal communication, such as holding hands with loved ones. Let us walk through the conditions of the rule of double effect:

- **Is it a good or morally neutral act?**
  Giving the patient medication to prevent observers from being disturbed is not a good act. At best, it is morally neutral. Some would contend that treating a patient to benefit the patient's medical providers or family is inadequately respecting his or her autonomy as an individual.
- **Is the provider acting with good intent?**
  The provider who attempts to alleviate potential suffering by a family whose loved one is dying or by the dying person's caregivers is acting with good intent.

- **Is the bad effect necessary to produce the good effect?**
  In the case of neuromuscular blocking agents, the bad effect, paralysis, is required to get the good effect, which is an external appearance of comfort.
- **Is the good effect more significant than the bad?**
  The good effect, protection of observers from the disturbing experience of seeing their loved one struggle with breathing, is significant. It does not, however, override the patient's right to avoid suffering. By making the patient unable to express discomfort or distress, using neuromuscular blocking agents in this situation prioritizes the rights of the family and medical team over those of the patient. In addition, it is likely to harm the patient if he or she is experiencing discomfort and pain that is not relieved because it is not recognized.

Therefore, the rule of double effect cannot be applied to the use of neuromuscular blocking agents to treat dyspnea in dying patients.

See Chapter 21 for a more-detailed discussion of symptom management during end-of-life care.

■■ While planning for Daniel's terminal extubation, he raises the possibility of organ donation. A coordinator from the local organ-procurement organization comes to your hospital to speak with him and his family about their options. Daniel states that he would like to be an organ donor if possible.

Organ Donation After Cardiac Death

The successful transplantation of organs from one person to another is one of the miracles of modern medicine. This success has not come without significant ethical issues, however. One of the current controversies in medical ethics is organ **donation after cardiac death (DCD)**, also called **non–heart-beating organ donation (NHBOD)**. Interestingly, prior to the late 1960s, all organ donors were non–heart-beating donors. With the establishment of death by neurological criteria, otherwise known as brain death or total brain death, transplantation moved to exclusively using organs from neurologically dead donors. This was because outcomes were better for the transplant recipients. As demand for transplanted organs has increased far past the supply, non–heart-beating donors have again been considered as a way to obtain more organs for patients who desperately need them. Since the late 1990s, many medical institutions have developed protocols to allow the procurement of organs from non–heart-beating donors, but this process has not been without controversy.

The typical process for DCD is as follows: A patient or the patient's family has requested planned withdrawal of life-sustaining therapy and has also requested that resuscitative measures (e.g., CPR, intubation) not be initiated. They have also requested that the patient be a candidate for organ donation. After the donation-consent process is complete, the patient undergoes the planned withdrawal of life-sustaining therapies. If he progresses to death within 1 hour after withdrawal, he is observed for a number of minutes (which varies by institutional policy) for return of spontaneous circulation or respiratory effort. If he is simultaneously unresponsive, apneic, and pulseless for the duration of the observation period, he is declared dead, and organ procurement will begin. If he does not die within the hour waiting period, he is no longer a donation candidate and continues receiving comfort measures during the dying process.

There are several reasons why this process is controversial. The first has to do with what is commonly known as the dead donor rule. This was developed in the 1960s to clearly state that organ procurement must always come after, and not cause, a patient's death. Cardiopulmonary death is defined as simultaneous and irreversible unresponsiveness, apnea, and absent circulation. The heart must stop beating. Patients who are dead by neurological criteria are declared dead because they no longer have any brain function, even though they may still have a heartbeat when kept on a ventilator. If the ventilator is removed, they will not breathe, and the heart will stop soon after. The patient may not die because the heart or other vital organs have been removed. The crux of the ethical debate on this issue centers on the ambiguity of irreversibility in this scenario. A patient who has a cardiac arrest and does not undergo CPR will die. If the patient in the next bed has a cardiac arrest and does undergo successful CPR, he or she will live. One could argue that the first patient might not be irreversibly dead, yet very few ethicists would require that this patient be resuscitated if she or her family/surrogates had chosen that she be allowed to die.

In 2008, *The New England Journal of Medicine* described several examples of pediatric cardiac transplant after NHBOD (48). In this article, three infants were non–heart-beating organ donors. Declaration of death occurred between 75 and 180 seconds after the cessation of cardiac circulation. In all three recipients, the heart was restarted, and all three recipients were alive at 6 months. Many readers of this report felt that this was an example of violation of the dead donor rule, as the heart was not irreversibly stopped. There was particular focus on the last two cases in which the period of asystole was shortened to 75 seconds.

The length of asystole has particular importance because it speaks to our uncertainty regarding when death occurs and when irreversibility sets in. Although the dead donor rule outlines criteria for death, it does not give a time frame. Some ethicists argue that this uncertainty is unacceptable, and therefore removal of organs within a time frame in which the patient may not be truly dead (defined by them as irreversibly despite intervention) is unethical. In fact, some go so far as to say that the organ-procurement process is the act that kills the patient (49).

Other ethicists take a different approach, claiming that there is a distinction between irreversible death and permanent death. Those who take this stance argue for the recognition of several stages of death after the initial end of vital functions. The first stage is a period in which autoresuscitation, or the return of breathing and pulse may occur. The second stage is one in which death is permanent without intervention but could be reversible if intervention occurs. The third stage is one in which death is permanent and irreversible. Irreversible death means that no matter what interventions are made, the patient will still be dead. Permanent death is death that applies to that person, not to the possible recoverable function of an individual organ. In this argument, if a person has chosen not to be resuscitated, then death after withdrawal of life-sustaining therapies is in fact permanent and will progress to irreversible. The fact that organs can function after removal and transplantation does not alter the fact of the donor individual's death. They further argue that NHBOD is ethically permissible during the second period, the period of permanent but not necessarily irreversible death (50). They agree that organ procurement during the time period where autoresuscitation is possible is not permissible.

To standardize practice and to address these ethical concerns, several professional organizations have created recommendations for the ethical practice of NHBOD. These groups include the Institute of Medicine (51), the American College of Critical Care Medicine (52), and the American Society of Transplant Surgeons (53). They make specific recommendations regarding the waiting period between the onset of unresponsiveness, apnea, and absent pulse and organ procurement; care of the dying patient who may be a donor; and care of the patient's family. This debate will continue, however, because organs remain in shortage and society continues to grapple with the best ways to meet the ongoing demand.

Clinical medicine and clinical research are both guided by principles of bioethics. Because of their professional skills at providing life-sustaining therapies such as MV, RTs are likely to encounter ethically complex clinical situations. Bioethics offers a way to think about not only what *can* be done for a patient, but also what *ought* to be done.

■■ The hospital team makes arrangements to allow Daniel's family to be with him at the time of extubation in a preanesthesia holding area of the hospital. Thirty minutes after extubation, Daniel dies peacefully. He is asystolic and apneic for 2 minutes in keeping with the hospital's protocol. His parents leave the holding area, and Daniel is taken to the operating room. His kidneys are transplanted into a 6-year-old girl and a 65-year-old man. His liver is transplanted into a 35-year-old woman.

■■ Critical Thinking Questions: Daniel Rogers

1. In your institution, how should an error in ventilator settings be reported?
2. If you do not agree with the chosen respiratory treatment ordered for Daniel, how could you engage in conscientious refusal?
3. Would there ever be a time in Daniel's care that consumerism would be an appropriate decision-making model?
4. What would be an appropriate course of action if Daniel was not asystolic within 1 hour after extubation during the attempted DCD?

▶● Case Studies and Critical Thinking Questions

■ Case 1: Baby Boy (BB) McGrath

You are working as the delivery room coverage RT at a 15-bed level IIB neonatal intensive care unit (NICU). The neonatologist and charge nurse are called by the labor and delivery department regarding a new admission. Katie McGrath is a 22-year-old who is 23 6/7 weeks into her pregnancy. She has been diagnosed with premature rupture of membranes and premature labor, and her cervix is currently 3 cm dilated. All attempts by the obstetric staff to stop contractions have been thus far unsuccessful. The neonatologist on service is going to discuss with the family current viability and presumed prognosis for BB McGrath if delivery occurs within the next few days or weeks. The neonatologist hopes to return with the family's preliminary decisions regarding resuscitation.

• Based on information from Chapters 2, 3, and 4, what is the likelihood of survival without long-term sequelae for BB McGrath?
• Using the guided decision-making for resuscitation, what is a reasonable deliberative decision for the neonatologist and parents to make?

• Is the plan set forth by the neonatologist a reasonable one, based on what you know about 23 6/7 week gestation neonates?
• Is it permissible to stop delivery room resuscitation once they have begun, without providing chest compressions or medications if they are warranted under Neonatal Resuscitation Program guidelines?

Two days later, you are once again on the delivery team when you are called to Katie McGrath's delivery. You, the neonatologist, a neonatal nurse practitioner (NNP), and the NICU admitting nurse respond to the delivery. The neonatologist greets the parents and takes a place between the delivery bed and radiant warmer in preparation for communicating with the parents during the resuscitation. BB McGrath is born 5 minutes later, limp and apneic. The NNP leads the resuscitation. The nurse places BB McGrath in a plastic bag up to his neck, and you begin bag-mask ventilation at 30 breaths per minute. The nurse auscultates the heart rate (HR) during positive-pressure ventilation (PPV) and determines the heart rate is about 70 beats per minute (bpm). The NNP prepares for the intubation, while the RN places a pulse oximeter on BB McGrath's right hand. The intubation is successful, with a 2.5-cm ETT placed 6.5 cm at the lip, with positive color change on end-tidal CO_2 monitor and bilateral breath sounds. However, during the intubation, the heart rate drops below 60 bpm, and you are unable to increase the HR with PPV. The neonatologist updates the McGraths regarding their son's status. They quickly decide not to escalate any further attempts at resuscitation measures but request that you continue ventilation. After another 2 minutes, the heart rate is still less than 60 bpm. The parents request that the team stop resuscitation so they can hold their son. The neonatologist conveys the parent's decision to the team and instructs resuscitation to stop. The neonatologist removes the ETT and plastic bag, places a bonnet on BB McGrath's head, and swaddles him, then hands him over to his parents. You and the rest of the team quietly leave the room to allow the parents time alone with their son. The neonatologist stays for an additional few minutes in the room to discuss potential physiological findings with the family and will stay on the delivery unit to document the time of death.

■ Case 2: Lucy Scanlon

Lucy Scanlon is a previously healthy 2-year-old who was admitted to your PICU 3 days ago. She was at a neighborhood party and walked into a pool, losing consciousness and aspirating chlorinated water. She was submerged for less than 5 minutes. Since admission, she has been on high-frequency oscillatory ventilation. Lucy's current ventilation settings are as follows: frequency of 5 hertz, change in pressure (δP) of 65 mm Hg, mean airway pressure of 33 mm Hg, inspiratory-time of 33%, FIO_2 of 1.0. Her last blood gas was pH, +7.32; partial pressure of carbon dioxide, +48 mm Hg; partial pressure of oxygen, +55 mm Hg; and HCO_3, +24.4 mEq/L.

- *What is Lucy's oxygenation index?*
- *What are some advanced respiratory therapies that could potentially improve Lucy's oxygenation?*

Lucy initially presented with atrial fibrillation, which has subsequently resolved, but throughout the last 18 hours, the pediatric intensivists have been struggling to maintain an adequate blood pressure. Despite starting and titrating dopamine and dobutamine drips, Lucy's blood pressure is consistently maintaining around 86/42 mm Hg (mean = 55.3 mm Hg). A family meeting is called with the parents, grandparents, bedside nurse, nurse manager, pediatric intensivist, ECMO coordinator, and RT. The discussion will clarify the cardiopulmonary issues that Lucy is now having. Decisions need to be made by the family in collaboration with the team regarding the next steps in Lucy's care, including whether to pursue ECMO.

- *What is it about Lucy's diagnosis and presentation that could make her a candidate for ECMO? Based on the prognosis for near-drowning and Lucy's current clinical picture, do you think she meets the criteria for ECMO?*

The pediatric intensivist explains Lucy's recent progress to her parents as well as the likely progression over the next few hours and days. ECMO is explained as a treatment option. The intensivist describes the merit of using ECMO as such: "ECMO will not heal Lucy's lungs. It may not make things better, and it can certainly make things worse. And I do not know if it will work or not. But it can buy us some time to figure out how to resolve the lung problems that Lucy is having without resorting to really aggressive ventilator strategies, which may be causing or contributing to her recent blood pressure instability." Lucy's parents would like the PICU team to "try everything" to heal Lucy's lungs. The PICU intensivist will activate the ECMO team and estimates that Lucy will be on ECMO within 1 hour.

- *Should an ethics committee be called in before Lucy is cannulated and placed on ECMO? If someone on the team does not agree with this decision, can the parents' decision be overridden?*

Multiple-Choice Questions

1. The four ethical principles that guide much of modern bioethics include:
   I. Justice.
   II. Autonomy.
   III. Fidelity.
   IV. Veracity.
   V. Compassion.
   VI. Informed consent.
   VII. Beneficence.
   VIII. Nonmaleficence.
   a. I, II, IV, VI
   b. II, III, IV, V
   c. I, II, VI, VII
   d. I, II, VII, VIII

2. In health care, the principle of justice refers to:
   a. A patient's right to equal access to medical care.
   b. Holding health-care providers accountable for errors made.
   c. A patient's right to make decisions based on his or her personal values.
   d. Providing care that is not harmful to the patient.

3. Interventions that can prevent medical errors include:
   a. Computerized medical records.
   b. Work duty hour limits.
   c. Patient education.
   d. Visibly marking surgical sites before the procedure.
   e. All of the above.

4. During a public health emergency, clinicians may have a duty to:
   I. Report to work.
   II. Comply with mandatory vaccination.
   III. Suspend professional autonomy and engage in resource allocation.
   IV. Not discuss resource limitations with patients.
   a. I, II, III, IV
   b. I, II, III
   c. I, III, IV
   d. I, II, IV

5. In pediatrics, *assent* indicates:
   a. Clinician agreement with parental decision-making.
   b. A child understands and agrees with a proposed medical treatment.
   c. Parental agreement with their child's desire for a medical treatment.
   d. Parental agreement with the physician's recommendations.

6. The role of the hospital ethics committee is to:
   a. Act as advisors to the health-care team.
   b. Make medical decisions in ethically complex cases.
   c. Act as legal counsel in ethically complex cases.
   d. Encourage patients to agree with physician recommendations.

7. According to the principle of double effect:
   a. Parents have a right to any medical treatment for their child, even if that treatment is medically ineffective.
   b. Patients have a right to receive any medical treatment, even if that treatment is medically ineffective.
   c. Patients have a right to adequate pain medication, even if that medication hastens death.
   d. Physicians have a right to refuse to provide medically ineffective treatments.

8. You need to suction the tracheostomy of Andrew, a 3-year-old with SMA type 1. Mom warned you that Andrew does not like suctioning and that he has been fussy all morning. What is an appropriate distraction strategy to use to improve Andrew's compliance with suctioning?
   a. Ask his mom to read Andrew a story while you suction.
   b. Tell Andrew that it will not hurt.
   c. Wrap Andrew's arms and legs in a blanket.
   d. Tell Andrew you willll turn on the TV if he lets you suction his airway.

9. For the last 4 years, you have been taking care of a patient with SMA type 2. He has had an increase in the number of admissions for pulmonary infections, and a family meeting is going to be held about whether to perform a tracheotomy. Which of the following principles could be used as a valid argument *in favor* of performing the procedure?
   a. Principle of double effect
   b. Quality of life
   c. Nonmaleficence
   d. None of these could be used as arguments in favor of tracheotomy.

10. Donation after cardiac death is a process of organ donation in which:
    a. Organs are procured after a patient is declared neurologically dead.
    b. Organ donation is considered after families have agreed to both withdrawal of life-sustaining therapies and noninitiation of resuscitation.
    c. Organs are procured after 1 hour of asystole.
    d. Organ procurement could be considered the cause of death.

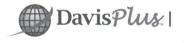 For additional resources login to Davis*Plus* (http://davisplus.fadavis.com/ keyword "Perretta") and click on the Premium tab. (Don't have a *Plus*Code to access Premium Resources? Just click the Purchase Access button on the book's Davis*Plus* page.)

REFERENCES

1. Miller G. *Pediatric Bioethics.* New York, NY: Cambridge University Press; 2010.
2. Veatch R. *The Basics of Bioethics.* 2nd ed. Upper Saddle River, NJ: Prentice Hall; 2003.
3. Beauchamp T, Childress J. *Principles of Biomedical Ethics.* 6th ed. New York, NY: Oxford University Press; 2009.
4. Committee on Bioethics, American Academy of Pediatrics. Informed consent, parental permission, and assent in pediatric practice. *Pediatrics.* 1995;95(2):314-317.
5. American Medical Association. Council on Ethical and Judicial Affairs Report G–A-92. Confidential care for minors. http://www.ama-assn.org/ama1/pub/upload/mm/369/40b.pdf. June, 1992. Accessed December 28, 2012.
6. The National Commission for the Protection of Human Subjects of Biomedical and Behavioral Research, Department of Health, Education, and Welfare. *The Belmont Report: Ethical Principles and Guidelines for the Protection of Human Subjects of Research.* DHEW publication OS 78-0014. Washington, DC: Department of Health, Education, and Welfare; 1979.
7. Berlinger N. *After Harm: Medical Error and the Ethics of Forgiveness.* Baltimore, MD: Johns Hopkins University Press; 2005:156.
8. U.S. Department of Health and Human Services, Office for Human Research Protections. *Code of Federal Regulations. Title 45: Public Welfare. Part 46: Protection of Human Subjects.* www.hhs.gov/ohrp/policy/ohrpregulations.pdf. Updated January 15, 2009. Accessed December 28, 2012.
9. American Association for Respiratory Care. *Position Statement: AARC Statement of Ethics and Professional Conduct.* Irving, TX: American Association for Respiratory Care; 2009. http://www.aarc.org/resources/position_statements/ethics.html. Accessed December 28, 2012.

10. Williams CT, Fost N. Ethical considerations surrounding first time procedures: a study and analysis of patient attitudes toward spinal taps by students. *Kennedy Inst Ethics J.* 1992;2(3):217-231.

11. Annas G. *The Rights of Patients: The Basic ACLU Guide to Patient Rights.* Totowa, NJ: Humana Press; 1992.

12. Institute of Medicine. *To Err is Human: Building a Safer Health System.* Washington, DC: Committee on Quality of Health Care in America; 2000.

13. The Joint Commission. *Improving America's Hospitals: The Joint Commission's Annual Report on Quality and Safety, 2007.* Oakbrook Terrace, IL: The Joint Commission; 2007.

14. Kachalia A, Kaufman SR, Boothman R, et al. Liability claims and costs before and after implementation of a medical error disclosure program. *Ann Intern Med.* 153(4): 213-221.

15. Gostin LO, Sapsin JW, Teret SP, et al. The Model State Emergency Health Powers Act: planning for and response to bioterrorism and naturally occurring infectious diseases. *JAMA.* 2002;288(5):622-628.

16. Simonds AK, Sokol DK. Lives on the line? Ethics and practicalities of duty of care in pandemics and disasters. *Eur Respir J.* 2009;34(2):303-309.

17. Rakita RM, Hagar BA, Lammert JK. Vaccination mandates vs opt-out programs and rates of influenza immunization. *JAMA.* 304(16):1786.

18. Poland GA. Mandating influenza vaccination for health care workers: putting patients and professional ethics over personal preference. *Vaccine.* 28(36):5757-5759.

19. Kind T, Genrich G, Sodhi A, Chretien KC. Social media policies at US medical schools. *Med Educ Online.* 2010;Sep15(15) .doi: 10.3402/meo.v15i0.5324.

20. Orzalesi M, Cuttini M. Ethical considerations in neonatal respiratory care. *Biol Neonate.* 2005;87(4):345-353.

21. Faden R, Beauchamp T. *A History and Theory of Informed Consent.* New York, NY: Oxford University Press; 1986.

22. Meyer EC, Burns JP, Griffith JL, Truog RD. Parental perspectives on end-of-life care in the pediatric intensive care unit. *Crit Care Med.* 2002;30(1):226-231.

23. Fraser J, Harris N, Berringer AJ, Prescott H, Finlay F. Advanced care planning in children with life-limiting conditions—the Wishes Document. *Arch Dis Child.* 2010; 95(2):79-82.

24. Sibbald R, Downar J, Hawryluck L. Perceptions of "futile care" among caregivers in intensive care units. *CMAJ.* 2007;177(10):1201-1208.

25. Schwenzer KJ, Wang L. Assessing moral distress in respiratory care practitioners. *Crit Care Med.* 2006;34(12): 2967-2973.

26. Peerzada JM, Richardson DK, Burns JP. Delivery room decision-making at the threshold of viability. *J Pediatr.* 2004;145(4):492-498.

27. Cadge W, Catlin EA. Making sense of suffering and death: how health care providers construct meaning in a neonatal intensive care unit. *J Relig Health.* 2006;45(2):248-263.

28. Brown-Saltzman K, Upadhya D, Larner L, Wenger NS. An intervention to improve respiratory therapists' comfort with end-of-life care. *Respir Care.* 2010;55(7):858-865.

29. Rocker GM, Cook DJ, O'Callaghan CJ, et al. Canadian nurses' and respiratory therapists' perspectives on withdrawal of life support in the intensive care unit. *J Crit Care.* 2005;20(1):59-65.

30. Back AL, Arnold RM. Dealing with conflict in caring for the seriously ill: "it was just out of the question." *JAMA.* 2005;293(11):1374-1381.

31. Robins PM, Meltzer L, Zelikovsky N. The experience of secondary traumatic stress upon care providers working within a children's hospital. *J Pediatr Nurs.* 2009;24(4): 270-279.

32. Meadors P, Lamson A, Swanson M, White M, Sira N. Secondary traumatization in pediatric healthcare providers: compassion fatigue, burnout, and secondary traumatic stress. *Omega (Westport).* 2009;60(2):103-128.

33. Committee on Bioethics, American Academy of Pediatrics. Policy statement—physician refusal to provide information or treatment on the basis of claims of conscience. *Pediatrics.* 2009;124(6):1689-1693.

34. Pope TM. Legal briefing: conscience clauses and conscientious refusal. *J Clin Ethics.* 2010;21(2):163-176.

35. Bell EF. Noninitiation or withdrawal of intensive care for high-risk newborns. *Pediatrics.* 2007;119(2):401-403.

36. Mercurio MR. The ethics of newborn resuscitation. *Semin Perinatol.* 2009;33(6):354-363.

37. Whittall H. Noninitiation or withdrawal of intensive care for high-risk newborns. *Pediatrics.* 2007;119(6):1267-1269.

38. Burd L, Short SK, Martsolf JT, Nelson RA. Prevalence of type I spinal muscular atrophy in North Dakota. *Am J Med Genet.* 1991;41(2):212-215.

39. Koul R, Al Futaisi A, Chacko A, et al. Clinical and genetic study of spinal muscular atrophies in Oman. *J Child Neurol.* 2007;22(10):1227-1230.

40. Ludvigsson P, Olafsson E, Hauser WA. Spinal muscular atrophy: incidence in Iceland. *Neuroepidemiology.* 1999; 18(5):265-269.

41. Thieme A, Mitulla B, Schulze F, Spiegler AW. Chronic childhood spinal muscular atrophy in Germany (West-Thuringen)—an epidemiological study. *Hum Genet.* 1994;93(3):344-346.

42. Wang CH, Finkel RS, Bertini ES, et al. Consensus statement for standard of care in spinal muscular atrophy. *J Child Neurol.* 2007;22(8):1027-1049.

43. Bach JR, Campagnolo DI, Hoeman S. Life satisfaction of individuals with Duchenne muscular dystrophy using long-term mechanical ventilatory support. *Am J Phys Med Rehabil.* 1991;70(3):129-135.

44. Bush A, Fraser J, Jardine E, Paton J, Simonds A, Wallis C. Respiratory management of the infant with type 1 spinal muscular atrophy. *Arch Dis Child.* 2005;90(7):709-711.

45. Emanuel EJ, Emanuel LL. Four models of the physician-patient relationship. *JAMA.* 1992;267(16):2221-2226.

46. Hardart MK, Truog RD. Spinal muscular atrophy—type I. *Arch Dis Child.* 2003;88(10):848-850.

47. *Vacco v Quill.* 521 US 793 (1997).

48. Boucek MM, Mashburn C, Dunn SM, et al. Pediatric heart transplantation after declaration of cardiocirculatory death. *N Engl J Med.* 2008;359(7):709-714.

49. Potts M, Byrne PA, Evans DW. Infant heart transplantation after cardiac death: ethical and legal problems. *J Clin Ethics.* 2010;21(3):224-228.

50. Antommaria AH. Dying but not killing: donation after cardiac death donors and the recovery of vital organs. *J Clin Ethics.* 2010;21(3):229-231.

51. Committee on Non-Heart-Beating Transplantation, Institute of Medicine. *Non-Heart-Beating Organ Transplantation: Practice and Protocols.* Washington, DC: National Academy Press; 2000.

52. Ethics Committee, American College of Critical Care Medicine, Society of Critical Care Medicine. Recommendations for nonheartbeating organ donation: a position paper by the Ethics Committee, American College of Critical Care Medicine, Society of Critical Care Medicine. *Crit Care Med.* 2001;29(9):1826-1831.

53. Shehab N, Schaefer MK, Kegler SR, Budnitz DS. Adverse events from cough and cold medications after a market withdrawal of products labeled for infants. *Pediatrics.* 2010;126(6):1100-1107.

Chapter 21

Palliative and End-of-Life Care

Wynne Morrison, MD, MBE

Key Terms

Advance directive
Concurrent care
Do not attempt resuscitation
  (DNAR) order
Euthanasia
Hospice agencies
Palliative care
Terminal extubation
Terminal sedation
Terminal weaning

Chapter Objectives

After reading this chapter, you will be able to:

1. Describe the role of the respiratory therapist in helping families with difficult pediatric end-of-life decision-making.
2. Discuss the range of reasonable decisions possible for a family deciding how to best care for their child with a life-threatening illness.
3. Explain the balance of burden and benefit in determining what respiratory support to offer at the end of life.
4. Outline the process of creating a "do not attempt resuscitation" order.
5. Describe at least two different approaches to discontinuing mechanical ventilation) at the end of life.
6. Name at least two nonpharmacological strategies for the treatment of dyspnea at the end of life.
7. Name three members of the palliative-care team and their respective roles.
8. Discuss the uses and side effects of narcotic and sedative agents at the end of life.
9. Help a family determine the ideal location of death, depending on the patient's and family's circumstances.
10. Discuss the services that are typically available from hospice agencies to support dying at home.
11. List five ways that the team can help support a family at the time of a patient's death.
12. Describe vital components of end-of-life care, including self-care and team support.

■■ Michael Simpson

Michael is 4 years old and has myotubular myopathy, a genetic disorder of muscle function, leading to profound weakness of his face, extremities, and respiratory muscles. His disease was diagnosed at a few months of age, when he was not rolling himself over or sitting when it would normally be expected. He cannot be fed by mouth owing to difficulty swallowing and frequent choking, so he has had a gastrostomy tube placed. Since the age of 8 months, he has required noninvasive positive-pressure ventilation (NIPPV) for 18 to 20 hours a day, but he has been cared for predominantly at home with frequent rehospitalizations for infections requiring an escalation of his respiratory support. He has been intubated for pneumonia three times in the past 2 years, each time spending 2 to 4 weeks in the intensive care unit (ICU), and he has now been readmitted with an adenovirus infection. For the past several days, he decompensates rapidly if taken off of positive pressure for even a few minutes, and he requires aggressive interventions from the respiratory therapy team on an almost hourly basis to help with his secretion clearance. This includes suctioning, adjusting his bi-level positive airway pressure device (BiPAP) interface, giving nebulized medications, and using a cough-assist device. You and his mother have just spent 45 minutes together at his bedside administering his treatments, and she turns to you and asks whether you think this is too much to put him through.

Modern medicine has been able to cure many diseases. Health-care professionals are able to save the lives of many children and relieve much suffering for patients who would have died at an early age even a few decades ago. Many of these life-saving interventions involve the support and treatment of respiratory failure, whether by mechanical ventilation (MV), secretion-management modalities, or even extracorporeal support until the cause of respiratory failure is either treated or stabilized. Some children are able to recover from critical illness, or even repeated episodes of such illnesses, to go on to lead happy, productive lives. Modern technology has also allowed health-care professionals to stabilize many children with chronic illnesses, helping them to live much longer lives than they would have in the past, even when the disease cannot be cured. With careful medical management, many children with diabetes, cystic fibrosis, congenital heart disease, or other chronic conditions can do very well.

There are other conditions that can be very difficult to manage, however, because they are likely to be life limiting. Children with these conditions often do not survive with a good quality of life into adulthood, yet health-care professionals are able to manage the life-threatening complications that arise so that there is much uncertainty regarding whether or not death is imminent. Even when faced with an illness for which the medical team is almost certain that short-term survival is not possible, such as with cancer that is no longer responding to treatment, health-care professionals are still faced with decisions regarding the possibility of using life-sustaining technology. These decisions are difficult because although such technology may prolong life, it sometimes only prolongs the dying process, without offering relief of suffering.

Patients and the public worry about this last possibility—that medical interventions can cause suffering and dehumanization when a patient is dying. It is perhaps not surprising then that the modern hospice and palliative-care movement has grown exponentially over the same period of time during which technology has become better and better at prolonging life indefinitely. **Palliative care** focuses on helping patients and families decide what medical interventions are most likely to be helpful, rather than harmful. It also focuses on managing pain and other symptoms so that, no matter what choices are made, patients can be as comfortable as possible at the end of life. The old adage is that good palliative care focuses on quality rather than quantity of life by "adding life to the years, rather than years to the life."

Providing the best care possible for families who have a child at the end of life can be challenging. Seeing a family in distress carries its own emotional toll, and staff members may struggle with feeling that they or the medical system have failed when a child dies. Yet, it is hoped, the staff can take advantage of its accumulated knowledge and experience to help a family cope and minimize a child's suffering through this last transition in life.

To aid respiratory therapists (RTs) helping families with difficult pediatric end-of-life decision-making, this chapter will provide an overview of the core principles of palliative and end-of-life care. Topics will include discussions regarding goals of care, the logistics of discontinuing MV, the pharmacological and nonpharmacological management of symptoms, and the typical support services available for patients, families, and the health-care team.

Please note that, throughout this chapter, the term *palliative care* will be used to refer to the sensitive, holistic, multidisciplinary management of symptoms and psychosocial distress at the end of life, rather than referring to care that is provided by a particular specialist or in any particular location. Expert opinion from those trained and/or certified in hospice and palliative medicine can be invaluable and should be sought when it can be useful (Table 21-1), but many other health-care professionals are also called upon to provide high-quality end-of-life care in their normal scope of practice.

Table 21-1	Palliative-Care Teams Are Comprised of Individuals From a Variety of Disciplines, Some Noted Here. Individual Team Structures Vary.
Discipline	**Role**
Physician/nurse practitioner	Assess and prescribe medications to treat pain and suffering; assist patients and families with decision-making; write orders to limit resuscitation
Nurse coordinator/case manager	Interface with insurance companies and hospice agencies to organize appropriate patient care and family support
Social worker	Interfaces with insurance companies and hospice agencies to organize appropriate patient care and family support; counsels patients and families on financial and psychosocial issues; provides bereavement support
Chaplain	Provides spiritual support to patients and families and coordinates specific religious rituals when desired
Child life therapist/art therapist/ music therapist	Work with patients and siblings to process distressing circumstances in a non-threatening manner; provide memory-making activities and family support around the time of a child's death
Psychologist	Provides support and counseling to patients and families and referrals to broader mental health support when needed
Bereavement coordinator/grief counselor	Organize hospital services or memorials for families; provide resources or referrals to counseling and support groups for families
Usually From an Outside Agency	
Hospice medical director (hospital physician will often function in this role for children)	Works with team to manage patient's symptoms at home
Hospice nurse	Provides phone and in-home support for patients and families to manage symptoms and facilitate remaining at home; usually may declare death at home
Hospice volunteer/nurse's aide	Assist with patient care needs at home

The hospice agency may also have its own social worker, chaplain, counselors, and bereavement support.

Framing the Discussion About Appropriate Goals of Care

Despite real strides in curing and managing childhood illnesses, more than 50,000 children still die every year in the United States (1, 2). Most of these children will die in the hospital (3, 4); thus, it is important for hospital staff members to be comfortable providing these patients and their families with the best possible care.

It is common for families to first share their concerns about "how much is too much" for their child with one of the therapists or nurses at the bedside rather than with the team of physicians. The nurses and therapists are the providers who are constantly present and may be the most aware of both the suffering and progress of their child. Parents may worry that voicing their thoughts to the medical team will lead to an overly rapid change in the treatments being provided when they are still uncertain about the right course of action. Or perhaps they are looking for an early validation from the nonphysician staff that these are appropriate questions to be asking.

It can put a therapist in an awkward position when a parent raises difficult questions about a child's care, particularly if the therapist already has thoughts about what would be the right choices for the child. When framing the discussion about appropriate goals of care, however, it is important to listen first before offering opinions. Although a mother may be asking you what you think, you do not yet know how she feels about the various options or whether she even knows the different choices that could be made at this point. It is also important to bring physician and nursing colleagues into the conversation early to make certain that the entire team agrees on the course of action that is offered or advised (Teamwork 20-1).

> ■ ■ Instead of answering Michael's mother's question, you ask her what she has been thinking—does she think Michael is suffering? Have she and her husband talked about these issues? You ask if she would be comfortable having you approach the team about setting up a time to talk with them about how Michael is doing and work out an appropriate plan of care. Mrs. Simpson says she would be grateful to have a chance to talk about her concerns.

Another reason it is important to listen first is that there may be factors other than the child's clinical condition that affect how a family looks at their situation. Perhaps the mother and father have disagreed on how much they feel their child is suffering. Perhaps a grandparent is telling them that they "can never give up" on their child. Maybe members of their spiritual community keep telling them that, if they pray hard enough, their child will be cured.

Teamwork 21-1 Active Listening

THE TERM *ACTIVE LISTENING* REFERS TO STATEMENTS AND BEHAVIORS THAT DO THE FOLLOWING:

- Acknowledge emotions and difficulties experienced by the person speaking
- Convey to the speaker that he or she is being heard
- Avoid prematurely closing a topic of conversation

These techniques can be useful if a family expresses distress or asks a team member difficult questions. They can be particularly useful if a team member wants to understand the issues and concerns but is not in a position to recommend a plan or negotiate an agreement until other team members are informed of the discussion as well.

There are important behaviors for active listening:

- Pause, if able, in the tasks at hand to give the patient or family your full attention when a concern is raised
- Make eye contact
- Nod or offer affirmatives when appropriate
- Repeat some word or phrases used by the speaker
- Do not attempt to leave the room as quickly as possible
- Let them know if and when you will be following up on the conversation

Possibly useful statements:

- "It must be really hard when …"
- "I think I hear you saying that …"
- "A lot of families worry about the same things."
- "So what you are most worried about now is that …"
- "I would like to talk about these questions with the rest of the team. Is that ok? Is there anything else you want me to make sure to tell them?"

Or perhaps they had another child die from the same disease and feel upset, angry, or guilty about how things went for him. It is also common that the hospital team members see the child only when he is at his worst, with an acute illness, and the child may have a much better quality of life at home than they realize (5). In trying to help a family decide about their child's care, therefore, it is helpful to ask them to tell you more about the child's quality of life at home.

When the team is having a discussion with the family about appropriate goals of care, it is important to avoid framing aggressive interventions such as intubation and ventilation or cardiopulmonary resuscitation as "doing everything" or alternatively framing a focus on comfort as "giving up" or "doing nothing." Few families would ever want to feel that they gave up on their child, and almost all will say "yes, do everything!" if that is the question put to them. A better approach is to counsel the family that there may come a point in a child's life when focusing on comfort and quality of life rather than invasive interventions is the most life-affirming choice they can make. Deciding that a child has suffered enough does not mean that a family values their child's life any less than if they had decided to continue medical therapy, and they may need reassurance from the team that choosing this path is also a caring decision—a way to cherish and protect their child. Interestingly enough, the "quality vs. quantity" of a child's remaining time may be a valid choice less often than clinicians think. In some adult populations, early referrals to palliative care have been shown to not only improve comfort and quality of life, but also to actually help patients live longer (6). It is unclear, however, whether this is because the patient is avoiding complications of escalating therapies or because focusing on quality of life actually improves health status.

Decision-making in pediatrics is more complicated when prognosis is uncertain. Some disease processes, such as cancer, may have an expected time course of disease progression, but many chronic conditions, such as neuromuscular or metabolic disorders, static encephalopathy, heart failure, and chronic lung disease, have a less-predictable course. Many families know that they would not want invasive procedures when their child is dying, but it can be very difficult to tell when the end is near. Recurrent complications such as pneumonia may be frequent. If the family has seen the child recover from many such episodes, it may be only logical to them to keep trying the next time there is a decompensation. In addition to determining whether a particular episode is treatable, it can be useful to help a family think about how burdensome the interventions are and whether the illness trajectory is one of increasingly difficult hospitalizations or whether the child recovers well after each illness to a reasonable quality of life. Over time, it may become clear whether aggressive management during such episodes benefits the child. If the child is spending more and more time in the hospital, with less "good time" at home, it may be time to reassess what is best for the child.

An **advance directive** (sometimes called a "living will") spells out specific interventions that a patient does or does not want to happen. Only competent, adult patients can have legally binding advance directives, but some patients who receive care in children's hospitals may have advance directives. Such documents can typically be used only as rough guidelines because it is difficult for an individual to anticipate the complexities of specific situations that might arise.

For example, patients who previously stated that they would not want invasive measures such as MV if diagnosed with a terminal condition might change their minds if the ventilation were required only to get them through a brief complication like pneumonia. Advance directives that name a health-care decision-maker or "durable power of attorney" can require the team to include that person in decision-making. The majority of patients in pediatric centers are younger than 18, so their parents are therefore the default decision-makers (Special Populations 20-1). Reasonable efforts should be made to include both parents in decision-making whenever possible, unless one of the parents has had parental rights legally terminated.

● **Special Populations 21-1**

Adult-Aged Patients in Pediatric Centers

Some patients in pediatric centers are older than 18 years but continue to receive care from the pediatric team either because they have been long-term patients or because they have diseases that are best understood by the pediatric specialists. Patients with cystic fibrosis and congenital heart disease fell into this category in the past, but now they often receive care in programs that facilitate the transition to adult centers. When adult patients are cared for in pediatric centers, the team sometimes forgets that they are independent decision-makers. A competent 20-year-old should be asked if it is acceptable for the team to speak with his parents before the parents are given information. A 24-year-old with a life-limiting illness should be offered the opportunity to complete an advance directive rather than have the team assume the parents would be the substituted decision-makers (51). Spouses or significant others of patients may have important points to contribute regarding decision-making. If a competent 20-year-old who is no longer able to speak for himself has identified his girlfriend as his health-care agent, then her opinions would take precedence over those of his parents.

Some adult patients are cognitively impaired and unable to make decisions for themselves. In these cases, it is usually appropriate for the parents to continue in the decision-making role. Such cases should be discussed with the social work or legal team at the hospital to determine if additional legal processes, such as paperwork assigning guardianship, are required.

For any competent adult patient, the patient's own current statements about what he or she wants done in any given situation would override wishes spelled out previously in a legal document. Even if the patient is critically ill or unable to speak, efforts should be made to communicate and ascertain current wishes whenever possible.

■■ You tell Michael's physicians and nurses about the questions his mother is raising, and a meeting is arranged with both parents the following day. The ICU attending physician, primary nurse, and you are all able to attend the meeting. During the discussion, Michael's parents confide that they worry that with each illness he requires so many interventions to help him handle his secretions and avoid plugging that he is often uncomfortable and agitated. Yet when he is at home and doing well, they feel that he is happy, comfortable, and loves interacting with his family and watching movies. After much discussion, the decision is made to intubate Michael if needed. Everyone hopes that he can return to baseline following this illness, but the medical team will reassess whether this outcome seems likely as events evolve.

The Simpsons also worry that he is often frightened when strangers come into the room, and his mother feels she can never leave his bedside. The team suggests posting signs at the bedside to make sure all staff members realize that Michael is cognitively intact and alert. They plan to encourage everyone to talk to him and prepare him before starting any procedures or therapy. They also decide to allow his dog to visit him in the hospital to attempt to improve his mood. In addition, the attending physician tells the family about the palliative-care team at the hospital ("a team that helps to support many families whose children have life-threatening conditions") and says that she plans to call this team so they can get to know Michael and his family.

Early Referral/Concurrent Care

Initiating palliative care should not wait until a decision is made not to escalate or to withdraw interventions. It is possible to focus on comfort and quality of life even while continuing potentially aggressive disease-focused or curative therapies. In hospitals where there is a specialized palliative-care team, it can be helpful for the team to get to know a patient and family early so that they may provide support and build an alliance even before difficult decisions need to be made. Doing so usually allows the development of a better relationship than that which occurs when patients and families meet the team for the first time right after making a decision not to escalate or to withdraw therapies.

There is a growing recognition that **concurrent care**, or the simultaneous pursuit of both palliative and curative measures, benefits most patients (7). Whereas in the past patients were required to forego therapies with curative intent (e.g., chemotherapy) in order to enroll in hospice, many payors are beginning to see the benefits of allowing more flexibility.

In fact, recent health-care reform legislation includes a provision that children whose health care is funded by Medicaid or by the Children's Health Insurance Program (CHIP) be eligible for simultaneous curative and palliative interventions, including hospice, by 2013 (8). Many private insurers are beginning to offer similar benefits. The advantage of encouraging early referrals and allowing concurrent care is that it avoids artificially forcing a family to make a difficult choice between supportive services and ongoing treatments.

It is also important to realize that intubation, ventilation, and tracheostomy are not necessarily incompatible with a palliative approach. There are some situations in which intubation and sedation might be more comfortable for a patient than trying to avoid intubation. In Michael's case, for example, it might be much easier to manage his secretions if he is intubated, and the team might be more willing to give him medications that will sedate him because they are less worried about suppressing his already-weak cough. He may be able to be more easily fed once intubated, and he would not have to be awakened hourly for chest physiotherapy. Yet, he is also likely to be fairly difficult to wean from the ventilator and could require intubation for weeks. Similarly, a tracheostomy sometimes makes sense for a patient who is approaching the end of life if it allows a significant amount of remaining quality time for the patient without the discomfort of an endotracheal tube (ETT). The advantages of such procedures always need to be weighed against the disadvantages, with consideration of whether the intervention promotes a high quality of life or prolongs suffering.

Michael's case is a good illustration of trying to consider ways to improve his life—educating the staff, letting him see his pet—even while he is undergoing aggressive interventions. His physician introduced the palliative-care team in a positive way, as a group who could help support Michael and his family, without making it seem that their only role is to care for children who are imminently dying. Some families also need reassurance that a palliative-care team will work alongside rather than replace the other providers (e.g., oncologists, pulmonologists) with whom the family already has a close relationship. It is also good practice to promote team communication by having the nursing and respiratory therapy staff members attend the family meeting. The nurses and therapists can be very helpful in raising concerns they have about what is difficult for the patient. Having everyone participate in the discussion and formulation of a plan presents a consistent message to the family. It is common for a family to ask the bedside nurse or therapist for their interpretation of what the doctor said following a meeting.

■ ■ Over the next week, Michael's secretions become thicker and more difficult to clear. One night, he becomes much more distressed and hypoxemic, and a chest radiograph shows that his entire left lung has collapsed, likely secondary to a mucus plug. He does not improve with suctioning and increasing his positive pressure and fractional concentration of inspired oxygen (FIO_2), and he is therefore intubated. Once he is intubated, his lung is able to be recruited, and his supplemental oxygen is slowly weaned.

Two weeks pass with continued support. He had initially improved, and his ventilator was weaned to minimal settings, but he rapidly failed the first attempt at extubation. He has now developed a fever, tachycardia, and hypotension, requiring fluid resuscitation and an epinephrine infusion. His lung disease worsens because of sepsis and fluid overload, leading to the need to switch him to high-frequency oscillatory ventilation (HFOV) to maintain oxygenation.

The team meets again with Michael's parents to consider how to best care for him at this point. In their discussions, the attending physician mentions that some families might choose to stop ventilation and focus on keeping Michael comfortable at this point, but that others would want to continue as long as there was a small chance that their child could recover. The physician also says that if Michael's septic shock progresses to the point that he suffers a cardiac arrest, it would be unlikely that he could be successfully resuscitated. Michael's parents say that they are still hoping Michael has a chance to recover but agree that, if his heart stops, "it is his time to go."

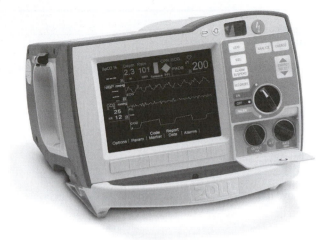

Figure 21-1 Zoll® R Series® Plus Defibrillator *(Courtesy of Zoll Corporation)*

Do Not Attempt Resuscitation Orders

A **do not attempt resuscitation (DNAR) order** specifies that certain interventions, such as MV, chest compressions, or defibrillation, will not be attempted if a patient's condition deteriorates (9) (Fig. 21-1). A specific order is required to forego these interventions because the default assumption is that all patients and families would want such life-sustaining interventions attempted in an emergent situation unless prior conversations between the medical team and the patient or family have occurred to determine that they are either not indicated or not desired. DNAR orders are not all alike. It is important that, when written, they specifically instruct the team what will and will not be done. It is fairly common to have an order to provide all interventions, such as MV, oxygen, antibiotics, fluids, and vasoactive infusions, up to the point of a cardiac arrest, but then to forego chest compressions, defibrillation, and arrest medications if the heart stops. In different situations,

an order might specify that a patient is not to be intubated. Again, staff members need to realize that a DNAR order does not mean that the patient's needs are ignored (see Fig. 21-2 for an example of a DNAR order). It is vitally important at this time to pay very close attention to ensuring that the patient is comfortable. The patient and family should not feel that they have been abandoned because they have decided that a handful of interventions are not beneficial. In Michael's case, for example, there remains a chance that he might survive the illness, so the team needs to maintain its intense focus on interventions that treat and prevent further organ failure.

Recent literature usually refers to limitations of life-sustaining treatments as "do not attempt resuscitation" orders rather than "do not resuscitate" (DNR) orders, the previously used term. The argument in favor of using the phrase "do not attempt resuscitation" is that it does not imply that resuscitation would have been successful, but only that attempts to resuscitate the patient would have been made. Because of frequent media depictions of successful cardiopulmonary resuscitation (10), the general public may have an overly optimistic assessment of how effective CPR can be. Education may therefore be necessary to correct this misperception. Table 21-2 shows the range of reported survival to hospital discharge following cardiopulmonary arrest, with only some of those survivors having a good neurological outcome. Some authors have advocated that orders to limit resuscitative efforts should be called "allow natural death" orders, so that they do not emphasize what will *not* be provided (11, 12).

Although the team members at the bedside will need detailed orders specifying which interventions are to be provided, it is usually best in family

I (patient name) _____ hereby request to forego the following resuscitative measures during my current hospital care:

(Select interventions that *will not* be performed in the event of respiratory or cardiac arrest):

☐ Non-invasive ventilation
☐ Manual positive pressure ventilation
☐ Intubation
☐ Mechanical ventilation
☐ Inotropic medications
☐ Chest compressions
☐ Defibrillation

I (have/have not) _____discussed this decision with my relatives and friends, describing the nature and justification for my decisions.

My physician, _____, has explained to me the nature of resuscitative measures, their risks and benefits, and the risks and benefits of refusing such interventions. I have had an opportunity to ask questions, and have had all of my questions answered by my physician.

After careful consideration of all I discussed with my physician, I request to forego the above-selected attempts at resuscitation.

Name: _____

Signature: _____

Date: _____

Time: _____

Witness: _____

Date: _____

Time: _____

Figure 21-2 Example of a DNAR Order

Table 21-2	Overall Success of Resuscitation Following Cardiopulmonary Arrest for Each Group in Published Studies (13-20)	
	Range of Survival to Hospital Discharge	
Population	**Out-of-Hospital Arrest**	**In-Hospital Arrest**
Adult	3%–16%	6%–22%
Pediatric	4%–16%	27%

conversations to avoid presenting a list of possible interventions and then asking them to say yes or no to each one. The family conversation should focus instead on the overall goals of care (e.g., comfort, prolonging life if at all possible, a time-limited trial of an intervention to see if there is a response), and the medical team can then determine what specific interventions meet those goals.

In Michael's case, the attending physician was offering his family a choice between several alternative paths, each of which would be reasonable from a medical standpoint. The use of the phrase "some families choose" may have helped the family realize that multiple options were available and that reasonable families could choose any of those options. The physician guided them toward setting limits on resuscitative efforts if Michael had a cardiac arrest, presumably because resuscitative efforts were unlikely to be successful when advanced ventilatory support and vasoactive medications were already in place. Although it was clear that the family had the ultimate decision, the physician provided them with medical expertise to help them make that decision.

Families will occasionally ask health-care providers for their opinion about the best course of action. How would you handle the question, "If this was your child, what would you do?" (21, 22). Providing an opinion can be helpful—and is preferable to leaving a family feeling that they have to take the burden of a decision entirely on their own shoulders—but it should be done in way that does not assume they share your values or that there is only one acceptable choice in the circumstances (Box 21-1) (23–25).

Box 21-1 Examples of Useful Phrases to Support a Family Making Difficult Decisions

"I know these are difficult discussions to have. But I can tell that you are working very hard to really think about what is best for your child."

"In situations like this, I have seen loving families that choose different paths depending on what life has been like for their child recently. Do you want me to talk about what some of those options might look like?"

"I wish that your child was not in this situation and that there were therapies that we had to offer to make it better. We will continue to do everything we can think of to take the best possible care of him. But considering that it may not be possible to cure his disease at this point, we also need to think about how to make sure that we do not make him suffer any more than necessary."

"Tell me about your child and what is important to him."

"You can really help us in this situation by letting us know what life is like for him when he is doing well and is not in the hospital. We only get to see him when he is ill. You know him best and can best tell us what quality of life he has."

"Given everything that we have discussed, I have some thoughts about which of the medical interventions we have to offer are most likely to be useful in your child's situation. Would it be helpful to you for me to make a recommendation about what I think might be the best path forward?"

For more examples, see essay by Dr. James Tulsky on communication (23).

■■ Michael improves following his episode of sepsis, and again his ventilatory support is able to be weaned over a 4-week period. Despite being on extubatable settings and daily "sprinting" exercises to continuous positive airway pressure (CPAP) and pressure support, he fails an extubation attempt to NIPPV because of weakness. He has been in the ICU for more than 3 months now, and the team begins discussions with the family regarding the possibility of a tracheostomy to provide ongoing mechanical support of his breathing.

After a few days of considering what has been said, Michael's parents tell the team that they would not want to proceed with a tracheostomy. They feel that Michael's activities would be so limited by being constantly ventilated with likely repeated hospitalizations that he would lose much of his enjoyment in life. They meet with another family who has a child with a tracheostomy at home to make sure they understand what is involved, but the Simpsons still agree that it is not what they want for Michael. The team therefore plans one more extubation attempt but decides that, if he fails, he will not be reintubated.

Discontinuing Mechanical Ventilation

Michael's case is different from that of some children for whom MV is discontinued because there is a moderately good chance that he could survive the extubation because he is on low ventilator settings. It is therefore very important to prepare the family for a range of possible outcomes of the extubation—he could breathe adequately with NIPPV (if all agree to provide this) and potentially be discharged home. However, it is also possible that he will struggle to breathe and require medications to help him be comfortable. Yet, even in this scenario, he could live for hours to days following the extubation. It is therefore important to avoid being overly certain in predicting a time from extubation to death, even for the sickest patients.

In Michael's case, the weaning of his ventilator to extubation would likely be fairly standard, and medications for dyspnea would be provided only if he demonstrated that he needs them. When a ventilator is being discontinued for a patient on higher settings with an expected inability to survive, it is important that there is a plan in place to ensure patient comfort during the process (26). Removing the ETT may improve comfort, but the loss of positive pressure may worsen work of breathing (WOB). If medications for comfort are going to be used, discuss with the team whether doses should be given or infusions started or increased prior to discontinuing the ventilator. The specific pharmacological treatment of dyspnea is discussed later in this chapter.

Terminal Extubation Versus Terminal Weaning

There are two commonly used approaches to discontinuing MV in a patient expected to die: terminal extubation and terminal weaning (27, 28). With **terminal extubation,** the ventilator is discontinued and the ETT removed without weaning the ventilator prior to doing so. This technique is often appropriate for a patient who is heavily sedated or obtunded and therefore not expected to experience much respiratory distress when the ventilator is discontinued. **Terminal weaning** is a method of slowly lowering ventilatory support over a period of hours (or days, in the early descriptions) prior to removing the ETT. Depending on the situation, some degree of weaning the ventilator may offer the advantage of assessing how comfortable the patient is with lower ventilatory pressures and oxygen supplementation prior to removing the ETT, which would allow the escalation of sedatives or narcotics as needed beforehand. Weaning also has a theoretical benefit of allowing the retention of carbon dioxide prior to the extubation because severe respiratory acidosis can have a sedative effect. Unfortunately, respiratory acidosis usually causes marked agitation until the partial pressure of carbon dioxide (PCO_2) rises significantly, so this is rarely a true benefit of slow weaning. Treating respiratory distress with medications is a better option. Slow weaning also has the disadvantage of delaying the extubation at a time when the family is likely ready to have the ventilator removed as soon as possible. A few minutes at lower settings is almost always enough to assess whether the patient is comfortable and if the use of medications is needed. If a patient is being extubated from an advanced mode of ventilation such as HFOV, it might be helpful to offer the family the possibility of switching to conventional ventilation prior to the extubation so that they can hold the child before or while the ETT is removed.

Preparing the Family

Prior to an extubation, the team should formulate a plan for the logistics of the process. The team should decide beforehand about whether other medical equipment, such as nasogastric tubes, central lines, and intravenous (IV) tubes or catheters, will be removed at the same time. Maintaining some form of IV access can be useful for administering medications to treat distress. Many families will want to be present if possible for the extubation, but they should not be forced to be at the bedside if they are more comfortable waiting elsewhere. Some families have cultural or spiritual traditions that they would like to follow prior to the withdrawal. Families may need time to gather or prepare relatives. Some family members prefer to hold their child or lie in bed with their child at the time of extubation. It is helpful to ask the parents directly how many other family members they would like to have present so that the team can help control how crowded a room gets if the parents prefer privacy. Conversely, some relaxation of limits on the number of visitors that can be present is also helpful for many families who benefit from the support of extended family members. Moving the child to a private room prior to the extubation, if one is available, is often helpful to give a grieving family privacy, avoid distressing other families that might be present in the unit, and help staff focus on the needs of the dying child.

Families should also be prepared for what their child might look like when the tube is removed.

Increased WOB, color changes, noisy breathing, and increased secretions can all be anticipated. Family members can be reassured that any signs of distress will be treated, but if they are bothered by unusual breathing patterns such as stridor or agonal breaths, they can be reassured that this is a normal occurrence and that their child is not alert or suffering. Staff members should check in frequently following an extubation to make sure that the child is comfortable and that the family feels supported. Turning off monitors and following vital signs from another monitor outside the room can minimize disturbances in the room.

Organ Donation

Prior to withdrawing MV, it is important to assess whether organ donation following cardiac death can be offered to the family. Most organ donation occurs following a neurological determination of death ("brain death"), in which case the ventilator does not need to be discontinued prior to organ procurement because the patient has already been declared dead. For patients who are not brain dead but are expected to die within 1 hour following discontinuation of ventilation, it may still be possible to donate after death is declared using cardiopulmonary criteria (see Chapter 20 for an in-depth discussion). Some disease processes, often infections or disseminated cancer, will prevent a patient from being a donor. Exploring these questions proactively with the local organ-procurement organization prior to the extubation is useful to determine if there is a possibility of offering this procedure to the family.

■■ Michael's parents ask to extubate him the day after the family meeting so that arrangements can be made to have his grandparents present as well. As there is a chance that Michael will survive his extubation, his family is preparing for all possibilities. They have decided to continue to use his BiPAP, which is reasonable because it is a baseline level of support for him. The team has planned with his parents that they would not increase his BiPAP pressures above his usual home baseline to avoid adding possible discomfort caused by using high pressures and the need for a tighter-fitting mask. They decided together, however, that they could use a higher FIO_2 than his baseline, at least temporarily, by using the ICU ventilator rather than his home BiPAP machine. The rationale was that the higher FIO_2 should not cause discomfort and would, it is hoped, help him make a transition back to his home level of support. If his home pressure settings are not enough to treat his dyspnea, the plan is to increase his pharmacological treatment of breathlessness until he is comfortable. An RT who has recently finished orientation has responsibility for his care for the day and asks you to help because he has never removed a ventilator from someone who may die following its discontinuation.

When the team and family are ready, you and the new therapist, along with one of the physicians, remove Michael's ETT. He has a very shallow respiratory effort. He is placed quickly onto his nasal mask BiPAP interface with his home settings (end-expiratory airway pressure [EPAP] of 6 and inspiratory positive airway pressure [IPAP] of 15) with 100% oxygen supplementation. His oxygen saturations then improve from the 70s to the low 90s, and his WOB is improved, but he continues to look somewhat anxious and distressed. His family asks if it is time to give him medication for comfort.

Treating Dyspnea

Often, a family and the medical team have to work closely together to determine when it is necessary to treat respiratory distress with medications at the end of life. For every intervention, it is necessary to weigh the burdens versus the benefits to determine whether it makes sense in the particular clinical situation. There are many factors to consider after terminal extubation, for example, particularly considering the degree of uncertainty regarding how quickly death will follow extubation. Is the patient experiencing more distress than usual following an extubation? Are the patient's symptoms improving over time with noninvasive positive pressure or are they worsening? In many patients, it is also important to distinguish whether the signs of respiratory distress are accompanied by a subjective feeling of air hunger, or dyspnea (29). Patients who are obtunded or comatose at the end of life may show some signs of distress, such as airway obstruction or difficulty handling secretions, but if the patient is not alert enough to be aware of the symptoms, it is usually only necessary to reassure family or staff members who are watching. Such symptoms are normal in the situation, and the patient is not in pain. In patients who are alert and distressed, however, there is a greater need to treat (Fig. 21-3).

Supplemental Oxygen and Nonpharmacological Therapies

One important question is whether to provide supplemental oxygen or mechanical supports, such as NIPPV or a nasopharyngeal airway, to a dying patient. Again, the burdens and benefits of such actions must be weighed for the specific case. If the patient is not accustomed to NIPPV, it may simply make him or her more uncomfortable because of the pressure on the patient's face, with little benefit added

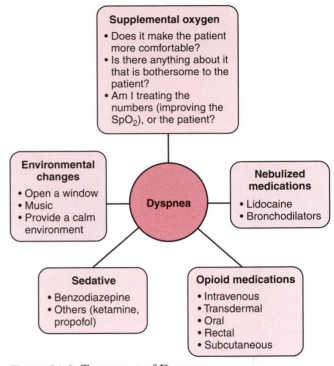

Figure 21-3 Treatment of Dyspnea

from prolonging the dying process. Yet Michael has spent much of his life on BiPAP, so he is less likely to be distressed by the mask itself. If he begins to have difficult-to-treat complications such as skin breakdown from the interface, it will be important for his family to realize that there is no moral imperative to continue the BiPAP. Even though he has been using NIPPV for a long time, it is still a medical intervention that can be discontinued if the situation warrants doing so.

Providing supplemental oxygen for dying patients is different from doing so in other circumstances. When deciding to treat dying patients with supplemental oxygen, whether at home or in the hospital, the following questions should be considered:

• Does it make the patient more comfortable?
• Is there anything about it that is bothersome to the patient?
• Am I treating the numbers (improving the saturation of oxygen) or the patient?

Sometimes, other physical measures can also help with breathlessness—consider opening a window, providing a calm environment, or music. Blowing a fan toward the patient's face may also relieve air hunger. When such interventions are inadequate, pharmacological agents can be used.

Pharmacological Treatment

A wide range of pharmacological treatments are available for the management of pain and suffering at the end of life. This section will focus predominantly on medications that may be useful when respiratory symptoms are severe and will cover various narcotic and sedative agents. In addition, the nebulized delivery of medications will be briefly addressed because RTs may be involved in administering medications by this route.

Opioid (Narcotic) Medications

Opioid or narcotic agents are usually the first-line therapy for the treatment of dyspnea or pain at the end of life (30). There are many formulations available, including IV medications given by infusions or as bolus doses, oral liquids or pills, sublingual or transdermal (patch) preparations, and agents for rectal administration. For those able to take tablets or capsules, oral preparations are available in both immediate and sustained-release formulations. Subcutaneous infusion catheters can be used in patients who are unable to take adequate doses of medication by mouth, but in whom maintaining IV access is either difficult or burdensome (31).

All opioids have effects at the μ-opioid receptor in the central nervous system (CNS) to cause analgesia (pain control), euphoria, and cough suppression. They also have predictable side effects such as suppression of the drive to breathe, itching, nausea, constipation, and urinary retention. Side effects can end up causing almost as much distress as the symptoms one is attempting to treat, so anticipation and treatment (e.g., a laxative regimen for constipation) are important. Changing from one agent to another can sometimes both decrease side effects and improve pain control. Duration of action of the narcotics varies notably, with the more lipid-soluble drugs, such as Fentanyl, having very short half-lives. Morphine is longer acting, but because it leads to a release of histamine, it may cause more itching than other narcotics. It can also cause bothersome neurological toxicities such as myoclonus (involuntary muscle twitches) when used at high doses for long periods, particularly in patients with multiorgan failure (32). Hydromorphone and oxycodone are useful alternatives if unmanageable side effects occur. Codeine can be particularly problematic because it is not effective until it is metabolized to morphine, and 10% of people are unable to metabolize it (30). In those patients, it can cause severe nausea without the benefit of pain relief. Meperidine should also be avoided because a metabolite can accumulate that has been reported to cause seizures in both adults and children. Methadone has a very long half-life that can make dosing adjustments difficult, but it has the advantage of NMDA receptor effects that sometimes help with neuropathic pain and has added benefits in patients who are opioid tolerant. Tolerance can develop over time to all opioids, requiring an escalation of doses. Withdrawal symptoms occur if these medications are abruptly discontinued or weaned too rapidly. Symptoms can include agitation, sweating, tachycardia, fever, tremors, yawning, vomiting, and diarrhea. Specific care should be taken in pediatrics when using combination agents (an opioid combined with acetaminophen, for instance); dose escalation of the opioid may become necessary for severe pain, but escalating could lead to toxicity and organ injury from the other agent. It is usually better, therefore, to dose opioids separately from acetaminophen or nonsteroidal anti-inflammatory agents to avoid this problem.

Rule of Double Effect

The respiratory-depressant effect of opioids is particularly worrisome to clinicians who use them to treat pain because they are concerned about causing or hastening death by increasing doses. The "rule of double effect," which is covered in depth in Chapter 20, justifies the use of opiates to treat severe pain, even if they do lead to respiratory depression. In patients who are not expected to die, the respiratory depression can be managed by lowering doses, using reversal agents, or providing MV if needed. In patients who are expected to die, it is possible that medications might hasten death, but this risk is justified by the importance of treating pain and dyspnea. In reality, clinicians are rarely confronted with a choice of this nature. If medication doses are increased incrementally until pain is controlled, they are highly unlikely to cause respiratory depression because the pain itself is a powerful respiratory stimulant. Eventually, doses much higher than the maximum recommended starting dose are commonly necessary, especially in patients who have been receiving these medications for some time. There is no upper limit on doses that can be administered, as long as the beneficial effects and side effects are balanced. Studies in adult patients at the end of life have shown, perhaps surprisingly, that those who receive the highest doses of narcotic and sedative agents often survive the longest following the withdrawal of life-sustaining therapies (33), suggesting that it is rare that these agents hasten death in usual practice. Even in neonates, high doses of narcotics—when appropriately titrated for control of symptoms—are not associated with time to death (34). Underdosing of pain medications at the end of life is unfortunately far more often a problem than overdosing (35).

Nebulized Medications

Nebulized medications such as morphine have been studied in an attempt to determine if this route of administration provides relief for subjective feelings of breathlessness without the side effects and respiratory depression that are seen with systemic administration of narcotics (36). Although case reports and case series have suggested that a high percentage of patients report relief with nebulized opioids (37), randomized controlled trials have not shown an improved benefit over placebo or subcutaneous morphine (38, 39). With conflicting data on the utility of nebulized opioids, a trial for any individual patient who requires treatment for dyspnea but wishes to remain as alert as possible may be warranted.

In some patients, particularly those with chronic lung disease, nebulized bronchodilators such as albuterol can also relieve symptoms of respiratory distress. Nebulized lidocaine is sometimes used, both as a possible treatment for dyspnea and for severe cough (40).

> ■■ Michael's parents were concerned that he would be anxious throughout the process of extubation, so the team decided that the IV administration of medications would be preferable to nebulized medications because they would have the additional benefit of calming him. He also has the advantage of having IV access already in place.

Sedatives

In many patients, breathlessness and anxiety can become a vicious cycle. Agitation worsens respiratory distress, and carbon dioxide accumulation causes panic and a feeling that it is impossible to get enough air. Opioids can often improve this distress but sometimes are inadequate alone. In patients with difficult-to-treat symptoms or with high levels of anxiety, sedative agents can be very helpful. The most commonly used in adults and children are the benzodiazepines, such as diazepam, lorazepam, or midazolam. These agents are usually calming and can also have an amnestic effect (decreasing the memory of stressful events). They can decrease WOB and may also help patients sleep in the acute setting, although long-term administration can cause disruption of normal sleep-wake cycles. It may be possible to use low-enough doses to relieve symptoms without causing mental status changes. In some patients, however, symptoms such as pain or dyspnea can become so difficult to manage that it is worth having a discussion regarding whether it would be better to provide sedation to the point of sleepiness or unconsciousness. Many patients and families will choose to tolerate some symptoms in order to have the patient remain as alert as possible at the end of life, but others have symptoms that are distressing enough that sedation is required. When sedation is added, opioids should not be discontinued.

Terminal sedation is a phrase sometimes used to refer to sedation to unconsciousness at the end of life,

when symptoms cannot be managed by other means. Sedation is titrated carefully until symptoms are controlled, with no intent of causing death. **Euthanasia** refers to the purposeful administration of medications to end life, and it is illegal in the United States. The use of any sedative agent, including propofol or ketamine, may be acceptable if symptoms are not controllable by any other means. Medications that only hasten death without relieving symptoms, such as neuromuscular blocking agents or potassium chloride, are not acceptable (see Chapter 20).

Managing Secretions

Many patients have difficulty managing secretions at the end of life, and the noise of breathing from accumulated secretions can be distressing to families. Most patients at this stage are no longer alert enough to be distressed by these symptoms themselves. It is important to reassure families that some accumulation of secretions and noisy breathing is normal at this stage. If the secretions are particularly disturbing, patients can be given anticholinergic agents such as atropine or glycopyrrolate to dry the secretions, although the secretions will likely not completely disappear. Although diphenhydramine can also dry secretions, it can have significant neurological side effects such as dizziness or confusion at the end of life, particularly when combined with other agents. Secretions may also be worsened by overly vigorous IV fluid administration, and decreasing supplemental fluid may be helpful. Many families need guidance to determine the appropriate degree of suctioning to provide. Excessive suctioning can be distressing and cause more suffering, but some amount may help patients handle their secretions and be more comfortable. Individual patient circumstances need to be considered, always keeping the overall goal of comfort in mind.

> ■■ Considering Michael's neuromuscular disease, the team was concerned that drying his secretions with medications would lead to worsening problems with plugging and an inability to cough and clear thickened mucus from his lungs. They therefore decided not to use anticholinergic agents and to continue his secretion-clearance therapies such as the cough-assist device, with a plan for frequent reassessment as to whether such interventions are causing undue distress. They also give Michael intermittent doses of morphine following his extubation, which seem to make him much more comfortable, and he is able to rest and be held by his family. His oxygen saturations remain in the 80s and higher for the first 24 hours. The following day, his saturations fall further despite good pulmonary toilet and continued noninvasive support.

Location of Death

Over time, more families of children with complex chronic conditions are choosing to take their children home at the end of their life (41–43). This choice is possible only because of the systems that have been developed for supporting families at home by providing nursing care and medications for comfort. Agencies that focus specifically on providing such care at home for dying patients are called **hospice agencies**. Most hospice agencies are able to provide a nurse on call who will respond to questions regarding how to manage symptoms and come to the home when needed. Medications such as opioids and benzodiazepines are kept in the home in case they are needed. Most agencies also provide a multidisciplinary support team, often including social workers, chaplains, nurse's aides, or grief counselors. Medical direction of a child's care at home may be provided by the medical director of the hospice, but because most hospices take care of far more adult than pediatric patients, the day-to-day management of the medications may instead be done by a pediatrician or pediatric subspecialist at the hospital. Most hospices are also able to provide some degree of respiratory support at home, with oxygen and suctioning equipment commonly available if needed. Hospice agencies may also be able to deliver medications to the home to help a family spend as much time with their loved one as possible, but they often are unable to provide particularly expensive medications because they would rapidly exceed the flat, per diem rate for care that the agency receives. Hospice staff members are experienced in managing a wide variety of symptoms in the home setting and usually see it as their mission to help a family stay at home if at all possible in order to avoid the overuse of technology at the time of their loved one's death.

Uncertainties in prognosis in pediatric patients sometimes lead to difficulty deciding when it is appropriate to refer a child to a hospice agency to assist with home care (44). For a patient to qualify for the Medicare hospice benefit in adult care, it is currently necessary for a physician to certify that the normal life expectancy for a patient with that terminal illness is less than 6 months, if the illness runs its normal course. The patient will likely still be eligible and can be reenrolled if he or she survives more than 6 months. Many hospices also require such a certification for children, with an understanding that there may be a fair degree of uncertainty regarding the time course. Yet, if a child lives for years longer than expected, it may become necessary for them to transition off of hospice to a home-care management plan more appropriate for a chronic illness.

Even though there are many reasons families may choose to take their child home to die, it is not the right choice in every circumstance. There may be symptoms that would be difficult to manage at home (Table 21-3) or family circumstances that would make it problematic. The optimal location may be determined by many issues, including how long the patient is expected to survive. A family's preference may also change over time if symptoms worsen or improve or if the time course is uncertain. Any family that takes a child home to die should be reassured that they can return to the hospital if needed.

Many families worry about how siblings might react. Often social workers and child life specialists can help parents talk to the siblings of the dying child and decide how to involve them to an appropriate degree in saying goodbye, whether at home or in the hospital. In Michael's case, he requires close attention to his secretion management, and remaining in the hospital lets his family focus more on being with him than on his medical care. Although in many cases it is appropriate to transfer a patient with a DNAR order out of the ICU, in some cases the ICU team knows the patient and family best because they have been there for months. In such cases, families often appreciate being able to stay with familiar staff members if possible.

If a patient who has previously had chronic medical care in the home is going home to die, it is important for the family or medical team to have an explicit conversation with home nurses about the goals of his care and anticipated course. As opposed to hospice nurses, home-shift nurses may or may not

| Table 21-3 | Symptoms That Can Be Difficult to Manage at Home and Strategies for Helping to Do So in Cases Where Families Are Committed to Staying Home |

Symptom/Problem	Management Strategy
Severe pain requiring IV medication	Continuous infusions at home
Bleeding/risk of severe bleeding	Have dark towels available so that blood is less visible/distressing
Seizures	Rectal administration of diazepam
Respiratory distress/anxiety	Calming environment/fan/sedatives and narcotics/oxygen (see text)
Sibling distress	Social worker/art therapist/child life specialist home visit
Family exhaustion/burnout	Respite stay in hospital or in-patient hospice

Hospitalization may be necessary.

have previously taken care of dying patients, and if they have been working with the patient and his family for a long time, they may be distressed by the circumstances as well. Discussing the plan and making sure that everyone is comfortable with it avoids problems such as an undesired call to emergency medical services by a home-care nurse who may be uncomfortable with the situation.

■ ■ The palliative-care team talks with the Simpsons about whether they would like to go home or whether they would be more comfortable staying in the hospital. After taking some time to think, his parents decide that, although they would have wanted to take him home if he were awake and aware of his environment, they feel that he is not likely to be very awake. They also worry about how his 7-year-old sister would handle his dying at home and feel that the assistance of the ICU team in managing his symptoms and pulmonary toilet is invaluable. They have also gotten to know the ICU team very well over the last few admissions and are therefore comfortable staying with the support of the familiar team.

Over the next day, Michael's saturations continue to fall. He has been placed on a morphine infusion at this point, and he looks comfortable and asleep. His mother has been sleeping in the bed next to him or holding him in her lap when she is awake. When Michael's oxygen saturations are no longer rising above the 60s, his parents ask if the BiPAP can be discontinued. The team agrees that this is reasonable. After he is given an additional dose of morphine to make sure that he is comfortable, you remove the BiPAP mask and help his mother clean his face. You stay with his parents to make sure that he continues to look comfortable, and he dies in their arms within 15 minutes.

Supporting the Family

In addition to providing good symptom management for children at the end of life, the team can help support the family in many other ways. For most families, it is very important to maintain contact with their child near the end of life (45). The team can help with this by letting the family hold the child or lie in bed with the child. As noted previously, moving to a private room if one is available and allowing more visitors than usual is also helpful. Even though the family can no longer anticipate the recovery of their child at this point, there are many other things they can hope for—that the child's suffering will soon end, that the death will have some meaning or perhaps contribute to medical knowledge, or that their family will survive

the ordeal intact (24). Staff members can also help with memory-making activities, such as providing handprints or footprints, clippings of hair, or photographs. Suggesting to the parents that they enlist other family and friends to take calls, update others, and bring food to the parents helps the parents spend as much time with the child as possible and helps the extended family and friends keep busy with tasks to do. Simply sitting with a family to talk about their child and their child's life can be a very caring act. Both before and after the time of death, staff members should check in with the family often to make sure the child is comfortable and to let the family know they are available to help, but it is also important to let the family have private time with the child.

Many families will have religious or spiritual rituals that they would like to have performed around the time of a child's death (46). Examples of possible rituals include specific prayers or procedures for caring for the body. Staff members can ask the family if there are any practices that the team should know about and can enlist help from a hospital chaplain or a family's own spiritual advisor when needed. Families report that their religious and spiritual beliefs are an important source of support for them following a child's death (47).

Support of the family should continue after the death of the child. Many hospitals have bereavement programs or committees that follow up by sending a card or making a phone call. Others have institutional memorial services that families are invited to attend. Some programs also have counseling or support groups available for families. Many staff members report that they attend funerals (48), and families usually appreciate some follow-up with them, particularly if the child was hospitalized for a long time. If an autopsy is going to be performed, the physician will often schedule a follow-up meeting to discuss the results. Follow-up meetings can be useful to families even if no autopsy has been done (49).

Supporting the Team

In caring for the patient and family, it is important to remember that the death of a patient can be a difficult and emotional experience for members of the health-care team as well. Team members often struggle with the balance between their own need to pause and acknowledge the death of a patient and the need to move on quickly to care for other children in the hospital who need their attention. The new RT who helped to extubate Michael may need to talk with someone more senior to process the experience. Some institutions may have counseling available for staff members through human resources offices or employee assistance programs. A staff debriefing may be useful for particularly difficult cases (50). Staff members can often reassure themselves that the child is no longer suffering and that they provided the best possible care for the child and his or her family at a difficult time.

Sometimes team members wonder how closely involved to get with a family on a personal level if they have spent a lot of time with them. While it may be reasonable to maintain contact with some families following the death of a patient, care should be taken to maintain a professional relationship. Before meeting a patient's mother for lunch or becoming friends with a family member on an online social network, it is a good idea to discuss such interactions with colleagues and supervisors to make sure a professional boundary is not being crossed.

Team members also wonder if it is acceptable to cry or show emotion in front of a family when they are distressed by a patient's death. Most families appreciate it when staff members show they care. Crying or expressing sadness may therefore be appropriate, particularly when there has been a long-term relationship with the family. A good rule of thumb is that it would be inappropriate to become so emotional that the child's family might begin to feel that they need to reassure the staff member. The staff member should maintain enough composure that he or she is able to be a source of support for the family.

End-of-life care for pediatric patients is challenging for clinicians in all disciplines. Emotions can run high, both among the family and staff members. Symptoms can be difficult to manage, and sorting through how aggressively to intervene takes patience, perspective, and skill. Yet, when such care is managed well, staff members can take pride in having helped a patient and the patient's family navigate one of the most difficult events imaginable in anyone's life. Learning how to do so as gracefully and competently as possible is one of our most critical responsibilities as health-care providers.

■■ Critical Thinking Questions: Michael Simpson

1. What could you have done if Michael's mother had not been receptive to your suggestion of a team conversation about Michael's plan of care?
2. How might you approach a staff member who you notice is not talking to Michael when providing bronchial hygiene?
3. What possible benefits to tracheostomy might there have been for Michael?
4. If Michael hadn't had an IV in place, what are some therapies (pharmacological and nonpharmacological) that could have been attempted to alleviate his dyspnea?
5. What additional considerations may have been needed if Michael had lived for another 3 days? Another 3 weeks?

❯● Case Studies and Critical Thinking Questions

■ Case 1: Stephen Cates

Stephen Cates is a 16-year-old with cystic fibrosis who has had progressive deterioration in his pulmonary function following a lung transplant 3 years ago. He has decided that he would not want to undergo a repeat transplant, and his parents support him in this decision. The team explains that a do not attempt resuscitation order, including a do not intubate order, would help achieve Stephen's goals of avoiding unwanted aggressive interventions at the end of life and of spending as much time at home as possible. He and his parents agree. Stephen uses BiPAP at night and several hours during the day to help his WOB and to let him spend more time with his friends and family before dying.

- How can you best help Stephen think about things he might want to do before dying? Memory-making for his family that he participates in? A special celebration of his life with his friends? Are there things Stephen wants to tell his loved ones or special tasks he wants to complete while he is still able?
- What considerations might be important for Stephen in determining when to be at home and when to be at the hospital?
- What strategies can be considered to help Stephen if he becomes severely short of breath as his respiratory distress worsens?
- Who is/are the legal decision-maker(s) regarding Stephen's medical care? Are there ways to facilitate the team and family listening to and respecting his thoughts on decisions made?

■ Case 2: Baby Girl (BG) Kemp

A 2-month-old 23-week gestation premature infant with severe respiratory distress syndrome and a large (grade IV) intraventricular hemorrhage has developed worsening hypoxemia despite an FIO_2 of 1.0, high-frequency ventilation, sedation, and neuromuscular blockade. When the neonatology team explains that they do not think the infant can survive, the parents tearfully state that they do not want to prolong her suffering.

- Would an agreement not to escalate therapies or a withdrawal of MV be appropriate in this case? What factors might be relevant in that decision?
- The parents have never been able to hold BG Kemp since her birth. What could the team do to help them hold her and spend time together as a family before her death? Are there ways that the physical environment

of the ICU might facilitate or impede this goal? What steps can be taken to overcome such limitations?

- *The parents ask if the ETT can be removed when the ventilator is discontinued so that they can see BG Kemp's face. What is your answer?*
- *Are there medications that you would increase prior to stopping the ventilator? Are there any that you would discontinue?*

■ Case 3: Sanjay Patel

Sanjay Patel is a 4-year-old child with Leigh's disease (progressive weakness with eventual respiratory failure and brain injury). He underwent a tracheostomy 2 years ago when he was severely hypotonic, but he is still able to laugh and interact with his family. He is cared for at home with 16 hours of home nursing care a day, and his parents have been trained to manage his tracheostomy and ventilator for the remaining hours. Sanjay's brain disease has now progressed to a

point that he is no longer aware of his environment and has frequent episodes of agitation with tachycardia and hypertension. The Patels feel that his quality of life is now so poor that they want to discontinue ventilation. They would prefer to have him die at home, surrounded by his family, rather than in the hospital.

- *Is it ethical to discontinue ventilation once it has been begun? Are there special considerations in a patient who has been chronically ventilated?*
- *What resources would be available to help the Patel family stay at home for a ventilator withdrawal?*
- *The Patel family does not want to have Sanjay stuck to place an IV. What other routes of medication administration are available if needed for his comfort?*
- *Sanjay has two siblings, ages 6 and 9. What resources are available to help them cope?*

Multiple-Choice Questions

1. A 14-year-old boy has sustained severe injuries after being struck by a car. Two days after the injury, his parents state that "he would never want to be hooked up to machines" and ask that the ventilator be discontinued. In what circumstances is it possible to do so?
   a. The patient would have to be "brain dead" to remove the ventilator.
   b. A judge would have to order the removal of the ventilator.
   c. The parents and medical team would have to agree that the prognosis was poor enough that continuing ventilation carried more burden than possible benefit.
   d. The parents' request alone is sufficient and must be honored.

2. Which of the following terms refers to care that is focused on relieving the suffering of patients?
   a. Hospice care
   b. Curative care
   c. Palliative care
   d. Concurrent care

3. A 24-year-old young man with cystic fibrosis still receives his care at the pediatric center. He has a legally documented advance directive naming his boyfriend as his decision-maker and stating that he does not want to be intubated for an acute event. He is brought to the emergency department by his mother in respiratory distress from pneumonia, and she demands that he be placed on a ventilator.

Reasonable courses of action include the following:
   a. Intubate him because his mother requests it.
   b. Attempt to discuss the situation with the patient and determine if he is able to express his wishes in the current situation.
   c. If the patient is unable to communicate, stabilize him with noninvasive ventilation while attempts are made to reach his boyfriend who is the legal decision-maker.
   d. Call his father to ask him what he wants done.
   e. b or c
   f. a or d

4. A 12-year-old with relapsed leukemia, sepsis, and multiorgan failure is mechanically ventilated and on high doses of a norepinephrine infusion. Her parents meet with the oncology team and decide to place a do not attempt resuscitation order because it is highly unlikely that she will be able to survive. The appropriate next step is to:
   a. Extubate her because she is now DNAR.
   b. Ask for clarification from the physician who had the conversation about whether current interventions are going to continue and whether medical care will be escalated if a cardiac arrest does not occur.
   c. Stop assessing her for wheezing and the need for PRN albuterol doses because other patients will benefit more from your time at this point.

5. A 6-year-old has a progressive brain tumor that has led to respiratory failure. His parents have accepted the physician's recommendation to have him extubated so that they can focus on his comfort at this time. In preparing to discontinue the ventilator, you lower the FIO_2, and he becomes cyanotic and anxious with wide, frightened eyes. An appropriate course of action would be to:
   a. Remove the tube quickly to see if he is more comfortable.
   b. Increase the FIO_2 temporarily and ask for additional medications so that he is comfortable prior to discontinuing the ventilator.
   c. Tell his parents that you think he will struggle far too much if the ventilator is discontinued and suggest that they pursue a tracheostomy instead.
   d. Ask that he receive a dose of paralytic prior to the extubation so that his WOB is not distressing to his parents.

6. Which of the following are options for parents during a terminal extubation?
   a. Holding the child while you extubate
   b. Complete a religious service before or during the extubation
   c. Wait in a family waiting room during the extubation
   d. Any of the above are options that should be offered to the family.

7. Narcotics (opioids) can cause the following signs or symptoms *except*:
   a. Diarrhea
   b. Relief of air hunger
   c. Relief of pain
   d. Itching
   e. Nausea

8. Hospice agencies typically:
   a. Provide 24-hour nursing care and rehabilitation services for a patient going home on a ventilator.
   b. Provide insurance coverage for a patient who is not eligible for Medicare or Medicaid.

   c. Facilitate comfort and family support so that a patient can remain home and avoid unwanted medical interventions at the end of life.
   d. Consult with the hospital to obtain a do not attempt resuscitation order on a patient.

9. You walk into the room of a 9-year-old girl with end-stage cancer to perform chest physiotherapy. She is sleeping, but her mom asks if you have a few minutes to talk about whether you think any of the respiratory treatments ordered for her daughter are "worth it." What strategies can you use to help you respond to this request?
   a. Offer to get the physician or bedside nurse to discuss these issues.
   b. Pause in what you're doing and give your full attention to the mom.
   c. Do not allow the conversation to go on too long and distress the family.
   d. Recommend to the mom a plan of changes to the respiratory order.

10. You are a home-care RT and receive a call from a father whose 4-year-old son, James, is receiving oxygen via nasal cannula as part of his hospice care. Dad called because James is looking more short of breath, and he was worried that perhaps the oxygen equipment isn't working correctly. You will come out to visit to be sure everything is working; what other things can you suggest for James to improve his dyspnea?
    I. Albuterol
    II. Quiet, calming environment
    III. Fan
    IV. Sedative
    V. Increase oxygen
    VI. Noninvasive ventilation
    a. I, II, III, IV
    b. II, III, IV, V
    c. I, IV, V
    d. II, III

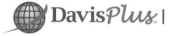

REFERENCES

1. Mathews TJ, Minino AM, Osterman MJ, et al. Annual summary of vital statistics: 2008. *Pediatrics.* 2011;127(1): 146-157.
2. National Center for Injury Prevention and Control, Centers for Disease Control and Prevention. WISQARS leading causes of death reports, 1999-2007. http://webappa .cdc.gov/sasweb/ncipc/leadcaus10.html. Updated June 1, 2010. Accessed January 3, 2013.
3. Feudtner C, Christakis DA, Zimmerman FJ, et al. Characteristics of deaths occurring in children's hospitals: implications for supportive care services. *Pediatrics.* 2002;109(5): 887-893.
4. Feudtner C, Connor SR. Epidemiology and health services research. In: Carter BS, Levetown M, eds. *Palliative Care for Infants, Children, and Adolescents: A Practical Handbook.* Baltimore, MD: Johns Hopkins University Press; 2004.
5. Janse AJ, Gemke RJ, Uiterwaal CS, et al. Quality of life: patients and doctors don't always agree: a meta-analysis. *J Clin Epidemiol.* 2004;57(7):653-661.
6. Temel JS, Greer JA, Muzikansky A, et al. Early palliative care for patients with metastatic non-small-cell lung cancer. *N Engl J Med.* 2010;363(8):733-742.
7. Corcoran AM, Casarett DJ. Improving communication and rethinking hospice care. *Chest.* 2010;137(6): 1262-1263.
8. National Hospice and Palliative Care Organization. Hospice wins big impact tournament. http://www.nhpco.org/ i4a/pages/index.cfm?pageid=5853. Published July 26, 2011. Accessed January 3, 2013.
9. Morrison W, Berkowitz I. Do not attempt resuscitation orders in pediatrics. *Pediatr Clin North Am.* 2007;54(5): 757-771.
10. Diem SJ, Lantos JD, Tulsky JA. Cardiopulmonary resuscitation on television: miracles and misinformation. *N Engl J Med.* 1996;334(24):1578-1582.
11. Cohen RW. A tale of two conversations. *Hastings Cent Rep.* 2004;34(3):49.
12. Knox C, Vereb JA. Allow natural death: a more humane approach to discussing end-of-life directives. *J Emerg Nurs.* 2005;31(6):560-561.
13. Nichol G, Thomas E, Callaway CW, et al. Regional variation in out-of-hospital cardiac arrest incidence and outcome. *JAMA.* 2008;300(12):1423-1431.
14. van Walraven C, Forster AJ, Parish DC, et al. Validation of a clinical decision aid to discontinue in-hospital cardiac arrest resuscitations. *JAMA.* 2001;285(12):1602-1606.
15. Tortolani AJ, Risucci DA, Rosati RJ, et al. In-hospital cardiopulmonary resuscitation: patient, arrest and resuscitation factors associated with survival. *Resuscitation.* 1990; 20(2):115-128.
16. Bloom HL, Shukrullah I, Cuellar JR, et al. Long-term survival after successful in-hospital cardiac arrest resuscitation. *Am Heart J.* 2007;153(5):831-836.
17. Young KD, Gausche-Hill M, McClung CD, et al. A prospective, population-based study of the epidemiology and outcome of out-of-hospital pediatric cardiopulmonary arrest. *Pediatrics.* 2004;114(1):157-164.
18. Nadkarni VM, Larkin GL, Peberdy MA, et al. First documented rhythm and clinical outcome from in-hospital cardiac arrest among children and adults. *JAMA.* 2006;295(1): 50-57.
19. Samson RA, Nadkarni VM, Meaney PA, et al. Outcomes of in-hospital ventricular fibrillation in children. *N Engl J Med.* 2006;354(22):2328-2339.
20. Girotra S, Nallamothu BK, Spertus JA, Li Y, Krumholz HM, Chan PS; American Heart Association Get with the Guidelines–Resuscitation Investigators. Trends in survival after in-hospital cardiac arrest. *N Engl J Med.* 2012; 367(20):1912-1920.
21. Truog RD. "Doctor, if this were your child, what would you do?" *Pediatrics.* 1999;103(1):153-154.
22. Kon AA. Answering the question: "Doctor, if this were your child, what would you do?" *Pediatrics.* 2006;118(1): 393-397.
23. Tulsky JA. Beyond advance directives: importance of communication skills at the end of life. *JAMA.* 2005;294(3): 359-365.
24. Feudtner C. The breadth of hopes. *N Engl J Med.* 2009; 361(24):2306-2307.
25. Sulmasy DP, Snyder L. Substituted interests and best judgments: an integrated model of surrogate decision making. *JAMA.* 2010;304(17):1946-1947.
26. Munson D. Withdrawal of mechanical ventilation in pediatric and neonatal intensive care units. *Pediatr Clin North Am.* 2007;54(5):773-785.
27. Truog RD, Cist AF, Brackett SE, et al. Recommendations for end-of-life care in the intensive care unit: The Ethics Committee of the Society of Critical Care Medicine. *Crit Care Med.* 2001;29(12):2332-2348.
28. Gianakos D. Terminal weaning. *Chest.* 1995;108(5): 1405-1406.
29. Ripamonti C, Bruera E. Dyspnea: pathophysiology and assessment. *J Pain Symptom Manage.* 1997;13(4):220-232.
30. Friedrichsdorf SJ, Kang TI. The management of pain in children with life-limiting illnesses. *Pediatr Clin North Am.* 2007;54(5):645-672.
31. Bruera E, Brenneis C, Michaud M, et al. Use of the subcutaneous route for the administration of narcotics in patients with cancer pain. *Cancer.* 1988;62(2):407-411.
32. Glare P, Walsh D, Sheehan D. The adverse effects of morphine: a prospective survey of common symptoms during repeated dosing for chronic cancer pain. *Am J Hosp Palliat Care.* 2006;23(3):229-235.
33. Chan JD, Treece PD, Engelberg RA, et al. Narcotic and benzodiazepine use after withdrawal of life support: association with time to death? *Chest.* 2004;126(1):286-293.
34. Partridge JC, Wall SN. Analgesia for dying infants whose life support is withdrawn or withheld. *Pediatrics.* 1997;99(1): 76-79.
35. Solomon MZ, O'Donnell L, Jennings B, et al. Decisions near the end of life: professional views on life-sustaining treatments. *Am J Public Health.* 1993;83(1):14-23.
36. Ullrich CK, Mayer OH. Assessment and management of fatigue and dyspnea in pediatric palliative care. *Pediatr Clin North Am.* 2007;54(5):735-756.
37. Coyne PJ, Viswanathan R, Smith TJ. Nebulized fentanyl citrate improves patients' perception of breathing, respiratory rate, and oxygen saturation in dyspnea. *J Pain Symptom Manage.* 2002;23(2):157-160.
38. Davis CL. The use of nebulized opioids for breathlessness. *Palliat Med.* 1995;9(2):169-170.
39. Bruera E, Sala R, Spruyt O, et al. Nebulized versus subcutaneous morphine for patients with cancer dyspnea: a preliminary study. *J Pain Symptom Manage.* 2005;29(6): 613-618.
40. Hagen NA. An approach to cough in cancer patients. *J Pain Symptom Manage.* 1991;6(4):257-262.
41. Siden H, Miller M, Straatman L, et al. A report on location of death in paediatric palliative care between home, hospice and hospital. *Palliat Med.* 2008;22(7):831-834.
42. Feudtner C, Silveira MJ, Christakis DA. Where do children with complex chronic conditions die? Patterns in Washington state, 1980-1998. *Pediatrics.* 2002;109(4): 656-660.

43. Feudtner C, Feinstein JA, Satchell M, et al. Shifting place of death among children with complex chronic conditions in the United States, 1989-2003. *JAMA*. 2007;297(24): 2725-2732.

44. Feudtner C, Kang TI, Hexem KR, et al. Pediatric palliative care patients: a prospective multicenter cohort study. *Pediatrics*. 2011;127(6):1094-1101.

45. Meert KL, Briller SH, Schim SM, et al. Examining the needs of bereaved parents in the pediatric intensive care unit: a qualitative study. *Death Stud*. 2009;33(8):712-740.

46. Lanctot D, Morrison W, Kock KD, et al. Spiritual dimensions. In: Carter BS, Levetown M, Friebert SE, eds. *Palliative Care for Infants, Children, and Adolescents: A Practical Handbook*. 2nd ed. Baltimore, MD: Johns Hopkins University Press; 2011:227-243.

47. Meyer EC, Burns JP, Griffith JL, et al. Parental perspectives on end-of-life care in the pediatric intensive care unit. *Crit Care Med*. 2002;30(1):226-231.

48. Borasino S, Morrison W, Silberman J, et al. Physicians' contact with families after the death of pediatric patients: a survey of pediatric critical care practitioners' beliefs and self-reported practices. *Pediatrics*. 2008;122(6):e1174-e1178.

49. Eggly S, Meert KL, Berger J, et al. A framework for conducting follow-up meetings with parents after a child's death in the pediatric intensive care unit. *Pediatr Crit Care Med*. 2011;12(2):147-152.

50. Serwint JR. One method of coping: resident debriefing after the death of a patient. *J Pediatr*. 2004;145(2):229-234.

51. Luce JM. End-of-life decision making in the intensive care unit. *Am J Respir Crit Care Med*. 2010;182(1):6-11.

Glossary

A

Accelerations: increase in fetal heart rate, associated with fetal movement; a sign of fetal well-being.

Acinar unit: lung unit consisting of a respiratory bronchiole, alveolar ducts, and alveolar sacs.

Activated clotting time (ACT): bedside laboratory test that detects how fast blood will begin to clot once a sample is taken from an extracorporeal life support circuit and introduced into the device; usual ACT is 180 to 220 seconds.

Active cycle of breathing (ACB): basic breathing exercise that cycles through three types of breathing: diaphragmatic breathing, thoracic expansion, and forced expiratory technique.

Active phase: period during labor when cervix dilates to approximately 8 to 9 cm; time of the most rapid cervical dilatation.

Acute lung injury: umbrella term used for lung damage displaying hypoxemic respiratory failure, characterized by bilateral pulmonary infiltrates rich in neutrophils, and in the absence of clinical heart failure.

Acute respiratory distress syndrome (ARDS): acute heterogeneous disease that causes an overwhelming pulmonary inflammation that leads to severe hypoxemia and respiratory failure.

Adenoid hypertrophy: enlargement of adenoid tissue.

Adrenergic: type of medication that produces bronchodilation by stimulating beta-2 receptors on airway smooth muscles, thus relaxing the muscle and reversing the airflow obstruction.

Advance directive: instructions that spell out specific interventions that a patient does or does not want to happen; sometimes called a living will.

Adverse drug event: injury resulting from medical intervention related to a drug. It can be attributable to preventable and nonpreventable causes.

Air-oxygen blender: device that brings compressed air and oxygen from a high-pressure source into a chamber and then sends the gases to a metering device that controls the mixing of the two gases.

Airway edema: swelling caused by fluid that accumulates in the interstitial spaces of the airway, limiting localized air flow.

Airway hyperresponsiveness: exaggerated bronchoconstrictor response to a wide variety of stimuli; a major feature of asthma.

Airway pressure release ventilation (APRV): alternative mode of ventilation that couples a high continuous airway pressure and intermittent time-cycled release to augment the patient's spontaneous ventilation.

Airway remodeling: caused by both the inflammation and repeated and continuous incidences of bronchoconstriction. These permanent changes in the airway can increase obstructions and decrease responsiveness and can cause a patient to be less responsive to therapy.

Airway resistance: friction that occurs between moving molecules in the gas stream and between these moving molecules and the wall of the respiratory system.

Allergic bronchopulmonary aspergillosis (APBA): fungal infection within the lungs, characterized by an exaggerated immune response or hypersensitivity to the fungus *Aspergillus*.

Alveolar phase: time in fetal lung development beginning about gestational week 36 and continuing up to the second year of life; a time of rapid alveolar proliferation.

Amnioinfusion: procedure in which normal saline or lactated Ringer's solution is placed into the uterus after rupture of the amniotic sac.

Analgesia: absence of a normal sense of pain.

Angioedema: allergic reaction that causes rapid swelling just below the skin, typically found around the lips and eyes.

Angioplasty: dilation and widening of a narrowed blood vessel.

Anticholinergics: pharmacological agents that act by blocking parasympathetic nerve fibers such as those seen in airway smooth muscle, thereby allowing relaxation of the muscle and reduction of the intrinsic vagal tone of the airway.

Anti-immunoglobulin E (IgE) therapy: pharmacological form of immunotherapy used to prevent asthma symptoms.

Antileukotrienes: pharmacological agents that act by preventing leukotrienes from causing airway inflammation in asthma.

Antipyretics: pharmacological agents that reduce fever.

Aortic stenosis: any discrete narrowing that occurs between the left ventricle and the aorta.

Apgar score: measurement used to describe the state of the newborn at various stages after birth to help guide early post-resuscitative care. Used by clinicians to assess the quality of their resuscitative efforts; evaluates appearance (color), pulse, grimace, activity, and respirations.

Apnea of prematurity (AOP): sudden cessation of breathing that lasts for at least 20 seconds or is accompanied by bradycardia or oxygen desaturation (cyanosis) in an infant younger than 37 weeks' gestation (wG).

Apoptosis: programmed cell death.

Applicability: usefulness in clinical practice.

Areflexia: absence of reflexes.

Arterial switch operation: a surgical procedure used to repair transposition of the great arteries; the aorta is removed from the right ventricle and connected to the proximal pulmonary artery to form a neo-aorta, and the pulmonary artery is removed from the left ventricle and connected to the proximal aorta to form the neo-pulmonary artery.

Aryepiglottic folds: prominent folds of mucous membranes stretching between the lateral margin of the epiglottis and the arytenoid cartilage.

Ascites: fluid in the peritoneal cavity.

Aspiration: material (volatile, solids, or oral secretions) passing the vocal cords and into the tracheobronchial tree.

Assent: agreement by a child who cannot legally give informed consent, but whom parents and providers believe to have some capacity for understanding the decision at hand and for expressing preferences.

Assist-control ventilation: form of patient-triggered ventilation that assumes the majority of the work of breathing, requiring minimal patient effort. The patient is only required to make an initial inspiratory effort and then will be provided with a full mechanical breath; if no spontaneous effort is made, a time-triggered mechanical breath will be given.

Asthma: common chronic disorder of the airways with a complex interaction of airflow obstruction, bronchial hyperresponsiveness, and an underlying inflammation.

Asthma action plan: Written patient disease-management tool that includes daily management strategies for asthma and guidelines on how to recognize and handle worsening symptoms.

Asthma severity: intrinsic intensity of disease.

Asymptomatic cyanosis: neonate who is blue, with saturations in the 75% to 85% range without respiratory distress.

Atelectasis: collapsed or airless condition of the lung caused by decreased lung compliance, inadequate tidal volume, or airway obstruction.

Atelectrauma: injury to the lung as a result of repeated collapse and re-expansion of alveoli.

Atopy: genetic predisposition for hypersensitivity to allergens.

Atresia: congenital absence or closure of a normal body opening or tubular structure.

Atrial septal defect (ASD): opening in the intra-atrial septum that creates an anatomical connection between the two uppermost chambers of the heart.

Atrial septostomy: creates a hole in the atrial wall, causing a wide-open atrial level shunt so that mixing can occur and saturations will stabilize; also known as a Rashkind procedure.

Auto-positive end expiratory pressure (PEEP): the gas trapped in the alveoli at the end of expiration, caused by inadequate time for exhalation.

Autogenic drainage: independent breathing technique in which patients breathe at various lung volumes to mobilize secretions.

Autonomy: represents a person's right to make decisions that are based on his or her personal values, without undue influence from others, including family members or clinicians.

B

Bacterial tracheitis: infection of the trachea causing marked subglottic edema and thick mucus or pus-containing secretions; also known as bacterial laryngotracheobronchitis, pseudomembranous croup, or bacterial croup.

Ball-valve obstruction: blockage of the airway that opens during inspiration, allowing air to enter the alveoli, but closes the airway during exhalation, causing localized air trapping.

Beneficence: obligates clinicians to provide care that will be beneficial to the well-being of the patient and will serve the best interests of the patient. Care provided in this context may include cure of disease, relief from pain, or enhancement of health and quality of life.

Best-interest standard: decisions should ideally maximize the child's welfare.

Bicuspid: a heart valve consisting of two functional leaflets.

Bidirectional Glenn (BDG) procedure: surgical intervention that changes pulmonary blood flow to a passive flow or drainage system, connecting the superior vena cava to the pulmonary artery, bypassing the right heart.

Bi-level positive airway pressure (BiPAP): method of respiratory support delivered via mask or nasal prongs that provides preset expiratory and inspiratory pressures, and allows for a preset respiratory rate.

Bioethics: discipline dedicated to the ethical and moral complexities that arise during the course of biomedical research and clinical patient care.

Biomarkers: biochemical, genetic, or molecular indicators that can be used to screen for diseases.

Biventricular hypertrophy: enlargement of both ventricles.

Blalock-Taussig (BT) shunt: surgical procedure wherein the right subclavian vein is connected to the right pulmonary artery to provide pulmonary blood flow.

Botulism: progressive neuroparalytic disease that has several distinct clinical presentations; results in acute symmetric descending flaccid paralysis.

Breath-actuated nebulizer: inhaled medication delivery device that only delivers medication during inspiration.

Breath-enhanced nebulizer: increases medication output when it senses an increase in inspiratory flow, then decreases medication delivery when inspiration concludes.

Bronchiolitis: viral airway infection that causes inflammation of the small bronchiolar airways.

Bronchoalveolar lavage (BAL): diagnostic technique used to determine the pathogenic agent in lung infections, particularly those due to opportunistic pathogens in an immunocompromised patient. Using sterile technique, a BAL catheter is placed down the endotracheal tube, guided by fiber-optic bronchoscopy. Saline is injected and then aspirated into a specimen trap using suction, without withdrawing the catheter. The process of injecting and aspirating saline is repeated until an adequate sample is obtained or the patient shows signs of intolerance.

Bronchoconstriction: bronchial smooth muscle contraction.

Bronchoprovocation: pulmonary function test that attempts to deliberately stimulate the bronchial smooth muscle to assess airway hyperresponsiveness.

Bronchopulmonary dysplasia (BPD): a type of chronic lung disease, currently defined as the need for supplemental oxygen for at least 28 days after birth, assessed at discharge or when the baby is close to his or her estimated full-term age; first described in 1967, but recent changes to the pathology and signs and symptoms have persuaded clinicians to change the definition to the one described above, and change the term to "new BPD."

C

Caffeine citrate: a type of methylxanthine used as a stimulant in the treatment of apnea of prematurity for its very wide therapeutic index.

Canalicular phase: lung growth occurring during gestation weeks 17 to 26; bronchioles continue to multiply, lung vascularization begins, and acinar units begin to form.

Capillary blood gas (CBG): arterialized blood sample drawn from a warmed heel or the sides of the tips of the fingers or toes.

Capnometry: measurement of the concentration of carbon dioxide in exhaled gas.

Carboxyhemoglobin: attachment of carbon monoxide to a hemoglobin, rendering a red blood cell useless for oxygen transport; occurs because carbon monoxide's affinity for hemoglobin is 200 times that of oxygen.

Cardiac murmur: abnormal heart sound resulting from turbulent blood flow across a cardiac structure.

Cardiomegaly: a heart silhouette occupying greater than 60% of the thoracic diameter on chest radiography.

Catastrophic deterioration: sudden change in the status of the infant, which can include hypotension, shocky appearance, need for increased ventilatory support, seizures, acidosis, or anemia.

Central apnea: absence of breathing that occurs when the respiratory center of the brainstem does not send normal periodic signals to the muscles of respiration.

Central chemoreceptors: found in the brainstem, they send signals to increase ventilation in response to low cerebrospinal fluid (CSF) pH, which is affected by the amount of CO_2 crossing the blood–brain barrier.

Cerebral perfusion pressure (CPP): equal to the difference between the mean arterial pressure (MAP), approximated by multiplying the diastolic blood pressure by two-thirds and adding that to one-third of the systolic pressure.

Cerebrum: largest part of the brain, controlling sensations, voluntary muscular activities, consciousness, and higher mental functions such as memory learning, reasoning, judgment, intelligence, and emotions.

CHARGE syndrome: set of congenital defects that include coloboma (hole in one of the structures of the eye), heart abnormalities, atresia choanae, retarded mental development, genital hypoplasia, and ear deformities.

Chemical pneumonitis: inflammation of and damage to the lungs caused by the inhalation of certain chemicals, atelectasis, and pulmonary hypertension.

Chest physiotherapy: airway clearance technique consisting of percussion, vibration, and postural drainage.

Chest wiggle factor: continuous, visible vibration of the thorax from the umbilicus to the nipple line; used by clinicians to evaluate adequacy of amplitude during HFOV. Vibrations are seen from the groin to the nipple line in prepubescent patients and from the mid-thighs to the nipple line in adults.

Choanal atresia: congenital condition in which the posterior portion of the nasal passage ends in a blind pouch, with complete obstruction of the passageway between the nose and the nasopharynx.

Choanal stenosis: occurs when the posterior portion of the nasal passages are narrowed but not completely obstructed.

Chorioamnionitis: infection of the amniotic fluid.

Chorionic villi: vascular projections that include the fetal portion of the placenta; responsible for the exchange of nutrients and waste.

Chronic lung disease (CLD): any pulmonary disease that results from a neonatal respiratory disorder; bronchopulmonary dysplasia (BPD) is the most commonly described form of CLD.

Cleft lip: failure of parts of the lip to completely fuse together during the first 12 weeks of gestation.

Cleft palate: failure of parts of the hard palate to completely fuse together during the first 12 weeks of gestation, leaving a connection between the oral and nasal cavities.

Clinical ethics: application of bioethical principles to patient care, research, and health policy.

Coarctation of the aorta: discrete narrowing of the descending thoracic aorta, usually distal to the takeoff of the left subclavian artery.

Columella: anterior, external aspect of the septum.

Compassion fatigue: results from ongoing stress in health-care providers who do not have adequate ability or time to engage in self-care practices. Symptoms of compassion fatigue can include apathy, anger, anxiety, self-doubt, difficulty focusing, work absences, and substance abuse.

Complete vascular ring: the abnormal growth and continuation of multiple aortic arches that are present in fetal development. They include double aortic arch and right aortic arch with aberrant left subclavian artery, which encircle and cause compression of both the esophagus and trachea.

Concurrent care: simultaneous pursuit of both palliative and curative measures, which benefits most patients.

Conduit: channel.

Confidentiality: clinician's duty to not reveal information disclosed to them by a patient or about a patient.

Congenital diaphragmatic hernia (CDH): a serious congenital malformation that occurs when the segments of the diaphragm fail to fuse by the eighth week of gestation, and the abdominal contents herniate, or protrude through the wall, into the thoracic cavity.

Congenital vascular malformations: abnormal development of arterial, venous, or lymphatic structures within the airway; their development can cause airway obstruction that necessitate surgical intervention.

Conscientious refusal: clinicians' moral and legal right to not provide care that they find ethically objectionable.

Consolidation: solidified alveoli causing decreased amounts of oxygen to reach the alveolar capillary membrane.

Consumerism: when the physician or medical provider simply performs whatever action the parent or family requests.

Continuous positive airway pressure (CPAP): method of noninvasive respiratory support provided by mask or nasal prongs that delivers a constant positive airway pressure maintained throughout the respiratory cycle.

Coronary sinus: where cardiac veins return blood flow to the right atrium.

Corticosteroids: group of hormones secreted by the adrenal cortex in the brain. Can also be manufactured synthetically, which acutely improves lung mechanics and gas exchange and reduce inflammatory cells and their products.

Cranial vault: portion of the skull where the brain is encased.

Cricoid pressure: pushing the cricoid cartilage against the cervical spine, compressing the esophagus to prevent passive regurgitation; also known as the Sellick maneuver.

Cricothyroidotomy: an emergency surgical airway procedure involving an incision between the cricoid and thyroid cartilages in the midline of the anterior neck; also known as a cricothyrotomy.

Critical opening pressure: pressure at which the lungs begin to expand or inflate.

Cromones: pharmacological agents that act to stabilize mast cells and interfere with chloride channel function, preventing the release of mediators and minimizing airway inflammation.

Croup: a viral-mediated inflammatory condition of the subglottic airway, which corresponds to the area between the true vocal folds and the trachea.

Cushing's triad: a clinical finding in brain injury in which bradycardia, hypertension, and irregular respirations are all present.

Cyanotic congenital heart disease: group of neonatal heart defects resulting from structural abnormalities that lead to significant mixing of oxygenated and deoxygenated blood and cause oxygen saturations less than 85%; should be suspected in cases in which a newborn's oxygen saturation is low and the baby is cyanotic despite adequate ventilation and oxygenation.

Cyanotic heart defects: congenital abnormalities that lead to significant mixing of oxygenated and deoxygenated blood and cause oxygen saturations less than 85%.

Cystic fibrosis transmembrane conductance regulator (CFTR) gene: mutation in both copies of this gene is the cause of cystic fibrosis.

Cytochrome oxidase: component of the electron transport chain that turns oxygen into energy for the body.

D

Dead space ventilation: area of the lung that is being ventilated but not perfused.

Decannulation: process of removing extracorporeal life-support cannulas and ligating the vessels.

Deceleration phase: time during labor when the cervix reaches complete dilatation (10 cm) and the presenting part of the fetus (usually the head) descends into the midpelvis (transition phase).

Deliberative decision-making: decisions about care determined through a discussion with care providers and family members.

Demyelination: loss of the myelin sheath on the nerve axon. The myelin sheath is essential in the rapid conduction of nerve impulses through the neuron.

Diffuse axonal injury: shearing injury to the deeper brain structures.

Discontinuing resuscitation efforts: medical decision to cease life-saving therapies; can be considered when a newborn's heart rate remains undetectable for 10 minutes during a resuscitation.

Disruption (in fetal development): during fetal development, an abnormally produced defect after normal structural development.

Disseminated intravascular coagulation (DIC): process that consumes the factors that clot blood; manifests as oozing or bleeding from any mucosal site, or into the skin (petechiae).

Do not attempt resuscitation (DNR) order: a written document specifying that certain interventions, such as mechanical ventilation, chest compressions, or defibrillation, will not be attempted if a patient's condition deteriorates.

Donation after cardiac death (DCD): also called non–heart-beating organ donation (NHBOD); determined by death within 1 hour of a planned withdrawal of life-sustaining therapies, with no subsequent signs of return of spontaneous circulation or respiratory effort.

Doppler interrogation: using ultrasound to determine blood flow velocity in different locations in the heart.

Double aortic arch: one of the more common types of aortic arch abnormality, in which the right and left aortic arches are present at birth and encircle the trachea and esophagus; the type most likely to cause clinical symptoms.

Drooling: saliva running from the mouth; a classic sign of epiglottitis that occurs because of dysphagia.

Dry drowning: laryngospasm that persists after the individual loses consciousness so that no fluid enters the lungs.

Duchenne's muscular dystrophy (DMD): most common, lethal, X-linked genetic disease, resulting in rapidly worsening muscle weakness and a decrease in muscle mass over time.

Ductus arteriosus: fetal vessel that connects the pulmonary artery to the aorta near the left subclavian artery; vents excess blood entering the pulmonary system, bypassing the left side of the heart.

Ductus venosus: first shunt encountered from the placenta in fetal circulation, which connects the umbilical vein to the inferior vena cava within the liver.

Dysfunctional swallowing: describes abnormalities in swallowing or managing oropharyngeal secretions; a well-recognized cause of aspiration in children.

Dysmotility: abnormality of smooth muscle function in gastrointestinal tract.

Dysphagia: painful and difficult swallowing; makes patients unable to manage secretions.

Dysphonia: hoarseness or difficulty with speech; a classic sign of epiglottitis due to pain.

Dyspnea: subjective feeling of shortness of breath.

E

Early decelerations: benign changes in fetal heart rate that represent head compression or changes in vagal tone after brief hypoxic episodes; begin with the onset of a contraction, reach the lowest point at the peak of the contraction, and return to baseline as the contraction ends.

Ebstein anomaly: malformation of the heart in which there are abnormal leaflets of the tricuspid valve, found between the right atrium and ventricle, as well as displacement of the leaflets into the right ventricle.

Echocardiogram: non-invasive tool using ultrasound to visualize cardiac structures.

Electrocardiogram (EKG): reading of the electrical activity of the heart.

Embryonic phase: phase of human development from conception to gestation week 6; the phase in which the respiratory epithelium begins to grow, including the lung buds and trachea.

Empyema: pus in the pleural cavity.

Endobronchial masses: unexpected growth within a bronchus; uncommon in children.

Endocarditis: inflammation of the heart valves.

Endoderm: innermost germ layer of the embryo.

Endoscopy: diagnostic test in which a camera is used on the end of a flexible tube inserted into the body for definitive diagnosis; can be used to augment successful intubation and airway protection.

Epiglottitis: bacterial infection of the epiglottis and the surrounding tissues, including the entire supraglottis (the portion of the larynx above the vocal cords), which can progress rapidly to life-threatening airway obstruction.

Epinephrine: in respiratory therapy, an inhaled pharmacological agent given to reduce upper airway inflammation; usually given as racemic epinephrine.

Epithelialization: healing by the growth of epithelium over an open wound surface.

Escharotomies: incisions in the skin that can release the pressure from the eschars and changes in surrounding tissues.

Eschars: areas of dead tissue that occur after severe burns.

Esophageal atresia (EA): congenital defect in which the esophagus ends in a blind-ended pouch rather than connecting normally to the stomach.

Euthanasia: purposeful administration of medications to end life; illegal in the United States.

Evidence-based medicine: conscientious, explicit, and judicious use of current best evidence in making decisions about the care of the individual patient.

Exacerbations: increase in symptoms.

Excision: resection; removal of a portion or all of a structure.

Exclusivity: patent protection that allows manufacturing a drug without competition from other suppliers for a period of time.

Exercise-induced asthma: symptoms present only during physical exertion.

Exhaled breath condensate: biomarker test for asthma. Exhaled air condenses when it comes into contact with a cooled collector, allowing the collection of respiratory particles, droplets, and water vapor; low exhaled breath condensate pH is a biomarker that indicates poorly controlled asthma.

Expressive language: a person's capacity to communicate his or her current thoughts and feelings.

Extracorporeal life support (ECLS): technique used to support the heart and/or lungs externally when the native heart and/or lungs are no longer able to provide adequate support.

Extracorporeal membrane oxygenation (ECMO): practice of placing an intensive care unit (ICU) patient on artificial support, giving the native lungs and/or heart a period of rest.

Extracorporeal membrane oxygenation (ECMO) heaters: heat blood before reinfusing it into the patient to preserve thermal regulation.

Extracorporeal membrane oxygenation (ECMO) pump: operates as a servo-controlled, positive displacement pump. Has two rollers that will optimally occlude or squeeze the tubing in the pump and direct blood through the tubing, creating pressure and flow through the system.

Exudative stage: first stage of acute respiratory distress syndrome; begins when the inflammatory cascade is triggered from a direct or indirect lung injury, resulting in damage to the cellular lung structure. Outpourings of inflammatory mediators increase the permeability of the alveolar capillary membrane.

Exudative tracheitis: bacterial infection of the trachea causing edema and oozing of fluid and cellular debris from the airway walls.

F

Fetal bradycardia: fetal heart rate (FHR) less than 110 beats per minute.

Fetal circulation: the circulatory pathway for blood in a fetus; includes a system of shunts and differences in normal blood pressures that diverts blood flow through alternative tracts compared with adult circulation.

Fetal heart rate (FHR) monitoring: continuous electronic monitoring used for intrapartum fetal surveillance.

Fetal lung fluid: fetal fluid that is secreted by epithelial cells of the lung to help maintain the patency of the airways and acinar units during their growth until delivery; chemically has a very low pH, bicarbonate, and protein levels, but higher sodium and chloride concentrations than amniotic fluid.

Fetal scalp blood sampling: used during labor when the fetal heart rate monitoring is nonreassuring to determine the acid-base status of the fetus; obtained from the scalp after the membranes have been ruptured.

Fetal tachycardia: fetal heart rate (FHR) greater than 160 beats per minute.

Fibrotic stage: third stage of acute respiratory distress syndrome; results in total lung remodeling, leading to widespread fibrosis and scarring.

Fixed split S2: heart murmur heard in a patient with an atrial septal defect who has more blood flow traveling across the pulmonary valve, thus causing the pulmonary valve to close after the aortic valve in inspiration and exhalation.

Flaccid paralysis: relaxed or absent muscular tone.

Flow inflating bag: type of manual resuscitation bag/bag valve mask; will fill with oxygen only when a compressed source of oxygen is attached and requires a tight seal between the mask and the patient to remain inflated.

Fomites: airway secretions that live on inanimate objects.

Fontan procedure: third stage of surgical treatment of hypoplastic left heart syndrome; routes inferior vena cava flow from the right atrium to the pulmonary artery via an intracardiac or extracardiac conduit.

Foramen ovale: fetal shunt that provides an opening between the right and left atria.

Forced expiratory technique (FET): creates an increased expiratory airflow and thereby mobilizes the mucus from the distal, small airways into the more central airways where it can then be expelled with a cough; also known as a huff.

Foreign antigen: substances from outside the body capable of eliciting an immune response.

Fractional exhaled nitric oxide (FeNO): most widely used exhaled biomarker of airway inflammation in asthma; measures the amount of nitric oxide in exhaled breath.

Functional residual capacity (FRC): volume of gas remaining in the lungs after a normal resting expiration.

Futility: concept that describes medical treatments that are not expected to result in any benefit to the patient.

G

Gangliosides: complex molecules that are in nerve cell membranes and are instrumental in recognition of cells and cell-to-cell communication.

Gastroschisis: abdominal wall defect characterized by protrusion of the intestines through the abdominal wall not covered by amnion.

Gentle ventilation: lung-protective strategy in which a peak inspiratory pressure is selected that provides adequate air entry and an respiratory rate of 20 to 40 breaths/min is initiated and adjusted to maintain a $PaCO_2$ of 40 to 60 mm Hg.

Germinal matrix: a weakly supported and highly vascularized area of the lateral ventricles in the developing brain; formed to assist in rapid cellular formation.

Gestation: time frame from conception to birth.

Glasgow coma scale (GCS): clinical tool often used to quickly assess consciousness and neurological status during the acute assessment of a patient who has suffered intracranial injury.

Glossoptosis: obstruction of the airway by the bulk of the tongue.

Glottic web: membrane spread between the vocal folds near the anterior commissure.

Glottis: sound-producing apparatus of the larynx, including the two vocal folds and the intervening space; opens to allow inspiration and closes to facilitate speech, airway protection, and increases in intrathoracic pressure.

Goals of care: the determination by family and clinician of desirable and undesirable patient outcomes.

Golden minute: the 60 seconds that neonatal resuscitation program (NRP) providers have to complete the initial assessment and interventions of resuscitation.

Grunting: noise produced by breathing against a partially closed glottis; a form of expiratory retard when neonates partially close their glottis at the end of expiration to create a back pressure in the lungs with the goal of stabilizing alveoli and terminal airways to prevent collapse; signifies significant respiratory distress in an infant.

Guillain-Barré syndrome: neurological condition that affects peripheral nerves and presents as progressive ascending weakness in both arms and legs and areflexia.

Gyri: numerous folds covering the two cerebrum hemispheres; along with sulci, serves to increase the surface area of the brain; begins to appear around 14 weeks of gestation.

H

Hamartomas: congenital masses that may occur in the posterior of the nose, near the internal opening of the eustachian tube orifice.

Heated, humidified, high-flow nasal cannula (HFNC): an oxygen delivery device that produces a high flow of gas at nearly 100% humidity gas, virtually free of droplets, at body temperature or above; this allows higher gas flows to be tolerated by patients.

Heliox: gas mixture of helium and oxygen used to treat hypoxemia during airway obstruction; is reported to be effective in a variety of respiratory conditions such as upper airway obstruction, status asthmaticus, decompression sickness, postextubation stridor, bronchiolitis, and acute respiratory distress syndrome.

Hemoptysis: expectoration of blood arising from the airway or lungs.

Herniate: to protrude abnormally from an enclosed cavity.

Heated, humidified, high-flow nasal cannula (HFNC): an oxygen delivery device produces a high flow of highly humidified air, virtually free of droplets, at body temperature or above. The high humidity allows for much higher flow rates to be tolerated by neonatal patients without the risk of nasal mucosal drying or bleeding.

High-frequency chest wall oscillation (HFCWO): technique to clear mucus using an inflatable jacket with an air pulse generator that rapidly fills and deflates the jacket at a set pressure.

High-frequency jet ventilation (HFJV): a method of mechanical ventilation that uses a transitional flow pattern of gas delivery that allows fresh, oxygen-rich gas to travel down the center of the airways at very high velocity in small bursts, getting downstream of restricted portions of the airways reaching the alveoli and bypassing damaged portions of the lung without leaking.

High-frequency oscillatory ventilation (HFOV): piston-diaphragm oscillator that uses rates of 180 to 900 coupled with a directly set mean airway pressure to manage oxygenation and ventilation.

High-frequency ventilation (HFV): uses rapid respiratory rates (>150 breaths/min) and very small tidal volume (usually less than anatomic dead space) to provide ventilation and lung protection.

Histamine: chemical mediator producing an immediate allergic response.

Hospice agencies: focus specifically on providing care at home for dying patients.

Hospital ethics committee: multidisciplinary committee composed of members from both the medical and lay communities.

Hyaline membrane disease (HMD): lung disease of premature infants first characterized in the early 20th century because of the unique cellular characteristics of the lung; more commonly called respiratory distress syndrome (RDS).

Hydrocarbons: chemical compounds made only of hydrogen and carbon.

Hydroxycobalamin: precursor to vitamin B12, which binds cyanide, forms cyanocobalamin, and is excreted without any toxic effects.

Hygiene hypothesis: the theory that, in early life, nature may "immunize" against the allergic march through microbial exposures of the respiratory tract, gastrointestinal tract, and possibly the skin.

Hyperbaric chambers: pressure chambers that allow the delivery of fractional concentration of inspired oxygen (FIO_2) of 1.0 at higher than atmospheric pressure.

Hyperoxia test: arterial blood gases are obtained from the right radial artery on room air and 1.0 fractional concentration of inspired oxygen (FIO_2) and compared to assess a patient's ability to oxygenate; cyanotic heart defects should be suspected when partial pressure of oxygen (PaO_2) is lower than 150 mm Hg on FIO_2 1.0; pulmonary disease should be suspected if PaO_2 is greater than 150 mm Hg on FIO_2 1.0.

Hypertrophy: increase in size of a vessel or anatomical structure.

Hypoplasia: increased distance between alveolar spaces and capillaries, which worsens gas exchange and lung tissue underdevelopment.

Hypoplasia: organ or tissue underdevelopment.

Hypoplastic: undeveloped veins.

Hypoplastic left heart syndrome (HLHS): cyanotic heart disease in which parts of the left side of the heart do not fully develop.

Hypoxic-ischemic encephalopathy: acute or subacute brain injury due to hypoxia and acidosis.

I

Iatrogenic: lung injury caused by medical interventions, such as mechanical ventilation.

Immunocompromised: a state in which the immune system's ability to fight infectious disease is deficient or entirely absent.

Immunotherapy: therapy involving subcutaneous injections of increasing amounts of a known allergen.

Incubator: used in the neonatal population to control environmental temperature and humidity; helps minimize heat loss via conduction and promotes a quiet, dark environment, reducing external stimuli that can be distressing to premature infants.

Induced hypothermia: deliberate lowering of body temperature with the goal of minimizing brain injury after severe and prolonged hypoxia; cooling is initiated within 6 hours of birth; the infant is cooled for 72 hours and then gradually warmed.

Informed consent: process that requires clear communication to family members about risks and benefits, adequate time for questioning and understanding, protection from undue influences, and transparency about the right to revoke consent at any point.

Inhaled antibiotics: nebulized form of pharmacological antibacterial agents, frequently used for patients with cystic fibrosis who have recurrent airway infections; the rationale for the inhaled route is that it delivers a high concentration of drug to the airway surface, where it is most needed, while minimizing systemic drug toxicity.

Inotropes: pharmacological agents used to improve cardiac contractility.

Insufflation-exsufflation device: mucus-clearing device that helps with airway clearance and prevents accumulation of mucus in the lungs and airways of patients with a weak cough; works by inflating the lungs with a positive pressure, followed by an active negative pressure exsufflation that creates a peak and sustained flow high enough to provide adequate shear and velocity to loosen and move secretions toward the mouth for suctioning or expectoration.

Intracranial pressure (ICP): pressure within the portion of the skull where the brain is encased.

Intrapulmonary percussive drainage: mucus-clearing device using a mask or mouthpiece that delivers small bursts of positive pressure (5 to 35 cm H_2O) at rates of 100 to 300 cycles/min, superimposed on a patient's own breathing; can be effective in treating atelectasis.

Intrapulmonary shunt: lung perfusion without ventilation.

Intraventricular hemorrhage (IVH): neonatal complication that occurs most commonly in premature infants, characterized by bleeding within the ventricles of the brain.

J

Justice: principle that requires health care to be delivered fairly so that no one patient group unduly suffers the burden of scarce resources. Justice means that all individuals have a right to equal access to medical care, and that individuals have a right to a minimum standard of health care.

K

Ketamine: anesthetic agent with strong analgesic action that mediates bronchodilation.

L

Labor: passage of the fetus and the placenta from the uterus to the extrauterine world (childbirth).

Laryngoceles: abnormal outpouchings of the laryngeal mucosa in the laryngeal ventricles.

Laryngomalacia: softening of the tissues of the larynx; the most common laryngeal anomaly and congenital cause of stridor.

Laryngopharyngeal reflux (LPR): reflux of gastric acid into the pharynx and larynx.

Laryngospasm: an involuntary muscle contraction of the laryngeal cords; helps to prevent fluid or other materials from entering the lungs.

Laryngotracheobronchitis (croup): a viral disease causing airway narrowing involving the subglottis, presenting with a "barky" cough, stridor, and occasionally hoarseness.

Late decelerations: indicative of uteroplacental insufficiency and, if recurrent, considered to represent fetal compromise and need further evaluation for delivery; the temporal relationship is variable to the onset of the contraction, occurring after the peak of the contraction, persisting after the contraction stops, and gradually returning to baseline.

Latent phase: first phase of labor, characterized by a time when contractions become more coordinated and the cervix reaches 4 cm dilatation.

Law of Laplace: states that volume will be preferentially delivered into segments of the lung that are partially open.

Leukocytosis: increase in the number of white blood cells.

Leukotrienes: potent bronchoconstrictors derived mainly from mast cells mediate the inflammatory response; inhibition of this mediator has been shown to improve lung function and reduce asthma symptoms.

Ligation: surgical tying to correct a malfunction, as provided in correcting a patent ductus arteriosus in neonatal life.

Limb-girdle muscular dystrophy (LGMD): describes a diverse group of muscular dystrophies that are caused by specific protein defects in muscle.

Lipoids: oils and animal fats; may result in an uncommon cause of respiratory distress in children.

Long-acting beta agonists (LABAs): pharmacological agents used for long-term control and prevention of symptoms in moderate or severe persistent asthma.

Lung transplantation: surgical technique that replaces a damaged lung with a healthy, donor lung or lobe.

M

Macroglossia: an enlarged tongue.

Magnesium: an ion found in abundance in the human body; when given intravenously, has been shown to have beneficial effects on smooth muscle relaxation and inflammation in the airway.

Maladaptation: pulmonary vascular bed is normally developed; however, adverse perinatal conditions cause active vasoconstriction and interfere with the normal postnatal reduction in pulmonary vascular resistance, causing persistent pulmonary hypertension of the newborn (PPHN).

Maldevelopment: situation in which the lungs develop normally, but the pulmonary arteriole muscle layer is abnormally thick and grows in smaller vessels that normally have no muscle cells, causing pulmonary hypertension.

Malformation: abnormal or anomalous formation or structure; deformity.

Mandatory vaccination: some health-care systems require personnel to be vaccinated against certain diseases, such as influenza.

Mast cells: concentrated beneath the mucous membranes of the respiratory tract; when covered with IgE molecules, they will bind with foreign antigens and stimulate degranulation, releasing such mediators as histamine, prostaglandin D_2, and leukotrienes. These mediators produce an immediate hypersensitivity reaction within the airway walls. Mast cells may also be activated by osmotic stimuli, such as during exercise-induced bronchospasm, and they may potentially continue to send signals stimulating inflammation even when exposure to allergens is limited.

Maximum expiratory pressure (MEP): The pressure obtained when a patient breathes out quickly and forcefully to residual volume.

Maximum inspiratory pressure (MIP): the pressure obtained when a patient quickly breathes in fully to total lung capacity.

Mean airway pressure (Paw): close reflection of mean alveolar pressure calculated on all mechanical ventilators; used to evaluate the amount of support provided to mechanically ventilated patients.

Meconium: newborns' first stool, which is the by-product or metabolic waste of gestation.

Meconium aspiration syndrome (MAS): respiratory distress occurring soon after delivery in a meconium-stained infant, which is not otherwise explainable and is associated with a typical radiographic appearance of patchy infiltrates or irregular streaky, linear densities and consolidation throughout the lung fields.

Meconium aspirator: device that allows for attachment of wall suction and use of the ETT as a large-bore suction device within the trachea at delivery in a nonvigorous newborn with meconium-stained amniotic fluid.

Meconium ileus: failure to pass meconium after birth, causing impaction of meconium in the large intestines.

Medical error: implies a preventable adverse event, a threat to patient safety that could have been avoided.

Medication error: any preventable event that occurs in the process of ordering or delivering a medication, regardless of whether an injury occurred or the potential for injury was present.

Mesenchyme: embryonic connective tissue.

Mesentery: the double-layer peritoneal fold attaching the small intestine to the posterior body wall.

Mesoderm: middle germ layer of the embryo.

Methacholine: parasympathomimetic broncho-constrictor that acts directly on smooth muscle receptors and will cause immediate bronchoconstriction; the inhalant of choice when performing bronchoprovocation testing.

Methemoglobin (MetHb): red blood cell that loses an electron from the ferrous ion and is no longer capable of binding with oxygen.

Methylxanthines: stimulant medications, generally stimulating the central nervous system and cardiac muscles; have also been known to stimulate the respiratory drive, increase diaphragm activity, increase minute ventilation, enhance chemoreceptor sensitivity to CO_2, reduce periodic breathing, reduce hypoxic respiratory depression, increase metabolic rate, increase oxygen consumption, and stimulate diuresis.

Micrognathia: abnormal smallness of the lower jawbone.

Mixed apnea: dysfunctional breathing that combines elements of obstructive and central sleep apneas.

Monro-Kellie doctrine: the total volume within the cranial vault is strictly limited by the fixed walls of the skull.

Moral distress: dilemma a clinician experiences when he or she is prevented from doing what the clinician feels is best for the patient, or when clinician feels obligated to do something not in the patient's best interest.

Morbidity: number of deceased patients.

Mucolytics: pharmacological therapies designed to thin airway secretions.

Mucus: viscous fluid normally made up of a combination of mucin, leukocytes, inorganic salts, water, and epithelial cells.

Muscle relaxant: pharmacological therapy used to eliminate patient spontaneous movement.

Myasthenia gravis (MG): autoimmune disorder characterized by fluctuating muscle weakness and fatigue.

Myelomeningocele: birth defect in which the backbone and spinal canal do not close before birth; a type of spina bifida.

Myocardial cells: cardiac muscle cells.

Myocardial ischemia: inadequate supply of blood and oxygen for the demands of the heart muscle.

N

Nasal endoscopy: procedure using a narrow fiber-optic or rigid telescope or otoscope to evaluate upper airway abnormalities.

Natural history of asthma: refers to its course over an individual's lifetime; its progression and symptoms can vary throughout an individual's life.

Necrosis: death of cells, tissues, or organs.

Necrotizing enterocolitis (NEC): serious complication of prematurity that primarily affects the gastrointestinal (GI) tract; the process of development includes hypoxic-ischemic and inflammatory damage that can result in death of the tissues in almost any region of the GI tract.

Needle decompression: emergency procedure in which a needle is inserted into the pleural cavity to relieve air pressure in the thoracic space, during a tension pneumothorax.

Negative pressure pulmonary edema: occurs when a person attempts to take deep breaths against a closed glottis, usually during submersion in water; the negative pressure generated can be very high and can damage the alveolar and capillary bed, leading to fluid being pulled into the lung parenchyma as with a vacuum.

Neonatal Resuscitation Program (NRP): an educational program jointly sponsored by the American Academy of Pediatrics and the American Heart Association (AHA); designed to teach an evidence-based approach to resuscitation of the newborn to hospital staff, including physicians, nurses, and respiratory therapists, who care for newborns at the time of delivery.

Neurogenic pulmonary edema (NPE): sudden increase in pulmonary interstitial fluid associated with numerous central nervous system insults.

Neuropathy: disease or malfunction of the nerves.

Newborn screening: blood test that identifies infants who may have cystic fibrosis (CF); not all infants with a positive newborn screen actually have CF. Infants with a positive newborn screening test must have additional testing before a definitive diagnosis of CF can be made.

Nitric oxide (NO): substance produced by nearly every cell and organ in the human body. NO performs many functions including vasodilation, platelet inhibition, immune regulation, enzyme regulation, and neurotransmission.

Nitrogen washout: caused by delivery of 1.0 fractional concentration of inspired oxygen (FIO_2), with the potential of causing absorption atelectasis. Nitrogen acts as an alveolar-stabilizing gas, preventing alveolar collapse or atelectasis during gas exchange. When FIO_2 is increased, the amount of nitrogen within the alveoli decreases (is "washed out of the alveoli"), and it is no longer available for alveolar stabilization.

Non–heart-beating organ donation (NHBOD): a process for organ procurement where organs are harvested if the patient progresses to death within one hour of withdrawal of life-sustaining therapy, and death is maintained for an established number of minutes.

Noninvasive positive-pressure ventilation (NIPPV): method of respiratory support delivered via mask or nasal prongs that provides preset expiratory and inspiratory pressures and allows for a preset respiratory rate.

Nonmaleficence: obligates clinicians to care for patients in a way that causes no harm.

Nonvigorous: having a depressed respiratory effort, poor muscle tone, and/or heart rate less than 100 beats per minute.

Normothermia: normal body temperature.

Norwood procedure: first stage of surgical treatment for hypoplastic left heart syndrome, which consists of four steps: creation of a neo-aorta using the pulmonary artery and homograft material to reconstruct the aortic arch in continuity with the right ventricle; removal of the atrial septum; providing a source of pulmonary blood flow via a systemic-to-pulmonary artery shunt (such as a Blalock-Taussig shunt or Sano modification); and ligation of the patent ductus arteriosus.

O

Obstructive apnea: absent or dysfunctional breathing that occurs when the upper airway is intermittently blocked.

Off-label use: term used when a medication is prescribed and delivered for an intended use other than that in the proposed labeling.

Omphalocele: a midline defect of the abdomen with the umbilical cord rising from the middle, encapsulated by the peritoneal sac; the small intestines, liver, and stomach are frequently the herniated organs.

Optimal positive end expiratory pressure (PEEP): pressure at which static lung compliance is maximized and oxygen transport is greatest.

Ostium primum ASD: defect in the septum primum that occurs directly superior to the atrioventricular valves.

Ostium secundum ASD: occurs when the septum primum does not grow to completely cover and fuse with the septum secundum.

Ostomies: surgically formed openings allowing a portion of the intestines to pass through a fistula to the skin surface.

Oxygen hood (oxyhood): clear plastic enclosure that is placed around a neonate's head and connected to a humidified gas source to provide a fixed oxygen concentration.

Oxygenation index (OI): equation that assesses the severity of lung dysfunction that is used frequently to help determine the need for escalating respiratory care.

Oxygenator: device for mechanically oxygenating the blood.

P

Palliation: treatment aimed to improve symptoms of a disease.

Palliative care: focuses on helping patients and families decide what medical interventions are most likely to be helpful, rather than harmful, and on managing pain and other symptoms so that no matter what choices are made, patients can be as comfortable as possible at the end of life. The old adage is that good palliative care focuses on quality rather than quantity of life, "adding life to the years, rather than years to the life."

Pancreatic insufficiency: pancreas does not secrete an adequate amount of enzyme to digest food appropriately.

Paradoxical split: heart murmur that signifies closure of the pulmonary valve; is always heard prior to the closure of the aortic valve.

Paresis: weakness in both arms and legs, progressing to partial or incomplete paralysis.

Partial obstruction: occlusion that may allow some passage of air into and out of the alveolar space.

Patent ductus arteriosus (PDA): failure of the ductus arteriosus to close after delivery, causing shunting of blood.

Paternalism: physician or other medical provider makes a decision alone, subsequently informing the patient or family of the provider's actions.

Patient-triggered ventilation: modes of mechanical ventilation in which a breath is provided in response to measured or presumed respiratory effort by the patient.

Peak expiratory flow (PEF): a pulmonary function test used to evaluate severity of asthma symptoms; measurement is taken by having the patient stand, take a deep breath to fill the lungs completely, then blow out as hard and as fast as possible in one single exhalation.

Pentamidine isethionate: antibiotic administered with a nebulizer or IV for *Pneumocystis jiroveci* pneumonia.

Penumbra: the at-risk area of the brain that surrounds injured tissue.

Percussion: part of chest physiotherapy; involves cupping the hands and rhythmically clapping over the chest wall; performed over the lung segment being drained to loosen mucus from the airway walls.

Perforation: act or process of making a hole.

Pericardiocentesis: emergency procedure in which a needle is inserted into the pericardial sac to evacuate air.

Perimembranous ventricular septal defect: congenital heart abnormality consisting of a hole in the ventricular wall located beneath the aortic annulus (the ring of fibrous tissue that anchors the valve leaflets).

Periodic breathing: a common but benign form of abnormal breathing in a neonate, characterized by cycles of hyperventilation followed by short apneic pauses of less than 3 seconds.

Peripheral chemoreceptors: found in the carotid body, between the internal and external carotid arteries, which are sensitive to O_2, CO_2, pH, glucose, and temperature changes.

Peritonsillar abscess: collection of pus in the area in the potential space superolateral to the tonsil; thought to be secondary to obstruction of the minor salivary glands.

Permissive hypercapnia: a method of mechanical ventilation that provides adequate oxygenation and accepts slightly high carbon dioxide to maintain ventilation while minimizing high airway pressures and barotrauma.

Persistent pulmonary hypertension of the newborn (PPHN): syndrome with severe hypoxemia and high pulmonary artery pressures that occurs when the pulmonary vascular resistance (PVR), normally high in utero, fails to decrease after birth.

Phagocytosis: engulfing and destroying of microorganisms, foreign antigens, or cell debris.

Pharmacodynamic: the action of a drug.

Pharmacokinetic: drug metabolism, particularly the duration of action, distribution in the body, and method of excretion.

Phenotype: observable symptoms of an organism.

Phosphatidylcholine (PC): a main phospholipid in surfactant; found starting at about 24 weeks' gestation; phospholipids serve to interact with air in the alveolar space, helping to reduce the surface tension of the lungs upon compression or exhalation.

Phosphatidylglycerol (PG): a phospholipid that makes up mature surfactant; appears at approximately 35 weeks' gestation; phospholipids serve to interact with air in the alveolar space, helping to reduce the surface tension of the lungs upon compression or exhalation.

Pilocarpine iontophoresis: commonly known as a "sweat test," it measures the amount of chloride in the sweat; high amounts of chloride in the sweat is an indicator of cystic fibrosis.

Placenta: structure in the uterus from which the fetus derives its nourishment and oxygen.

Plateau pressure: amount of pressure applied to the alveoli, measured by creating a short inspiratory pause during a mechanical breath.

Pleurodesis: creation of adhesions between the two thoracic pleura, to prevent recurrence of pneumothoraces.

Pneumatosis: air within the intestinal wall.

Pneumocytes: lung cells.

Pneumomediastinum: condition in which extra-alveolar air dissects through the lung interstitium and ruptures into the mediastinum.

Pneumonia: inflammation of the lung parenchyma, usually due to infection with bacteria, viruses, or other pathogenic causes.

Pneumopericardium: air within the pericardial sac.

Pneumoperitoneum: free air in the abdomen.

Pneumothorax: air in the pleural cavity.

Poiseuille's law: used to calculate endotracheal tube resistance, it states that resistance is a function of the tube length divided by the radius of the tube to the fourth power.

Polyhydramnios: abnormally high volume of amniotic fluid.

Polysomnogram: a sleep study.

Pores of Kohn: minute openings thought to exist between adjacent alveoli.

Positive end expiratory pressure (PEEP): mechanical ventilation setting that maintains a pressure within the alveoli throughout the respiratory cycle, measured at the end of exhalation.

Positive expiratory pressure (PEP): airway clearance strategy in which positive pressure is created in the airways by resisting expiration.

Post-ductal SpO₂: oxygen saturation taken from an area of the body whose arterial blood supply is after the ductus arteriosus; typically from the lower limbs.

Postural drainage: chest physiotherapy technique that uses gravity to mobilize mucus from different lung segments.

Preductal SpO₂: oxygen saturation taken from an area of the body whose arterial blood supply comes prior to the ductus arteriosus, including the head and the right upper limb.

Pressure control ventilation: method of mechanical ventilation that allows the pressure delivered to the lungs to remain constant, and volume delivery will change with lung characteristics; a volume of gas is delivered to the lungs over a specified time period until a clinician-chosen "safe pressure" is reached.

Pressure support ventilation: an assisted form of ventilation that provides a constant pressure during ventilation when it senses a patient's inspiratory effort.

Preterm: live birth occurring before 37 week's gestation.

Primary apnea: absence of breathing at birth; stimulation will result in resumption of breathing.

Professional competence: professional ethics require that clinicians attain professional competency via an appropriate level of training relevant to their area of expertise.

Professional ethics: address the interactions among professionals, individuals, and society.

Proliferating: growing

Proliferative stage: second stage of acute respiratory distress syndrome; characterized by the proliferation (rapid increase) of type II pneumocytes and fibroblasts (cells that play a role in wound healing).

Prone positioning: placement of a patient "face-down," which may be considered for a mechanically ventilated patient if he or she continues to have difficulty oxygenating or ventilating.

Prostaglandin E (PGE): hormone-like substances that perform a variety of functions in the body.

Pseudoglandular phase: phase of fetal lung development occurring during weeks 7 to 17; named so for the gland-like appearance of the lung during this stage; a time of rapid airway proliferation, larynx and vocal cord development, and completion of the oropharynx and nasopharynx.

Ptosis: drooping eyelids.

Pulmonary atresia: abnormal development of the pulmonary valve, which sits between the right ventricle and the pulmonary artery.

Pulmonary edema: leaking of fluid from the capillaries in the lungs into the interstitium and alveolar sac.

Pulmonary exacerbation: characterized by increased airway secretions, infection, and inflammation.

Pulmonary function testing (PFT): one of several different tests used to evaluate the condition of the respiratory system; they are direct measurements of airflow and lung volumes.

Pulmonary hypertensive crisis: characterized by a rapid increase in pulmonary vascular resistance, which results when the pulmonary artery pressure exceeds systemic blood pressure and right heart failure ensues.

Pulmonary hypoplasia: congenital underdevelopment of lung tissue during fetal growth.

Pulmonary interstitial emphysema (PIE): dissection of air into the tissue of the lungs surrounding the pulmonary vasculature.

Pulmonary vascular resistance (PVR): amount of resistance there is to blood flow through the lungs, caused by dilation or constriction of the pulmonary arteries.

Pulmonary vein confluence: location where the pulmonary veins come together.

Pulmonic stenosis: narrowing in the right ventricular outflow tract between the right ventricle and the main pulmonary artery.

Pulse pressure: difference between systolic blood pressure and diastolic blood pressure.

Pulsus paradoxus: a greater than 15 mm Hg drop in systolic blood pressure during inspiration.

R

Rapid sequence intubation (RSI): introduction of an endotracheal tube with minimal passage of time between anesthetic drug delivery and the onset of ideal intubating conditions.

Receptive language: a person's ability to comprehend what is being said to him or her.

Recurrent respiratory papillomatosis (RRP): a viral disease caused by the human papillomavirus (HPV); generally transmitted from the child's mother, who may be asymptomatic; causes tumor-like legions to grow on the larynx.

Refractory hypoxemia: continued hypoxemia despite increasing oxygen demands.

Regurgitation: backflow of blood into the atrium during diastole.

Resection: to cut off or cut out a portion of an organ.

Respiration: diffusion of oxygen and elimination of carbon dioxide through the alveolar-capillary membrane.

Respiratory distress syndrome (RDS): form of lung disease of premature infants characterized by severe impairment of respiratory function primarily caused by lack of surfactant, but is compounded by decreased surface area for gas exchange, thick alveolar-capillary membrane, and underdeveloped (and thus insufficient) vascularization.

Respiratory syncytial virus (RSV): viral pathogen; most common cause of bronchiolitis in young children.

Reticulogranular: rough, grainy-appearing lung tissue on a chest radiograph.

Retinopathy of prematurity (ROP): a complication of prematurity and one of the major causes of blindness in children in the developed world; occurs when the normal development of retinal vessels is disrupted by premature delivery and the extrauterine environment.

Retropharyngeal abscess: occurs when a pocket of purulence develops behind the posterior pharyngeal wall, causing symptoms of neck stiffness, neck pain, fever, and cervical adenopathy.

Ribavirin: a broad-spectrum antiviral medication used in the treatment of children with severe RSV, delivered through a small particle aerosol generator.

Right ventricular outflow tract obstruction (RVOTO): decrease in pulmonary blood flow caused by blood being unable to leave the right side of the heart and progress to the pulmonary arteries.

Robin sequence: consists of a triad of a small mandible (micrognathia or retrognathia), glossoptosis (obstruction of the airway by the bulk of the tongue) and cleft palate.

Rule of double effect: action that is known to have two possible effects, where the intended one is beneficial and the unintended one is not beneficial; can be morally permissible under specific circumstances.

Rule of nines: common formula used to calculate the percentage of skin burned.

S

Saccular cysts: abnormal outpouchings of the laryngeal mucosa in the laryngeal ventricle.

Saccular phase: period in fetal lung development beginning at about 30 weeks; when true alveoli begin to appear in the airways distal to the terminal bronchioles.

Saccules: short, shallow sacs that form in the saccular phase; function as an alveolar-capillary membrane, but are structurally more simple than alveoli.

Saltatory syndrome: gradual change in neurological status, tone, and spontaneous movements.

Sano modification: surgical modification that connects the right ventricle to the pulmonary artery via a conduit.

Scaphoid abdomen: hollowed-out or convex belly.

Scoliosis: lateral curvature of the spine; may accelerate decline in lung function by worsening lung restriction.

Secondary apnea: absence of breathing at birth; no amount of stimulation will restart breathing.

Secondary drowning: temporal delay of edema that can occur up to 24 hours after a near-drowning event.

See-saw breathing pattern: during breathing attempts, the stomach and chest are moving out of synch with each other.

Seldinger technique: a method of percutaneous introduction of a device (such as an artificial airway) in which a guide is placed in an opening first, and a larger, more permanent structure is threaded over it, to ensure proper placement of an invasive device; described by Sven I. Seldinger in 1921 as a method for placement of a catheter into a vessel and used frequently in the placement of central venous catheters.

Self-inflating bag: type of manual resuscitation bag/bag-valve-mask; does not need a compressed gas source in order to inflate, because it fills spontaneously with air after being squeezed; requires a reservoir attachment to deliver 1.0 FIO_2 when connected to an oxygen source.

Septa: a dividing wall or partition, such as the space between saccules or alveoli.

Septum: wall that divides two cavities.

Septum primum: thin area of tissue connected to the endocardial cushions.

Septum secundum: muscular structure that grows downward from the upper portion of the embryological atria.

Serosanguineous: body fluid that consists of blood and serum.

Shock: Hypotension with decreased systemic perfusion.

Short-acting beta agonist (SABA): pharmacological agent that relaxes airway smooth muscles during bronchoconstriction to reverse the signs and symptoms of acute airflow obstruction, namely cough, chest tightness, and wheezing.

Silent aspiration: aspirating without eliciting reflex to cough to remove material from the airway.

Sinus venosus: located directly inferior to the junction of the superior vena cava and the right atrium; almost always associated with partial anomalous pulmonary venous return.

Sinusoidal FHR pattern: fetal heart rate pattern associated with severe fetal hypoxia, acidosis, or anemia; consisting of regular, smooth oscillations of the baseline variability; typically lasts for at least 10 minutes.

Sniffing position: airway positioning so that the patient's head and chin are thrust slightly forward, with the intent to open the airway

Sodium thiosulfate: pharmacological agent used in cyanide poisonings that can help increase the conversion of cyanide to specific nitrates. This prevents the binding with cytochrome oxidase so that aerobic metabolism will continue.

Spinal cord injury (SCI): partial or complete fracture, compression, or stretching of the spinal cord.

Spinal muscular atrophy (SMA): characterized by lower motor neuron degeneration, and respiratory muscle strength is disproportionately weaker than the diaphragm muscle; a leading cause of death in children younger than 2 years of age.

Spirometry: measurement of airflow and lung volumes.

Starling's forces: vaginal squeezes of the chest as an infant progresses through the birth canal.

Static compliance: measurement of lung distensibility taken under conditions of no airflow.

Status asthmaticus: severe, persistent, and intractable asthma that does not respond to initial short-acting beta-agonist therapy.

Subglottic: the lower part of the larynx just below the vocal cords to the top of the trachea.

Subglottic cysts: a closed sac or pouch that contains fluid, semifluid, or solid material, found in the area below the glottis.

Subglottic hemangiomas: an abnormal buildup of blood vessels in the subglottic tissue, which can cause airway obstruction.

Subglottic stenosis: narrowing of the airway below the vocal folds.

Sulci: furrows separating gyri in the brain.

Supraglottic larynx: portion of the larynx above the vocal cords.

Supraglottis: portion of the larynx just above the glottis, including the epiglottis, bilateral false vocal folds, bilateral arytenoids, and the bilateral aryepiglottic folds, which serve to protect the airway from aspiration.

Supravalvar stenosis: narrowing of the vessel above the heart valve at the suture line of the connection site of the great vessels.

Surfactant: a chemically complex agent whose main function is to stabilize the air-liquid interface of the alveoli and bronchioles and to lower surface tension.

Surfactant-replacement therapy: installation of artificially derived surfactant directly into the lungs.

Synchronized intermittent mandatory ventilation (SIMV): form of patient-triggered mechanical ventilation that will deliver a preset number of mechanical ventilator breaths, attempting to synchronize them with patient efforts; any additional patient effort beyond the preset mandatory respiratory rate will be monitored by the ventilator but not supported in any way; if no spontaneous effort is sensed, a time-triggered mechanical breath will be delivered.

Systemic vascular resistance (SVR): the resistance to blood flow through the peripheral system.

T

Tamponade: accumulation of fluid or air in the pericardial sac that impairs the filling of the heart during diastole and impedes cardiac output.

Target effect: method of drug delivery in which a drug is dosed until the desired effect is achieved or until unacceptable side effects or toxicity occur.

Team support: services provided to health-care team members to assist them in coping with a patient's death.

Tension pneumothorax: life-threatening accumulation of air in the pleural cavity; each breath forces new air through the rupture that does not escape through the route of entry.

Terminal extubation: ventilator is discontinued and the endotracheal tube removed without weaning the ventilator prior to doing so.

Terminal sedation: refers to sedation to unconsciousness at the end of life, when symptoms cannot be managed by other means.

Terminal weaning: method of slowly lowering ventilatory support over hours (or days) prior to removing the endotracheal tube.

Tet spell: occurs in patients with tetralogy of Fallot; a sudden increase in right ventricular outflow tract obstruction causing a period of hypercyanosis.

Tetanus: neurological disease caused by a neurotoxin produced by the anaerobic bacterium *Clostridium tetani.*

Tetralogy of Fallot (TOF): congenital cyanotic heart defect caused by a combination of four conditions: ventricular septal defect (VSD); an aorta that overrides the VSD; obstruction of the right ventricular outflow tract; and right ventricular hypertrophy.

Time-cycled pressure-limited (TCPL) ventilation: the historically most common form of mechanical ventilation for neonates, providing positive pressure ventilation at a regular frequency without regard to patient respiratory effort; mechanical breaths will be delivered to a preset mandatory pressure and initiated and terminated based on preset time.

Time-triggered breaths: mandatory ventilator breaths.

Tissue test: an evaluation method used to identify choanal atresia, whereby the practitioner holds a piece of tissue or wisp of cotton in front of each nare—if choanal atresia is present, the tissue (or cotton wisp) will not move with respiration.

Tocolytic drugs: pharmacological agents used to inhibit or dampen uterine contractions.

Tonsillar hypertrophy: palatine tonsils (commonly referred to as tonsils), situated between the anterior and posterior tonsillar pillars, become enlarged, causing airway obstruction.

Total anomalous pulmonary venous return (TAPVR): type of congenital cyanotic heart defect that results when there is no connection between the pulmonary vein confluence and the left atrium.

Total obstruction: airway occlusion that will not allow inhalation or exhalation and leads to atelectasis and hypoventilation.

T-piece resuscitator: a mechanical device designed to deliver manual breaths at a set flow that provides consistent peak inspiratory pressure and positive end expiratory pressure.

Tracheal masses: unexpected growth within a trachea; uncommon in children.

Tracheal occlusion: placing a tracheal plug in utero into the fetus for a period of time to promote lung growth.

Tracheoesophageal fistula (TEF): a form of esophageal atresia involving the connection between the esophagus and the trachea. It can lead to severe pulmonary complications requiring a multidisciplinary approach to manage both digestive and respiratory malformations.

Tracheostomy: permanent opening created during a tracheotomy to provide and secure an open airway.

Tracheotomy: surgical procedure to create an opening in the trachea for long-term airway stabilization; incision into the trachea through the skin and soft tissues of the neck.

Transcutaneous monitoring: method of electrochemically measuring skin-surface partial pressure of oxygen (PO_2) and partial pressure of carbon dioxide (PCO_2) by heating localized areas of the skin to induce hyperperfusion.

Transient tachypnea of the newborn (TTN): condition of term or near-term infants, characterized by mild respiratory distress during the first few hours of life. It is caused by failure to clear fetal lung fluid prior to delivery.

Transillumination: placement of a high-intensity light source on the thorax to diagnose or rule out a pneumothorax in a neonate.

Transposition of the great arteries (TGA): congenital cyanotic heart defect that occurs when the two main arteries leaving the heart have changed places so that the aorta arises from the right ventricle and the pulmonary artery arises from the left ventricle.

Traumatic brain injury (TBI): caused by a bump, blow, or jolt to the head or a penetrating head injury that disrupts the normal function of the brain.

Trismus: facial rigidity that often starts with the facial muscles related to chewing and smiling; commonly described as lockjaw.

Truncus arteriosus: congenital cyanotic heart defect in which a single great vessel leaves the heart and supplies the systemic and pulmonary circulation.

Type I cells: alveolar cells that form the structure of the alveolar capillary membrane.

Type II cells: alveolar cells that make, store, and secrete things such as type I cells, fetal lung fluid, and pulmonary surfactant.

U

Underdevelopment: persistent pulmonary hypertension of the newborn characterized by hypoplastic pulmonary vasculature from pulmonary hypoplasia, which produces a relatively fixed level of pulmonary hypertension.

V

Validity: closeness to the truth.

Valleculae: spaces between the base of tongue and the epiglottis.

Vallecular cysts: a closed sac or pouch that contains fluid, semifluid, or solid material, found in the vallecula.

Valvotomy: cardiac surgical procedure that consists of division of the valve leaflets or valve replacement.

Valvuloplasty: cardiac procedure wherein a catheter with a balloon at the tip is passed into the valve orifice and inflated to enlarge the opening.

Variable decelerations: most common form of decelerations and represent umbilical cord compression; no temporal relationship to the onset of the contraction.

Vascular endothelial growth factor (VEGF) inhibitors: intravitreal (into the eye) medication that reduces the effect of VEGF on the developing retina, halting the development of retinopathy of prematurity.

Vascular resistance: resistance to flow that must be overcome in order to push blood through the circulatory system.

Venoarterial extracorporeal membrane oxygenation: form of extracorporeal support in which two large cannulas are inserted by a surgeon, one into the right internal jugular vein and a second into the right common carotid artery. The cannulas are connected to the extracorporeal membrane oxygenation circuit, creating a cardiopulmonary bypass system that parallels the native cardiopulmonary system.

Venovenous extracorporeal membrane oxygenation: a double-lumen cannula is placed by the surgeon in the right internal jugular vein to remove deoxygenated blood from the right atrium, cycle the blood though an artificial lung oxygenator, and then pump it back into the right atrium where the patient's native heart will be responsible for pumping the blood throughout the body.

Ventilation: transport of gas in and out of the lungs.

Ventilator-associated pneumonia (VAP): pneumonia that occurs in patients being given mechanical ventilation; term does not imply that ventilation is the cause of the pneumonia

Ventricular septal defect (VSD): opening in the intraventricular septum that causes a connection between the right and left ventricles.

Vestibular stenosis: constriction or narrowing of the soft tissue in the nares; can develop as an uncommon consequence of using nasal prongs.

Viability: ability to survive outside of the uterus.

Vibration: chest physiotherapy technique performed by gently shaking the chest wall with hands or a mechanical device during expiration to help mobilize secretions by oscillating the airways and increasing expiratory flow rates.

Viscous: sticky, gummy, gelatinous mucus that blocks peripheral airways and is difficult to expectorate.

Vitamin A (retinol): essential for the optimal growth of cells and tissues. A deficiency may contribute to the development of bronchopulmonary dysplasia.

Vocal fold paralysis: interruption of laryngeal nerve impulse, which controls vocal cord movement.

Vocal fold nodules: callus-like lesions that develop at the junction between the anterior and middle third of the vocal folds.

Volume-control ventilation: delivers a consistent volume with each breath, which allows for better control of minute ventilation.

Volume-targeted ventilation: allows clinicians to deliver a pressure-style breath while targeting a specific tidal volume.

Volutrauma: overdistension of the lung, causing tissue injury.

Volvulus: twisting of the bowel on itself, causing obstruction.

Vomer: posterior aspect of the nasal septum.

W

Westley croup score: tool commonly used to characterize the severity of respiratory impairment in children with croup.

Wet drowning: when the laryngeal cords no longer contract, typically after a person loses consciousness, and fluid is aspirated into the lungs.

Withholding resuscitation efforts: a conscious decision not to initiate some or all forms of life-sustaining therapy after delivery; may be appropriate in cases in which gestation, birth weight, and/or congenital anomalies are associated with high mortality and poor outcomes.

Work of breathing (WOB): force generated by a patient to overcome the frictional resistance and static elastic forces that oppose lung expansion.

X

Xanthines: pharmacological stimulants, classified as bronchodilators, although they are less potent than beta-2 agonists.

Index

Note: Page numbers followed by "b" denote boxes; "f" denote figures; "t" denote tables.